Medical Pharmacology and Therapeutics

THIRD EDITION

DEREK G. WALLER BSc (HONS), DM, MBBS (HONS), FRCP

Consultant Physician and Senior Lecturer in Medicine and Clinical Pharmacology
Southampton University Hospitals NHS Trust

ANDREW G. RENWICK OBE, BSc, PhD, DSc

Emeritus Professor
School of Medicine
University of Southampton

KEITH HILLIER BSc, PhD, DSc

Visiting Senior Lecturer in Pharmacology
School of Medicine
University of Southampton

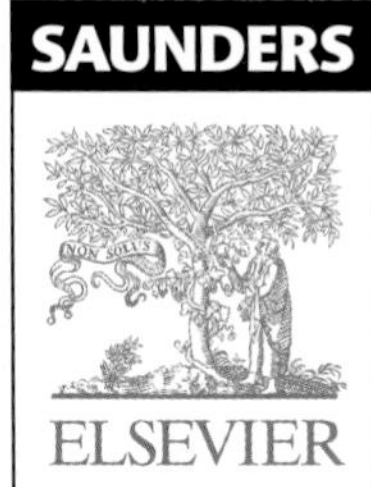

Edinburgh London New York Oxford Philadelphia St Louis Sydney Toronto 2010

SAUNDERS
ELSEVIER

ISBN 978 0 7020 2991 2

British Library Cataloguing in Publication Data
A catalogue record for this book is available from the British Library

Library of Congress Cataloging in Publication Data
A catalog record for this book is available from the Library of Congress

Notice
Knowledge and best practice in this field are constantly changing. As new research and experience broaden our knowledge, changes in practice, treatment and drug therapy may become necessary or appropriate. Readers are advised to check the most current information provided (i) on procedures featured or (ii) by the manufacturer of each product to be administered, to verify the recommended dose or formula, the method and duration of administration, and contraindications. It is the responsibility of the practitioner, relying on their own experience and knowledge of the patient, to make diagnoses, to determine dosages and the best treatment for each individual patient, and to take all appropriate safety precautions. To the fullest extent of the law, neither the Publisher nor the Authors assumes any liability for any injury and/or damage to persons or property arising out of or related to any use of the material contained in this book.

The Publisher

Printed in China

Contents

SECTION 8 The immune system

SECTION 9 The endocrine system and metabolism

SECTION 10 The skin and eyes

SECTION 11 Chemotherapy

SECTION 12 General features: toxicity and prescribing

Preface

The third edition of *Medical Pharmacology and Therapeutics* has been extensively revised and updated while preserving the widely popular approach of the second edition. The text is structured to reflect the ways that drugs are used in clinical practice. It provides information suitable for all healthcare professionals who require a sound knowledge of the basic science and clinical applications of drugs.

As before, a disease-based approach has been taken wherever possible with the aim of explaining clinical pharmacology and therapeutics and the principles of drug use for the management of common diseases. *Medical Pharmacology and Therapeutics* provides sound basic pharmacology background material sufficient to underpin the clinical context. New sections on pulmonary hypertension, attention deficit hyperactivity disorder, narcolepsy and macular degeneration have been added, reflecting the growing therapeutic options in these conditions. Many of the diagrams are new or modified to further clarify complex areas of pharmacology.

Each chapter in this *Third Edition* includes:

- An updated and succinct explanation of the major pathogenic mechanisms of the disease and consequent clinical symptoms and signs, helping the reader to put into context the actions of drugs and the consequences of their therapeutic use.
- An updated comprehensive review of major drugs classes relevant to the disease in question. Example drugs are used to illustrate pharmacological principles and to introduce the reader to drugs currently in widespread clinical use.
- Basic pharmacology and mechanisms of drug action, key pharmacokinetic properties and important unwanted effects associated with individual drugs and drug classes.
- A structured approach to the principles of disease management, outlining core principles of drug choice and planning a therapeutic regimen for many common diseases.
- An updated and reorganised drug compendium giving details of most drugs in the classes discussed in the chapter that have not been used as specific examples. For easy reference these tables set out key similarities and differences among drugs in each class and complement the information provided in the chapter.
- Additional and new style self- assessment exercises and case studies to enable the reader to test their understanding of the principles covered in each chapter.

Chapters covering generic concepts of pharmacology and therapeutics have been extensively updated and simplified and include: how drugs work at a cellular level, drug development, drug metabolism and pharmacokinetics, the autonomic nervous system, drug toxicity and drug prescribing. Information about genetic variations in both drug handling and drug responses, areas of increasing interest in drug development, has been expanded.

It is our intention that the third edition of this book will encourage readers to develop a deeper understanding of the principles of drug usage that will help them to become safe and effective prescribers and to carry out basic and clinical research and to teach. As medical science advances these principles should underpin the life-long learning essential for the maintenance of these skills.

DGW
AGR
KH

Drug dosage and nomenclature

Drug nomenclature

In the past, the non-proprietary (generic) names of some drugs have varied from country to country, leading to potential confusion. Progressively, international agreement has been reached to rationalise these variations in names and a single recommended International Non-proprietary Name (rINN) given to all drugs.

Where the previously given British Approved Name (BAN) and the rINN have differed, the rINN is now the accepted name and is used through this book.

A source of minor irritation, however, is that in most authoritative publications issuing from the UK the internationally accepted name is still being called its BAN or new BAN, and this is likely to continue. For full information on this, the reader is referred to:

http://www.mhra.gov.uk/Howweregulate/Medicines/Namingofmedicines/ChangestomedicinesnamesBANstorINNs/CON009669

A special case has been made for two medicinal substances: adrenaline (rINN – epinephrine) and noradrenaline (rINN – norepinephrine). Because of the clinical importance of these substances and the widespread European use and understanding of the terms adrenaline and noradrenaline, manufacturers have been asked to continue to dual-label products adrenaline (epinephrine) and noradrenaline (norephinephrine). In this book where the use of these agents as administered drugs is being described dual names are given. In keeping with European convention, however, adrenaline and noradrenaline alone are used when referring to the physiological effects of the naturally occurring substances.

Drug dosages

Medical knowledge is constantly changing. As new information becomes available, changes in treatment, procedures, equipment and the use of drugs become necessary. The authors and the publishers have taken care to ensure that the information given in the text is accurate and up to date. However, readers are strongly advised to confirm that the information, especially with regard to drug usage, complies with the latest legislation and standards of practice.

1

General principles

1 Principles of pharmacology and mechanisms of drug action

STUDYING PHARMACOLOGY

A drug is a chemical administered in an attempt to prevent, treat or diagnose disease. Natural substances are considered to be drugs when they are administered for such purposes (e.g. herbal medicines). The term 'drug' is used for all medicinal substances and not only illicit substances.

Pharmacology is a study of the effect of chemicals on biological systems. This book is confined to pharmacology as it relates to human medicine. Some of the objectives of learning about pharmacology related to human medicine are:

- to realise that medicines should be prescribed safely and effectively; this also requires the development of numeracy skills for accurately calculating drug doses and dilutions
- to understand the ways that drugs work to affect biological systems
- to appreciate that pharmacology cannot be understood comprehensively without the parallel understanding of related biological and clinical sciences such as biochemistry, physiology and pathology
- to provide a suitable framework to allow comparison of the relative benefits and risks of different drugs (drug selection)
- to be able to comprehend and to participate in research studies advancing knowledge of better treatment of patients.

The frequently asked question 'What do I need to know?', has no single answer. This will depend upon the individual requirements of the course you are studying and the examinations you will be taking. Your year of study (both pre- and post-graduation) is also of relevance; you should be aware that the depth of knowledge required in different areas and topics may vary as you progress through your studies; for example, early in the course you might not be required to have detailed knowledge of drug monitoring, but you should know if the drug has a narrow therapeutic index (when the plasma concentration of the drug that will cause unwanted effects is only slightly higher than the therapeutic plasma concentration). Your personal enthusiasm for pharmacology is also of importance!

We suggest that the following list provides guiding principles. For a drug you are studying in depth, you should know:

- the non-proprietary (generic) drug name *(not trade name)*
- the class to which the drug belongs
- whether the drug is available without prescription and, if so, what problems may be associated with such uncontrolled usage – for example, a patient may not report that he or she is taking a non-prescribed drug; this could interact with a subsequently prescribed drug
- the main reasons for using the drug
- the way the drug works
- how the drug is given (route, drug monitoring)
- absorption, distribution and elimination of the drug
- unwanted effects and unusual characteristics of the drug.
- propensity to cause drug interactions
- are there non-pharmacological treatments that are effective alternatives or will complement the drug treatment?

The drug formulary that is the bible for prescribers in the UK is the *British National Formulary* (BNF), available online at *http://www.bnf.org/bnf*

This contains entries for all drugs licensed for use in the UK. The appendix given at the end of this chapter provides a limited formulary list of core drugs taken from each drug class, which, although exhaustive, should provide students in the early stages of training with reference points to know which key drugs they should be learning about.

RECEPTORS AND RECEPTOR-MEDIATED MECHANISMS OF TRANSMITTER AND DRUG ACTION

The activities of most cellular processes are closely controlled in order to optimise homeostatic conditions in relation

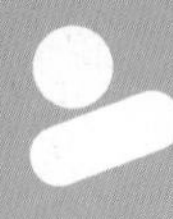

to physiological and metabolic requirements. Control can be divided into three main areas:

1. **The generation of a biological signal.** Homeostasis is maintained by communications between cells, tissues and organs in order to optimise bodily functions and responses to external changes. Communication is usually by signals in the form of chemical messengers, such as neurotransmitters or hormones.
2. **Cellular recognition sites (receptors).** The signal is recognised by responding cells via interaction of the signal with a site of action, binding site or receptor, which may be in the cell membrane, the cytoplasm or the nucleus.
3. **Cellular changes.** Interaction of the signal and its site of action in responding cells results in functional changes within the cell that give rise to an appropriate biochemical or physiological response to the original homeostatic stimulus.

Each of these three steps provides important targets for drug action and this chapter will outline the principles underlying drug action mainly in areas 2 and 3.

ACTIONS OF DRUGS AT BINDING SITES (RECEPTORS)

As shown in the receptor table at the end of this chapter, receptors tend to occur in different families (different receptor types). Within any one family of receptors there are different family members (receptor subtypes). As might be expected, distinct families of receptors have different characteristics. However, although individual members (receptor subtypes) of each family share some common traits inherent in the 'family', it is also possible for some subtypes to produce distinct different biological effects.

The search for the 'holy grail' in pharmacology is for a 'perfect drug' that binds to only one type of receptor/binding site and produces only one desired biological effect without unwanted effects. Although perfection has not been attained, it has proved possible to develop drugs that bind to one type of receptor to produce a desired effect but that have *less* (but not zero) ability to bind to other receptors which might produce unwanted effects.

Where a drug binds to one type of receptor in preference to another it is said to show *selectivity of binding* or *selectivity of drug action*. Selectivity is never absolute but can be high with some drugs and low with others. A drug with a high degree of selectivity is likely to show a greater difference between the dose required for its biological action and the dose required for an unwanted or toxic action. Examples of these are given in later sections.

For most drugs the first step in producing a biological effect is by interaction of the drug with special recognition or binding site(s) [receptors] either on the cell membrane or inside the cell and it is this binding that triggers the cellular response. The chemical signal is termed a *ligand*, because it ligates to (ties itself to) the specialised cellular macromolecule. The cellular macromolecule is termed a *receptor*, because it receives the ligand.

Receptors may be either in the cell membrane, in order to react with extracellular ligands that cannot readily cross the cell membrane (such as peptides), or in the cytoplasm, for lipid-soluble ligands that can cross the cell membrane.

MAJOR TYPES OF RECEPTORS

Despite the great structural diversity of drug molecules, *most* act on the following types of protein binding sites (loosely called superfamilies of receptors) to bring about biological change.

- **Transmembrane ion channels.** These control the passage of ions across membranes and are widely distributed.
- **G-protein-coupled receptors.** This is a family of transmembrane receptors named because of their interaction with **G**uanine nucleotides. Following activation by a drug, second messenger substances are formed which can bring about cellular molecular changes including the opening of transmembrane ion channels.
- **Kinase-linked receptors.** This is a large family of transmembrane receptors with a cytosolic enzymic component. They signal changes in cells by phosphorylating or dephosphorylating enzymes, thereby altering their activity.
- **Nuclear receptors.** This group of receptors responds to ligands by modification of gene transcription, to increase or decrease the expression of specific cellular proteins.

It should be noted that some mechanisms, such as the opening of ion channels, can be operated by direct interactions of drugs with the channel or by the G-protein-coupled mechanisms occurring as a first step and subsequent intracellular events may then activate transmembrane ion channels.

Transmembrane ion channels

Channels (pores) that cross lipophilic membranes (transmembrane channels) are ubiquitous and allow the transportation of ions into and out of cells. The intracellular concentrations of ions are controlled by a combination of ion pumps, which transport specific ions from one side of the membrane to the other, and ion channels (or gates), which open to allow the selective transfer of ions down their concentration gradients. Based on concentration gradients across the cell membrane:

- both Na^+ and Ca^{2+} will diffuse into the cell if the channels are open, making the cytosol more positive and causing depolarisation of excitable tissues
- K^+ will diffuse out of the cell, making the cytosol more negative and inhibiting depolarisation
- Cl^- will diffuse into the cell, making the cytosol more negative and inhibiting depolarisation.

The two major types of channel are superfamilies of *ligand-gated ion channels (LGICs)* and *voltage-gated ion channels (VGICs, also called ionotropic receptors)*. LGICs are opened by the binding of a ligand to an extracellular part of the channel, and VGICs are opened at particular membrane potentials by voltage-sensing segments of the channel. Both channel types are the targets for drug action. Both LGICs and VGICs can control the transportation of a single ion (e.g. K^+ channels – see Table 8.1); as an added complexity, types of LGICs for K^+ exist that function in response to different ligands and different VGICs for K^+ exist that respond to different membrane potentials.

Ligand-gated ion channels (LGICs) are a superfamily of receptors including nicotinic acetylcholine receptors,

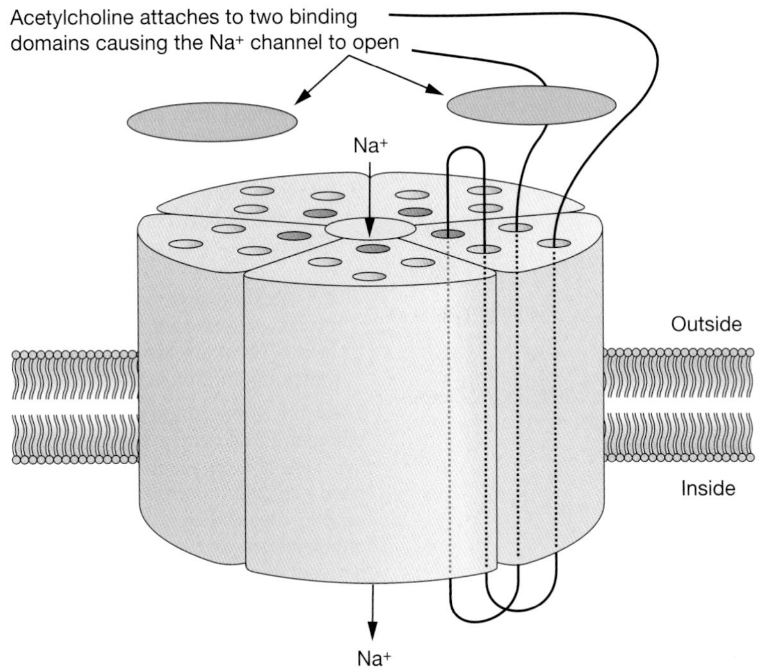
Acetylcholine attaches to two binding domains causing the Na+ channel to open
Na+
Outside
Inside
Na+

Fig. 1.1 **Typical ligand-gated transmembrane ion channel**. The diagram is based on the acetylcholine nicotinic receptor, which consists of five subunits (each of which comprises four transmembrane segments, M1–M4 – shown as dashed lines) surrounding the central ion channel and has two acetylcholine-binding sites (shown as red circles). For clarity, the transmembrane structure of only one of the five subunits is illustrated. Each acetylcholine-binding site is formed by the extracellular domains of two adjacent α_1 subunits. The M2 transmembrane segment of each subunit (shown in blue) is part of the ion channel and undergoes conformational change on ligand binding that allows selective ion flow down its concentration gradient. The ligand-gated GABA-linked Cl^- channel is shown in Figure 20.1.

gamma-aminobutyric acid (GABA) receptors, glycine receptors and $5HT_3$ receptors. They consist of a number of transmembrane subunits, which cluster around a central channel. Each peptide subunit is orientated so that hydrophilic chains face towards the channel and hydrophobic chains towards the membrane lipid bilayer. Binding of an agonist to the receptor causes a conformational change in the protein and results in extremely fast opening of the ion channel. The nicotinic acetylcholine receptor is a good example of this type of structure (Fig. 1.1). It requires the binding of two molecules of acetylcholine for channel opening. Channel opening lasts only milliseconds because the ligand rapidly dissociates and is inactivated. Ion channels may be influenced by ligand-operated G-protein-coupled receptors (see below) in two ways:

- indirectly, via the second messenger system affecting the status of the channel
- directly, via the G-protein subunits (α or $\beta\gamma$, see below) interacting with the channel.

Voltage-gated ion channels (VGICs) consist of several subunits, each of which is a transmembrane protein that crosses the membrane in a number of loops. The central unit contains the pore through which the ions pass and is largely responsible for the selectivity of the channel for a particular ion. Ion selectivity is determined by the amino acid composition of a short segment of the pore, which is different for each type of ion channel. Both Na^+ and K^+ channels show fast inactivation after opening; this is produced by an intracellular loop of the channel, which blocks the open channel from the intracellular end. The activity of voltage-gated channels may be modulated by drugs, either indirectly via intracellular events, such as second messenger-mediated changes (see Fig. 5.5) or directly, for example by local anaesthetics (see Ch. 18) binding to and blocking activated Na^+ channels.

The ability of the transmembrane subunits to exist in a number of configurations leads to the existence of many different subtypes of channel for a single ion. For example, there are many different voltage-gated Ca^{2+} channels (L, N, P/Q, R and T) and voltage-gated K^+ channels (see Table 8.1).

G-protein-coupled receptors (GPCRs) and second messenger systems

This is an extremely important type of receptor since the human genome has about 1000 sequences for G-protein-coupled receptors. The structure of a hypothetical G-protein-linked transmembrane receptor is shown in Figure 1.2. Most G-protein-coupled transmembrane receptors have the N-terminals on the extracellular side and cross the membrane seven times with helical segments (heptahelical), so that the C-terminal is on the inside of the cell.

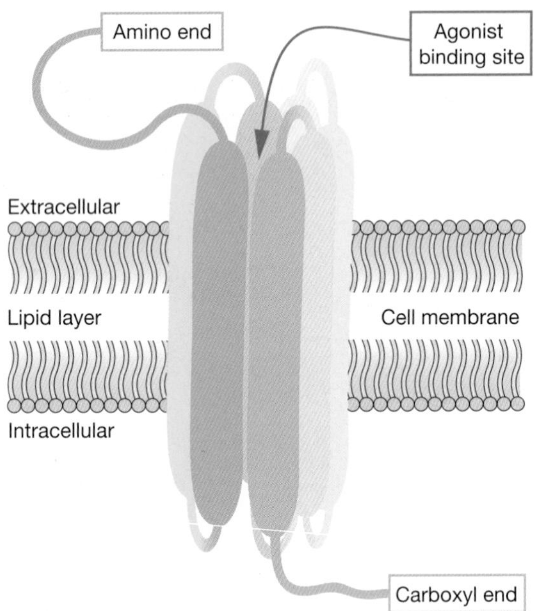

Fig. 1.2 **Hypothetical seven-transmembrane receptor.** The receptor is a glycoprotein in which sites of glycosylation are present on intracellular loops. The orientation of the receptor within the membrane is achieved by folding of the polypeptide chain resulting in seven transmembrane segments (shown as thick regions), which orientate the peptide within the cell membrane. The receptor is stabilised across the membrane by the presence of polar groups where the chains leave the lipid bilayer. The ligand-binding site represents a small volume in space in which regions of the polypeptide are orientated in such a way as to bind appropriate ligands only. Other possible ligands may be too large for the site or may show much weaker binding characteristics.

They are therefore universally called seven-transmembrane receptors (7TM receptors). The outer loops produce the active site for ligand binding and the inner loops are involved in coupling to the second messenger system, usually via a G-protein (Figs 1.3 and 1.4). The binding of an appropriate agonist (natural ligand or agonist drug) to the ligand-binding site, on the extracellular side of the membrane, alters the three-dimensional conformation of the receptor protein. The consequences of the change in conformation depend on the nature of the receptor, the intracellular enzymes and other systems to which it is linked, and to some extent on the substrate. The intracellular enzyme systems produce an intracellular signal, the second messenger, which alters the functioning of the cell.

Second messenger systems

Second messengers can be considered as the 'foot soldiers' of the extracellular signal, since they are released into the cytosol and are responsible for affecting a wide variety of enzymes, ion channels, transporters, etc. There are two complementary second messenger systems (Figs 1.3 and 1.5).

Cyclic nucleotide system

One system is based on cyclic nucleotides such as:

- cyclic adenosine monophosphate (cAMP), which is synthesised from adenosine triphosphate (ATP) via the enzyme adenylyl cyclase, and is involved in numerous cellular functions by activating protein kinase A, which phosphorylates proteins, many of which are enzymes; phosphorylation can either activate or suppress cell activity
- cyclic guanosine monophosphate (cGMP), which is synthesised from guanosine triphosphate (GTP) via guanylyl cyclase; cGMP exerts most of its actions through protein kinase G, which, when activated by cGMP, phosphorylates target proteins.

There are many isoforms of adenylyl cyclase; these show different tissue distributions and could be important selective sites of drug action in the future, although this has not been exploited successfully to date. The cyclic nucleotide second messenger is inactivated by hydrolysis by phosphodiesterase enzymes to give AMP or GMP. There are 11 different families of phosphodiesterase enzymes, which provide a potential site for selective drug action and a focus for successful drug development (Table 1.1).

The phosphatidylinositol system

The other system is based on inositol 1,4,5-triphosphate (IP_3) and diacylglycerol (DAG), which are synthesised from the membrane phospholipid phosphatidylinositol 4,5-bisphosphate (PIP_2) by the enzyme phospholipase C (Figs 1.3 and 1.5). There are a number of isoenzymes of phospholipase C, which may be activated by the α-subunits of G-proteins or the $\beta\gamma$-subunits of G-proteins (see below). The second messengers produced by phospholipase C (IP_3 and DAG) are inactivated and then converted back to PIP_2. The main function of IP_3 is to mobilise Ca^{2+} in cells. With the increase in Ca^{2+} brought about by IP_3, DAG is able to activate protein kinase C and phosphorylate target proteins.

The G-protein system

The G-protein system (Fig. 1.4) consists of three different subunits (i.e. it is a heterotrimer).

- *The α-subunit.* Twenty-three different types have been identified that belong to four families (α_s, α_i, α_q and α_{12}). The α-subunit is important because it binds GDP/GTP; it also has GTPase activity, which is involved in terminating the activity. When an agonist binds to the receptor, GDP (which is normally present) is replaced by GTP and the α-subunit dissociates from the $\beta\gamma$-subunits. The α-subunit/GTP complex is active while GTP is bound to it, but it is inactivated when the GTP is hydrolysed to GDP.
- *The β-subunit.* Five closely related forms have been identified. The β-subunit remains associated with the γ-subunit when the receptor is occupied and the combined $\beta\gamma$-subunit may activate cellular enzymes, such as phospholipase C.
- *The γ-subunit.* Ten different forms are known. The γ-subunit remains associated with the β-subunit when the receptor is occupied.

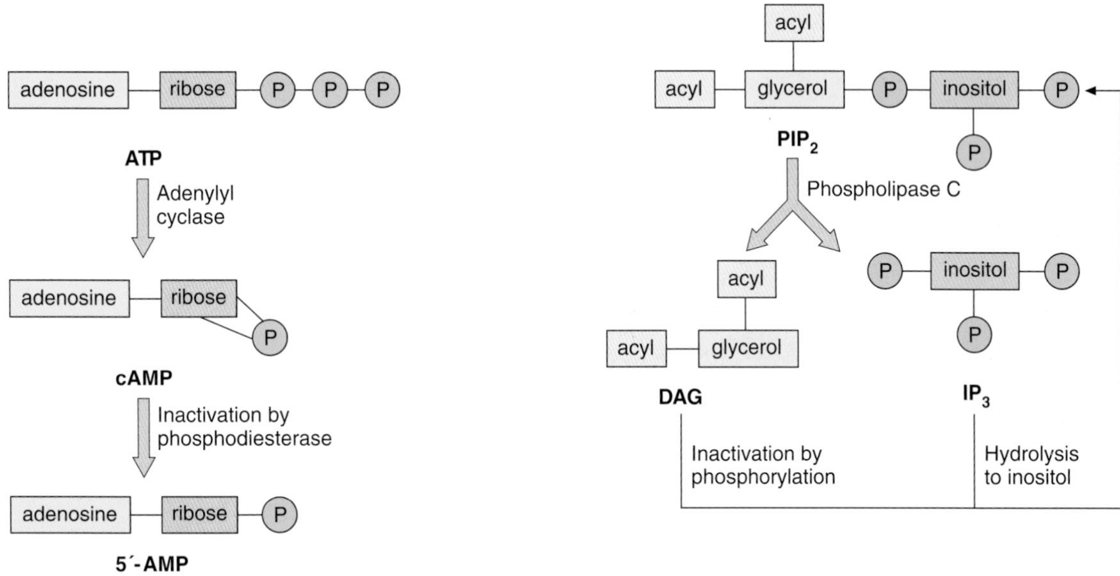

Fig. 1.3 **Second messenger systems.** Stimulation of transmembrane receptors (see Fig. 1.2 and text) produces intracellular changes by activating or inhibiting cascades of second messengers. Examples are cyclic adenosine monophosphate (cAMP), diacylglycerol (DAG) or inositol triphosphate (IP_3) formed from phosphatidyl inositol 4,5 biphosphate (PIP_2). (See also Fig. 1.5). As described in the text, second messengers then go on to influence diverse cellular proteins and induce cellular responses.

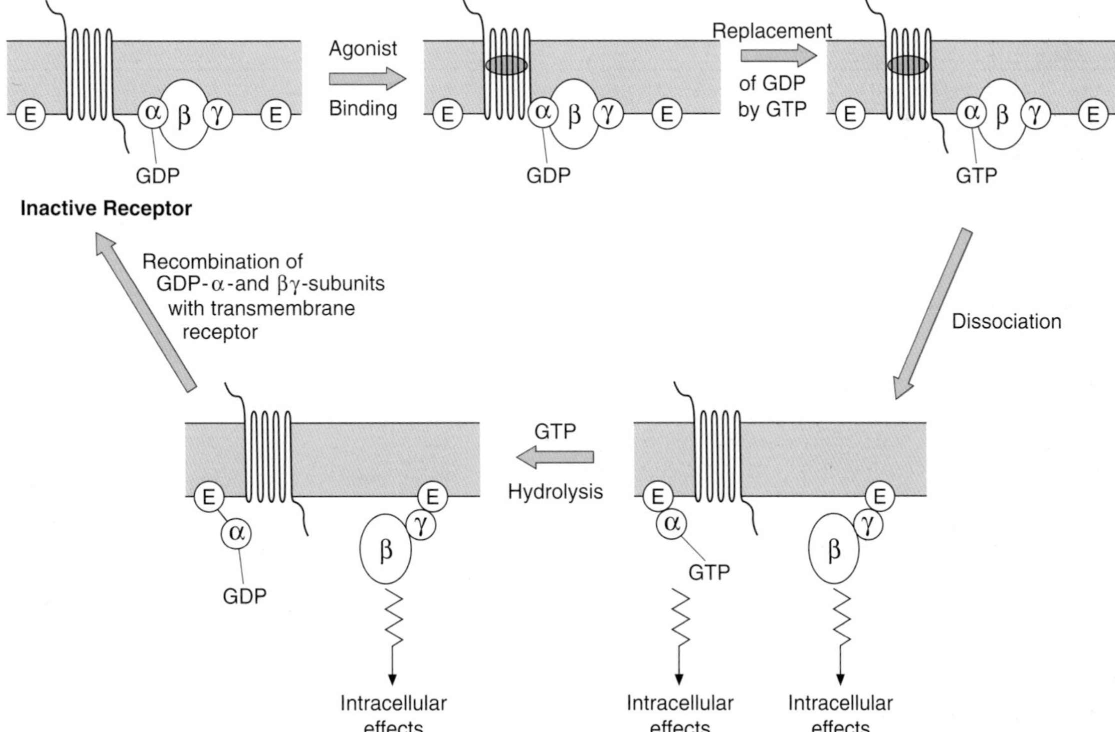

Fig. 1.4 **The functioning of G-protein subunits**. Ligand (agonist) binding results in replacement of GDP on the α-subunit by GTP and this is followed by dissociation of the α- and βγ-subunits, which affect a range of intracellular systems (shown as E on the figure) such as second messenger systems (e.g. adenylyl cyclase and phospholipase C), other enzymes and ion channels (see Fig. 1.5). Hydrolysis of GTP inactivates the α-subunit, which then reforms the inactive transmembrane receptor.

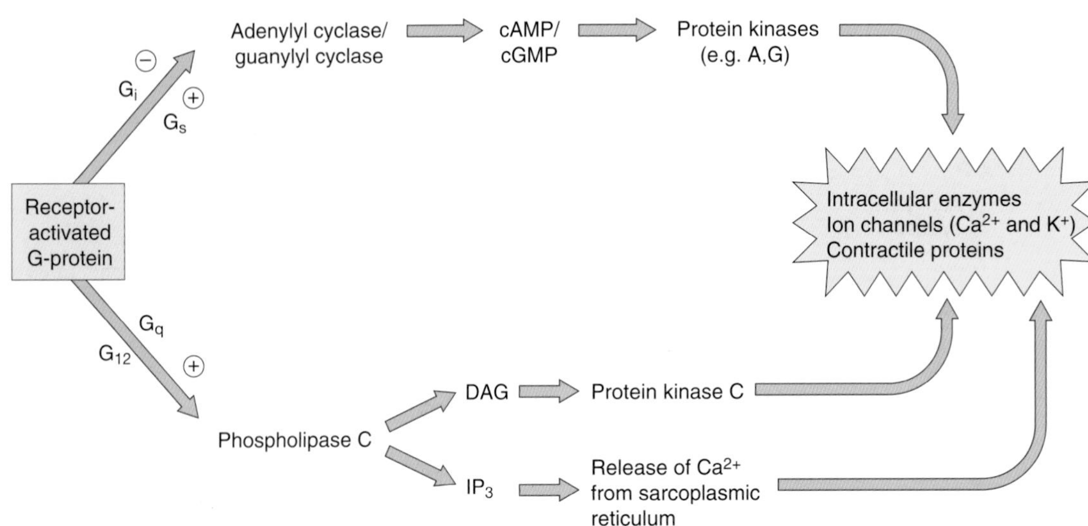

Fig. 1.5 **The intracellular consequences of receptor activation and G-protein dissociation**. The G-proteins affect the second messenger systems (Fig. 1.3); cAMP, cGMP, diacylglycerol (DAG) and inositol triphosphate (IP_3) produce a number of intracellular changes either directly, or indirectly via actions on protein kinases (which change the activities of other proteins by phosphorylation), or by actions on ion channels (Fig. 5.5). The pathways can be activated or inhibited depending upon the type of receptor and G-protein and the particular ligand stimulating the receptor. The effect of the same second messenger can vary enormously depending upon the biochemical functioning of the cell type in different tissues.

Table 1.1 Isoenzymes of phosphodiesterase (PDE)

Enzyme	Main substrate	Main site(s)	Drug(s)	Therapeutic potential
PDE1	cAMP + cGMP	Heart, brain, lung, smooth muscle	Under development; (vinpocetine)	Undefined
PDE2	cGMP	Adrenal gland, heart, lung, liver, platelets	Under development	Undefined
PDE3	cAMP	Heart, lung, liver, platelets, adipose tissue, inflammatory cells, smooth muscle	Aminophylline Enoximone Milrinone Cilostazol	Asthma (Ch. 12) Congestive heart failure (see Ch. 7); peripheral vascular disease (Ch. 10)
PDE4	cAMP	Sertoli cells, kidney, brain, liver, lung, inflammatory cells	Aminophylline	Asthma (Ch. 12) Inflammation COPD, IBD
PDE5	cGMP	Smooth muscle, endothelium, neurons, lung, platelets	Sildenafil Dipyridamole	Erectile dysfunction (Ch. 16)
PDE6	cGMP	Photoreceptors	Dipyridamole	Undefined
PDE7	cAMP	Skeletal muscle, heart, kidney, brain, pancreas, T-lymphocytes	Under development	Inflammation (combined with PDE4 inhibitor)
PDE8	cAMP	Testes, eye, liver, skeletal muscle, heart, kidney, ovary, brain, T-lymphocytes	Under development	Undefined
PDE9	cGMP	Kidney, liver, lung, brain	Under development	Undefined
PDE10	cGMP	Testes, brain	Under development	Schizophrenia?
PDE11	cGMP	Skeletal muscle, prostate, kidney, liver, pituitary and salivary glands, testes	Under development	Undefined

cAMP, cyclic adenosine monophosphate; cGMP, cyclic guanosine monophosphate; COPD, chronic obstructive pulmonary disease; IBD, inflammatory bowel disease.

The sequence from receptor binding to activation of second messenger systems is illustrated in Figure 1.4. Binding of an agonist to the receptor results in the replacement of GDP by GTP, and the α- and $\beta\gamma$-subunits of the G-protein are activated. GDP binds more strongly than GTP to the non-activated receptor, but the reverse is true once the ligand binds to the receptor. The subunits dissociate from the receptor protein and exert their intracellular effects via enzymes, ion channels and transporters that respond to the presence of the second messengers. The α-subunit has GTPase activity, which converts the active α-subunit/GTP complex to an inactive α-subunit/GDP complex; the GTPase activity is regulated by a family of proteins, which may provide additional future sites for selective drug actions. The GDPα- and $\beta\gamma$-subunits recombine with the receptor protein to give the inactive form of the receptor/G-protein complex.

There are three main types of G-proteins, the properties of which are largely determined by the nature of the α-subunit:

- G_s: stimulates membrane-bound adenylyl or guanylyl cyclase to increase cAMP or cGMP
- G_i (and G_o): inhibits adenylyl or guanylyl cyclase to decrease cAMP or cGMP
- G_q (and G_{12}): activates phospholipase C.

Activation of the receptor/G-protein complex can produce a number of intracellular events (Fig. 1.5) which affect many cellular processes such as enzyme activity (via the enzyme protein per se or via gene transcription), contractile proteins, ion channels (affecting depolarisation of the cell) and cytokine production. The intracellular effects are mediated by the GTP-α-subunit or the $\beta\gamma$-subunit. Depending on the type of G-protein, the GTP-α-subunit may close K^+ channels, activate phospholipase C or activate adenylyl cyclase, while the $\beta\gamma$-subunit may open K^+ channels, close Ca^{2+} channels, activate phospholipase A or C, activate or inhibit adenylyl cyclase, activate receptor kinases or activate the transmembrane Ca^{2+} pump. The effects on ion channels may be:

- *direct*, for example the $\beta\gamma$-subunit of the acetylcholine muscarinic receptor acts directly to open K^+ channels in the sinoatrial node to hyperpolarise the cell, or
- *indirect*, for example the opening of a K^+ channel via phosphorylation of channels through cAMP-mediated activation of protein kinase A.

The intracellular concentration of Ca^{2+} is important for many processes and this is affected by G_i and G_o proteins, which inhibit N and P/Q type Ca^{2+} channels, G_s proteins, which stimulate L and P/Q channels, and G_q and G_{12} proteins, which release Ca^{2+} from intracellular stores via the action of IP_3 on its receptors on the endoplasmic reticulum.

Protease-activated receptors (PARs)

Protease-activated receptors (also called proteinase-activated receptors) are recently identified transmembrane G-protein-coupled receptors which are stimulated by cleavage of the N-terminal of the receptor by a serine protease, rather than by the usual receptor occupancy (as described above). Proteolysis by proteases such as thrombin and trypsin produces a new N-terminal sequence of the receptor protein that can act as a ligand, which becomes 'tethered' back onto the receptor within extracellular loop-2 (Fig. 1.6). To date, four protease-activated receptors (PAR 1–4) have been identified, each with distinct N-terminal cleavage sites and different tethered ligands (Table 1.2). The receptors appear to play roles in platelet activation and clotting (Ch. 11), and act to transfer information on extracellular changes to intracellular functions, such as occurs during inflammation and tissue repair. They may also be involved in brain development, detecting noxious stimuli at sensory nerve endings, and regulation of intestinal secretions and permeability. The processes of receptor inactivation and intracellular events have not been fully defined, but are probably similar to those outlined above for other G-protein-coupled receptors. Clinically useful and selective drugs for these receptors are currently under development.

Kinase-linked transmembrane receptors

Kinase-linked transmembrane receptors, which bind extracellular peptide signalling substances such as insulin, are similar to the G-protein-linked receptors in that they have a ligand-binding domain on the surface of the cell membrane, traverse the membrane and have an intracellular 'effector' region (Fig. 1.7). However, they differ in a number of important respects:

- the extracellular region associated with the ligand-binding domain is very large; this is related to the size of the endogenous ligands, which are peptides such as insulin and cytokines
- there is a single transmembrane helical region
- the intracellular region possesses tyrosine kinase activity; different receptors have different intracellular effector regions.

Ligand binding is accompanied by dimerisation of two kinase-linked receptors, and these phosphorylate each other. This activated 'pair of receptors' then phosphorylates specific intracellular protein(s). The phosphorylated intracellular proteins are active enzymes, such as kinases or phospholipases, which can then bring about the relevant intracellular changes appropriate to the biological activities of the extracellular ligand. The phosphorylated intracellular kinases can either act directly on metabolising enzymes or alter the gene transcription of enzymes. Phosphorylation and dephosphorylation are important regulatory steps in the activation/deactivation of numerous intracellular proteins, such as enzymes and transporters.

Intracellular (nuclear) hormone receptors

Many hormones produce long-term changes in cellular activity by altering the genetic expression of enzymes, cytokines or receptor proteins. Such actions on DNA expression are mediated by interactions with intracellular receptors. The sequence of hormone binding and actions for most nuclear receptors are shown in Figure I.8. The cytosolic hormone receptor is usually in an inactive form linked to a protein called heat shock protein (HSP). Binding of the hormone causes dissociation of the HSP and the

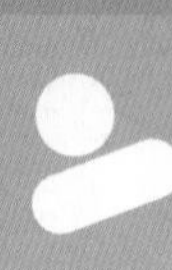

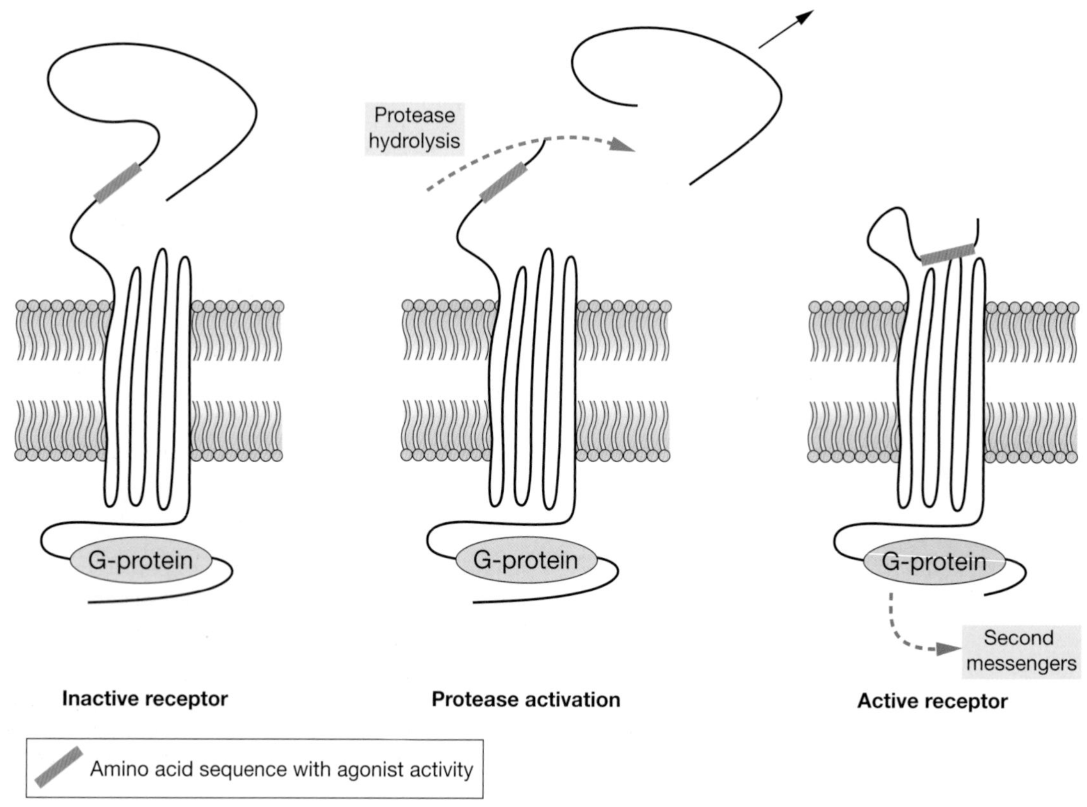

Fig. 1.6 **Protease-activated receptor.** The G-protein-coupled receptor is activated by a protease (see Table 1.2) which hydrolyses the extracellular peptide chain to expose a segment that acts as a ligand (shown in red) and activates the G-protein-coupled receptor. The activated receptor is inactivated by phosphorylation of the intracellular (C-terminal) part of the receptor protein.

Table 1.2 Protease-activated G-protein-coupled receptors

Receptor	Main sites	Functions	Activating protease[a]	*Possible* future therapeutic uses of specific inhibitors
PAR-1	Inflammatory cells, platelets and endothelium; gastrointestinal tract; respiratory epithelium	Regulation of inflammation; angiogenesis; thrombin signalling	Thrombin, plasmin, cathepsin-G	Atherosclerosis, cancer, fibrotic diseases
PAR-2	Inflammatory cells; gastrointestinal tract; kidney; respiratory epithelium	Regulation of inflammation; ion transport	Trypsin, tryptase, cathepsin-G	Allergic airway inflammation, arthritis
PAR-3	Inflammatory cells	Regulation of inflammation	None known	Accessory receptor to PAR-1 or PAR-4
PAR-4	Inflammatory cells	Regulation of inflammation	Thrombin, trypsin, cathepsin-G	Inflammation

[a]Main enzymes.

hormone binds to its receptor. The hormone/receptor complex passes through pores in the nuclear membrane and interacts with hormone response elements on the genome to modify the expression of downstream genes. Translocation and binding to DNA involves a variety of different chaperone, co-activator and co-repressor proteins, and the system is considerably more complex than indicated in Figure 1.8. Binding of the hormone/receptor complex to the hormone response element usually activates genes (transactivation), but binding sometimes silences gene expression and results in a decrease in mRNA synthesis (transrepression). Co-activators are transcrip-

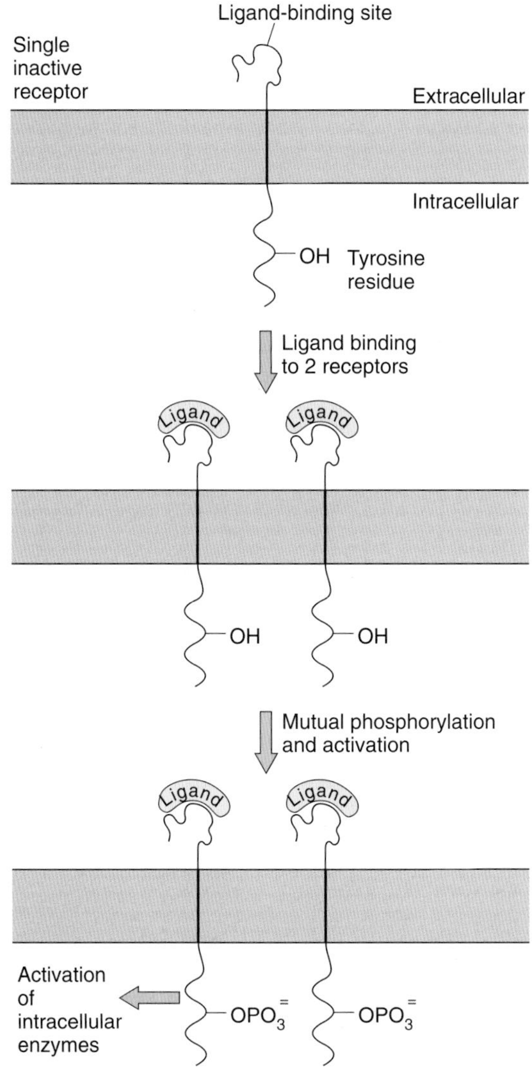

Fig. 1.7 **Kinase-linked transmembrane receptor**. The receptor has a large extracellular domain, a single transmembrane segment and an intracellular tyrosine kinase domain which is responsible for intracellular effects (see text for details).

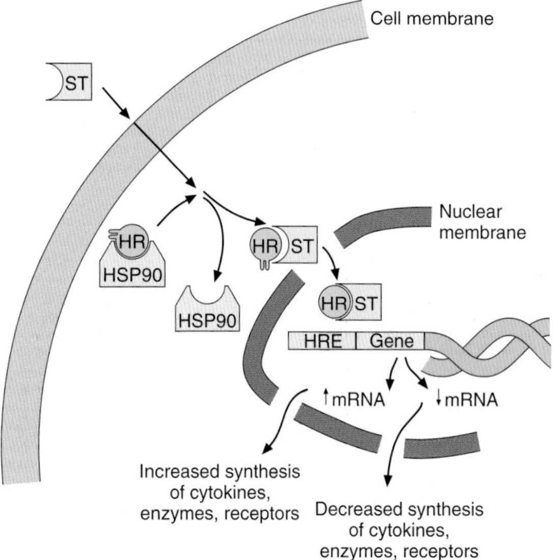

Fig. 1.8 **The activation of intracellular hormone receptors**. Steroid hormones (ST) are lipid-soluble compounds which readily cross membranes and bind to intracellular receptors (HR). This binding displaces a protein called heat shock protein (HSP90) and the hormone/receptor complex enters the nucleus, where it can either increase or decrease gene expression by binding to hormone response elements (HRE) on DNA.

Box 1.1 Some families of intracellular receptors

Oestrogen receptor	ER
Progesterone receptor	PR
Androgen receptor	AR
Glucocorticoid receptor	GR
Mineralocorticoid receptor	MR
Thyroid hormone receptor	TR
Vitamin D receptor	VDR
Retinoic acid receptor	RAR
9-*cis*-Retinoic acid receptor	RXR
Peroxisome proliferator-activated receptor	PPAR

tional cofactors that also bind to the receptor and increase the level of gene induction; an example is histone acetylase, which facilitates transcription by increasing the ease of unravelling of DNA. Co-repressors also bind to the receptor and repress gene activation; an example is histone deacetylase, which prevents further transcription. Steroid hormones (and some other hormones) are recognised by specific members of the steroid/thyroid receptor superfamily (Box 1.1). In some cases, for example peroxisome proliferator-activated receptor (PPAR), the receptor is present within the nucleus and binding of the ligand (usually a lipid molecule) occurs without the translocation step. The PPARs (PPAR-γ, PPAR-α and PPAR-δ) function as lipid sensors and regulate the expression of genes that influence metabolic events (see Chs 29, 40, 48 for more details of PPARs).

Steroids, and synthetic steroid analogues, show selectivity for different receptors, which then determines the spectrum of gene expression that is affected. Frequently, the hormone response element needs two hormone/receptor complexes to form a dimer in order to alter gene expression. Some steroid hormone/receptor complexes (e.g. involving ER, PR, AR, GR and MR – see Box 1.1) form homodimers (two molecules of the same hormone/receptor complex, e.g. ER–ER) while the others, especially receptors present within the nucleus (TR, VDR, RAR and RXR), form heterodimers (molecules of two different hormone/receptor complexes, e.g. RAR–RXR).

The intracellular receptor protein that binds steroids is made up of five regions with different functions (Table 1.3).

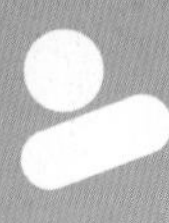

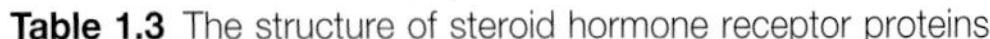

Table 1.3 The structure of steroid hormone receptor proteins

Section of protein	Action	Role
N-terminus		
A/B	Transactivation	Activates target genes and gives the specificity of the receptor response
C	DNA binding and dimerisation	Binds receptor to DNA by two zinc finger regions
D	Nuclear localization	Hinge region to allow correct conformation
E	Ligand binding	Ligand specificity of receptor; a large complex region; this region also binds heat shock protein
F	Unknown	Deletion of this region does not alter functioning
C-terminus		

Different regions of the receptor are involved in hormone binding, DNA binding and DNA modulation.

Hormone drugs act primarily by mimicking the endogenous hormone (i.e. as an agonist) but often the drug has a longer half-life (Ch. 2) than the endogenous ligand and produces a long-term change. Some drugs act as antagonists by blocking the binding of the normal ligand.

OTHER SITES OF DRUG ACTION

Probably every protein in the human body has the potential to have its structure or activity altered by foreign compounds, so that the list of 'other sites' is almost limitless. In addition to the sites and mechanisms of actions discussed above, drugs may also bind to and either activate or inhibit other sites.

- *Cell membrane ion pumps.* For example, Na^+/K^+-ATPase in the brain is activated by the anticonvulsant phenytoin whereas that in cardiac tissue is inhibited by digoxin; K^+/H^+-ATPase in gastric parietal cells is inhibited by proton pump inhibitors (e.g. omeprazole, Ch. 33).
- *Enzymes.* For example, a number of anticancer drugs inhibit enzymes involved in purine, pyrimidine or DNA synthesis. Some drugs act on the enzymes that synthesise or degrade the endogenous ligands for extracellular or intracellular receptors, or second messenger molecules (Table 1.1).
- *Organelles.* For example, some antibiotics interfere with the functioning of the bacterial ribosome.
- *Transport proteins.* For example, diuretics affect Na^+ transport in the renal tubules, and probenecid inhibits renal tubular secretion of anions (see Ch. 2 and Ch. 14).

PROPERTIES OF RECEPTORS

Receptor binding

The binding of the ligand to the receptor is normally reversible; consequently, the intensity and duration of the intracellular changes are dependent on the continuing presence of the ligand. The extent of drug binding to the receptor (receptor occupancy) is proportional to the drug concentration; the higher the concentration, the greater the occupancy. The interaction between the ligand and its receptor does not usually involve permanent covalent chemical bonds but weaker, reversible forces such as:

- ionic bonding between ionisable groups in the ligand (e.g. NH_3^+) and in the receptor (e.g. COO^-)
- hydrogen bonding between amino-, hydroxyl-, keto-functions, etc, in the drug and the receptor
- hydrophobic interactions between lipid-soluble sites in the ligand and receptor
- van der Waals forces, which are very weak interatomic attractions.

The receptor protein is not a rigid structure: binding of the ligand alters its conformation and the biological properties of the protein, leading to the intracellular changes that are described above.

Receptor selectivity

There are numerous possible extracellular and intracellular chemical signals produced in the body, which can affect different processes. Therefore, a fundamental property of a receptor is its *selectivity*, i.e. the extent to which it can recognise and respond to only one ligand or a group of related ligands (such as adrenaline and noradrenaline). Some receptors show high selectivity and bind a single endogenous ligand (e.g. acetylcholine is the only endogenous ligand that binds to N_1 nicotinic receptors; see Ch. 4), whereas other receptors are less selective and will bind a number of related endogenous ligands (e.g. the β_1-adrenoceptors on the heart will bind noradrenaline, adrenaline and to some extent dopamine, which are all catecholamines).

The ability of receptors to recognise and bind the appropriate ligand depends on an interaction between the receptor molecule and certain characteristics of the chemical structure of the ligand. The formulae of a few representative endogenous ligands that bind to different receptors are shown in Figure 1.9; differences in structure that determine selectivity of action between receptors may be subtle. Receptor selectivity occurs because the three-dimensional organisation of the different sites for reversible binding interactions (such as anion and cation sites, lipid centres and hydrogen bonding sites; see above) corresponds to the three-dimensional structure of the endogenous ligand. Receptors are proteins that are folded into a tertiary structure such that the necessary specific arrangement of bonding centres is brought together within a small volume – the receptor site (Fig. 1.10). Binding of the natural ligand alters the three-dimensional conformation of the protein, which triggers the receptor activity.

There may be a number of subtypes of a receptor, each of which specifically recognises or binds the same ligand. For example, α_1-, α_2-, β_1-, β_2- and β_3-adrenoceptors all bind adrenaline, but they occur to a different extent in different tissues, and produce different intracellular changes when

(a)

$CH_2CH_2NH_2$ / OH / OH

Dopamine

OH / $CHCH_2NH_2$ / OH / OH

Noradrenaline

HO / $CH_2CH_2NH_2$ / N / H

5-Hydroxytryptamine (5HT)

HN / N / $CH_2CH_2NH_2$

Histamine

(b)

NH_2 / CH_2 / COOH

Glycine

O / NH_2 / C—CH_2CH_2CH / HO / COOH

Glutamate

O / NH_2 / C—CH_2—CH / HO / COOH

Aspartate

O / NH_2 / C—$CH_2CH_2CH_2$ / HO

ɣ - aminobutyrate (GABA)

(c)

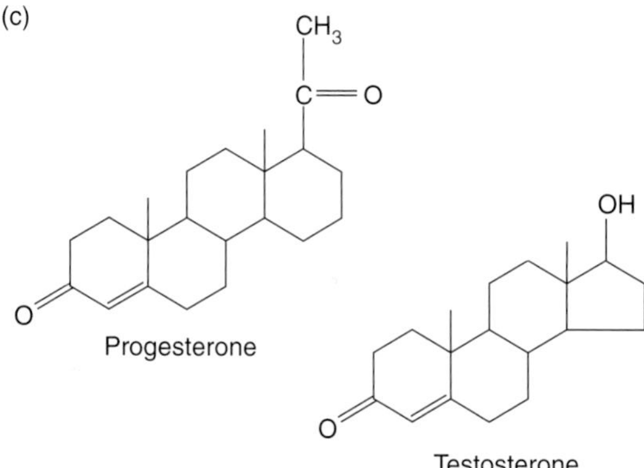

Fig. 1.9 **Groups of chemicals that show preference for different receptors in spite of similar structure.** (a) Biogenic amines; (b) amino acids; (c) steroids.

stimulated or blocked (see Ch. 4). The different characteristics of the receptor subtypes allow a drug (or natural hormone) with a particular three-dimensional structure to show selective actions by recognising and then acting preferentially on one particular receptor, with fewer unwanted effects from stimulation of related receptors. It should be noted that although ligands may have a high affinity for one receptor subtype, this is never absolute. For example, the neurotransmitter acetylcholine stimulates acetylcholine receptors on ganglia (nicotinic N_1 receptor subtype), the neuromuscular junction of skeletal muscle (nicotinic N_2 receptor subtype) and at smooth muscle (muscarinic receptor subtype); these receptors all respond to acetylcholine at low concentrations but have been shown to be structurally different by using a variety of pharmacological techniques. However, synthetic drugs have been produced which show selectivity of action between these different receptors (due to different affinities/efficacies – see later) and are used for different clinical purposes. This aspect is discussed in detail in Chapter 4. Until recently, receptor subtypes were 'discovered' when a pharmaceutical company developed a new agonist or antagonist that was found to alter some, but not all, of the activities of a currently known receptor class. Recent developments in molecular biology have enhanced our abilities to detect receptor subtypes. Based on genetic information it is now recognised that there are multiple types of most receptors, and also that there is genetic variation between individuals in the properties or abundance of these receptors (pharmacogenetics – see the end of this chapter). The recognition and cloning of subtypes of receptors is important in that it should facilitate the development of drugs showing greater selectivity and hopefully fewer unwanted effects. Greater understanding of genetic differences underlying human variability in drug responses offers the potential for individualisation of the mode of treatment and selection of the correct drug and dosage (see Ch. 3).

Drug stereochemistry and activity

Receptors have a three-dimensional organisation in space and, therefore, the ligand has to be presented to the receptor in the correct configuration (rather like fitting a right hand into a right-handed glove). Because some drugs are a mixture of stereoisomers (the same chemical structures but with different three-dimensional configurations), the different isomers may show very different binding characteristics and biological properties. For example, the different stereoisomers of the α- and β-adrenoceptor antagonist drug labetalol bind to different types of receptor. A drug that is an equal mixture of levo- and dextro-isomers (or S- and R- forms; a racemate) could be a mixture of 50% active compound plus 50% inactive, or, in some cases, a mixture of 50% therapeutic drug and 50% inactive but toxic compound. In addition, the different isomers may show different rates of metabolism (see Ch. 2). In consequence, there has been a trend in recent years for the development of single isomers for therapeutic uses; one of the earliest examples was the use of levodopa (the levo-isomer of dopa) in Parkinson's disease (Ch. 24).

Receptor numbers

The number of receptors present in a cell is not static, and there is a high turnover of receptors which are being formed and removed continuously. Cell membrane receptor

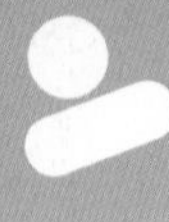

ADRENOCEPTOR

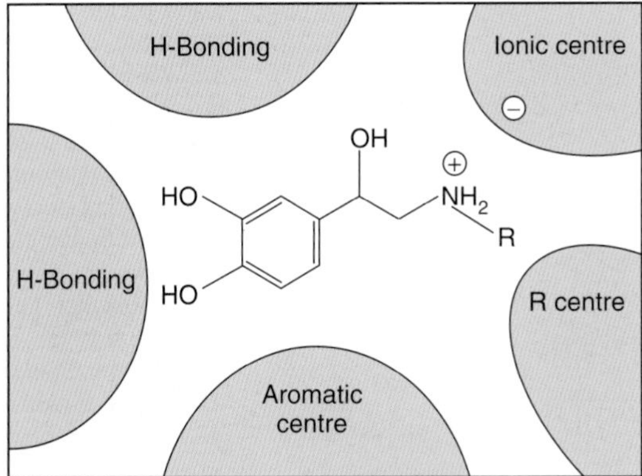

MUSCARINIC RECEPTOR

VII VI
OH OH HO
HO
I
N
O
V
O
HO
II
O O⁻
C
OH
III IV

Fig. 1.10 **Receptor ligand-binding sites.** The coloured areas are schematic cross-sections of the seven transmembrane segments of the receptor protein (labelled I to VII). Different segments provide different properties (hydrogen bonding, anionic site, etc.) to make up the active binding site.

proteins are synthesised in the endoplasmic reticulum and transported to the membrane; regulation of functioning receptor numbers in the membrane occurs via both transport to the membrane (often as homo- or heterodimers) and removal by internalisation. The numbers of receptors within the cell membrane may be altered as a consequence of exposure of the receptor to the drug being used for treatment, with either an increase (*upregulation*) or a decrease (*downregulation*) in receptor numbers. Changes in receptor numbers following treatment with some drugs can be an important part of the therapeutic response. A well-recognised example is the therapeutic benefit of tricyclic antidepressants (Ch. 22); although they produce an almost immediate increase in the availability of monoamine neurotransmitters, it is the subsequent relatively slow adaptive downregulation in monoamine receptor numbers that takes many days or weeks which is associated with the time taken to produce a therapeutic response. Tolerance to the effects of some drugs (e.g. opioids) may arise from downregulation of opioid receptor numbers; as a result, there is the need for increased doses to produce the same analgesic activity (Ch. 19).

COMPONENTS OF DRUG ACTION

Drug actions can show a number of important properties:

- selectivity
- potency
- efficacy.

Selectivity

Many drugs may act preferentially on particular receptor types or subtypes, such as β_1- and β_2-adrenoceptors, to different extents (see above) but no drug is specific, i.e. 100% selective, for only one receptor subtype. It is important to be able to measure the degree of selectivity of a drug and to be able to express numerically the extent to which a drug affects one receptor in relation to another. For example, it is therapeutically important in understanding therapeutic efficacy and unwanted effects that the bronchodilator salbutamol is approximately ten times more effective in stimulating the β_2-adrenoceptors in the airways smooth muscle than the β_1-adrenoceptors in the heart.

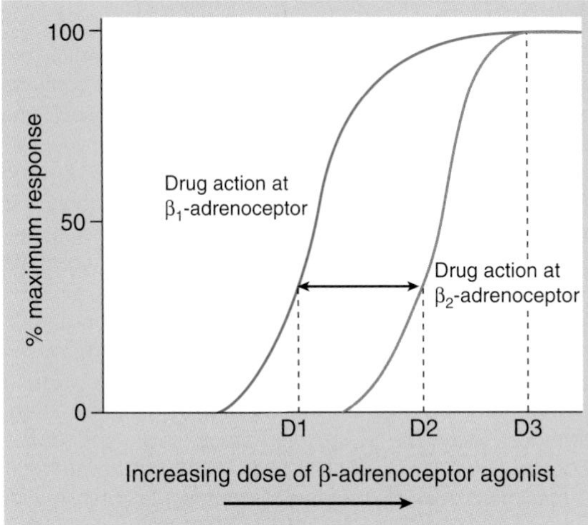

***Fig. 1.11* Selectivity of action of a β-adrenoceptor agonist.** This illustrates the relative selectivity of action for the β_1-adrenoceptor of a hypothetical drug and that selectivity is maintained only over a particular dose range. The drug shows β_1-adrenoceptor selectivity, because at low doses it produces dose-related β_1-adrenoceptor stimulation with less effect on β_2-adrenoceptors. If dose D1 was 10 times less than dose D2, the selectivity ratio for the β_1-adrenoceptor is 10. This selectivity diminishes at the higher end of the dose–response curve and is completely lost at doses that produce a maximum response of the drug on both β_1- and β_2-adrenoceptors (D3).

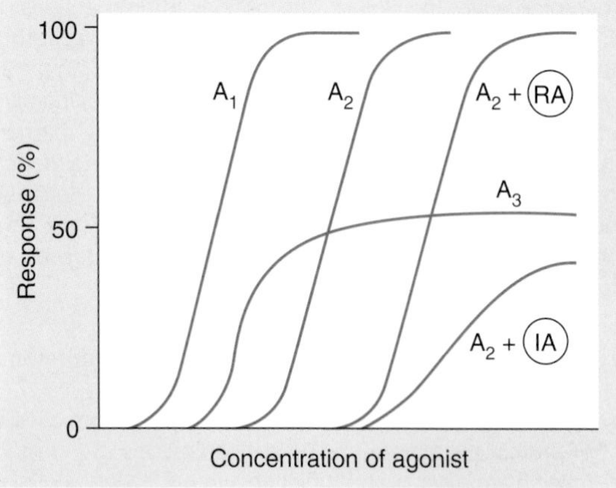

***Fig. 1.12* Dose–response curves for agonists in the absence or presence of reversible (competitive) or irreversible (non-competitive) antagonists.** A_1, A_2, two different agonists (A_1 more potent than A_2); A_3, partial agonist; RA, reversible antagonist; IA, irreversible antagonist.

Under many circumstances it is possible to determine for an individual drug the relationship between the dose applied and the biological effect (response) on different receptor subtypes by constructing dose–response curves (Fig 1.11). In modern pharmacological studies it is likely that this type of experiment would be performed by studying the effects of the drugs on isolated cell lines expressing the particular receptor being studied. In Figure 1.11, smaller concentrations of the drug being tested are required to stimulate the β_1-adrenoceptor compared with those required to stimulate the β_2-adrenoceptor and the drug is therefore said to have selectivity of action at the β_1-adrenoceptor. The degree of receptor selectivity is given by the ratio of the levels of response by each receptor type when measured at equimolar doses or concentrations. It is clear from Figure 1.11 that the ratio is highly concentration-dependent and is not apparent at high concentrations, when a maximal stimulation at both receptor subtypes occurs.

Potency

The potency of a drug in vitro is largely determined by the strength of its binding to the receptor, which is a reflection of the receptor affinity, and the ability of the receptor/drug complex to elicit downstream events. The more potent a drug, the lower will be the concentration needed to bind to the receptor and to give a response for an agonist (or to block a response for an antagonist). The potency of a drug in vivo is the amount or dose of drug necessary to produce a specified level of effect, and is dependent on receptor density, efficiency of the stimulus response mechanism, affinity and efficacy (as well as pharmacokinetic variables (Ch. 2) that determine the delivery of the drug to its site of action). Therefore, the in vivo potencies of a series of related drugs may not reflect their in vitro receptor-binding properties.

Potencies of different drugs *have* to be compared using the ratio of the doses required to produce (or block) *the same percentage response*. Because dose–response curves are usually parallel in part (for drugs that share a common mechanism of action), the ratio is the same at different response values, e.g. 10%, 20% or 50% response, but not at 100% response.

Efficacy

The efficacy of a drug is its ability to produce the maximal response possible and relates to the extent of functional change imparted to the receptor. For example, agonists can be divided into two groups (Fig. 1.12):

- full agonists, which give an increase in response with increase in concentration until the maximum possible response is obtained (curves A_1 and A_2)
- partial agonists, which also give an increase in response with increase in concentration but cannot produce the maximum possible response (curve A_3).

CLASSIFICATION OF DRUG ACTION

Different types of drug action will be introduced throughout this book. They can be classified as:

- agonists
- antagonists
- partial agonists
- inverse agonists
- allosteric modulators
- enzyme inhibitors/activators
- non-specific.

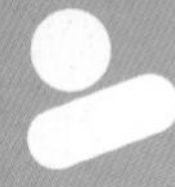

These represent the classic descriptions of drug actions. It is now recognised that many G-protein-linked receptors can show basal, agonist-independent activity. The G-protein can exist in two different low energy states, inactive and active, which are separated by an energy barrier. Receptors with a low energy barrier show a higher tendency for spontaneous activity, in the absence of a ligand. Because the receptors exist as an equilibrium between active and inactive forms, the basal activity can be either increased or decreased by different types of ligands as follows:

- *agonists* fully activate the receptor
- *antagonists* have no effect on basal activity, but competitively block the access of other ligands
- *partial agonists* induce submaximal activation of the G-protein even at saturating concentrations
- *inverse agonists* inhibit basal activity.

Agonists

An agonist whether a therapeutic drug (ligand) or the endogenous agonist (also a ligand), binds to the receptor or site of action, and changes the conformation of the receptor to its active state. An agonist shows both *affinity* (the strength of binding for the receptor) and *efficacy* (the extent of functional change imparted to the receptor). Drugs may differ in their affinity and efficacy.

The affinity or strength of binding of the drug to the receptor

This determines the concentration necessary to produce a response and, therefore, is directly related to the potency of the drug. In the examples in Figure 1.12, drug A_1 is more potent than drug A_2, but both are capable of producing a maximal response (they have the same efficacy). For some compounds a maximal response may require all of the receptors to be occupied, but for most drugs/receptors the maximal response is produced while some receptors remain unoccupied, that is, there may be *spare receptors*. The presence of spare receptors becomes important when considering changes in receptor numbers owing to adaptive responses during chronic treatment (tolerance) or caused by irreversible binding of an antagonist (see below).

The rate of binding/dissociation

This is usually of negligible importance in determining the rates of onset or termination of effect in vivo, because these depend mainly on the rates of delivery to and removal from the target organ, that is, on the overall absorption or elimination rate of the drug from the body (see Ch. 2).

Changes in the number of receptors

The effect of changes in the numbers of receptors on dose–response relationships is complex. With downregulation of receptors, the response obtained depends upon the extent of downregulation and also on the extent of occupancy that is necessary to produce a maximal response. In practice, maximal drug effects are normally produced at concentrations that do not give 100% receptor occupancy; with downregulation, the same maximal response may be produced but only with higher percentage occupancy of the reduced number of receptors and hence with higher concentrations/doses.

Antagonists

An antagonist binds to the receptor (i.e. has affinity) but does not cause the conformational change that converts the receptor to its active state (i.e. has zero efficacy). The compound will, however, block access to the receptor-binding site of the naturally occurring agonist. The drug effect may only be detectable when the natural agonist is present (e.g. β-adrenoceptor antagonists lower heart rate, particularly when the rate is increased by stimulation of the sympathetic nervous system). The binding of most clinically useful antagonists is reversible and competitive; in consequence, the receptor blockade can be overcome by an increase in the concentration of the naturally occurring receptor agonist or by the administration of an agonist drug. Therefore, reversible antagonist drugs move the dose–response curve for an agonist to the right but do not alter the maximum possible response (as shown in curve A_2+RA when compared with A_2 alone in Fig. 1.12). Antagonists also exhibit selectivity of action. For example, the β-adrenoceptor antagonist propranolol is a non-selective antagonist acting equally on β_1- and β_2-adrenoceptors, whereas atenolol shows selective antagonism of β_1-adrenoceptors and has less effect on β_2-adrenoceptors.

Irreversible antagonists, such as phenoxybenzamine, bind covalently to their site of action, and a full response cannot be achieved even by a very large increase in agonist concentration (as shown in curve A_2+IA compared with A_2 alone in Fig. 1.12).

Partial agonists

A drug showing both agonist and antagonist properties is known as a partial agonist: the activity expressed at any time is dependent on the concentration of the natural ligand or agonist. Partial agonism is responsible for the therapeutic efficacy of several drugs, including buspirone, buprenorphine, pindolol and salbutamol. Even maximal occupancy of a partial agonist at all available receptors produces a submaximal response, for example because of incomplete amplification of the receptor signal via the G-proteins. A partial agonist will show agonist activity at low concentrations of the natural ligand, but the dose–response will not reach the maximal activity even when all receptors are occupied (see Fig. 1.12, drug A_3). At high concentrations of the naturally occurring agonist, a partial agonist will behave as an antagonist, because it will prevent access of the naturally occurring agonist to the receptor and thereby result in a submaximal response. As a consequence, these drugs can be thought of as stabilisers of cell communication, by enhancing deficient systems while simultaneously blocking excessive activity.

Inverse agonists

The concept of an inverse agonist arose because some compounds were found to show 'negative efficacy' – in other words, they acted on unoccupied receptors to produce a change opposite to that caused by an agonist. The presence of an inverse agonist shifts the receptor equilibrium towards the inactive state, thereby reducing the level of basal activity; in consequence, significant effects will occur only if there is a high level of basal (spontaneous) activity. The role of inverse agonist activity in the therapeutic effects of drugs remains to be fully elucidated, but a number

Table 1.4 Drugs that show inverse agonist activity

Receptor	Drugs
α_1-Adrenoceptor	Prazosin, terazosin
β_1-Adrenoceptor	Metoprolol
Muscarinic M_1	Pirenzepine (not available for clinical use in the UK)
Histamine H_1	Cetirizine, loratadine
Histamine H_2	Cimetidine, ranitidine, famotidine
Dopamine D_2	Haloperidol, clozapine, olanzapine
Angiotensin II receptor subtype AT_1	Losartan, candesartan, irbesartan
Cysteinyl leukotriene CysLT1	Montelukast, zafirlukast

of drugs exhibit this type of activity (Table 1.4). Antagonists (see above) bind to the receptor and block the activity of both agonists and inverse agonists. The mechanism of action of inverse agonists is not well characterised, but they may destabilise the receptor/G-protein coupling, or they may preferentially bind to the inactivated form of the receptor, thereby shifting the equilibrium away from the active form. A final complication is that some drugs, for example β-adrenoceptor antagonists, which act as an antagonist at some tissue receptors, may be an inverse agonist when the receptor is expressed on a different tissue (possibly due to association of the receptor protein with different G-proteins).

Allosteric modulators

An allosteric modulator does not act directly on the ligand/receptor site (also called the orthosteric site) but binds to a different (allosteric) site on the receptor. Binding to the allosteric site can change receptor activity by altering the conformation of the protein so as to affect the normal (orthosteric) binding site and thereby enhance or decrease the binding of the natural ligand to its receptor. An example is the benzodiazepine drugs, which alter the affinity of Cl^- channels for the neurotransmitter GABA (Ch. 20). Alternatively, allosteric modulators may change the conformation of the receptor protein so that it alters the receptor signalling (second messenger) domain without affecting the orthosteric site.

Enzyme inhibitors/activators

Some drugs have a site of action that is an enzyme; the drug acts either on the catalytic site or at an allosteric site. An example is the anticholinesterase group of drugs (see Ch. 4).

Non-specific actions

Some compounds produce their desired therapeutic outcome without interaction with a specific site of action on a protein – for example, the action of osmotic diuretics on the kidney.

TOLERANCE TO DRUG EFFECTS

Tolerance to drug effects is characterised by a decrease in response with repeated doses. Tolerance may occur through:

- a decrease in the concentrations of drug at the receptor
- a decrease in response produced by the receptor to the same concentration of drug
- a decrease in the number of receptors (so that an increased % occupancy is necessary to produce the same response).

The relationship between drug dosage and the concentrations delivered to the receptor is discussed in Chapter 2: some drugs stimulate their own metabolism, and, as a result, they are eliminated more rapidly on repeated dosage and lower concentrations of drug are available to produce a response. However, most clinically important examples of tolerance arise from changes in receptor numbers and concentration–response relationships.

Desensitisation is used to describe both long-term and short-term changes in dose–response relationships arising from a decrease in response of the receptor. Desensitisation can occur by a number of mechanisms:

- decreased receptor numbers (downregulation): a slow process taking hours or days
- decreased receptor binding affinity
- decreased G-protein coupling
- modulation of the downstream response to the initial signal.

Extracellular receptors coupled to G-proteins show rapid desensitisation (within minutes) during continued activation, which occurs through three mechanisms.

- **Homologous desensitisation.** The enzymes activated following ligand binding to a receptor/G-protein complex include G-protein-coupled receptor kinases (GRKs), which interact with the βγ-subunit of the G-protein and inactivate the occupied receptor protein by phosphorylation; a related peptide, β-arrestin, enhances the GRK-mediated desensitisation.
- **Heterologous desensitisation.** The receptor (whether occupied or not) is inactivated through phosphorylation by a cAMP-dependent kinase (protein kinase A or protein kinase C), which causes uncoupling of the G-protein and can be switched on by a variety of signals that increase cAMP.
- **Receptor internalisation.** Endocytosis of the agonist-coupled receptor can occur within minutes of constant activation of G-protein-coupled receptors and makes the receptor unavailable for further agonist actions by uncoupling the G-protein from the receptor. The phosphorylated receptor protein may then be internalised and undergo intracellular dephosphorylation prior to re-entering the cytoplasmic membrane.

Downstream modulation of the signal may also occur through feedback mechanisms or simply through depletion of some essential cofactor. An example of the latter is the depletion of the SH groups necessary for the generation of nitric oxide during chronic administration of organic nitrates (see angina, Ch. 5); high doses of indirectly acting

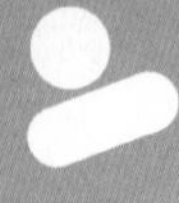

sympathomimetic amines may cause depletion of neuronal noradrenaline, which is necessary for their activity (see Ch. 4).

PHARMACOGENOMICS, PHARMACOGENETICS AND DRUG RESPONSES

There are person-to-person variations for any biological property, including the responses to drug administration. The nature of the response is usually similar in all individuals, because they share the same underlying biology, but the magnitude of the response to the same dose of a drug can differ markedly within a group of individuals. For many responses, this variation is reflected in a single Gaussian distribution (Fig. 1.13a), and such variability is an inherent part of the need to individualise dosage for the person. The presence of a genetic polymorphism in a receptor, site of action, enzyme or transporter (Fig. 1.13b) can give rise to much wider person-to-person variation in response, such that some individuals may have no response to a standard dose while others show toxicity. The genetic origins of many polymorphisms is of increasing importance in relation to drug development (see Ch. 3) and also because it allows the future possibility for genetic screening to be used to optimise drug and dosage selection.

Pharmacogenetics has been defined as 'the influence of variations in DNA sequence on drug response', and relates to how genetic differences between individuals affect the response to a drug or the fate of a drug in the body (Ch. 2). Pharmacogenetic research has been undertaken for more than four decades, largely in relation to in vivo variability, and has often used classic genetic techniques such as studies in twins and patterns of inheritance.

Pharmacogenomics has been defined as 'the investigation of variations of DNA and RNA characteristics as related to drug response', and relates to genome-wide approaches that define the presence of single-nucleotide polymorphisms (SNPs) in the genes which affect the activity of the gene product. Molecular biological techniques have allowed recognition of more than 1.4 million SNPs in the human genome. SNPs can be:

- in the upstream regulatory sequence of a coding gene, which can result in increased or decreased expression of the gene in response to the regulatory transcription factors that control the gene product; the gene product will be the same as the normal or 'wild' type of gene product
- in the coding region of the gene, which will result in a gene product with an altered amino acid sequence that may have higher activity (although this is unlikely), similar activity, lower activity or no activity at all.

In addition, there can be inactive SNPs because they are in non-coding or silent regions of the genome, or because the base change does not alter the amino acid encoded. In consequence, a major challenge for the future is not in identifying SNPs and the presence of genotypic differences, but rather in defining the functional consequences of the genetic difference and the magnitude of phenotypic differences. Future research will also focus on the importance of different combinations of genetic variants (haplotypes) rather than on single gene differences. The rapid advances in molecular biology have allowed analysis of person-to-person differences in the sequences of the genes involved

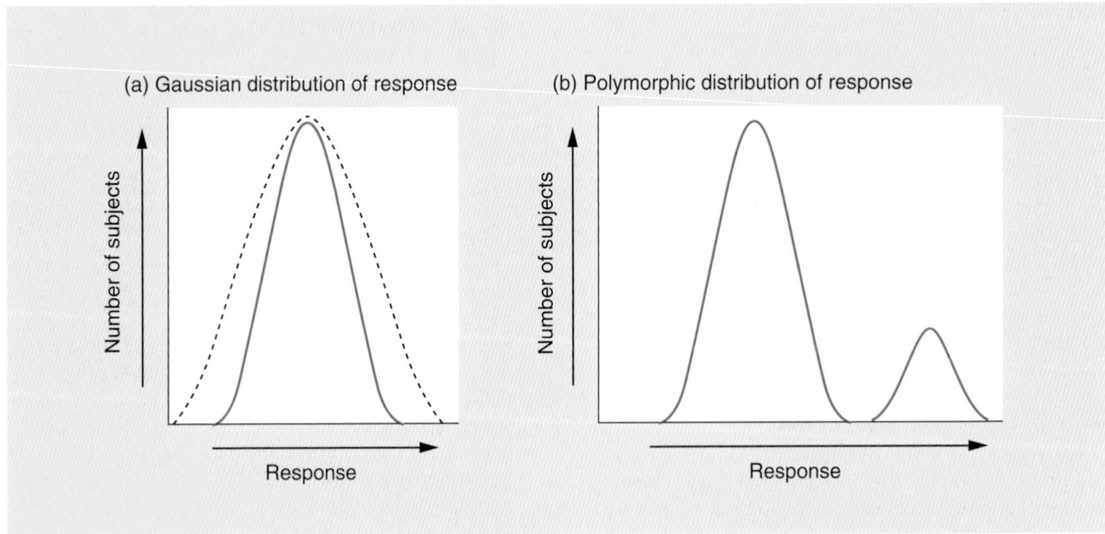

Fig. 1.13 **Inter-individual variation in response to a single dose.** The graphs show the numbers of individuals in a population showing a particular level of response to a single dose of a drug against the magnitude of the response. In Figure 1.13a, most individuals show the average response and the overall shape is a normal distribution. In a normal monomorphic distribution (Fig. 1.13a), the magnitude of inter-individual variability is indicated by the coefficient of variation (the dotted line in Fig. 1.13a is for a response showing wider inter-individual variation). Both the coefficient of variation and the magnitude of the difference between phenotypes affect the variation in a polymorphic distribution (Fig. 1.13b).

in receptors (pharmacodynamics – this chapter) and in drug metabolism and drug transport (pharmacokinetics – Ch. 2). Knowledge of the precise nature of the differences (SNPs) that result in genetic polymorphisms is beyond the scope of an undergraduate text, and is not necessary to understand or appreciate either the current position or possible future developments in the area of pharmacogenomics.

Genetic polymorphisms in receptors and second messenger systems are likely to be of increasing importance in the future. While polymorphisms in pharmacokinetics (see Ch. 2) are likely to have an important impact on dosage selection, polymorphisms in receptors may be more important for drug selection. For example, discovery of a major polymorphism that caused a functional deficit in the angiotensin (AT_2) receptor would mean that neither an angiotensin-converting enzyme (ACE) inhibitor (Ch. 6) nor an AT_2 receptor antagonist would be a good choice to lower blood pressure in such subjects, whereas a β-adrenoceptor antagonist would still be effective. In contrast, a functional deficit in the β_1-adrenoceptor could make an ACE inhibitor a better choice than a β-adrenoceptor antagonist for treating cardiovascular conditions. Genomic studies have identified SNPs in nearly every receptor type found in the autonomic system, some of which have been linked to abnormal cardiovascular or respiratory drug responses; however, a genetic variant of major clinical importance has yet to be identified.

Genetic polymorphisms have been reported in many receptor types, and these have been a major focus of research in relation to the aetiology of diseases. To date, few studies have been performed on the influence of genetic differences in receptor structure on drug responses. Polymorphisms of various G-protein receptors have been found in different domains of the protein with a range of different effects (given in parentheses): the N-terminal domain (altered ligand binding or downregulation), the transmembrane domain (altered ligand binding or coupling to G-protein), the intracellular loop (altered ligand binding or coupling to G-protein) and the C-terminal domain (altered coupling to G-protein). However, despite the large number of variants identified, the clinical and therapeutic implications of few of these have been characterised.

Sixteen different human α_{1A}-adrenoceptor isoforms have been identified, including five full-length and 11 truncated versions (which are incapable of ligand binding and signal transduction). Polymorphisms have been reported for each of the three main α_2-adrenoceptor types (α_{2A}, α_{2B} and α_{2C}), but the consequences for drug activities in clinical practice have not been defined. Nine polymorphisms have been identified in the β_2-adrenoceptor, and certain genetic variants have been associated with different asthma phenotypes and also with differences in drug responses. Polymorphisms in dopamine D_2 receptors have been observed and studied in various conditions, such as alcohol and drug dependency, but, in general, clear relationships of variants of the different dopamine receptors to diseases have not been established, despite the vast amount of research undertaken.

Pharmacogenetic variability will be increasingly important to optimise drug responses and to minimise adverse effects in individuals. Exploitation of genetic differences will require specific individual genetic information. Until such information is available routinely, careful monitoring of the subject's response will remain the best guide to successful treatment.

Information on genetic polymorphisms in different receptors can be found on the OMIM® (Online Mendelian Inheritance in Man®; Johns Hopkins University) database, available at *http://www.ncbi.nlm.nih.gov/omim*

CONCLUSIONS

The selectivity of drugs arises from their ability to interact with and affect certain target sites within a cell. In principle, high selectivity should result in safer drugs with fewer adverse effects. Our increasing knowledge of the complexity of receptor pharmacology offers the promise of safer drugs in the future, especially when genetic differences in pharmacokinetics (Ch. 2) and receptors can be taken into account using individual genetic information, prior to the subject being administered any drug. However, it should be remembered that:

- not all effects seen following drug administration are caused by the drug (a 'placebo effect' can be produced just by a clinical consultation)
- nearly all drugs show multiple effects no matter how receptor-selective they are
- not all effects produced by a drug will be therapeutically beneficial.

FURTHER READING

Ackerman MJ, Clapham DE (1997) Ion-channels – basic science and clinical disease. *N Engl J Med* 336, 1575–1586

Alexander SPH, Mathie A, Peters JA (2008) Guide to receptors and channels (GRAC), 3rd edition (2008 revision). *Br J Pharmacol* 153(suppl 2), S1–S209

Berger JP, Akiyama TE, Meinke PT (2005) PPARs: therapeutic targets for metabolic disease. *Trends Pharmacol Sci* 26, 244–251

Boswell-Smith V, Spina D, Page CP (2006) Phosphodiesterase inhibitors. *Br J Pharmacol* 147, S252–S257

Bourguet W, Germain P, Gronemeyer H (2000) Nuclear receptor ligand-binding domains: three-dimensional structures, molecular interactions and pharmacological implications. *Trends Pharmacol Sci* 21, 381–388

Catterall WA (1995) Structure and function of voltage-gated ion channels. *Annu Rev Biochem* 64, 493–531

Catterell WA, Goldin AL, Waxman SG (2003) International Union of Pharmacology. XL. Compendium of voltage-gated ion channels: sodium channels. *Pharmacol Rev* 55, 575–578

Catterall WA, Striessnig J, Snutch TP et al (2003) International Union of Pharmacology. XL. Compendium of voltage-gated ion channels: calcium channels. *Pharmacol Rev* 55, 579–581

Chuang TT, Iacovelli L, Sallese M, de Blasi A (1996) G protein-coupled receptors: heterologous regulation of homologous desensitization and its implications. *Trends Pharmacol Sci* 17, 416–421

Costa T, Cotecchia S (2005) Historical review: Negative efficacy and the constitutive activity of G-protein coupled receptors. *Trends Pharmacol Sci* 26, 618–624

Dohlman HG, Thomer J, Caron MG, Lefkowitz RJ (1991) Model systems for the study of seven-transmembrane-segment receptors. *Annu Rev Biochem* 60, 653–688

Dolphin A (2003) International Union of Pharmacology. XL. Compendium of voltage-gated ion channels: G protein modulation of voltage-gated calcium channels. *Pharmacol Rev* 55, 607–627

Essayan DM (2001) Cyclic nucleotide phosphodiesterases. *J Allergy Clin Immunol* 108, 671–680

Ferguson FFG (2001) Evolving concepts in G protein-coupled receptor endocytosis: the role in receptor desensitization and signaling. *Pharmacol Rev* 53, 1–24

Fredholm BB, IJzerman AP, Jacobson KA, Klotz KN, Linden J (2001) International Union of Pharmacology. XXV. Nomenclature and classification of adenosine receptors. *Pharmacol Rev* 53, 527–552

Gudermann T, Kalkbrenner F, Schultz G (1996) Diversity and selectivity of receptor–G-protein interaction. *Annu Rev Pharmacol Toxicol* 36, 429–459

Gutman GA, Chandy KG, Adelman JP et al (2003) International Union of Pharmacology. XL. Compendium of voltage-gated ion channels: potassium channels. *Pharmacol Rev* 55, 583–586

Hanoune J, Defer N (2001) Regulation and role of adenylyl cyclase isoforms. *Annu Rev Pharmacol Toxicol* 41, 145–174

Hawrylyshyn KA, Michelotti GA, Coge F, Guenin S-P, Schwinn DA (2004) Update on human α1-adrenoceptor subtype signaling and genomic organization. *Trends Pharmacol Sci* 25, 449–455

Hirano K, Yufu T, Hirano M, Nishimura J, Kanaide H (2005) Physiology and pathophysiology of proteinase-activated receptors (PARs): regulation of the expression of PARs. *J Pharmacol Sci* 97, 31–37

Hofmann F, Biel M, Kaupp UB (2003) International Union of Pharmacology. XL. Compendium of voltage-gated ion channels: cyclic nucleotide modulated channels. *Pharmacol Rev* 55, 587–589

Hollinger S, Hepler JR (2002) Cellular regulation of RGS proteins: modulators and integrators of G protein signaling. *Pharmacol Rev* 54, 527–559

Kenakin T (2004) Principles: Receptor theory in pharmacology. *Trends Pharmacol Sci* 25, 186–192

Kirstein SL, Insel PA (2004) Autonomic nervous system pharmacogenomics: a progress report. *Pharmacol Rev* 56, 31–52

Kobilka BK, Deupi X (2007) Conformational complexity of G-protein-coupled receptors. *Trends Pharmacol Sci* 28, 397–406

Koenig JA, Edwardson JM (1997) Endocytosis and recycling of G protein-coupled receptors. *Trends Pharmacol Sci* 18, 276–287

Lefkowitz RJ (2004) Historical review: A brief history and personal retrospective of seven-transmembrane receptors. *Trends Pharmacol Sci* 25, 413–422

Lucas KA, Pitari GM, Kazerounian S et al (2000) Guanylyl cyclases and signaling by cyclic GMP. *Pharmacol Rev* 52, 375–413

McLeod HL, Evans WE (2001) Pharmacogenomics: unlocking the human genome for better drug therapy. *Annu Rev Pharmacol Toxicol* 41, 101–121

Milligan G, Bond RA, Lee M (1995) Inverse agonism: pharmacological curiosity or potential therapeutic strategy? *Trends Pharmacol Sci* 16, 10–13

Polson JB (1996) Cyclic nucleotide phosphodiesterases and vascular smooth muscle. *Annu Rev Pharmacol Toxicol* 36, 403–427

Privalsky ML (2004) The role of corepressors in transcriptional regulation by nuclear hormone receptors. *Annu Rev Physiol* 66, 315–360

Rana BK, Shiina T, Insel PA (2001) Genetic variations and polymorphisms of G protein-coupled receptors: functional and therapeutic implications. *Annu Rev Pharmacol Toxicol* 41, 593–624

Simon MI, Strathmann MP, Gautam N (1991) Diversity of G proteins in signal transduction. *Science* 252, 802–808

Strader CD, Fong TM, Tota MR, Underwood D, Dixon RAF (1994) Structure and function of G-protein-coupled receptors. *Annu Rev Biochem* 63, 101–132

Strange PG (2003) Mechanisms of inverse agonism at G-protein-coupled receptors. *Trends Pharmacol Sci* 23, 89–95

Streetman DS (2007) Clinical pharmacogenetics of the major adenosine triphosphate-binding cassette and solute carrier drug transporters. *J Pharm Pract* 20, 219–233

Sunahara RK, Dessauer CW, Gilman AG (1996) Complexity and diversity of mammalian adenylyl cyclases. *Annu Rev Pharmacol Toxicol* 36, 461–480

Tsai M-J, O'Malley BW (1994) Molecular mechanisms of action of steroid/thyroid receptor superfamily members. *Annu Rev Biochem* 63, 451–486

Wei LN (2003) Retinoid receptors and their coregulators. *Annu Rev Pharmacol Toxicol* 43, 47–72

Wess J (1993) Molecular basis of muscarinic acetylcholine receptor function. *Trends Pharmacol Sci* 14, 308–313

Wong AHC, Buckle CE, Van Tol HHM (2000) Polymorphisms in dopamine receptors: what do they tell us? *Eur J Pharmacol* 410, 183–203

Examples of some types of receptors and their properties (some of this information was derived from Alexander, Mathie and Peters 2008)

Type	Typical location(s)	Principal transduction mechanism	Biological actions	Agonists[1]	Antagonists[1]
7-transmembrane receptors					
Acetylcholine					
Muscarinic[a]					
M_1	CNS and autonomic ganglia (minor role), gastric	G_q	Neurotransmission in CNS, gastric secretion	***non-selective*** *for all M receptors*-bethanecol, pilocarpine, carbachol	Pirenzepine ***non-selective*** *for all M receptors* – atropine, hyoscine, propantheline
M_2	Heart, CNS	G_i	Bradycardia, smooth muscle contraction (GI, airways, bladder)		
M_3	Smooth muscles, secretory glands	G_q	Contraction, secretion	I	Darifenacin
Adrenergic					
α-Adrenoceptors[b]					
α_1 ($\alpha_{1A}\alpha_{1B}\alpha_{1D}$)	CNS and postsynaptic in sympathetic nervous system human prostate (α_{1A})	G_q	Contraction of arterial smooth muscle, decrease in contractions of gut, contraction of prostate tissue	Phenylephrine, methoxamine (tamsulosin α_{1A})	Prazosin, indoramin
α_2 ($\alpha_{2A}\alpha_{2B}\alpha_{2C}$)	Presynaptic (in both α- and β-adrenergic neurons)	G_i	Decreased noradrenaline release	Clonidine (oxymetazoline α_{2A})	Yohimbine
β-Adrenoceptors[c]					
β_1	CNS and heart (nodes and myocardium)	G_s	Increased force and rate of cardiac contraction	Dobutamine NA > AD	Atenolol, metoprololol
β_2	Widespread	G_s	Bronchial dilation, decrease in contraction of gut, metabolic effects	Salmeterol, terbutaline, AD > NA	Butoxamine
β_3	Adipocytes	G_s	Mobilisation of fat stores	AD = NA	–
Cannabinoids					
CB_1, CB_2	Cortex,hippocampus, amygdala, basal ganglia, cerebellum	Gi/G_0	Behaviour, pain, nausea, stimulation of appetite, depression	*N*-arachidonoylethanolamine (anandamide), 2-arachidonylglyceryl	
Cholecystokinin					
CCK_1, CCK_2	CCK_1, primarily GI CCK_2 primarily in CNS	G_q/G_s	CCK_1, gall bladder emptying, inhibits gut motility; CCK_2 CNS nociception, anxiety, appetite	CCK-4, CCK-8, CCK-33, gastrin	
Calcitonin–gene related peptide					
CGRP	Sensory nerve endings	G_q/G_s	Vasodilation, nociception, inflammation	CGRP	

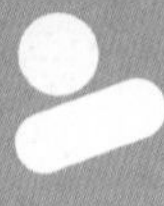

Examples of some types of receptors and their properties (some of this information was derived from Alexander, Mathie and Peters 2008)

Type	Typical location(s)	Principal transduction mechanism	Biological actions	Agonists[1]	Antagonists[1]
Dopamine[d]					
D_1	CNS (N, O, P, S), kidney,[d] heart[d]	G_s	Vasodilation in kidney (see notes)	Fenoldopam	
D_2	CNS (C, N, O, SN), pituitary gland, chemoreceptor trigger zone gastrointestinal tract	G_i↑ K^+ channels, ↓ Ca^{2+} channels	Linked to schizophrenia, prolactin secretion, movement control, memory	Bromocriptine, pergolide	Butyrophenones, sulpiride, renoxipride, domperidone
D_3	CNS (F, Me, Mi) (limbic system)	G_i	Cognition emotion		Sulpiride
D_4	CNS, heart	G_i	Linked to schizophrenia		Clozapine
D_5	CNS (Hi, Hy)	G_s			
5-Hydroxytryptamine (5HT), serotonin)[e]					
$5HT_{1A}$	CNS	G_i	Anxiety sleep, appetite, nerve inhibition	Buspirone	
$5HT_{1B}$	CNS blood vessels	G_i	Vasoconstriction presynaptic inhibition	Sumatriptan, eletriptan	
$5HT_{1D}$	CNS, blood vessels	G_i	Vasoconstriction behaviour	Sumatriptan, eletriptan	Metergoline
$5HT_{1E}$	CNS	G_i			
$5HT_{1F}$	CNS	G_i			
$5HT_{2A}$	CNS platelets, smooth muscle	G_q	Schizophrenia, platelet aggregation, vasodilation/ vasoconstriction	LSD	Ketanserin
$5HT_{2B}$	Stomach	G_q	Contraction, morphogenesis		
$5HT_{2C}$	CNS	G_q	Satiety		
$5HT_4$	CNS, myenteric plexus, smooth muscle	G_s	Anxiety, memory, gut motility	Metoclopramide, renzapride	
$5HT_{5A}$	CNS	G_i			
$5HT_{5B}$	CNS	?			
$5HT_6$	CNS	G_s			
$5HT_7$	CNS GI blood vessels	G_s		LSD	Clozapine
Histamine					
H_1	CNS, endothelium, smooth muscle	G_q	Sedation, sleep, vascular permeability, inflammation		Mepyramine
H_2	CNS, cardiac muscle, stomach	G_s	Gastric acid secretion	Dimaprit	Cimetidine, ranitidine

Examples of some types of receptors and their properties (some of this information was derived from Alexander, Mathie and Peters 2008)

Type	Typical location(s)	Principal transduction mechanism	Biological actions	Agonists[1]	Antagonists[1]
H_3	CNS (presynaptic), myenteric plexus	G_i	Appetite, cognition		Thioperamide
H_4	Eosinophils, basophils, mast cells	G_i			
Gamma-aminobutyric acid receptor type B ($GABA_B$)					
$GABA_B$	Brain neurons, glial cells, spinal motor neurons and interneurons	G_i effects on Ca^{2+} channel (closes) and K^+ channel (opens)	Widespread reduction of impulse transmission in CNS, suppression of polysynaptic reflexes in spine, generation of spike and wave discharges in absence epilepsy	Baclofen	
Glutamate (metabotropic)[f]					
Group I ($mglu_1$ and $mglu_5$)		G_q	Multiple possible roles; memory, learning, pain perception, anxiety, modulation of transmission (e.g. DA and NA) ?schizophrenia		
Group II ($mglu_2$ and $mglu_3$)		G_i			
Group III ($mglu_4$, $mglu_6$, $mglu_7$ and $mglu_8$)		G_i			
Peptides					
Angiotensin II					
AT_1	Blood vessels, adrenal cortex, brain	G_q/G_0	Vasconstriction, salt retention, aldosterone synthesis, increased noradrenergic activity, cardiac hypertrophy		Losartan, valsartan
AT_2	Blood vessels, endothelium, adrenal cortex brain	Tyrosine phosphatases	Weak vasodilation, fetal development, vascular growth. Stimulates NO synthesis in endothelium		
Bradykinin					
B_1 (induced)	Widespread (induced by injury, cytokines)	G_q	Acute inflammation. Stimulates NO synthesis	ACE inhibitors (indirect via BK stimulation)	
B_2 (constitutive)		G_q	Chronic inflammation. Most actions of kinins, vasodilation, pain response		
Endothelins					
ET_A	Endothelium	G_q	Vasoconstriction, proliferation blood vessels		Sitaxentan, bosentan

Examples of some types of receptors and their properties (some of this information was derived from Alexander, Mathie and Peters 2008)

Type	Typical location(s)	Principal transduction mechanism	Biological actions	Agonists[1]	Antagonists[1]
ET_B	Endothelium (Ch. 6)	G_q	Release of nitric oxide (indirect vasodilation), direct vasoconstriction, natriuresis		Bosentan
Ghrelin	Stomach, endocrine cells; ghrelin receptors are widespread	G_q	Ligand for GH secretagogue receptor, induces appetite	[D-Arg^1, D-Phe^5, D-Trp^{7,9}, Leu^{11}]-substance P	
Melanocortin receptor family [MC_1-MC_5] (Ch. 37)		G_s	MSH skin pigmentation, feeding behaviour. ACTH (specifically at MC_2) skin pigmentation HPA function	Melanocyte stimulating hormone (MSH)	agouti-related protein (AGRP) (Ch. 37)
Natriuretic peptides					
ANP_A		G-protein, guanylyl cyclase	Increase Na^+ excretion		
ANP_B		G-protein, guanylyl cyclase	Increase Na^+ excretion		
Neuropeptide Y (NPY) receptor family Y_1–Y_6) (Ch. 37)	Y receptors wide distribution in CNS hypothalamus. NPY secreted into blood from stomach	G_i	Increases appetite; stress; memory learning		
Tachykinins (neurokinins)					
NK_1		G_q: slow build-up of response	Nociception (substance P)	Substance P	
NK_2		G_q: slow build-up of response	Nociception (neurokinin A)	Substance P	
NK_3		G_q	(Neurokinin B)	Substance P	
Opioids					
δ, κ, μ, N/OFQ (nociceptin/ orphanin)		G_i			
Orexin (OX_1 OX_2) (also known as hypocretins) (Ch. 37)	Hypothalamus and other areas of brain	G_q	Increases food intake, wakefulness, body temperature. Activated by orexin-A and B		
Proteinase activated receptors (PAR_1, PAR_2, PAR_3, PAR_4)	Platelets, endothelial cells, myocytes, neurons	G_q, G_i	Activated by proteolytic cleavage	Trypsin, thrombin	

Examples of some types of receptors and their properties (some of this information was derived from Alexander, Mathie and Peters 2008)

Type	Typical location(s)	Principal transduction mechanism	Biological actions	Agonists[1]	Antagonists[1]
Vasopressin and Oxytocin					
V_{1a}	Pituitary, brain	G_q	Vasoconstriction, platelet aggregation	Arginine vasopressin > oxytocin	
V_{1b}	Pituitary, brain	G_q plus G_i,	Modulates ACTH secretion	Arginine vasopressin > oxytocin	
V_2	Kidney	G_s	Antidiuretic effect on collecting duct and ascending limb of loop of Henle	Arginine vasopressin > oxytocin	
OT	Breast, brain uterus	G_q	Lactation, uterine contraction, CNS actions	Oxytocin > arginine vasopressin	
Purinergic receptors (purinoreceptors)					
Adenosine					
A_1		G_i↑ K^+ conduction in heart	Decreased glomerular filtration rate, cardiac depression, vasoconstriction, decreased CNS activity, bronchoconstriction	–	Methylxanthines
A_{2A}		G_s	Vasodilation, decreased CNS activity, inhibition of platelet aggregation, bronchodilation		Methylxanthines
A_{2B}		G_q	Action on intestine and bladder	–	Enprofylline
A_{2B}		G_s Ca^{2+} influx	Release of mediators from mast cells?		
A_3		G_i	Wide tissue distribution; release of mediators from mast cells		
P2Y-receptors ($P2Y_1$, $P2Y_2$, $P2Y_4$, $P2Y_6$)	A family of peptides present in almost all tissues	G_q, G_s	Biological effect depends upon G protein coupling	Activated by ATP, ADP, UTP, UDP and UDP-glucose.	
Ligand-gated receptors or channels (also called transmitter-gated receptors or channels)					
Nicotinic N_1	Autonomic ganglia	Ligand-gated ion channel	Postganglionic activation	Carbachol, nicotine	Trimetaphan, mecamylamine
Nicotinic N_2	Neuromuscular junction	Ligand-gated ion channel	Muscle contraction	Nicotine	Gallamine, vecuronium
$5HT_3$	CNS (A), enteric nerves, sensory nerves	Ligand-gated Na^+/K^+ channels	Emesis		Granisetron, ondansetron
$GABA_A$[h]	Brain neurons, spinal motor neurons and interneurons	Ligand-gated Cl^- channel (open)[g]	Widespread reduction of impulse transmission in CNS, inhibition of sensory signals at spinal level	Muscimol (benzodiazepines) (zolpidem)	(Picrotoxin) (flumazenil)

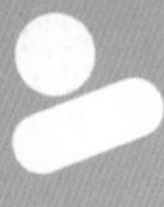

Examples of some types of receptors and their properties (some of this information was derived from Alexander, Mathie and Peters 2008)

Type	Typical location(s)	Principal transduction mechanism	Biological actions	Agonists[1]	Antagonists[1]
Glycine	Brain neurons, spinal motor neurons and interneurons	Ligand-gated Cl^- channel (open)[g]	Widespread reduction of impulse transmission in CNS, inhibition of sensory signals at spinal level	Intravenous anaesthetics	Strychnine, tropisetron, endocannabinoids
Ionotropic glutamate-like receptors (AMPA, NMDA, kainate)[f]					
N-Methyl D-aspartate(NMDA)[i]	CNS (B, C, sensory pathways)	Ligand-gated Ca^{2+} channel (slow)	Synaptic plasticity, excitatory transmitter release, excessive amounts may cause neuronal damage	Aspartate	Ketamine, phenyclidine (inhibit Ca^{2+} flux)
Kainate	CNS (Hi)	Ligand-gated Ca^{2+} channel (fast)	Synaptic plasticity, transmitter release	Kainate	
a-amino-3-hydroxy-5-methyl-4-isoxazole propionic acid (AMPA)	CNS (similar to NMDA receptors)	Ligand-gated Ca^{2+} channel (fast)	Synaptic plasticity, transmitter release		
Purinergic P2X family ($P2X_1$-$P2X_7$)	$P2X_1$ smooth muscle; $P2X_{2\text{-}3}$ ganglia	Ligand-gated ion channels (Na^+, Ca^{2+} and K^+ and exceptionally Cl^-)	Neuronal depolarisation, influx of Na^+ and Ca^{2+} > efflux of K^+	Endogenous ligand ATP	
Ryanodine receptors (RyR1, RyR2, RyR3)	RyR (skeletal muscle), RyR2 (heart), RyR3 (widespread, brain)	Cytosolic Ca^{2+}, ATP	Intracellular Ca^{2+} concentrations, ?myasthenia gravis	Ryanodine, caffeine	>100 mM Ca^{2+}, Mg^{2+} dantrolene

[1]Only selected agonists and antagonists are included. Many of these are investigational tools and have no clinical use.

The transduction processes are G_s = ↑ adenylyl cyclase, increased protein kinase A; G_i = ↓ adenylyl cyclase, decreased protein kinase A; G_q = ↑ phospholipase C, increased IP_3, diacylglycerol.

AD – adrenaline; NA – noradrenaline; LSD – lysergic acid diethylamide.

[a]Additional muscarinic receptors (M_4 (G_i) and M_5 (G_q)) have been identified recently but their clinical importance is unclear.
[b]Three α_1-adrenoceptors have been identified (α_{1A}, α_{1B}, α_{1D}), all of which act via G_q proteins: α_{1A}-adrenoceptors have a higher affinity for noradrenaline than for adrenaline, α_{1B}- and α_{1D}-adrenoceptors do not show selectivity.
[c]The β-adrenoceptors differ in their affinities for noradrenaline (NA) and adrenaline (AD): β_1, NA > AD; β_2, AD > NA: β_3, NA = AD.
[d]Commonly divided into D_1-like (D_1 and D_5) and D_2-like (D_2, D_3,D_4). The type of receptor in heart and kidney remains questionable as the mRNA for D_1 receptors has not been found (it could be D_5). CNS areas: A, area postrema; B, basal ganglia; C, caudate putamen; Ch, choroid; Co, cortex; F, frontal cortex; G, globus pallidus; Hi, hippocampus; Hy, hypothalamus; Me, medulla; Mi, midbrain: N, nucleus accumbens; 0, olfactory tubercle; P, putamen; R, raphe nucleus; S, striatum; SN, substantia nigra; T, thalamus.
[e]There are many experimental drugs that are selective agonists and antagonists for receptors subtypes and some are undergoing clinical trials for various conditions. Only clinically useful examples are given. The identification and classification of 5HT receptors is a complex and rapidly changing field. 5HT is involved in numerous pathways within the CNS and the roles of the different receptor types has not been fully characterised. Effects associated with the different receptors are not well established, with the exception of $5HT_3$ and emesis.
[f]Glutamate produces increased neuronal activity in many regions of the CNS; the different receptors are formed from subunits that can exist in different isoforms; a number of variants have been demonstrated for each.
[g]Part of response to vascular damage.
[h]GABA produces inhibition of neurotransmission widely throughout the brain.The $GABA_A$ receptor Cl^- channel has a binding site for GABA and also adjacent binding sites for benzodiazepines (which affect the response to GABA), barbiturates, picrotoxin and steroids.

APPENDIX

LIMITED STUDENT FORMULARY

This formulary has been derived from the formulary put together by Maxwell and Walley (2003), the Southampton University Hospitals Trust formulary and the Southampton Medical School Pharmacology Course documents.

Its purpose is to introduce students in the early years of their undergraduate course in medicine to representative examples of core drugs and their uses in major areas of medicine. It is not exhaustive.

GASTROINTESTINAL SYSTEM	
Therapeutic problem	**Core drugs**
Dyspepsia and gastro-oesophageal reflux disease	Antacids *e.g. magnesium and aluminium-containing antacids, eg aluminium hydroxide and magnesium carbonate* Acid secretion inhibition e.g. proton pump inhibitors and H2 receptor antagonists (see peptic ulcer disease drugs); Anti-reflux drugs, *e.g. gaviscon*
Motility stimulants	These may be used in gastrointestinal reflux disease *e.g. metoclopramide*
Peptic ulcer disease	Proton-pump inhibitors, *e.g. omeprazole* H2 receptor antagonists, *e.g. ranitidine, cimetidine;* other drugs *e.g. sucralfate, misoprostil*
Helicobacter pylori eradication	Antibiotics, *e.g. clarithromycin, amoxicillin, metronidazole*
Inflammatory bowel disease (ulcerative colitis, Crohn's disease)	Corticosteroids, *e.g. prednisolone* Other drugs *e.g. sulfasalazine, mesalazine* Cytokine inhibitors, *e.g. infliximab*
Clostridium difficile colitis	Antibiotics for *C. difficile*, *metronidazole* *Vancomycin*
Diarrhoea	Oral rehydration therapy; Antimotility drugs, *e.g. loperamide, codeine*
Constipation	Bulk forming laxatives, *e.g. ispaghula* Stimulant laxatives, *e.g. senna* Osmotic laxatives, *e.g. magnesium hydroxide, lactulose* Faecal softeners, *e.g. docusate*
Bowel cleansing	*Sodium picosulfate*
Antispasmodics	Antimuscarinics, *e.g. hyoscine* Other antispasmodics, *mebeverin*

CARDIOVASCULAR SYSTEM	
Therapeutic problem	**Core drugs**
Hypertension	β-adrenoceptor antagonists, *e.g. atenolol* α-adrenoceptor antagonists, *e.g. doxazosin.* Centrally-acting antihypertensives, *e.g. clonidine, moxonidine* Angiotensin-converting enzyme inhibitors, *e.g. captopril* Angiotensin-II receptor antagonists, *e.g. candesartan, losartan* Thiazide and related diuretics, *e.g. bendroflumethazide, metolazone.* Loop diuretics, *e.g. furosemide* Potassium-sparing diuretics, *e.g. amiloride, spironolactone* Calcium channel blockers, *e.g. amlodipine* Potassium channel openers, *e.g. minoxidil, nicorandil*
Heart failure	Many drugs used for hypertension are of benefit, in addition positive inotropic drugs: cardiac glycosides, *e.g. digoxin*. Phosphodiesterase inhibitors, e.g. milrinone β-adrenoceptor antagonists, *e.g. bisoprolol*

CARDIOVASCULAR SYSTEM	
Therapeutic problem	**Core drugs**
Acute coronary syndrome (angina, myocardial infarction)	Many drugs listed under hypertension; in addition: *Glyceryl trinitrate, isosorbide mononitrate* inhibitors of platelet aggregation, *e.g. aspirin, dipyridamole, clopidogrel, abciximab* Thrombolytics, *e.g. streptokinase, tenecteplase* Heparins, *unfractionated* heparins, *low molecular weigh heparins* Oral anticoagulants, *e.g. warfarin* Lipid-regulating drugs, *e.g. simvastatin*
Arrhythmias	Antiarrhythmic drugs, *e.g. digoxin, adenosine, amiodarone, lidocaine, β-adrenoceptor antagonists, calcium channel blockers*
Cardiac arrest, deep vein thrombosis, pulmonary embolus, **Pulmonary oedema, stroke treatment and prevention, hyperlipidaemia**	Appropriate drugs chosen from the classes already described for the Cardiovascular System
RESPIRATORY SYSTEM	
Therapeutic problem	**Core drugs**
Asthma (acute and chronic), chronic obstructive pulmonary disease, respiratory failure	Oxygen; Bronchodilators: β_2-adrenoceptor agonists, *e.g. salbutamol, salmeterol* Antimuscarinc bronchodilators, *e.g. ipratropium* Leukotriene receptor antagonists, *e.g. montelukast* Other drugs, *e.g. aminophylline, cromoglicate, magnesium sulphate* Corticosteroids, e.g. *beclometasone*
CENTRAL NERVOUS SYSTEM	
Therapeutic problem	**Core drugs**
Insomnia, anxiety	Benzodiazepines and other drugs, *e.g. diazepam* Other drugs, *e.g. buspirone*, *propranolol*
Schizophrenia, mania	Antipsychotic drugs, *e.g. chlorpromazine, clozapine* Mood stablisers, *e.g. lithium*
Depression	Tricyclic and related antidepressants, *e.g. amitriptyline* Selective serotonin re-uptake inhibitors, *e.g. fluoxetine* Monoamine oxidase inhibitors, *e.g. phenelzine*
Analgesia	Simple analgesics without anti-inflammatory properties, *e.g. paracetalmol.* Nonsteroidal analgesics – see section on Musculoskeletal and Joint Diseases Compound analgesics *e.g. co-codamol* Opioid analgesics, *e.g. codeine, morphine, diamorphine*
Nausea and vertigo	Dopamine antagonists, *e.g. metoclopramide* Serotonin type 3 ($5HT_3$) receptor antagonists, *e.g. ondansetron* Muscarinic receptor antagonists, *e.g. hyoscine* Other agents, *betahistine*
Acute and chronic migraine *Acute migraine* *Prophylaxis of chronic migraine*	Serotonin type 1 receptor agonists, *e.g. sumatriptan* Serotonin type 2 receptor antagonists, *e.g. pizotifen*
Epilepsy	Anticonvulsant therapy, *e.g. diazepam, phenytoin, carbamazepine, sodium valproate, gabapentin*
Status epilepicus	*e.g. diazepam*
Parkinson's disease	Drugs enhancing dopaminergic activity, *e.g. L-dopa* and dopa decarboxylase inhibitor combinations, *e.g. co-careldopa* Other drugs influencing dopamine or dopamine receptors, *e.g. bromocriptine, entacapone, ropinirole* Antimuscarinic drugs, *e.g. procyclidine*
Dementia (Alzheimer's disease)	Anticholinesterases, *e.g. donepizil* *NMDA receptor antagonists, e.g. memantine*

INFECTIOUS DISEASES	
Therapeutic problem	**Core drugs**
Community and hospital acquired infections (bacteria, fungi, viruses)	Penicillins, *e.g. benzyl penicillin, amoxicillin, co-amoxiclav, flucloxacillin* Cephalosporins, *e.g. cefalexin* Tetracyclines *e.g. oxytetracycline* *Trimethoprim* Aminoglycosides, *e.g. gentamicin* *Vancomycin* Macrolides, *e.g. erythromycin* *Chloramphenicol* Quinolones, *e.g. ciprofloxacin* *Metronidazole* Antituberculosis drugs, *e.g. isoniazid, rifampicin, ethambutol* Antifungal drugs, *e.g. amphotericin, fluconazole* Antiviral drugs, e.g. *acyclovir* Nucleoside reverse transcriptase inhibitor, *e.g. abacavir* Protease inhibitors, *e.g. saquinavir* Antimalarial drugs, *e.g. mefloquine, proguanil*

ENDOCRINE SYSTEM	
Therapeutic problem	**Core drugs**
Diabetes mellitus, thyroid disease, osteoporosis, hormone deficiencies and excess	Diabetes, *e.g. long and short-acting insulins* Sulphonylureas, *e.g. gliclazide* Biguanides, *e.g. metformin* The glitazones, *e.g. rosiglitazone* Thyroid disease, *e.g. levothyroxine, propranolol, carbimazole* Bisphosphonates, *e.g. alendronic acid, calcium, vitamin D* Hypothalamic, pituitary hormones and anti-oestrogens: Anti-oestrogens, *e.g. clomifene* Anterior pituitary hormones, *e.g. somatotropin* Hypothalamic hormones, *e.g. gonadorelin (LHRH)* Posterior pituitary hormones and antagonists, *e.g. desmopressin, vasopressin*
Genito-urinary disorders	
Urinary retention	α-blockers, *e.g. doxazosin*
Benign prostatic hypertrophy	5α-reductase inhibitors, *e.g. finasteride*
Urinary frequency and incontinence	Antimuscarinic drugs, e.g. *oxybutynin*
Erectile dysfunction	Phosphodiesterase inhibitors, e.g. *sildenafil*

OBSTETRICS AND GYNAECOLOGY	
Therapeutic problem	**Core drugs**
Steroid oral contraception	Combined oral contraceptives, progestogen-only contraceptives Emergency contraception, progestin
Injectable contraception	Injectable steroidal contraceptives, e.g. *medroxyprogesterone acetate*
Intrauterine contraception	Intra-uterine progestogen containing device
Menstrual disorders	
Dysmenorrhoea	Mefenamic acid
Menorrhagia	Progestogens Antifibrinolytic agent, *e.g. tranexamic acid*
Endometriosis	*Combined contraceptive; danazol*
Hormone replacement therapy (menopause)	*Oestrogens (natural and synthetic), progestins*
Induction of labour	Oxytocics, *e.g. prostaglandins, oxytocin*
Prevention of pre-term labour and myometrial relaxation	Calcium channel blockers, *e.g. nifedipine* *β-adrenoceptor agonists, e.g. terbutaline*
Induction of abortion	*Oxytocics, mifepristone*
Post-partum haemorrhage	*Oxytocics, ergometrine*

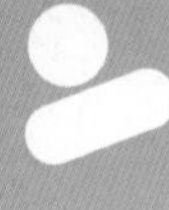

MALIGNANT DISEASE AND IMMUNOSUPPRESSION	
Therapeutic problem	**Core drugs**
Anti-cancer and immunosuppression	Anti-cancer drugs: alkylating agents, *e.g. cyclophosphamide* Cytotoxic antibiotics, *e.g. doxorubicin* Antimetabolites, *e.g. methotrexate* Vinca alkaloids, *e.g. vinblastin* Other drugs, *e.g. asparaginase, cisplatin* Anti-oestrogens, *e.g. tamoxifen, anastrazole, herceptin* Immunosuppressant agents acting in a variety of ways, *e.g. azathioprine, corticosteroids, cyclosporine* Anti CD20 monoclonal antibody, *e.g. rituximab* *Interferon alfa*
Musculoskeletal and joint disease	
Rheumatoid arthritis	Simple analgesic *e.g. paracetamol*, Nonsteroidal anti-inflammatory drugs, *e.g. indometacin, diclofenac* Corticosteroids *e.g. prednisolone* Disease modifying drugs, *e.g. methotrexate, gold, penicillamine, anti-malarials (hydroxychloroquine), azathioprine, sulfasalazine, cytokine inhibitors, e.g. infliximab*
Impaired neuromuscular transmission, e.g. myasthenia gravis	Anticholinesterases, *e.g. pyridostigmine*
Spasticity	Skeletal muscle relaxants, *e.g. baclofen*
Ophthalmology	
Glaucoma	β-Blockers, *e.g. timolol* Prostaglandin analogues, *e.g. latenoprost* Sympathomimetics, *e.g. brimonidine* Carbonic anhydrase inhibitors, *e.g. acetazolamide* Miotics, *e.g. pilocarpine*
Mydriatics and cycloplegics	Mydriatics, *e.g. phenylephrine* Mydriatics and cycloplegics, *e.g. atropine, tropicamide*
Surgery, anaesthetics and intensive care	Many drugs listed from other sections would be used including opioids, sympathomimetics, anti-emetics Intravenous anaesthetics for induction, *e.g. thiopental, propofol* Inhalation anaesthetics, *e.g. isoflurane* Muscle relaxants, *e.g. suxamethonium, atracurium* Antimuscarinics, *e.g. atropine, glycopyrronium* Anticholinesterases, *e.g. neostigmine* Local anaesthesia, *e.g. lidocaine, bupivacaine* Analgesics, *e.g. morphine, fentanyl*

Maxwell S, Walley T. Teaching safe and effective prescribing in UK medical schools: a core curriculum for tomorrow's doctors. Br J Clin Pharmacol 2003;55:496-503.

2 Pharmacokinetics

The type of response of an individual to a particular drug (for example a decrease in blood pressure) depends on the inherent pharmacological properties of the drug at its site of action. However, the time delay between drug administration and response, and the intensity and duration of response, usually depend on parameters such as:

- the rate and extent of uptake of the drug from its site of administration
- drug distribution to different tissues, including the site of action
- the rate of elimination from the body.

Overall, the response of the patient represents a combination of the effects of the drug at its site of action in the body (*pharmacodynamics*) and the way the body influences drug delivery to its site of action (*pharmacokinetics*) (Fig. 2.1). Both pharmacodynamic and pharmacokinetic aspects are subject to a number of variables (Fig. 2.1), which affect the dose–response relationship. Pharmacodynamic aspects are determined by processes such as drug–receptor interaction and are specific to the class of the drug (e.g. β-adrenoceptor antagonists). Pharmacokinetic aspects are determined by general processes, such as transfer across membranes, xenobiotic (foreign compound) metabolism and renal elimination, which apply irrespective of the pharmacodynamic properties.

Pharmacokinetics may be divided into three basic processes:

- **absorption**: the transfer of the drug from its site of administration to the general circulation
- **distribution**: the transfer of the drug from the general circulation into the different organs of the body
- **elimination**: the removal of the drug from the body, which may involve either excretion or metabolism.

Each of these can be described in biological terms, involving biochemical and physiological processes, and also in mathematical terms. The mathematical description of pharmacokinetic processes determines many of the quantitative aspects of drug prescribing:

- why oral and intravenous treatments may require different doses
- the interval between doses during chronic therapy
- the dosage adjustment that may be necessary in hepatic and renal disease
- the calculation of dosages for the very young and the elderly.

THE BIOLOGICAL BASIS OF PHARMACOKINETICS

Drug structures bear little resemblance to normal dietary constituents such as carbohydrates, fats and proteins, and they are handled in the body by different processes. Drugs that bind to the receptor for a specific endogenous neurotransmitter rarely resemble the natural ligand in chemical structure, and they do not usually share the same carrier processes or metabolising enzymes with the natural ligand. Consequently, the movement of drugs around the body is mostly by simple passive diffusion rather than by specific transporters, while metabolism is usually by 'drug-metabolising enzymes', which have low substrate specificity and can handle a wide variety of drug substrates.

GENERAL CONSIDERATIONS

Passage across membranes

With the exception of direct intravenous or intra-arterial injections, a drug must cross at least one membrane in its movement from the site of administration into the general circulation. Drugs acting at intracellular sites must also cross the cell membrane to exert an effect. The main mechanisms by which drugs can cross membranes (Fig. 2.2) are:

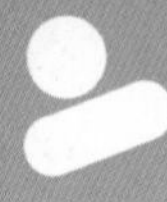

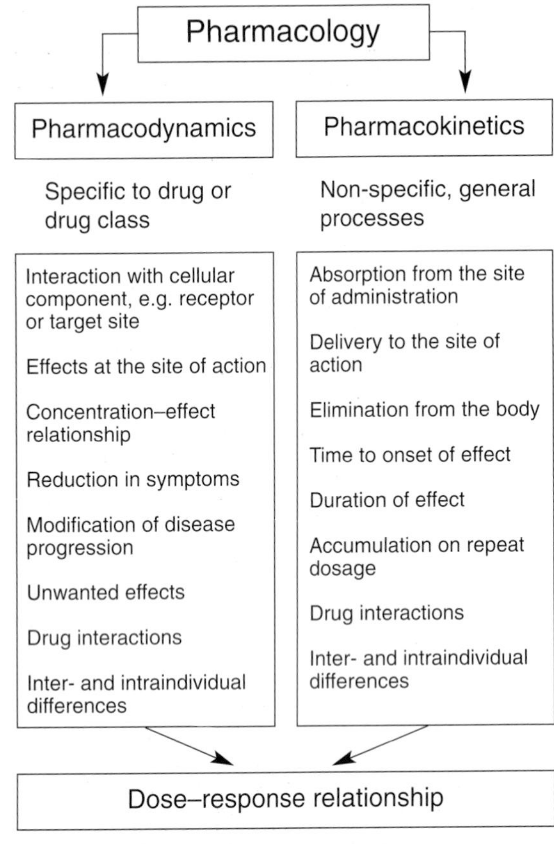

Fig. 2.1 **Factors determining the response of an individual to a drug.**

- passive diffusion
- carrier-mediated processes: facilitated diffusion and active transport
- through pores or ion channels
- pinocytosis.

1. Passive diffusion

Passive movement down a concentration gradient occurs for all drugs. To cross a membrane, the drug must pass into the phospholipid bilayer (Fig. 2.2) and therefore has to have a degree of lipid solubility. Eventually a state of equilibrium will be reached in which equal concentrations of the diffusible form of the drug are present in solution on each side of the membrane.

2. Carrier-mediated processes

Two carrier-mediated processes are of widespread importance in the transport of drugs across lipid membranes.

- *Active transportation* utilises energy and transports drugs into or out of cells against their concentration gradient. It is performed by a family of non-specific carriers termed the ATP-binding cassette (ABC) superfamily of membrane transporters (Fig. 2.2, Table 2.1).
- *Facilitated transportation* does not utilise energy and drugs are transported only down their concentration gradients using the solute carrier (SLC) superfamily of transporters (Fig. 2.2, Table 2.1).

In humans, the ABC active-transporter superfamily contains 49 members, which are organised into seven subfamilies (A–G) based on their relative sequence homology. Interest in this area has exploded since the discovery of the P-glycoprotein (PGP) (also known as multidrug resistance 1

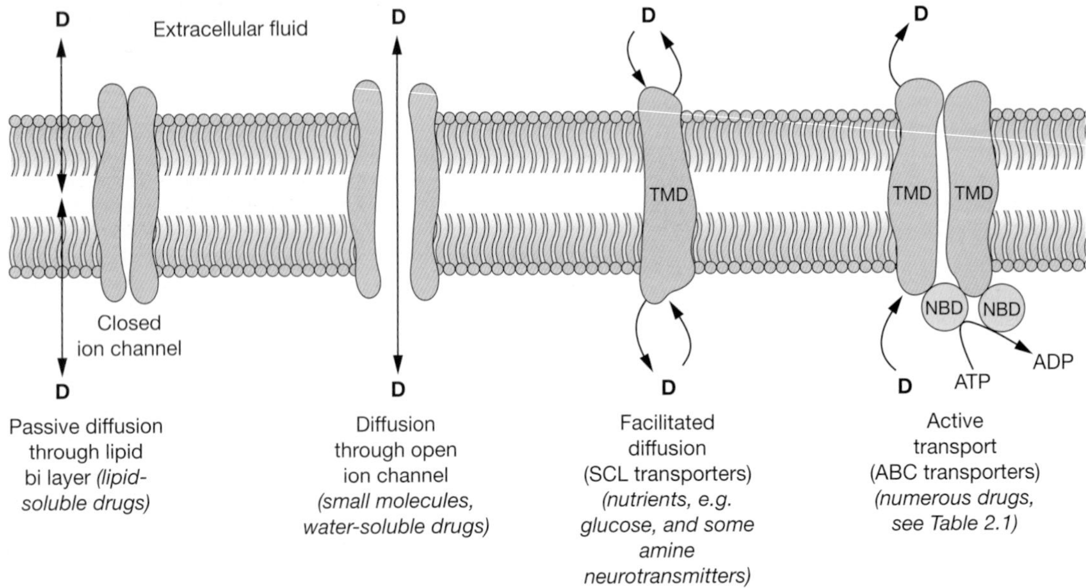

Fig. 2.2 **The passage of drugs across membrane bilayers.** D, drug; TMD, transmembrane domain; NBD, nucleotide-binding domain; ABC, ATP-binding cassette superfamily of transport proteins; SCL, solute carrier superfamily of transporters (see Table 2.1). Some drugs have an affinity for and bind to a transporter but are not released, so that they inhibit the transport of other drug substrates.

Table 2.1 Drug transporters

Transporter	Typical substrates	Sites in the body
ABC superfamily	**A**TP-**B**inding **C**assette superfamily of transport proteins. Although there are a number of transporters in each family, the four ABC transporters listed below can explain multidrug resistance in all cell lines analysed to date. Utilise ATP for active transport	
MDR1[a] or P-glycoprotein (ABCB1)	Hydrophobic and cationic (basic) molecules; numerous drugs, including anticancer drugs	Apical surface of membranes of epithelial cells of intestine, liver, kidney, blood–brain barrier, testis, placenta and lung
MRP1[a] (ABCC1)	Numerous, including anticancer drugs, glucuronide and glutathione conjugates	Basolateral surface of membranes of most cell types with high levels in lung, testes, and kidney and in blood:tissue barriers
MRP2[a] (ABCC2)	Numerous, including anticancer drugs, glucuronide and glutathione conjugates	Apical surface of membranes; mainly in liver, intestine, and kidney tubules
BRCP (ABCG2) Breast cancer resistance protein	Anticancer, antiviral drugs, fluoroquinolones, flavonoids	Apical surface of breast ducts and lobules, small intestine, colon epithelium, liver, placenta, brain barrier and lungs
SLC superfamily	**SoLute Carrier** superfamily of transporters. Comprises **o**rganic **a**nion **t**ransporters (OATs) and **o**rganic **c**ation **t**ransporters (OCTs)	
OAT1 (SLC22A6)	Numerous, including PAH, NSAIDs, penicillins, diuretics and phase II drug metabolites	Kidney (basolateral), brain, placenta, smooth muscle
OAT2 (SLC22A7)	Salicylate, acetylsalicylate, PGE_2, dicarboxylates and PAH	Kidney (basolateral), liver
OAT3 (SLC22A8)	Similar to OAT1	Kidney (basolateral), liver, brain, smooth muscle
OAT4 (SLC22A11)	Steroid sulphate conjugates	Kidney (apical), placenta
OCT1 (SLC22A1)	Serotonin, noradrenaline, histamine, agmatine, aciclovir, ganciclovir	Mainly in the liver, but also in kidney, small intestine, heart, skeletal muscle and placenta
OCT2 (SLC22A2)	Serotonin, noradrenaline, histamine, agmatine, amantadine, cimetidine	Mainly in the kidney, but is also in placenta, adrenal gland, neurons and choroid plexus
OCT3 (SLC22A3)	Serotonin, noradrenaline, histamine, agmatine	Liver, kidney, intestine, skeletal and smooth muscle, heart, lung, spleen, neurons, placenta and the choroid plexus

[a]PGP, MRP1 and MRP2 have all been described as 'multidrug resistance protein' in some publications.
NSAIDs, non-steroidal anti-inflammatory drugs; PAH, para-amino hippurate.

[MDR1] or ABCB1 transporter), which transports a wide range of drug substrates, including anticancer drugs, from the basolateral to the apical side of the cell membrane, and therefore acts as an efflux transporter. ABCB transporter proteins contain two hydrophobic transmembrane domains, which consist of different numbers of membrane-spanning α-helices (12 in PGP), and two intracellular hydrophilic nucleotide (ATP)-binding domains, which bind and hydrolyse ATP. The transporter is on the apical surface and acts as an efflux pump that transports substrates from the cell into the bile, urine or gut lumen. ABCC or multidrug resistance-associated protein (MRP-related) transporters have a common core structure that contains two or three membrane-spanning domains, each comprising five or six transmembrane α-helices, plus two intracellular nucleotide-binding domains. MRP1 is on the basolateral membrane and therefore pumps substrates into the interstitial space rather than the lumen of the gut, kidney or bile duct. Breast cancer resistance protein (BCRP) is a member of the ABCG family; it consists of a single transmembrane domain of six α-helices with a single terminal ATP-binding domain but may function as a dimer (making the functioning structure similar to the ABCB and ABCC types).

The solute carrier (SLC) superfamily comprises organic anion transporters (OATs) and organic cation transporters (OCTs). Organic anion transporters (OAT1 to OAT4) are present in various tissues; OAT1 (Table 2.1) is the classic organic anion transporter in the kidney (Ch. 14). The transporters consist of 12 membrane-spanning domains with a large glycosylated but largely hydrophobic loop between the first and second domain. This loop determines the requirement that substrates must show a combination of both hydrophobic and highly polar characteristics. The OATs probably act as organic anion–dicarboxylate exchangers since OAT1-mediated uptake of substrates is stimulated by an outwardly directed concentration gradient of dicarboxylates such as α-ketoglutarate. Organic cation transporters (OCT1, OCT2 and OCT3) have a predicted membrane topology of 12 α-helical transmembrane domains and large substrate-binding pockets. They effect facilitated diffusion and can transport cations in both directions across the membrane; the driving forces that determine the direction

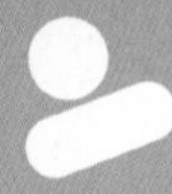

of transport are the concentration gradient of the transported substrate and the membrane potential. Substrates common to all three transporters are serotonin (5-hydroxytryptamine, 5-HT), noradrenaline, histamine and agmatine; although some drugs can act as substrates, many basic drugs act as inhibitors.

The therapeutic actions of a number of drugs result from the fact that they bind to carrier proteins and act as inhibitors of the transporter; examples are probenecid, which inhibits the secretion of anions, such as penicillins, by OAT1, and verapamil, which increases the intracellular concentrations of anticancer drugs by inhibiting PGP (MDR1) (Ch. 52).

3. Passage through membrane pores or ion channels

Movement occurs down a concentration gradient and can only occur for extremely small water-soluble molecules (<100 Da). This is applicable to therapeutic ions such as lithium and radioactive iodine.

4. Pinocytosis

This can be regarded as a form of carrier-mediated entry into the cell cytoplasm. Pinocytosis is normally concerned with the uptake of macromolecules; however, successful attempts have been made to utilise it for targeted drug uptake by incorporating the drug into a lipid vesicle or liposome (e.g. amphotericin and doxorubicin; Ch. 51).

Transmembrane concentration gradients

A number of reversible and irreversible processes can influence the total concentration of drug present on each side of the membrane at equilibrium (Fig. 2.3). Ionisation is a fundamental property of most drugs which are either weak acids, such as aspirin, or weak bases, such as propranolol. The presence of an ionisable group(s) is essential for the mechanism of action of most drugs, because ionic forces represent a key part of ligand–receptor interactions (Ch. 1).

The overall polarity of the drug and its extent of ionisation determine the extent of distribution (for example, entry into the brain), accumulation in adipose tissue, and mechanism and route of elimination from the body.

In general terms, the ionised form of the molecule can be regarded as the water-soluble form and the un-ionised form as the lipid-soluble form. Drugs with ionisable groups exist in equilibrium between charged and uncharged forms. The extent of ionisation can affect both the pharmacodynamics (for example, the affinity for the receptor) and the pharmacokinetics (for example, the extent of uptake by adipose tissue and the route of elimination). The ease with which a drug can diffuse across a lipid bilayer (Fig. 2.2) is determined by the lipid solubility of its un-ionised form. Drugs that are fixed in their ionised form at all pH values, such as the quaternary amine suxamethonium (Ch. 27), cross membranes extremely slowly or not at all; they have limited effects on the brain (because of lack of entry) and are given by injection (because of lack of absorption from the intestine).

The extent of ionisation of a drug depends on the strength of the ionisable group and the pH of the solution. The extent of ionisation is given by the acid dissociation constant K_a.

$$K_a = \frac{[\text{conjugate base}][H^+]}{[\text{conjugate acid}]} \tag{2.1}$$

The term conjugate acid refers to a form of the drug able to *release a proton* such as:

- an un-ionised acidic drug (Drug–COOH) or
- an ionised basic drug (Drug–NH_3^+).

The conjugate base is the corresponding equilibrium form of the drug that has *lost a proton*, such as:

- an ionised acidic drug (Drug–COO^-) or
- an un-ionised basic drug (Drug–NH_2).

For acidic drugs, the value of K_a is normally low (e.g. 10^{-5}) and therefore it is easier to compare compounds using the negative logarithm of the K_a, which is called the pK_a (e.g. 5). For acidic functional groups, a strong acid (such as an –SO_3H group) will have a high value for K_a (e.g. 10^{-1} or 10^{-2}) and numerically a low pK_a (e.g. 1 or 2), whereas weakly acidic groups (such as a phenolic–OH) have a pK_a of 9–10.

In contrast, for basic functional groups, the stronger the base, the greater will be its ability to retain the H^+ as a conjugate acid, resulting in a low K_a and a high pK_a. Thus, strongly basic groups (such as R–NH_2 where R is an alkyl group) have a pK_a of 10–11, while weakly basic groups (such as R_3N) have a pK_a of 2–3.

The pH of body fluids is controlled by the buffering capacity of the ionic groups present in endogenous mole-

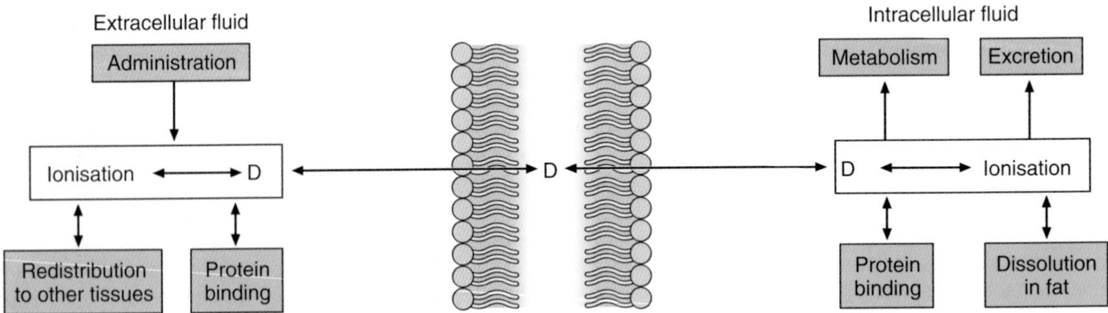

Fig. 2.3 **Passive diffusion and the factors that affect the concentrations of drug freely available in solution (as an equilibrium between un-ionised and ionised forms).**

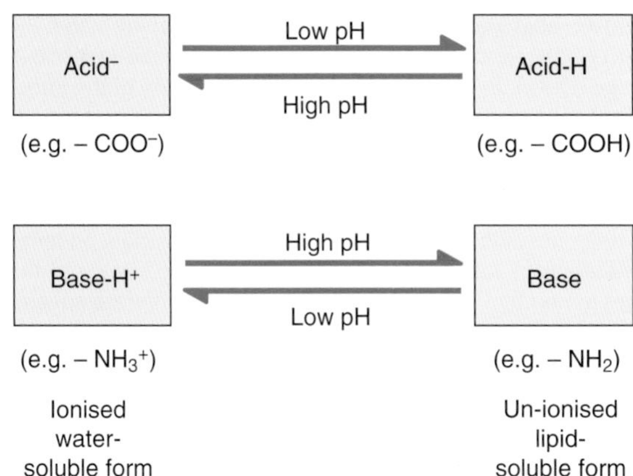

Fig. 2.4 **The effect of pH on drug ionisation.**

Urine (pH 6) Membrane Plasma (pH 7.4)

For an acidic drug (DH)

$D^{\ominus}$ ⇄ DH ⇄ DH ⇄ DH ⇄ $D^{\ominus}$

Overall →

For a basic drug (D)

$DH^{\oplus}$ ⇄ D ⇄ D ⇄ D ⇄ $DH^{\oplus}$

Overall ←

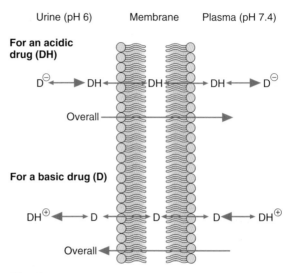

Fig. 2.5 **Partitioning of acidic and basic drugs across a pH gradient.**

cules such as phosphate ions and proteins. When the fluids on each side of a membrane have the same pH values, there will be equal concentrations of both the diffusible, un-ionised form and the polar ionised form of the drug on each side of the membrane at equilibrium. When the fluids on each side of a membrane are at different pH values, the concentrations of the diffusible, un-ionised form on each side of the membrane at equilibrium will be equal, but the concentrations of the ionised drug in equilibrium with the un-ionised will be determined by the pH of the solution and the pK_a of the drug. This results in pH-dependent differences in drug concentration on each side of a membrane (pH partitioning). The pH differences between plasma (pH 7.4) and stomach contents (pH 1–2) and urine (pH 5–7) can influence drug absorption and drug elimination.

Drugs are 50% ionised when the pH of the solution equals the pK_a of the drug. Acidic drugs are most ionised when the pH of the solution exceeds the pK_a, whereas basic drugs are most ionised when the pH is lower than the pK_a (Fig. 2.4). The practical importance is that the total concentration of drug will be higher on the side of the membrane where it is most ionised (Fig. 2.5), which has implications for drug absorption from the stomach and the renal elimination of some drugs. In drug overdose, increasing the pH of the urine can enhance the renal elimination of acidic drugs, such as aspirin, by retaining the ionised drug in the urine (see below), whereas a decrease in urine pH can be useful for basic drugs, such as dexamfetamine. It is important to realise that changing urine pH in the wrong direction for the type of drug taken in overdose (e.g. making the urine more acid in aspirin overdose) will make matters worse!

The low pH of the stomach contents (usually pH 1–2) means that most acidic drugs are present largely in their un-ionised (proton-associated) form and pH partitioning allows the drug to pass into plasma (pH 7.4) where it is more ionised. In contrast, basic drugs are highly ionised in the stomach and absorption is negligible until the stomach empties and the drug can be absorbed from the lumen of the duodenum (pH about 8).

ABSORPTION

Absorption is the process of transfer of the drug from the site of administration into the general or systemic circulation.

Absorption from the gut

The easiest and most convenient route of administration of medicines is orally by tablets, capsules or syrups. The large surface area of the small intestine, combined with its high blood flow, can give rapid and complete absorption of orally administered drugs. However, this route presents a number of barriers for the drug prior to reaching the systemic circulation. A number of factors can affect the rate and extent to which a drug can pass from the gut lumen into the general circulation.

Drug structure

Drug structure is a major determinant of absorption, distribution and elimination. Drugs need to be lipid-soluble to be absorbed from the gut. Therefore, highly polar acids and bases tend to be absorbed only slowly and incompletely, with much of the dose not absorbed but voided in the faeces. High polarity may be useful for delivery of the drug to the lower bowel (see Ch. 34). The structures of some drugs can make them unstable either at the low pH of the stomach (e.g. benzylpenicillin) or in the presence of digestive enzymes (e.g. insulin). Such compounds have to be given by injection, but administration by other routes may be possible (e.g. inhalation for insulin).

Drugs that are weak acids or bases may undergo pH partitioning between the gut lumen and mucosal cells. Acidic drugs will be least ionised in the stomach lumen, and most absorption would be expected at this site. However, the potential for absorption in the stomach is decreased by its low surface area and the presence of a zone at neutral

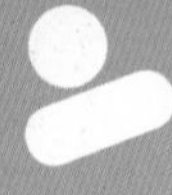

pH on the immediate surface of the gastric mucosal cells (the mucosal bicarbonate layer – see Ch. 33). In consequence, even weak acids, such as aspirin, tend to be absorbed mainly from the small intestine. Basic drugs are highly ionised in the stomach; as a result, absorption does not occur until the drug has passed from the stomach to the small intestine.

Formulation

Drugs cannot be absorbed until the administered tablet/capsule disintegrates and the drug is dissolved in the gastrointestinal contents to form a *molecular solution*. Most tablets disintegrate and dissolve quickly and completely and the whole dose rapidly becomes available for absorption. However, some formulations are produced that disintegrate slowly so that the rate at which the drug is absorbed is limited by the rate of release and dissolution of drug from the formulation, rather than by the transfer of the dissolved drug across the gut wall. This is the basis for modified-release formulations (e.g. slow-release) in which the drug either is incorporated into a complex matrix from which it diffuses, or is administered in a crystallised form that dissolves only slowly. Dissolution of a tablet in the stomach can be prevented by coating it in an acid-insoluble layer, producing an enteric-coated formulation, for example omeprazole (Ch. 33) and aspirin, which allows delivery of intact drug to the duodenum.

Gastric emptying

The rate of gastric emptying determines the rate at which a drug is delivered to the small intestine, which is the major site of absorption. A delay between dose administration and the detection of the drug in the circulation is seen frequently after oral dosing, and is usually caused by delayed gastric emptying. The co-administration of drugs that slow gastric emptying, for example antimuscarinics, can alter the rate of drug absorption.

Food has a complex effect on drug absorption since it reduces the rate of gastric emptying and delays absorption, but it can also alter the total amount of drug absorbed.

First-pass metabolism

Metabolism of drugs (see below) can occur prior to and during absorption, and this can limit the amount of parent compound that reaches the general circulation. Drugs taken orally have to pass four major metabolic barriers before they reach the general circulation.

Intestinal lumen

This contains digestive enzymes secreted by the mucosal cells and pancreas that are able to split amide, ester and glycosidic bonds. Intestinal proteases prevent the oral administration of peptide drugs, which are the usual products derived from molecular biological approaches to drug development. In addition, the lower bowel contains large numbers of aerobic and anaerobic bacteria that are capable of performing a range of metabolic reactions, especially hydrolysis and reduction.

Intestinal wall

The cells of the wall of the upper intestine are rich in enzymes such as monoamine oxidase (MAO), L-aromatic amino acid decarboxylase, CYP3A4 (see below) and the enzymes responsible for the phase 2 conjugation reactions (see below). In addition, the luminal membrane of the intestinal cells (enterocytes) contains the efflux transporter PGP (see above), which limits the absorption of some drugs by transporting them back into the intestinal lumen. Drug molecules that enter the enterocyte may undergo three possible fates – i.e. diffuse into the hepatic portal circulation, undergo metabolism within the cell, or be transported back into the gut lumen by PGP. There are overlapping substrate specificities of CYP3A4 and PGP, and for common substrates the combined actions can prevent the majority of an oral dose reaching the portal circulation.

Liver

Blood from the intestine is delivered, by the splanchnic circulation, directly to the liver, which is the major site of drug metabolism in the body (see metabolism, below).

Lung

Cells of the lung have high affinities for many basic drugs and are the main site of metabolism for many local hormones via MAO or peptidase activity.

If there is extensive metabolism at one or more of these sites, only a fraction of the administered oral dose may reach the general circulation as the parent compound. This process is known as first-pass metabolism because it occurs at the first passage through these organs. The liver is generally the most important site of first-pass metabolism. Hepatic metabolism can be avoided by administration of the drug to a region of the gut from which the blood does not drain into the hepatic portal vein, for example the buccal cavity and rectum; a good example of this is the buccal administration of glyceryl trinitrate (Ch. 5).

Absorption from other routes

Percutaneous (transcutaneous) administration

The human epidermis (especially the stratum corneum) represents an effective permeability barrier to water loss and to the transfer of water-soluble compounds. Although lipid-soluble drugs are able to cross this barrier, the rate and extent of entry are very limited. In consequence, this route is only really effective for use with potent non-irritant drugs, such as glyceryl trinitrate (Ch. 5) or fentanyl (Ch. 19), or to produce a local effect. The slow and continued absorption from dermal administration (e.g. via adhesive patches) can be used to produce low, but relatively constant, blood concentrations, e.g. the use of nicotine patches.

Intradermal and subcutaneous injection

Intradermal or subcutaneous injection avoids the barrier presented by the stratum corneum, and entry into the general circulation is limited largely by the blood flow to the site of injection. However, these sites only allow the administration of small volumes of drug and tend to be used for local effects, such as local anaesthesia, or to limit the rate of drug absorption, for example insulin. Slow uptake from the site of injection, as seen with some insulin preparations, can result in an increased duration of action.

Intramuscular injection

The rate of absorption from an intramuscular injection depends on two variables: the local blood flow and the water solubility of the drug, increases in either of which enhance the rate of removal from the injection site. Absorption of drugs from the injection site can be prolonged intentionally either by incorporation of the drug into a lipid vehicle or by formation of a sparingly soluble salt, such as benzathine benzylpenicillin (Ch. 51), thereby creating a depot formulation.

Intranasal administration

The nasal mucosa provides a good surface area for absorption, combined with low levels of proteases and drug-metabolising enzymes compared with the gastrointestinal tract. In consequence, intranasal administration is used for the administration of some drugs, such as desmopressin (Ch. 43), sumatriptan and zolmitriptan for migraine (Ch. 26), and insulin for diabetes (although currently withdrawn; Ch. 40), as well as for drugs that are designed to produce local effects, such as nasal decongestants and locally active corticosteroids (Ch. 39).

Inhalation

Although the lungs possess the characteristics of a good site for drug absorption (a large surface area and extensive blood flow), inhalation is rarely used to produce systemic effects. The principal reasons for this are the difficulty of delivering non-volatile drugs to the alveoli and the potential for local toxicity to alveolar membranes. Therefore, drug administration by inhalation is largely restricted to:

- volatile compounds, such as general anaesthetics (Ch. 17)
- locally acting drugs, such as bronchodilators and corticosteroids used in asthma (Ch. 12)
- potent agents, such as ergotamine for migraine (which, however, has been withdrawn; Ch. 26), since this route avoids the gastric stasis that is a common feature of a migraine attack.

The last two groups present technical problems for administration because the drugs are not volatile and have to be given either as aerosols containing the drug or as fine particles of the solid drug (see Ch. 12). Particles greater than 10 μm in diameter settle out in the upper airways, which are poor sites for absorption, and the drug then passes back up the airways via ciliary motion and is eventually swallowed. The optimum particle size for airways deposition is 2–5 μm. It has been estimated that only 5–10% of the dose may be absorbed from the airways, even when the administration technique generates mostly small particles (i.e. 5 μm or less). Particles less than 1 μm in diameter are not deposited in the airways and are exhaled.

Minor routes

Although drugs may be applied to all body surfaces and orifices, this is usually to produce a local and not a systemic effect. However, absorption from the site of administration may be important in limiting both the duration of action and the production of unwanted systemic actions.

DISTRIBUTION

Distribution is the process by which the drug is transferred reversibly from the general circulation into the tissues as the concentrations in blood increase, and from the tissues into blood when the blood concentrations decrease. For most drugs this occurs by passive diffusion of the un-ionised form across cell membranes (Fig. 2.2) until equilibrium is reached (Fig. 2.3). At equilibrium, any process that removes the drug from one side of the membrane results in movement of drug across the membrane to re-establish the equilibrium (Fig. 2.3).

After an intravenous injection, there is a high initial plasma concentration, and the drug may rapidly enter and equilibrate with well-perfused tissues such as the brain, liver and lungs (Table 2.2), giving relatively high concentrations in these tissues. However, the drug will continue to enter poorly perfused tissues, and this will lower the plasma concentration. The high concentrations in the rapidly perfused tissues then decrease in parallel with the decreasing plasma concentrations, which results in a transfer of drug back from those tissues into the plasma (Fig. 2.6). In most cases, the uptake into well-perfused tissues is so rapid that these tissues may be assumed to equilibrate instantaneously with plasma and represent part of the 'central' compartment (see below). Redistribution from well-perfused to poorly perfused tissues is of clinical importance for terminating the action of some drugs that are given as a rapid intravenous injection or bolus. For example, thiopental produces rapid anaesthesia after intravenous dosage, but effects in the brain are short lived because continued

Table 2.2 Relative organ perfusion rates in humans[a]

Organ	Cardiac output (%)	Blood flow (ml min^{-1} 100 g^{-1} tissue)
Well-perfused organs		
Lung	100	1000
Adrenals	1	550
Kidneys	23	450
Thyroid	2	400
Liver	25	75
Heart	5	70
Intestines	20	60
Brain	15	55
Placenta (full term)	–	10–15
Poorly perfused organs		
Skin	9	5
Skeletal muscle	16	3
Connective tissue	–	1
Fat	2	1

[a]Except for the placenta, the data are for an adult male under resting conditions.

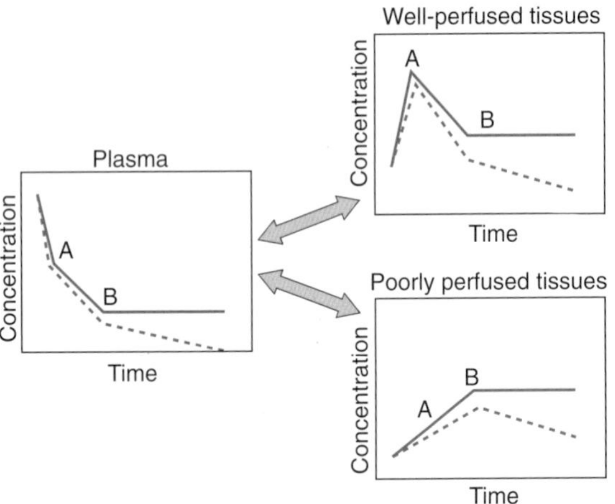

Fig. 2.6 **A simplified scheme for the redistribution of drugs between tissues.** The initial decrease in plasma concentrations results from uptake into well-perfused tissues, which essentially reaches equilibrium at point A. Between points A and B, the drug continues to enter poorly perfused tissues, which results in a decrease in the concentrations in both plasma and well-perfused tissues. At point B, all tissues are in equilibrium. N.B. The scheme has been simplified by representing the phases as discrete linear steps and also by the omission of any removal process. The presence of a removal process would produce a parallel decrease in all tissues from point B (shown as ----).

uptake into muscle lowers the concentrations in the blood and therefore in the brain (section A to B in Fig. 2.6; see also Fig. 17.2).

The processes of elimination (such as metabolism and excretion) are of major importance and are discussed in detail below. Elimination processes lower the concentration of the drug within the cells of the organ that eliminates the drug; the lower intracellular concentration results in a transfer from plasma into the drug-eliminating cells in order to maintain the equilibrium. The concentration of drug in plasma therefore decreases and this results in drug transfer from other tissues into plasma in order to maintain their equilibria. Thus, there is a net transfer from other tissues via the circulation to the organ(s) of elimination. Figure 2.6 illustrates how elimination (shown as a dashed line) produces a parallel decrease in drug concentrations in both plasma and tissues.

Reversible protein binding

Many drugs show an affinity for specific sites on non-receptor proteins, which results in a reversible association or binding:

$$\text{Drug} + \text{protein} \rightleftharpoons \text{Drug–protein complex}$$

The drug–protein complex is not biologically active.

Binding sites occur with circulating proteins, such as albumin and α_1-acid glycoprotein (Table 2.3), and with intracellular proteins (Fig. 2.3). The drug–protein binding interaction resembles the drug–receptor interaction since it is an extremely rapid, reversible and saturable process and different ligands can compete for the same site. However, it differs in two extremely important respects:

- drug–protein binding is of low specificity and does not result in any pharmacological effect but serves simply to lower the concentration of free drug in solution; such non-receptor protein binding lowers the concentration of drug available to act at receptors
- large amounts of drug may be present in the body bound to proteins such as albumin; in contrast, the amount of drug actually bound to receptors at the site of pharmacological activity is only a minute fraction of the total body load (but is in equilibrium with the total body load – see later).

Table 2.3 Examples of drugs that undergo extensive plasma protein binding and may show therapeutically important interactions

Bound to albumin	Bound to α_1-acid glycoprotein
Digitoxin	Chlorpromazine
Furosemide	Propranolol
Ibuprofen	Quinidine
Indometacin	Tricyclic antidepressants
Phenytoin	Lidocaine
Salicylates	
Sulphonamides	
Thiazides	
Tolbutamide	
Warfarin	

The rapidly reversible nature of protein binding is important because protein bound drug can act as a depot. If the intracellular concentration of unbound drug decreases, for example through metabolism, then this will affect all the equilibria shown in Figure 2.3. Drug will dissociate from intracellular protein binding sites, and some will transfer across the membrane from plasma until the various intracellular equilibria are re-established. As a result, the extracellular (plasma) concentration of unbound drug will decrease, and the drug will dissociate from plasma protein-binding sites. The ratio of the total amount of drug in the extracellular and intracellular compartments is determined largely by the relative affinity of the intra- and extracellular binding proteins.

Competition for protein binding can occur between different drugs (drug interaction; see Ch. 56), and also between drugs and natural, endogenous ligands. Administration of a highly protein-bound drug (such as aspirin) to an individual who is already receiving maintenance therapy with a drug that binds reversibly to plasma proteins (such as warfarin; see Ch. 11) will result in displacement of the already bound drug from its binding sites; this increases the unbound concentration and therefore the biological activity of the displaced drug. In practice, such protein-binding interactions are frequently of limited duration because the extra free drug is removed by metabolism or excretion.

An important interaction involving the displacement of an endogenous compound occurs in infants given highly protein-bound drugs such as sulphonamides: drugs that compete for the same albumin binding sites as endogenous

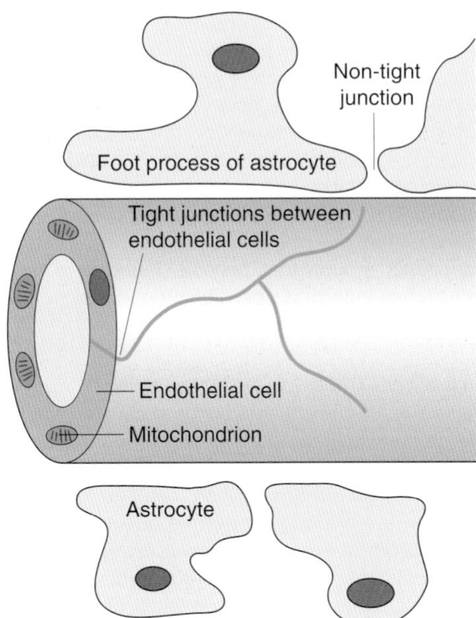

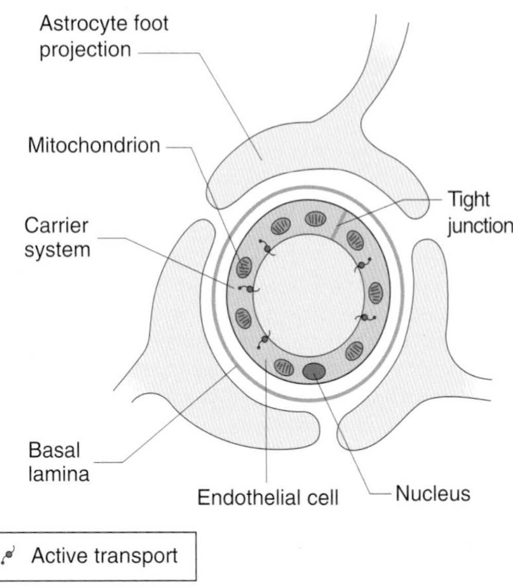

Fig. 2.7 **The blood–brain barrier**. The barrier arises from the low number of membrane pores, the tight junctions between adjacent cells, and the presence of efflux transporters that remove any drug that enters the endothelial cell. The presence of astrocytes is the stimulus for these changes in endothelial structure and function. Astrocytes are one of the several types of cells found in the CNS that make up the glia. They have numerous sheet-like processes and may provide nutrients to neurons.

bilirubin can displace the bilirubin and cause a potentially dangerous increase in its plasma concentration, which can cause kernicterus.

Irreversible protein binding

Certain drugs, because of chemical reactivity of the parent compound or a metabolite, undergo covalent binding to plasma or tissue components, such as proteins or nucleic acids. When the binding is irreversible, as for example the interaction of some cytotoxic agents with DNA, then this should be considered as equivalent to elimination, because the parent drug cannot re-enter the circulation, as occurs after simple distribution to tissues. In contrast, the covalent binding of thiol-containing drugs, such as the ACE inhibitor captopril (Ch. 6), to proteins via the formation of a disulphide bridge, may be slowly reversible. In such cases, the covalently bound drug will not dissociate in response to a rapid decrease in the concentration of unbound drug and such binding represents a slowly equilibrating reservoir of drug.

Distribution to specific organs

Although the distribution of drugs to all organs is covered by the general considerations discussed above, two systems require more detailed consideration: the brain, because of the difficulty of drug entry, and the fetus, because of the potential for toxicity.

Brain

Lipid-soluble drugs, such as the intravenous general anaesthetic thiopental, readily pass from the blood into the brain, and for such drugs the brain represents a typical well-perfused tissue (see Fig. 2.6, Table 2.2). In contrast, the entry of water-soluble drugs into the brain is much slower than into other well-perfused tissues, and this has given rise to the concept of a blood–brain barrier, since only lipid-soluble compounds can readily enter the brain. The functional basis of the barrier (Fig. 2.7) is reduced capillary permeability owing to:

- tight junctions between adjacent endothelial cells (capillaries are composed of a single-cell-thick endothelial layer without smooth muscle)
- a decrease in the size and number of pores in the endothelial cell membranes
- the presence of a surrounding layer of astrocytes.

In addition, efflux transporters such as PGP in the endothelial cells are an important part of the blood–brain barrier, and serve to return drug molecules that have entered the cell back into the circulation, thereby preventing their entry into the brain and reducing any effects in the central nervous system.

Water-soluble endogenous compounds needed for normal brain functioning, such as carbohydrates and amino acids, enter the brain via specific uptake transporters of the SLC superfamily (Table 2.1). Some drugs, for example levodopa, may enter the brain using these transport processes, and in such cases the rate of transport of the drug will be influenced by the concentrations of competitive endogenous substrates.

There is limited drug-metabolising ability in the brain and drugs leave by diffusion back into plasma, by active transport processes in the choroid plexus, or by elimination in the cerebrospinal fluid. Organic acid transporters (SLC

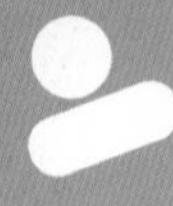

superfamily – Table 2.1) are important in removing polar neurotransmitter metabolites from the brain.

Fetus

Lipid-soluble drugs can readily cross the placenta and enter the fetus. The placental blood flow is low compared with that in the liver, lung and spleen (Table 2.2); consequently, the fetal concentrations equilibrate slowly with the maternal circulation. Highly polar and large molecules (such as heparin; see Ch. 11) do not readily cross the placenta. The fetal liver has only low levels of drug-metabolising enzymes. It is maternal elimination processes that predominantly control fetal concentrations of drug; lowering of maternal concentrations allows drug to diffuse back across the placenta from fetal to maternal circulation.

After delivery, the baby may show effects from drugs given to the mother close to delivery (such as pethidine for pain control; see Ch. 19): such effects may be prolonged because the infant now has to rely on his/her own immature elimination processes (Ch. 56).

ELIMINATION

Elimination is the removal of drug from the body and may involve metabolism in which the drug molecule is transformed into a different molecule, and/or excretion in which the drug molecule is expelled in the body's liquid, solid or gaseous 'waste'.

Metabolism

Lipid solubility is an essential property of most drugs, since it allows the compound to cross lipid barriers and hence to be given via the oral route. Metabolism is essential for the elimination of lipid-soluble chemicals from the body, because it converts a lipid-soluble molecule (which would be reabsorbed from urine in the kidney tubule – see later) into a water-soluble species (which is capable of rapid elimination in the urine, often via an anion transporter). The drug itself is eliminated as soon as metabolism converts it into a different chemical structure. However, the elimination of the unwanted carbon skeleton of the drug may involve a complex series of biotransformation reactions (see below).

Metabolism of the parent drug produces a new chemical entity, which may show different pharmacological properties:

- *complete loss of biological activity*: the most common result of drug metabolism; arises from increased polarity (especially phase 2 metabolism – see below) which prevents receptor binding
- *decrease in activity*: the metabolite retains some activity
- *increase in activity*: the metabolite is more potent than the parent drug; a prodrug is an inactive parent compound that is converted by metabolism into the active molecular species
- *change in the nature of the activity*: the metabolite shows different pharmacological or toxicological properties.

The various steps of drug metabolism can be divided into two phases (Fig. 2.8). Although many compounds undergo both phases of metabolism, it is possible for a chemical to undergo only a phase 1 or a phase 2 reaction. Phase 1 metabolism (oxidation, reduction and hydrolysis) is often described as preconjugation, because it produces a molecule that is a suitable substrate for a phase 2 or conjugation reaction. The enzymes involved in these reactions have low substrate specificities and can metabolise a vast range of drug substrates (as well as most environmental pollutants). In this section, drug metabolism is discussed in terms of the functional groups that may be found in different drugs, rather than individual specific compounds.

Phase 1

Oxidation reactions (Table 2.4) are by far the most important of the phase 1 reactions and can occur at carbon, nitrogen or sulphur atoms within the drug structure. In most cases, an oxygen atom is retained in the metabolite, although some reactions, such as dealkylation, result in loss of the oxygen atom in a small fragment of the original molecule. Oxidation reactions are catalysed by a diverse group of enzymes, of which the cytochrome P450 system is the most important. Cytochrome P450 is a superfamily of membrane-bound enzymes (Table 2.5) that are present in the smooth

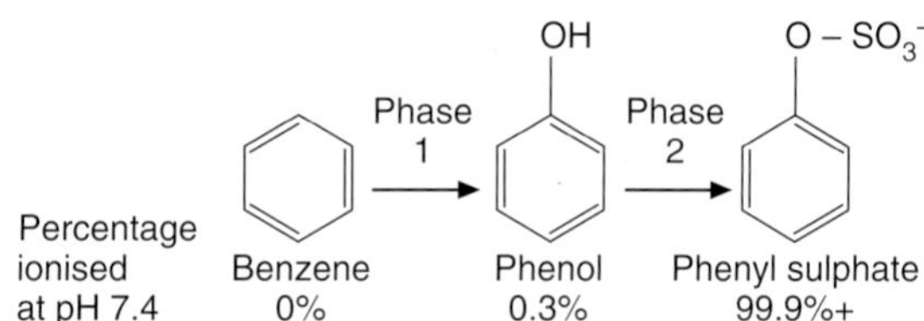

Fig. 2.8 **The two phases of drug metabolism.** Reactions of phase 1 and phase 2 metabolism are also called 'preconjugation' and 'conjugation' reactions, respectively.

Table 2.4 Oxidation reactions

Oxidation at carbon atoms	
Aromatic	$ArH \rightarrow ArOH$
Alkyl	$RCH_3 \rightarrow RCH_2OH \rightarrow RCHO \rightarrow RCOOH$
Dealkylation	$ROCH_3 \rightarrow ROH + HCHO$ $RNHCH_3 \rightarrow RNH_2 + HCHO$
Deamination	$RCH_2NH_2 \rightarrow RCHO + NH_3$ $RCH(CH_3)NH_2 \rightarrow RCO(CH_3) + NH$
Oxidation at nitrogen atoms	
Secondary amines	$R'-N(H)-R \rightarrow R'-N(OH)-R$
Tertiary amines	$R_3N \rightarrow R_3N \rightarrow O$
Oxidation at sulphur atoms	
Thioethers	$R{-}S{-}R \rightarrow R{-}S(\rightarrow O){-}R$

R, aliphatic or aromatic group; Ar, aromatic group.

endoplasmic reticulum of cells (Fig. 2.9). The liver is the major site of drug oxidation. The amounts of cytochrome P450 in extrahepatic tissues are low compared with those in liver.

Cytochrome P450 is a haemoprotein that can bind both the drug and molecular oxygen (Fig. 2.10). It catalyses the transfer of one oxygen atom to the substrate while the other oxygen atom is reduced to water:

Table 2.5 The cytochrome P450 superfamily

Isoenzyme	Comments
CYP1A	Important for methylxanthines and paracetamol; induced by smoking
CYP2A	Limited number of substrates; significant inter-individual variability
CYP2B	Limited number of substrates
CYP2C	CYP2C9 is an important isoform; CYP2C19 shows genetic polymorphism
CYP2D	Major isoform; metabolises numerous drugs; CYP2D6 shows genetic polymorphism
CYP2E	Metabolises alcohol; induced by alcohol
CYP3A	Main isoform in liver and intestine; metabolises about 60% of current drugs
CYP4	Metabolises fatty acids

Human liver contains at least 20 isoenzymes of cytochrome P450. Families 1–4 are related to drugs and their metabolism; families 17, 19, 21 and 22 are related to steroid biosynthesis.

$$RH + O_2 + NADPH + H^+ \rightarrow ROH + H_2O + NADP^+$$

The reaction involves initial binding of the drug substrate to the ferric (Fe^{3+}) form of cytochrome P450 (Fig. 2.10), followed by reduction (via a specific cytochrome P450 reductase) and then binding of molecular oxygen. Further reduction is followed by molecular rearrangement, with release of the reaction products (drug metabolite(s) and water) and regeneration of ferric cytochrome P450.

Oxidations at nitrogen and sulphur atoms are frequently performed by a second enzyme of the endoplasmic reticulum, the flavin-containing mono-oxygenase, which also requires molecular oxygen and NADPH. A number of other enzymes, such as alcohol dehydrogenase, aldehyde oxidase and MAO, may be involved in the oxidation of specific functional groups.

Reduction reactions (Table 2.6) can occur at unsaturated carbon atoms and at nitrogen and sulphur centres; such reactions are less common than oxidation. Reduction reactions can be performed both by the body tissues and also by the intestinal microflora. The tissue enzymes include cytochrome P450 and cytochrome P450 reductase.

Hydrolysis and hydration reactions (Table 2.7) involve addition of water to the drug molecule. In hydrolysis, the drug molecule is split by the addition of water. A number of enzymes that are present in many tissues, are able to hydrolyse ester and amide bonds in drugs. The intestinal bacteria are also important for the hydrolysis of esters and amides and of drug conjugates eliminated in the bile (see below). In hydration reactions, the water molecule is retained in the drug metabolite. Hydration of an epoxide ring, by epoxide hydrolase, produces a dihydrodiol (Table 2.7); this is an important reaction in the metabolism and

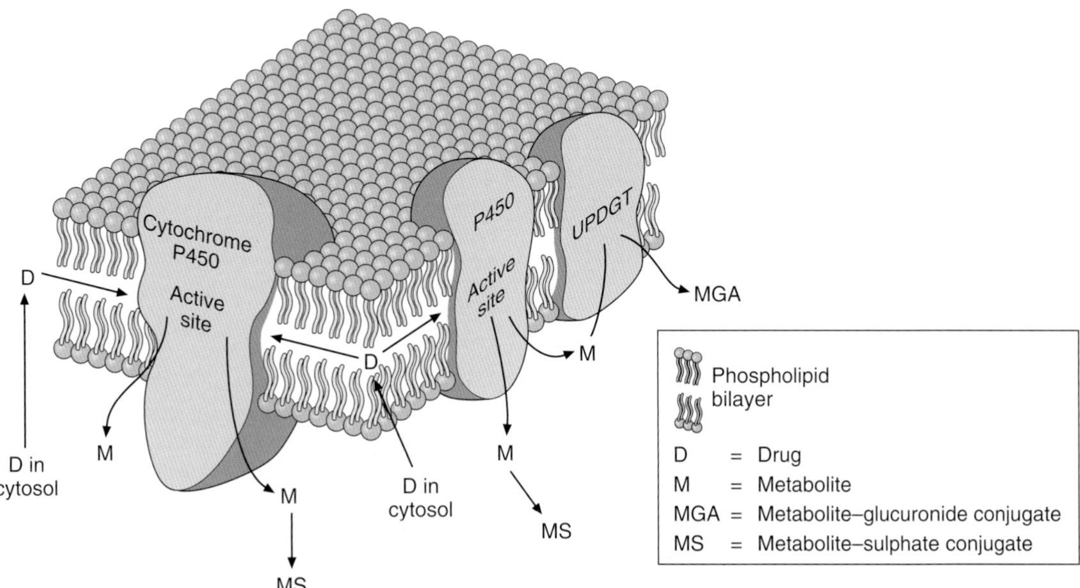

Fig. 2.9 **Drug metabolism in the smooth endoplasmic reticulum.** The lipid-soluble drug (D) partitions into the lipid bilayer of the endoplasmic reticulum. The cytochrome P450 oxidises the drug to a metabolite (M) that is more water-soluble and diffuses out of the lipid layer. The metabolite may undergo a phase 2 (conjugation) reaction with UDP-glucuronyl transferase (UDPGT) in the endoplasmic reticulum or sulphate in the cytosol, to give a glucuronide conjugate (MGA) or a sulphate conjugate (MS), respectively.

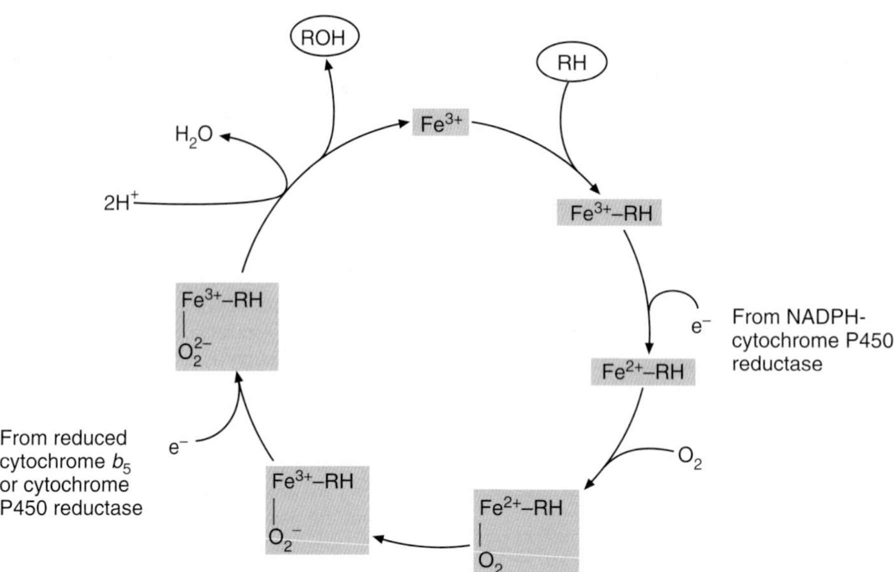

Fig. 2.10 **The oxidation of substrate (RH) by cytochrome P450**. Fe^{3+}, the active site of cytochrome P450 in its ferric state; RH, drug substrate; ROH, oxidised metabolite. Cytochrome b_5 is present in the endoplasmic reticulum and can transfer an electron to cytochrome P450 as part of its redox reactions.

Table 2.6 Reduction reactions

Reduction at carbon atoms	
Aldehydes	$RCHO \rightarrow RCH_2OH$
Ketones	$RCOR \rightarrow RCHOHR$
Reduction at nitrogen atoms	
Nitro groups	$ArNO_2 \rightarrow ArNO \rightarrow ArNHOH \rightarrow ArNH_2$
Azo group	$ArN{=}NAr' \rightarrow ArNH_2 + H_2NAr'$
Reduction at sulphur atoms	
Sulphoxides	$R\text{–}\overset{\overset{O}{\uparrow}}{S}\text{–}R \rightarrow R\text{–}S\text{–}R$
Disulphides	$R\text{-}S\text{-}S\text{-}R' \rightarrow RSH + HSR'$

R, aliphatic or aromatic group; Ar, aromatic group.

Table 2.7 Hydrolysis and hydration reactions

Hydrolysis reactions
Esters
$RCO.OR' \rightarrow RCOOH + HOR'$
Amides
$RCO.NHR' \rightarrow RCOH + H_2NR'$
Hydration reactions
Epoxides
H–C(–O–)–C–H (epoxide) → H–C(OH)–C(OH)–H

R, R′, different aliphatic/aromatic groups.

toxicity of a number of aromatic compounds, for example the drug carbamazepine (Ch. 23).

Phase 2

Phase 2 or conjugation reactions involve the formation of a covalent bond between the drug, or its phase 1 metabolite, and a normal body constituent (endogenous substrate). Energy to synthesise the bond is supplied by activation of either the endogenous substrate or the drug. Table 2.8 shows the types of phase 2 reactions, the functional group necessary in the drug molecule and the activated species for the reaction. The products of conjugation reactions are usually highly water-soluble and without biological activity.

The activated endogenous substrate for glucuronide synthesis is uridine-diphosphate glucuronic acid (UDPGA), which is synthesised from UDP-glucose (the precursor used for glycogen synthesis). The enzymes that transfer the glucuronic acid moiety to the drug (UDP-glucuronyl transferases) occur in the endoplasmic reticulum close to the cytochrome P450 system (Fig. 2.9). Glucuronide synthesis occurs in many tissues, especially the gut wall and liver, where it is important in the first-pass metabolism of substrates such as simple phenols.

Sulphate conjugation is performed by a cytosolic enzyme, which utilises high-energy sulphate (3′-phosphoadenosine-5′-phosphosulphate or PAPS) as the

Table 2.8 Major conjugation reactions

Reaction	Functional group	Activated species	Product
Glucuronidation	–OH –COOH $-NH_2$	UDPGA (uridine diphosphate glucuronic acid)	COOH O O–Drug
Sulphation	–OH $-NH_3$	PAPS (3′-phosphoadenosine 5′-phosphosulphate)	$-O-SO_3H$ $-NH-SO_3H$
Acetylation	$-NH_2$ $-NHNH_2$	Acetyl-CoA	$-NH-COCH_3$ $-NHNH-COCH_3$
Methylation	–OH $-NH_2$ –SH	S-Adenosyl methionine	$-OCH_3$ $-NHCH_3$ $-SCH_3$
Amino acid	–COOH	Drug-CoA	CO-NHCHRCOOH
Glutathione	Various	–	Glutathione conjugate

endogenous substrate. The capacity for sulphate conjugation is limited by the availability of PAPS, and sulphate conjugation is dose-dependent. Saturation of sulphate conjugation contributes to the metabolic events involved in the liver toxicity seen with overdose of paracetamol (acetaminophen in the USA) (see Ch. 53).

The reactions of acetylation and methylation often decrease polarity because they block an ionisable functional group (Table 2.8). These reactions mask potentially active functional groups such as amino and catechol moieties, and the enzymes are primarily involved in the inactivation of neurotransmitters such as noradrenaline or of local hormones such as histamine.

The conjugation of drug carboxylic acid groups with amino acids is unusual because the drug is converted to a high-energy form (a CoA derivative) prior to the formation of the conjugate bond. The enzymes involved in the formation of the drug CoA derivatives are involved in the metabolism of intermediate-chain-length fatty acids. Conjugation of the drug CoA derivative with an amino acid is catalysed by transferase enzymes.

Conjugation with the tripeptide glutathione (GSH or L-α-glutamyl-L-cysteinylglycine) is important in drug toxicity. This reaction is catalysed by a family of transferase enzymes and the product has a covalent bond between the drug, or its metabolite, and the thiol group in the cysteine (Fig. 2.11). The substrates are often reactive drugs or activated metabolites, which are inherently unstable (see Ch. 53), and the reaction can also occur non-enzymatically. Glutathione conjugation is a detoxication reaction in which glutathione acts as a scavenging agent to protect the cell from toxic damage. The initial glutathione conjugate undergoes a series of subsequent metabolic reactions, which illustrates the complexity of drug metabolism (Fig. 2.11). Glutathione conjugates (and endogenous cysteine conjugates such as leukotriene C_4 [LTC_4]) are transported out of cells by the MRP1 transporter (Table 2.1) and glutathione acts as a co-substrate for the transport of drugs via MRP1 (Fig. 2.2).

A good example of a drug that undergoes a complex array of biotransformation reactions is diazepam

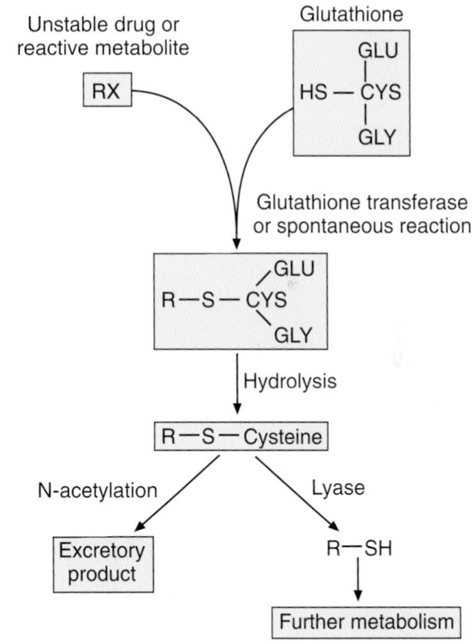

Fig. 2.11 **The formation and further metabolism of glutathione conjugates.**

(Fig. 2.12). Cytochrome P450-mediated oxidation and removal of the N-methyl group (see Table 2.4) produces N-desmethyldiazepam, which retains biological activity at $GABA_A$ receptors. Both diazepam and N-desmethyldiazepam undergo ring oxidation, giving temazepam and oxazepam, respectively, which are also used as anxiolytics and sedatives (see Ch. 20). Oxazepam and temazepam contain an aliphatic hydroxyl group, which is conjugated with glucuronic acid, giving an inactive, water-soluble excretory product. In addition, temazepam can undergo N-demethylation to give oxazepam.

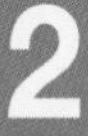
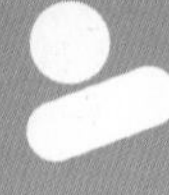

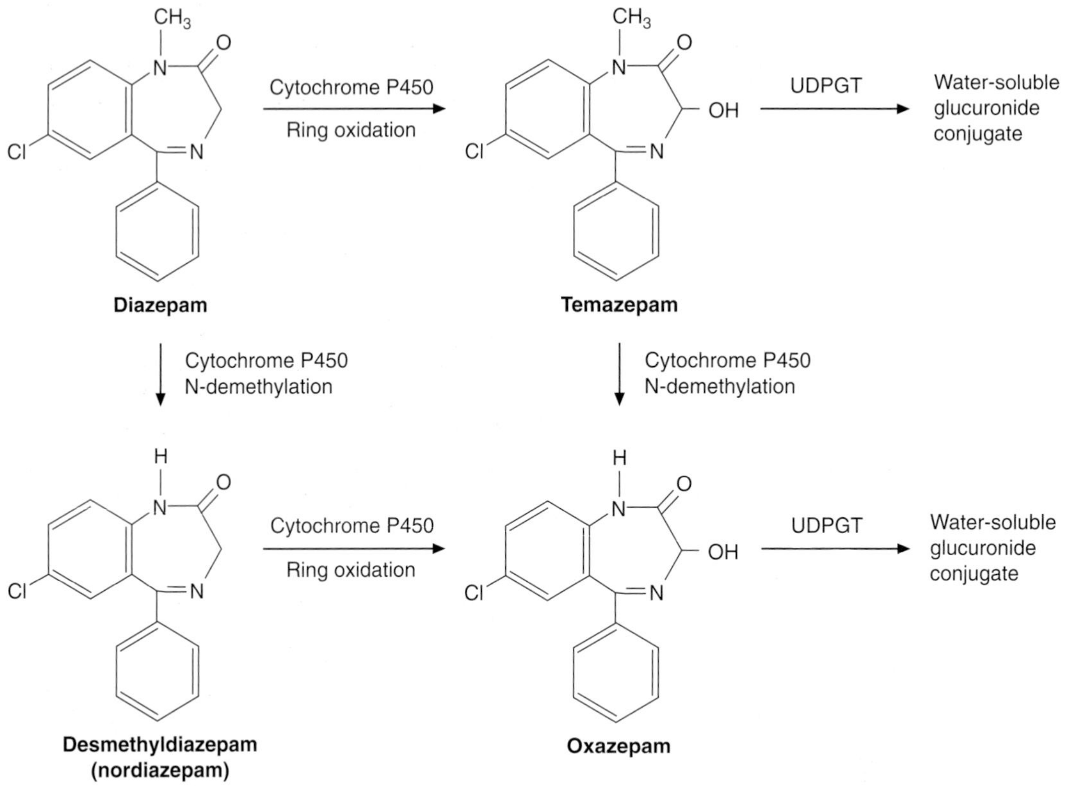

Fig. 2.12 **The pathways of metabolism of diazepam in humans**. This figure illustrates that a single drug may generate a number of metabolites, which may possess similar pharmacological properties. UDP-glucuronyl transferase (UDPGT) is the enzyme that transfers glucuronic acid from UDPGA to the alicyclic OH group.

Factors affecting drug metabolism

The liver is the main site of drug metabolism; the large surface area of the sinusoids, combined with the high enzyme activity in hepatocytes, can result in very rapid drug uptake and metabolism by hepatocytes as the blood flows through the liver (see Ch. 56 for normal sinusoid architecture and the effects of liver disease on hepatic drug uptake). The ability of individuals to metabolise drugs is determined by their genetic constitution, their environment and their physiological status.

Genetic constitution

This is an increasingly important area of pharmacology and is presented at the end of this chapter under 'Pharmacogenomics, pharmacogenetics and drug kinetics'.

Environmental influences

The activity of drug-metabolising enzymes, especially the cytochrome P450 system, can be increased or inhibited by foreign compounds such as environmental contaminants and therapeutic drugs. Induction of cytochrome P450 results in increased intracellular concentrations of the enzyme following exposure to the inducing agent. Environmental contaminants such as organochlorine compounds (e.g. dioxins) and polycyclic aromatic hydrocarbons (e.g. benzo[a]pyrene in cigarette smoke) induce CYP1A (Table 2.9). Therapeutic drugs can induce members of the CYP2 and CYP3 families (Table 2.9). Chronic consumption of alcohol induces CYP2E. Induction of cytochrome P450 isoenzymes occurs over a period of a few days, during which the inducer interacts with nuclear receptors to increase the transcription of the mRNA, following which the additional enzyme is synthesised. The increased amounts of the enzyme last for a few days after the removal of the inducing agent, and the extra enzyme is removed by normal protein turnover. In contrast, inhibition of drug-metabolising enzymes is by direct reversible competition for the enzyme site and the time course follows closely the absorption and elimination of the inhibitor substance. A number of drugs (Table 2.9) produce clinically significant drug interactions because of their induction or inhibition of cytochrome P450 enzymes. Such changes in hepatic metabolism can affect both the bioavailability and clearance of drugs undergoing hepatic elimination (see below).

Physiological status

The functional capacity of the drug-metabolising enzymes is dependent on both the intrinsic enzyme activity and the delivery of drug to the site of metabolism via the circulation. Drug metabolism, and hence clearance and half-life (see below), for most drugs, are affected significantly by age (noteworthy are the very young and the elderly) and by liver disease. This is discussed further in Chapter 56.

Table 2.9 Common substrates, inhibitors and inducers of cytochrome P450 (CYP) isoenzymes

Isoenzyme	Substrates (examples)	Inhibitors (examples)	Inducers (examples)
CYP1A2	Caffeine, PAHs, paracetamol, theophylline	Cimetidine, clarithromycin, erythromycin, grapefruit juice, isoniazid, ketoconazole	Omeprazole, charbroiled foods, cigarette smoke, TCDD
CYP2A6	Coumarin, halothane, nicotine	Grapefruit juice, ketoconazole, tranylcypromine	Dexamethasone, phenobarbital, rifampicin
CYP2B6	Bupropion, cyclophosphamide, efavirenz, ifosfamide	Fluoxetine, orphenadrine, paroxetine	Carbamazepine, phenobarbital, phenytoin, rifampicin
CYP2C9	Glibenclamide, ibuprofen, losartan, tolbutamide, S-warfarin	Amiodarone, cimetidine, fluconazole, fluoxetine, ketoconazole, omeprazole, valproic acid	Carbamazepine, dexamethasone, phenobarbital, rifampicin
CYP2C19	Omeprazole	Cimetidine, fluvoxamine, moclobemide, omeprazole	Carbamazepine, rifampicin
CYP2D6	Amitriptyline, bisoprolol, codeine, desipramine, encainide, many SSRIs, methamphetamine, metoprolol, ondansetron, propafenone, propranolol	Amiodarone, cimetidine, fluoxetine, haloperidol, methadone, quinidine	Carbamazepine, phenobarbital, phenytoin, rifampicin
CYP2E	Chlorzoxazone, ethanol, paracetamol	Disulfiram, isoniazid	Ethanol
CYP3A4	Numerous drugs of different classes, e.g. alfentanil, amiodarone, carbamazepine, cisapride, clonazepam, diazepam, diltiazem, erythromycin, felodipine, fluconazole, lidocaine, midazolam, nifedipine, saquinavir, tamoxifen, terfenadine, verapamil	Cimetidine, clarithromycin, clotrimazole, erythromycin, fluconazole, grapefruit juice, ketoconazole, saquinavir	Carbamazepine, dexamethasone, ethosuximide, isoniazid, phenobarbital, phenytoin, rifampicin

SSRIs, selective serotonin reuptake inhibitors; TCDD, tetrachlorodibenzodioxin (dioxin) – an environmental pollutant.
The above lists are not comprehensive, but give the more important examples.

Excretion

Drugs and their metabolites may be eliminated from the circulation by various routes:

- **in fluids (urine, bile, sweat, tears, milk, etc.):** these routes are most important for low-molecular-weight polar compounds, and the urine is the major route; milk is important because of the potential for exposure of the breastfed infant
- **in solids (faeces, hair, etc.):** drugs enter the gastrointestinal tract by various mechanisms (see below) and faecal elimination is most important for high-molecular-weight compounds that are excreted in bile; the sequestration of foreign compounds into hair is not of quantitative importance, because of the slow growth of hair, but distribution of a drug along the hair shaft can be used to indicate the history of drug intake during the preceding weeks
- **in gases (expired air):** this route is only of importance for volatile compounds.

Excretion via the urine

There are three processes involved in the handling of drugs and their metabolites in the kidney: glomerular filtration, reabsorption and tubular secretion. The total urinary excretion of a drug depends on the balance of these three processes:

$$\text{Total excretion} = \text{glomerular filtration} + \text{tubular secretion} - \text{reabsorption}$$

Glomerular filtration

All molecules less than about 20 kDa undergo filtration under positive hydrostatic pressure through the pores of 7–8 nm in the glomerular membrane. The glomerular filtrate contains about 20% of the plasma volume delivered to the glomerulus, and about 20% of all water-soluble, low-molecular-weight compounds in plasma, including non-protein-bound drugs, enter the filtrate. Plasma proteins and protein-bound drug are not filtered; therefore, the efficiency of glomerular filtration for a drug is influenced by the extent of plasma protein binding.

Reabsorption

The glomerular filtrate contains numerous constituents that the body cannot afford to lose. There are specific tubular uptake processes for carbohydrates, amino acids, vitamins, etc., and most of the water is also reabsorbed (see Ch. 14). Drugs may pass back from the tubule into the plasma if they are substrates for these specific uptake processes (very rare) or if they are lipid-soluble. The urine is concentrated on its passage down the renal tubule; as the tubule-to-plasma concentration gradient increases, only the most polar molecules remain in the urine. Because of extensive

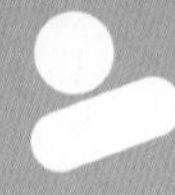

reabsorption, lipid-soluble drugs are not eliminated via the urine, and are retained in the circulation until they are metabolised to water-soluble products (see above), which are efficiently removed from the body. The pH of urine is usually less than that of plasma; consequently, pH partitioning, between urine (pH 5–6) and plasma (pH 7.4), may either increase or decrease the tendency of the compound to be reabsorbed (Fig. 2.5).

Tubular secretion

The renal tubule has secretory transporters (Table 2.1) on both the basolateral and apical membranes for compounds that are acidic (organic anion transporters – OATs 1–4) or basic (organic cation transporters – OCTs 1–3). In addition, there are multidrug resistance-associated proteins (MRPs), which were originally identified in a cell line resistant to anticancer drugs but have since been found as important transporters in various tissues. Drugs and their metabolites (especially the glucuronic acid and sulphate conjugates) may undergo an active carrier-mediated elimination, primarily by OATs but also by MRPs. Because secretion rapidly lowers the plasma concentration of unbound drug, there will be a rapid dissociation of any drug–protein complex; as a result, even highly protein-bound drugs may be cleared almost completely from the blood in a single passage through the kidney.

Excretion via the faeces

Uptake into hepatocytes and subsequent elimination in bile is the principal route of elimination of larger molecules (those with a molecular weight greater than about 500 Da). Conjugation with glucuronic acid increases the molecular weight of the substrate by almost 200 Da, and therefore bile can be an important route for the elimination of glucuronide conjugates. Once the drug, or its conjugate, has entered the intestinal lumen via the bile (Fig. 2.13), it passes down the gut and may eventually be eliminated in the faeces. However, some drugs may be reabsorbed from the lumen of the gut and re-enter the hepatic portal vein. As a result, the drug is recycled between the liver, bile, gut lumen and hepatic portal vein. This is described as an enterohepatic circulation; it can maintain the drug concentrations in the general circulation, because some of the reabsorbed drug will escape hepatic extraction and pass through the sinusoids from the hepatic portal vein into the hepatic vein. Highly polar glucuronide conjugates of drugs or their oxidised metabolites that are excreted into the bile undergo little reabsorption in the upper intestine. However, the bacterial flora of the lower intestine can hydrolyse the conjugate back to the original drug, or its oxidised metabolite, and glucuronic acid. The original drug, or its primary metabolite, will have greater lipid solubility than the glucuronic acid conjugate and will be absorbed from the gut lumen and enter the hepatic portal vein (Fig. 2.13).

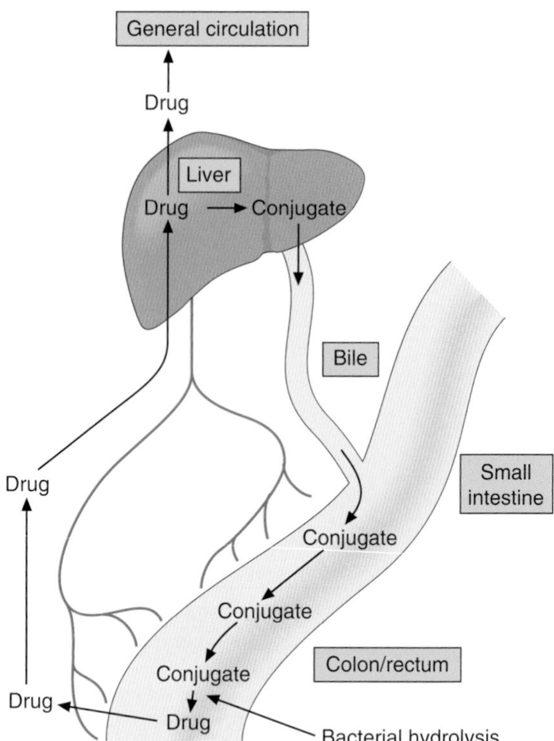

Fig. 2.13 **Enterohepatic circulation of drugs.**

THE MATHEMATICAL BASIS OF PHARMACOKINETICS

The use of mathematics to describe the fate of a drug in the body can be complex and rather daunting for undergraduates. Nevertheless, a basic understanding is essential for an appreciation of many aspects of drug handling and for the rational prescribing of drugs. The following account gives the mathematics for the absorption, distribution and elimination of a single dose of a drug, before brief consideration of chronic (repeat-dose) administration and the factors that can affect pharmacokinetic processes.

GENERAL CONSIDERATIONS

Three basic processes, absorption, distribution and elimination, need to be described in mathematical terms. For each process, it is important to know the rate or speed with which the drug is processed and also the extent of the process, i.e. the amount or proportion of drug that undergoes that process.

For nearly all physiological and metabolic processes, the rate of reaction is proportional to the amount of substrate (drug) available: this is described as a **first-order reaction**. Diffusion down a concentration gradient and glomerular filtration are examples of first-order reactions. Protein-mediated reactions, such as metabolism and active transport, are also first-order at low concentrations, because if the concentration of the substrate is doubled, then the formation of product is doubled. However, as the substrate concentration increases, the enzyme or transporter can become saturated with substrate and the rate of reaction cannot increase in response to a further increase in concentration. The process then occurs at a fixed maximum rate that is independent of substrate concentration, and the reaction is described as a **zero-order reaction**; examples

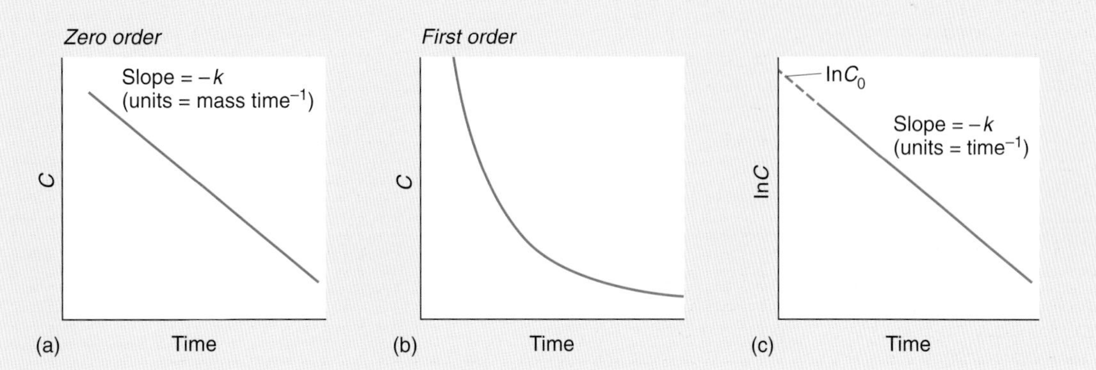

Fig. 2.14 **Zero- and first-order kinetics**. *C*, concentration; *k*, rate constant.

are the metabolism of ethanol (Ch. 54) and phenytoin (Ch. 23). When the substrate concentration has decreased sufficiently for protein sites to become available again, then the change in concentration will proceed at a rate proportional to the concentration available – in other words, the reaction will revert to first-order.

Zero-order reactions

If a drug is being processed (absorbed, distributed or eliminated) according to zero-order kinetics, then the change in concentration with time (dC/dt) is a fixed amount per time – independent of concentration:

$$\frac{dC}{dt} = -k \qquad (2.2)$$

The units of k (the reaction rate constant) will be an amount per unit time (e.g. mg min^{-1}). A graph of concentration against time will produce a straight line with a slope of $-k$ (Fig. 2.14a).

First-order reactions

In first-order reactions, the change in concentration at any time (dC/dt) is proportional to the concentration present at that time:

$$\frac{dC}{dt} = -kC \qquad (2.3)$$

The units of the rate constant, k, are time^{-1} (e.g. h^{-1}), and k may be regarded as the proportional change per unit of time. The rate of change will be high at high concentrations but low at low concentrations (Fig. 2.14b), and a graph of concentration against time will produce an exponential decrease. Such a curve can be described by an exponential equation:

$$C = C_0 e^{-kt} \qquad (2.4)$$

where C is the concentration at time t and C_0 is the initial concentration (when time = 0). This equation may be written more simply by taking natural logarithms:

$$\ln C = \ln C_0 - kt \qquad (2.5)$$

and a graph of $\ln C$ against time will produce a straight line with a slope of $-k$ and an intercept of $\ln C_0$ (Fig. 2.14c).

The units of k (which are time^{-1}, e.g. h^{-1}) are difficult to use practically, and therefore the rate of a first-order reaction is usually described in terms of its half-life (which has units of time). The half-life is the time taken for a concentration to decrease to one-half. The half-life is independent of concentration (Fig. 2.15) and is a characteristic for that particular first-order process and that particular drug. The decrease in plasma concentration after an intravenous bolus dose is shown in Figure 2.15, which has been plotted such that the concentration is halved every hour.

The relationship between the half-life and the rate constant is derived by substituting $C_0 = 2$ and $C = 1$ into the above equation, when the time interval t will be one half-life ($t_{1/2}$), giving:

$$\ln 1 = \ln 2 - kt_{1/2}$$
$$0 = 0.693 - kt_{1/2} \qquad (2.6)$$
$$t_{1/2} = \frac{0.693}{k}$$

(Note: $0.693 = \ln 2$)

A half-life can be calculated for any first-order process (e.g. for absorption, distribution or elimination). In practice, the 'half-life' normally reported for a drug is the half-life for the elimination rate (i.e. the slowest, terminal phase of the plasma concentration–time curve; see below).

ABSORPTION

The mathematics of absorption apply to all 'non-intravenous' routes – for example, oral, inhalation, percutaneous, etc. – and are illustrated by absorption from the gut lumen.

Rate of absorption

Following oral doses of some drugs, it is possible to see three distinct phases in the plasma concentration–time curve that reflect absorption, distribution and elimination (Fig. 2.16a). However, for most drugs, slow absorption masks the distribution phase (Fig. 2.16b). The rate of absorption after oral administration is determined by the rate at which the drug is able to pass from the gut lumen

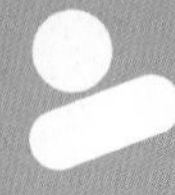

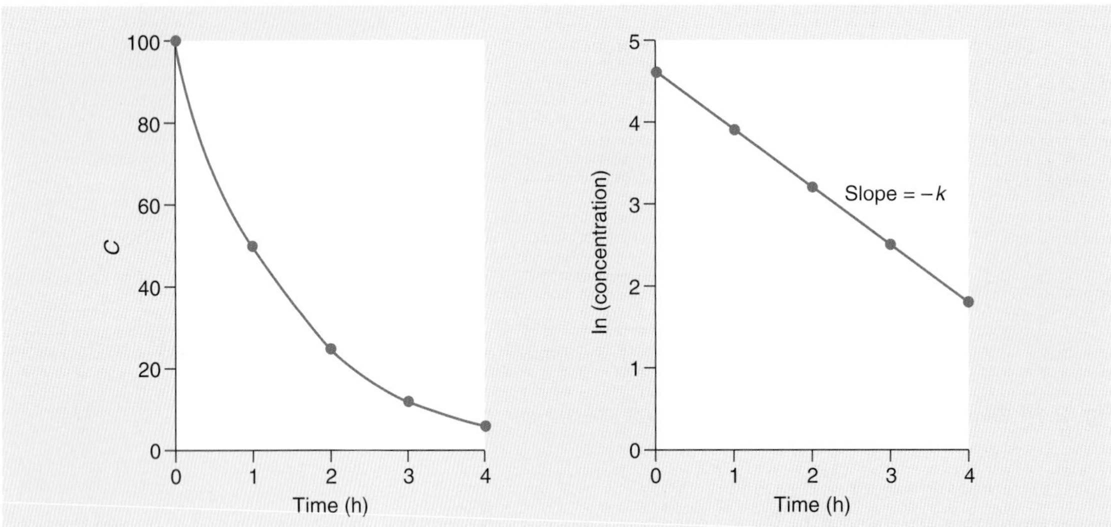

Fig. 2.15 **The elimination half-life of a drug in plasma**. Here the concentration (*C*) decreases by 50% every hour, i.e. the half-life is 1 h.

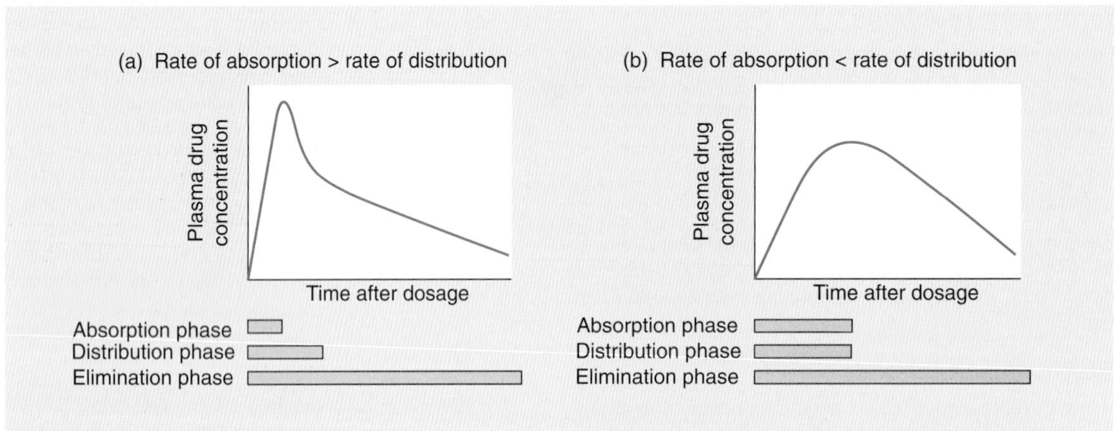

Fig. 2.16 **Plasma concentration–time profiles after oral administration**. The processes of distribution and elimination start as soon as some of the drug has entered the general circulation. A clear distribution phase is seen if the rate of absorption is extremely rapid, so that absorption is complete before distribution is finished (Fig. 2.16a). For most drugs, the rate of absorption is slow compared with the rate of distribution, and distribution occurs as rapidly as the drug is absorbed; therefore, distribution is complete when absorption is complete, and a clear distribution phase is not seen (Fig 2.16b).

into the systemic circulation. The rate of absorption influences the shape of the plasma concentration–time curve after an oral dose, as shown in Figure 2.17. For lipid-soluble drugs, there is an initial steep increase, from which the absorption rate constant (k_a) can be calculated, and a slower decrease, from which the elimination rate constant (k) can be calculated. In Figure 2.17a, the absorption is essentially complete by point B since the subsequent data are fitted by a single exponential rate constant (the elimination rate) (see below).

A number of factors can affect this apparently simple pattern.

- **Gastric emptying**. Basic drugs undergo negligible absorption from the stomach (see above). In consequence, there can be a delay of up to an hour between drug administration and the detection of drug in the general circulation (Fig. 2.17b).
- **Food**. The pattern of absorption can be affected by changes in gastric emptying (Fig. 2.17b) and food can alter the absorption rate, i.e. value of k_a (Fig. 2.17c).
- **Decomposition or first-pass metabolism prior to or during absorption**. This will reduce the amount of drug that reaches the general circulation but will not affect the rate of absorption (which is usually determined by lipid

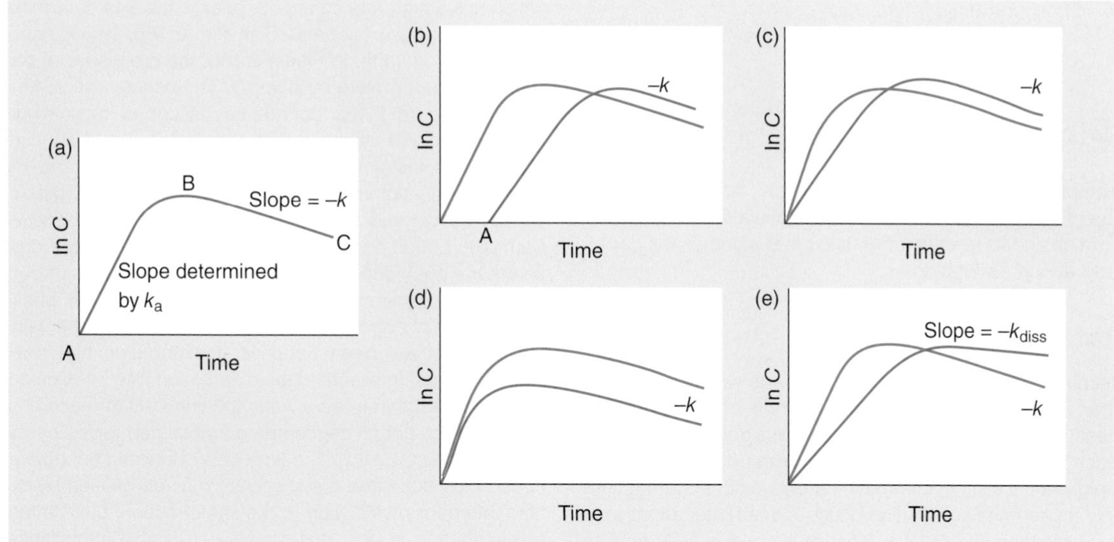

Fig. 2.17 **Plasma concentration–time curves following oral administration**. (a) General profile (A, start of absorption; B, end of absorption; B–C, elimination [rate = k]) (this 'normal' profile is repeated as a green line in panels b–e). (b) Influence of gastric emptying: there is a delay between $t = 0$ and A. (c) Influence of food: slower absorption results in a reduction in the absorption rate constant (k_a) derived from A–B. (d) Decrease in bioavailability (owing to incomplete dissolution of formulation, decomposition, increased first-pass metabolism). (e) Slow-release formulation: the rate at which the drug can be eliminated is limited by the rate at which the formulation disintegrates (k_{diss}).

solubility). Therefore, the curve is parallel but at lower concentrations (Fig. 2.17d).

- **Modified-release formulation**. If a drug is eliminated rapidly, the plasma concentrations will show rapid fluctuations during regular oral dosing, and patients may have to take the drug at very frequent intervals. This can be avoided by giving a tablet that releases drug at a slow and predictable rate over many hours: a modified-release formulation. The profile is affected by continuing absorption from the intestine, and the terminal slope of the concentration–time curve is then determined by the dissolution rate of the oral formulation, not by the elimination of the drug from the circulation (Fig. 2.17e).

Extent of absorption

The parameter that measures the extent of absorption is termed the *bioavailability* (F). This is defined as *the fraction of the administered dose that reaches the systemic circulation as the parent drug* (not as metabolites). For oral administration, incomplete bioavailability ($F < 1$) may result from:

- *incomplete absorption and loss in the faeces*, either because the molecule is too polar to be absorbed or because the tablet did not release all of its contents
- *first-pass metabolism*, in the gut lumen, during passage across the gut wall or by the liver prior to the drug reaching the systemic circulation.

The bioavailability of a drug has important therapeutic implications, because it is the major factor determining the dosage requirements for different routes of administration. For example, if a drug has an oral bioavailability of 0.1, the oral dose needed for therapeutic effectiveness will need to be 10 times higher than the corresponding intravenous dose.

The bioavailability is a characteristic of the drug and is independent of dose (providing that the processes of absorption and elimination are not saturated). Bioavailability is normally determined by comparison of plasma concentration data obtained after oral administration (when the fraction F enters the general circulation as the parent drug) with data following intravenous administration (when, by definition, 100% enters the general circulation as the parent drug). The amount in the circulation cannot be compared at a single time point, because intravenous and oral dosing show different concentration–time profiles. This is avoided by using the total area under the plasma concentration–time curve (AUC) from $t = 0$ to t = infinity (which is a reflection of the total amount of drug that has entered the general circulation): if the oral and intravenous (iv) doses are equal

$$F = \frac{AUC_{oral}}{AUC_{iv}} \tag{2.7}$$

or if different doses are used

$$F = \frac{AUC_{oral} \times Dose_{iv}}{AUC_{iv} \times Dose_{oral}} \tag{2.8}$$

This calculation assumes that the elimination is first-order. The AUC is a reflection of overall body exposure and is discussed below under clearance.

An alternative method to calculate F is to measure the total urinary excretion of the parent drug (Aex) following oral and intravenous doses (even in situations where the urine is a minor route of elimination); if the oral and intravenous (iv) doses are equal

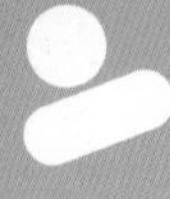

$$F = \frac{Aex_{oral}}{Aex_{iv}} \tag{2.9}$$

DISTRIBUTION

Distribution of a drug is the reversible movement of the parent drug from the blood into the tissues during administration and its re-entry from tissue into blood as the parent drug during elimination.

Rate of distribution

Because a distinct distribution phase is not usually seen after oral dosage (Fig. 2.16b), the rate of distribution is measured following an intravenous bolus dose. Some drugs reach equilibrium between blood/plasma and tissues very rapidly and a distinct distribution phase is not apparent, and only the terminal elimination phase is seen after an intravenous injection (Fig. 2.18a). Most drugs take a finite time to distribute into, and equilibrate with, the tissues, which results in a rapid distribution phase (slope A–B in Fig. 2.18b, which has a high rate constant), prior to the slower terminal elimination phase (slope B–C in Fig. 2.18b, which has a lower rate constant). In Figure 2.18b, the processes of distribution are complete by point B. The concentration–time curve in Figure 2.18b cannot be described by a single exponential term, and two first-order rates occur. By convention, the faster (distribution) rate is termed α and the slower (elimination) rate β. The distribution rate constant (α) cannot be derived directly from the slope A–B, because both distribution and elimination start as soon as the drug enters the body and A–B represents the summation of both processes. Back extrapolation of the terminal (β) phase gives an initial concentration at point D, which is the value that would have been obtained if distribution had been instantaneous. In practice, the distribution rate (α) is calculated for the difference between the line D–B for each time point and the actual concentration measured (given by the line A–B in Fig. 2.18b). The time delay between an intravenous bolus dose and the response may be caused by the time taken for distribution to the site of action, but the rate of distribution is only occasionally of clinical importance. Redistribution of intravenous drugs, such as thiopental (Ch. 17), may limit the duration of action (see Fig. 2.6).

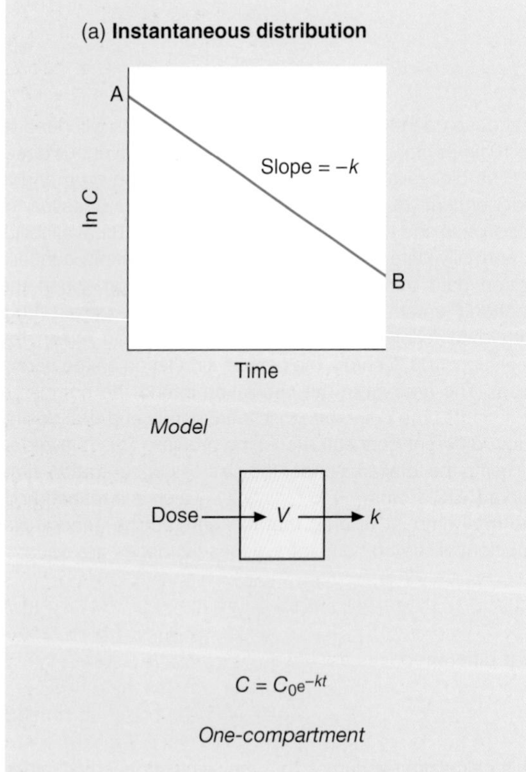

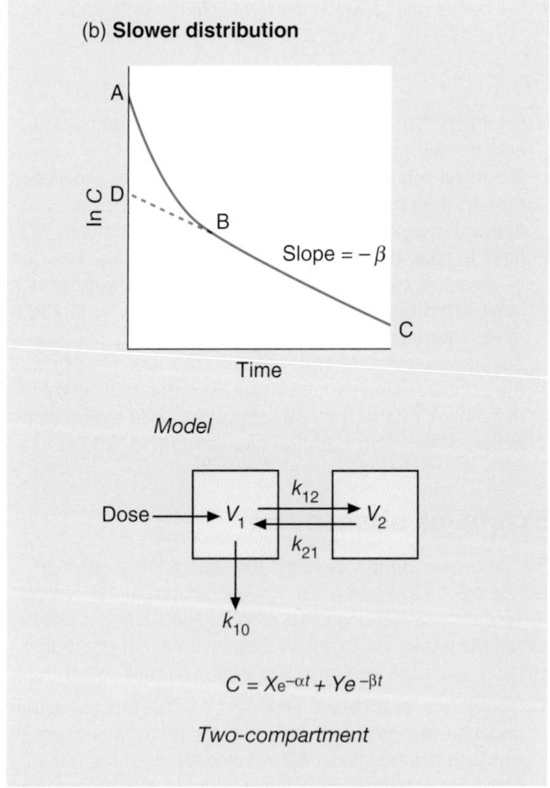

Fig. 2.18 **Plasma concentration–time curves for the distribution of drugs into one- and two-compartment models.** The terms k, α, β, k_{10}, k_{12}, k_{21}, are rate constants; α and β are composite rate constants which define the distribution and elimination rates. The terms α and β relate to distribution (k_{12} or k_{21}) and elimination (k_{10}) processes and are determined by k_{10}, k_{12} and k_{21}. V are volumes of distribution, and X and Y are constants. (Note: the equation for a two-compartment system is usually written as $C = Ae^{-\alpha t} + Be^{-\beta t}$, where A and B are constants equivalent to X and Y; X and Y were used to avoid confusion with points A and B on the graph.)

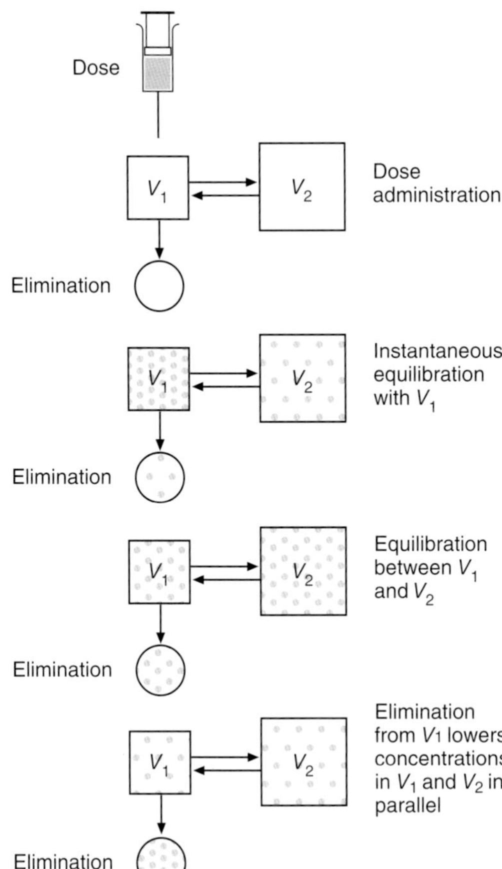

Fig. 2.19 **Schematic diagram of drug distribution.** (Note, at equilibrium, the total concentrations in V_1 and V_2 may be different, because of protein binding, etc.)

Instantaneous and slow distributions are described by different mathematical models: the former is described as a *one-compartment model* (Fig. 2.18a), in which all tissues are in equilibrium instantaneously; the latter is described as a *two-compartment model* (Fig. 2.18b), in which the drug initially enters and reaches instantaneous equilibrium with one compartment (blood and possibly well-perfused tissues) prior to equilibrating more slowly with a second compartment (possibly poorly perfused tissues; refer back to Fig. 2.6). This is shown schematically in Figure 2.19.

The rate of distribution is dependent on two main variables:

- for *water-soluble drugs*, the rate of distribution depends on the rate of passage across membranes, i.e. the diffusion characteristics of the drug
- for *lipid-soluble drugs*, the rate of distribution depends on the rate of delivery (the blood flow) to those tissues, such as adipose, that accumulate the drug.

For some drugs, the natural logarithm of the plasma concentration–time curve shows three distinct phases; such curves require three exponential rates and represent a *three-compartment model*. Although two- or three-compartment models may be necessary to give a mathematical description of the data, they are of limited practical value.

Extent of distribution

The extent of distribution of a drug from plasma into tissues is of clinical importance because it determines the relationship between the concentration present in the blood or plasma and the total amount of drug in the body (body burden). In consequence, the extent of distribution determines the amount of a drug that has to be administered in order to produce a particular plasma concentration (see below).

The distribution of a drug between blood or plasma and tissues can be determined directly in animals, but in humans only the concentration in blood or plasma can be measured. Therefore the extent of distribution has to be estimated from the amount remaining in blood, or more usually plasma, after completion of distribution.

The parameter that describes the extent of distribution is the *apparent volume of distribution* (V), where:

$$V = \frac{\text{Total amount of drug in the body}}{\text{Plasma concentration}} \tag{2.10}$$

The apparent volume of distribution is a characteristic property of the drug and is independent of dose. In the simple example shown by Figure 2.18a, if a dose of 50 mg of a particular drug is injected, this will mix instantaneously into the apparent volume of distribution V. If the initial plasma concentration is 1 μg mL^{-1} (equivalent to point A in Fig. 2.18a), then the apparent volume of distribution will be given by:

$$V = \frac{\text{Total amount (dose)}}{\text{Plasma concentration}} = \frac{50\,000\ \mu\text{g}}{1\ \mu\text{g mL}^{-1}}$$
$$= 50\,000\ \text{mL} = 50\ \text{L}$$

In other words, after giving the dose, it appears that the drug has been dissolved in 50 L of plasma. However, the plasma volume in adult humans is only 3 L and, therefore, much of the drug must have left the plasma and entered tissues, in order to give the low plasma concentration present (1 μg mL^{-1}). The clinical relevance of V is apparent when a physician needs to calculate how much drug should be given to a patient in order to produce a specific, desired plasma concentration. If an initial plasma concentration of 2.5 μg mL^{-1} of the same drug were needed for a clinical effect, this would be produced by giving an intravenous dose of [plasma concentration × V] or [2.5 μg mL^{-1} × 50000 mL] – that is, 125000 μg or 125 mg.

In the more complex example shown in Figure 2.18b, the dose of 50 mg will distribute instantaneously only into V_1 (the central compartment usually comprising plasma and well-perfused tissues). Measurement of the initial concentration (point A in Fig. 2.18b) will not represent distribution into V_2 and the volume calculated using point A will under-represent the true extent of distribution (see Fig. 2.19). Distribution into V_2 (the peripheral compartment usually comprising poorly perfused tissues) is not complete until point B in Figure 2.18b. However, by the time point B is reached, there will have been considerable elimination, and so the total amount of drug in the body is no longer known. This can be overcome by back-extrapolating the elimination

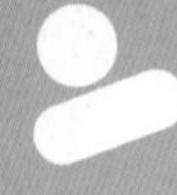

phase (B–C in Fig. 2.18b) to the intercept (point D), which is the concentration that would have been obtained if distribution into V_2 had been instantaneous (see Equation 2.10):

$$V = \frac{\text{Dose}}{\text{Concentration at point D}} \quad (2.11)$$

Alternative equations for the calculation of *V* are presented below.

V is not a physiological volume but simply a reflection of the amount of drug remaining in the blood or plasma after distribution. It provides no information on which tissues the drug has entered. For example, a high value for *V* could result from either reversible accumulation in adipose tissue (owing to dissolution in fat) or reversible accumulation in liver and lung (owing to high intracellular protein binding). The actual tissue distribution can be determined only by measurement of tissue concentrations.

The term *V* reflects the relative affinity of plasma and tissues for a drug. The value of *V* is usually calculated using the total concentration in plasma – that is, free (unbound) drug plus protein-bound drug. A low value for *V* can result if a drug is highly bound to plasma proteins but not to tissue proteins, but there is no simple relationship between plasma protein binding and *V* (Table 2.10).

If the tissues have a very high affinity for the drug, the value of *V* will be extremely high and may greatly exceed the body weight. Chloroquine is a good example of such a drug (Table 2.10) and the value illustrates clearly that *V* should be regarded as a mathematical ratio (not as an indication of physiological distribution to an actual volume of plasma!).

The term *V* indicates the volume of plasma that has to be cleared of drug by the organs of elimination, such as the liver and kidneys, which extract the drug from the plasma and remove it from the body by metabolism or excretion. It is independent of dose or concentration. Because *V* is constant, a twofold increase in plasma concentration will be accompanied by a twofold increase in the concentrations of drug in tissues and also in the total amount of drug in the body (body burden) (Equation 2.10).

Although the apparent volume of distribution may seem a rather abstract (and possibly even irrelevant) parameter, it is important for two reasons. Firstly, it is the parameter that relates the total body drug load present at any time to the plasma concentration. Secondly, together with clearance, it determines the overall elimination rate constant (*k*) and therefore the half-life: the half-life determines the duration of action of a single dose, the time interval between doses on repeated dosage and the potential for accumulation (see below).

Table 2.10 The apparent volume of distribution (*V*) and plasma protein binding of selected drugs

Drug	*V* (L kg^{-1})	Binding (%)
Warfarin and furosemide	0.1	99
Aspirin	0.2	49
Gentamicin	0.3	<10
Propranolol	3.9	93
Nortriptyline	18.5	95
Chloroquine	185.7	61

Note: *V* is given in litres per kilogram body weight; therefore, for chloroquine, the total volume of distribution will be 13 000 L per 70-kg patient.

ELIMINATION

The rate at which the drug is eliminated is important because it usually determines the duration of response, the time interval between doses and the time to reach equilibrium during repeated dosing.

Rate of elimination

The rate of elimination is usually indicated by the terminal half-life – that is, the half-life for the final (slowest) rate (*k* in Fig. 2.18a; β in Fig. 2.18b). The elimination half-lives of drugs range from a few minutes to many days (and, in rare cases, weeks).

The rate at which a drug can be eliminated from the body, and therefore the half-life, is determined by two independent, biologically determined variables: the activity of the mechanisms responsible for metabolising/excreting the drug and the extent of movement of drug from the blood into tissues.

The activity of the metabolising enzymes or excretory mechanisms

The organs of elimination (usually the liver and kidneys) remove drug that is delivered to them via the blood. Providing that first-order kinetics apply (in other words, the process is not saturated), a constant proportion of the drug carried in the blood will be removed on each passage through the organ of elimination, independent of the concentration in the blood. In effect, this is equivalent to a constant proportion of the blood flow to the organ being cleared of drug. The more active the process (e.g. hepatic metabolism), the greater will be the proportion of the blood flow cleared of drug on one passage through the organ. For example, if 10% of the drug carried to the liver by the plasma (at a flow rate of 800 mL min^{-1}) is cleared, by uptake and metabolism, this is equivalent to a clearance of 10% of the plasma flow (80 mL min^{-1}); if the drug is metabolised more readily and 20% of the drug is cleared, this gives a clearance of 160 mL min^{-1}. The proportion of the blood flow cleared of drug will have units of volume per time (e.g. mL min^{-1}). The plasma clearance (CL) of the drug is the sum of all clearance processes (metabolism + renal + bile + exhalation + etc.) and is the volume of plasma cleared of drug per unit time; it is the best indication of the overall activity of the elimination processes.

$$\text{CL} = \frac{\text{Rate of elimination from the body}}{\text{Plasma concentration}} \quad (2.12)$$

$$\text{For example } \frac{\mu\text{g min}^{-1}}{\mu\text{g mL}^{-1}} = \text{mL min}^{-1}$$

The plasma clearance is a characteristic value for a particular drug (see Table 2.11), is a constant for first-order (non-saturated) reactions, and is independent of dose or concentration. Because clearance is constant (Equation 2.12), a twofold increase in plasma concentration will be accompanied by a twofold increase in the rate at which the drug is eliminated from the body. The greater the value of plasma clearance, the greater will be the rate at which the drug will be removed from the body, i.e. the elimination rate constant (*k*) is proportional to plasma clearance.

Reversible passage of drug from the blood into tissues

The organs of elimination can only act on drug that is delivered to them via the blood supply. If, after equilibration with tissues, the blood or plasma concentration is very low, then the apparent volume of distribution (*V*) is very high. The low plasma concentration will result in a low rate of elimination from the body; in other words, the rate at which the drug can be eliminated will be limited by the extent of tissue distribution. Therefore, the elimination rate constant (*k*) is inversely proportional to the apparent volume of distribution.

$$k \propto \frac{1}{V} \tag{2.13}$$

Plasma clearance

The overall rate of elimination is dependent on the two variables, the volume of plasma cleared per minute (CL) and the total apparent volume of plasma that has to be cleared (*V*):

$$k = \frac{\text{CL}}{V} \tag{2.14}$$

or

$$t_{1/2} = \frac{0.693V}{\text{CL}} \quad \text{since } t_{1/2} = \frac{0.693}{k}$$

This is illustrated in Figure 2.20 and Table 2.11. The elimination rate constant (or half-life) is the best indication of changes in drug concentration with time, and for many drugs this will relate to the decrease in therapeutic activity following a single dose. Clearance is the best measurement of the ability of the organs of elimination to remove the drug and determines the average plasma concentrations (and therefore therapeutic activity) at steady state (see below). Clearance is usually determined using the area under the plasma concentration–time curve (AUC).

$$\text{CL} = \frac{\text{Dose}}{\text{AUC}} \tag{2.15}$$

This simple equation is used to calculate clearance (one of the most important pharmacokinetic parameters) under the following conditions:

1. The dose must be given intravenously so that it is all available to the organs of elimination (i.e. CL = Dose/AUC_{iv}). For the oral route, only a fraction (*F*; see above) may reach the general circulation and therefore the dose used in the calculation should be the corrected dose (the administered dose × *F*, as applied in Equation 2.8). Equation 2.8 is based on the fact that the clearance processes reflect what happens to the drug once it is in the general circulation and do not depend on the route of administration, and is a rearrangement of

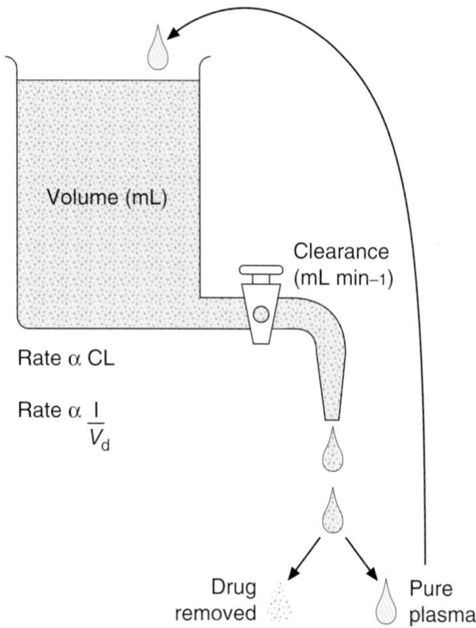

Fig. 2.20 **The relationship between clearance, apparent volume of distribution and overall elimination rate.** The drug is eliminated by the clearance process, which removes drug from a fixed volume of plasma per unit time. The drug is then separated and the pure plasma added back to the tank to maintain a constant volume (the apparent volume of distribution, *V*). The fluid, therefore, continuously recycles via the clearance process and the concentration of drug decreases exponentially. The time taken for one cycle is equal to the volume divided by the clearance (the greater the volume, the greater the time needed; however, the greater the clearance, the shorter the time).

Table 2.11 Pharmacokinetic parameters of selected drugs

Drug	Clearance (mL min^{-1})	Apparent volume of distribution (L per 70 kg)	Half-life (h)
Warfarin	3	8	37
Digitoxin	4	38	161
Diazepam	27	77	43
Valproic acid	76	27	5.6
Digoxin	130	640	39
Ampicillin	270	20	1.3
Amlodipine	333	1470	36
Nifedipine	500	80	1.8
Lidocaine	640	77	1.8
Propranolol	840	270	3.9
Imipramine	1050	1600	18

Note: The drugs are arranged in order of increasing plasma clearance. A long half-life may result from a low clearance (e.g. digitoxin), a high apparent volume of distribution (e.g. amlodipine) or both.

$$\mathrm{CL} = \frac{\mathrm{Dose_{iv}}}{\mathrm{AUC_{iv}}} = F \times \frac{\mathrm{Dose_{oral}}}{\mathrm{AUC_{oral}}}$$

2. The AUC should be the area under the concentration–time curve, not the logarithm of the concentration–time curve.
3. The AUC should be extrapolated to infinity.

V can be calculated using Equations 2.14 and 2.15, and is more reliable than the extrapolation method given in Fig. 2.18b:

$$\mathrm{CL} = \frac{\mathrm{Dose}}{\mathrm{AUC}} = kV$$

$$V = \frac{\mathrm{Dose}}{\mathrm{AUC} \times k} \quad \text{or} \quad \frac{\mathrm{Dose}}{\mathrm{AUC} \times \beta} \qquad (2.16)$$

Plasma clearance, as defined above, is the sum of all clearance processes. Measurement of specific processes such as metabolic clearance or renal clearance would require specific measurement of the rate of elimination by that process. In practice, this is only really possible for renal clearance ($\mathrm{CL_r}$).

Renal clearance can be calculated from the rate of excretion in urine (as the parent drug) during a urine collection and the mid-point plasma concentration:

$$\mathrm{CL_r} = \frac{\text{Rate of excretion in urine (as the parent drug)}}{\text{Plasma concentration (mid-point)}} \qquad (2.17)$$

$$\frac{\mu\mathrm{g\ min^{-1}}}{\mu\mathrm{g\ mL^{-1}}} = \mathrm{mL\ min^{-1}}$$

Measurement of renal clearance can be useful in a number of ways.

- Comparison of renal clearance with plasma clearance will show the importance of the kidney in the overall elimination of the compound; this can be of value in predicting the potential impact of renal disease.
- The difference between plasma and renal clearance is normally equivalent to **metabolic clearance** (which cannot be measured directly), and this can be of value in predicting the potential impact of liver disease.
- Comparison of renal clearance with the glomerular filtration rate (GFR), after allowance for protein binding, provides an estimate of the extent of either reabsorption (if clearance is less than GFR) or active secretion (if clearance is greater than GFR).
- Renal clearance can be changed by altering kidney function, for example by changing the urine pH, which can be useful in treating drug overdose (see Ch. 53).

Biliary clearance of a drug can be measured using the above approach, but in practice is seldom done, because of the difficulty of collecting bile samples.

Extent of elimination

The extent of elimination is of limited value because eventually all the drug will be removed from the body. Measurement of total elimination in urine, faeces and expired air as parent drug and metabolites can give useful insights into the extent of absorption, metabolism, and renal and biliary elimination.

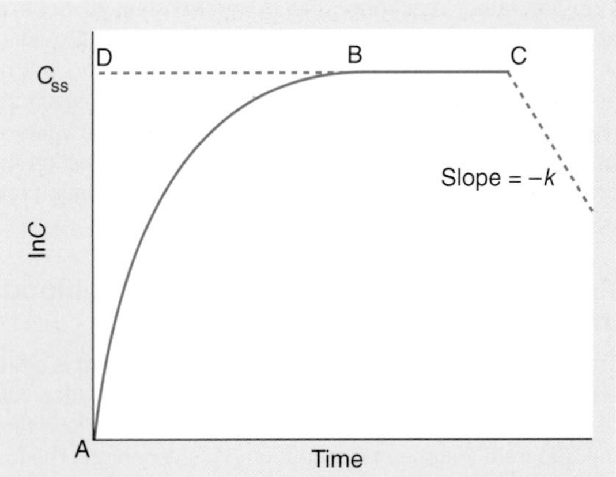

Fig. 2.21 **Constant intravenous infusion (between points A and C).** Steady state is reached at point B and the steady-state concentration (C_{ss}; given by D) can be used to calculate clearance: CL = rate of infusion/C_{ss} (see text). Clearance can also be calculated from the area under the total curve (AUC) and the total dose infused between A and C. The slope on cessation of infusion is the terminal elimination phase (k or β). The distribution phase is not usually detected because distribution is occurring throughout the period A to C. The apparent volume of distribution can be calculated as: V = Dose/(AUC × k). The increase to steady state is determined by the elimination rate constant and it takes approximately four to five half-lives to reach steady state.

CHRONIC ADMINISTRATION

Long-term or chronic drug therapy is designed to maintain a constant concentration of the drug in blood and all tissues of the body, including the site of action. In practice, a constant concentration can only be achieved by a constant intravenous infusion that has continued long enough to reach a steady-state balance between drug input and drug elimination (Fig. 2.21).

Time to reach steady state

During constant infusion, the time to reach steady state is dependent on the elimination half-life, and steady-state is approached after four or five times the elimination half-life. Intuitively, it may seem peculiar that the elimination half-life determines the time required to reach equilibrium during constant input. The proportion of the daily dose that is eliminated each day during constant intake is determined by the elimination rate constant and therefore the half-life (Equation 2.6). For a drug with a half-life of 6 h most of each daily dose will be eliminated within the same 24-h period, and the steady-state balance between input and output will be reached on the first or second day of treatment. In contrast, for a drug with a half-life of 2 days only about 25% of the first dose will be eliminated within the first 24-h period and the drug will continue to accumulate in the body until the amount eliminated balances out the daily input. The amount eliminated each day is given by Equation 2.12 and is the plasma concentration multiplied by the clearance (expressed per day).

Since the elimination half-life is dependent on both CL and *V*, each of these can contribute to any delay in achieving steady state. A drug with a large *V* will have a long half-life and, therefore, it will take a longer time to reach steady state. It is easy to envisage the slow 'filling' of such a high volume of distribution during regular administration.

Plasma concentration at steady state (C_{ss})

Once steady state has been reached, the plasma and tissues are in equilibrium, and the distribution rate constant and *V* will not affect the plasma concentration. The value of C_{ss} is determined solely by the balance between the rate of infusion and the rate of elimination (or clearance): from Equation 2.12, the rate of elimination equals CL × C_{ss}, so that CL × C_{ss} = Rate of infusion or

$$C_{ss} = \frac{\text{Rate of infusion}}{\text{CL}} \qquad (2.18)$$

This relationship for an intravenous infusion can be used to calculate plasma clearance:

$$\text{CL} = \frac{\text{Rate of infusion}}{C_{ss}} \qquad (2.19)$$

Clearance and volume of distribution can also be calculated using the AUC between zero and infinity and the terminal slope after cessation of the infusion (see Fig. 2.21).

Oral administration

Most chronic administration is via the oral route, and the rate and extent of absorption affect the shape of the curve. Because oral therapy is by intermittent doses there will be a series of peaks and troughs between doses (Fig. 2.22).

The rate of absorption will influence the inter-dose profile, since very rapid absorption will exaggerate fluctuations, while slow absorption will dampen down the peak.

The extent of absorption, or bioavailability (*F*), will influence the average steady-state concentration, because it determines the dose entering the circulation. The rate of input during chronic oral therapy is given by:

$$\frac{D \times F}{t} \qquad (2.20)$$

where *D* is the administered dose, *F* is bioavailability, and *t* is the interval between doses. At steady state, the rate of input is balanced by the rate of elimination, that is:

$$\frac{D \times F}{t} = \text{CL} \times C_{ss} \qquad (2.21)$$

Therefore:

$$C_{ss} = \frac{D \times F}{t \times \text{CL}} \qquad (2.22)$$

This is an important equation and reflects the balance between input and output. In reality the balance is between:

- the input of drug, which is determined by the prescriber, who can change C_{ss} by altering either the dose or the dose interval (and sometimes the bioavailability of the drug formulation), and
- the removal of drug, which is determined by the characteristics of the individual taking the drug: metabolism/renal function can change C_{ss} by altering bioavailability and/or clearance.

Loading dose

A therapeutic problem may arise when a rapid effect is required for a drug that has a long or very long half-life; for example, if the half-life of the drug is 12–24 h the steady-state conditions will not be reached until 2–4 days, but if the half-life is 1 week it will take over 4 or 5 weeks. Increasing the dose rate does not reduce the time to reach steady state; a higher dose rate will reduce the time taken to reach any particular concentration, but plasma concentrations will continue to increase to give a higher steady-state level (after the same time interval of about four or five half-lives).

Any delay between the initiation of treatment and the attainment of steady state may be avoided by the administration of a *loading dose*. A loading dose is a high initial or first dose that, as the name implies, is designed to 'load up' the body. In principle, this is done by giving a first dose that is equivalent to the total body load which would be produced at steady state by the intended chronic dosage regimen. This will avoid the slow build-up to steady state,

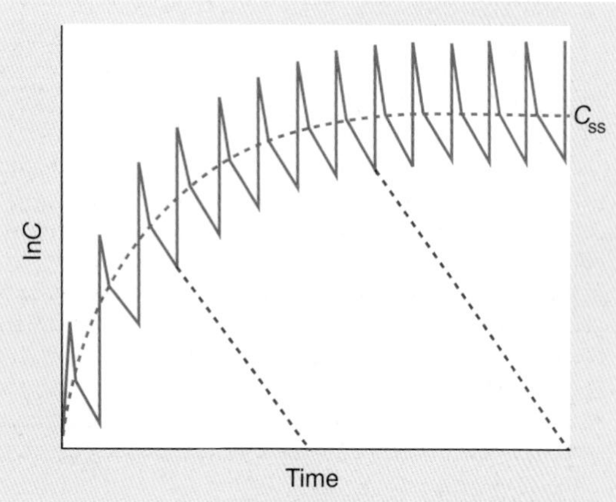

Fig. 2.22 **Chronic oral therapy (——) compared with intravenous (----) infusion at the same dosage rate.** The oral dose shows very rapid absorption and distribution followed by a more slow elimination phase within each dose interval. Cessation of therapy after any dose would produce the line shown in blue.

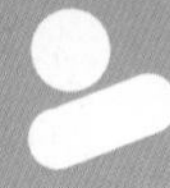

and the steady-state body load can then be maintained by giving the dosage regimen that would eventually have resulted in the same steady-state concentration. The amount of drug equivalent to the steady-state body load is the target C_{ss} multiplied by V (see Equation 2.10).

$$\text{Loading dose} = C_{ss} \times V \qquad (2.23)$$

In cases where C_{ss} or V are not known, the loading dose can be calculated based on the proposed maintenance regimen by replacing C_{ss} with Equation 2.22 and V by CL/k (Equation 2.14):

$$\text{Loading dose} = \frac{D \times F}{t \times CL} \times \frac{\text{CL}}{k} \qquad (2.24)$$

$$= \frac{D \times F}{t \times k}$$

$$= \frac{D \times F \times 1.44 \times t_{1/2}}{t}$$

It is clear from this last equation that the magnitude of any loading dose compared with the maintenance dose is proportional to the half-life.

Loading doses may need to be given in two or three fractions over a period of about 24–36 h. The reason is that during tissue distribution of the loading dose, there are higher (non-steady-state) concentrations in the blood and rapidly equilibrating tissues, and lower (non-steady-state) concentrations in the slowly equilibrating tissues (see Fig. 2.6). The excessive concentrations in rapidly equilibrating tissues may give rise to toxicity. This can be minimised by giving the loading dose in fractions, which would allow tissue distribution of one fraction before the next was given.

FACTORS AFFECTING PHARMACOKINETICS

A number of factors can affect the physiological processes of absorption, distribution and elimination. Aspects such as pregnancy, age, and diseases of the organs of elimination are discussed in Chapter 56. Clinically important variability in plasma drug concentrations can arise from inter-individual differences in bioavailability, V and CL of the drug:

- **drug interactions**: see Chapter 56, and the induction and inhibition of P450 discussed above
- **age**: see Chapter 56
- **diseases**, especially of the liver and kidneys: see Chapter 56
- **environmental factors**, for example alcohol and smoking
- **genetics**: this is becoming an increasingly important area and is discussed in detail below in relation to pharmacokinetics and in Chapter 1 in relation to receptors.

PHARMACOGENOMICS, PHARMACOGENETICS AND DRUG KINETICS

The earliest studies on pharmacogenetics were performed in relation to enzymes involved in drug metabolism. N-Acetyltransferase was one of the first drug metabolism pathways found to show a genetic polymorphism that influenced both plasma concentrations of a drug (isoniazid) and the therapeutic response. Individuals with low enzyme activity, so-called 'slow acetylators', had higher blood concentrations of isoniazid and a better response but a greater risk of toxicity than did 'fast acetylators'. Because N-acetylation is a minor pathway of drug metabolism, pharmacogenetics remained of largely academic interest until the late 1970s, when it was found that CYP2D6 – one of the isoforms of cytochrome P450, the major drug-metabolising enzyme – showed a functionally important genetic polymorphism that could affect a wide variety of different drugs. It was found that the basic genotypic difference relates to the coding of an inactive enzyme in those without appreciable CYP2D6 activity – 'poor metabolisers'. Developments in genotyping have now allowed the identification of 75 different alleles and also variations in the number of copies of the coding region, with normal 'extensive metabolisers' having one copy of the normal gene, although individuals with up to 13 copies have been identified. Cytochrome P450 was one of the earliest enzyme systems to be a focus of research in the field of human genomics.

Knowledge of the precise nature of the differences, single-nucleotide polymorphisms (SNPs, Ch. 1) that result in genetic polymorphisms is beyond the scope of an undergraduate text, and is not necessary to understand or appreciate either the current position or possible future developments in the area of pharmacogenomics. There is a well-established database on genetic differences in many of the major pathways of foreign compound metabolism (Table 2.12).

- Ethnic origin may influence drug metabolism; for example, subjects from the Indian subcontinent show a two- to threefold lower systemic clearance of nifedipine (a CYP3A4 substrate) compared with Caucasians
- have different proportions of the population showing a genetic deficiency or polymorphism (see Table 2.12).

There is an increasing interest in pharmacogenetics of transporter proteins. Although in its infancy, compared with pharmacogenetics of drug metabolism, the available data indicate that there are functionally important polymorphisms in some ABC transporter proteins (see Table 2.1). A number of SNPs have been identified in the *MDR1* gene, which codes for PGP, although the consequences of this for drug transport and for the aetiology of diseases are not clear. There are splice variants for the OAT transporters in the kidneys, but, again, the incidence and consequences of these for humans have not been defined.

Genetic polymorphisms are likely to be of greatest clinical significance when the polymorphic enzyme is the main pathway affecting bioavailability and/or elimination and when the drug has a narrow therapeutic index (Ch. 53).

Information on genetic polymorphisms and genetic variants of the enzymes and transporters involved in drug metabolism and biodisposition can be found on the OMIM® (Online Mendelian Inheritance in Man®; Johns Hopkins University) database, available at *http://www.ncbi.nlm.nih.gov/omim*

Table 2.12 Pharmacogenetic differences in drug-metabolising enzymes

Enzyme	Incidence of deficiency or slow-metaboliser phenotype[a]	Typical substrates	Consequences of deficiency or slow-metaboliser status
Phase I reactions			
Pseudocholinesterase (butyrylcholinesterase, plasma cholinesterase)	1 in 3000	Suxamethonium (succinylcholine)	Prolonged paralysis and apnoea for up to 3 h after a dose
Alcohol dehydrogenase	5–10% (approx. 90% in Asians)	Ethanol	Profound vasodilation on ingestion of alcohol
CYP1A1	10%?	PAHs	Increased risk of low birth weight in smokers
CYP2A6	15%	Nicotine, coumarin	Reduced nicotine metabolism
CYP2B6	?	Ifosfamide, efavirenz	Numerous SNPs identified; significance unclear; reduced bioactivation of cyclophosphamide
CYP2C9[b]	About 10% in white and 3% in black subjects	Tolbutamide, diazepam, warfarin	Increased response if parent drug is active, e.g. increased risk of haemorrhage with warfarin
CYP2C19	5% (about 20% in Asians)	Omeprazole	Increased response if parent drug is active
CYP2D6	5–10%	Nortriptyline, codeine	Increased response if parent drug is active, but reduced response if oxidation produces the active form, e.g. codeine
Dihydropyrimidine dehydrogenase	1% are heterozygous	Fluorouracil	Enhanced drug response
Phase II reactions			
N-Acetyltransferase	50% (10–20% in Asians)	Isoniazid, hydralazine, procainamide	Enhanced drug response in slow acetylators
Glucuronyl-transferase 1A1	10% (1–4% Asians)	Irinotecan (bilirubin)	Enhanced effect (Gilbert's syndrome; increased bilirubin)
Glutathione transferase family[c]		Reactive compounds or metabolites	Increased risk of cancer from environmental carcinogens; therapeutic implications unclear
Thiopurine S-methyl transferase	0.3%	Mercaptopurine, azathioprine	Increased risk of toxicity (because the doses normally used are close to toxic)
Catechol-O-methyltransferase	25%	Levodopa	Slightly enhanced drug effect
Transporters			
ABCB1 (PGP)	A number of SNPs have been identified (incidences vary with ethnic origins)	Digoxin, anticancer drugs, dihydropyridine, calcium channel blockers	Possibly higher drug levels with some SNPs, but lower drug levels due to increased activity with other SNPs

[a]Incidence for Caucasians.
[b]There is more than one abnormal allele that can result in a deficient activity phenotype.
[c]There are multiple glutathione transferase (GST) isoenzymes, e.g. GSTalpha(1–5), GSTmu(1–5), GSTpi, GSTtheta, many of which can exist in multiple isoforms; most research has investigated links between polymorphisms and the risks of different diseases, especially cancer.
PAHs, polycyclic aromatic hydrocarbons; PGP, P-glycoprotein; SNP, single-nucleotide polymorphism.

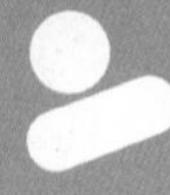

FURTHER READING

Abdel-Rahman SM, Kauffman RE (2004) The integration of pharmacokinetics and pharmacodynamics: understanding dose–response. *Annu Rev Pharmacol Toxicol* 44, 111–136

Altman RB, Klein TE (2002) Challenges for biomedical informatics and pharmacogenomics. *Annu Rev Pharmacol Toxicol* 42, 113–133

Aweeka F, Greenblatt RM, Blaschke TF (2004) Sex differences in pharmacokinetics and pharmacodynamics. *Annu Rev Pharmacol Toxicol* 44, 499–523

Burckhardt BC, Burckhardt G (2003) Transport of organic anions across the basolateral membrane of proximal tubule cells. *Rev Physiol Biochem Pharmacol* 146, 95–158

Cholerton S, Daly AK, Idle JR (1992) The role of individual human cytochromes P450 in drug metabolism and clinical response. *Trends Pharmacol Sci* 13, 434–439

Choudhuri S, Klaassen CD (2006) Structure, function, expression, genomic organization, and single nucleotide polymorphisms of human ABCB1 (MDR1), ABCC (MRP), and ABCG2 (BCRP) efflux transporters. *Int J Toxicol* 25, 231–259

Cole SPC, Deeley RG (2006) Transport of glutathione and glutathione conjugates by MRP1. *Trends Pharmacol Sci* 27, 438–446

Daly AK (2003) Pharmacogenetics of the major polymorphic metabolizing enzymes. *Fundam Clin Pharmacol* 17, 27–41

de Boer AG, van der Sandt ICJ, Gaillard PJ (2003) The role of drug transporters at the blood–brain barrier. *Annu Rev Pharmacol Toxicol* 43, 629–656

Evans WE, McLeod HL (2003) Pharmacogenomics – drug disposition, drug targets, and side effects. *N Engl J Med* 348, 538–549

Fromm MF (2004) Importance of P-glycoprotein at blood–tissue barriers. *Trends Pharmacol Sci* 25, 423–429

Gonzalez TJ (1992) Human cytochromes P450: problems and prospects. *Trends Pharmacol Sci* 13, 346–352

Gurwitz D, Weizman A, Rehavi M (2003) Education: teaching pharmacogenomics to prepare future physicians and researchers for personalised medicine. *Trends Pharmacol Sci* 24, 122–125

Handschin C, Meyer UA (2003) Induction of drug metabolism: the role of nuclear receptors. *Pharmacol Rev* 55, 649–673

Ingelman-Sundberg M (2004) Pharmacogenetics of cytochrome P450 and its applications in drug therapy: the past, present and future. *Trends Pharmacol Sci* 25, 193–200

Koepsell H (2004) Polyspecific organic cation transporters: their functions and interactions with drugs. *Trends Pharmacol Sci* 25, 375–381

Lee G, Dallas S, Hong M, Bendayan R (2001) Drug transporters in the central nervous system: brain barriers and brain parenchyma considerations. *Pharmacol Rev* 53, 569–596

Lee W, Kim RB (2004) Transporters and renal drug elimination *Annu Rev Pharmacol Toxicol* 44, 137–166

Lin JH, Lu AY (2001) Interindividual variability in inhibition and induction of cytochrome P450 enzymes. *Annu Rev Pharmacol Toxicol* 41, 535–567

McLeod HL, Evans WE (2001) Pharmacogenomics: unlocking the human genome for better drug therapy. *Annu Rev Pharmacol Toxicol* 41, 101–121

Marzolini C, Paus E, Buclin T, Kim RB (2004) Polymorphisms in human MDR1 (P-glycoprotein): recent advances and clinical relevance. *Clin Pharmacol Ther* 75, 13–33

Miyazaki H, Sekine T, Endou H (2004) The multispecific organic anion transporter family: properties and pharmacological significance. *Trends Pharmacol Sci* 25, 654–662

Nebert DW, Vesell ES (2007) Can personalised drug therapy be achieved? A closer look at pharmaco-metabonomics. *Trends Pharmacol Sci* 27, 581–586

Pirmohamed M, Park BK (2001) Genetic susceptibility to adverse drug reactions. *Trends Pharmacol Sci* 22, 298–305

Schwab M, Eichelbaum M, Fromm MF (2003) Genetic polymorphisms of the human MDR1 drug transporter. *Annu Rev Pharmacol Toxicol* 43, 285–307

Tukey RH, Strassburg CP (2000) Human UDP-glucuronosyltransferases: metabolism, expression, and disease. *Annu Rev Pharmacol Toxicol* 40, 581–616

Weinshilboum R (2003) Inheritance and drug response. *N Engl J Med* 348, 529–537

Xie H-G, Kim RB, Wood AJJ, Stein MC (2001) Molecular basis of ethnic differences in drug disposition and response. *Annu Rev Pharmacol Toxicol* 41, 815–850

SELF-ASSESSMENT

1. The following statements describe drug pharmacokinetics. Are they true or false?
   a. The plasma clearance of a drug usually decreases with increase in the dose prescribed.
   b. First-pass metabolism may limit the bioavailability of orally administered drugs.
   c. Drugs that show high first-pass metabolism in the liver also have a high systemic clearance.
   d. The half-life of many drugs is longer in infants than in children or adults.
   e. A decrease in renal function may affect both systemic clearance and oral bioavailability.
   f. Benzathine benzylpenicillin has a prolonged half-life because the renal extraction of penicillin is reduced.
   g. Nifedipine is eliminated more rapidly in cigarette smokers.
   h. Chronic treatment with phenobarbital can increase the systemic clearance and oral bioavailability of co-administered drugs.
   i. A loading dose is not necessary for drugs that have short half-lives.
   j. An obese person is likely to show an increased volume of distribution and decreased clearance of prescribed drugs and would require higher dosage than a non-obese subject during chronic drug therapy.
   k. Drugs are always taken with meals in order to reduce unwanted effects.
2. Figure 2.23 shows the changes in plasma levels of two drugs, A and B, given as 10-mg doses by oral and intravenous routes. From the plasma concentration–time curves, compare the two drugs for the following properties (do not perform detailed calculations):
   a. Absorption from the gut.
   b. Oral bioavailability.

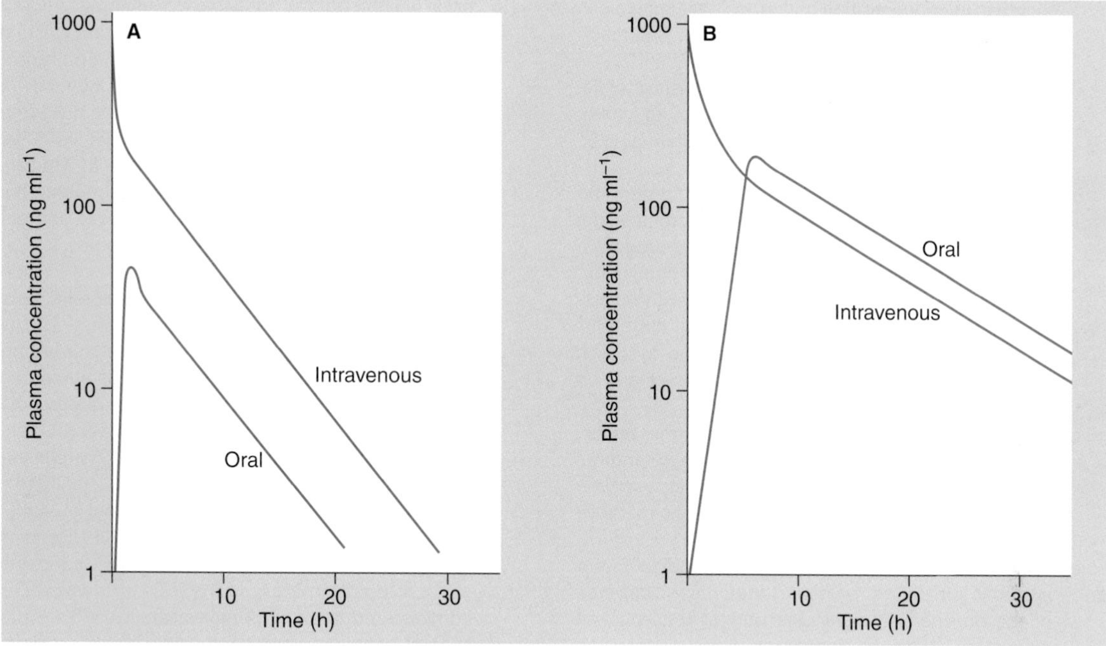

Fig. 2.23 **Plasma concentration–time curves for two drugs.**

c. Distribution to tissues.
d. Elimination half-life.
e. Extent of accumulation during daily administration of each drug.

3. A man weighing 70 kg was admitted to hospital with a serious infection and was treated with two antibiotics. Gentamicin is not absorbed on oral administration and is given by intravenous administration. Cefalexin is given orally and the bioavailability is 90% ($F = 0.9$).

Volume of distribution (V) (L/70 kg):	gentamicin, 18;	cefalexin, 18.
Clearance (CL) (L/h/70 kg):	gentamicin, 5.4;	cefalexin, 18.
Half-life (h):	gentamicin, 2–3;	cefalexin, 0.9.

Additional information: gentamicin is very toxic and its use has to be monitored carefully; gentamicin is not metabolised and it is excreted unchanged by the kidneys. The maximum therapeutic plasma concentrations should not exceed 5 mg/L, since higher concentrations can lead to ototoxicity (damage to the ear) and nephrotoxicity (damage to kidneys).

a. You have calculated that you will give him 900 mg of gentamicin by injection as a bolus (single) dose, in order to achieve a plasma concentration that will not exceed the toxic plasma concentration. Is this a safe dose?
b. Because of the short half-life of gentamicin you then decide that it will be best to give him a continuous intravenous infusion to maintain a steady-state plasma concentration of 2500 μg/L. What rate of infusion should be given?
c. What maximum plasma concentration would be obtained if a single oral loading dose of 500 mg cefalexin was given?

4. Mrs J, weighing 70 kg, was diagnosed with congestive heart failure and atrial fibrillation. She was started on digoxin.

Volume of distribution (V) (L/70 kg):	640
Clearance (CL) (L/h/70 kg):	7.2
Half-life (h):	42

Additional information: the plasma concentrations for therapeutic effectiveness are 800–2000 ng/L. Toxic effects occur above 2000 ng/L.

a. How long would it take to reach a steady-state concentration in plasma?
b. What dose should be given as a loading dose to achieve a plasma level of 800 ng/L?

5. A 7-year-old girl weighing 31 kg was admitted to A&E with asthma. Treatment was started with theophylline. The desired steady-state concentration is 15 μg/mL plasma. The apparent volume of distribution (V) is 0.5 L/kg and the oral bioavailability is 60% ($F = 0.6$). What would be the most appropriate oral loading dose?
A. 139 mg
B. 232 mg
C. 387 mg
D. 644 mg

ANSWERS

1. a. **False.** Clearance, like bioavailability and apparent volume of distribution, is independent of dose and is a characteristic for the drug (providing that the processes are not saturated). An increase in dose results in an increase in the concentrations of the drug in plasma and body tissues. A twofold increase in drug concentrations gives twofold higher concentrations available to elimination processes; consequently, the rate of elimination increases twofold. Since clearance is given by the rate of elimination/plasma concentration, this ratio is not altered. A decrease in clearance with increase in dose occurs when the elimination process is saturated and an

increase in concentration cannot give an increase in the rate of elimination. Few drugs show saturation kinetics (zero order) at therapeutic doses.

b. **True**. This statement is true for all 'pre-systemic' sites of metabolism of the oral dose, e.g. gut lumen, intestinal wall and liver. Low bioavailability may also arise from poor absorption.
c. **True**. If the liver is able to 'mop up' a high proportion of the drug as it is absorbed from the gastrointestinal tract, it will also clear a high proportion of drug from the blood after it has entered the general circulation. For example, if 80% of an oral dose undergoes first-pass liver metabolism during absorption, then 80% of all drug delivered to the liver via the systemic blood flow will also be cleared; systemic clearance will equal 80% of liver blood flow.
d. **True**. A longer half-life can arise from a higher apparent volume of distribution or a lower clearance; babies (under 6–12 months) show lower systemic clearance because of both reduced hepatic metabolism and lower renal excretion.
e. **False**. A decrease in renal function could affect systemic clearance, providing that renal clearance of the drug was a significant part of total plasma clearance. However, bioavailability is simply the fraction of the oral dose that reaches the general circulation, and the kidneys are not part of the route between gut lumen and general circulation. (Although the AUC of an oral dose may be increased in renal disease, the AUC of an intravenous dose will also show a similar increase and bioavailability is not altered.)
f. **False**. Benzathine benzylpenicillin is a depot injection of penicillin in which the prolonged half-life results from prolonged and sustained release from the site of injection. Once absorbed into the blood, the circulating penicillin is handled by the kidneys as normal.
g. **False**. Nifedipine is metabolised by CYP3A4; no interaction would occur, because smoking induces CYP1A2. Our increased understanding of the cytochrome P450 isoenzymes has allowed more rational predictions of 'drug–drug' and 'drug–environmental chemical' interactions (see Table 2.9).
h. **False**. Phenobarbital is a potent inducer of cytochrome P450 enzymes, which can increase the ability of the liver to extract the drug from the blood. This can increase the systemic clearance but decreases the oral bioavailability of co-administered drugs.
i. **True**. A loading dose is designed to produce the body load that will be present during chronic treatment (at steady state) without the time delay while the body accumulates the drug at the start of chronic treatment. Drugs with short elimination half-lives do not accumulate significantly and therefore the body load after the first normal (non-loading) dose will be the same as during chronic treatment.
j. **False**. The influence of body composition on the apparent volume of distribution depends on the nature of the drug. Lipid-soluble drugs would show an increased apparent volume of distribution (V) in an obese patient (when expressed per kilogram body weight) but the converse would apply to water-soluble drugs. However, the V and clearance (CL) of drugs are independent variables; there is no reason why the different distribution in the body should affect the ability of the liver to extract the drug from the blood. Students sometimes can get confused about V and CL and think that if more of the drug enters the fat this will lower the blood concentration and hence must lower CL. It is important to appreciate that V and CL are independent variables. If more drug enters adipose tissue (because there is more of it), then plasma concentration (C) will tend to be lower and V, which equals the amount in the body/C_p, will be higher. Because the plasma concentration at any time is lower and CL is a constant for that drug, then the rate of elimination at any point in time will be lower (CL = rate of elimination/C_p and therefore rate of elimination = CL × C). The elimination half-life is related to both V and CL (half-life is 0.693 V/CL) and an increase in V without a change in CL would result in an increase in half-life. Because the steady-state plasma concentration (C_{ss}) depends on CL but not on V ($C_{ss} = D \times F/CL \times t$, where D is administered dose, F is bioavailability and t is the interval between doses), C_{ss} would not be affected and there would not be any need to modify a chronic dosage regimen because of an increase in V. However, the steady-state body load ($C_{ss} \times V$) would be higher and, therefore, it could take longer to reach steady-state conditions (as indicated by the increase in half-life). *[If you have understood this answer, then you have 'cracked' pharmacokinetics!]*
k. **False**. This statement is true for some drugs but not for all drugs: it depends on the drug. Administration of drugs with food will generally decrease the rate of absorption (because of effects on gastric emptying and/or absorption rate) and this will often reduce the peak plasma concentration. This may, in some cases, reduce unwanted effects. Another advantage of taking medicines with meals is that it can increase compliance with a three-times-daily (tds) dosage schedule. Potential disadvantages are the delay in absorption and, in some cases, interference with absorption, giving a decrease in bioavailability; for example, the absorption of tetracycline antimicrobials is almost completely abolished if they are taken with milk.

2. a. The rate of absorption is determined by the rate of increase after oral dosing. Drug A is absorbed very rapidly, while drug B takes about 6 h to reach a peak concentration.
b. The extent of absorption (bioavailability or F) is determined by the AUC_{oral}/AUC_{iv}. For drug A, the AUC_{oral} is much smaller than AUC_{iv} and therefore F is much less than 1. In contrast, for drug B, the AUC_{oral} approximately equals the AUC_{iv} and so F is approximately 1.
c. The rate of distribution is given by the rate of decrease between the administration of the intravenous bolus dose (at time 0) and the establishment of the terminal elimination phase. The terminal phase for drug A starts at about 1 h, whereas that for drug B starts at about 4 h. Therefore, A distributes more

rapidly. The extent of distribution is given by the apparent volume of distribution, V, which is indicated by the intravenous dose divided by the intercept (C_0) obtained on back-extrapolation of the terminal phase of the plasma concentration–time curve (intravenous dose/C_0). Both A and B give a similar intercept and, therefore, have similar apparent volumes of distribution.

d. The elimination half-life is given by 0.693/terminal slope (0.693/k or 0.693/β) and it is obvious that drug B has a longer half-life than drug A. The reason for the longer half-life of B is the lower clearance (CL) of B (since the volume of distribution is similar for A and B). This is also apparent by visual inspection of the graphs; CL = $\text{Dose}_{iv}/\text{AUC}_{iv}$ and the AUC_{iv} for B is much greater than that for A (the doses were the same).

e. The potential for accumulation depends on the difference between half-life and dose interval. It is clear that nearly all of drug A has been removed from the plasma (and therefore the body) by 24 h, whereas considerable amounts of B remain at 24 h. Therefore, B would show significant accumulation on daily dosage.

3. a. No, it is not safe, it is 10 times too high.
The relationship between plasma concentration and body burden is given by Equation 2.10, which defines the apparent volume of distribution. This equation can be rearranged into:

amount in body (or intended dose) $= C \times V$
(For a single dose this describes the relationship between the dose and initial or peak plasma level)

$$\text{Dose (mg)} = 5\,(\text{mg/L}) \times 18\,(\text{L}) = 90\text{ mg}$$

(Note – pharmacokinetic parameters such as clearance and apparent volume of distribution are sometimes expressed per person and sometimes per kilogram body weight. In this example V is given per person and so the doses are per person not per kilogram body weight. Always put the units into the equation and make sure they cancel out to give the correct final units – in the above example the dose is milligrams per person not milligrams per kilogram.)

b. At steady state the rate of infusion = CL (clearance) × C_{ss} (rearranging Equation 2.18). Therefore for a plasma concentration of 2500 μg/L you will need to give an infusion rate of 5.4 (L/h) × 2500 (μg/L) = 13 500 μg/h. (Note – since there are 1000 μg in 1 mg this equals 13.5 mg/h.)

c. For a single dose the peak concentration is approximately equal to the administered oral dose times bioavailability divided by the apparent volume of distribution (V) (rearranging Equation 2.10 and correcting oral dose for bioavailability):

$$C = (\text{dose} \times F)/V = 500\,(\text{mg/70 kg}) \times 0.9/18\,(\text{L/70 kg}) = 25\text{ mg/L}$$

(Note – because the dose is given orally some of the dose will have been eliminated before the peak concentration is reached. In consequence, the body burden at the time of the peak concentration will not be the complete 500-mg dose and the concentration will be less than 25 mg/L. In clinical practice this could be ignored.)

4. a. It takes up to about five times the elimination half-life to reach steady state, i.e. 4–5 × 42 h or about 7 days (hence the need for a loading dose).

b. The relationship between dose (body burden) and plasma concentration is given by Equation 2.10.

$$\text{Loading dose} = C \times V = 800\,(\text{ng/L}) \times 640\,(\text{L}) = 512000\text{ ng} = 512\ \mu\text{g}$$

(Note there are 1000 ng in 1 μg and 1000 μg in 1 mg).

5. The answer is **C**.
In this example you need to be careful about the units used in the equation and the bioavailability. Because V is given in units of litres per kilogram it is important to make all units equivalent and convert V into litres per person (31 kg in this case); also, the desired plasma concentration of 15 μg/mL has to be converted to 15 mg/L.

$$\text{Body burden (loading dose)} = C \times V$$

$$V = 0.5\,(\text{L/kg}) \times 31\,(\text{kg}) = 15.5\text{ L}$$

If the oral bioavailability was 100%, then the loading dose = 15 (mg/L) × 15.5 (L) = 232 mg. However, the bioavailability is only 60% and therefore the oral dose has to be increased appropriately to give the same plasma level and should be 232/0.6 mg, or 387 mg, in order to give an *absorbed dose of 232 mg.* (See answer to question 3c about the effect of elimination of part of the dose prior to the peak concentration.)

3 Drug discovery, safety and efficacy

Initially, most medicines were of botanical or zoological origin. During the 20th century there was an enormous increase in the use of synthetic organic chemicals, while the 21st century is likely to see the increasing use of the products derived using data from the human genome project. The introduction of recombinant DNA technology has extended medicines to include peptides identical to those of human origin, such as epoetin (recombinant erythropoietin) and human insulin preparations. The major benefit of drugs for the treatment of disease is illustrated most dramatically with antimicrobial chemotherapy, which revolutionised the chances of patients surviving severe infections such as lobar pneumonia, the mortality from which was 27% in the pre-antimicrobial era but fell to 8% (and subsequently less) following the introduction of sulphonamides and then penicillins.

Early medicines were often naturally occurring inorganic salts such as mercury compounds or plant extracts, often containing a mixture of complex organic compounds, more than one of which may have been the active constituent. The active constituents of many plant-derived preparations are nitrogen-containing organic molecules, which are also known as alkaloids; for example, laudanum is an alcohol extract of opium which contains high concentrations of the alkaloid morphine. Early therapeutic successes included the use of foxgloves (which contain cardiac glycosides) for the treatment of 'dropsy' (fluid retention); however, there was also considerable toxicity, because the plant preparations contained variable amounts of the active glycoside and such compounds have a narrow therapeutic index (Ch. 7).

A major advance in the safety of plant-derived medicines was the isolation, purification and chemical characterisation of the active component. This had three main advantages:

- The administration of controlled amounts of the purified active compound removed biological variability in potency of the crude plant preparation.
- The administration of the purified active compound removed the unwanted and potentially toxic effects of contaminating substances in the crude preparations.
- The identification and isolation of the active component allowed the mechanism of action to be defined, leading to the synthesis and development of drugs based on the structure of the active component with the same action but with greater potency, greater selectivity, fewer unwanted effects, altered duration of action, better absorption, etc.

Thus, although drug therapy has natural and humble origins, it is the application of scientific principles which has given rise to the clinical safety and efficacy of modern medicines. In the age of 'scientific reason' it is surprising that so many people believe that 'natural' medicinal products offer equivalent therapeutic effectiveness with advantages of greater safety and fewer unwanted effects.

A major advantage of modern drugs is their ability to act selectively, i.e. to affect only certain specific body systems or processes. For example, a drug which both lowered blood glucose and reduced blood pressure may not be suitable for the treatment of someone with diabetes (because of unwanted hypotensive effects) or a person with hypertension (because of unwanted hypoglycaemic effects) or even those with both conditions (because different doses may be needed for each effect).

DRUG DISCOVERY

The discovery of a new drug can be achieved in several different ways (Fig. 3.1). The simplest method is to subject new chemical entities (novel chemicals not previously synthesised) to a battery of screening tests that are designed to detect different types of biological activity. These include in vitro studies on isolated tissues, as well as in vivo studies of complex and integrated systems, such as animal behaviour. Novel chemicals for screening may be produced by direct chemical synthesis or may be isolated from biological sources, such as plants, and then purified and characterised. This approach has been revolutionised in recent years by developments in 'high-throughput screening', which takes advantage of laboratory robotics combined with in vitro cell lines that express cloned human receptors or enzymes. Solid-phase peptide synthesis combined with knowledge from the human genome project allows the rapid synthesis of large libraries of potential candidate molecules. Active compounds can then be selected based on interactions with cell lines that express a range of possible sites of action, such as G-protein-coupled or nuclear receptors, enzymes important in drug metabolism, and cells derived from human cancers. Such methods allow the screening of hundreds of compounds each day and allow selection of suitable 'lead compounds', which are then subjected to more labour-intensive and detailed tests.

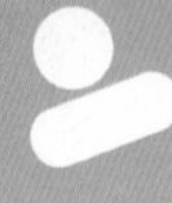

A second approach involves the synthesis and testing of chemical analogues of existing medicines; generally, the products of this research show only minor advances in absorption, potency or a more selective action. However, unexpected additional properties may become evident when the compound is tried in humans; for example, minor modifications of the sulphanilamide antimicrobial molecule gave rise to the thiazide diuretics and the sulphonylurea hypoglycaemics.

More recently, attempts have been made to design substances to fulfil a particular biological role, which may entail the synthesis of a naturally occurring substance (or a structural analogue), its precursor or an antagonist. Good examples include levodopa, used in the treatment of Parkinson's disease, the histamine H_2 receptor antagonists, and omeprazole, the first proton pump inhibitor. Logical drug development of this type depends on a detailed understanding of human physiology both in health and disease. High-throughput screening is particularly useful in such a focused approach. In silico (computer-based) approaches to the modelling of receptor binding sites has facilitated the development of ligands with high binding affinities and, often, high selectivity.

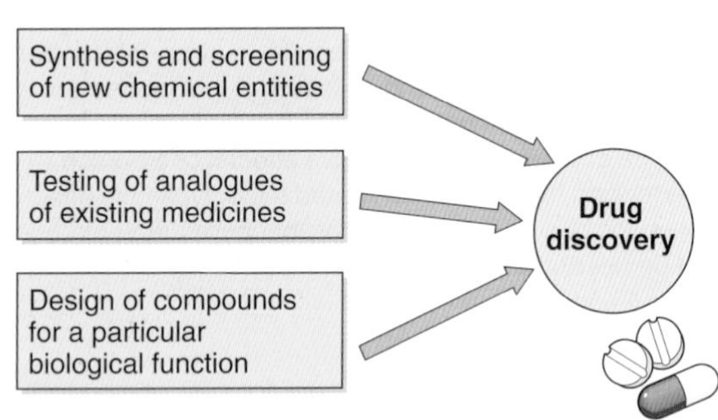

Fig. 3.1 **Approaches to drug discovery.**

The recent phenomenal advances in molecular biology have led to the increasing use of genomic techniques, both to identify genes associated with pathological conditions and subsequently to develop compounds that can either mimic or interfere with the activity of the gene product. Such compounds are often proteins, which gives rise to problems of drug delivery to the relevant tissue and to the site of action, which may be intracellular, and raise issues related to safety testing (see below). The potential of genomic research is enormous but currently under-exploited in relation to the development of marketed drugs. However, given the time and cost involved in getting a new drug approved (see below), it can be anticipated that we are currently seeing only the tip of the iceberg of drugs that will be developed based on these methods. A good example of the potential of genomic research is the drug imatinib (Ch. 52), which was developed to inhibit the enzyme Bcr-Abl tyrosine protein kinase, which was identified in chronic myeloid leukaemia cells by molecular biological methods; imatinib is a typical non-protein organic molecule with a high oral bioavailability, and is eliminated by CYP3A4-mediated metabolism.

Information on genetic polymorphisms and genetic variants in possible targets for drug action can be found on the OMIM® (Online Mendelian Inheritance in Man®; Johns Hopkins University) database, available at *http://www.ncbi.nlm.nih.gov/omim*

DRUG APPROVAL

Each year, many thousands of synthetic novel compounds (new chemical entities) and pure compounds isolated from plant sources are screened for useful and/or novel pharmacological activities. Potentially valuable compounds are then subjected to a sequence of in vitro and in vivo animal studies and clinical trials, which provide essential information on safety and therapeutic benefit (Fig. 3.2).

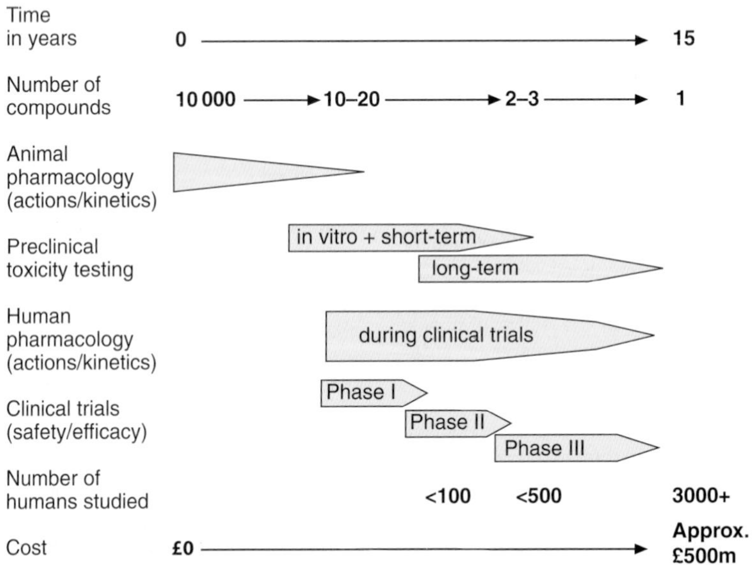

Fig. 3.2 **The development of a new drug to the point at which a licence is approved.** Post-marketing surveillance will continue to add data on safety and efficacy.

All drugs and formulations licensed for sale in the UK have to pass a rigorous evaluation of:

- safety
- quality
- efficacy.

In the European Union (EU), new drugs are now approved under a harmonised procedure of drug regulation. The European Medicines Evaluation Agency (EMEA – *http://www.emea.europa.eu*) is a decentralised body of the European Union, with headquarters in London, which is responsible for the regulation of medicines in the EU. It receives advice from the Committee for Medicinal Products for Human Use (CHMP), which is a body of international experts who evaluate data on the safety, quality and efficacy of medicines. Under the current systems, new drugs are evaluated by the CHMP, and national advisory bodies have an opportunity to assess the data before a final CHMP conclusion is reached.

The UK Commission on Human Medicines (CHM) was established in 2005 to replace both the Medicines Commission and the Committee on Safety of Medicines which previously had evaluated medicines regulated in the UK under the Medicines Act (1968). The CHM is one of a number of committees established under the Medicines and Healthcare products Regulatory Agency (MHRA – *http://www.mca.gov.uk*). The MHRA provides advice to the Secretary of State for Health.

Safety

Historically, the introduction of new drugs has been bought at a price of significant toxicity, and regulatory systems have arisen as much to protect people taking drugs from toxicity as to ensure benefit. The Food and Drugs Administration (FDA – *http://www.fda.gov/default.htm*) was established in the USA in 1937. This followed a dramatic incident in 1937, when 76 people died of renal failure after taking an elixir of sulphanilamide which contained the solvent diethylene glycol. Similarly, some 30 years later, the occurrence of limb malformations (phocomelia) and cardiac defects in infants born to mothers who had taken thalidomide for the treatment of nausea in the first trimester of pregnancy led to the establishment of the precursor of the UK CSM (*http://www.mhra.gov.uk/Aboutus/index.htm*).

Today, major tragedies are avoided by a combination of in vitro studies and animal toxicity tests (preclinical testing) and careful observation during clinical studies on new drugs (see below). The development and continuing refinement of preclinical toxicity testing has increased the likelihood of identifying chemicals with direct organ toxicity. During clinical trials, immunologically mediated effects are likely to be seen at the lower end of the dose ranges that are used in such trials (see Ch. 53).

Quality

An important function of regulatory bodies is to ensure the consistency of prescribed medicines. Drugs have to comply with defined criteria for purity, and limits are set on the content of any potentially toxic impurities. The stability – and, if necessary, sterility – of the drug also has to be established. Similarly, licensed formulations have to contain a defined and approved amount of the active drug, which has to be released at a specified rate. There have been a number of cases in the past where a simple change to the manufactured formulation has affected tablet disintegration, the release of drug, and the therapeutic response. The quality of drugs for human use is defined by the specifications in the European Pharmacopoeia and the British Pharmacopoeia.

Efficacy

All medicines, apart from homeopathic products, must have evidence of efficacy for their licensed indications. Efficacy, the ability to produce a predefined level of clinical response, can be established only by trials in people with the disease, for whom the medicine is intended, and therefore the demonstration of efficacy is a major aim of the later phases of clinical research (Fig. 3.2).

ESTABLISHING SAFETY AND EFFICACY

Regulatory bodies such as the CHMP and CHM require supporting data from in vitro studies, animal studies and clinical investigations before a new drug is approved. Although there is some overlap, the basic aims and goals are:

- **preclinical studies**: to establish the basic pharmacology, pharmacokinetics and toxicological profile of the drug and its metabolites, using animals and in vitro systems
- **phase I clinical studies**: to establish the human pharmacology and pharmacokinetics, together with a simple safety profile
- **phase II clinical studies**: to establish the dose–response and to develop the dosage protocol for clinical use, together with more extensive safety data
- **phase III clinical studies**: to establish the efficacy and safety profile of the drug in people with the proposed disease for which the drug will be indicated
- **pharmacovigilance**: to monitor adverse events following approval and the more widespread use of the drug.

PRECLINICAL STUDIES

Preclinical studies must be carried out before a compound can be administered to humans. These studies investigate three areas:

- **pharmacological effects**: in vitro effects using isolated cells/organs; receptor-binding characteristics; in vivo effects in animals and/or animal models of human diseases; prediction of potential therapeutic use
- **pharmacokinetics**: identification of metabolites (since these may be the active form of the compound); evidence of bioavailability (to assist with the design of both clinical trials and in vivo animal toxicity studies); establishment of principal route and rate of elimination
- **toxicological effects**: a battery of in vitro and in vivo studies undertaken with the aim of identifying toxicity as

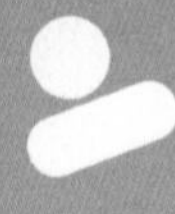

early as possible, and before there is extensive in vivo exposure of animals or, subsequently, of humans.

Toxicity testing

Toxicity testing has two primary goals: identification of hazards and prediction of the likely risk of that hazard occurring in humans receiving therapeutic doses of the new medicine. A wide range of doses is studied; high doses are required to increase the ability to detect hazards, and lower doses are needed to analyse dose–response relationships in order to predict the risk at doses producing the anticipated therapeutic effect. Toxicity tests include the following (*http://www.emea.europa.eu/htms/human/humanguidelines/nonclinical.htm*):

- **Mutagenicity**: a variety of in vitro tests using bacteria and mammalian cell lines are employed at an early stage to define any potential damage to DNA that may be linked to carcinogenicity or teratogenicity; in vivo studies may be undertaken to investigate the mechanism of genotoxicity.
- **Acute toxicity**: a single dose is given by the route proposed for human use; this may reveal a likely site for toxicity and is essential in defining the initial dose for human studies. Acute toxicity data, including information on the doses causing lethality, are essential for safe manufacture; the LD_{50} (a precise estimate of the dose required to kill 50% of an animal population) has been replaced by simpler and more humane methods that define the dose range associated with acute toxicity.
- **Subacute toxicity**: repeated doses are given for 14 or 28 days; this will usually reveal the target for toxic effects, and comparison with single-dose data may indicate any potential for accumulation.
- **Chronic toxicity**: repeated doses are given for up to 6 months; this reveals the target for toxicity (except cancer). The aim is to define dose regimens associated with adverse effects and a no-observed adverse effect level ('safe' dose).
- **Carcinogenicity**: repeated doses are given throughout the lifetime of the animal (usually 2 years in a rodent bioassay).
- **Reproductive toxicity**: repeated doses are given from prior to mating and throughout gestation to assess any effect on fertility, implantation, fetal growth, the production of fetal abnormalities (teratogenicity) and neonatal growth.

The extent of animal toxicity testing required prior to the first administration to humans is related to the proposed duration of human exposure and the population to be treated. All drugs are subjected to an initial in vitro screen for mutagenic potential: if satisfactory, this is followed by acute and subacute studies for up to 14 days of administration to two animal species. Doses studied are usually a low dose (sufficient to cause the pharmacological/therapeutic effect), a high dose (sufficient to cause target organ toxicity), and an intermediate dose, together with a control (untreated) group of animals. Teratogenicity and reproductive toxicity studies are required if the drug is to be given to women of childbearing age; since the thalidomide tragedy, rabbits have been used for teratogenicity studies because, unlike rodents, they show fetal abnormalities when treated with thalidomide. Carcinogenicity testing is necessary for drugs that may be used for long periods, for example over 1 year.

Table 3.1 European Medicines Agency (EMEA) guidelines for the length of animal toxicity studies necessary to support phase I and phase II studies in humans

Duration of clinical trial	Minimum duration of repeat-dose animal toxicity studies	
	Rodents	*Non-rodents*
Single dose	2 weeks	2 weeks
Up to 2 weeks	2 weeks	2 weeks
Up to 1 month	1 month	1 month
Up to 3 months	3 months	3 months
More than 3 months	6 months	6 months

Adapted from EMEA guidance at: *http://www.emea.europa.eu/pdfs/human/ich/028695en.pdf*

An international review of the extent of in vivo animal testing necessary prior to phase I and phase II clinical trials has concluded that the duration of animal toxicity tests should be the same as proposed human exposure (Table 3.1). The same advice applies for phase III studies in Japan and the USA, but the EU recommends more extensive animal studies, i.e. 1-month studies in rodents and non-rodents for a 2-week phase III human trial, 3 months in rodents and non-rodents for a 1-month phase III study in humans, and 6 months in rodents and 3 months in non-rodents for a 3-month phase III human trial (*http://www.emea.europa.eu/pdfs/human/ich/028695en.pdf*). Dogs are the 'non-rodent species' usually studied.

The use of animals for the establishment of chemical safety is an emotive issue, and there is extensive current research to replace in vivo animal studies with in vitro tests based on known mechanisms of toxicity. However, toxicology as a predictive science is still in its infancy, and at present it is impossible to replicate the complexity of mammalian physiology and biochemistry by in vitro systems. In vivo studies remain essential to investigate interference with either integrative functions or complex homeostatic mechanisms. Carefully controlled safety studies in animals are an essential part of the current procedures adopted to prevent extensive human toxicity, which would inevitably result from the use of untested compounds. Although toxicology has failed in the past to prevent some tragedies (see above), these have led to improvements in methods, and current tests provide an effective predictive screen. However, it is worth noting that there have been examples of approved drugs which have had to be withdrawn because of severe reactions that were not detected in preclinical studies, for example the cyclo-oxygenase type 2 (COX-2)-selective non-steroidal anti-inflammatory drug rofecoxib and the 'statin' cerivastatin. This may become increasingly important in the future because drugs developed, using molecular biological methods, to act specifically at human receptors may show limited or no activity at the analogous rodent receptors; however, animal studies will still provide a useful screen for non-specific, non-receptor-mediated effects.

Students should be aware that not all hazards detected at very high doses in experimental animals are of relevance to human health. An important function of expert advisory bodies such as the CHMP is to assess the relevance to human health of effects detected in experimental animals at doses that may be two orders of magnitude (or more) above human exposures. Many 'chemical scare' stories in the media are based on a hazard detected at high experimental doses in animals rather than the relevant risk estimated for human exposures.

PRE-MARKETING CLINICAL STUDIES: PHASES I–III

The purposes of pre-marketing clinical studies are:

- to establish that the drug has a useful action in humans
- to define any toxicity at therapeutic doses in humans
- to establish the nature of common (type A) unwanted effects (see Ch. 53).

Traditionally, pre-marketing clinical studies have been subdivided into three phases, although the distinction between these is blurred; the following classification system provides a useful framework (*http://www.emea.europa.eu/htms/human/humanguidelines/efficacy.htm*).

Phase I studies

Phase I is the term used to describe the first few administrations of a new drug to humans. A principal aim of these studies is to define basic properties, such as route of administration, pharmacokinetics and metabolism, and tolerability. The studies are usually carried out by the pharmaceutical company, often using a specialised contract research organisation. Subjects taking part in phase I studies are often healthy volunteers recruited by open advertisement, especially when the compound is of low predicted toxicity and has wide potential use, for example an antihistamine. In some cases, people suffering from the condition in which the drug will be used may be studied, for example cytotoxic agents used for cancer chemotherapy.

The first few administrations are usually by mouth in a dose that may be as low as one-fiftieth of the minimum required to produce a pharmacological effect in animals (after scaling for differences in body weight). Depending upon what is found, the dose may be then built up, either in small increments or by doubling, until a pharmacological effect is observed or an unwanted action occurs. During these studies, toxic effects are looked for by means of routine haematology and biochemical investigations of liver and renal function; other tests, including an electrocardiogram, will be performed as appropriate. It is also usual to study the disposition, metabolism and main pathways of elimination of the proposed new drug in humans at this stage. Such studies help to identify the most suitable dose and route of administration for future clinical studies; all guidelines suggest that metabolism data may assist in the choice of appropriate animal species for further toxicity studies, but in reality the massive database on rats, mice and dogs means that these are the usual species studied. Investigations of drug metabolism and pharmacokinetics often necessitate the use of radioactively labelled compounds containing carbon-14 or tritium (^3H) as part of the drug molecule.

Peptide drugs have to be given intravenously in clinical trials, in order to mimic the route of proposed clinical use. Very low doses should be studied in the first instance, especially with peptides that are designed to interact specifically with human homeostatic or signalling systems, because studies in animals may not reveal the full biological activities. Despite these safeguards, TGN 1412, a new immodulatory compound, caused significant toxicity in its first human phase I trial in March 2006. The severe toxicity occurred at a dose 500 times lower than the dose found to be safe in animals.

Phase II studies

During phase II studies, the detailed clinical pharmacology of the new compound is determined in groups of individuals with the intended clinical condition. A principal aim of these studies is to define the relationship between dose and pharmacological and/or therapeutic response in humans. Evidence of a beneficial effect will normally emerge during phase II studies. However, the large subjective element in human illness may make it difficult to distinguish between pharmacological and placebo effects. Additional studies may be undertaken at this stage in special groups such as elderly people, if it is intended that the drug will be used in that population. Other studies may investigate the mechanism of action or test for potential interactions with other drugs. The optimum dosage regimen should be defined in the phase II studies, and this is then used in large clinical trials, which aim to demonstrate the efficacy and safety of the drug.

Phase III studies

Phase III studies are the main clinical trials and usually involve comparison with a placebo that looks (and tastes) similar to the active compound. However, it is difficult to justify the use of a placebo once an effective form of treatment has been established for a condition, and lack of treatment may result in risk to the individual. It is normal to establish the advantages and disadvantages of the new compound by comparison with the best available treatment or the leading drug in the class. In these trials, the drug under evaluation may be used alone or given with other established treatment for the disease being treated. In some circumstances (e.g. cancer chemotherapy), the new agent or placebo is added to the best available current treatment.

Clinical trials are of two main types (Fig. 3.3): within-subject and between-subject comparisons. In within-subject trials, an individual is randomly allocated to commence treatment with either the new compound or its comparator (or placebo) before 'crossing over' to the alternative therapy. In contrast, between-subject comparisons involve randomisation to receive one of two (or more) treatments for the duration of the study.

Within-subject comparisons can usually be performed on a smaller number of subjects (about half that required for between-subject studies), since the individual acts as his or her own control and most non-treatment-related

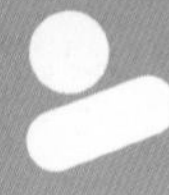

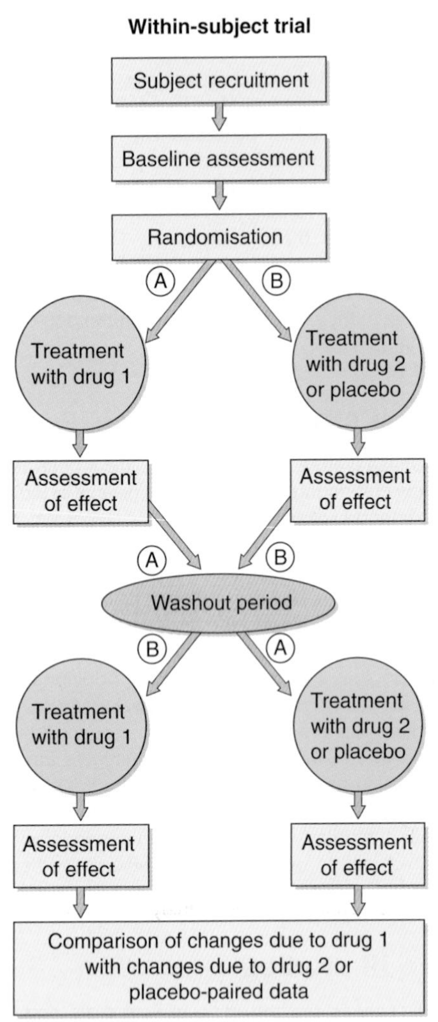

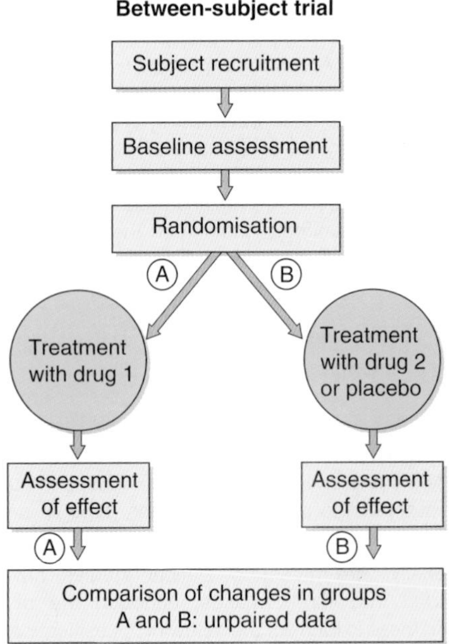

Fig. 3.3 **The design of clinical trials.** Subjects are randomly allocated to group A or group B.

variables are eliminated. However, such studies often require longer involvement of each individual. Also there may be carry-over effects from one treatment that affect the apparent efficacy of the second treatment, although statistical analysis should be able to deal with this problem. Studies of this type may be difficult to interpret when there is a pronounced seasonal variation in the severity of a condition, such as Raynaud's phenomenon or hayfever. Cross-over studies (Fig. 3.3) cannot be used if the treatment is curative – for example, an antibiotic for treating acute infections.

Between-subject comparisons require roughly twice as many participants but have the advantages that each subject will usually be studied for shorter periods of time and carry-over effects are avoided. Although it is not possible to provide a perfect match between subjects entering the two (or more) different treatment groups, this approach to the evaluation of new drugs is preferred by many drug regulatory authorities.

Whichever form of comparison is made, measurements of benefit (and adverse effects) are made at regular intervals using a combination of objective and subjective techniques (Table 3.2). Throughout these studies, careful attention is paid to detecting and reporting both unwanted effects (type A reactions) and other unpredictable type B reactions (Ch. 53). Type B reactions are rarely seen prior to the marketing of a new drug, because they may occur only once in every 1000–10 000 or more individuals treated with the drug. It is salutary to note that by the time a new medicine is marketed, only 2000–3000 people may have taken the drug, usually for short periods. Only a few hundred people may have 6 months or more of exposure to the new compound and the total experience may amount to no more than 500 patient-years (1000 people taking the drug for 6 months is 500 person-years).

POST-MARKETING SURVEILLANCE: PHASE IV (PHARMACOVIGILANCE)

Phase IV studies involve pharmacovigilance (post-marketing surveillance) and further post-marketing studies

Table 3.2 Examples of response measurements during clinical trials

New drug type	Measurement techniques	
	Objective	*Subjective*[a]
Antianginal	Exercise tolerance Blood pressure Heart rate GTN use	Fatigue Frequency of anginal attacks Pain intensity
Antiarthritic	Grip strength Joint size Paracetamol use	Duration of morning stiffness Pain intensity

[a]Subjective effects are often quantified by the use of a 10-cm visual analogue scale, e.g. 0 cm = no pain at all; 10 cm = the worst pain I have ever had.
GTN, glyceryl trinitrate.

of efficacy, sometimes for additional indications to those licensed. Pharmacovigilance describes the identification and responses to risk/benefit issues emerging for authorised medicines, arising from their use in clinical practice, and includes the effective dissemination of information to optimise the safe and effective use of medicines (*http://www.mhra.gov.uk/SearchHelp/Glossary/GlossaryP*).

The full spectrum of benefits and risks of medicines may not become clear until after marketing. Reasons for this include the low frequency of certain adverse drug reactions, and the tendency to avoid the inclusion of children, the elderly and women of childbearing age in pre-marketing clinical studies. Another factor is the widespread use of other medicines in normal clinical practice, which could produce an unexpected interaction with the new drug.

Two main systems of pharmacovigilance, or post-marketing surveillance, are in use in the UK. The first and most important is known as the yellow card system; it depends upon doctors reporting suspected serious adverse reactions directly to the MHRA (see MHRA website at *http://www.mhra.gov.uk*) using postage prepaid cards (available in the *British National Formulary* [BNF], and the *Monthly Index of Medical Specialties* [MIMS]). In addition to reporting suspected serious adverse effects of established drugs, doctors are asked to supply information about all unwanted effects of medicines that have been marketed recently. Each year, the MHRA receives some 20 000 yellow cards/slips. In return for their efforts, doctors are supplied at regular intervals with an information circular about current drug-related problems.

The second form of pharmacovigilance involves systematic post-marketing surveillance of recently marketed medicines. This may be organised by the pharmaceutical company responsible for the manufacture of the new drug (companies also receive information via their representatives). The MHRA administers the General Practice Research Database (GPRD – *http://www.gprd.com/home*) which comprises the anonymised records from 450 GP practices. It is used in conjunction with the yellow card scheme to provide a warning system for approved medicines. To date, the database has been used to assess the safety of the oral combined hormone contraceptive, the MMR vaccine, antidepressants, hormone replacement therapy, and non-steroidal anti-inflammatory drugs such as aspirin and ibuprofen.

Prescription event monitoring (PEM) provides a method for the detailed further study of observations or possible associations provided by pharmacovigilance programmes. This involves

- identification of a possible health problem associated with an approved medicine
- identification by the Prescription Pricing Authority of individuals who have been prescribed a drug of interest
- the subsequent distribution of 'green cards' to those individuals' GPs, with a request that they complete all details about the person and events that occurred.

The cards are then returned to the coordinating unit in Southampton, where the data are analysed. PEM has the advantage that it does not require doctors to make a value judgement concerning a link between the prescription of a drug and any medical event that occurs in the subject while receiving the drug. At first sight, a broken leg may be thought an unlikely drug-related adverse effect, but it could be the result of drug-induced hypotension, ataxia or metabolic bone disease.

Finally, detailed monitoring of adverse reactions to drug therapy takes place in some hospitals. These data contribute further to our overall knowledge. The future linkage of computerised medical records, including drug prescribing, offers the promise of more rapid identification of adverse events and a greater ability to investigate possible associations between prescription and adverse events.

Recent developments in information about the beneficial and adverse effects of drugs have been:

- the use of systematic meta-analyses of clinical trials' data
- the establishment in the UK of the National Institute for Health and Clinical Excellence (NICE).

Combining the data from a number of similar clinical trials can provide an overview of the validity and reproducibility of clinical findings. The statistical method used, meta-analysis, is complex and only trials of a similar design, including outcome measures, sensitivity, duration, etc., should be combined. The Cochrane database (*http://www.update-software.com/publications/Cochrane*) provides a regularly updated collection of evidence-based medicine; the abstracts in the database can be searched without charge.

NICE (*http://www.nice.org.uk*) was established in 1999 as an independent organisation responsible for providing national guidance on treatments and care for people using the NHS in England and Wales. It provides advice on the clinical value and cost-effectiveness of new treatments, but also on existing treatments if there is uncertainty about their use. NICE produces guidance on:

- the use of new and existing medicines and treatments within the NHS in England and Wales (technology appraisals)
- the appropriate treatment and care of people with specific diseases and conditions within the NHS in England and Wales (clinical guidelines)
- whether interventional procedures used for diagnosis or treatment are safe and work well enough for routine use (interventional procedures).

FURTHER READING

Austin CP (2004) The impact of the completed human genome sequence on the development of novel therapeutics for human disease. *Annu Rev Med* 55, 1–13

Dollery C (2003) The clinical pharmacologist's view; drug discovery and early development. In: Wilkins MR (ed) Experimental Therapeutics. London: Martin Dunitz, Taylor and Francis; pp 3–24

Kerwin R (2004) The National Institute for Clinical Excellence and its relevance to pharmacology. *Trends Pharmacol Sci* 25, 346–348

Lynch A, Connelly J (2003) The toxicologist's view; non-clinical safety assessment. In: Wilkins MR (ed) Experimental Therapeutics. London: Martin Dunitz, Taylor and Francis; pp 25–50

McLeod HL, Evans WE (2001) Pharmacogenomics: unlocking the human genome for better drug therapy. *Annu Rev Pharmacol Toxicol* 41, 101–121

Marchetti S, Schellens JH (2007) The impact of FDA and EMEA guidelines on drug development in relation to Phase 0 trials. *Br J Cancer* 97, 577–581

Persidis A (1998). High-throughput screening. Advances in robotics and miniturization continue to accelerate drug lead identification. *Nat Biotechnol* 16, 488–489

Shah RR, Branch SK, Steele C (2003) The regulator's view; regulatory requirements for marketing authorizations for new medicinal products in the European Union. In: Wilkins MR (ed) Experimental Therapeutics. London: Martin Dunitz, Taylor and Francis; pp 51–75

Walker DK (2004) The use of pharmacokinetic and pharmacodynamic data in the assessment of drug safety in early drug development. *Br J Clin Pharmacol* 58, 601–608

4 The nervous system, neurotransmission and the peripheral autonomic nervous system

This chapter deals predominantly with details of the peripheral autonomic nervous system; the general principles relating to the central nervous system and the somatic nervous system are similar, but specific details are dealt with in later chapters.

ARRANGEMENT OF THE CENTRAL AND PERIPHERAL NERVOUS SYSTEMS

There are two principal neuronal control systems in the body. Functionally they are highly integrated and should be considered holistically. However, for educational clarity they are introduced separately.

- The *central nervous system* (CNS) comprises neuronal networks of the brain, brainstem and spinal cord.
- The *peripheral nervous systems*, which interconnect the CNS to the organs of the body, include:
  - the autonomic (automatic or involuntary) nervous system, which comprises sympathetic and parasympathetic nervous systems and also includes the enteric nervous system of the gut.
  - the somatic (voluntary) nervous system, which innervates skeletal muscle and is dealt with in Chapter 27.

The CNS integrates, processes and responds to sensory messages.

- It receives sensory information from all parts of the body, including visceral sensory afferent nerves (e.g. from viscera, smooth muscle and cardiac muscle) and somatic sensory afferents (e.g. from skeletal muscle).
- It responds by sending instructions via the autonomic efferent nerves of the sympathetic and parasympathetic nerves (e.g. to glands, smooth muscle and cardiac muscle) and somatic motor efferents (to skeletal muscle).

PRINCIPLES OF NEUROTRANSMISSION

Action potentials passing along axons provide instructions to other separate neurons or non-neuronal cells (e.g. smooth muscle cells) (Fig. 4.1). Instructions are transferred by the release of chemical neurotransmitters from the presynaptic endings of the neuron, which then diffuse through a small physical space, called the synaptic cleft, and stimulate the receiving (postsynaptic) cells via recognition proteins (receptors) (Fig. 4.1). The instructions may be to tell the receiving cells to increase (excitatory) or reduce (inhibitory) their activity.

Figure 4.1 shows schematically an excitatory neuronal unit innervating postsynaptic cells.

Neurotransmitters, which are the chemical signals, can be either synthesised within the presynaptic region (e.g. noradrenaline) or transported from the cell body to the synaptic region (e.g. peptides). The neurotransmitter is taken up from the cytosol, using specific transporters within the nerve ending, and stored within membrane vesicles. The transmitter within the vesicle may form a complex; for example, noradrenaline forms a complex with adenosine triphosphate (ATP), which reduces the free concentration of noradrenaline within the vesicle.

The release of the neurotransmitter can be 'fine-tuned' by axo-axonic connections and by presynaptic receptors (which are discussed below). A generalised scheme for neurotransmission is as follows (Fig. 4.1):

a) The cell body (or soma) responds to an appropriate stimulus by generating an action potential (AP).
b) The AP is conducted along the axon by the opening of voltage-gated Na^+ channels and the influx of Na^+; when the AP reaches the presynaptic nerve terminal it results in an influx of Ca^{2+} through voltage-dependent channels.
c) Ca^{2+}-dependent processes result in fusion of neurotransmitter-containing vesicles with the presynaptic membrane and release of stored chemical transmitter into the synaptic space.

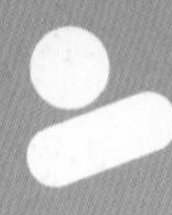

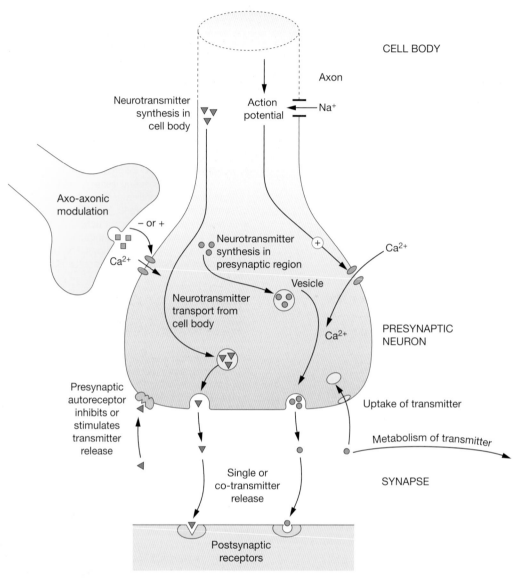

Fig. 4.1 **Illustration of the principles of neurotransmission at a synapse.** Basic principles of synthesis, storage, release, action and inactivation of a neurotransmitter are shown and described in the text. At many synapses co-transmission of different neurotransmitters occurs.

d) The released neurotransmitter binds to and stimulates the appropriate receptors in the postsynaptic membranes and generates (transduces) biochemical changes in the recipient cells; these may be functional changes in cells (e.g. smooth muscle contraction) or excitation or inhibition of another neuron (e.g. transmission of the AP to postsynaptic nerve fibres).
e) The released neurotransmitter may also stimulate autoreceptors in the presynaptic membranes, and thereby modulate the further release of the neurotransmitter.
f) The transmitter is degraded by enzymes or taken back into the presynaptic neuron for reuse.

Neurons may release a single transmitter, but often more than one transmitter may be released; there are many examples of *co-transmission*, which are described later in this book.

PRESYNAPTIC RECEPTORS AND MODULATION OF TRANSMITTER RELEASE

An important characteristic of neurons is the presence of presynaptic receptors (Fig. 4.2, Fig. 4.4 and Table 4.1). Presynaptic receptors may either increase or decrease the release of the neurotransmitter and are described as facilitatory and inhibitory, respectively. There are two main sources of ligands for presynaptic receptors:

Table 4.1 The control of transmitter release by presynaptic receptor mechanisms

Neurotransmitter	Presynaptic receptors inhibiting release	Presynaptic receptors facilitating release
Acetylcholine	M_2, α_2, D_2/D_3, $5HT_3$	N_1, NMDA
Dopamine	D_2/D_3, M_2	N_1, NMDA
Gamma-aminobutyric acid (GABA)	$GABA_B$	–
Histamine	H_3	–
Serotonin (5-hydroxytryptamine; 5-HT)	$5HT_{1D}$, α_2	$5HT_3$
Noradrenaline	α_2, H_3, M_2, D_2, opioid	β_2, N_1, angiotensin II

NMDA, N-methyl-D-aspartate.

- neurotransmitter released from the vesicles that can act presynaptically (autoreceptors)
- neurotransmitter released from other neurons, usually by axo-axonal synapses (Fig. 4.1), involving a different neurotransmitter to that released by the neuron itself (heteroreceptors).

Inhibition of transmitter release is usually achieved by limiting Ca^{2+} entry through voltage-gated ion channels into the neuron.

The first recognition of a clinically important presynaptic receptor came with the discovery that the antihypertensive agent clonidine lowers blood pressure via stimulation of presynaptic α_2-adrenoceptors, with subsequent inhibition of the release of vasoconstricting noradrenaline. Presynaptic receptors (Table 4.1) are increasingly being recognised as having important roles in the clinical effects produced by many drugs.

Box 4.1 Targets for drug action within the ANS

- Muscarinic receptors at postganglionic nerve endings in the parasympathetic nervous system (muscarinic receptor subtypes)
- Adrenergic receptors for noradrenaline and adrenaline in the sympathetic nervous system (α- and β-adrenoceptor subtypes)
- Presynaptic receptors in the parasympathetic and sympathetic nervous systems
- Modification of synthesis, storage, release and inactivation of acetylcholine
- Modification of synthesis, storage, release and inactivation noradrenaline

THE PERIPHERAL AUTONOMIC NERVOUS SYSTEM (ANS)

The ANS is an important site for drug action because:

- the ANS either controls or contributes to the control of the functioning of nearly all of the major organ systems of the body
- ANS dysfunction is present in many diseases
- ANS dysfunction can occur as an unwanted effect of drug treatment
- the ANS utilises two major different neurotransmitters and a number of receptor subtypes; this provides a variety of sites for drug action (Box 4.1), which allows modification of particular body functions with some degree of selectivity.

The peripheral ANS is subdivided into two main branches (Fig. 4.2, Box 4.2):

- *parasympathetic nervous system*, which utilises acetylcholine (ACh) as the final transmitter at muscarinic receptors on the cells that are being stimulated (called the innervated or effector cells or organs)
- *sympathetic nervous system*, which utilises noradrenaline as the transmitter at adrenoceptors on most, but not all, effector organs; the release of adrenaline and noradrenaline from the adrenal medulla during sympathetic nervous system stimulation is also an important and integral part of the sympathetic nervous system response.

Anatomically, in both branches of the ANS, the efferent neurons innervating effector organs are linked to neurons in the CNS via ganglia. The distribution and neuronal interconnections differ between the two branches (Fig. 4.2).

- The parasympathetic efferents give more discrete innervation of organs; the ganglia are close to the innervated organs and they therefore have long preganglionic fibres; there are few or no interconnections between ganglia, so that innervated organs can be affected independently.
- The sympathetic efferents are classically described as being involved in the 'flight or fight' response and affect many body systems simultaneously. Many of the ganglia are close to the spinal column, in the paravertebral sympathetic ganglion chain that lies along each side of the spinal column, and have many interconnections; these nerves have long postganglionic fibres. All neurons in the sympathetic system can be activated simultaneously because of numerous neuronal interconnections within the paravertebral chain; also, axons passing though the chain without synapsing can interconnect with ganglia such as the inferior mesenteric ganglion and can then diversify to innervate several organs (Fig. 4.2).

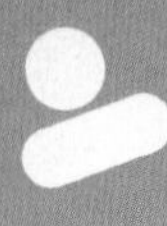

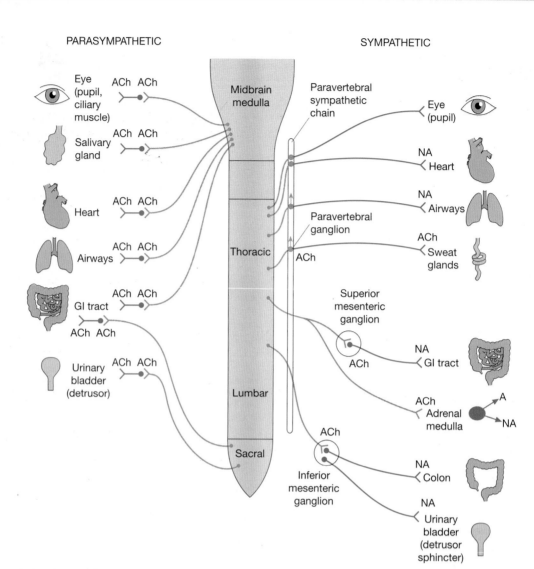

Fig. 4.2 **Organisation of the parasympathetic and sympathetic autonomic nervous systems.** Activation of the sympathetic nervous system leads to widespread release of noradrenaline supplemented by release into the circulation of adrenaline and noradrenaline from the adrenal medulla, whereas stimulation of the parasympathetic nervous system is more localised to particular organs. Airways have sparse sympathetic innervation and dilation is mainly a result of circulating adrenaline. The ganglia innervating some organs are not part of the paravertebral chain but are grouped together to form the coeliac, superior mesenteric or inferior mesenteric ganglia. At all ganglia the transmitter is acetylcholine and the receptors are nicotinic type 1. ACh, acetylcholine; NA, noradrenaline; A, adrenaline; GI, gastrointestinal.

Box 4.2 Organisation of the autonomic nervous system

- Parasympathetic and sympathetic efferent nerves from the spinal cord synapse at intermediate ganglia before synapsing with the effector cells at their postganglionic nerve endings
- Acetylcholine and noradrenaline are the principal neurotransmitters in the ANS but other transmitters also have neurotransmitter roles
- Stimulation of the sympathetic nervous system has a widespread effect in the body because of interconnections between efferent fibres, whereas the parasympathetic nervous system is more organ-specific (Fig. 4.2)
- The neurotransmitters are synthesised in the presynaptic neuron, stored, and released into the synapse in response to depolarization and Ca^{2+} influx caused by an action potential
- At all ganglia, the neurotransmitter is acetylcholine, acting on nicotinic N_1 receptors, which then elicits an action potential in the postganglionic nerve
- Parasympathetic efferents have muscarinic receptors at neuroeffector synapses
- Most sympathetic efferents have noradrenergic receptors at neuroeffector synapses
- Adrenaline and noradrenaline are synthesised and released in the adrenal medulla in response to sympathetic stimulation and enhance the effects of local noradrenaline release

Many organs are innervated by both the parasympathetic and sympathetic nervous systems, which act in concert and may have opposite effects on the organ function. The concept of opposing actions, although imperfect, can be useful in remembering the effects that each part of the nervous system has on tissue function. Tables 4.2 and 4.3 show the effects that stimulation of the sympathetic or parasympathetic nervous systems have on major tissues and the primary receptors that are involved. Under resting conditions, the predominant drive to many organs is from the parasympathetic nervous system.

Physiological functions often require coordination of sympathetic and parasympathetic activities; for example, urination is brought about by a decreased adrenergic drive to the sphincter muscle and an increased muscarinic drive to the detrusor muscle (see urinary bladder; Tables 4.2 and 4.3 and Ch. 15).

Students should familiarise themselves with the ANS and the possible sites of drug action (Tables 4.2 and 4.3). Such knowledge is fundamental to understanding both the principal mechanisms of action for some drugs and the source of unwanted effects for others.

THE SYMPATHETIC NERVOUS SYSTEM AND NORADRENERGIC TRANSMISSION

Noradrenaline and adrenaline are members of a group of amine transmitters called catecholamines (a catechol is a benzene ring with two adjacent hydroxyl groups; Fig. 4.3a). Both the catechol and amino groups are important for receptor binding. The receptors that noradrenaline and adrenaline stimulate are described as adrenoceptors and the effects of noradrenaline and adrenaline at these receptors are described as noradrenergic and adrenergic effects.

Table 4.2 Effects of stimulation of the sympathetic nervous system (via adrenoceptor subtypes) in major tissues[a]

Tissue	Effect	Receptor type[a]
Heart rate	Increase	β_1 (β_2 in heart disease)
Contractility	Increase	β_1 (β_2 in heart disease)
AV conduction	Increase	β_1
Blood vessels in skin/gut	Constriction	α_1, α_2[b]
Blood vessels in skeletal muscle	Dilation[c]	β_2
Bronchial smooth muscle	Dilation[c]	β_2
GI motility	Relaxation	α_1, β_2
GI sphincter tone	Contraction	α_1
Uterine smooth muscle	Contraction Relaxation	α_1, β_2
Bladder detrusor	Relaxation	β_2
Bladder sphincter	Constriction	α_1
Penis	Ejaculation	α_1
Pilomotor muscles	Constriction	α_1
Sweat glands	Secretion	M
Pupil (radial muscle)	Contraction dilates pupil	α_1
Hepatic glycogenolysis	Increase	β_2, α
Skeletal muscle glycogenolysis	Increase[c]	β_2
Fat cell lipolysis	Increase[c]	β_1, α, β_3
Pancreas insulin secretion	Decrease	α
Platelets	Aggregation	α_2
Presynaptic nerve terminal (noradrenergic)	Inhibition of NA release Increased NA release	α_2 β_2
Presynaptic nerve terminal (muscarinic)	Inhibition of ACh release	α_2
Kidney (JGA) renin release	Increase	β_1

[a]Only the principal receptor types are shown.
[b]Variable distribution.
[c]Respond to circulating adrenaline; little noradrenergic innervation.
JGA, juxtaglomerular apparatus; M, muscarinic receptor.

Table 4.3 Effect of stimulation of parasympathetic nerves (via muscarinic receptor subtypes) in major tissues

Tissue	Effect	Receptor type[a]
Heart rate	Decrease	M_2
Contractility of atria	Decrease	M_2
AV conduction velocity	Decrease	M_2
Vascular endothelium	Dilates blood vessel – NO release	M_1, M_3
Bronchial smooth muscle	Constriction	M_2, M_3
Gut motility	Contraction, relaxation	M_2, M_3
Gut sphincter tone	Increased	M_3
Gut secretions	Increased	M_3
Bladder detrusor	Contraction	M_3
Bladder sphincter	Relaxation	M_3
Penis	Erection	M_3
Eye pupil circular muscle	Contraction (miosis)	M_3
Ciliary muscle	Contraction (accommodates for near vision)	M_3
Pancreatic insulin secretion	Increased	M_1, M_3
Salivary glands	Secretion	M_1, M_3
Emesis	Increased	M_3

[a]Only the principal receptor types are shown. Other subtypes may play a functional role in particular conditions.
M, muscarinic receptor.

The approved European names of noradrenaline and adrenaline solely when they are formulated and used therapeutically as medicines are *norepinephrine* and *epinephrine*, respectively; however, when the physiological actions are being described, the terms noradrenaline and adrenaline are used. Most preparations of adrenaline and of noradrenaline in Europe are dual-labelled with both terms. In contrast, the terms epinephrine and norepinephrine are used in the USA for both therapeutic and physiological descriptions, but US texts also use the term adrenoceptor, so that norepinephrine acts on adrenoceptors!

Synthesis of catecholamines: noradrenaline, adrenaline and dopamine

Catecholamine neurotransmitters are synthesised from inactive precursors (Fig. 4.3b). The basic carbon skeleton of catecholamines is derived from phenylalanine or tyrosine, which are aromatic amino acids. Phenylalanine has an unsubstituted benzene ring, while tyrosine has a 4-hydroxyl (phenolic) group. Both phenylalanine and tyrosine are used in protein synthesis. To convert tyrosine to a catecholamine requires oxidation at the aromatic ring (to produce a catechol which has two hydroxyl groups in the positions shown) and decarboxylation at the amino acid group (to produce an amine).

The sequence of synthesis of adrenaline (via dopamine and noradrenaline) is given in Figure 4.3b. The oxidation of tyrosine to levodopa by tyrosine hydroxylase, which occurs within the neuron, commits the molecule to become a neurotransmitter. This step is subject to negative feedback by the catecholamines that are subsequently produced, thereby regulating supply. Conversion of levodopa to dopamine is catalysed by a cytosolic enzyme, L-aromatic amino acid decarboxylase (usually known as dopa decarboxylase), which is able to decarboxylate a range of aromatic amino acids. The amine product, dopamine, is then taken up by vesicles via a specific transporter. In neurons that use dopamine as their primary transmitter, this is the end of the synthetic pathway. Dopamine is a vital neurotransmitter in some parts of the peripheral nervous system and also widely in the CNS (Chs 7, 21 and 24).

The vesicles present in noradrenergic neurons contain the enzyme dopamine-β-hydroxylase, which oxidises the β-carbon (i.e. that next to the CH_2NH_2 group). This enzyme is largely present in the membranes of the vesicles, but on exocytosis some is lost into the synapse, following which it diffuses into the bloodstream and is slowly cleared. Dopamine-β-hydroxylase in blood can be used as an indication of peripheral noradrenaline release. In noradrenergic neurons, this is the end of the synthetic pathway.

The adrenal medulla contains an additional enzyme (phenylethanolamine-N-methyl transferase), which converts noradrenaline to adrenaline by the addition of a methyl group to the nitrogen atom (Fig. 4.3b).

Noradrenaline storage

Noradrenaline (or dopamine) is stored in the vesicles as a complex with ATP and proteoglycans. There is a specific catecholamine transporter (Fig. 4.4) that transfers noradrenaline (or dopamine) from the cytoplasm into the vesicles.

Noradrenaline release

Release, in response to a nerve impulse, occurs following Ca^{2+} influx and Ca^{2+}-mediated fusion of the noradrenaline vesicle with the cytoplasmic membrane.

Noradrenaline present in the cytoplasm of the presynaptic neuron may also be released by so-called 'indirectly acting sympathomimetic amines', which are low-molecular-weight basic compounds – for example, food constituents (such as tyramine), therapeutic drugs (such as

(a)

HO, HO (catechol ring) —CH(X)—CH_2NHY

	X	Y
Dopamine	H	H
Noradrenaline	OH	H
Adrenaline	OH	CH_3

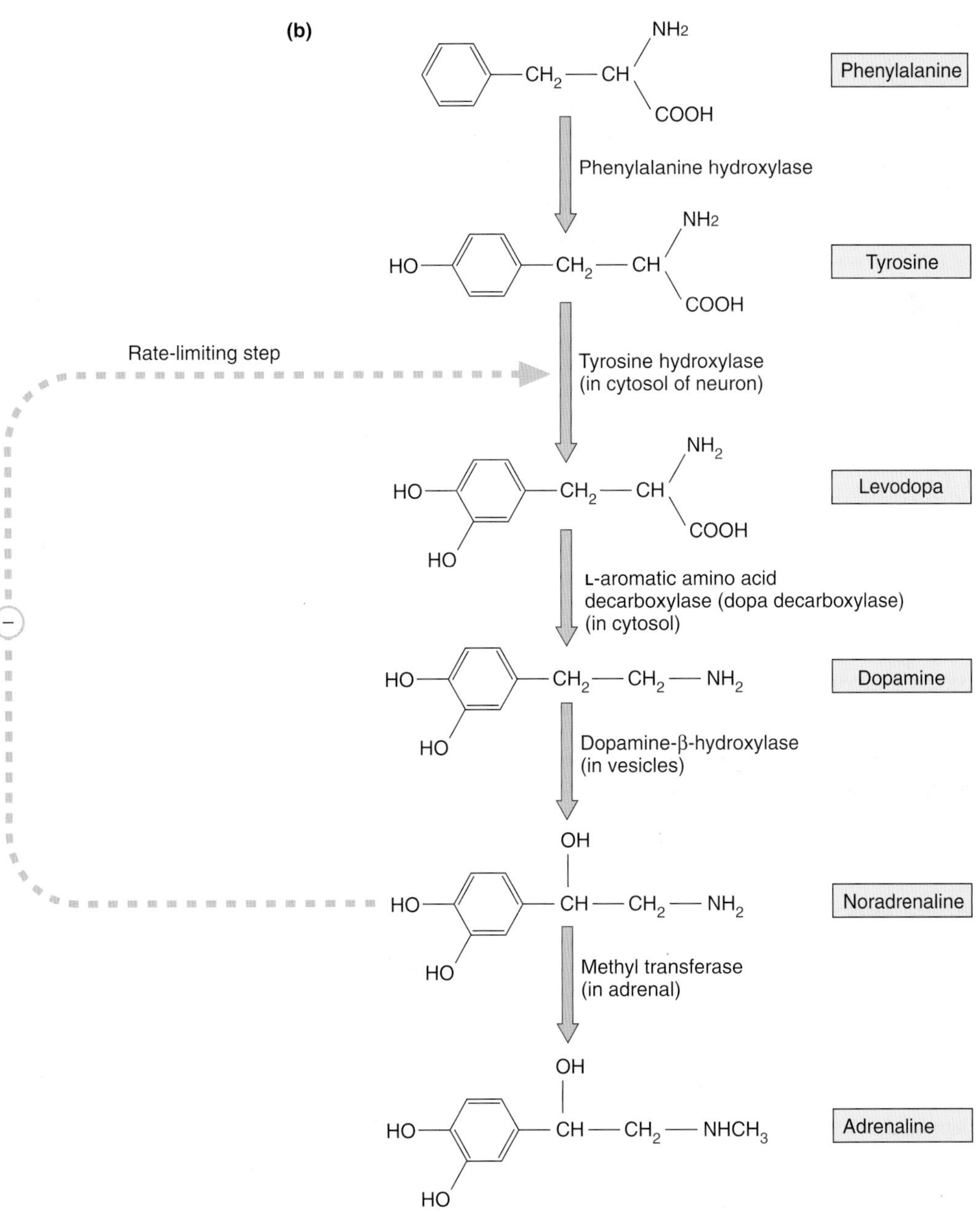

Fig. 4.3 **The structure of the main physiological catecholamines (a) and their synthesis from amino acid precursors (b).**

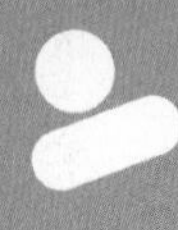

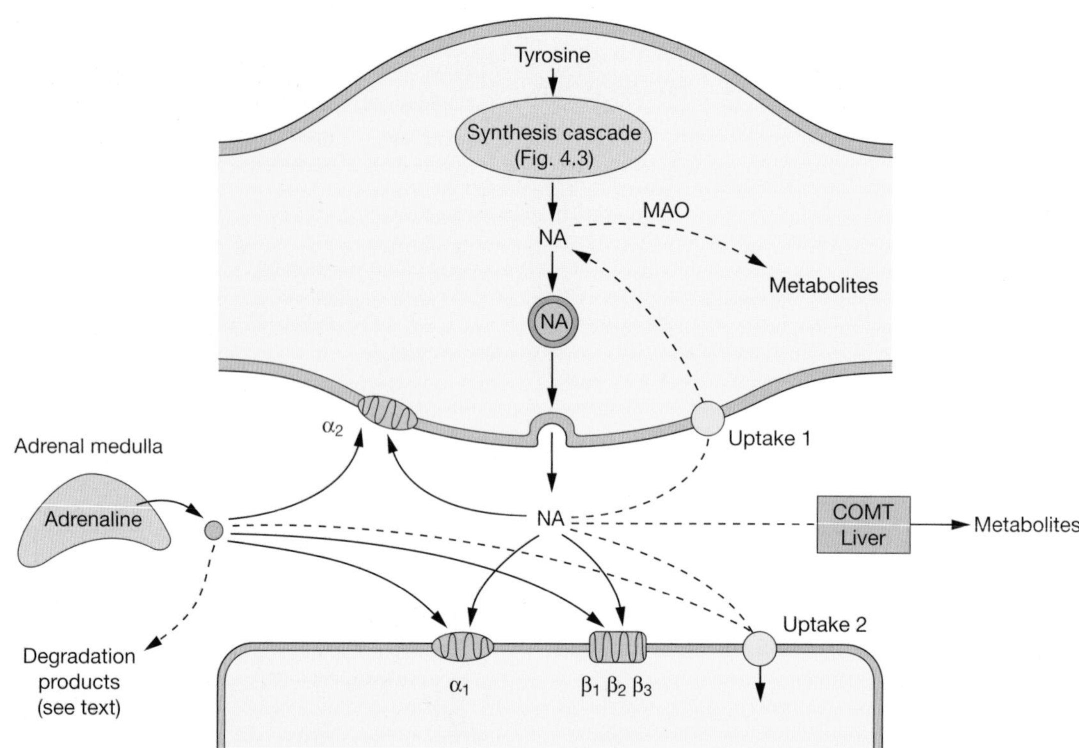

Fig 4.4 **A noradrenergic nerve terminal (varicosity) showing the processes involved in the synthesis and inactivation of noradrenaline and adrenaline.** Solid lines illustrate the sites of action of released noradrenaline and adrenaline, and dotted lines show the ways that the actions of noradrenaline are curtailed. COMT, catechol-O-methyltransferase; MAO monoamine oxidase; NA, noradrenaline.

ephedrine) and some drugs of abuse (such as amfetamine and methamphetamine). Such compounds are taken into the presynaptic cytosol by uptake 1 (Fig. 4.4) and into the vesicles, from which they displace noradrenaline. Consequently, there is an increased amount of noradrenaline in the cytoplasm, available for release. The increased noradrenaline release into the synapse is responsible for the biological effects produced by ingestion of compounds like tyramine, ephedrine and amfetamine.

Reuptake and metabolism of released noradrenaline

The principal mechanism for the removal of noradrenaline from the synapse is reuptake (approximately 70–90%) into the presynaptic neuron via a specific high-affinity carrier called uptake 1; it does not transport adrenaline (Fig. 4.4). Some of the remaining noradrenaline in the synapse is taken up into non-neuronal tissues by a low-affinity carrier called uptake 2 which also transports adrenaline; some of the remaining noradrenaline and the majority of any adrenaline released into the circulation as a co-transmitter is metabolised. Separate uptake-1 type transporters exist for serotonin (5-hydroxytryptamine, 5-HT) and dopamine released from their respective neurons. Therapeutic agents that selectively block the noradrenaline or serotonin uptake-1 transporters and increase the amount of neurotransmitter in the synapse are used in treating depression (Ch. 22). Cocaine also blocks the reuptake of noradrenaline by uptake 1.

There are two main enzymes involved in the initial steps in the metabolism of noradrenaline: monoamine oxidase (MAO) and catechol-O-methyltransferase (COMT).

Monoamine oxidase

MAO is present on the surface of the mitochondria of the presynaptic neuron, where it oxidises free cytoplasmic noradrenaline. It is also present in many other sites such as the gastrointestinal epithelium and liver. Oxidative removal of the amino group on noradrenaline via MAO is the major pathway of metabolism of noradrenaline and other aminergic neurotransmitters, and converts the primary amino group (–CH_2NH_2; see Fig. 4.3b) into an aldehyde (–CHO). Loss of the amino group prevents binding to the postsynaptic receptor, and therefore is an inactivation process. In the periphery, metabolism results in the formation of vanillylmandelic acid, which is the main urinary metabolite. In the CNS, the aldehyde is reduced to an alcohol (CH_2OH), which is conjugated with sulphate (see Ch. 2) before being excreted in the urine. There are two main forms of MAO, MAO-A and MAO-B (Table 4.4), which differ in their organ distribution and substrate affinities. The uses and unwanted effects of inhibitors of MAO-A and/or MAO-B isoenzymes are discussed in Chapter 22 (depression) and Chapter 24 (Parkinson's disease).

Table 4.4 Monoamine oxidase (MAO) and its inhibitors

Isoenzyme	Location in human tissues	Main substrates	Examples of inhibitors	
			Irreversible	*Reversible*
MAO-A	Gastrointestinal tract, placenta	Serotonin, noradrenaline		Moclobemide
MAO-B	Brain[a], liver[a], platelets	Phenylethylamine, tyramine	Selegiline, rasagiline	
MAO-A or MAO-B		Tyramine, dopamine, adrenaline	Isocarboxazid, phenelzine, tranylcypromine	

[a]Both isoenzymes are present, but in humans the amount of MAO-B exceeds that of MAO-A.

Catechol-O-methyltransferase

COMT occurs only at low levels in noradrenergic neurons, but is present in many other tissues, including the adrenal gland and liver. The enzyme catalyses the transfer of a methyl group onto the phenolic group at position 3 of the aromatic ring (see Fig. 4.3b) to convert the –OH group into $-OCH_3$. This removes the catechol centre and prevents binding to the postsynaptic receptor. COMT is a minor route of inactivation of both dopamine and noradrenaline. Inhibitors of COMT are used as an adjunct to levodopa therapy for Parkinson's disease (Ch. 24).

The main metabolites of noradrenaline excreted in urine are:

- 3,4-dihydroxymandelic acid (formed by oxidation of the $-CH_2NH_2$ to –CHO and then –COOH) and vanillylmandelic acid (its 3-O-methyl analogue)
- 3,4-dihydroxyphenylglycol (formed by oxidation of the $-CH_2NH_2$ to –CHO and then reduction to $-CH_2OH$), 3-methoxy-4-hydroxyphenylglycol (its 3-O-methyl analogue) and their sulphate conjugates.

Sympathetic nervous system receptors

All ganglia utilise ACh as a neurotransmitter, acting predominantly on nicotinic type 1 (N_1) receptors to elicit an action potential in the postganglionic axon. The receptor type at most postganglionic nerve endings in the sympathetic nervous system are adrenergic receptors (adrenoceptors).

Based on the effects of a number of adrenoceptor agonists and antagonists, the adrenoceptor family was divided into two types, α and β; it was soon recognised that there are a number of subtypes, categorised as α-subtypes (α_1 and α_2) and β-subtypes (β_1, β_2 and β_3) (see drug receptor table at the end of Ch. 1 and Table 4.2). It is now understood that there are multiple forms of some of these main subtypes (i.e. α_{1A}, α_{1B} and α_{1D}, and α_{2A}, α_{2B} and α_{2C}) and these are discussed where clinically relevant in later chapters. Different receptor subtypes (see drug receptor table at the end of Ch. 1) show different affinities for the endogenous catecholamines, noradrenaline and adrenaline:

α_1: noradrenaline $\geq$ adrenaline
α_2: adrenaline > noradrenaline
β_1: noradrenaline $\geq$ adrenaline
β_2: adrenaline > noradrenaline
β_3: noradrenaline = adrenaline.

Selective stimulation or blockade of individual adrenoceptor subtypes forms the basis of significant areas of pharmacology and therapeutics and is dealt with in relevant chapters.

THE PARASYMPATHETIC NERVOUS SYSTEM AND CHOLINERGIC TRANSMISSION

Synthesis of acetylcholine

Acetylcholine (ACh) $[(CH_3)_3N^+CH_2CH_2OCOCH_3]$ is synthesised within the cytosol of the cholinergic neuron from choline $[(CH_3)_3N^+CH_2CH_2OH]$ and acetyl-CoA (Fig. 4.5). Choline is a highly polar, quaternary amino compound that is also present in phospholipids (e.g. phosphatidylcholine); it is obtained largely from the diet. Because of its fixed positive charge, it does not readily cross cell membranes and there are specific transporters to allow uptake into the presynaptic neuron (Fig. 4.5) and from the gastrointestinal tract and across the blood–brain barrier (Ch. 2). Acetylation of the hydroxyl group of choline to form ACh is catalysed by the enzyme choline acetyltransferase. The rate of synthesis of ACh is controlled closely and is related to ACh turnover, so that rapid release of ACh stores is associated with enhanced synthesis.

Storage of acetylcholine

The cytosolic ACh is taken up into membrane vesicles by a specific transmembrane transporter and is stored in the vesicles in association with ATP and acidic proteoglycans (which are also released on exocytosis of the vesicles). Each vesicle contains 1000 to 50 000 ACh molecules and neuromuscular junctions (Ch. 27) contain about 300 000 vesicles.

Release of acetylcholine

Release occurs by Ca^{2+}-mediated fusion of the vesicle membrane with the cytoplasmic membrane and exocytosis (Fig. 4.5). This process can be inhibited by botulinum toxin and stimulated by the toxin from the black widow spider. The numbers of vesicles released depends on the site of the synapse, with between 30 and 300 vesicles undergoing exocytosis, releasing from 30 000 to over 3 million ACh molecules into the synaptic cleft. Neurons within the CNS

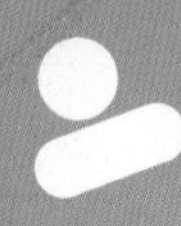

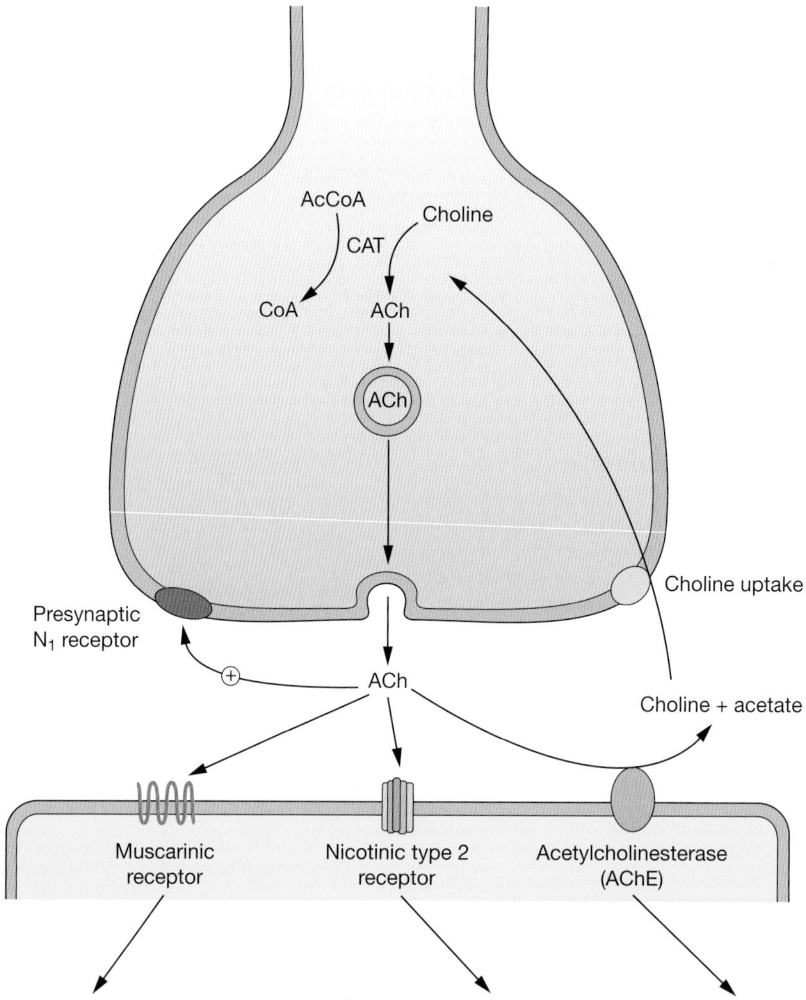

AcCoA
CAT
Choline
CoA
ACh
ACh
Choline uptake
Presynaptic N_1 receptor
ACh
Choline + acetate
Muscarinic receptor
Nicotinic type 2 receptor
Acetylcholinesterase (AChE)

Stimulants	Inhibitors
glaucoma (Ch. 50)	dilate pupil (Ch. 50) dilate airway (Ch. 12) stabilise bladder (Ch. 15) reduce gut motility (Ch. 35) prevent bradycardia (Ch. 8) antiemetic (Ch. 32) antiparkinsonian (Ch. 24)

Stimulants	Inhibitors
muscle relaxant (Ch. 27)	muscle relaxant (Ch. 27)

Inhibitors
glaucoma (Ch. 50) dementias (Ch. 9)

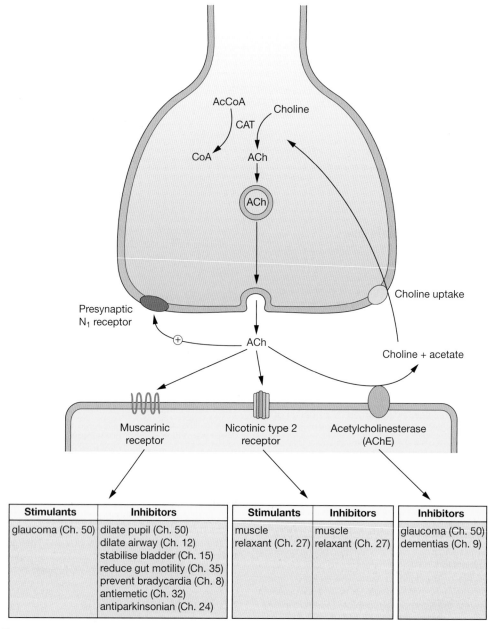

Fig. 4.5 **Illustration of the mechanisms involved in the synthesis, release and inactivation of acetylcholine.** The actions of agonists and inhibitors of muscarinic receptors, nicotinic type 1 (N_1) receptors and acetylcholinesterase are shown with the relevant chapters detailing with their pharmacology. ACh, acetylcholine; AcCoA, acetyl CoA; CAT, choline acetyltransferase.

are more sensitive to ACh release and require fewer ACh molecules to be released to stimulate a recipient axon compared with the neuromuscular junction, which requires millions of molecules to be released for skeletal muscle contractility to occur.

Metabolism and inactivation of released acetylcholine

Both presynaptic and postsynaptic membranes are rich in acetylcholinesterase (AChE), and the released ACh is hydrolysed very rapidly (usually <1 ms) to give choline and acetate. This rapid hydrolysis, and the rapid equilibration between ACh bound to the receptor and free in the synapse, means that the 'receptor phase' of the transmission process only lasts for 1–2 ms (the postsynaptic changes may be more prolonged; see below).

AChE is an important target for drug action and for the toxic effects of some chemicals; the active site of the esterase enzyme has two critical features involved in the metabolism of ACh (Fig. 4.6):

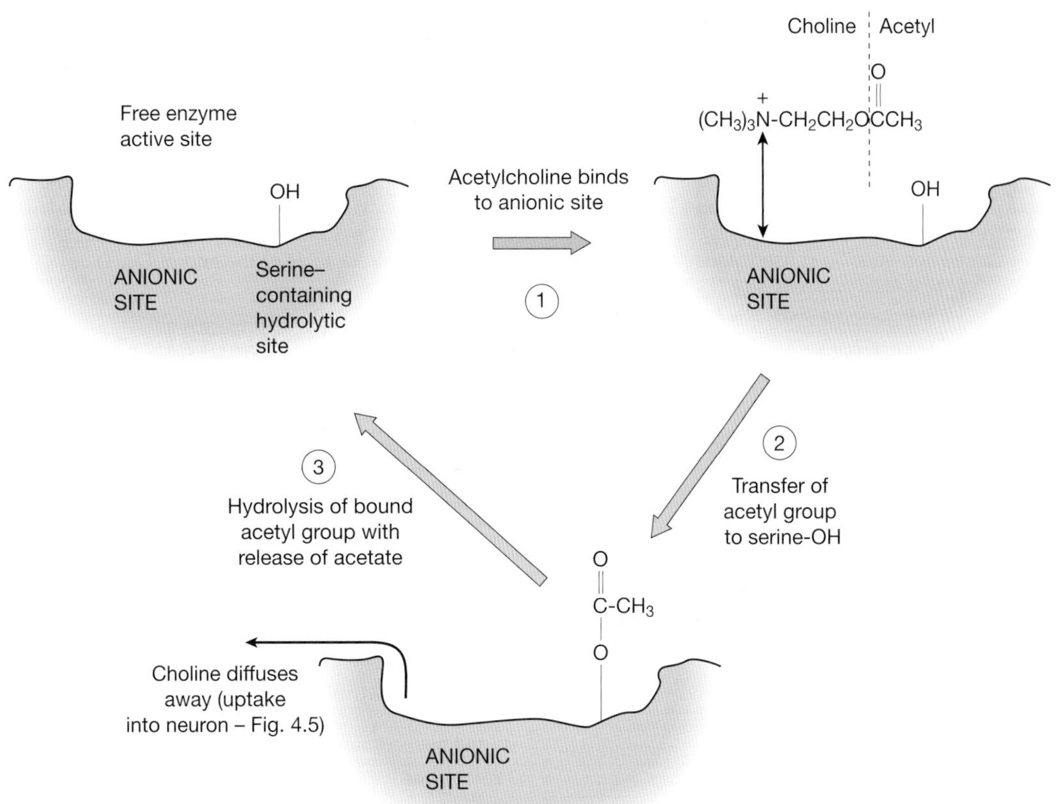

Fig 4.6 **The mechanism of hydrolysis of acetylcholine by acetylcholinesterase.**

- an anionic site, which forms an ionic bond to the quaternary nitrogen of the choline part of ACh
- a hydrolytic site, which contains a serine moiety; the hydroxyl group of the serine accepts the acetyl group (CH_3CO–) from ACh and very rapidly transfers it to water to complete the hydrolysis reaction.

Inhibition of AChE will prevent the breakdown of ACh and lead to prolonged receptor occupancy, the consequences of which depend on the nature of the receptor and the innervated cell/tissue.

AChE inhibitors can be divided into three types.

- **AChE inhibitors that bind to the anionic site**. The enzyme can be inhibited by an agent binding reversibly to the anionic site, for example edrophonium (Ch. 28).
- **AChE inhibitors that carbamylate the serine group**. Some inhibitors bind to the anionic site and transfer a carbamoyl group [$(CH_3)_2NCO$–] instead of an acetyl group (CH_3CO–) from the drug to the serine hydroxyl group. The carbamoyl group is hydrolysed more slowly from the serine than is an acetyl group and, as a result, prolonged and profound (but reversible) inhibition of the enzyme occurs; this occurs, for example, with neostigmine and pyridostigmine These are used in treating myasthenia gravis and reversing neuromuscular block by non-depolarising blockers (Chs 27 and 28).
- **Acetylcholinesterase inhibitors that phosphorylate the serine hydroxyl group**. Some inhibitors react with the serine hydroxyl group (with or without binding to the anionic site) to produce a phosphorylated enzyme. The phosphorylated enzyme is stable to hydrolysis and, therefore, inhibitors such as the organophosphates, which inhibit AChE in this way, cause irreversible inhibition of the enzyme (or very slowly and only partially reversible inhibition). Such permanent changes in enzyme activity are of limited clinical use. The drug ecothiopate acts via phosphorylation of AChE and has limited clinical use in ophthalmology. Compounds in this group may also be encountered clinically in people suffering accidental or intentional poisoning with organophosphates. Organophosphates are important environmental chemicals due to their use as pesticides, and there has been concern in recent years over the exposure of agricultural workers to such compounds, for example in sheep dips. Organophosphates have also been used as nerve gases for chemical warfare. The active serine hydroxyl group may be regenerated early after exposure by administration of the drug pralidoxime, which is an antidote to organophosphate poisoning. However, a few hours after exposure the phosphorylated enzyme undergoes changes, known as ageing, and pralidoxime cannot reactivate the enzyme after ageing has occurred.

Unlike many other neurotransmitters, ACh is not inactivated by a specific reuptake process, but because choline is a limited resource, there is a specific reuptake mechanism to allow choline to re-enter the presynaptic neuron and to be reused rather than simply to diffuse away. No such process occurs for acetate because it is readily available from intermediary metabolism. Presynaptic uptake of choline can be inhibited by structural analogues, such as hemicholinium, but such drugs are not useful clinically because of the widespread and non-specific consequences of impairment of ACh uptake, synthesis and release.

Cholinergic receptors

The cholinergic receptors can be divided into nicotinic and muscarinic types. Two nicotinic and five muscarinic subtypes have been characterised (see drug receptor table at the end of Ch. 1). The receptors were originally named after nitrogen-containing basic compounds (alkaloids) present in plants (**nicotine**) or fungi (**muscarine**). Figure 4.5 gives information about the general effects of stimulants and inhibitors of muscarinic and nicotinic type 1 receptors and anticholinesterase inhibitors and identifies the chapter(s) that describe the clinical relevance of these actions.

Nicotinic (N_1) receptors

These occur within the CNS and on the postsynaptic membranes of all ganglia of both the sympathetic and parasympathetic branches of the ANS.

Nicotinic (N_2) receptors

These occur at the junction between the somatic motor nerves and skeletal muscles (the neuromuscular junction; see Ch. 27).

The nicotinic receptor is a ligand-gated ion channel of five subunits (see Fig. 1.1), with disulphide cross-linking between adjacent subunits; there are different types of subunit (α, β, γ and δ), and different combinations give rise to neuronal N_1 receptors or neuromuscular junction N_2 receptors. The differences between N_2 and N_1 receptors in their agonist/antagonist binding characteristics are clinically very important, because they allow neuromuscular blockade (paralysis) without major effects on the ANS.

Muscarinic (M) receptors

These are G-protein-coupled receptors widely distributed in the CNS and in pre- and postganglionic fibre/effector organ junctions of the parasympathetic branch of the ANS. These receptors are also present on most sweat glands (other than the palms of the hands), which are, however, innervated by the sympathetic branch of the ANS. Table 4.3 shows the effect of stimulation of the muscarinic receptors in major tissues and the principal muscarinic receptor subtype that is involved. Application of molecular biology has identified five subtypes of muscarinic receptor (M_1–M_5) (see drug receptor table at the end of Ch. 1). The distribution and functions of receptors M_1, M_2 and M_3 have been well characterised (Table 4.3).

In addition to occurring on postsynaptic sites, N_1 and M receptors are also found presynaptically; recent data suggest that the main role of N_1 receptors in the CNS may be as a presynaptic neuromodulator.

It should be appreciated that AChE inhibitors increase the concentrations of ACh at all nicotinic and muscarinic receptor sites, and therefore produce a diverse array of effects. For example, when an AChE inhibitor is used to overcome reversible neuromuscular blockade (see Ch. 27), it increases ACh-mediated effects produced via the parasympathetic nervous system, for example on the gastrointestinal tract and heart. These unwanted effects of ACh can be blocked by co-administration of an antimuscarinic agent (see drug receptor table at the end of Ch. 1).

OTHER TRANSMITTERS IN THE PERIPHERAL NERVOUS SYSTEM

In addition to acetylcholine and noradrenaline, there are other mediators that have roles in neurotransmission and function in the peripheral nervous system. Many of these are also of considerable importance in the central nervous system. The different mediators are dealt with in the chapters that describe their clinical importance, and include:

- amines, e.g. dopamine, histamine, serotonin
- amino acids, e.g. glutamate, glycine, gamma-aminobutyric acid (GABA)
- peptides, e.g. opioids, substance P
- purines, e.g. adenosine, ATP.

Nitric oxide, calcitonin gene-related peptide, vasoactive intestinal peptide (VIP), neuropeptide Y, ghrelin and others are described later in the book

AMINES

Dopamine

Dopamine is a very important neurotransmitter both within the CNS and in the periphery, and subsequent chapters cover its actions (Chs 7, 21, 24 and 32).

Synthesis

Synthesis has been described above under noradrenaline (Fig. 4.3a).

Storage

Storage has been described above under noradrenaline.

Release

Nerve stimulation causes release of dopamine present in vesicles (see noradrenaline). Dopaminergic neurons are not important in the clinical responses to indirectly acting sympathomimetics, although certain behavioural responses to amphetamines are linked to dopamine D_2 receptor activity. The antiviral drug amantadine, which is of some value in Parkinson's disease, causes release of dopamine.

Removal of activity of released dopamine

Dopamine is removed by similar mechanisms to those described above for noradrenaline, with reuptake representing the major pathway. Metabolism yields primarily 3,4-dihydroxyphenylacetic acid and its 3-methyl analogue (homovanillic acid).

Receptors

It is now recognised that there are a number of types of dopamine receptors, and relatively selective therapeutic agents are available for some of these (see drug receptor table at the end of Ch. 1). Dopamine receptors are classified into those that increase cAMP (D_1 and D_5) and those that decrease cAMP (D_2, D_3 and D_4). The D_4 receptor shows polymorphic expression; subtypes D_2 and D_4 are associated with schizophrenia and relatively selective antagonists of each are valuable antipsychotic drugs and have some different biological properties (Ch. 21).

Serotonin (5-Hydroxytryptamine)

Serotonin (or 5-HT; Fig. 4.7a) is a neurotransmitter in the CNS and periphery that shows characteristics similar to the catecholamines.

Synthesis

Serotonin is synthesised from the amino acid tryptophan by two reactions that are similar to those used in the conversion of tyrosine to dopamine. The first reaction is oxidation of the benzene ring of tryptophan to form 5-hydroxytryptophan, which is catalysed by the enzyme tryptophan hydroxylase (which is the rate-limiting step and is only found in serotonin-producing cells). Conversion of the amino acid function to an amine is catalysed by aromatic amino acid decarboxylase (see noradrenaline synthesis).

Serotonin is present in the diet but undergoes essentially complete first-pass metabolism by MAO in the gut wall and liver. Serotonin is not synthesised by blood platelets, but they have a very efficient transporter, which allows them to accumulate high concentrations of serotonin from the circulation which can be released when platelets aggregate and during migraine.

Storage

Major sites of serotonin storage in the body are the enterochromaffin cells of the gastrointestinal tract and platelets. Neurons utilizing serotonin are widely distributed in the brain. In presynaptic neurons serotonin is stored in vesicles as a complex with ATP, and there is an active uptake process of serotonin which transfers cytoplasmic serotonin into the storage vesicle.

Release

The release of serotonin vesicles is by Ca^{2+}-mediated exocytosis. A rise in intraluminal pressure in the gastrointestinal tract stimulates the release of serotonin from the chromaffin cells. Release of serotonin from chromaffin cells contributes to nausea following cancer chemotherapy with cytotoxic drugs, by stimulating sensory receptors in the gastrointestinal tract and by stimulating the chemoreceptor trigger zone (Ch. 32). There is a significant release of platelet serotonin in migraine (Ch. 26).

Metabolism and removal of activity

The principal mechanism of inactivation of released serotonin is via its reuptake into the presynaptic nerve. The process shows a high affinity for serotonin, and is different from that on adrenergic neurons, which has allowed selective inhibitors to be developed. Selective serotonin reuptake inhibitors (SSRIs) are useful antidepressants (Ch. 22).

Metabolism within the neuron is by MAO, which converts the $-CH_2NH_2$ group to an aldehyde ($-CHO$), which is then oxidised to a carboxylic acid ($-COOH$), producing

(a) HO $CH_2CH_2NH_2$ N H

5 HT

(b) $CH_2CH_2NH_2$ HN N

Histamine

(c) O NH_2 C — $CH_2CH_2CH_2$ HO

γ-Aminobutyric acid (GABA)

(d) NH_2 HOOC CH_2CH_2CH COOH

Glutamate

(e) NH_2 CH_2 COOH

Glycine

(f)

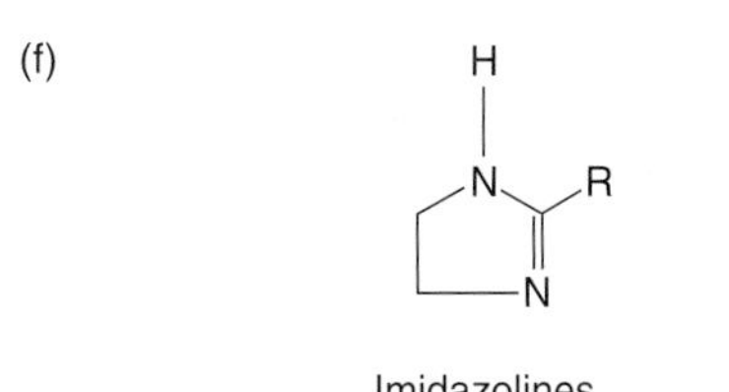

Imidazolines

(g) H_2N NH $CH_2CH_2CH_2CH_2NH_2$ NH

Agmatine

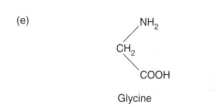

Fig. 4.7 **The structures of some of the diverse amine, amino acid and imidazoline neurotransmitters.**

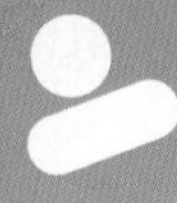

the excretory product 5-hydroxyindoleacetic acid (5-HIAA). There is a considerable turnover of serotonin in the chromaffin and nerve cells, and 5-HIAA is a normal constituent of human urine.

Receptors

There is a family of serotonin receptors, which has allowed the development of selective drugs (see drug receptor table at end of Ch. 1). Thus far, the different serotonin receptors comprise 13 different 7TM G-protein-coupled receptors and one ligand-gated ion channel, which are divided into seven classes ($5HT_1$ to $5HT_7$) on the basis of their structural and operational characteristics. Not all of the subtypes of receptors have recognised physiological roles. Receptors in the $5HT_1$ group are mostly presynaptic and inhibit adenylyl cyclase, whereas those in the $5HT_2$ group are mostly postsynaptic in the periphery and activate phospholipase C. Identification of receptor subtype functions and selective inhibitors or stimulants has facilitated progress in the treatment of diseases (e.g. migraine Ch. 26, depression Ch 22).

Histamine

Histamine (Fig. 4.7b) is an important transmitter both in the CNS and in the periphery, as well as being a mediator released from mast cells and basophils.

Synthesis

The amino acid histidine is converted to histamine through decarboxylation by histidine decarboxylase. In addition to the synthesis and storage of histamine by mast cells and basophils, there is continual synthesis, release and metabolic inactivation by growing tissues and in wound healing.

Storage

Most attention has focused on the storage of histamine in mediator-releasing cells, such as mast cells, basophils and enterochromaffin cells in the gut (Chs 12 and 33). In such cells, it is present in granules, associated with heparin. The presence of histidine decarboxylase and the storage of histamine in neurons in the CNS, although less well explored, appears to be associated mainly with the hypothalamus, where projections run to many parts of the brain. Histamine plays a role in wakefulness, memory, appetite and many other functions.

Release

The release of histamine from mast cells and basophils has been studied extensively in relation to allergic reactions (Chs 12 and 39). The release of histamine from neurons may be similar to the release of other amine neurotransmitters, but this has not been demonstrated unequivocally.

Removal of activity

Histamine is rapidly inactivated by oxidation of the amino group ($–CH_2NH_2$) to an aldehyde and then an acid (–COOH), imidazoleacetic acid. Histamine is not a substrate for MAO and the oxidation is catalysed by diamine oxidase (or histaminase). A second, minor route of metabolism is methylation of the cyclic –NH group by histamine-N-methyltransferase, and the product is then a substrate for MAO, producing N-methylimidazoleacetic acid. Histamine is also eliminated as an N-acetyl conjugate.

Receptors

There are four receptors for histamine (see drug receptor table at the end of Ch. 1). H_1 receptors have been studied extensively in relation to inflammation and allergy (Chs 12 and 39). The discovery of H_2 receptors affecting the release of gastric acid led to the development of important selective inhibitors that reduce acid secretion and contribute to the treatment of dyspepsia and to ulcer healing (Ch. 33). Histamine-containing neurons are found in the brain, particularly in the brainstem, with pathways projecting into the cerebral cortex. H_1 receptors are probably important in these pathways, because sedation is a serious problem with H_1 receptor antagonists (Ch. 39) that are able to cross the blood–brain barrier (Ch. 2). The so-called second-generation antihistamines produce less sedation. H_1 receptors are also involved in emesis (Ch. 32). H_2 receptors are present in the brain and are probably responsible for the confusional state associated with the use of the H_2 receptor antagonist cimetidine (Ch. 33).

AMINO ACIDS

Gamma-aminobutyric acid

GABA ($HOOCCH_2CH_2CH_2NH_2$) is an important inhibitory neurotransmitter responsible for about 40% of all inhibitory activity in the CNS (Fig. 4.7c).

Synthesis

GABA is formed by the decarboxylation of glutamate via the enzyme glutamate decarboxylase, which is present in GABAergic neurons.

Storage

GABA is stored in membrane vesicles in the brain and in interneurons within the spinal cord (particularly laminae II and III).

Release

GABA is released by Ca^{2+}-mediated exocytosis. Co-transmitters, such as glycine, metenkephalin and neuropeptide Y, are stored in GABA vesicles and released with GABA.

Removal of activity

Uptake is the principal mechanism for the removal of GABA from the synaptic cleft. The antiepileptic drug tiagabine may act as an inhibitor of GABA uptake (Ch. 23).

GABA is metabolised by transamination with α-ketoglutarate, which forms the corresponding aldehyde (succinic semialdehyde) and amino acid (glutamic acid). The antiepileptic drug vigabatrin inhibits GABA transamination.

Receptors

There are two main GABA receptors, with different mechanisms of action (see drug receptor table at the end of Ch. 1). Stimulation of both receptors produces hyperpolarisation of the cell membrane, with $GABA_A$ causing rapid inhibition and $GABA_B$ producing a slower and more prolonged response. The $GABA_A$ receptor comprises a number of subunits. There are multiple forms of each subunit and numerous possible combinations (see Fig. 20.1); consequently, the $GABA_A$ receptor should be regarded as a family of receptors. Hyperpolarisation following $GABA_A$ receptor stimulation results from the opening of Cl^- channels and influx of Cl^-. $GABA_B$ receptors are G-protein-linked receptors that hyperpolarise the cell indirectly by closing Ca^{2+} channels and opening K^+ channels. In addition, there is a third receptor, $GABA_C$, which is linked to changes in Cl^- conductance associated with retinal function, but its physiological and clinical significance remain unclear. Both $GABA_A$ and $GABA_B$ receptors are found presynaptically and inhibit neurotransmitter release by hyperpolarising the cell (via opening Cl^- or K^+ channels) and reducing release of the vesicles of the innervating cell (via closing Ca^{2+} channels). Many important drugs act by altering GABA breakdown or by enhancing GABA activity at its receptor (Chs 20 and 23).

Glutamate

Glutamate (Fig. 4.7d) is an important excitatory amino acid neurotransmitter with wide-reaching actions in physiological and pathological conditions. The functions of glutamate are described in later chapters. Aspartate (which is similar to glutamate but has only one CH_2 group) acts at the same receptors. Administration of glutamate or aspartate causes CNS excitation, tachycardia, nausea and headache, and convulsions at very high doses. Hyperactivity at glutamate receptors has been proposed as a factor in the generation of epilepsy (Ch. 23).

Synthesis

Glutamate (glutamic acid) is an amino acid that is formed in most cells and is widely distributed within the CNS.

Storage

Glutamate is stored in presynaptic vesicles in the neurons.

Release

Exocytosis of vesicles is mediated via the influx of Ca^{2+} into the presynaptic nerve terminal, as occurs for other neurotransmitters. Some antiepileptic drugs, for example lamotrigine and valproate (Ch. 23), inhibit glutamate release.

Removal of activity

The action of glutamate in the synapse is terminated by a specific carrier, which transports glutamate into the neuron and surrounding glial cells.

Receptors

There are two major types of glutamate receptor that are described as either metabotropic or ionotropic and which have a range of biological actions (see drug receptor table at the end of Ch. 1).

Glycine

Glycine (Fig. 4.7e) is a widely available amino acid that acts as an inhibitory neurotransmitter. It is released in response to nerve stimulation and acts in the spine, lower brainstem and retina.

Synthesis

Glycine is present in all cells and is accumulated by neurons.

Storage

Glycine is stored within neurons in vesicles.

Release

Vesicle release accompanies an action potential, as described above for other neurotransmitters. Tetanus toxin prevents glycine release, and the decrease in glycine-mediated inhibition results in reflex hyperexcitability.

Removal of activity

Released glycine is inactivated by a high-affinity uptake process.

Receptors

Glycine receptors are ligand-gated Cl^- channels similar in structure to $GABA_A$ channels: they are present mainly on interneurons in the spinal cord. Strychnine produces convulsions through the blockade of glycine receptors. Glycine is important for the activity of NMDA (N-methyl-D-aspartate) receptors (see drug receptor table at the end of Ch. 1).

PEPTIDES

The importance of peptides as neurotransmitters has been appreciated in recent years, largely because of the development of highly specific and sensitive probes, combined with histochemical techniques, which has allowed their detection and measurement. Unlike other classes of neurotransmitter, peptides are synthesised in the cell body as precursors, which are transported down the axon to the site of storage. There are specific receptors for different peptides (see drug receptor table at the end of Ch. 1). An action potential causes the release of the peptide from its precursor; inactivation is probably via hydrolysis by a local peptidase.

Peptide neurotransmitters are often found stored in the same nerve endings as other transmitters (described above) and undergo simultaneous release (co-transmission).

Peptides do not cross the blood–brain barrier readily. A major problem for exploiting our increasing knowledge of the importance of peptides is devising ways to deliver the novel products derived from molecular biology to the sites within the brain where they can have an effect.

Substance P is released from C-fibres (Ch. 19) by a Ca^{2+}-linked mechanism and is an important neurotransmitter for sensory afferents in the dorsal horn. It is also present in the substantia nigra, associated with dopaminergic neurons, and may be involved in the control of movement.

Opioid peptides are a range of peptides that are the natural ligands for opioid receptors (known formerly as the 'morphine' receptor); the receptor was recognised in the brain and gastrointestinal tract for many years before the natural ligand was identified. These are discussed in Chapter 19.

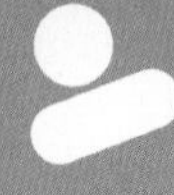

A number of other peptides are detectable in the CNS particularly in the hypothalamus and/or pituitary gland (e.g. neurotensin, oxytocin, somatostatin, vasopressin; see Chs 43 and 45) or in the gastrointestinal tract (e.g. cholecystokinin and vasoactive intestinal peptide).

PURINES

Adenosine and guanosine are endogenous purines and exist in the body in the free form, attached to ribose or deoxyribose (as nucleosides) and as mono-, bi- or triphosphorylated nucleotides. Purines within cells are usually incorporated into nucleotides, which are involved in the energetics of biochemical processes (e.g. ATP), act as intracellular signals (e.g. cAMP and cGMP – Ch. 1) and are involved in the synthesis of RNA and DNA. ATP is present in the presynaptic vesicles of some other neurotransmitters and is released along with the primary neurotransmitter, following which it may act on postsynaptic receptors (co-transmission). Extracellular ATP is rapidly hydrolysed via adenosine diphosphate (ADP) to adenosine. Adenosine itself is very rapidly metabolised and inactivated.

There is a family of purine receptors that show individual selectivity for different purines and give different responses (see drug receptor table at the end of Ch. 1). The adenosine receptors (A_1–A_3) show very high selectivity for adenosine itself. Adenosine is used therapeutically to terminate supraventricular tachycardia. Purinergic receptors (P_2) are specific for the adenosine phosphates, and ADP causes platelet aggregation via P_2 type receptors. The effect of ADP can be inhibited with clopidogrel, which has important antiaggregatory actions (Ch. 11)

IMIDAZOLINES

The realisation that there may be an additional, unrecognised group of neurotransmitters/receptors involved in the control of blood pressure arose from studies on α_2-adrenoceptor agonists. The unwanted effects produced by the drug clonidine, an early imidazoline α_2-adrenoceptor agonist, led to the development of moxonidine and rilmenidine. These imidazolines possessed fewer unwanted effects, but not all of their actions could be interpreted by actions on the α_2-adrenoceptor. A specific imidazoline-binding site was identified in the rostral ventrolateral medulla, and an endogenous 'ligand' that would displace clonidine from this site was proposed (see Ch. 6).

This led to the suggestion that there is an imidazoline receptor that has a high affinity for imidazoline compounds (Fig. 4.7f). There are three imidazoline receptors (I_1, I_2 and I_3). Agmatine (Fig. 4.7g), which is a metabolite of arginine, is an endogenous ligand for I receptors, but is also a ligand at the α_2-adrenoceptor. This compound occurs in synaptosomes and is a postulated natural transmitter.

Binding sites of the I_1 type are present in the brainstem, kidneys, liver and prostate. The contribution of the I_1 receptor to the overall control of blood pressure is not clearly established. The I_2 binding site is associated with MAO and is an allosteric modulating region on the enzyme, not a neurotransmitter receptor. The I_3 site appears to modulate the action of K_{ATP} channels and is linked to insulin release from the pancreas.

FURTHER READING

Abrams P, Andersson K-E, Buccafusco J et al (2006) Muscarinic receptors: their distribution and function in body systems, and the implications for treating overactive bladder. *Br J Pharmacol* 148, 565–578

Barnes NM, Sharp T (1999) A review of central 5-HT receptors and their function. *Neuropharmacology* 38, 1083–1152

Berg KA, Maayani S, Clarke WP (1998) Interactions between effectors linked to serotonin receptors. *Ann NY Acad Sci* 861, 111–120

Bloom FE, Morales M (1998) The central 5-HT_3 receptor in CNS disorders. *Neurochem Res* 23, 653–659

Bousquet P, Dontenwill M, Greney H, Feldman J (1998) I1-Imidazoline receptors: an update. *J Hypertens* 16(suppl), S1–S5

Bousquet P, Monassier L, Feldman J (1998) Autonomic nervous system as a target for cardiovascular drugs. *Clin Exp Pharmacol Physiol* 25, 446–448

Bowery NG, Bettler B, Froestl W et al (2002) International Union of Pharmacology. XXXIII. Mammalian gamma-aminobutyric acid (B) receptors: structure and function. *Pharmacol Rev* 54, 247–264

Buckley NJ, Bachfischer U, Canut M et al (1999) Repression and activation of muscarinic receptor genes. *Life Sci* 64, 495–499

Burgen AS (2000) Targets of drug action. *Annu Rev Pharmacol Toxicol* 40, 1–16

Buscher R, Herrmann V, Insel PA (1999) Human adrenoceptor polymorphisms: evolving recognition of clinical importance. *Trends Pharmacol Sci* 20, 94–99

Cartmell J, Schoepp DD (2000) Regulation of neurotransmitter release by metabotropic glutamate receptors. *J Neurochem* 75, 889–907

Dajas-Bailador F, Wonnacott S (2004) Nicotinic acetylcholine receptors and the regulation of neuronal signalling. *Trends Pharmacol Sci* 25, 317–324

Docherty JR (1998) Subtypes of functional alpha I- and alpha 2-adrenoceptors. *Eur J Pharmacol* 361, 1–15

Eglen RM, Reddy H, Watson N, Challiss RAJ (1994) Muscarinic acetylcholine receptor subtypes in smooth muscle. *Trends Pharmacol Sci* 15, 114–119

Eglen RM, Choppin A, Dillon MP, Hegde S (1999) Muscarinic receptor ligands and their therapeutic potential. *Curr Opin Chem Biol* 3, 426–432

Frishman WH, Kotob F (1999) Alpha-adrenergic blocking drugs in clinical medicine. *J Clin Pharmacol* 39, 7–16

Grace AA, Gerfen CR, Aston-Jones G (1998) Catecholamines in the central nervous system. Overview. *Adv Pharmacol* 42, 655–670

Green AR, Hainsworth AH, Jackson DM (2000) GABA potentiation: a logical pharmacological approach for the treatment of acute ischaemic stroke. *Neuropharmacology* 39, 1483–1494

Hieble JP (2000) Adrenoceptor subclassification: an approach to improved cardiovascular therapeutics. *Pharm Acta Helv* 74, 163–171

Hoyer D, Hannon JP, Martin GR (2002) Molecular, pharmacological and functional diversity of 5-HT receptors. *Pharmacol Biochem Behav* 71, 533–554

Insel PA (1996) Adrenoceptors – evolving concepts and clinical implications. *N Engl J Med* 334, 580–585

Kennedy C (2000) The discovery and development of P2 receptor subtypes. *J Auton Nerv Syst* 81, 158–163

Kirstein SL, Insel PA (2004) Autonomic nervous system pharmacogenomics: a progress report. *Pharmacol Rev* 56, 31–52

Mayersohn M, Guentert TW (1995) Clinical pharmacokinetics of the monoamine oxidase-A inhibitor moclobemide. *Clin Pharmacokinet* 29, 292–332

Noll G, Wenzel RR, Binggeli C, Corti C, Luscher TF (1998) Role of sympathetic nervous system in hypertension and effects of cardiovascular drugs. *Eur Heart J* 19(suppl), F32–F38

Piascik MT, Perez DM (2001) Alpha1-adrenergic receptors: new insights and directions. *J Pharmacol Exp Ther* 298, 403–410

Rana BK, Shiina T, Insel PA (2001) Genetic variations and polymorphisms of G protein-coupled receptors: functional and therapeutic implications. *Annu Rev Pharmacol Toxicol* 41, 593–624

Rangachari PK (1998) The fate of released histamine: reception, response and termination. *Yale J Biol Med* 7l, 173–182

Robidoux J, Martin TL, Collins S (2004) Beta-adrenergic receptors and regulation of energy expenditure: a family affair. *Annu Rev Pharmacol Toxicol* 44, 297–323

Romanelli MN, Gualtieri F (2003) Cholinergic nicotinic receptors: competitive ligands, allosteric modulators, and their potential applications. *Med Res Rev* 23, 393–426

Rudolph U, Crestani F, Möhler H (2001) $GABA_A$ receptor subtypes: dissecting their pharmacological functions. *Trends Pharmacol Sci* 22, 188–194

Satchell D (2000) Purinergic nerves and purinoceptors: early perspectives. *J Auton Nerv Syst* 81, 2l2–217

Shaikh S, Kerwin RW (2002) Receptor pharmacogenetics: relevance to CNS syndromes. *Br J Clin Pharmacol* 54, 344–348

Sherwin AL (1999) Neuroactive amino acids in focally epileptic human brain: a review. *Neurochem Res* 24, 1387–1395

Simons FE, Simons KJ (1999) Clinical pharmacology of new histamine H_1 receptor antagonists. *Clin Pharmacokinet* 36, 329–352

Small KM, McGraw DW, Liggett SB (2003) Pharmacology and physiology of human adrenergic receptor polymorphisms. *Annu Rev Pharmacol Toxicol* 43, 381–411

Takana K (2000) Functions of glutamate transporters in the brain. *Neurosci Res* 37, 15–19

Thibonnier M, Coles P, Thibonnier A, Shoham M (2001) The basic and clinical pharmacology of nonpeptide vasopressin receptor antagonists. *Annu Rev Pharmacol Toxicol* 41, 175–202

Vanden Broeck J, Torfs H, Poels J et al (1999) Tachykinin-like peptides and their receptors. A review. *Ann NY Acad Sci* 897, 374–387

Wallukat G (2002) The beta-adrenergic receptors. *Herz* 27, 683–690

Williams M (2000) Purines: from premise to promise. *J Auton Nerv Syst* 81, 285–288

Yanai K Tashiro M (2007) The physiological and pathophysiological roles of neuronal histamine: an insight from human positron emission tomography studies. *Pharmacol Ther* 113, 1–15

Youdim MBH, Edmondson D, Tipton K (2006) The therapeutic potential of monoamine oxidase inhibitors. *Nat Rev Neurosci* 7, 295–309

Zhang D, Pan Z-H, Awobuluyi M, Lipton SA (2001) Structure and function of $GABA_C$ receptors: a comparison of native versus recombinant receptors. *Trends Pharmacol Sci* 22, 121–132

SELF-ASSESSMENT

1. In the following questions, the first statement, in italics, is true. Is the accompanying statement also true?
   a. *The autonomic nervous system (ANS) is only one of the neuronal systems controlling bodily functions.* The sympathetic division of the ANS utilises adrenaline as its primary transmitter substance.
   b. *Drugs acting at the ganglia affect both sympathetic and parasympathetic nervous systems.* Ganglion-blocking drugs also block the neuromuscular junction.
   c. *Acetylcholine is metabolised extremely rapidly by acetylcholinesterase in the synaptic cleft.* Acetylcholinesterase is not the only enzyme in the body that breaks down acetylcholine.
   d. *Dopamine and noradrenaline are synthesised from the intermediate precursor levodopa.* Dopamine is a transmitter in the peripheral autonomic nervous system.
   e. *There are two major monoamine oxidase isoenzymes, MAO-A and MAO-B.* Both isoenzymes metabolise tyramine.
   f. *The differentiation of adrenoceptors into several subtypes is of clinical importance.* Both α_1- and α_2-adrenoceptor antagonists can be used to lower blood pressure.
   g. *Botulism periodically causes fatalities and is caused by poisoning by the bacterial toxin from Clostridium botulinum.* Botulinum toxin enhances acetylcholine release from cholinergic neurons.
   h. *There are three major types of β-adrenoceptor: β_1, β_2 and β_3.* The β_3-adrenoceptor is the most widespread.
   i. *Stimulation of presynaptic adrenoceptors controls noradrenaline release.* Propranolol inhibits noradrenaline release.
   j. *The major route by which the action of synaptic noradrenaline and serotonin is curtailed is by reuptake into presynaptic neurons by an uptake mechanism.* The reuptake of noradrenaline and serotonin can be inhibited selectively.
   k. *The parasympathetic and sympathetic nervous systems often have opposite effects in an organ.* Sympathetic nervous stimulation to the gut inhibits gut motility and sphincter tone.
   l. *The vagal cranial nerve to the eye decreases pupil size and limits accommodation to near vision.* Administration of adrenaline (epinephrine) decreases pupil size.

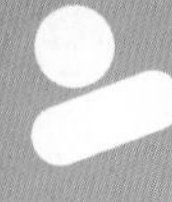

2. Which one of the following statements concerning neurotransmission is **correct**?
   A. All neurotransmitters are synthesised at sites close to the presynaptic nerve ending.
   B. The uptake of released neurotransmitter into the presynaptic nerve endings is by passive diffusion.
   C. Receptors on the presynaptic membrane can enhance or inhibit acetylcholine release.
   D. All nerves in the peripheral sympathetic nervous system release a single neurotransmitter at their postganglionic nerve endings.
   E. When an action potential arrives at the postganglionic nerve ending, fusion of vesicles containing neurotransmitter with the presynaptic membrane of the neuron is facilitated by an influx of K^+.

ANSWERS

1. a. **False**. Noradrenaline is the transmitter substance at the postganglionic nerve endings. Adrenaline is released only from the adrenal medulla and acetylcholine is the transmitter in sweat glands and hair follicles.
   b. **False**. Although acetylcholine is the transmitter at all ganglia and the neuromuscular junction, at sensible doses ganglion-blocking drugs block the nicotinic N_1 receptors in autonomic ganglia but not N_2 receptors at the neuromuscular junction.
   c. **True**. Pseudocholinesterase (butyrylcholinesterase, plasma cholinesterase; see Ch. 2) can also metabolise acetylcholine but does so more slowly. Pseudocholinesterase, however, has a broader spectrum of activity and can metabolise drugs such as suxamethonium (succinylcholine).
   d. **True**. Dopamine is predominantly an important transmitter in the CNS but is also a transmitter in selected situations in the periphery, e.g. the renal vascular smooth muscle.
   e. **True**. This is important, as selective inhibitors of MAO-A used in the treatment of depression leave MAO-B unaffected and this is available to metabolise tyramine in food, therefore avoiding the 'cheese reaction'.
   f. **False**. Stimulation of α_1-adrenoceptors on resistance vessels causes constriction; therefore, their blockade lowers blood pressure. However, α_2-adrenoceptor (presynaptic) stimulation reduces noradrenaline release and blockade of these receptors would raise blood pressure.
   g. **False**. Botulinum toxin inhibits acetylcholine release and can be used locally where there is skeletal muscle spasm or excessive sweating.
   h. **False**. The β_3-adrenoceptor has been found in adipocytes, the heart, colon and some other tissues, but is less widespread than the β_2-adrenoceptor. The β_3-adrenoceptor on adipocytes is being investigated to see if its stimulation will be effective to treat obesity.
   i. **True**. Propranolol is a non-selective antagonist of β-adrenoceptors, and the role of the presynaptic β_2-adrenoceptor is to increase noradrenaline release.
   j. **True**. Selective reversible inhibitors of the uptake of noradrenaline or serotonin (e.g. fluoxetine) are available and are used in the treatment of depression.
   k. **False**. Sympathetic nervous stimulation releases noradrenaline and inhibits motility but increases the tone of the sphincters.
   l. **False**. When the sympathetic supply to the radial muscle of the iris is stimulated, the muscle contracts and the pupil size increases. This effect can be used to facilitate retinal examination.
2. Answer **C**.
   A. Incorrect. Peptides are synthesised in the cell body and transported to the postganglionic nerve ending.
   B. Incorrect. Active transporters transfer released neurotransmitters, e.g. noradrenaline and serotonin, back into the presynaptic neuron.
   C. Correct. On parasympathetic nerve endings, stimulation of presynaptic N_1 receptors increases acetylcholine release whereas stimulation of presynaptic M_2 receptors decreases acetylcholine release.
   D. Incorrect. Co-transmission is common. For example, noradrenaline and vasoactive intestinal polypeptide are released from sympathetic nerve endings to the gut.
   E. Incorrect. An influx of Ca^{2+} is associated with transmitter release.

2

The cardiovascular system

5 Ischaemic heart disease

The heart receives about 5% of the cardiac output at rest via the coronary arteries, and extracts about 75% of the oxygen from the blood perfusing the coronary vasculature. When the metabolic demand from the myocardium becomes greater (for example with exercise), coronary artery blood flow increases by up to three- to fourfold, to supply the necessary oxygen; there is no increase in the percentage of oxygen extracted from the blood passing through the myocardium. Myocardial perfusion occurs largely during diastole, when the muscle of the heart is relaxed and not compressing the intramyocardial vessels. Therefore, unlike for other organs, cardiac perfusion is reliant on the diastolic blood pressure.

Ischaemic heart disease most frequently arises as a result of restriction of blood flow to cardiac muscle by atheroma in the large epicardial coronary arteries. Atheromatous plaques tend to form in areas of flow disturbance, such as bends in the vessels or near branching vessels. A brief overview of the mechanisms involved in atheroma formation and plaque rupture is given in Figure 5.1. The plaques are often confined to a small segment of the coronary artery, but atheroma can diffusely involve a long segment of the vessel. Localised plaques frequently involve only part of the circumference of the arterial wall, leaving the rest free of significant disease and still able to respond to vasoconstrictor and vasodilator influences. Flow disturbances, and the consequent changes in shear stress, at the site of an atheromatous plaque impair endothelial function and reduce local generation of vasodilator substances such as nitric oxide (see organic nitrates below). Therefore, diseased segments of an artery are particularly prone to vasospasm, which produces dynamic flow limitation superimposed on the fixed atheromatous narrowing. If the coronary artery disease is longstanding, then collateral vessels can develop around the atheromatous narrowing, and improve perfusion distal to the diseased segment of the artery.

The major risk factors for coronary artery disease (in common with atheroma in other parts of the vascular tree) are male gender, smoking, hypertension, hypercholesterolaemia and diabetes mellitus. The effects of these risk factors are additive, and when several are present coronary atheroma occurs more extensively and at a younger age. There are two morphological types of atheromatous plaque. Some have a lipid-rich core, with a substantial infiltration of inflammatory cells and a thin fibrous cap. Such plaques are relatively unstable ('vulnerable' plaques) and are more prone to plaque disruption by ulceration or rupture of the cap, leading to thrombus formation (see below). Other plaques have a fibrotic core, with a thick fibrous cap, and are more stable. The reasons why both stable and unstable plaques can coexist in the coronary circulation is not well understood.

Myocardial ischaemia can sometimes occur in the presence of structurally normal epicardial coronary arteries. In this situation, it arises either from abnormal regulation of the microvascular circulation within the myocardium, or from intense vasoconstriction of an epicardial artery (coronary vasospasm).

CLINICAL MANIFESTATIONS OF MYOCARDIAL ISCHAEMIA

STABLE ANGINA

Angina pectoris is pain arising from heart muscle after it switches to anaerobic metabolism, and is a symptom of reversible myocardial ischaemia. Ischaemia is the consequence of an imbalance between oxygen supply and oxygen demand in a part of the myocardium (Fig. 5.2). This results from an inability to increase coronary blood flow sufficiently to meet the metabolic demands of the heart, usually because of a fixed atheromatous narrowing of an epicardial coronary artery. Early atheromatous plaques enlarge by stretching the medial smooth muscle (remodelling) and do not narrow the lumen of the vessel until 40–50% of the cross-sectional area of the vessel is diseased. Once luminal narrowing occurs, symptoms arise when 75% of the cross-sectional area of the vessel lumen is occluded.

Stable angina is most frequently experienced as chest pain on exertion or with emotional stress and is relieved by rest. Reversible myocardial ischaemia can also present with shortness of breath (due to diastolic stiffening of the left ventricle when a reduced cellular energy supply impairs the uptake of Ca^{2+} by the sarcoplasmic reticulum [see also diastolic heart failure Ch. 7]), or it can occur without symptoms (silent ischaemia). Stable angina is an indication that there is significant coronary artery narrowing (usually as a consequence of an atheromatous plaque) but there is no

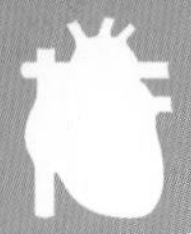

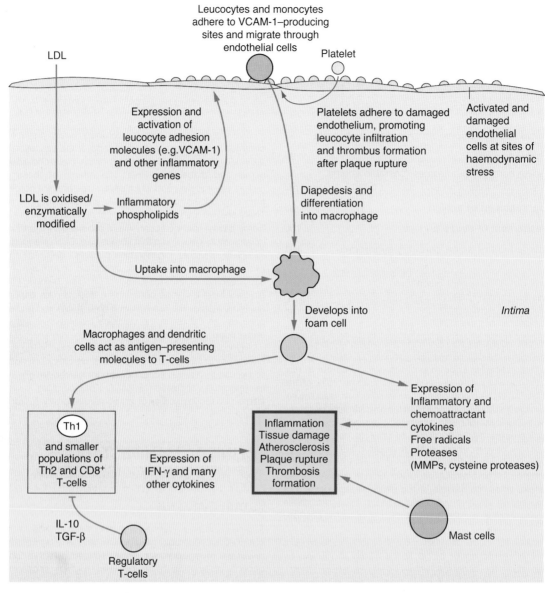

Fig. 5.1 **Aspects of inflammatory processes that contribute to coronary heart disease**. Multifactorial processes contribute to coronary heart disease; endothelium is damaged and activated; platelets adhere and promote leukocyte infiltration and thrombus formation; low-density lipoprotein (LDL) is oxidised and is taken up into macrophages, subsequently forming foam cells. Dysfunctional expression of a host of cytokines, free radicals and metalloproteinases occurs. Overall there is exacerbation of inflammation, endothelial damage, atheroma formation, plaque rupture and thrombus formation. These processes are influenced by risk factors such as smoking, heredity, hypercholesterolaemia, hypertension, obesity, diabetes, age and gender. IFN-γ, interferon-gamma; IL-10, interleukin-10; MMPs, metalloproteinases; TGF-β, tumour growth factor beta; Th, T helper cell; VCAM-1, vascular cell adhesion molecule 1.

plaque disruption. Vasospasm at the site of an atheromatous plaque accentuates the reduction in flow produced by a fixed atheromatous obstruction, and when it is present angina occurs at a lower work load.

People with stable angina have an increased risk of subsequent myocardial infarction or sudden cardiac death, due to rupture of an atheromatous plaque (see below). On average, the annual rate of such events is about 2%.

ACUTE CORONARY SYNDROMES (UNSTABLE ANGINA, MYOCARDIAL INFARCTION AND SUDDEN DEATH)

Acute coronary syndromes have a common pathophysiological origin, arising from disruption of an unstable atheromatous plaque in a coronary artery. This can be precipitated by sudden stresses on the cap produced by pulsatile blood

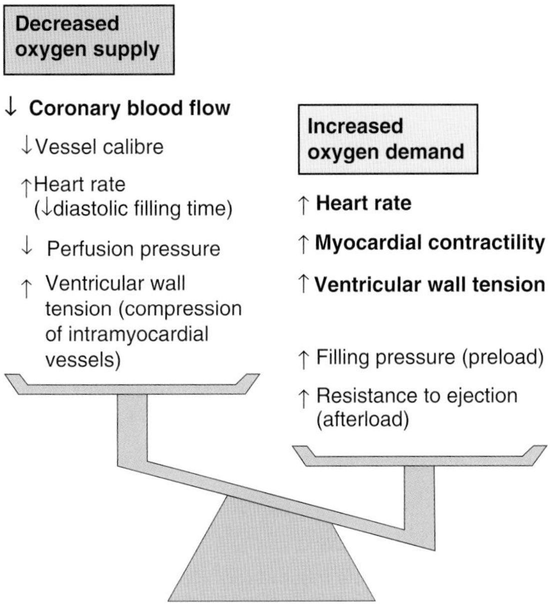

Decreased oxygen supply

↓ **Coronary blood flow**

↓Vessel calibre

↑Heart rate (↓diastolic filling time)

↓ Perfusion pressure

↑ Ventricular wall tension (compression of intramyocardial vessels)

Increased oxygen demand

↑ **Heart rate**

↑ **Myocardial contractility**

↑ **Ventricular wall tension**

↑ Filling pressure (preload)

↑ Resistance to ejection (afterload)

Fig. 5.2 **Factors affecting the balance of oxygen supply and demand in angina.**

flow across the plaque, by elastic recoil of the vessel in diastole or by vasospasm. As a consequence of these stresses, the thin cap over the plaque fissures or ulcerates, leading to plaque rupture and exposure of the core of the plaque to circulating blood. This promotes platelet aggregation (Ch. 11), thrombus formation and local vasospasm and therefore a sudden reduction in blood flow. Platelet–thrombin microemboli can break off from the thrombus and impact in small distal vessels downstream from the thrombus.

Unstable angina

If there is incomplete occlusion of the coronary artery following plaque rupture, angina may occur on minimal exertion; if the vessel is almost completely occluded, then angina occurs at rest. A sudden change in severity of ischaemic symptoms is known as unstable angina. Unlike myocardial infarction, symptoms of unstable angina are usually relieved by glyceryl trinitrate (see below), or resolve spontaneously within 30 min.

Unstable angina is distinguished pathologically from other acute coronary syndromes because perfusion of the ischaemic tissue remains sufficient to prevent necrosis of myocytes. More complete coronary artery occlusion leads to myocardial infarction. Following an episode of unstable angina, the thrombus may become incorporated into the plaque or bleeding may occur into the plaque. After healing, the plaque is substantially larger, leading to greater long-term luminal narrowing.

Myocardial infarction and sudden cardiac death

Myocardial infarction is usually associated with intense, prolonged chest pain and sympathetic nervous stimulation which increases cardiac work. However, about 15% of infarctions do not present with pain, and may go unrecognised (silent infarction). Myocardial infarction most commonly arises from complete coronary artery occlusion following disruption of an unstable atheromatous plaque (see unstable angina above). Occlusion often occurs at the site of an atheromatous lesion that previously was only producing mild or moderate stenosis of the artery and may not have caused symptoms prior to disruption. Muscle necrosis begins if the occlusion lasts for longer than 20–30 min. The diagnosis of acute myocardial infarction requires a rise in the plasma concentrations of sensitive cardiac markers, such as troponin I or troponin T, that are released from necrotic myocytes. Cell death begins in the subendocardial muscle which is furthest from the epicardial blood supply (the endocardium receives its oxygen from the ventricular cavity), and, unless perfusion is restored, it extends across the full thickness of the myocardium (transmurally) over the next few hours. Activation of endogenous fibrinolysis (Ch. 11) and the presence of a good collateral circulation are factors that favour reperfusion of the ischaemic area and naturally limit the size of the infarct. If very early reperfusion occurs, the damage is usually confined to the subendocardial myocardium.

Prolonged occlusion of a major coronary artery usually produces a full-thickness (or transmural) myocardial infarction. This often produces characteristic changes on the electrocardiograph (ECG), with early ST-segment elevation and eventually pathological Q waves. The resulting infarction is referred to as an ST-elevation myocardial infarction (STEMI). A subendocardial infarction often presents without diagnostic ECG changes. In these cases the ECG may show ST-segment depression or T-wave inversion (consistent with myocardial ischaemia), or even be normal. The resulting infarction is classified as a non-ST-segment elevation infarction (NSTEMI), because of the absence of the characteristic ST-segment changes found with more extensive myocardial damage.

Myocardial infarction principally affects left ventricular muscle, and the amount of muscle lost correlates well with both early and late survival. Infarction of the anterior muscle of the left ventricle (usually resulting from an occlusion in the left coronary artery system) causes greater myocardial loss than does inferior infarction of the ventricle (usually from right coronary artery occlusion). The amount of muscle loss also determines the extent of left ventricular remodelling (a geometrical change in the left ventricle that begins with healing of the infarct) which determines the risk of subsequent heart failure. Sudden cardiac death results when fatal ventricular arrhythmias arise from ischaemic tissue.

DRUG TREATMENT OF ANGINA

Drug treatment for angina is directed either:

- to reduce oxygen demand by decreasing cardiac work, and/or
- to increase oxygen supply by improving coronary blood flow.

Drugs can be taken to relieve the ischaemia rapidly during an acute attack or as regular prophylaxis to reduce the risk

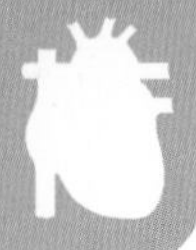

of subsequent episodes. Several classes of drug are used to treat angina.

Organic nitrates

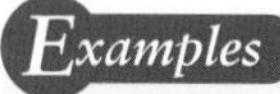

glyceryl trinitrate, isosorbide dinitrate, isosorbide mononitrate

Mechanism of action and effects

The organic nitrates are vasodilators that relax vascular smooth muscle by mimicking the effects of endogenous nitric oxide. Enzymatic degradation of the nitrate releases nitric oxide, which combines with thiol groups in vascular endothelium to form nitrosothiols. Nitrosothiols activate guanylyl cyclase, which generates the second messenger cyclic guanosine monophosphate (cGMP, Fig. 5.3). cGMP activates protein kinase G, which reduces the availability of intracellular Ca^{2+} to the contractile mechanism of vascular smooth muscle, causing relaxation and vasodilation. Vasodilation is produced in three main vascular beds.

- **Venous capacitance vessels**, leading to peripheral pooling of blood and reduced venous return to the heart. This lowers left ventricular filling pressure (preload), which decreases ventricular wall tension and therefore reduces myocardial oxygen demand. Venous dilation is produced at moderate plasma nitrate concentrations, and tolerance to this action occurs rapidly during continued treatment.
- **Arterial resistance vessels**, leading to reduced resistance to left ventricular emptying (afterload). This lowers blood pressure, decreases cardiac work and contributes to a reduced myocardial oxygen demand. Arterial dilation requires higher plasma nitrate concentrations than does venodilation, but tolerance occurs less readily during long-term treatment.
- **Coronary arteries**: nitrates have little effect on total coronary blood flow in angina; indeed, flow may be reduced because of a decrease in perfusion pressure. However, blood flow through collateral vessels may be improved, and nitrates also relieve coronary artery vasospasm. The net effect is increased blood supply to ischaemic areas of the myocardium. Coronary artery dilation occurs at low plasma nitrate concentrations, and tolerance is slow to develop.

Pharmacokinetics

Glyceryl trinitrate is the most widely used organic nitrate. It is well absorbed from the gut but undergoes extensive first-pass metabolism in the liver to inactive metabolites. To increase its bioavailability, glyceryl trinitrate is given by one of four routes that avoid first-pass metabolism.

- **Sublingual**: the tablet is placed under the tongue and is absorbed rapidly across the buccal mucosa. The very short half-life of glyceryl trinitrate (less than 5 min) limits the duration of action to approximately 30 min. Tablets

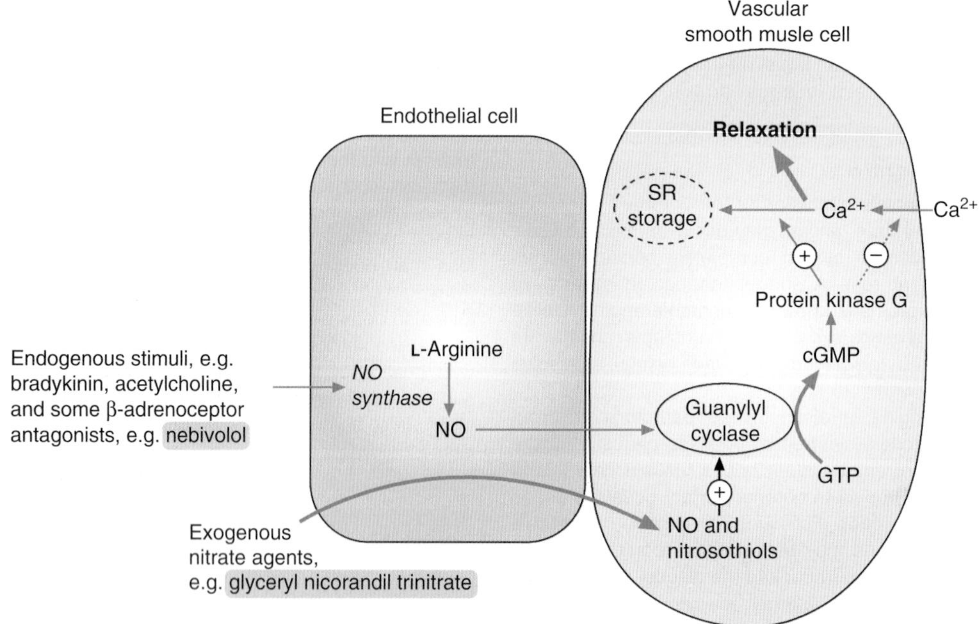

Fig 5.3 **Actions of endogenous and exogenous nitric oxide (NO).** Endogenous NO from endothelial cells relaxes smooth muscle by the following steps: NO activates guanylyl cyclase with subsequent formation of cGMP, which activates protein kinase G, which decreases Ca^{2+} influx into the cell and increases Ca^{2+} storage in the sarcoplasmic reticulum and increases myosin light-chain dephosphorylation. Exogenous agents such as organic nitrates react with tissue thiols, generating NO or nitrosothiols, which then activate guanylyl cyclase and increase cGMP (see also Fig. 6.4).

lose their potency with prolonged storage, and a metered-dose aerosol spray is a more stable delivery mechanism.

- **Buccal**: a tablet containing glyceryl trinitrate in an inert polymer matrix is held between the upper lip and gum, which permits slow release of drug to prolong the duration of action.
- **Transdermal**: glyceryl trinitrate is absorbed well through the skin and can be delivered from an adhesive patch via a rate-limiting membrane or matrix. Steady release of the drug maintains a stable blood concentration for at least 24 h after application of the patch.
- **Intravenous**: the short duration of action of glyceryl trinitrate is an advantage for intravenous dose titration.

Isosorbide dinitrate is well absorbed orally and is biologically active, but this is limited by its short half-life (0.5–2 h) and extensive first-pass metabolism. Variable amounts of a major active metabolite, isosorbide 5-mononitrate, are formed. Isosorbide mononitrate has a longer half-life than dinitrate (3–7 h) and is responsible for the majority of the sustained clinical effect. Modified-release formulations are often used to prolong the duration of action of isosorbide dinitrate. Isosorbide dinitrate is also used via an aerosol spray for a rapid onset of action, or can be given by intravenous infusion (although the longer half-life makes dose titration less easy than with glyceryl trinitrate).

Isosorbide 5-mononitrate is not subject to first-pass metabolism and can be used orally as an alternative to isosorbide dinitrate, since it gives a more predictable clinical response.

Unwanted effects

- Venodilation can produce postural hypotension, dizziness, syncope and reflex tachycardia. Tachycardia can be reduced by concurrent use of a β-adrenoceptor antagonist.
- Arterial dilation causes throbbing headaches and flushing, but tolerance to these effects is common during treatment with long-acting nitrates.
- Tolerance to the therapeutic effects of nitrates develops rapidly if there is a sustained high plasma nitrate concentration. Tolerance is therefore a particular problem with delivery of glyceryl trinitrate via transdermal patches or with the long-acting nitrates. The cause is incompletely understood, but an important mechanism may be production of oxygen free radicals (superoxides, generated in response to the excess NO production) which degrade NO. There is limited evidence that co-administration of an angiotensin-converting enzyme (ACE) inhibitor, angiotensin receptor antagonist or hydralazine (Ch. 6) may reduce nitrate tolerance by impairing superoxide formation. Activation of the sympathetic nervous system and the renin–angiotensin system in response to hypotension may also counteract the vasodilator actions of the nitrates. Tolerance can be avoided by a 'nitrate-low' period of several hours in each 24 h. This is preferable to a 'nitrate-free' period, which carries a risk of rebound angina. A nitrate-low period is achieved by asymmetric dosing with conventional formulations of isosorbide mononitrate or dinitrate (e.g. twice daily at 8 a.m., 1 p.m.) or by using a once-daily formulation of isosorbide mononitrate that allows plasma nitrate concentrations to fall overnight. Transdermal nitrate patches must be removed for part of each 24 h (e.g. overnight) to prevent tolerance, thereby creating a nitrate-free period.
- Drug interactions are most troublesome with phosphodiesterase inhibitors, such as sildenafil, used in the treatment of erectile dysfunction. These inhibit cGMP metabolism (Ch. 16) and co-administration can result in marked hypotension.

Beta-adrenoceptor antagonists (β-blockers)

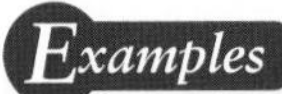

atenolol, bisoprolol, carvedilol, labetalol, metoprolol, nebivolol, pindolol, propranolol

Mechanism of action and effects in angina

All β-adrenoceptor antagonists (often simply referred to as β-blockers) act as competitive antagonists of catecholamines at β-adrenoceptors. They achieve their therapeutic effect in angina by blockade of the cardiac β_1-adrenoceptor with reduced generation of intracellular cAMP. As a result they:

- decrease heart rate (by inhibition of the cardiac I_f pacemaker current in the sinoatrial node; see Ch. 8); this is most marked during exercise, when the rate of rise in heart rate is blunted
- reduce the force of cardiac contraction (see Ch. 7)
- lower blood pressure by reducing cardiac output (a consequence of both the decreased heart rate and force of myocardial contraction).

The overall effect is to reduce myocardial oxygen demand. The slower heart rate also lengthens diastole and gives more time for coronary perfusion, which effectively improves myocardial oxygen supply.

Certain β-adrenoceptor antagonists have additional properties, which might reduce the incidence of unwanted effects or enhance their blood pressure-lowering actions (see below and also Chs 6 and 8):

- **Cardioselectivity**. Some β-adrenoceptor antagonists, for example atenolol, bisoprolol and metoprolol, are selective antagonists at the β_1-adrenoceptor. They are usually called cardioselective drugs since the most important site of action on β_1-adrenoceptors is the heart. Other β-adrenoceptor antagonists, for example propranolol, have equal or greater antagonist activity at β_2-adrenoceptors; these drugs are referred to as 'non-selective' β-adrenoceptor antagonists. The cardioselectivity of all β-adrenoceptor antagonists is dose-related, and they produce progressively more β_2-adrenoceptor blockade at higher doses (Ch. 1).
- **Partial agonist activity (PAA) or intrinsic sympathomimetic activity (ISA).** Certain β_1-adrenoceptor antagonists, such as pindolol, also have ISA and therefore act as partial agonists. For example, pindolol is a non-selective β-adrenoceptor antagonist that also has weak

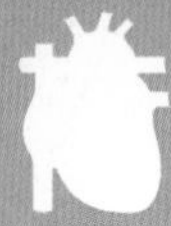

agonist properties, mainly at β_2-adrenoceptor (Ch. 1 and Fig. 6.7). If the drug is a partial agonist at the β_2-adrenoceptor, it will produce vasodilation in some vascular beds (see Fig. 6.7). However, drugs with PAA at the β_1-adrenoceptor have less inhibitory effect on heart rate and force of contraction and may be less effective than full antagonists in the treatment of severe angina. In contrast they are less likely to cause a resting bradycardia. Beta-adrenoceptor antagonists with PAA are not widely used.

- **Vasodilator activity**. Pure β-adrenoceptor antagonists do not cause vasodilation. Indeed, the reflex response to β-adrenoceptor blockade is vasoconstriction, mediated in part by the sympathetic nervous system stimulation of α_1-adrenoceptors in response to the fall in cardiac output. However, some β-adrenoceptor antagonists have additional properties that produce arterial vasodilation. Mechanisms of vasodilation include β_2-adrenoceptor partial agonist activity (e.g. pindolol), α_1-adrenoceptor blockade (e.g. carvedilol, labetalol), or an increase in endothelial nitric oxide synthesis (e.g. nebivolol) (Fig. 6.7). Nebivolol (like sotalol [Ch. 8] and propranolol) is a racemic mixture; the D-isomer of nebivolol is responsible for both β-adrenoceptor blockade and vasodilation, but the L-isomer has only vasodilator properties. Vasodilation does not have any proven advantage for the treatment of angina, but may be useful when β-adrenoceptor antagonists are given for the treatment of hypertension (Ch. 6).

Pharmacokinetics

Highly lipophilic β-adrenoceptor antagonists, such as propranolol and metoprolol, are well absorbed from the gut but undergo extensive first-pass metabolism in the liver, with considerable variability among individuals. Reduction in heart rate during exercise is closely related to the plasma concentration of a β-adrenoceptor antagonist. Consequently, dose titration of lipophilic β-adrenoceptor antagonists is usually necessary to achieve an optimal clinical response. Most lipophilic β-adrenoceptor antagonists have short half-lives (see compendium), and are often available in modified-release formulations to prolong their duration of action.

Water-soluble (hydrophilic) β-adrenoceptor antagonists, such as, pindolol, and celiprolol, are incompletely absorbed from the gut. They are subject to limited or negligible first-pass metabolism and are eliminated unchanged in the urine. The dose range to maintain effective plasma concentrations is narrower than for those drugs that undergo metabolism. The half-lives of hydrophilic β-adrenoceptor antagonists are usually longer than those of lipophilic drugs (see compendium).

Unwanted effects

- **Blockade of β_1-adrenoceptors**. Beta-adrenoceptor antagonists can precipitate acute heart failure if there is pre-existing poor left ventricular function, when high sympathetic nervous activity is necessary to maintain cardiac output. However, there is a paradox that when used at low doses with gradual dose titration they are part of the core therapy of heart failure (Ch. 7). The reduction in cardiac output can also impair blood supply to peripheral tissues, which can be detrimental in critical leg ischaemia (Ch. 10) or can provoke Raynaud's phenomenon (Ch. 10). Excessive bradycardia occasionally occurs, and β-adrenoceptor antagonists should be used with caution or avoided in the presence of advanced atrioventricular conduction defect (heart block). Drugs with partial agonist activity are less likely to cause bradycardia or to reduce cardiac output.
- **Blockade of β_2-adrenoceptors.**
  - *Bronchospasm* can be precipitated in people with asthma and in some people with chronic obstructive pulmonary disease; even cardioselective drugs are not completely safe.
  - *Hypoglycaemia* may be prolonged by non-selective β-adrenoceptor antagonists in people with diabetes who are treated with insulin (Ch. 40). Gluconeogenesis, a component of the metabolic response to hypoglycaemia, is dependent upon β_2-adrenoceptor stimulation in the liver. Beta-adrenoceptor antagonists also blunt the autonomic response that alerts the diabetic person to the onset of hypoglycaemia.
- **Effects on blood lipid levels**. Most β-adrenoceptor antagonists raise the plasma concentration of triglycerides and lower the concentration of high-density lipoprotein cholesterol (Ch. 48). These changes are modest, but are potentially atherogenic. They are most marked with non-selective β-adrenoceptor antagonists, and do not occur if the drug has partial agonist activity.
- **Central nervous system effects**. These include sleep disturbance, vivid dreams and hallucinations, and are more common with lipophilic drugs, which readily cross the blood–brain barrier. Fatigue and more subtle psychomotor effects, for example lack of concentration and sexual dysfunction, are less frequent.
- **Sudden withdrawal syndrome**. Upregulation of β-adrenoceptors (Ch. 1) during long-term treatment makes the heart more sensitive to catecholamines. Beta-adrenoceptor antagonists should be stopped gradually in people with ischaemic heart disease, to avoid precipitating unstable angina or myocardial infarction.
- **Drug interactions**. The calcium channel blockers verapamil and, to a lesser extent, diltiazem (see below) have potentially hazardous additive effects with β-adrenoceptor antagonists, since both reduce the force of cardiac contraction and slow heart rate.

Calcium channel blockers (calcium antagonists)

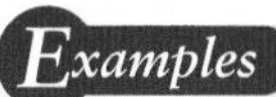

amlodipine, diltiazem, nifedipine, verapamil

Mechanism of action and effects

Calcium is essential for excitation–contraction coupling in muscle cells. The following controls of intracellular free Ca^{2+} levels are important pharmacologically (Figs 5.4 and 5.5):

- Ca^{2+} can enter cells through transmembrane voltage-gated or ligand-gated channels (Figs 5.4 and 5.5).

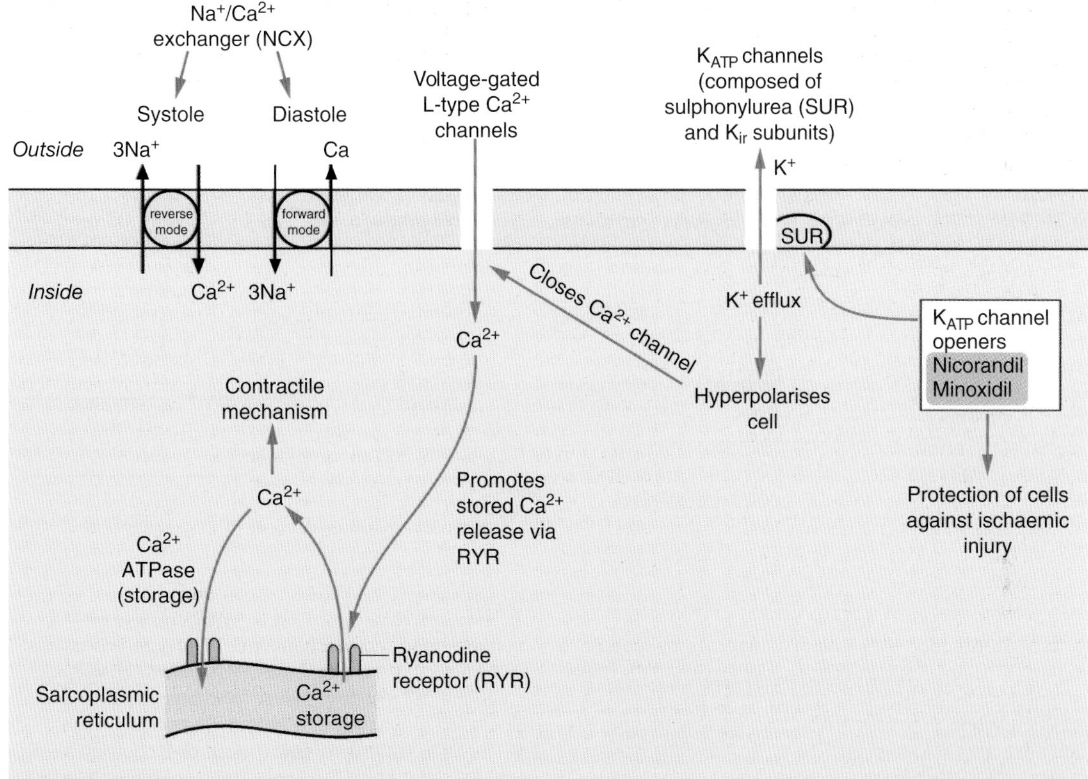

Fig. 5.4 **Aspects of the control of calcium regulation and actions of potassium channel openers in cardiac myocytes and blood vessels.** Cation regulation in cardiac cells and in vascular smooth muscle is under the control of a number of different mechanisms. Calcium entry through voltage-gated L-type Ca^{2+} channels can further amplify free Ca^{2+} (Ca^{2+}-induced release of Ca^{2+}) by stimulating diverse ryanodine receptors in the sarcoplasmic reticulum, releasing stored Ca^{2+}. Intracellular Ca^{2+} can also be regulated by exchange with Na^+ via the Na^+/Ca^{2+} exchangers (NCX). Hyperpolarisation of the cell by drugs which open K^+ channels acts to close voltage-gated L-type Ca^{2+} channels.

- A rise in intracellular free Ca^{2+} promotes release of Ca^{2+} from the sarcoplasmic reticulum through actions at ryanodine receptors (Figs 5.4 and 5.5).
- Ligand-gated channels, linked to G-protein-coupled receptors, release Ca^{2+} from intracellular stores in the sarcoplasmic reticulum.
- Ca^{2+} can exit cells in exchange for Na^+ via the Na^+/Ca^{2+} exchanger (Fig. 5.4).

There are at least five different types of Ca^{2+} channel, two of which are found in cardiovascular tissues.

- **Voltage-operated L-type (long-acting, high-threshold-activated, slowly inactivated) Ca^{2+} channels**: these are important therapeutically and are found in the cell membranes of a large number of excitable cells, including cardiac and vascular smooth muscle. Ca^{2+} enters the cell through these channels when the cell membrane is depolarised. The cardiac and vascular L-type Ca^{2+} channels have different subunit structures.
- **Voltage-operated T-type (transient, low-threshold-activated, fast inactivated) Ca^{2+} channels**: these are found in pacemaker cells of the sinoatrial and atrioventricular nodes, and are also present in vascular smooth muscle.

Calcium channel blockers (often referred to as calcium antagonists) have widely different chemical structures, but act principally by reducing Ca^{2+} influx through voltage-operated L-type Ca^{2+} channels. None of the currently available calcium channel blockers affect T-type channels to any important extent, or influence receptor (ligand)-mediated Ca^{2+} channels (which are involved in neurotransmitter release and respond to endogenous agonists such as noradrenaline [Fig. 5.5]).

There are clinically important differences among the calcium channel blockers, which bind to discrete receptors on the L-type Ca^{2+} channel. The receptor for verapamil is intracellular, while diltiazem and the dihydropyridines (such as nifedipine) have extracellular binding sites; however, the receptor domains for verapamil and diltiazem overlap. The various classes of calcium channel antagonists have different binding properties with their receptors: verapamil and diltiazem exhibit frequency-dependent receptor binding and gain access to the Ca^{2+} channel when it is in the open state (Ch. 1); in contrast, the dihydropyridines (e.g. nifedipine, amlodipine) preferentially bind to the channel in its inactivated state (Ch. 1). More Ca^{2+} channels are inactive in relaxed smooth muscle and dihydropyridines show relative selectivity for binding to

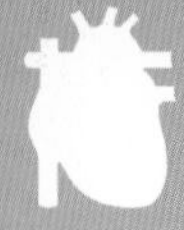

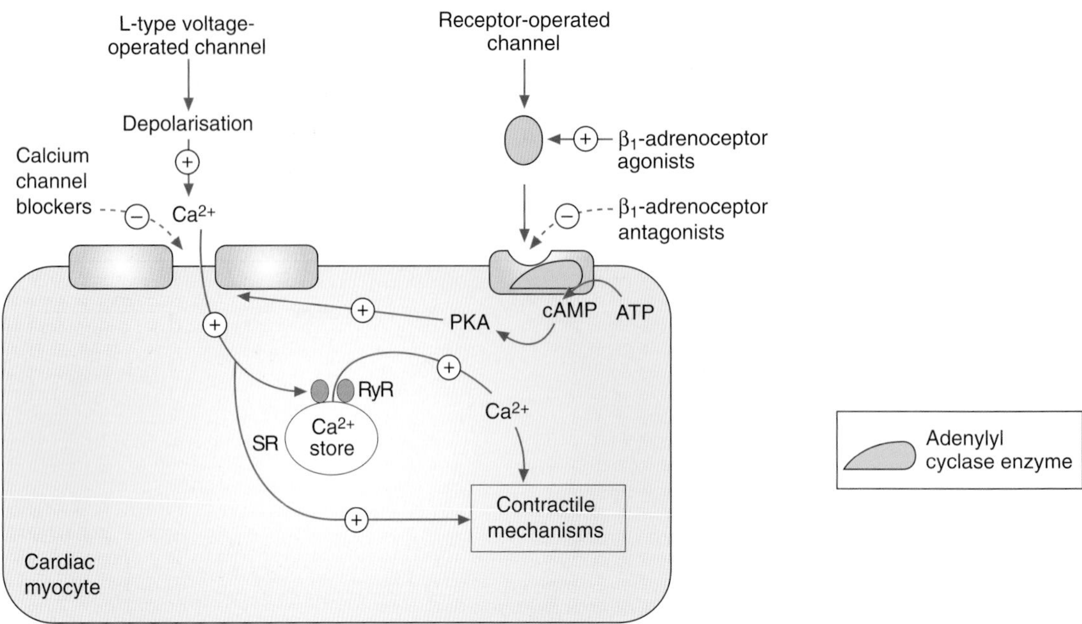

Fig. 5.5 **Contraction of the cardiac myocyte by receptor and voltage-operated mechanisms**. This figure illustrates some aspects of a complex system. Depolarisation during the action potential activates the L-type voltage-operated channels which are located in tubules and the plasma membrane. The influx of Ca^{2+} into the cell results in myosin phosphorylation and muscle contraction. It also promotes further Ca^{2+} release from the SR via stimulation of ryanodine receptors. Stimulation of the β_1- and β_2-adrenoceptors activates adenylyl cyclase and the generated cAMP binds to subunits of PKA, which phosphorylates L-type Ca^{2+} channels, increasing their opening time and facilitating Ca^{2+} entry. Block of L-type Ca^{2+} channels by calcium channel blockers or blockade of β_1-adrenoceptors will reduce activity of the voltage-operated channels. Other mechanisms exist (not shown). For example, stimulation of α-adrenoceptors stimulates PLC, which, via IP_3 and DAG generation, can release Ca^{2+} and phosphorylate L-type Ca^{2+} channels. DAG, diacylglycerol; IP_3, inositol 1,4,5 triphosphate; PKA, protein kinase A; PLC, phospholipase C; SR, sarcoplasmic reticulum; RyR, ryanodine receptor; +, stimulates activity; –, inhibits activity.

channels in vascular smooth muscle. These factors are important in determining the different pharmacological effects of the calcium channel blockers, and account for the relative vascular selectivity of the dihydropyridines and the antiarrhythmic properties of verapamil and diltiazem (Ch. 8).

Calcium channel blockers produce a number of effects that are important in the treatment of angina.

- **Arteriolar dilation**. Although all calcium channel blockers are vasodilators, dihydropyridine derivatives, such as nifedipine or amlodipine, are the most potent and show the greatest vascular selectivity. Arterial dilation reduces peripheral resistance and lowers the blood pressure. This reduces the work of the left ventricle, and therefore reduces myocardial oxygen demand. Short-acting dihydropyridines (e.g. nifedipine) produce a rapid drop in blood pressure after oral dosing, and reflex sympathetic nervous system activation leads to tachycardia (Fig. 5.6). Longer-acting compounds (e.g. amlodipine) or modified-release formulations of short-acting dihydropyridines gradually reduce blood pressure and cause little reflex tachycardia.
- **Coronary artery dilation**. Prevention or relief of coronary vasospasm improves myocardial blood flow.
- **Negative chronotropic effect**. Verapamil and diltiazem (but not the dihydropyridines) slow the rate of firing of the sinoatrial node and slow conduction of the impulse through the atrioventricular node (see also Ch. 8). Thus, reflex tachycardia is not seen with these drugs and they also slow the rate of rise in heart rate during exercise.
- **Reduced cardiac contractility**. Most calcium channel blockers (but particularly verapamil) have a negative inotropic effect. Amlodipine does not impair myocardial contractility.

A comparison of the cardiovascular uses of the different calcium channel blockers is shown in the drug compendium table at the end of this chapter.

Pharmacokinetics

Most calcium channel blockers are lipophilic compounds with similar pharmacokinetic properties. They are almost completely absorbed from the gut lumen, and undergo variable first-pass metabolism. Nifedipine is inactivated by metabolism, while verapamil and diltiazem have active, although less potent, metabolites. Their half-lives are mostly in the range of 2 to 12 h, and modified-release formulations are widely used to prolong their duration of action. Nifedipine is also available in a liquid-containing capsule formula-

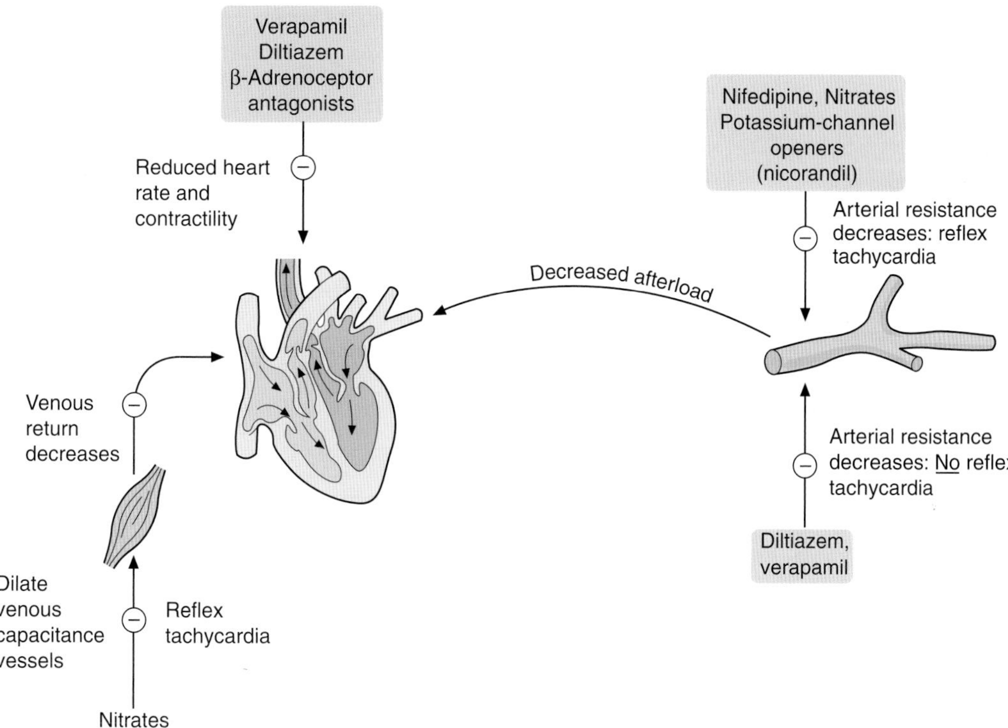

Fig. 5.6 **The complementary major sites of action of some antianginal drugs and the reflex response of the heart to their actions.** Reflex tachycardia results from the actions of nifedipine and potassium channel openers. Nifedipine causes a rapid fall in blood pressure, triggering the reflex. This is not a problem with diltiazem and verapamil, which slow heart rate. Reflex tachycardia can be minimised by using modified-release formulations of nifedipine or long-acting and more slowly acting compounds such as amlodipine.

tion; biting the capsule and swallowing the contents leads to a rapid onset of action. Verapamil can be given intravenously, a route that is usually reserved for the treatment of arrhythmias (Ch. 8).

Amlodipine differs from other calcium channel blockers in that it is slowly, but more completely, absorbed and does not undergo first-pass metabolism. It has a high volume of distribution (Ch. 2), due to extensive membrane partitioning in cells, and slower metabolism by the liver, which together result in a very long half-life of about 1–2 days.

Unwanted effects

- Arterial dilation can produce headache, flushing and dizziness, although tolerance often occurs with continued use. Ankle oedema, which is frequently resistant to diuretics, probably arises from increased transcapillary hydrostatic pressure. Tolerance to oedema does not occur. All these unwanted effects are most common with the dihydropyridines.
- Reduced cardiac contractility can precipitate heart failure in people with pre-existing poor left ventricular function, particularly with verapamil. Amlodipine, a dihydropyridine, does not depress cardiac contractility.
- Tachycardia and palpitations with dihydropyridines, especially with rapid-release formulations.
- Bradycardia and heart block with verapamil and diltiazem.
- Altered gut motility: constipation is most common with verapamil, less so with diltiazem. Nifedipine and related dihydropyridine drugs can cause nausea and heartburn.
- Gum hyperplasia.
- Drug interactions: verapamil and diltiazem can slow the heart rate excessively if they are used in combination with other drugs that have similar effects on atrioventricular nodal conduction, for example digoxin (Ch. 8) or β-adrenoceptor antagonists. Metabolism of many calcium channel blockers can be inhibited or accelerated by drugs that affect the liver P450 cytochrome enzymes.

Potassium channel openers

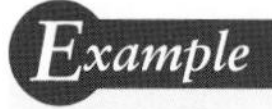

nicorandil

Mechanism of action

There are many different K^+ channels in cell membranes (Ch. 8, Table 8.1). They impact on several aspects of cellular function in health and disease. The K_{ATP} channels exist in

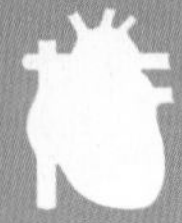

different tissues in a variety of configurations of subunits, making tissue specificity of drug action on the channels possible. The vascular adenosine triphosphate (ATP)-sensitive channel provides an inward rectifying current, and, when opened, K^+ exits the cell and results in hyperpolarisation. The channel is inhibited by ATP. Nicorandil opens the ATP-sensitive channel (Fig. 5.4). The hyperpolarisation produced in vascular smooth muscle cells inhibits opening of the voltage-dependent L-type Ca^{2+} channels, leading to vasodilation in systemic and coronary arteries (Fig. 5.4). In addition, enhanced K^+ channel function may provide protection of myocardial cells against ischaemic injury.

Nicorandil also carries a nitrate moiety, and part of its vasodilator action is via generation of nitric oxide in vascular smooth muscle (see organic nitrates above). This may account for the venodilation produced by the drug.

Pharmacokinetics

Nicorandil is rapidly and almost completely absorbed from the gut. It is eliminated by hepatic metabolism and has a short half-life of 1 h. However, the tissue effects correlate poorly with the plasma concentration and the biological effect lasts up to 12 h.

Unwanted effects

- Arterial dilation causes headache in 25–50% of people, but tolerance usually occurs with continued use. Palpitations (caused by reflex activation of the sympathetic nervous system) and flushing are less common than headache (Fig. 5.6).
- Dizziness.
- Nausea, vomiting.

Specific sinus node inhibitors

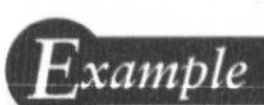

ivabradine

Mechanism of action

In cardiac pacemaker cells (such as the sinoatrial node) the pacemaker I_f current is responsible for diastolic depolarisation (Ch. 8). This is an inward current produced by the opening of channels permeable to both Na^+ and K^+ that are opened by the negative intracellular potential occurring in diastole. Ivabradine is a specific inhibitor of this current, and its major effect is to slow heart rate. The degree of channel inhibition is use-dependent, since ivabradine binds to the open channel from the internal side of the cell membrane. As a result, the efficacy of ivabradine increases with the frequency of channel opening and is greatest at higher heart rates. Unlike β-adrenoceptor antagonists, ivabradine has no effect on myocardial contractility.

Pharmacokinetics

Ivabradine is well absorbed from the gut, and undergoes extensive first-pass metabolism in the gut wall and liver. It is oxidised by CYP3A4 to a metabolite that retains activity. It has a half-life of 2 h.

Unwanted effects

- Bradycardia, first-degree heart block. It is recommended that the resting heart rate should not be allowed to fall below 50 beats min^{-1}.
- Headache, dizziness.
- Dose-related ocular symptoms, including phosphenes (flashes of light), photopsia, stroboscopic effects and blurred vision from inhibition of the I_f in the eye.

Late sodium current inhibitors

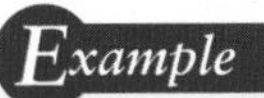

ranolazine

Mechanism of action

Transmembrane Na^+ channels are activated during the initial electrical excitation of myocardial cells, and are mainly inactivated during the plateau phase of the action potential. However, a small proportion of the Na^+ channels remain open, giving rise to the late Na^+ current. This current is increased in the presence of hypoxia, with a consequent increase in the intracellular Na^+ concentration. The rise in intracellular Na^+ activates the reverse mode of the Na^+/Ca^{2+} exchanger in the cell membrane, leading to removal of Na^+ from the cell, intracellular Ca^{2+} accumulation and increased diastolic myocardial tension (Fig. 5.4). Ranolazine attenuates the late transcellular Na^+ current in ischaemic myocardial cells, and reduces Ca^{2+} accumulation. There are two potentially beneficial consequences of this effect. The lower wall tension in the ventricles should reduce myocardial oxygen demand, and will also reduce compression of small intramyocardial coronary vessels, thus improving myocardial perfusion.

Pharmacokinetics

Ranolazine is partially absorbed from the gut, and extensively metabolised in the liver by CYP3A and to a limited extent CYP2D6. It has a short elimination half-life of about 2 h and a modified-release formulation is available.

Unwanted effects

- Nausea, dyspepsia, constipation
- Headache, dizziness, lethargy
- Prolongation of the QT interval on the ECG (Ch. 8), with the potential to provoke cardiac arrhythmias if used with other drugs that have the same effect.

MANAGEMENT OF STABLE ANGINA

The principal aims of treatment for stable angina are to relieve symptoms and to improve prognosis. Angina has a pronounced circadian rhythm and occurs most frequently in the hours after waking, so a drug given for prevention of symptoms should ideally be effective at this time. However, there is no convincing evidence that control of symptoms will affect either survival or the risk of a subsequent myocardial infarction. Improvement in prognosis is achieved mainly by using drugs that do not directly affect symptoms.

There are several important principles of management.

- Lifestyle changes: stopping smoking reduces coronary vasospasm, and may improve symptoms, but importantly reduces the risk of developing an acute coronary syndrome by up to 50%. Weight loss in people with obesity will reduce cardiac work, and regular exercise will improve fitness and attenuate the rise in heart rate on exercise.
- Reduction of high blood pressure to reduce cardiac work and to reduce progression of atheroma, and control of diabetes to reduce progression of atheroma.
- Reduction or elimination of provoking or exacerbating factors, such as anaemia, arrhythmias or thyrotoxicosis.
- Sublingual glyceryl trinitrate remains the treatment of choice for an acute anginal attack. It relieves symptoms within minutes, but gives only short-lived protection (20–30 min). Glyceryl trinitrate can also be taken for short-term prophylaxis before an activity that is likely to produce angina. For people who cannot tolerate a nitrate, a capsule of rapid-release nifedipine can be bitten and the contents swallowed to achieve a rapid effect.
- If anginal attacks are frequent, a longer-acting prophylactic antianginal drug should be used. A rise in heart rate is one of the main precipitating factors for angina, and a drug that lowers heart rate, such as a β-adrenoceptor antagonist, verapamil or diltiazem, may be most effective for first-line treatment. Nitrates are less suitable as first-line prophylactic agents because of the risk of tolerance. If symptoms are not controlled by optimal doses of a single drug, then a combination of a β-adrenoceptor antagonist with a calcium channel blocker (not verapamil), or either a β-adrenoceptor antagonist or calcium channel blocker with a long-acting nitrate, can be used. 'Triple therapy' (e.g. β-adrenoceptor antagonist, calcium channel blocker and a nitrate) has not been shown convincingly to be better than two agents, but the combination may sometimes give further symptomatic benefit. Nicorandil is generally used in combination therapy. The roles of ivabradine and ranolazine are less certain, particularly as their efficacy in combination with other antianginal drugs is unclear.
- Low-dose aspirin reduces the risk of subsequent myocardial infarction by about 35% (see Ch. 11).
- Lowering the total plasma cholesterol to <4.0 mmol L^{-1} by diet and by drugs (especially statins) (Ch. 48) reduces the risk of subsequent non-fatal myocardial infarction, cardiac death and the need for a coronary artery revascularisation procedure by more than 30%.
- ACE inhibitors (Ch. 6) have no antianginal action, but reduce the risk of subsequent myocardial infarction, especially in people at high risk of an event.
- Coronary artery bypass grafting (CABG) improves long-term prognosis compared with medical treatment in people with a left mainstem coronary artery stenosis, and in those with 'triple vessel disease' (significant stenoses of the left anterior descending, left circumflex and right coronary arteries) who have impaired left ventricular function. In less severe disease, it is used for symptom relief.
- Percutaneous coronary intervention (PCI; angioplasty, usually with insertion of a stent to maintain patency) is currently used for symptom relief only. Angioplasty alone is followed by a restenosis rate of about 40% at 6 months. This is reduced to about 20% by the use of a bare-metal stent, but with no difference in the risk of myocardial infarction or sudden death. Drug-eluting stents are coated with a polymer matrix containing an antiproliferative drug such as sirolimus or tacrolimus (Ch. 38). Their use has further reduced the risk of restenosis at 6 months to about 6%, but some have been associated with an increased risk of myocardial infarction. Insertion of a coronary artery stent requires intensive antiplatelet therapy with a combination of aspirin and clopidogrel to minimise early in-stent thrombosis. Short-term use of a glycoprotein IIb/IIIa antagonist such as abciximab (Ch. 11) further improves outcome for high-risk procedures.

Symptoms, and their response to treatment, are a poor guide to the severity of coronary artery disease, and exercise stress testing is a more accurate predictor. A poor performance during exercise testing, or failure to respond to two prophylactic drugs in adequate dosages, should lead to consideration of coronary angiography, with a view to CABG or PCI.

MANAGEMENT OF ACUTE CORONARY SYNDROMES

MANAGEMENT OF ACUTE CORONARY SYNDROMES WITHOUT ST-SEGMENT ELEVATION

Acute coronary syndromes require urgent treatment even if there is no initial evidence of myocardial infarction, since there is about a 10% risk of progression from unstable angina to myocardial infarction or death. A rise in the plasma concentrations of a sensitive marker of myocardial damage, such as troponin I or troponin T, is used to differentiate unstable angina from myocardial infarction, and to identify those at highest risk of a subsequent myocardial infarction or death. The management of an acute coronary syndrome is initially determined by the ECG. In the absence of ST-segment elevation on the ECG, management is intensive until a plasma troponin is obtained about 12 h after the onset of pain. If this is not raised and the ECG does not show ischaemic changes, then the risk of a subsequent cardiac event is much lower and treatment is then less intensive.

- Initial treatment is with sublingual glyceryl trinitrate and supplementary oxygen. Analgesia with an intravenous opioid such as morphine (Ch. 19), together with an antiemetic, is used for prolonged pain that does not settle with a nitrate.
- A loading dose of aspirin, followed by low-dose aspirin for maintenance (Ch. 11), should be given. Full anticoagulation with intravenous heparin or, more commonly, subcutaneous low-molecular-weight heparin (enoxaparin; Ch. 11) produces additive benefit. The risk of myocardial infarction or death within 14 days is reduced by about 60% using combined treatment with aspirin and heparin. Fondaparinux (Ch. 11) given subcutane-

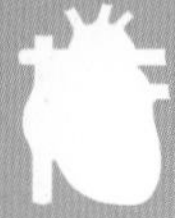

ously is as effective as low-molecular-weight heparin, and with a lower risk of bleeding. Dual platelet inhibition with clopidogrel and aspirin for at least a month and up to 1 year reduces the risk of myocardial infarction by a further 20% in non-ST-segment elevation myocardial infarction (NSTEMI) compared to aspirin alone, but is of no benefit in unstable angina. In people with NSTEMI who undergo percutaneous coronary intervention (PCI), the direct thrombin inhibitor bivalirudin (Ch. 11) further reduces the risk of ischaemic events during and after the procedure in combination with clopidogrel and aspirin. Heparin and a glycoprotein IIb/IIIa antagonist such as tirofiban (Ch. 11) can be used instead of bivalirudin, but there is a higher risk of bleeding.

- A β-adrenoceptor antagonist is the first-choice antianginal treatment, although a heart rate-limiting calcium channel blocker, such as verapamil or diltiazem, can be used if a β-adrenoceptor antagonist is contraindicated or not tolerated. A β-adrenoceptor antagonist reduces the risk of myocardial infarction by about 15% compared with no antianginal treatment. If the symptoms do not settle, then a dihydropyridine calcium channel blocker such as nifedipine, or nicorandil or a nitrate via a buccal tablet or by intravenous infusion can be used with a β-adrenoceptor antagonist. While these drugs often relieve symptoms, there is no evidence that they improve prognosis in acute coronary syndromes.
- In the acute phase of an acute coronary syndrome, angiography (followed when appropriate by CABG or PCI) is carried out for the 10% of people who are refractory to full medical treatment. If the unstable symptoms settle, those who had evidence of myocardial damage during the acute episode (an increase in the plasma concentration of troponin I or troponin T), or those who develop symptoms or ECG changes at an early stage during a standardised exercise test, should also be investigated by angiography.
- Cholesterol reduction to <4.0 mmol L^{-1} should be initiated by diet and a statin at the time of the event (Ch. 48). This reduces the long-term risk of myocardial infarction or cardiac death by 25–30%.

MANAGEMENT OF ST-SEGMENT ELEVATION MYOCARDIAL INFARCTION

The presence of ST-segment elevation on the ECG usually heralds a more extensive myocardial infarction, and, in contrast to non-ST-segment elevation myocardial infarction, assisted early opening of the occluded artery to reperfuse the myocardium limits the extent of myocardial damage and improves long-term outcomes.

- For pain relief, an intravenous opioid analgesic such as morphine (Ch. 19) is given, together with an antiemetic. Intramuscular injection should be avoided, since a low cardiac output and poor tissue perfusion often delay absorption. A nitrate (sublingual or intravenous) can also reduce pain by relief of coronary artery vasospasm at the site of the arterial occlusion, with restoration of some blood flow. An intravenous β-adrenoceptor antagonist can be given to reduce cardiac work, especially if there is hypertension, but should be avoided if there are signs of heart failure.
- Natural fibrinolysis can be enhanced by intravenous fibrinolytic therapy (Ch. 11) to rapidly reperfuse the occluded artery and limit the size of the infarct. Fibrinolysis is used only if there are clear ECG changes of ST-segment elevation acute myocardial infarction (characteristic ST-segment elevation in two or more contiguous leads) or left bundle branch block on the ECG and a good history of acute myocardial infarction. In the latter situation, an acute myocardial infarction cannot be easily diagnosed from the ECG but mortality is high. The greatest reduction in mortality is achieved in people at highest risk of death (i.e. anterior infarcts rather than inferior), the elderly (>65 years of age) and those with a presenting systolic blood pressure below 100 mmHg. Of the available agents, alteplase (rt-PA) produces more rapid reperfusion and opens a greater percentage of occluded vessels than does streptokinase, with better myocardial salvage and a consequent reduction in mortality. The synthetic rt-PA analogues such as tenecteplase achieve a similar outcome to alteplase, but are easier to administer and are increasingly used. Streptokinase is less commonly used now, since it produces symptomatic hypotension during about 10% of administrations. Alteplase and related drugs are less likely to lower blood pressure. Streptokinase should not be given if it has previously been used, since high titres of streptokinase-neutralising antibodies often persist for several years and may make repeat administration ineffective (Ch. 11). Alteplase and related compounds are relatively short-acting, and anticoagulation with heparin (preferably low-molecular-weight heparin) for 48 h after their use reduces reocclusion of the artery. As an alternative, fondaparinux (Ch. 11) for 8 days may further reduce mortality and reinfarction by up to 25% compared with heparin. Anticoagulation is not usually given after streptokinase because of its longer duration of action. Fibrinolytic therapy significantly reduces mortality if given within 12 h of the onset of pain, but the survival advantage is greater the earlier treatment is given. Treatment within 6 h of the onset of pain saves 30 lives per 1000 people treated, whereas only 20 lives per 1000 are saved if treatment is delayed to 6–12 h after the onset of pain.
- Percutaneous coronary intervention (PCI: coronary angioplasty, usually with insertion of a stent) can reduce mortality more than a fibrinolytic drug. It is the treatment of choice for reperfusion in ST-segment elevation myocardial infarction ('primary' PCI) if it can be started within 120 min of presentation, or if there are contraindications to fibrinolysis. 'Rescue' PCI can be considered if fibrinolysis has failed to reperfuse the infarct-related vessel.

In addition to the management discussed above, complications of myocardial infarction may need specific treatment (Box 5.1).

Secondary prophylaxis after myocardial infarction

Secondary prophylaxis to reduce late mortality after myocardial infarction can be achieved with several approaches.

Box 5.1 Complications after myocardial infarction

Heart failure
Cardiogenic shock
Cardiac rupture
  Free wall rupture
  Ventricular septal defect
Arrhythmias
  Ventricular fibrillation
  Ventricular tachycardia
  Supraventricular tachycardias
  Sinus bradycardia and heart block
Pericarditis
Intracardiac thrombus

- Stopping smoking is of major benefit, since it reduces the mortality after a myocardial infarction by up to 50%. Rehabilitation programmes, which include exercise, also reduce mortality by up to 25% and improve psychological recovery.
- Low-dose aspirin (Ch. 11) inhibits platelet aggregation and reduces mortality in the first few weeks when started within 24 h of the onset of pain, and reduces later mortality by up to 25%. Concurrent use of clopidogrel with aspirin for up to 1 year after the infarction reduces reinfarction after both ST- and non-ST-segment elevation myocardial infarction, compared with aspirin alone.
- Beta-adrenoceptor antagonists, started orally soon after the infarct, reduce both death and reinfarction by about 25%, although the mechanism is unknown. Greatest benefit is seen in those at highest risk, for example following anterior infarction and in those who have had serious post-infarct arrhythmias or post-infarct angina or heart failure. Heart failure should be controlled before a β-adrenoceptor antagonist is given (Ch. 7).
- An ACE inhibitor (Ch. 6) is of greatest benefit if there is clinical or radiological evidence of heart failure after myocardial infarction, with a reduction in mortality of about 25% over the subsequent year. There is a smaller survival advantage if there is significant left ventricular dysfunction after the infarction (an ejection fraction of 40% or less) but no clinical evidence of heart failure. In this group, a 20% reduction in mortality over 3–5 years after the event is accompanied by a significant reduction in non-fatal reinfarction (although the mechanism of this effect is unknown). ACE inhibitors also reduce both non-fatal reinfarction and death when there is well-preserved left ventricular function, although the absolute benefits are smaller. The effects of an ACE inhibitor are greatest with high doses, and are additional to those of a β-adrenoceptor antagonist. An angiotensin receptor antagonist (Ch. 6) has similar efficacy following myocardial infarction, and should be considered if an ACE inhibitor is poorly tolerated.
- Verapamil and diltiazem produce a small reduction in reinfarction, but do not reduce mortality. They may be detrimental if there have been symptoms or signs of heart failure. These drugs should be considered as an option only for those at high risk who cannot tolerate a β-adrenoceptor antagonist and who do not have significant left ventricular dysfunction. Nifedipine and similar calcium channel blockers do not improve prognosis after myocardial infarction.
- Long-term anticoagulation with warfarin (Ch. 11) reduces mortality and reinfarction to a similar extent to low-dose aspirin. In combination with aspirin, warfarin produces a further reduction in both fatal and non-fatal events but with an increased risk of bleeding.
- Cholesterol reduction to <4.0 mmol L^{-1} should be attempted by diet and usually cholesterol-lowering drugs, especially the statins (Ch. 48). Statins reduce reinfarction and cardiac death by 25–30%. Fibrates are less effective, but may be useful if the total cholesterol is not greatly raised but the high-density lipoprotein cholesterol is low.
- A Mediterranean diet reduces mortality after myocardial infarction. A further reduction in mortality can be achieved with supplementary omega-3 fatty acids. An antiarrhythmic effect may be responsible for these benefits (Ch. 48).

FURTHER READING

General

Hansson GK (2005) Inflammation, atherosclerosis and coronary heart disease. *N Engl J Med* 352, 1685–1695

Szewczyk A, Skalska J, Glab M et al (2006) Mitochondrial potassium channels: from pharmacology to function. *Biochim Biophys Acta* 1757, 715–720

Tamargo J, Caballero R, Gomez R et al (2004) Pharmacology of cardiac potassium channels. *Cardiovasc Res* 62, 9–33

Van der Hayden MAG, Wijnhoven TJM, Opthof T (2005) Molecular aspects of adrenergic modulation of cardiac L-type Ca^{2+} channels. *Cardiovasc Res* 65, 28–39

Stable angina

Abrams J (2005) Chronic stable angina. *N Engl J Med* 352, 2524–2533

Bales AC (2004) Medical management of chronic ischemic heart disease. Selecting specific drug therapies, modifying risk factors. *Postgrad Med* 115, 39–46

Belardinelli L, Shrycock JC, Fraser H (2006) The mechanism of ranolazine action to reduce ischemia-induced diastolic dysfunction. *Eur Heart J* 8(suppl A), A10–A13

Ben-Dor I, Battler A (2007) Treatment of stable angina. *Heart* 93, 868–874

Borer JS (2004) Drug insight: I_f inhibitors as specific heart-rate-reducing agents. *Nat Clin Pract Cardiovasc Med* 1, 103–109

Fayers KE, Cummings MH, Shaw KM et al (2003) Nitrate tolerance and the links with endothelial dysfunction and oxidative stress. *Br J Clin Pharmacol* 56, 620–628

Feher MD (2003) Lipid lowering to delay the progression of coronary artery disease. *Heart* 89, 451–458

Heidenreich PA, McDonald KM, Haslie T et al (1999) Meta-analysis of trials comparing β-blockers, calcium antagonists and nitrates for stable angina. *JAMA* 281, 1927–1936

Knight CJ (2003) Antiplatelet treatment in stable coronary artery disease. *Heart* 89, 1273–1278

Ko DT, Hebert PR, Coffey CS et al (2002) β-blocker therapy and symptoms of depression, fatigue, and sexual dysfunction. *JAMA* 288, 351–357

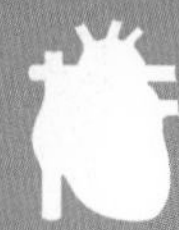

Nash DT, Nash SD (2008) Ranolazine for chronic stable angina. *Lancet* 372, 1335–1341

Ong HT (2007) β blockers in hypertension and cardiovascular disease. *BMJ* 334, 946–949

Opie LH, Commerford PJ, Gersh BJ (2007) Controversies in stable coronary heart disease. *Lancet* 367, 69–78

Toda N (2003) Vasodilating β-adrenoceptor blockers as cardiovascular therapeutics. *Pharmacol Ther* 100, 215–234

Weisman SM, Graham DY (2002) Evaluation of the benefits and risks of low-dose aspirin in the secondary prevention of cardiovascular and cerebrovascular events. *Arch Intern Med* 162, 2197–2202

Unstable angina and non-ST-segment elevation myocardial infarction

Bavry AA, Kumbhani DJ, Quiroz R et al (2004) Invasive therapy along with glycoprotein IIb/IIIa inhibitors and intracoronary stents improves survival in non-ST-segment elevation acute coronary syndromes: a meta-analysis and review of the literature. *Am J Cardiol* 93, 830–835

Chan MY, Becker RC, Harrington RA et al (2008) Noninvasive, medical management for non-ST-elevation acute coronary syndromes. *Am Heart J* 155, 397–407

Eikelboom JW, Anand SS, Malmberg K (2000) Unfractionated heparin and low molecular weight heparin in acute coronary syndrome without ST elevation: meta analysis. *Lancet* 355, 1936–1942

Jneid H, Bhatt DL, Corti R et al (2003) Aspirin and clopidogrel in acute coronary syndromes. Therapeutic insights from the CURE study. *Arch Intern Med* 163, 1145–1153

Kong DF, Hasselblad V, Harrington RA et al (2003) Meta-analysis of survival with platelet glycoprotein IIb/IIIa antagonists for percutaneous coronary interventions. *Am J Cardiol* 92, 651–655

Peters RJG, Mehta S, Yusuf S (2007) Acute coronary syndromes without ST segment elevation. *BMJ* 334, 1256–1259

Rothberg MB, Celestin C, Fiore LD et al (2005) Warfarin plus aspirin after myocardial infarction or acute coronary syndrome: meta-analysis with estimates of risk and benefit. *Ann Intern Med* 143, 241–250

Turpie AGG, Antman EM (2001) Low-molecular-weight heparins in the treatment of acute coronary syndromes. *Arch Intern Med* 161, 1484–1491

ST-segment elevation myocardial infarction

Boersma E, Mercado N, Poldermans D et al (2003) Acute myocardial infarction. *Lancet* 361, 847–858

Brouwer MA, Clappers N, Verheugt FWA (2004) Adjunctive treatment in patients treated with thrombolytic therapy. *Heart* 90, 581–588

COMMIT (ClOpidogrel and Metoprolol in Myocardial Infarction Trial) collaborative group (2005) Addition of clopidogrel to aspirin in 45 852 patients with acute myocardial infarction: randomised placebo-controlled trial. *Lancet* 366, 1607–1621

Dalal H, Evans PH, Campbell JL (2004) Recent developments in secondary prevention and cardiac rehabilitation after acute myocardial infarction. *BMJ* 328, 693–697

Gersh BJ, Antman EM (2006) Selection of the optimal reperfusion strategy for STEMI: does time matter? *Eur Heart J* 27, 761–763

Keeley EC, Hillis LD (2007) Primary PCI for myocardial infarction with ST-segment elevation. *N Engl J Med* 356, 47–54

Klein L, Gheorghiade M (2004) Management of the patient with diabetes mellitus and myocardial infarction. *Am J Med* 116(5A), 47s–63s

Lee VC, Rhew DC, Dylan M et al (2004) Meta-analysis: angiotensin-receptor blockers in chronic heart failure and high-risk acute myocardial infarction. *Ann Intern Med* 41, 693–704

Mendoza CE, Bhatt MR, Virani S et al (2006) Management of failed thrombolysis after acute myocardial infarction: an overview of current treatment options. *Int J Cardiol* 114, 291–299

Smalling RW (2006) Role of fibrinolytic therapy in the current era of ST-segment elevation myocardial infarction management. *Am Heart J* 151, S17–S23

Ting HH, Yang EH, Rihal CS (2006) Narrative review: Reperfusion strategies for ST-elevation myocardial infarction. *Ann Intern Med* 145, 610–617

White HD, Chew DP (2008) Myocardial infarction. *Lancet* 372, 570–584

SELF-ASSESSMENT

1. In the following questions, the first statement, in italics, is an important true statement. Is the accompanying statement true or false?
   a. *The mechanism by which glyceryl trinitrate causes vasodilation is through its ability to release nitric oxide.* Nitric oxide causes vasodilation by increasing cyclic adenosine monophosphate (cAMP) synthesis in vascular smooth muscle cells.
   b. *Glyceryl trinitrate has a more rapid onset of action when given sublingually than when given via a transdermal patch.* Transdermal absorption of glyceryl trinitrate from a patch avoids first-pass metabolism.
   c. *The increased oxygen demand of a rise in workload in the heart is met by an increase in coronary blood flow.* In angina, glyceryl trinitrate increases total coronary blood flow.
   d. *Glyceryl trinitrate can be administered safely with a β-adrenoceptor antagonist.* The benefit of glyceryl trinitrate in angina is primarily a result of its effect on coronary arteries.
   e. *Recombinant tissue-type plasminogen activator (rt-PA) is a genetically engineered copy of an endogenous fibrinolytic agent.* rt-PA inhibits the formation of plasmin.
2. From the following statements about angina and myocardial infarction, choose the one **incorrect** statement.
   A. Isosorbide 5-mononitrate is an active metabolite of isosorbide dinitrate and has the advantage that it does not undergo first-pass metabolism.
   B. Verapamil can reduce arterial blood pressure without causing reflex tachycardia.
   C. Platelet inhibitors such as the glycoprotein IIb/IIIa antagonist tirofiban can reduce the risk of myocardial infarction in high-risk individuals with unstable angina.
   D. Cholesterol reduction is of little benefit in reducing the risk of recurrence of myocardial infarction.
   E. Nifedipine does not improve prognosis after myocardial infarction.
3. Tolerance can develop when using isosorbide dinitrate. Which one of the following changes to the treatment regimen would reduce the likelihood of tolerance developing?

A. Switch to the longer-acting isosorbide mononitrate
B. Switch to using a continuously applied modified-release transdermal patch containing glyceryl trinitrate
C. Give glyceryl trinitrate in addition by the buccal route when necessary
D. Schedule doses so that there is period of low plasma concentration of isosorbide dinitrate each day
E. Administer isosorbide dinitrate together with a β-adrenoceptor antagonist

4. A combination of drugs was being prescribed for a person suffering from angina. Which one of the following combinations is **most likely** to have an adverse effect on cardiac function?
   A. Glyceryl trinitrate with the β-adrenoceptor antagonist atenolol
   B. Verapamil with the β-adrenoceptor antagonist atenolol
   C. Amlodipine with the β-adrenoceptor antagonist atenolol
   D. Glyceryl trinitrate with nicorandil
   E. Glyceryl trinitrate with low-dose aspirin

5. Case history questions

TK, a 65-year-old man who was a landscape gardener, had been having episodes of chest pain that he likened to indigestion. They were brought on by moderately strenuous exercise and relieved by rest but were not relieved by antacids. The symptoms had been present for approximately 1 year, but recently the frequency and intensity of the pains had become worse and they were now occurring several times a week. He was hypertensive and his serum cholesterol level was 6.6 mmol L^{-1}. He smoked 40 cigarettes per day and was overweight. He drank about 10 units of alcohol a week. He had a good exercise tolerance during a diagnostic exercise test but his ECG showed anterolateral ST-segment depression at peak exercise. There was no evidence of heart failure. A diagnosis of angina was made, and medical treatment started.

Despite continuing medication, 6 months later TK awoke with severe chest pains and dyspnoea that was not relieved by glyceryl trinitrate. Examination, biochemical tests and ECG recordings all led to the diagnosis of an acute ST-segment elevation myocardial infarction.

a. How could his acute attacks of angina have been treated?
b. The frequency of his attacks required prophylactic treatment. What options were available to reduce the frequency of anginal attacks?
c. What other drugs could have been useful to improve his prognosis?
d. Would lifestyle changes help Mr TK?
e. In unstable angina, which drug treatments would have been likely to reduce the progression of the episodes to myocardial infarction or sudden death?
f. What was the likely cause of the myocardial infarction?
g. Why was it important to give fibrinolytic therapy as quickly as possible?
h. TK was given the fibrinolytic agent recombinant tissue-type plasminogen activator (rt-PA; alteplase) because of fears that he would get an allergic response to streptokinase. Was this justified?
i. He was given 150 mg aspirin orally, after an initial loading dose. Would this have any added benefit if fibrinolytic therapy was also given?
j. The normal therapeutic dose of aspirin for headache is about 650 mg. Why was the dose given to TK so small?
k. Consideration was given to administering intravenous heparin to TK, but this was considered unnecessary because he had been given rt-PA. Was this decision correct?
l. Following his myocardial infarction, long-term prophylactic treatment of his condition was considered. Which of the following drugs would have been likely to be of benefit: low-dose aspirin, a β-adrenoceptor antagonist, an ACE inhibitor, verapamil, diltiazem or warfarin?

ANSWERS

1. a. **False**. Nitric oxide increases cGMP synthesis to bring about reduced intracellular free Ca^{2+} and vasodilation.
   b. **True**. Glyceryl trinitrate undergoes extensive first-pass metabolism after oral dosing, since initial entry into the systemic circulation is via the portal circulation and the liver. Transdermal patches or sublingual administration avoids the portal circulation and the drug gains direct access to the systemic circulation.
   c. **False**. Glyceryl trinitrate does not increase total coronary blood flow. It can, however, treat angina by increasing flow to the ischaemic areas by dilating collateral blood vessels or reducing coronary vasospasm.
   d. **False**. A major component of the benefit of glyceryl trinitrate is its peripheral vasodilator action, reducing preload and, to a lesser extent, peripheral vascular resistance, and afterload. These reduce workload on the heart. The reflex tachycardia that occurs through a fall in peripheral resistance can be reduced by concomitant treatment with a β-adrenoceptor antagonist.
   e. **False**. rt-PA cleaves plasminogen to increase the formation of plasmin, which results in the degradation of the fibrin that forms the framework of the thrombus (see Ch. 11).
2. Answer **D**.
   A. Correct – and can therefore give a more predictable response of greater duration.
   B. Correct. Unlike the dihydropyridines, verapamil also acts on the heart and reflex tachycardia does not occur. Modified-release formulations of dihydropyridines or the long-acting dihydropyridine amlodipine also reduce the incidence of reflex tachycardia.
   C. Correct. Platelet inhibition with an intravenous glycoprotein IIb/IIIa antagonist such as tirofiban reduces the risk of myocardial infarction or death in those at

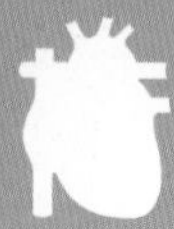

high risk (see also Ch. 11). These agents are most effective when there is a raised plasma concentration of the markers of myocardial damage, troponin I or troponin T.

D. Incorrect. Cholesterol reduction to <4.0 mmol L^{-1} should be attempted. Statins reduce reinfarction and cardiac death by 25–30%. Fibrates are less effective, but may be useful if the total cholesterol is normal or only modestly increased but the high-density lipoprotein cholesterol is low.

E. Correct. Nifedipine and similar dihydropyridine calcium channel antagonists do not improve prognosis after myocardial infarction. Verapamil and diltiazem produce a small reduction in reinfarction, but do not reduce mortality. They may be detrimental if there are signs of heart failure. These drugs should only be considered as an option for those at high risk who cannot tolerate a β-adrenoceptor antagonist and who do not have significant left ventricular dysfunction.

3. Answer **D**.
The only way to reduce tolerance is to allow periods with low plasma organic nitrate. Tolerance will develop to all the organic nitrates independent of the route given if plasma concentrations remain high continuously. A β-adrenoceptor antagonist will reduce reflex tachycardia but not the development of tolerance.

4. Answer **B**.
Verapamil and atenolol both have a negative inotropic effect and this could be problematic, particularly if there are signs of heart failure. They also have a negative chronotropic effect and the combination can cause severe bradycardia and heart block. It is possible that amlodipine and atenolol could cause excessive hypotension, but this is less likely. The other combinations are frequently given together:
   A. atenolol prevents reflex tachycardia caused by the nitrate
   D. nicorandil does not have any direct effect on the heart
   E. aspirin will reduce the likelihood of development of myocardial infarction.

5. Case history answers
   a. For acute attacks, sublingual glyceryl trinitrate is the first-choice drug to give rapid relief, although protection is only short-lived.
   b. For prophylaxis, a β-adrenoceptor antagonist is often the treatment of first choice, or a calcium channel blocker if this is contraindicated. A combination of both, or addition of a long-acting nitrate (but tolerance is a problem), could be used if symptoms are not well controlled with a single agent, but the benefit of triple therapy is not convincing. For example, atenolol and diltiazem given together significantly decrease the number of angina attacks compared with either used alone. These drugs will also lower blood pressure and heart rate, which are precipitating factors for angina. Their use together should be carefully monitored, however, because of the dangers of compounding bradycardia or heart failure.
   c. Additional therapy to improve prognosis includes low-dose aspirin (75–150 mg), which has been shown to reduce the risk of subsequent myocardial infarction. Lowering plasma cholesterol concentration by diet or by drugs such as simvastatin can also reduce the risk of subsequent myocardial infarction.
   d. Smoking, lack of exercise and obesity are all risk factors for coronary heart disease. TK is exposed to these increased risks and should address these by lifestyle changes.
   e. The most consistent evidence is for combined use of heparin and aspirin in unstable angina. Addition of a β-adrenoceptor antagonist produces a small additional benefit.
   f. Coronary artery occlusion at the site of an atheroma, causing myocardial necrosis.
   g. The benefit of fibrinolytic therapy is strongly dependent upon the delay between symptoms and administration. The benefit is particularly great if fibrinolytic therapy can be administered within 6 h from the onset of pain, but there is good evidence for benefit until at least 12 h.
   h. Allergic reactions to streptokinase are extremely rare. TK had not had a previous myocardial infarction and had not previously been administered streptokinase, so would be unlikely to have high titres of streptokinase-neutralising antibodies. It would, therefore, be safe to give TK streptokinase unless he had severe symptomatic hypotension. However, alteplase or a derivative is usually preferred.
   i. Aspirin and fibrinolytic therapy have been shown to have additive benefit for treating acute myocardial infarction, reducing subsequent reinfarction or death.
   j. Low doses of aspirin reduce the production of the platelet-aggregating agent thromboxane A_2 by platelets, while having less effect on the production of the platelet-disaggregating agent prostaglandin I_2 from endothelial cells. Large doses of aspirin do not produce any additional benefit, and the risk of gastric irritation or ulceration is increased.
   k. This is incorrect. Streptokinase has a longer duration of action than rt-PA and it is generally unnecessary to administer heparin when streptokinase has been given. However, it is necessary after the short-acting rt-PA, when it improves the long-term patency of the artery.
   l. Low-dose aspirin, β-adrenoceptor antagonists and ACE inhibitors all reduce mortality and the risk of reinfarction. The β-adrenoceptor antagonist will need to be given under close observation, since it carries a risk of worsening heart failure. In people who have signs of heart failure, verapamil and diltiazem may also be detrimental. Warfarin reduces mortality and reinfarction to a similar extent as low-dose aspirin, so is not required unless aspirin is poorly tolerated.

Drugs used to treat ischaemic heart disease

Drug	Half-life (h) and kinetics	Comments
Beta-adrenoceptor antagonists		
All drugs are given orally unless otherwise indicated. Beta-adrenoceptor antagonists are used in a wide variety of indications in addition to ischaemic heart disease, including hypertension and arrhythmias. For completeness, all oral or parenteral β-adrenoceptor antagonists are listed in this chapter, irrespective of their specific licensed clinical uses		
Acebutolol	7 [M + R] Oral bioavailability is 50–70%; active acetylated metabolite	β_1-Adrenoceptor selective; 10% β_1-adrenoceptor selective PAA; drug-induced lupus reported
Atenolol	7 [R] Eliminated by glomerular filtration	β_1-Adrenoceptor selective; given orally, or by injection or intravenous infusion
Betaxolol	13–24 [M + R] High oral bioavailability (80–90%); oxidised in liver and metabolites eliminated in urine	Also used topically for glaucoma; β_1-adrenoceptor selective
Bisoprolol	11 [M + R] Oral bioavailability is 90%; eliminated equally by glomerular filtration and secretion, and by metabolism in the liver	β_1-Adrenoceptor selective (less than atenolol)
Carvedilol	6 [M] Oral bioavailability is 20–30% owing to first-pass metabolism; metabolites eliminated in bile and urine	β-Adrenoceptor non-selective; vasodilator action from α_1-adrenoceptor blockade
Celiprolol	5 [R + some bile] Polar compound that has an oral bioavailability of 30–70% because of poor absorption	β_1-Adrenoceptor-selective; vasodilator action because of β_2-adrenoceptor PAA
Esmolol	0.15 [M] Rapidly hydrolysed in erythrocytes	β_1-Adrenoceptor selective; given by intravenous infusion
Labetalol	3 [M] Oral bioavailability is variable (10–90%) owing to first-pass metabolism; metabolised by glucuronidation	β_1-Adrenoceptor selective; vasodilator action through α-adrenoceptor blockade; α:β selectivity is 1:2 orally and 1:7 intravenously; given orally, or by intravenous injection or intravenous infusion
Metoprolol	3–10 [M + R] Oral bioavailability is about 50%; wide variability in metabolism by CYP2D6	β_1-Adrenoceptor selective (less than atenolol); given orally, or by injection or intravenous infusion
Nadolol	17–24 [R + bile] Poor absorption (30%)	β-Adrenoceptor non-selective
Nebivolol	10 [M] Metabolised by oxidation	β_1-Adrenoceptor selective; vasodilator from generation of NO
Oxprenolol	2 [M] Oral bioavailability is 20–80% owing to first-pass metabolism; hydroxy metabolite also active	β-Adrenoceptor non-selective; 18% β-adrenoceptor non-selective PAA
Pindolol	4 [M + R] High oral bioavailability (>90%); approximately equal elimination in urine and by metabolism	β-Adrenoceptor non-selective; vasodilator because of 35% β-adrenoceptor non-selective PAA
Propranolol	4 [M] Oral bioavailability is 10–50% owing to first-pass metabolism; oxidised by P450 and conjugated with glucuronic acid (17%)	β-Adrenoceptor non-selective; given orally or by intravenous injection
Sotalol	7–18 [R]	See under class III drugs (Ch. 8); uses restricted to life-threatening arrhythmias
Timolol	2–5 [M + some R] Oral bioavailability is 30–50%; eliminated by metabolism and renal excretion (20%)	Also used topically for glaucoma; β-adrenoceptor non-selective

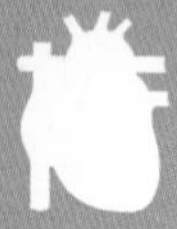

Drugs used to treat ischaemic heart disease

Drug	Half-life (h) and kinetics	Comments
Calcium channel blockers		
All are given orally unless stated otherwise; indications include angina, hypertension, Raynaud's phenomenon, arrhythmias and subarachnoid haemorrhage (see Chs 6 and 8–10)		
Dihydropyridines		
Metabolites are generally inactive; modified-release formulations are available for many of these drugs and are preferred for the treatment of angina and hypertension as they reduce fluctuations in blood pressure and reflex tachycardia. They have no antiarrhythmic activity		
Amlodipine	30–60 [M] Oral bioavailability is 60–80%; oxidised in liver	No detrimental effect in heart failure; used once daily
Felodipine	12–25 [M] Oral bioavailability is about 15% owing to first-pass metabolism; oxidised by CYP3A4	No detrimental effect in heart failure; used once daily
Isradipine	2–6 [M] Oral bioavailability is 20% owing to first-pass metabolism	
Lacidipine	7–8 [M] Low and variable oral bioavailability (4–52%) (common to many dihydropyridines owing to variable intestinal and hepatic CYP3A4 activity)	
Lercanidipine	3–5 [M] Oral bioavailability is 44% and is increased by a fatty meal; eliminated by CYP3A4-mediated oxidation to inactive metabolites	Long duration of action (24 h), by an undefined mechanism; used once daily
Nicardipine	1–12 [M] Oral bioavailability is dose-dependent owing to first-pass metabolism (5–10% at low doses and 30–45% at high doses); metabolised in liver	
Nifedipine	2–4 [M] Oral bioavailability is about 40% owing to first-pass metabolism by CYP3A4 in gut wall and liver	
Nimodipine	8–9 [M] Oral bioavailability is 5–10%; eliminated by oxidation in the liver	Selective for cerebral arteries; use is confined to the prevention and treatment of ischaemic neurological deficits following subarachnoid haemorrhage; given orally or by intravenous infusion
Nisoldipine	2–4 [M] Oral bioavailability is low (5–10%) and variable owing to intestinal and hepatic CYP3A4 metabolism; numerous metabolites	
Non-dihydropyridines		
In contrast to dihydropyridines, these drugs are also used for treatment and prevention of supraventricular arrhythmias, but are less effective for Raynaud's phenomenon. Modified-release formulations are available		
Diltiazem	2–5 [M] Oral bioavailability is about 50% owing to first-pass metabolism; a number of metabolites, mostly inactive	Reduces heart rate; some negative inotropic effect and should be avoided in heart failure
Verapamil	2–5 [M] Oral bioavailability is about 20% owing to first-pass metabolism; oxidised by CYP3A4; metabolites retain activity but are rapidly eliminated by conjugation; half-life is longer after chronic dosing (5–12 h)	Reduces heart rate; marked negative inotropic effect and should be avoided in heart failure; given orally or by slow intravenous injection (over 2 min)

Drugs used to treat ischaemic heart disease

Drug	Half-life (h) and kinetics	Comments
Nitrates		
Used for treatment of angina and in the management of heart failure		
Glyceryl trinitrate	1–3 min [M] Essentially complete first-pass metabolism if swallowed; the dinitrate metabolites have 10% of the activity but half-lives of about 40 min	Given sublingually, buccally, topically or as an intravenous infusion
Isosorbide dinitrate	0.5–2 [M] Low bioavailability from sublingual (30–60%) and topical (10–30%) administration; the active mononitrate metabolite inhibits clearance of the dinitrate during chronic treatment; high first-pass metabolism	Given sublingually, orally (as normal or modified-release tablets), topically or by intravenous infusion
Isosorbide mononitrate	3–7 [M] Oral bioavailability approaches 100%; metabolised by denitration and glucuronide conjugation; low first-pass metabolism	Given orally
Potassium channel activators		
Nicorandil	1 [M] Essentially complete oral bioavailability; oxidised and denitrated in the liver; biological effect much longer than predicted by half-life	Used for angina; given orally
Specific sinus node inhibitor		
Ivabradine	2 [M + R] Has an active N-dealkylated metabolite	Used for angina; given orally
Late sodium current inhibitor		
Ranolazine	1.4–1.9 [M + 5%R] Oral bioavailability is about 35–50%; metabolised largely by CYP3A4 and to a limited extent by CYP2D6	Approved for treatment of stable angina (in combination with amlodipine, β-adrenoceptor antagonists or nitrates) in those who have not achieved an adequate response or are intolerant of other antianginal agents

[M], metabolism; [R], renal excretion; PAA, partial agonist activity.

6 Systemic and pulmonary hypertension

SYSTEMIC HYPERTENSION

The cause of systemic hypertension in the majority of people is unknown, but abnormal regulation of the physiological mechanisms that normally control arterial blood pressure may be an important factor.

CIRCULATORY REFLEXES AND THE CONTROL OF SYSTEMIC BLOOD PRESSURE

Systemic blood pressure (BP) is determined by the cardiac output (CO) and by total peripheral resistance (TPR).

$$BP = CO \times TPR$$

Blood pressure is maintained within fairly narrow limits by a series of physiological reflexes that respond to both acute and chronic changes in blood pressure. There are both short-term and long-term control mechanisms. Important regulatory systems are:

- the autonomic nervous system
- the renin–angiotensin–aldosterone system
- local chemical mediators at the vascular endothelium.

The autonomic nervous system regulates arterial blood pressure by several mechanisms.

- *In the heart*, sympathetic impulses act mainly through β_1-adrenoceptors to increase myocardial contractility and heart rate, generating a greater cardiac output and increasing blood pressure (Ch. 4).
- *In arterial resistance vessels*, sympathetic stimulation of postsynaptic α_1-adrenoceptors produces arteriolar vasoconstriction. This raises blood pressure and redistributes blood flow to selected vascular beds to maintain perfusion of vital organs. This redistribution is helped by β_2-adrenoceptor-mediated vasodilation in skeletal muscle. Arterial vasoconstriction produces an increase in afterload on the heart, but, in the healthy heart, cardiac output is maintained by an increase in cardiac contractility.
- *In venous capacitance vessels*, sympathetic stimulation of postsynaptic α_1-adrenoceptors produces venous constriction. This increases venous return to the heart (preload), raises cardiac output and increases blood pressure (Fig. 7.1).
- *Stimulation of the parasympathetic nervous system* mainly acts by increasing the vagal output to the heart, slowing heart rate and reducing cardiac output. This reduces blood pressure (Ch. 4).

The autonomic nervous system provides immediate control of blood pressure. Change in systemic blood pressure is detected by baroreceptors (stretch receptors) in the aorta and carotid arteries. When blood pressure rises, stretch of the baroreceptors causes an increase in afferent nerve firing to the coordinating area in the medulla. This results in reflex inhibition of the sympathetic nervous system output and heightened parasympathetic outflow to the cardiovascular system, returning the blood pressure to normal. The opposite occurs when blood pressure falls (Fig. 6.1).

A slower compensatory mechanism in response to a reduction in blood pressure is initiated by the release of renin from the juxtaglomerular apparatus of the kidney (Fig. 6.2). The major stimuli leading to renin release are reduced renal blood flow (often as a result of a decrease in blood pressure), decreased Na^+ in the renal distal tubule, and direct sympathetic stimulation via β_1-adrenoceptors at the juxtaglomerular apparatus.

Renin is a protease that acts on circulating renin substrate (angiotensinogen) to release the decapeptide angiotensin I. This is cleaved by angiotensin-converting enzyme (ACE) to release the octapeptide angiotensin II. There are also several other enzymatic pathways for generating angiotensin II that do not involve ACE (Fig. 6.9). Angiotensin II acts on various tissues via its receptors, principally receptor types AT_1R and AT_2R (Fig. 6.2). Action at the AT_1R causes potent vasoconstriction, and also enhances sympathetic nervous tone by facilitating presynaptic neuronal release of

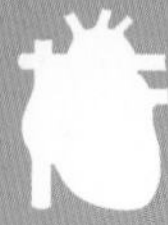

noradrenaline and through stimulation of central sympathetic outflow. Angiotensin II has a number of additional properties which promote salt and water retention (Fig. 6.3), one of the most powerful being the release of aldosterone from the adrenal cortex. Aldosterone acts at the distal renal tubule to conserve salt and water at the expense of K^+ loss (Ch. 14). Thus, angiotensin II and aldosterone raise blood pressure by vasoconstriction and by increasing circulating blood volume. Some actions of angiotensin II at the AT_2R appear to oppose those at the AT_1R (Fig. 6.2). Not all of the actions of stimulation of the AT_1R elevate blood pressure; its stimulation will enhance nitric oxide production in endothelium, resulting in vasodilation and dampening the pressor effects of angiotensin II (Fig. 6.4).

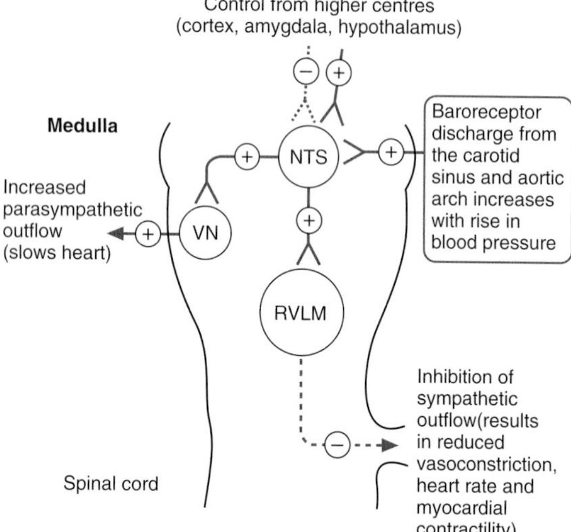

Fig. 6.1 **The role of baroreceptors**. Increased discharge from the baroreceptors in the carotid sinus and aortic arch results from stretch caused by increased blood pressure. This results in both a compensatory inhibition in sympathetic outflow from the medulla and an increase in the parasympathetic outflow. Both effects act to lower blood pressure; centrally acting drugs that lower blood pressure mimic the effect of increased baroreceptor outflow to the medullary centres (Fig. 6.8). NTS, nucleus of the tractus solitarius; RVLM, rostral ventrolateral medulla; VN, vagal nucleus (cardioinhibitory centre); +, stimulation; – , inhibition.

The integration of the fast-responding sympathetic nervous system and the slower-responding renin–angiotensin–aldosterone system in response to a fall in blood pressure is shown in Figure 6.3. These mechanisms prevent hypotension due to peripheral pooling of blood on standing and during exercise.

Additional mechanisms involved in controlling vascular tone and blood volume include circulating or local endothelial hormones and metabolites, such as natriuretic peptides, prostaglandins, bradykinin, nitric oxide, endothelin and adenosine (Fig. 6.4). Their relative importance may differ in health and disease states.

AETIOLOGY AND PATHOGENESIS OF SYSTEMIC HYPERTENSION

Hypertension is a common condition, found in 20–30% of the population of the developed world. It is usually asymptomatic but produces progressive structural changes in the heart and circulation. These predispose to clinical complications that are often referred to as 'target organ damage'. The principal complications of hypertension are ischaemic heart disease (especially in middle-aged Europeans and Americans), and cerebrovascular disease (especially in Asian and older people), which usually presents as thromboembolic stroke or, less commonly, as cerebral haemorrhage (Ch. 9). Ischaemic complications of hypertension are

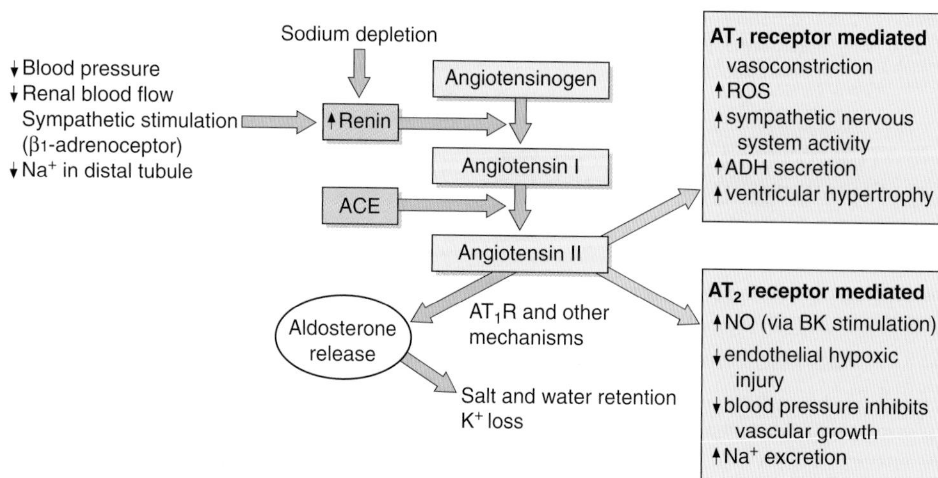

Fig. 6.2 **Formation and actions of angiotensin II**. Angiotensin II acts on a number of receptor subtypes. The type 1 (AT_1R) and type 2 (AT_2R) only are described. Currently, therapeutic drugs act predominantly to block the AT_1R type. The number of AT_2R is low relative to that of AT_1R but increases in pathological conditions. ACE, angiotensin-converting enzyme; ADH, antidiuretic hormone; BK, bradykinin, NO nitric oxide; ROS, reactive oxygen species.

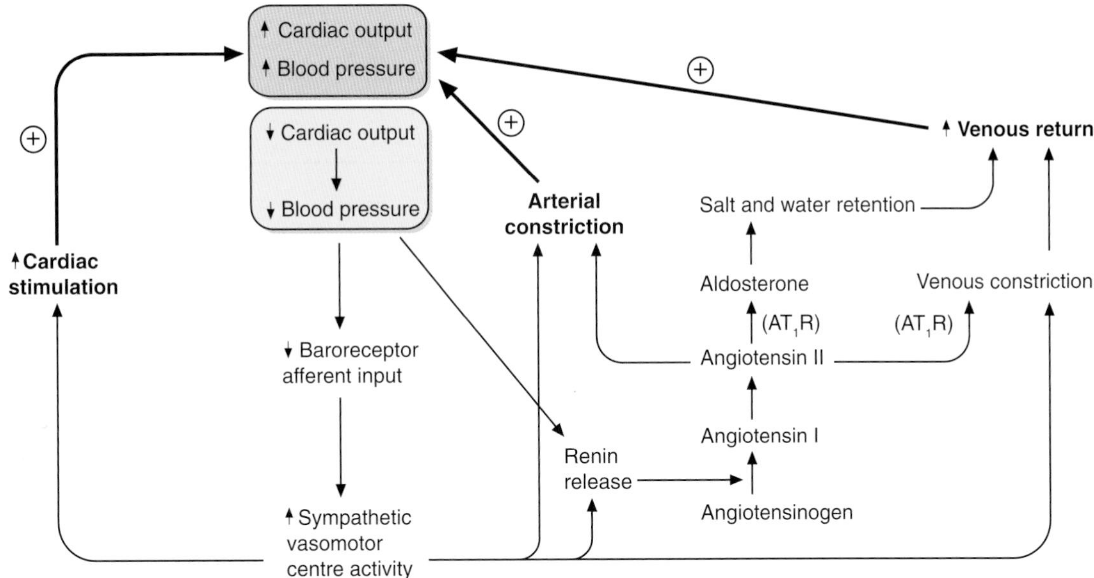

Fig. 6.3 **The control of blood pressure via the sympathetic and angiotensin/aldosterone cascades.** The integrated physiological compensatory mechanisms that occur in response to a fall in cardiac output or blood pressure (start at the yellow box). The sympathetic-mediated responses in the diagram are generally considered to be more rapidly responding events, whereas the angiotensin/aldosterone events are slower events. The final outcomes are increased venous return, increased arterial constriction and increased cardiac stimulation. Other events that may be important in controlling blood pressure at the level of the endothelium are shown in Figure 6.4. AT_1R, angiotensin type-1 receptor.

more common if it is accompanied by hypercholesterolaemia, diabetes and smoking. The underlying vascular lesions that occur in hypertension and their resulting complications are shown in Figure 6.5.

Sustained hypertension predisposes to left ventricular muscle hypertrophy (LVH). LVH is an independent risk factor for the complications of hypertension, particularly ischaemic heart disease (since the muscle outgrows its blood supply), diastolic heart failure (Ch. 7) and arrhythmias leading to sudden death (Ch. 8).

There is no absolute cut-off between normal and high blood pressure. Blood pressure in all populations is 'normally' distributed with a slight skew because of a small number of individuals with very high blood pressures. The risk of complications is also a continuous variable, increasing as blood pressure rises. Defining a point at which blood pressure is 'high' is, therefore, somewhat arbitrary, but is usually set at values greater than 140/90 mmHg. If target organ damage or diabetes is present, treatment reduces complications when introduced at blood pressures above this level. However, if there is no target organ damage, treatment may not alter outcome until the systolic pressure is sustained above 160 mmHg, or the diastolic blood pressure is sustained above 100 mmHg.

The diagnosis of sustained hypertension requires at least two, and preferably more, blood pressure readings over a time interval determined by the initial height of the blood pressure, unless target organ damage gives a clear indication that earlier treatment is necessary. Sometimes, the blood pressure is raised only when the measurement is taken by a doctor or, to a lesser extent, by a nurse. This phenomenon is termed 'white coat' or 'office' hypertension and appears to carry little risk of complications over the subsequent few years. It can usually be detected by repeated blood pressure readings that gradually approach the normal range, by measuring the blood pressure at home, or by use of an ambulatory 24-h blood pressure monitor. White coat hypertension often persists despite drug treatment, which can then result in quite troublesome *hypotension* away from the surgery or clinic. There is also a phenomenon of 'masked' hypertension, when blood pressure is normal in the clinic but high at home. This may carry a greater risk of complications than white coat hypertension.

Malignant or accelerated hypertension is an infrequently encountered condition, produced by very high blood pressure or a rapid rise in blood pressure. It is characterised pathologically by arterial fibrinoid necrosis, and identified clinically by the presence of flame-shaped haemorrhages, hard exudates, and 'cotton wool' spots in the retina, which can lead to visual disturbance. Papilloedema can also occur. If untreated, it usually leads to death within 5 years from renal failure, heart failure or stroke.

Hypertension is usually associated with increased peripheral arterial resistance, which arises from arteriolar smooth muscle constriction and hypertrophy of the arteriolar wall with an increase in the wall-to-lumen ratio and a smaller lumen (vascular remodelling). Cardiac output is often normal in younger people with hypertension, but reduced in the elderly. The cause of the inappropriately raised peripheral resistance is unknown in the majority of people with hypertension, who are said to have 'essential' hypertension. Essential hypertension probably has a polygenic inheritance, leading to several clinical subtypes with different underlying pathogenic mechanisms. Environmental influences and factors such as diet, level of exercise,

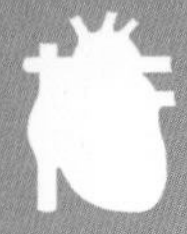

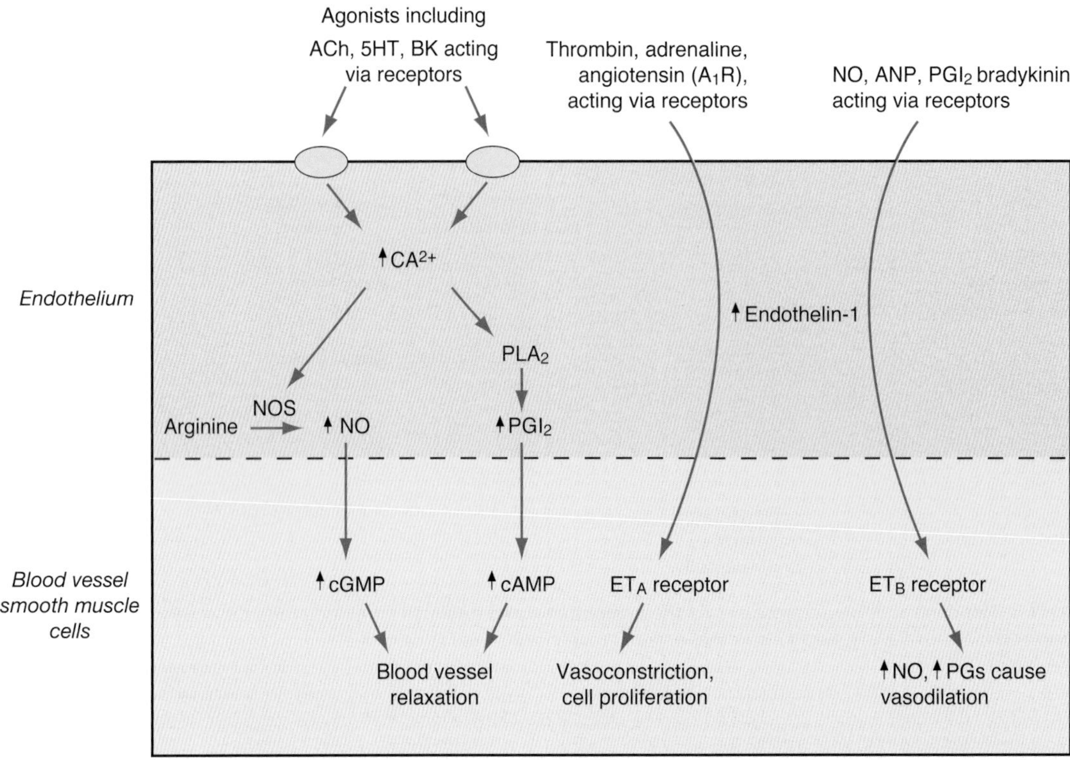

Fig. 6.4 **Influences of endothelial cells on blood vessel smooth muscle cell contractility.** Endothelial cells respond to a number of mediators and drugs resulting in the synthesis of second messengers and vascular smooth muscle cell modulators that can pass to the underlying vascular smooth muscle and result in relaxation or contraction. Precise mechanisms of control may vary in different vascular beds. The production of endothelial vasoactive nitric oxide (NO), prostaglandin PGI_2 (prostacyclin) and endothelin-1 can be influenced by many natural mediators and drugs as shown. Endothelial cells also contain angiotensin-converting enzyme (ACE), which breaks down bradykinin to inactive peptides. This is reduced by ACE inhibitor drugs, amplifying the effects of bradykinin on the synthesis of endothelial vasodilators. Endothelin is a potent vasoconstrictor acting on ET_A receptors but also can act via a generally smaller population of receptors (ET_B) to generate nitric oxide and prostaglandins and subsequent relaxation. Other substances such as adenosine also cause vasodilation. Atrial natriuretic peptide (ANP) is released from atrial cells and has effects to increase natriuresis and to increase cGMP, causing relaxation of blood vessels and a fall in blood pressure. Mechanical shear stress can also act to increase NO, PGI_2, and endothelin, thus potentially influencing relaxation or contraction.
ACh, acetylcholine; ANP, atrial natriuretic peptide; BK, bradykinin; 5-HT, serotonin; ET, endothelin receptor; NO, nitric oxide; NOS, nitric oxide synthase; PLA_2, phospholipase A_2; PGI_2, prostacyclin.

obesity and alcohol intake all interact with the genetic programming to determine the final level of blood pressure. There is evidence that reduced renal Na^+ excretion plays a central role in the pathogenesis of essential hypertension, and the kidney requires a higher than normal blood pressure to maintain a normal extracellular fluid volume. However, the disturbance in essential hypertension is much more widespread than the kidney, with cell membrane abnormalities in many organs.

Isolated systolic hypertension, usually found in older people, is the consequence of stiffening of large arteries. These vessels normally expand to accommodate the blood expelled from the heart in systole, which slows the pulse wave and increases the time taken for it to reach the peripheral resistance vessels. The pulse wave is normally reflected back from the peripheral vessels in diastole, and supports the diastolic blood pressure and therefore coronary artery perfusion. If the compliance of the large arteries is reduced, then the pulse wave reaches the peripheral vessels early and is reflected back in systole. This increases systolic blood pressure and reduces diastolic pressure. In isolated systolic hypertension, coronary artery perfusion can be impaired, while cardiac work is increased.

A secondary underlying cause of the high blood pressure, which often has a renal or endocrine origin, can be identified in about 5% of people with hypertension (Table 6.1).

Not surprisingly, since the cause of hypertension is unclear, treatment cannot be directed precisely at the underlying mechanism(s). Most antihypertensive drugs are vasodilators. They often modulate the natural hormonal or neuronal mechanisms responsible for blood pressure regulation. Less commonly, a hypotensive action is achieved by reducing cardiac output. The principal classes of antihypertensive drugs and their sites of action are shown in Table 6.2 and Figure 6.6.

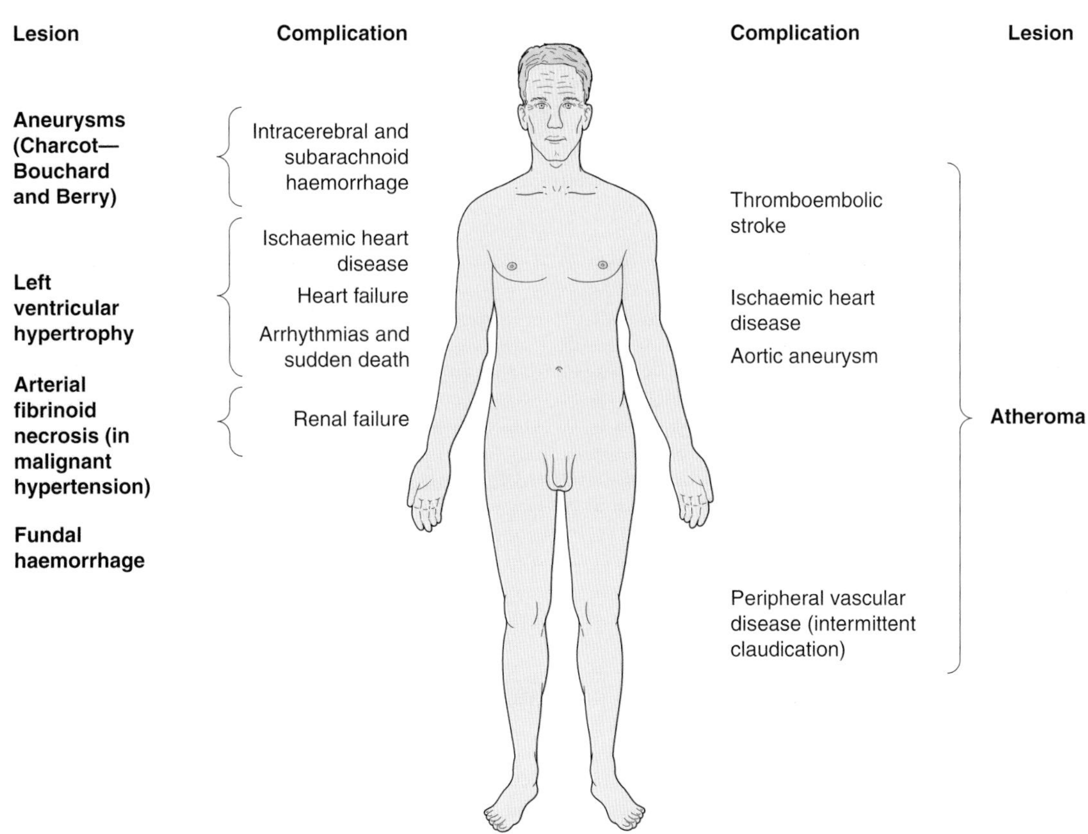

Fig. 6.5 **Complications of hypertension**. Hypertension causes vascular lesions and damage throughout the body.

Table 6.1 Principal causes of secondary hypertension

	Causes
Renal	Renal artery stenosis, glomerulonephritis, interstitial nephritis, arteritis, polycystic disease, chronic pyelonephritis
Endocrine	Conn's syndrome (aldosterone excess), Cushing's syndrome (glucocorticoid excess), phaeochromocytoma (catecholamine excess), acromegaly
Pregnancy	Pre-eclampsia and eclampsia
Drugs	Oestrogen, corticosteroids, non-steroidal anti-inflammatory drugs (NSAIDs), ciclosporin

Table 6.2 Principal classes of antihypertensive drugs and their sites of action

Sites of action	Drugs
Sympathetic nervous system	β-Adrenoceptor antagonists (β-blockers) α_1-Adrenoceptor antagonists (α_1-blockers) Selective imidazoline receptor agonists Centrally acting α_2-adrenoceptor agonists[a] Adrenergic neuron blockers[a] Ganglion blockers[a]
Hormonal control (renin–angiotensin system)	Angiotensin-converting enzyme (ACE) inhibitors Angiotensin II receptor antagonists Direct renin inhibitors
Vasodilation by other mechanisms	Diuretics Calcium channel blockers Potassium channel openers Nitrovasodilators[a] Endothelin-1 receptor antagonists

[a]Restricted use.

ANTIHYPERTENSIVE DRUGS

DRUGS ACTING ON THE SYMPATHETIC NERVOUS SYSTEM

Beta-adrenoceptor antagonists (β-blockers)

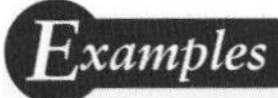

atenolol, nebivolol, propranolol

Mechanism of action in hypertension

Beta-adrenoceptor antagonists reduce blood pressure in several ways (Fig. 6.7). Selective β_1-adrenoceptor antagonists are as effective as non-selective drugs, indicating that β_2-adrenoceptor blockade makes little contribution. The more important actions are probably:

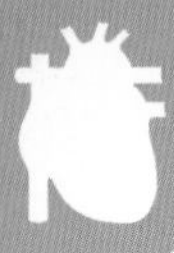

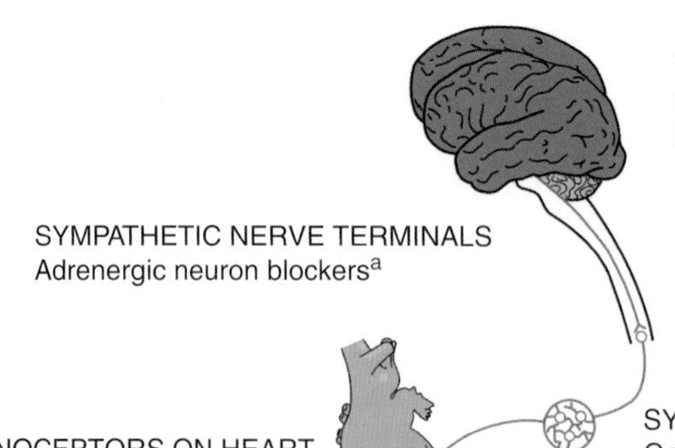

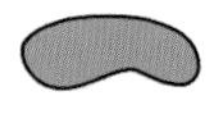
ADRENAL CORTEX
ACE inhibitors of angiotensin II formation
AT_1 receptor antagonists

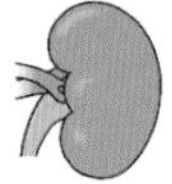

Fig. 6.6 **The classes of antihypertensive drug and their sites of action.**[a] Classes of drug that are rarely used now. ACE, angiotensin-converting enzyme.

- reduction of heart rate and myocardial contractility, which decrease cardiac output
- blockade of renal juxtaglomerular β_1-adrenoceptors, which reduces renin secretion
- peripheral vasodilation, but only with compounds that have a hybrid action, such as nebivolol, which produce vasodilation by mechanisms other than β_1-adrenoceptor antagonism (Fig. 6.7c and Ch. 5).
- blockade of presynaptic β-adrenoceptors in sympathetic neurons supplying arteriolar resistance vessels; this may reduce the release of noradrenaline and thus attenuate reflex arterial vasoconstriction, but the clinical importance of this effect is uncertain.

For further details about β-adrenoceptor antagonists and their many uses, see Chapters 5 and 8, and Box 6.1.

Alpha-adrenoceptor antagonists (α-blockers)

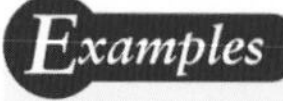

α_1-adrenoceptor selective antagonists: doxazosin, prazosin
non-selective antagonists: phenoxybenzamine (irreversible), phentolamine (reversible)

Mechanisms of action

Alpha-adrenoceptor antagonists (often referred to as α-blockers) lower blood pressure by blockade of postsynaptic α_1-adrenoceptors, leading to:

- reduced tone in arteriolar resistance vessels, and lower peripheral resistance
- dilation of venous capacitance vessels, which reduces venous return and therefore cardiac output.

When blood pressure falls, this is detected by arterial baroreceptors, which initiate a reflex increase in sympathetic discharge from the medulla, causing a reflex tachycardia (Figs 6.1 and 6.3). However, because noradrenaline released from cardiac sympathetic nerve terminals also stimulates inhibitory α_2-adrenoceptors on the presynaptic sympathetic neuron, the degree of sympathetic stimulation and reflex tachycardia is attenuated (Fig. 6.7a). Selective α_1-adrenoceptor antagonists do not block the presynaptic α_2-adrenoceptors on sympathetic nerve terminals; therefore reflex tachycardia is unusual. By contrast, non-selective α-adrenoceptor antagonists block both postsynaptic α_1-adrenoceptors and presynaptic α_2-adrenoceptors, and their use is accompanied by a marked reflex tachycardia. Non-selective agents now have little place in clinical practice except for the perioperative management of phaeochromocytoma.

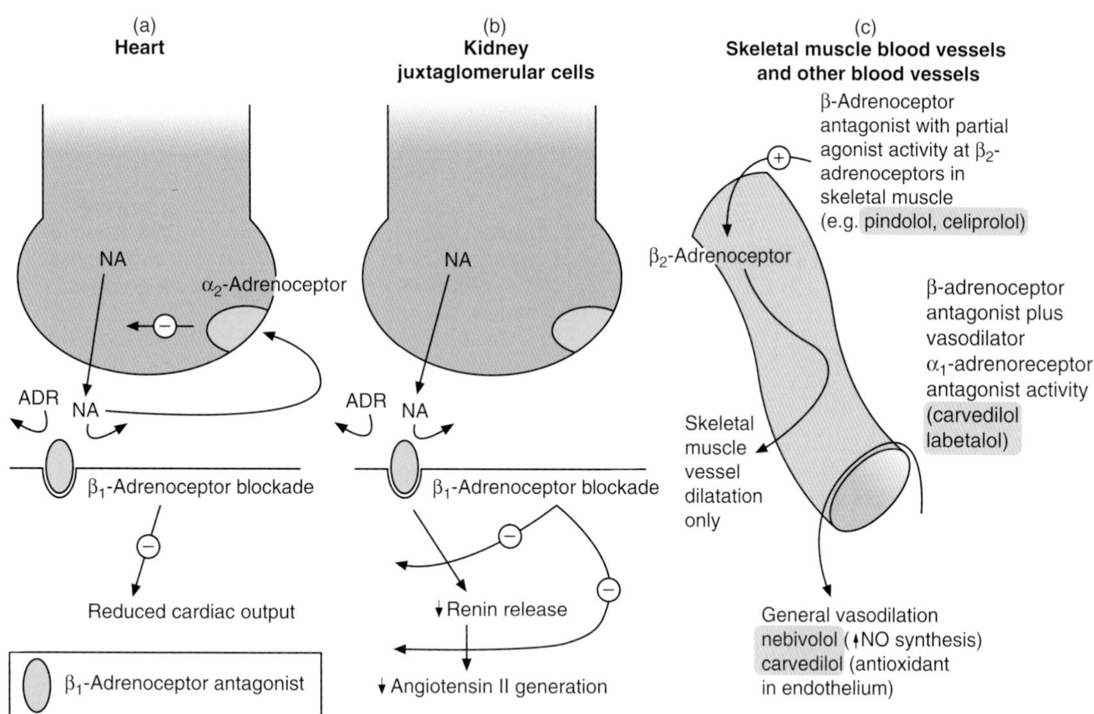

Fig. 6.7 **Sites of action of the β-adrenoceptor antagonists relevant to their use as antihypertensive agents.** (a) In the heart, the β_1-adrenoceptor antagonist drugs reduce noradrenaline- and adrenaline-induced stimulation of the β_1-adrenoceptors. The presynaptic stimulation of α_2-adrenoceptors, which inhibit noradrenaline release, still functions normally. (b) In the kidney, β_1-adrenoceptor blockade reduces the activity of the angiotensin II system. (c) Some selective β_1-adrenoceptor antagonists have hybrid activity: pindolol and celiprolol also have intrinsic sympathomimetic activity, acting as partial agonists stimulating the β_2-adrenoceptors in skeletal muscle blood vessels, which leads to vasodilation and a lowering of peripheral resistance. These drugs reduce heart rate and cardiac output less than do those without partial agonist properties. Nebivolol may dilate blood vessels more generally by releasing nitric oxide (NO). Carvedilol and labetalol also have α_1-adrenoceptor antagonist activity. ADR, adrenaline; NA, noradrenaline.

Box 6.1 Clinical uses of β-adrenoceptor antagonists

Treatment of hypertension (this chapter)
Prophylaxis of angina (Ch. 5)
Secondary prevention after myocardial infarction (Ch. 5)
Prevention and treatment of arrhythmias (Ch. 8)
Control of symptoms in thyrotoxicosis (Ch. 41)
Alleviation of symptoms in anxiety (Ch. 20)
Prophylaxis of migraine (Ch. 26)
Topically for treatment of glaucoma (Ch. 50)

Alpha-adrenoceptor antagonists produce a potentially beneficial effect on plasma lipids; they increase high-density lipoprotein cholesterol and reduce triglycerides (Ch. 48). Whether this has any relevance for the prevention of atheroma in individuals with hypertension is uncertain.

Pharmacokinetics

Selective α_1-adrenoceptor antagonists are well absorbed from the gut and undergo extensive first-pass metabolism and subsequent elimination by the liver. The compounds differ principally in their half-lives and, therefore, duration of action; for example, prazosin has a half-life of 3 h whereas doxazosin has a half-life of 9–12 h.

Unwanted effects

- Postural hypotension caused by venous pooling; this can be particularly troublesome after the first dose
- Lethargy, headache, dizziness
- Nausea
- Rhinitis
- Urinary frequency or incontinence (see also Ch. 15)
- Palpitation from reflex cardiac stimulation; this occurs more commonly with non-selective drugs.

CENTRALLY ACTING ANTIHYPERTENSIVE DRUGS

Selective imidazoline receptor agonists

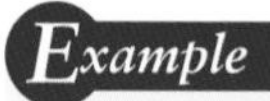

moxonidine

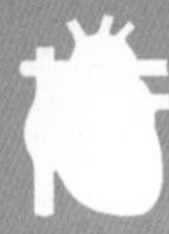

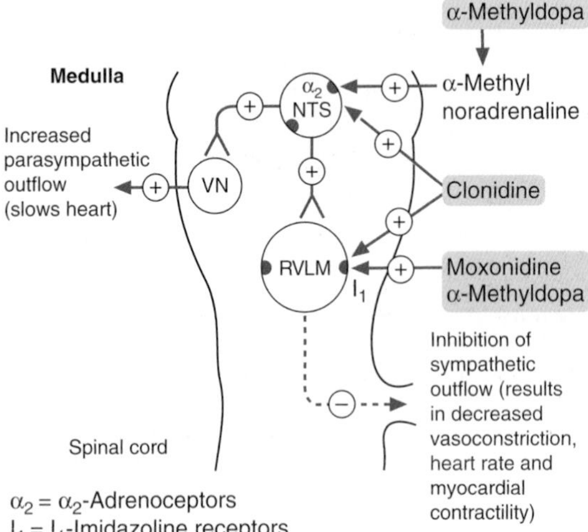

***Fig. 6.8* Mechanisms of centrally acting drugs in the control of blood pressure.** Methyldopa and moxonidine stimulate the same centres in the medulla that respond to raised blood pressure. They stimulate α_2-adrenoceptors in the nucleus of the tractus solitarius (NTS) and/or imidazoline receptors (perhaps also a subtype of α-adrenoceptor) in the rostral ventrolateral medulla (RVLM). Clonidine may also act through stimulating imidazoline receptors. VN, vagal nucleus (cardioinhibitory centre).

Mechanism of action

Imidazoline I_1 receptors are important for the regulation of sympathetic drive (Figs 6.1 and 6.8). They are concentrated in the rostral ventrolateral medulla, a part of the brainstem involved in control of blood pressure. Increased neuronal activity in this area, either through baroreceptor stimulation or by direct stimulation of I_1 receptors, will decrease sympathetic outflow, which results in a fall in blood pressure with no reflex tachycardia. Unlike other centrally acting drugs (clonidine and methyldopa), moxonidine has a low affinity for presynaptic α_2-adrenoceptors.

Pharmacokinetics

Moxonidine is well absorbed from the gut, and its principal route of elimination is the kidney. It has a short half-life (2–3 h) but a prolonged duration of action, which may reflect its high affinity for I_1 receptors.

Unwanted effects

- Dry mouth
- Nausea
- Fatigue, headache, dizziness.

Centrally acting α_2-adrenoceptor agonists

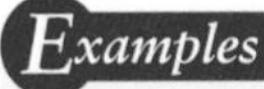

clonidine, methyldopa

Unwanted effects limit the use of the centrally acting α_2-adrenoceptor agonists, although methyldopa is a drug of choice in the treatment of hypertension in pregnancy (see below).

Mechanisms of action

The α_2-adrenoceptor agonists act at presynaptic autoreceptors in the central nervous system (CNS) to reduce sympathetic nervous outflow and increase vagal outflow from the medulla (Fig. 6.8). This reduces both peripheral arterial and venous tone.

Methyldopa is a prodrug that is metabolised in the nerve terminal as a 'false substrate' in the biosynthetic pathway for noradrenaline, to produce α-methylnoradrenaline. This metabolite is a potent α_2-adrenoceptor agonist. Clonidine is a direct-acting α_2-adrenoceptor agonist that is also an agonist at imidazoline I_1 receptors (see moxonidine). Clonidine has some peripheral postsynaptic α_1-adrenoceptor agonist activity, which produces direct peripheral vasoconstriction; this initially offsets some of the central blood pressure-lowering effect.

Pharmacokinetics

Methyldopa is incompletely absorbed from the gut and undergoes dose-dependent first-pass metabolism to an inactive derivative. It is eliminated by hepatic metabolism and the kidney, and has a half-life of 1–2 h.

Clonidine is completely absorbed from the gut and is eliminated partly by the kidney and partly by hepatic metabolism. It has a half-life of about 24 h.

Unwanted effects

- Sympathetic blockade: failure of ejaculation, and postural or exertional hypotension (unusual with clonidine, owing to its direct peripheral action)
- Unopposed parasympathetic action: diarrhoea
- Dry mouth
- CNS effects: sedation and drowsiness occur in up to 50% of people who take methyldopa; depression is occasionally seen
- Fluid retention with peripheral oedema
- Methyldopa induces a reversible positive Coombs' test in 20% of people, resulting from production of IgG to red cell membrane constituents; however, haemolytic anaemia is rare
- Sudden withdrawal of clonidine can produce severe rebound hypertension with tachycardia, sweating and anxiety.

DRUGS AFFECTING THE RENIN–ANGIOTENSIN SYSTEM

Angiotensin-converting enzyme (ACE) inhibitors

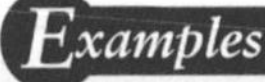

captopril, enalapril, lisinopril, ramipril

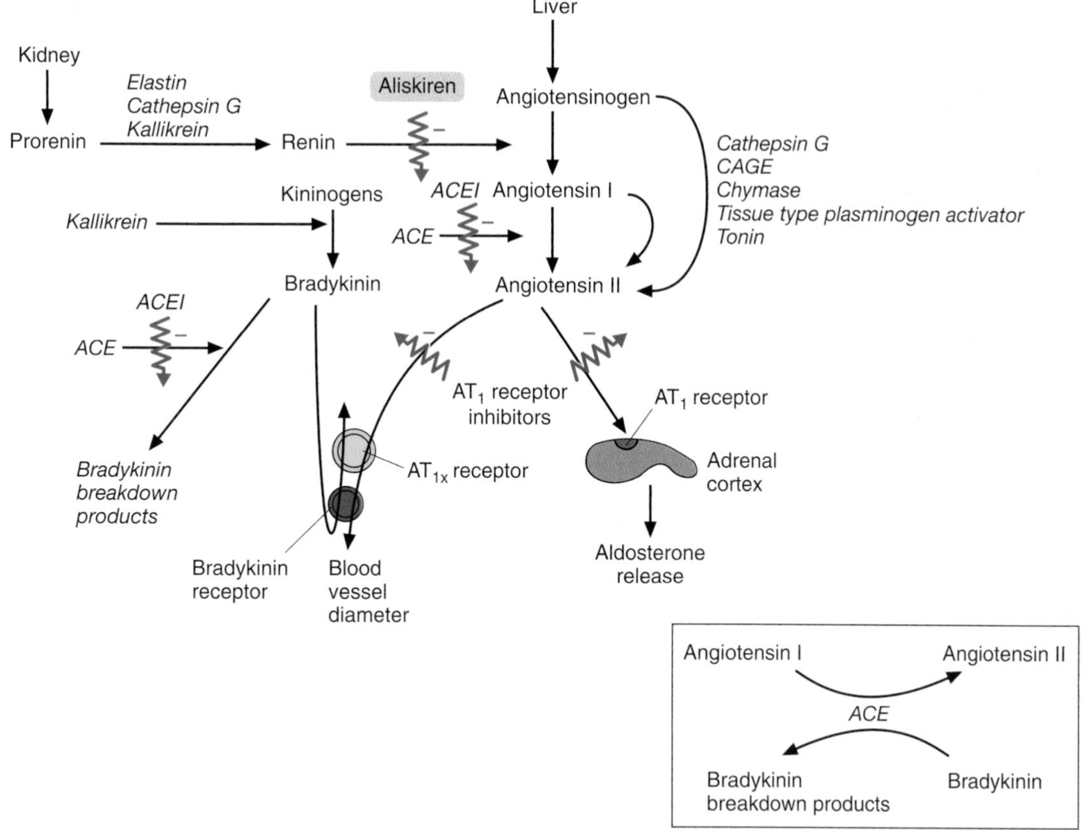

***Fig. 6.9* The biological actions of bradykinin and angiotensin II and drugs that modify these actions.** Bradykinin causes vasodilation by acting on vascular smooth muscle and on the endothelial cell (Fig. 6.4). Angiotensin II causes vasoconstriction by stimulating AT_1 receptors in the blood vessels and causes Na^+ retention by stimulating AT_1 receptors in the adrenal cortex, which results in aldosterone release. Angiotensin-converting enzyme inhibitors (ACEI) block angiotensin II formation from angiotensin I, although an alternative pathway still remains that can result in some angiotensin II formation from angiotensinogen or angiotensin I. Angiotensin receptor antagonists such as losartan act by inhibiting AT_1 receptors in blood vessels and the adrenal cortex. A newly introduced drug, aliskiren, directly inhibits the actions of renin on angiotensinogen. CAGE, chymotrypsin-like angiotensin-II-generating enzyme.

Mechanisms of action

The ACE inhibitors lower blood pressure by several mechanisms (see Figs 6.2, 6.4, 6.6, 6.9).

- Competitive inhibition of plasma ACE reduces generation of circulating angiotensin II and consequently reduces the release of aldosterone (Fig. 6.9).
- Inhibition of tissue ACE in the vascular wall is central to the hypotensive effect of these drugs (Fig. 6.9). Reduced tissue concentrations of angiotensin II lead to arterial dilation and, to a lesser extent, venous dilation. Angiotensin II production is not completely inhibited owing to alternative pathways for its generation that will be enhanced as a result of the counter-regulatory synthesis and release of renin (as a consequence of the reduction in blood pressure) after ACE inhibition.
- Reduction in angiotensin II-mediated potentiation of the sympathetic nervous system (Figs 6.2 and 6.3) prevents reflex tachycardia.
- Angiotensin II is implicated in the development of arterial remodelling and left ventricular hypertrophy (LVH) in hypertension. ACE inhibitors are more effective for regressing LVH than are diuretics or β-adrenoceptor antagonists.
- ACE also degrades vasodilator kinins and substance P (Fig. 6.9). Increased kinins (and vasodilator prostaglandins and nitric oxide) in the vascular wall may contribute to the hypotensive actions of ACE inhibitors. Perversely, some studies have shown that angiotensin II can also increase nitric oxide production in the endothelium and this may dampen the direct vasoconstrictor effects of angiotensin II on vascular smooth muscle (Fig 6.4).

There are many clinical uses of these drugs apart from hypertension; these are listed in Box 6.2.

Pharmacokinetics

Many ACE inhibitors are given as prodrugs, because the active forms are polar and poorly absorbed from the gut.

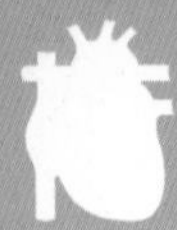

Box 6.2 Clinical uses of ACE inhibitors and angiotensin receptor blockers

Treatment of hypertension (this chapter)
Treatment of heart failure (Ch. 7)
Secondary prevention after myocardial infarction (Ch. 5)
Diabetic nephropathy (Ch. 40 and this chapter)

The prodrugs are converted in the liver to the active agent; for example, ramipril is converted to the active compound ramiprilat. In contrast, captopril and lisinopril are absorbed adequately as an active molecule. For most compounds, the active form is excreted unchanged by the kidney. The half-lives range from about 2 h (captopril and ramiprilat) to about 30–35 h (the active metabolites of cilazapril, enalapril and perindopril).

Unwanted effects

- Persistent dry cough that is not dose-related and may be caused by accumulation of kinins in the lung. This occurs in 10–30% of people who take ACE inhibitors, is more common in women, and can develop after many months of treatment.
- Postural hypotension, which is rare unless there is salt and water depletion, for example as a result of therapy with diuretics. Profound hypotension can occur in such individuals, particularly after the first dose. This is rarely a problem in the treatment of hypertension, but can be in the treatment of severe heart failure (Ch. 7).
- Renal impairment, especially in those with severe bilateral renal artery stenosis who rely on angiotensin-mediated efferent glomerular arterial vasoconstriction to maintain glomerular perfusion pressure.
- Disturbance of taste (which may be permanent), nausea, vomiting, dyspepsia or bowel disturbance.
- Rashes.
- Angioedema–more frequent in people of Afro-Caribbean origin.

Angiotensin receptor antagonists

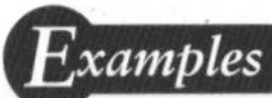

candesartan, losartan, valsartan

Mechanism of action

The angiotensin receptor antagonists are selective for the AT_1 receptor subtype (Fig. 6.2), which is found in the heart, blood vessels, kidney, adrenal cortex, lung and brain (Fig. 6.2). Actions of angiotensin II via this receptor include vasoconstriction, cell growth and proliferation, aldosterone release, sympathetic stimulation, salt and water retention, inhibition of renin concentrations and increase in reactive oxygen species. Angiotensin receptor antagonists have less effect at the AT_2 receptor subtype, *some* of the actions of which are the opposite of those seen at the AT_1 receptor (Fig. 6.2). In contrast to the use of ACE inhibitors, kinin degradation is unaffected by angiotensin receptor antagonists and inhibition of the effects of angiotensin II is more complete (Fig. 6.9). There are many clinical uses of these drugs apart from hypertension; these are listed in Box 6.2.

Pharmacokinetics

Losartan is well absorbed from the gut but has a low oral bioavailability because of first-pass metabolism. It is partially converted to an active metabolite, which is believed to be responsible for most of the pharmacological effects, and to several inactive metabolites. The half-life of losartan is about 2 h, while that of the active metabolite, which is largely excreted by the kidney, is longer (about 6 h)). Losartan is a competitive AT_1 receptor antagonist, but the active metabolite is a non-competitive antagonist.

Candesartan is given as a prodrug (candesartan cilexetil). This is rapidly hydrolysed in the liver to the active candesartan, which is eliminated by metabolism and renal excretion and has a half-life of 9–12 h. Valsartan is poorly absorbed from the gut. It is metabolised in the liver and has a half-life of 5–7 h.

Unwanted effects

Drugs in this class are usually well tolerated. Their major advantage over ACE inhibitors is the low incidence of cough. Angioedema is also rare. Unwanted effects include:

- Headache, dizziness
- Arthralgia or myalgia
- Fatigue.

Direct renin inhibitors

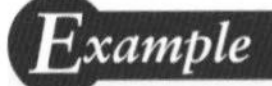

aliskiren

Mechanism of action

Aliskiren is a selective renin inhibitor with low affinity for other proteases. It binds competitively to the active site of the enzyme and inhibits the generation of angiotensin I (Fig. 6.9). Vasodilation is achieved by reduced angiotensin II synthesis, without the compensatory increase in plasma renin activity that occurs with an ACE inhibitor or angiotensin receptor antagonists. The place of aliskiren in the treatment of hypertension remains to be established.

Pharmacokinetics

Aliskiren is poorly absorbed from the gut and is excreted unchanged in the bile. It has a very long half-life (40 h).

Unwanted effects

With wider use, a more reliable indication of reported unwanted effects will be apparent. To date, unwanted effects include:

- Diarrhoea
- Cough.

VASODILATORS

Diuretics

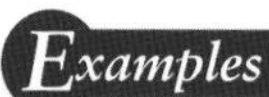

thiazide and thiazide-like diuretics: bendroflumethiazide, chlortalidone
loop diuretics: furosemide
potassium-sparing diuretics: spironolactone

Thiazide diuretics are most frequently used to lower blood pressure, but loop and potassium-sparing diuretics are used in some situations.

Mechanism of action in hypertension

Full details of the sites and mechanisms of action of diuretics on the kidney and unwanted effects are considered in Chapter 14. There are several actions involved in lowering blood pressure.

- An initial hypotensive effect is produced by intravascular salt and water depletion. However, compensatory mechanisms such as activation of the renin–angiotensin–aldosterone system largely restore plasma and extracellular fluid volumes (see Fig. 6.3) (unless salt and water retention was a major component of the initial hypertension, e.g. in advanced renal failure or as a consequence of other antihypertensive treatment).
- Direct arterial dilation is responsible for the longer-term reduction in blood pressure. The mechanism of vasodilation is not well understood, but may result from reduced Ca^{2+} entry into the smooth muscle of the arteriolar resistance vessel walls (perhaps as a consequence of intracellular Na^{+} depletion) and from synthesis of vasodilator prostaglandins.

Thiazide and thiazide-like diuretics

These produce their maximum blood pressure-lowering effect at doses lower than those required for significant diuretic activity. This is an advantage, since most unwanted effects are dose-related.

Loop diuretics

Unless used in a modified-release formulation, loop diuretics are usually less effective than thiazides in the treatment of essential hypertension. Despite having a more powerful diuretic action, their duration of action is too short. However, hypertension with advanced renal impairment or hypertension resistant to multiple drug treatment is more likely to be associated with fluid retention and often responds better to a loop diuretic than to a thiazide.

Potassium-sparing diuretics

Spironolactone, a specific aldosterone antagonist, is most effective for hypertension caused by primary hyperaldosteronism (Conn's syndrome), but is increasingly used to treat resistant hypertension. Amiloride and triamterene are less effective than thiazides in essential hypertension.

Box 6.3 Clinical uses of calcium channel blockers

Treatment of hypertension (this chapter)
Prophylaxis of angina (Ch. 5)
Treatment of Raynaud's phenomenon (Ch. 10)
Prevention and treatment of supraventricular arrhythmias (Ch. 8)
Subarachnoid haemorrhage (Ch. 9)

Calcium channel blockers (calcium antagonists)

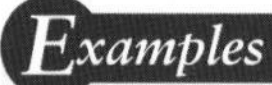

amlodipine, diltiazem, nifedipine, verapamil

The calcium channel blockers lower blood pressure principally by arterial vasodilation. For clinical uses, see Box 6.3. For further details, see Chapter 5.

Potassium channel openers

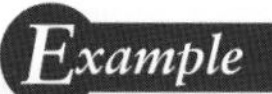

minoxidil

Mechanism of action

Vascular smooth muscle possesses ubiquitous ATP-sensitive K^{+} channels (K_{ATP}) (see also Ch. 8). Minoxidil acts on an ATP-sensitive K_{ir} subunit to open K_{ATP} channels, causing an efflux of K^{+} from the cell. This hyperpolarises the cell and leads to closure of voltage-gated Ca^{2+} channels and muscle relaxation (see also potassium channel openers, Fig. 5.4). Minoxidil is one of the most powerful peripheral arterial dilators.

Pharmacokinetics

Minoxidil is well absorbed from the gut, and mainly metabolised in the liver. It has a short half-life (3–4 h).

Unwanted effects

- Arterial vasodilation produces flushing and headache.
- The reflex sympathetic nervous system response to vasodilation causes tachycardia and palpitation (which can be blunted by concurrent use of a β-adrenoceptor antagonist, ACE inhibitor or angiotensin receptor antagonist).
- Salt and water retention occur through stimulation of the renin–angiotensin–aldosterone system (Fig. 6.2). This, along with increased transcapillary pressure from vasodilation, can produce peripheral oedema, which can be reduced by the concurrent use of diuretics.
- Hirsutism; therefore rarely used for treatment of women.

Hydralazine

Mechanism of action

The mechanism of action of hydralazine is uncertain, but it may activate guanylyl cyclase, leading to the intracellular

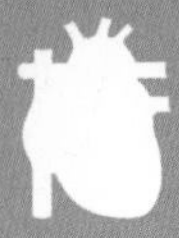

production of cGMP. This will produce smooth muscle relaxation by a mechanism similar to that of organic nitrates (Fig. 6.4 and Fig. 5.3).

Pharmacokinetics

Hydralazine is well absorbed from the gut and then undergoes extensive first-pass metabolism in the gut wall and liver, principally by N-acetylation. Some individuals, who are genetically determined slow acetylators (Ch. 2), require lower doses of hydralazine to achieve a clinical effect but are more susceptible to some of the unwanted effects. The half-life of hydralazine is about 4 h.

Unwanted effects

- Arterial vasodilation with reflex sympathetic activation produces tachycardia, flushing, hypotension and fluid retention.
- Headache, dizziness.
- A systemic lupus erythematosus (SLE)-like syndrome, which usually occurs after several months of treatment, is dose-related and is more common in slow acetylators. It resembles the naturally occurring disease but does not produce renal or cerebral damage and is slowly reversed if treatment is stopped. A positive antinuclear antibody is found in many individuals who do not develop the syndrome.

Nitrovasodilators

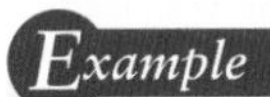

sodium nitroprusside

Mechanism of action

Nitroprusside is a nitrovasodilator with a mechanism of action similar to that of organic nitrates (Ch. 5). It produces dilation of arterioles and veins, reducing both peripheral resistance and venous return. Its use is limited to the emergency management of some hypertensive states.

Pharmacokinetics

Nitroprusside is given by intravenous infusion and its duration of action is less than 5 min. Metabolism to cyanide within red blood cells (by electron transfer from haemoglobin iron) terminates its effect. The cyanide is partly bound in the erythrocyte and partly liberated, when it is taken up by cells and inhibits intracellular cytochrome oxidase. Free cyanide is converted in the liver to less toxic thiocyanate. Thiocyanate accumulates with prolonged infusion; therefore, treatment is usually limited to a maximum of 3 days.

Unwanted effects

- Headache, dizziness
- Nausea, retching, abdominal pain
- Thiocyanate accumulation causes tachycardia, sweating, hyperventilation, arrhythmias and metabolic acidosis from inhibition of aerobic metabolism in cells.

TREATMENT OF HYPERTENSION

Morbidity and premature deaths associated with untreated hypertension are considerable (Fig. 6.5), and increase with advancing age. Therefore, treatment of older people with hypertension prevents more events in the short term than treating a similar number of younger people. However, early treatment will prevent vascular damage occurring in the younger individuals with hypertension – an important consideration since the vascular changes are not completely reversible once established.

The optimal target blood pressure is a systolic pressure below 140 mmHg and a diastolic pressure (phase V Korotkoff sound) below 90 mmHg in uncomplicated hypertension. When there is target organ damage or diabetes, a lower target of 130/80 mmHg is recommended, to minimise the risk of progressive vascular disease. There is no lower limit for blood pressure reduction, except in people with significant coronary artery disease. In this situation, lowering the diastolic blood pressure below 70 mmHg may reduce coronary artery perfusion and increase the risk of myocardial infarction. Even if the target pressures cannot be achieved, any blood pressure reduction in severe hypertension will reduce the risk of complications. Treating isolated systolic hypertension (systolic >160 mmHg, diastolic <90 mmHg) in the elderly gives similar benefits to the treatment of diastolic hypertension in this age group.

It is rarely possible to correct the underlying cause of hypertension. Lifestyle modifications such as weight loss, restriction of alcohol and salt intake, and increasing exercise may be enough to lower the blood pressure satisfactorily in some individuals with mild hypertension. In people with more severe hypertension, these measures can produce a substantial reduction in blood pressure but rarely restore it to normal values. It is important to advise all those with hypertension not to smoke, because smoking doubles the risk of cardiac and cerebrovascular events at any level of blood pressure.

The decision to treat hypertension with drugs should be determined largely by an assessment of the overall risk of complications in that individual. Drug treatment is usually started if blood pressure remains higher than the levels discussed above despite non-pharmacological approaches.

DRUG REGIMENS IN HYPERTENSION

Lowering blood pressure by a very modest amount with drugs (even if the target levels described above are not achieved) produces a substantial (≈40%) reduction in the risk of stroke, as well as reducing the risk of heart failure by 50% and reducing the incidence of renal failure. Drug treatment also reduces the risk of coronary artery disease in the elderly by about 25%; evidence for a similar reduction in the young is less convincing, which may reflect the short duration of the trials (up to 5 years). In people with evidence of left ventricular hypertrophy, regression of left ventricular mass during treatment of hypertension will reduce cardiovascular events by 60% compared to those in whom left ventricular mass is unchanged. ACE inhibitors, angiotensin receptor antagonists and calcium channel blockers may be most effective in this regard.

Choosing drugs for patients newly diagnosed with hypertension

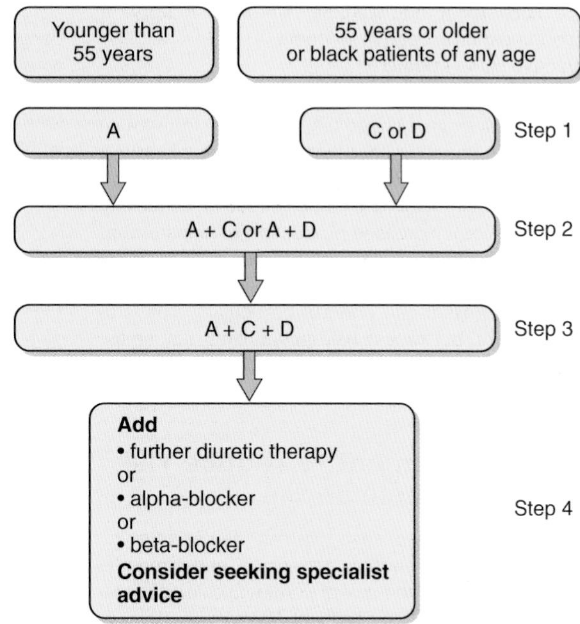

Fig. 6.10 **The British Hypertension Society recommendations for combining blood pressure-lowering drugs.** Combination therapy involving both B (a β-adrenoceptor antagonist) and D (a diuretic) may induce more new-onset diabetes.

Treatment regimens that are based on diuretics, calcium channel blockers, ACE inhibitors or angiotensin receptor antagonists have generally shown equal efficacy for reducing events. In contrast, β-adrenoceptor antagonists are less effective at preventing the complications of hypertension and are no longer recommended as first-line therapy. Treatment of hypertension should follow a 'stepped care' approach (Fig. 6.10). A single drug will achieve good blood pressure control in about one-third of people with hypertension. If the initial choice of drug fails to produce a reduction in blood pressure, then a change in therapy to an alternative first-line drug may be recommended. However, if the fall in blood pressure with the first drug is substantial but the target pressure is not reached, then the first drug should be continued and a second drug should be added.

The British Hypertension Society has endorsed the 'A/CD' protocol for combining blood pressure-lowering drugs which is based on their mode of action (Fig. 6.10). The underlying principle is that younger people with hypertension are more likely to have high plasma renin concentrations, and therefore a drug that suppresses the renin–angiotensin–aldosterone system is most likely to be effective. Conversely, elderly people with hypertension are more likely to have 'low renin' hypertension and a diuretic or calcium channel blocker is more likely to produce a substantial reduction in blood pressure. Use of a drug that suppresses the renin–angiotensin system creates the equivalent of a low renin state, while diuretics and calcium channel antagonists increase plasma renin. This provides the rationale for combination therapy with drugs from complementary classes. The recommendations are based on the probability of achieving optimal blood pressure control and the evidence that the achieved blood pressure, rather than the means by which it was achieved, is important for improving outcome. The exception is β-adrenoceptor antagonists, which are no longer recommended as first-line treatment for uncomplicated hypertension. Several studies have shown that atenolol is less effective at preventing complications of hypertension than are other classes of drugs, and there is little information on outcome with other β-adrenoceptor antagonists.

If three drugs with complementary actions, taken in adequate dosage, are insufficient to control the blood pressure, then the person is said to have 'resistant' hypertension.

Both diuretics and β-adrenoceptor antagonists increase the risk of developing new-onset diabetes, particularly when used together. This combination is not recommended for those who are at increased risk of glucose intolerance, such as people who are obese, those with a strong family history of type 2 diabetes, or people of South Asian or Afro-Caribbean origin, who have a higher risk of developing diabetes. In contrast, both ACE inhibitors and angiotensin receptor antagonists reduce the risk of developing diabetes.

Resistant hypertension

There are several possible causes of apparently resistant hypertension. These include:

- poor adherence to prescribed therapy (see Ch. 55)
- 'white coat' hypertension, which responds poorly to drug treatment

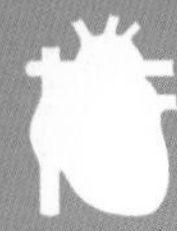

- secondary hypertension, most often caused by renal artery stenosis or Conn's syndrome
- drugs, such as a non-steroidal anti-inflammatory, a glucocorticoid or excessive alcohol
- obstructive sleep apnoea
- intravascular volume expansion.

Some people with resistant hypertension benefit from treatment with a loop diuretic rather than a thiazide, which will help if expansion of the plasma volume is contributing to drug resistance. Spironolactone can be effective, especially if there is evidence of increased production of aldosterone. An α-adrenoceptor antagonist or β-adrenoceptor antagonist are options as the fourth drug for resistant hypertension. In men, minoxidil can prove a particularly powerful hypotensive agent, but excess hair growth limits its use for women. In a few individuals, treatment with five drugs may be necessary.

Additional treatment to reduce risk of vascular complications

The use of aspirin at low dosage reduces the risk of myocardial infarction in people with hypertension, and is recommended when the predicted risk of cardiovascular disease is greater than 20% in the subsequent 10 years. A statin is also recommended for primary prevention of cardiovascular disease in people with hypertension at a similar level of risk, or in those with diabetes (Ch. 48).

HYPERTENSION IN SPECIAL GROUPS

There are reasons for selecting particular classes of drugs under certain specific conditions or when other conditions are present (Table 6.3). Ethnic differences may also be important: for example, people of Afro-Caribbean origin respond less well to β-adrenoceptor antagonists or ACE inhibitors as first-line therapy than do Caucasians, since at all ages they are more likely to have low-renin hypertension.

Malignant or accelerated hypertension

Early treatment is important for people with hypertension who have retinal haemorrhages and exudates or papilloedema. Rapid blood pressure reduction is potentially dangerous, since it can lead to cerebral underperfusion and ischaemic cerebral damage. Intravenous drugs should usually be avoided, and oral atenolol or nifedipine are the most widely recommended treatments, which gradually reduce the blood pressure over 24 h or more.

Renal artery stenosis

ACE inhibitors or angiotensin receptor antagonists usually produce an excellent reduction in blood pressure if hypertension is caused by renal artery stenosis, but they can lead to deterioration in renal function, especially if there are bilateral stenoses. Renal artery angioplasty with insertion of a stent is usually recommended to preserve renal function if there is renal impairment. However, this rarely results in a normalisation of blood pressure, although fewer drugs may subsequently be required to achieve target blood pressures.

Diabetic nephropathy

ACE inhibitors and angiotensin receptor antagonists appear to protect the kidney more than other classes of antihypertensive drug in diabetic nephropathy. In particular, they reduce progression from microalbuminuria to overt nephropathy, and can be more effective when combined than using either drug alone. There is probably an effect of these drugs that is additional to blood pressure reduction and reflects a reduction in glomerular perfusion pressure. Other complications of hypertension in those with diabetes are prevented equally well by β-adrenoceptor antagonists, thiazide diuretics or calcium channel blockers.

Table 6.3 Selection of antihypertensive drugs for coexisting conditions

	Diuretic	β-Adrenoceptor antagonist	ACE inhibitor	Calcium channel blocker	α_1-Adrenoceptor antagonist
Angina	+/–	+	+/–	+	+/–
After myocardial infarction	+/–	+	+	–	+/–
Congestive heart failure	+	+	+	–	+/–
Diabetes mellitus (with or without nephropathy)	+/–	+/–	+	+/–	+/–
Raynaud's phenomenon	+/–	–	+	+	+
Gout	–	+/–	+/–	+/–	+/–
Prostatism	–	+/–	+/–	+/–	+
Supraventricular arrhythmias	+/–	+	+/–	+[a]	+/–
Migraine	+/–	+	+/–	+/–	+/–

[a]Diltiazem or verapamil only.
ACE, angiotensin-converting enzyme; +, treatment of choice; +/–, no obvious advantage/not preferred; –, usually contraindicated.

Phaeochromocytoma

Hypertension in this condition is caused by excessive release of catecholamines from a tumour that often arises in the adrenal glands. Noradrenaline-secreting tumours most often lead to sustained hypertension, through vasoconstriction mediated by α_1-adrenoceptor stimulation. Treatment is always started with an α-adrenoceptor antagonist (usually phenoxybenzamine) to prevent the excessive vasoconstriction, followed by a β-adrenoceptor antagonist to block the arrhythmogenic effects of the catecholamines on the heart. Definitive treatment, whenever possible, is by surgical removal of the tumour.

Primary hyperaldosteronism

This can be caused by bilateral adrenal hyperplasia or, less commonly, by an adrenal tumour (Conn's syndrome). The drug treatment of choice is spironolactone, to directly block the effects of aldosterone at its renal tubular receptor. If there is a tumour, surgical excision should be considered.

Pregnancy

There are two issues peculiar to pregnancy.

- **Pre-existing chronic hypertension.** The risk of hypertension to mother and fetus is probably not great until the systolic blood pressure reaches 150 mmHg, or the diastolic blood pressure reaches 95 mmHg. Treatment at lower levels carries a risk of impairment of fetal growth. The drugs with the best safety record in this situation are methyldopa, nifedipine and labetalol. Certain drugs given to the mother can be teratogenic (Ch. 56). In the second trimester, although the risk of malformations is lower, diuretics and β-adrenoceptor antagonists are still contraindicated, because they may retard fetal growth and cause electrolyte imbalance in the newborn. ACE inhibitors or angiotensin receptor antagonists may cause oligohydramnios (reduced amniotic fluid production), renal failure and hypotension in the fetus, or intrauterine death and should be avoided at all stages of pregnancy.
- **Pre-eclampsia**. This usually occurs after 20 weeks of gestation. It presents as hypertension with oedema and proteinuria or hyperuricaemia in women whose blood pressure had previously been normal. There is a risk to the mother of convulsions, cerebral haemorrhage, abruptio placentae, pulmonary oedema and renal failure if this condition is untreated, and a risk to the fetus of severe growth retardation or even death. Once the diagnosis is established, bed rest is supplemented by antihypertensive drugs as described above for pre-existing hypertension in pregnancy. Labetalol given by intravenous infusion is favoured in severe pre-eclampsia.

PULMONARY HYPERTENSION

Pulmonary hypertension usually arises secondary to other diseases. It is most commonly found in people with chronic obstructive lung disease and other lung disorders, where it arises as a result of destructive changes affecting the structure of the vascular bed. It also occurs with multiple small pulmonary emboli which silt up the peripheral pulmonary arteries and increase vascular resistance. However, some people develop increased pulmonary vascular resistance for unknown reasons. The condition is then classified as primary pulmonary hypertension (PPH), and the pathology is associated with either the formation of plexiform vascular lesions or thrombotic arteriopathy. The most common presenting complaint in PPH is shortness of breath, although fatigue, chest pain, syncope, peripheral oedema and palpitation also frequently occur. The sustained increase in pulmonary vascular resistance leads to progressive right heart failure.

DRUGS FOR TREATING PULMONARY HYPERTENSION

Endothelin receptor antagonists

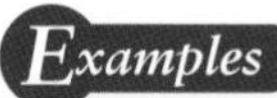

bosentan, sitaxentan

Mechanism of action

In PPH the expression of endothelin is increased in the pulmonary vasculature. Endothelin-1 is a powerful vasoconstrictor and smooth muscle mitogen which exerts its effects via two receptors, ET_A and ET_B. ET_A primarily mediates vasoconstriction and cell proliferation, while ET_B mediates vasodilation via nitric oxide release and is responsible for clearance of endothelin from the circulation (Fig. 6.4). Bosentan is an antagonist at both endothelin receptors. Sitaxentan is a selective antagonist at ET_A receptors, which has some theoretical advantages.

Pharmacokinetics

Bosentan is metabolised in the liver and has a half-life of 5 h. Sitaxentan is well absorbed from the gut, is metabolised in the liver, and has a half-life of 9 h.

Unwanted effects

- Gastrointestinal disturbances, including rectal haemorrhage with bosentan
- Vasodilator effects, including flushing, hypotension, palpitation, oedema
- Headache, fatigue
- Hepatic dysfunction
- Drug interactions: excessive anticoagulation with warfarin, since both bosentan and sitaxentan inhibit the metabolism of warfarin by CYP2C9.

Prostaglandins

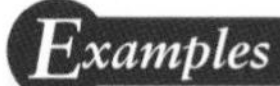

epoprostenol, iloprost

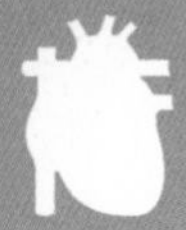

Epoprostenol is naturally occurring prostacyclin (PGI_2) and iloprost is a synthetic analogue of prostacyclin. Prostacyclin is a vasodilator that also inhibits platelet aggregation (Ch. 11), and both effects may be useful in the management of PPH. Initial studies used continuous intravenous infusion of epoprostenol, but there is now evidence for the use of inhaled iloprost. The main disadvantage is the need for inhalations every 2–3 h, and the high incidence of flushing, headache, jaw pain and cough. Longer-acting prostacyclin analogues are under development.

Phosphodiesterase inhibitors

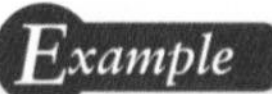

sildenafil, tadalafil

Cyclic GMP production in the pulmonary vasculature may be a protective mechanism against PPH. Oral phosphodiesterase type 5 inhibitors that inhibit breakdown of cGMP, such as sildenafil and tadalafil (Ch.16), reduce pulmonary artery pressure, and the effects are additive to those of inhaled iloprost.

MANAGEMENT OF PULMONARY HYPERTENSION

Secondary pulmonary hypertension in chronic lung disease is most effectively managed by alleviating hypoxaemia when possible. There is no specific drug therapy. Chronic embolic disease is treated by life-long anticoagulation with warfarin.

About 25% of people with PPH maintain a vasoactive pulmonary vascular bed (defined as a 20% decrease in pulmonary vascular resistance on acute challenge with a vasodilator). In this situation, treatment with a calcium channel blocker such as nifedipine will improve both symptoms and survival. However, most people with PPH show little evidence of vascular reactivity, and conventional vasodilators tend to produce excessive systemic hypotension before useful pulmonary vasodilation is achieved. For such individuals, there is now a choice of an endothelin antagonist, inhaled prostaglandin, or a phosphodiesterase inhibitor. All these drugs can improve symptoms and quality of life but have not been shown to improve survival. The role of combination therapy is under investigation.

FURTHER READING

Schneider MP, Boesen LI, Pollock DM (2007) Contrasting actions of endothelin ET_A and ET_B receptors in cardiovascular disease. *Annu Rev Pharmacol Toxicol* 47, 731–759

Toda N, Ayajiki K, Okamura T (2007) Interaction of endothelial cell nitric oxide and angiotensin in the circulation. *Pharmacol Rev* 59, 54–87

Systemic hypertension

August P (2003) Initial treatment of hypertension. *N Engl J Med* 348, 610–617

Blood Pressure Lowering Treatment Trialists' collaboration (2003) Effects of different blood pressure lowering regimens on major cardiovascular events: second cycle of prospectively designed overviews. *Lancet* 362, 1527–1535

Brown MJ, Cruickshank JK, Dominiczak AF et al (2003) Better blood pressure control: how to combine drugs. *J Hum Hypertens* 17, 81–86

Chiong JR, Aronow WS, Khan IA et al (2008) Secondary hypertension: current diagnosis and treatment. *Int J Cardiol* 124, 6–21

Ferrario C, Levy P (2002) Sexual dysfunction in patients with hypertension: implications for therapy. *J Clin Hypertens* 4, 424–432

Kaplan N, Opie LH (2006) Controversies in hypertension. *Lancet* 367, 168–176

Lindholm LH, Carlberg B, Samuelsson O (2005) Should beta blockers remain first choice in the treatment of primary hypertension? A meta-analysis. *Lancet* 366, 1545–1553

Messerli FH, Grossman E, Lever A (2003) Do thiazides confer specific protection against strokes? *Arch Intern Med* 163, 2557–2560

Moser M, Setaro JF (2006) Resistant or difficult-to-control hypertension. *N Engl J Med* 355, 385–392

Ong HT (2007) β blockers in hypertension and cardiovascular disease. *BMJ* 334, 946–949

Oparil S, Zaman A, Calhoun DA (2003) Pathogenesis of hypertension. *Ann Intern Med* 139, 761–776

Psaty B, Lumley T, Furberg CD et al (2003) Health outcomes associated with various antihypertensive therapies used as first-line agents: a network meta-analysis. *JAMA* 289, 2534–2544

Safar ME, Smulyan H (2004) Hypertension in women. *Am J Hypertens* 17, 82–87

Shafiq MM, Menon DV, Victor RG (2008) Oral direct renin inhibition: premise, promise, and potential limitations of a new antihypertensive drug. *Am J Med* 121, 265–271

Snow V, Weiss KB, Mottur-Pilson C et al (2004) The evidence base for tight blood pressure control in the management of type 2 diabetic mellitus. *Ann Intern Med* 138, 587–592

Sowers JR (2004) Treatment of hypertension in patients with diabetes. *Arch Intern Med* 164, 1850–1857

Staessen JA, Wang J, Bianchi G et al (2003) Essential hypertension. *Lancet* 361, 1629–1641

The Task Force for the Management of Arterial Hypertension of the European Society of Hypertension (ESH) and of the European Society of Cardiology (ESC) (2007) 2007 guidelines for the management of arterial hypertension. *J Hypertens* 25, 1105–1187

Vijan S, Hayward RA (2003) Treatment of hypertension in type 2 diabetes mellitus: blood pressure goals, choice of agents, and setting priorities in diabetes. *Ann Intern Med* 138, 593–602

Williams B (2005) Recent hypertension trials: implications and controversies. *J Am Coll Cardiol* 45, 813–827

Williams B, Poulter NR, Brown MJ et al (2004) British Hypertension Society guidelines for hypertension management 2004: summary. *BMJ* 328, 634–640

Williams B, Poulter NR, Brown MJ et al (2004) Guidelines for management of hypertension: report of the fourth working party of the British Hypertension Society, 2004 – BHS IV. *J Hum Hypertens* 18, 139–185

Yoder SR, Thomberg LL, Bisognano JD (2009) Hypertension in pregnancy and women of childbearing age. *Am J Med* 122, 890–895

Pulmonary hypertension

Badesh DB, Abman SH, Simmonneau G et al (2007) Medical therapy for pulmonary arterial hypertension. *Chest* 131, 1917–1928

Humbert M, Sitbon O, Simmoneau G (2004) Treatment of pulmonary hypertension. *N Engl J Med* 351, 1425–1436

Macchia A, Marchioli R, Marfisi RM et al (2007) A meta-analysis of pulmonary hypertension: a clinical condition looking for drugs and research methodology. *Am Heart J* 153, 1037–1047

McLaughlin VV, McGoon MD (2006) Pulmonary arterial hypertension. *Circulation* 114, 1417–1431

Rich S (2006) The current treatment of pulmonary arterial hypertension: time to redefine success. *Chest* 130, 1198–1202

SELF-ASSESSMENT

1. In the following questions, the first statement, in italics, is true. Is the accompanying statement also true?
   a. *Thiazide diuretics reduce sodium and water reabsorption in the distal convoluted tubule.* They are the drugs of choice for treating pregnancy-related hypertension.
   b. *Nifedipine shows selectivity for vasodilation over cardiac depression.* Nifedipine lowers blood pressure principally by arterial vasodilation.
   c. *Moxonidine stimulates imidazoline receptors in the medulla.* This increases sympathetic outflow and decreases vagal tone, lowering blood pressure.
   d. *Propranolol lowers blood pressure.* It does so by (i) decreasing cardiac output, (ii) reducing renin secretion, and (iii) peripheral vasodilation.
   e. *Amiloride and spironolactone are potassium-sparing diuretics.* Their diuretic action is through different mechanisms in the distal tubule and early collecting duct.
   f. *Stretch of baroreceptors increases the afferent impulses to the vasomotor centre.* This results in enhanced sympathetic nervous outflow and a rise in blood pressure.
   g. *Stimulation of presynaptic α-adrenoceptors in arteriolar resistance vessels inhibits noradrenaline release.* α_1-Adrenoceptor blockade by prazosin increases noradrenaline release.
   h. *Thiazide diuretics initially lower blood pressure by depleting salt and water.* The long-term reduction in blood pressure by thiazide diuretics is achieved with doses that do not cause diuresis and natriuresis.
   i. *ACE inhibitors prevent the conversion of angiotensin I to the vasoconstrictor angiotensin II.* ACE inhibitors also prevent the breakdown of the vasodilator bradykinin.
   j. *Minoxidil opens K^+ channels in smooth muscle cell membranes.* This K^+-channel opening destabilises the cell membrane, leading to vasoconstriction.
   k. *The antihypertensive effect of nitroprusside is limited to emergency management of some hypertensive states.* It can be administered for up to 2 months.
2. Choose the one **incorrect** option from the following statements concerning drugs used in the treatment of hypertension.
   A. Thiazide diuretics reduce blood pressure at doses lower than those required for diuresis.
   B. ACE inhibitors cause cough by inhibiting the formation of bradykinin.
   C. Combinations of antihypertensive drugs are commonly used in the treatment of hypertension.
   D. Angiotensin receptor antagonists lower blood pressure by blocking the angiotensin type-1 receptor (AT_1R).
   E. Nifedipine is more selective than verapamil for blockade of Ca^{2+} channels in the arteries compared with Ca^{2+} channels in the heart.
3. Endothelial-derived mediators can influence vascular smooth muscle function and dysfunction and can contribute to disease. Which one of the following **most correctly** describes an interaction between endothelium and smooth muscle?
   A. Bradykinin stimulates the release of nitric oxide and consequent elevation of cAMP, relaxing vascular smooth muscle.
   B. ACE inhibitors stimulate the formation of endothelin-1 in the endothelium.
   C. Part of the blood pressure-lowering effect of diuretics is due to stimulation of prostacyclin (PGI_2) in the endothelium.
   D. Mechanical stress reduces the synthesis of nitric oxide by the endothelium.
   E. Angiotensin inhibits the synthesis of endothelin-1 in the endothelium.
4. Extended-matching questions
   Choose which of the following drugs (A–D) would be a poor choice to use for the INITIAL treatment of a person newly diagnosed with hypertension in the scenarios beneath (4.1–4.4). Each drug may be used more than once.
   A. A non-selective β-adrenoceptor antagonist
   B. A thiazide diuretic
   C. An ACE inhibitor
   D. A calcium channel blocker
   4.1. A black, clinically obese male aged 75 years with a blood pressure of 150/100 mmHg and no other pathology
   4.2. A white female aged 40 years with type 1 diabetes and a blood pressure of 150/100 mmHg
   4.3. A white male aged 60 years with a blood pressure of 150/100 mmHg and elevated plasma triglycerides and cholesterol
   4.4. A woman 24 weeks pregnant with pre-existing chronic hypertension and a blood pressure of 150/100 mmHg

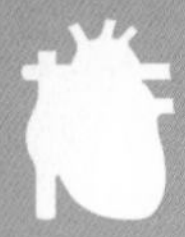

5. Case history questions

A 60-year-old man with non-insulin-dependent diabetes smoked 20 cigarettes a day. His plasma lipid levels were normal and there was no proteinuria. His ECG was normal. His height was 5′8″ (1.70 m) and his weight 210 lb (95.5 kg). He had his blood pressure checked three times over a period of weeks and it was consistently 175/110 mmHg. He had no evidence of fluid retention or heart failure. The doctor considered initiating treatment with atenolol or a calcium channel blocker.

a. What would you recommend?

Following several months of treatment with your chosen regimen, his blood pressure was still 155/95 mmHg and he then suffered a small myocardial infarction.

b. What changes in his therapy would you consider?

ANSWERS

1. a. **False**. Thiazide diuretics cause growth retardation of the fetus and are not recommended. Methyldopa, nifedipine and labetalol are most often used.
   b. **True**. Calcium channel blockers act by opening L-type voltage-gated Ca^{2+} channels, and nifedipine, a dihydropyridine, is relatively selective for these channels in smooth muscle. Verapamil and diltiazem, which are not dihydropyridines, have intermediate selectivity and therefore have both vascular and cardiodepressant properties that may contribute to their blood pressure-lowering actions.
   c. **False**. Selective stimulation of imidazoline receptor type I_1 in the ventrolateral medulla is the principal mechanism of action of moxonidine, which lowers blood pressure in hypertension by decreasing sympathetic outflow and increasing vagal outflow.
   d. **True** for (i) and (ii); **false** for (iii). Only β-adrenoceptor antagonists with ancillary properties, such as pindolol, which has partial agonist activity at β_2-adrenoceptors, produce peripheral vasodilation.
   e. **True**. Spironolactone blocks the aldosterone receptor, which stimulates the Na^+/K^+-ATPase pump, facilitating uptake of Na^+ into the interstitium from the tubule. Spironolactone therefore conserves K^+ in exchange for Na^+ loss. Amiloride, however, directly blocks the Na^+ channel on the luminal side of the tubule (see Ch. 14).
   f. **False**. Baroreceptor impulses to the vasomotor centre are inhibitory. Increased impulses, therefore, reduce sympathetic outflow, enhance vagal outflow and lower blood pressure.
   g. **False**. Prazosin is a selective α_1-adrenoceptor antagonist and therefore dilates blood vessels. It does not block the presynaptic receptor, which is α_2-adrenoceptor subtype, and stimulation of this receptor to limit further noradrenaline release can still take place.
   h. **True**. Longer-term vasodilation and blood pressure lowering may be because of inhibition of Ca^{2+} entry into vessel cells and synthesis of vasodilator prostaglandins.
   i. **True**. ACE breaks down bradykinin, which is found in endothelial cells and is a potent vasodilator.
   j. **False**. Minoxidil causes extrusion of K^+ from the cell, which results in the stabilisation of the membrane potential and vasodilation.
   k. **False**. Nitroprusside is converted to cyanide and then to thiocyanate. The toxicity of these limits its use to 3 days.
2. Answer **B**.
   A. Due to the vasodilator actions of the diuretics.
   B. ACE contributes to bradykinin catabolism and the inhibitor therefore increases bradykinin levels, which can result in cough.
   C. Satisfactory lowering of blood pressure can only be achieved with a single drug in about 40% of people with hypertension.
   D. The AT_1 receptor is relevant to the vasoconstrictor and aldosterone secretory actions of angiotensin II. The AT_2 receptor is involved in vascular growth and is less affected by the receptor antagonists such as losartan.
   E. Nifedipine is less cardiodepressant than verapamil because of its greater arterial selectivity.
3. Answer **C**.
   A. Bradykinin stimulates NO and consequently cGMP formation.
   B. ACE inhibitors result in elevated bradykinin and reduced angiotensin II; both actions will reduce endothelin-1 formation.
   C. True.
   D. Shear stress increases NO formation.
   E. Angiotensin II stimulates endothelin-1 formation.
4. Extended-matching answers
   4.1. Answer **A**, **B**, **C**.
   An ACE inhibitor, a β-adrenoceptor antagonist or a thiazide diuretic would not be first-choice treatment. The elderly and black people have low plasma levels of renin, and obesity increases the risk for diabetes, which may be exacerbated by a β-adrenoceptor antagonist or a thiazide diuretic.
   4.2. Answer **A**, **B**.
   A β-adrenoceptor antagonist or a thiazide diuretic may exacerbate the diabetes. For this age group, an ACE inhibitor would be an appropriate initial choice.
   4.3. Answer **A**, **B**.
   A β–adrenoceptor antagonist can increase plasma triglycerides and lower high-density lipoprotein cholesterol. A calcium channel blocker would be an appropriate first choice
   4.4. Answer **A**, **B**, **C**.
   Only a calcium channel blocker would be an acceptable choice from the list of drugs. All the others can cause unwanted effects on the fetus.
5. Case history answers
   a. A calcium channel blocker. NICE and the British Hypertension Society have compared the effect of β-adrenoceptor antagonists against other blood pressure-lowering drugs in terms of ability to prevent

cardiovascular complications and unwanted effects. They have made the general recommendation that β-adrenoceptor antagonists should not be the first choice for the initial treatment of newly diagnosed hypertension in the absence of a compelling reason for their use, such as angina. If possible, in diabetes the use of a β-adrenoceptor antagonist should be avoided. Because of his history (he had no evidence of angina), a calcium channel blocker would be the drug to try first (Fig. 6.10).

b. Blood pressure has not reached the target level and he has had a myocardial infarction. His blood pressure may be reduced further by introducing an ACE inhibitor. ACE inhibitors reduce angiotensin II formation and improve survival after a myocardial infarction, especially when there is left ventricular impairment. ACE inhibitors appear to protect the kidney in diabetic nephropathy and could be considered in this situation. Despite the comments earlier, the addition of a β-adrenoceptor antagonist could also be considered for additional long-term prognostic benefit, particularly if there is left ventricular impairment.

Drugs used to treat hypertension

Drug	Half-life (h) and kinetics	Comments
β-Adrenoceptor antagonists		
All β-adrenoceptor antagonists, except esmolol and sotalol, are used for hypertension; see Ch. 5 for individual drugs		
Calcium channel blockers		
All calcium channel blockers except nimodipine are used for treatment of hypertension; see Ch. 5 for individual drugs		
Diuretics		
Can be used to lower blood pressure; see Ch. 14 for individual drugs		
α_1-Selective adrenoceptor antagonists		
All drugs are given orally		
Doxazosin	9–12 [M] Oral bioavailability is 65% owing to incomplete absorption; metabolised by oxidation	Used for hypertension and benign prostatic hyperplasia
Indoramin	5 [M] Oral bioavailability is 10–25%; eliminated by oxidation (CYP2D6) to an active hydroxyl metabolite	Used for hypertension and benign prostatic hyperplasia
Prazosin	3 [M] Oral bioavailability is 60% owing to first-pass metabolism; high hepatic extraction and clearance by cytochrome P450	Used for hypertension, congestive heart failure, Raynaud's phenomenon and benign prostatic hyperplasia
Terazosin	12 [M] High oral bioavailability (>90%); mostly eliminated by hepatic metabolism but some eliminated unchanged in urine (5%) and faeces (25%)	Used for hypertension and benign prostatic hyperplasia
Non-selective α-adrenoceptor antagonists		
Used in phaeochromocytoma only		
Phenoxybenzamine	24 [M] Low oral bioavailability (20–30%); metabolised in the liver	Used for hypertensive episodes associated with phaeochromocytoma; given orally or by intravenous infusion
Phentolamine	1.5 [M + R] Eliminated by poorly defined metabolism and unchanged via renal excretion (10%)	Used for hypertensive episodes in and diagnosis of phaeochromocytoma; given by intravenous injection
Angiotensin-converting enzyme inhibitors		
These drugs are used for hypertension, heart failure, prophylaxis of ischaemic heart disease and diabetic nephropathy. All are given orally; many are prodrugs that undergo bioactivation by hepatic metabolism		
Captopril	2 [M + R] Good absorption (70–80%) with limited first-pass metabolism (10%); eliminated by renal filtration plus secretion, and formation of inactive metabolites	

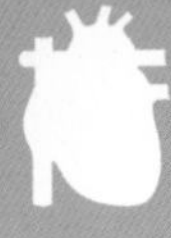

Drugs used to treat hypertension

Drug	Half-life (h) and kinetics	Comments
Cilazapril	30 [R cilazaprilat][a] Prodrug, which is well absorbed (60%); converted in liver to cilazaprilat, which shows biphasic elimination with half-lives of 1–2 and 30–50 h	
Enalapril	35 [R enalaprilat][a] Prodrug, which is well absorbed (60%); converted in liver to enalaprilat, both enalapril and enalaprilat are eliminated in the urine	
Fosinopril	12 [R fosinoprilat][a] Poorly absorbed prodrug of which about 30% is converted in the intestine and liver to fosinoprilat; fosinoprilat is eliminated unchanged in urine and faeces	
Imidapril	8 [imidaprilat][a] [M] Prodrug, which is well absorbed and rapidly hydrolysed (half-life 2 h) to the active imidaprilat, which is excreted in urine	
Lisinopril	12 [R] Incompletely absorbed from gut; excreted unchanged in urine (30%) and faeces (70%)	
Moexipril	10 [R moexiprilat][a] Poorly absorbed prodrug; converted in liver to moexiprilat; significant amounts (50%) are excreted in faeces as moexiprilat (possibly formed in gut lumen from unabsorbed compound)	
Perindopril	29 (perindoprilat)[a] [R perindoprilat] Well-absorbed prodrug; about 20% is converted in liver to perindoprilat, which is eliminated in urine	
Quinapril	2 (quinaprilat)[a] [R quinaprilat] Well-absorbed prodrug; converted in liver to quinaprilat, which is eliminated rapidly by renal tubular secretion	
Ramipril	1–5 (ramiprilat)[a] [R ramiprilat] Well-absorbed prodrug; converted in liver to ramiprilat, which is excreted in urine	
Trandolapril	16–24 (trandolaprilat)[a] [R + M] Well-absorbed prodrug; converted in liver to trandolaprilat and inactive metabolites; trandolaprilat is eliminated in urine and by metabolism and has a slow minor terminal half-life of 50–100 h (which is not clinically significant)	
Angiotensin II receptor antagonists acting at AT_1R receptor subtype		
Used for hypertension, heart failure, prophylaxis after myocardial infarction, and diabetic nephropathy. All drugs are given orally		
Candesartan	9–12 [R + M] Given as the prodrug, candesartan cilexetil, which is rapidly hydrolysed during absorption to the active candesartan (15%); candesartan is eliminated by renal excretion (26%) and in faeces (possibly as metabolites)	Highly selective blockade of AT_1 receptors
Eprosartan	5–9 [R] Rapidly absorbed but with a low bioavailability (13%); eliminated largely unchanged in urine plus some conjugation with glucuronic acid	
Irbesartan	11–15 [M + R] Oral bioavailability is 60–80%; metabolised by oxidation (CYP2C9) and conjugation; parent drug plus conjugates eliminated in urine and bile	Highly selective blockade at AT_1 receptors

Drugs used to treat hypertension

Drug	Half-life (h) and kinetics	Comments
Losartan	2 [M] Extensive first-pass metabolism (50%) to inactive metabolites plus an active metabolite	Highly selective blockade at AT_1 receptors; active metabolite gives prolonged non-competitive selective blockade at AT_1 receptors
Olmesartan	13 [R + bile] Given as medoxomil prodrug, which is rapidly and quantitatively converted to olmesartan in the gastrointestinal tract; olmesartan is eliminated unchanged	
Telmisartan	16–23 [bile + M] Good oral bioavailability (50%); eliminated unchanged in faeces, possibly after biliary excretion of the glucuronide conjugate	Highly selective blockade at AT_1 receptors
Valsartan	5–7 [M] Oral bioavailability is 25%; oxidised in liver to a hydroxy metabolite; duration of action is 24 h, allowing once-daily dosing	Highly selective blockade at AT_1 receptors
Direct renin inhibitors		
Aliskiren	40 h [faeces]] Poorly absorbed nonapeptide; oral bioavailability is only 3%	Given orally
Endothelin receptor inhibitors		
Used for pulmonary arterial hypertension		
Bosentan	5 [M] Extensively metabolised by, and an inducer of, CYP2C9 and CYP3A4; blood levels change during the early stages of treatment due to autoinduction of metabolism; metabolites eliminated in bile	Endothelin-A receptor antagonist; given orally
Sitaxentan	9 [R + faecal] 10% of administered dose metabolised	Highly selective endothelin-A receptor antagonist: possible effect on warfarin levels via inhibition of CYP2C9
Potassium channel openers		
Minoxidil	3–4 [M + R] Complete oral bioavailability; mainly eliminated as a glucuronide conjugate	Used for severe hypertension; given orally
Vasodilators		
Drugs used under special circumstances		
Diazoxide	28 [R + M] Given in emergencies by intravenous bolus injection; eliminated largely by glomerular filtration; long half-life is a result of high protein binding	Used for severe hypertension
Hydralazine	4 [M] Undergoes first-pass metabolism by N-acetylation with a bioavailability of 10–15% in fast acetylators and 30–35% in slow acetylators; eliminated by acetylation and oxidation; slow acetylators have high circulating concentrations of hydralazine	Used as an adjunct for treating moderate or severe hypertension, for heart failure and for hypertensive crisis; given orally, by slow intravenous injection or by intravenous infusion
Sodium nitroprusside	Seconds [decomposition + R] Decomposes to NO and CN, which are eliminated largely in the urine as nitrite and thiocyanate ions; the clinical responses (owing to NO) are very rapid and short-lived	Used for hypersensitive crisis, for controlled hypertension in anaesthesia and for acute heart failure

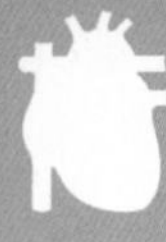

Drugs used to treat hypertension

Drug	Half-life (h) and kinetics	Comments
Centrally acting antihypertensive drugs		
Clonidine	20–25 [R + M] Good oral bioavailability (70%+); eliminated unchanged in urine (60%) and as hydroxyl metabolites	Selective α_2-adrenoceptor agonist; used for hypertension, migraine and menopausal flushing; given orally or by slow intravenous injection; sudden withdrawal may give hypertensive crisis
Methyldopa	1–2 [R + M] Oral bioavailability is 10–60% owing to conjugation with sulphate in the intestinal wall; eliminated by glomerular filtration and sulphate conjugation	Selective α_2-adrenoceptor agonist; used particularly for hypertension in pregnancy; given orally
Moxonidine	2–3 [R + M] Oral bioavailability is about 90%; eliminated largely in the urine unchanged	Selective imidazoline I_1 receptor agonist; given orally
Guanethidine	2 days [R] Eliminated by renal excretion and metabolism; very slow terminal phase (4–8 days) reported in some studies	Used only for hypertensive crisis; given by intramuscular injection

[a]The half-life and route of elimination [ ] relate to the active metabolite, which is named in square brackets.
[M], metabolism; [R], renal excretion.

7 Heart failure

MAINTENANCE OF CARDIAC OUTPUT

There are four major determinants of cardiac output:

- *preload*: this is governed by the ventricular end-diastolic volume, which in turn is related to ventricular filling pressure and, therefore, to venous return
- *heart rate*
- *myocardial contractility*
- *afterload*: the systolic wall tension in the ventricle; this reflects the resistance to ventricular emptying within both the heart and the peripheral circulation.

These factors normally balance the output from both sides of the heart. In the healthy heart, cardiac output is regulated mainly by changes in heart rate and preload. Heart rate is mainly modulated by the autonomic nervous system, with sympathetic nervous stimulation increasing heart rate.

The relationship between preload and stroke volume (the amount of blood ejected from the ventricle during systole with each contraction) is shown in Figure 7.1. The degree of stretch of the ventricular muscle (preload) determines the force of cardiac contraction (the Frank–Starling phenomenon). The curve describing this relationship is governed by intrinsic myocardial contractility: thus, the curve is shifted upwards and to the left when contractility is augmented, for example by sympathetic nervous stimulation. The normal physiological response to changes in left ventricular filling pressure in a healthy heart with normal contractility falls on the steep part of the curve, making stroke volume very sensitive to small changes in preload.

The relationship between afterload and stroke volume is shown in Figure 7.2. Afterload is determined largely by peripheral resistance but also by the size of the ventricle. Enlargement of the left ventricular cavity (e.g. as a result of increased venous return or preload) increases wall tension, and the heart must generate greater pressure both to initiate and to maintain contraction. Preload and afterload are therefore interrelated. In the healthy ventricle, a rise in afterload is met by an increase in myocardial contractility to maintain stroke volume.

PATHOPHYSIOLOGY OF HEART FAILURE

There is no universally accepted definition, but the heart failure syndrome is usually said to exist when the output of the heart is insufficient to meet the metabolic needs of the body. Heart failure has several underlying causes (Box 7.1), and can arise suddenly or develop gradually. In most causes of heart failure, the primary problem is a reduction in the stroke volume ejected from the left ventricle into the aorta due to impaired myocardial function.

The syndrome of heart failure arises largely from neurohumoral counter-regulation in response to the low blood pressure and low renal perfusion pressure (Fig. 7.3). The consequences of these compensatory mechanisms are vasoconstriction of both arteries and veins and excessive salt and water retention by the kidneys. These arise in an attempt to increase the blood pressure, but in the setting of a failing heart can exacerbate the cardiac dysfunction.

In the failing ventricle, the Frank–Starling curve is shifted downwards (failing ventricle curve: Fig. 7.1) and the maximal achievable stroke volume is reduced. The curve is also flatter, indicating that stroke volume is less dependent on changes in preload. Salt and water retention expands plasma volume, which, combined with venoconstriction that enhances venous return to the heart, increases the filling pressure of the left ventricle in an attempt to restore the resting stroke volume. Cardiac output may also be maintained by an increase in heart rate. If these responses are successful in preserving cardiac output, the heart failure is said to be *'compensated'*. *Decompensation* arises when the combination of the increases in preload and heart rate fail to restore a normal resting cardiac output (Fig. 7.3). The hydrostatic pressure in the pulmonary veins rises as the central blood volume continues to increase; pulmonary oedema occurs when the pressure exceeds the plasma colloid osmotic (oncotic) pressure, which holds fluid in the

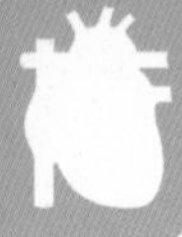

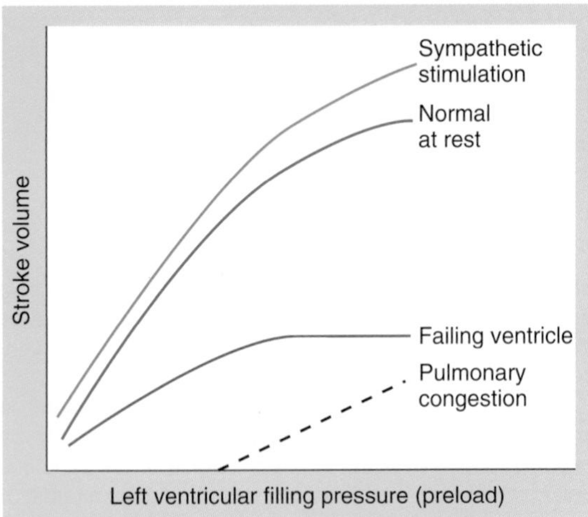

Fig. 7.1 **The relationship between preload (left ventricular filling pressure) and stroke volume (the Frank–Starling phenomenon) in the healthy and failing heart.** In the failing heart, if an increase in filling pressure and heart rate are insufficient to restore cardiac output, then pulmonary congestion will occur.

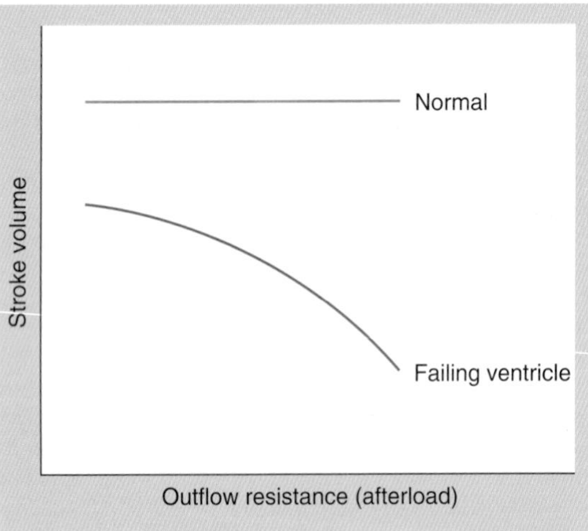

Fig. 7.2 **The relationship between afterload (outflow resistance) and stroke volume in the presence of normal and reduced myocardial contractility.**

blood vessel (Fig. 7.2). Eventually, the raised pulmonary vascular pressure leads to right heart failure (producing biventricular failure, previously called congestive cardiac failure), and oedema develops in the peripheral and splanchnic tissues. As described above, the compensatory mechanisms also increase peripheral arterial resistance (afterload) (Fig. 7.2). In the failing ventricle, an inability to augment contraction when afterload rises leads to a fall in stroke volume (Fig. 7.2) with further cardiac decompensation.

Heart failure arising from myocyte loss (such as occurs with myocardial infarction or cardiomyopathies) leads to

Box 7.1 Causes of heart failure

Coronary artery disease
Hypertension
Myocardial disease: cardiomyopathies, myocarditis
Valvular heart disease
Constrictive pericarditis
Congenital: atrial septal defect, ventricular septal defect, aortic coarctation
Infiltrative: amyloid, sarcoid, iron
Iatrogenic: β-adrenoceptor antagonists, antiarrhythmics, calcium channel blockers, cytotoxics, alcohol, irradiation
Arrhythmias, especially incessant tachyarrhythmias

adaptive changes in the surviving cells and extracellular matrix, known as remodelling. This eventually produces a more globular, dysfunctional left ventricle.

In aortic or mitral valve regurgitation, heart failure arises because the heart must accommodate the normal forward stroke volume and also the regurgitant volume (the volume leaking back into the left ventricle or left atrium). Eventually, the left ventricle cannot enlarge sufficiently to maintain an effective stroke volume. Regardless of the cause, the onset of symptomatic heart failure is due to a fall in cardiac output and therefore blood pressure.

Heart failure can also arise from impaired diastolic relaxation (diastolic heart failure). If the left ventricle fails to relax adequately, it will not accommodate the venous return, leading to pulmonary venous congestion and a low cardiac output, activating the same compensatory neurohumoral responses. Diastolic heart failure characteristically occurs in elderly people in association with left ventricular hypertrophy, but it also contributes to heart failure in ischaemic left ventricular dysfunction (see Ch. 5).

Symptoms in heart failure are caused by a reduced cardiac output ('forward failure') or venous congestion ('backward failure'). The most common complaint is breathlessness from increased pulmonary venous pressure, while fatigue, resulting from the reduced cardiac output and impaired skeletal muscle perfusion, is frequent. In response to the reduced perfusion, biochemical changes also occur in skeletal muscle, making it less efficient. Other symptoms, such as the discomfort of peripheral oedema and anorexia due to bowel congestion, are attributable to a high systemic venous pressure.

In the heart, β_1-adrenoceptors mediate enhanced contractility and hasten relaxation in response to sympathetic nervous stimulation. β_1- and to a lesser extent β_2-adrenoceptors mediate an increase in heart rate. In heart failure, chronic activation of these receptors also increases the chances of serious cardiac arrhythmias. However, if stimulation is excessive, β_1-adrenoceptors are down-regulated, which blunts the effects of chronic activation.

ACUTE LEFT VENTRICULAR FAILURE

Acute left ventricular failure usually results from a sudden inability of the heart to maintain an adequate cardiac output and blood pressure. This leads to reflex arterial and venous constriction (Fig. 7.3). There is a rapid rise in filling pressure of the left ventricle as a result of increased venous return.

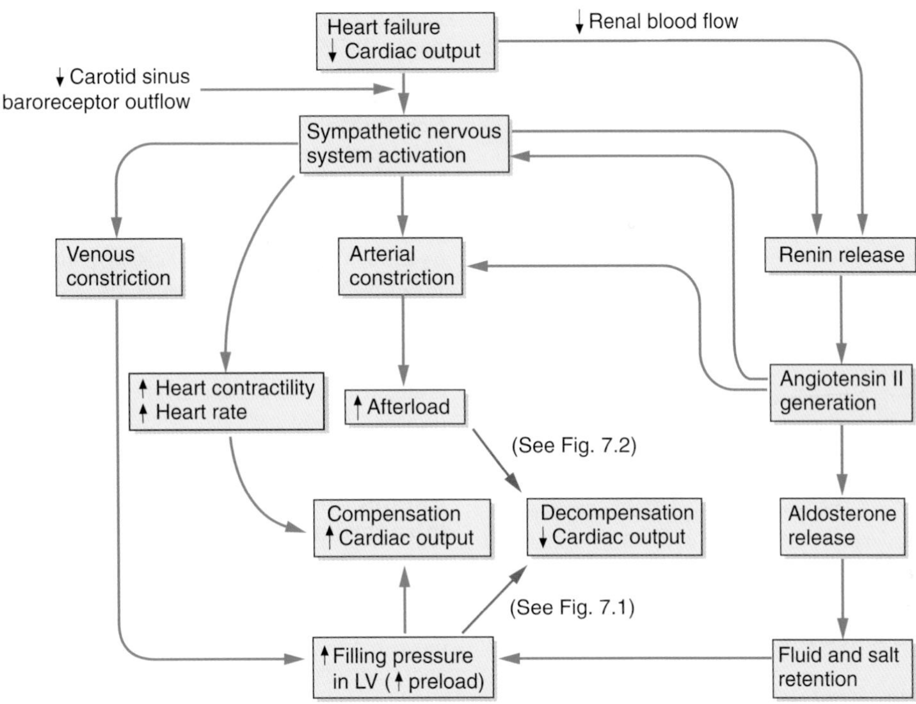

Fig. 7.3 **Neurohumoral consequences of heart failure**. Starting at the box at the top of the diagram, in the mildly impaired heart a fall in cardiac output results in a cascade of compensatory events (green arrows); overall these result in *compensation* and the consequent increase in preload can improve cardiac performance as shown in the bottom box in the diagram (see also Fig. 7.1 – normal curve). However, if cardiac function is significantly impaired (red lines), an increased preload cannot restore an adequate stroke volume (decompensation) (see Fig. 7.1 – failing ventricle curve). The increased afterload will also put additional strain on the failing heart and can further decrease cardiac output (see Fig. 7.2). Chronic heart failure is also associated with elevated activity in the sympathetic nervous system, angiotensin II and endothelin-1 and a downregulation in nitric oxide synthesis. These effects are compounded by downregulation of cardiac β_1-adrenoceptors.

If the heart is unable to expel the extra blood, the hydrostatic pressure in the pulmonary veins rises until it exceeds the plasma oncotic pressure and produces pulmonary oedema. The principal symptom is breathlessness, occurring on exertion in the early stages, then at rest with orthopnoea. Left ventricular failure can follow acute myocardial infarction, acute mitral or aortic valvular regurgitation, or arise from the onset of a brady- or tachyarrhythmia if there is pre-existing poor left ventricular function.

CARDIOGENIC SHOCK

The syndrome of cardiogenic shock arises when the systolic function of the left ventricle is suddenly impaired to such a degree that there is insufficient blood flow to meet resting metabolic requirements of the tissues. This definition excludes shock caused by hypovolaemia. The clinical hallmarks are a low systolic blood pressure (usually <90 mmHg), with a reduced cardiac output and an elevated left ventricular filling pressure. Cardiogenic shock can follow acute myocardial infarction, and in this situation usually indicates loss of at least 40% of the left ventricular myocardium. Other mechanical disturbances, such as acute mitral regurgitation or ventricular septal rupture, can produce cardiogenic shock in association with a lesser degree of myocardial damage. Less commonly, the syndrome is associated with right ventricular infarction. The mortality of cardiogenic shock, even with intensive treatment, is in excess of 70%.

CHRONIC HEART FAILURE

Myocardial damage from ischaemic heart disease is the most common cause of chronic heart failure, but potentially correctable causes such as valvular lesions, as well as treatable exacerbating factors such as anaemia or arrhythmias, may be identified. In most people with heart failure, there are signs of both right and left ventricular failure (biventricular or congestive heart failure). Chronic heart failure is not a trivial complaint. People with left ventricular systolic dysfunction who have symptoms only on exertion have a 2-year mortality risk of about 20%, while the 1-year mortality is 80% if there are symptoms at rest. In systolic heart failure, the degree of left ventricular dysfunction is a guide to prognosis. Death is either from progressive heart failure or from sudden arrhythmias. The mortality in heart failure due to left ventricular diastolic dysfunction is less than that of systolic heart failure, but still four times that of the general population.

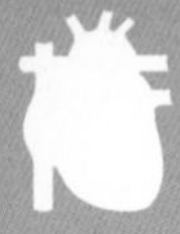

POSITIVE INOTROPIC DRUGS IN THE TREATMENT OF HEART FAILURE

Myocardial contractility can be improved by increasing the availability of free intracellular Ca^{2+} to interact with contractile proteins, or by increasing the sensitivity of the myofibrils to Ca^{2+}. Only drugs that increase myocardial intracellular Ca^{2+} are established in clinical use; they work by one of two distinct mechanisms:

- an action on the cell membrane Na^+/K^+-ATPase pump (e.g. digoxin)
- by increasing intracellular cyclic adenosine monophosphate (cAMP) (e.g. phosphodiesterase inhibitors).

An additional advantage of the positive inotropic drugs that increase myocardial cAMP is their ability to enhance the reuptake of Ca^{2+} by the sarcoplasmic reticulum in diastole. This improves diastolic relaxation in addition to augmenting systolic contractility.

DIGITALIS GLYCOSIDES

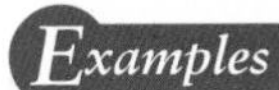

digitoxin, digoxin

Mechanism of action and effects

Effect on myocardial contractility

Digitalis glycosides are compounds with a steroid nucleus that were originally isolated from a species of foxglove (*Digitalis purpura*). They bind to the energy-dependent Na^+ pump (Na^+/K^+-ATPase) in the myocyte membrane. This pump establishes and maintains the Na^+ and K^+ gradients across the cell (Fig. 7.4), producing low intracellular Na^+ and high intracellular K^+ concentrations. A separate passive transmembrane exchange of Na^+ and Ca^{2+} occurs down their concentration gradients, with Na^+ entering the cell while Ca^{2+} is translocated out. The rate of this exchange is dependent on the intracellular Na^+ concentration. Digitalis glycosides produce partial inhibition of the Na^+/K^+-ATPase, which increases the intracellular Na^+ concentration. This lowers the concentration gradient for Na^+ across the cell membrane, and therefore Na^+/Ca^{2+} exchange is reduced so that Ca^{2+} is retained in the cell. The excess intracellular Ca^{2+} is stored in the sarcoplasmic reticulum during diastole and released during cell membrane excitation, leading to enhanced myocardial contraction.

Effects on cardiac action potential and intracardiac conduction

Digitalis glycosides are arrhythmogenic, but also have actions that are useful for treating certain arrhythmias.

Direct actions of digitalis glycosides on the heart can provoke arrhythmias by increasing myocardial excitability and automaticity (Ch. 8). The mechanisms that provoke arrhythmias are as follows.

- **Reduction of the resting membrane potential**: the cell membrane Na^+/K^+-ATPase pump extrudes three Na^+ out of the cell for every two K^+ that enter, which increases the resting negative intracellular electrical potential and hyperpolarises the cell (see Ch. 8). Inhibition of this membrane pump by digitalis glycosides leads to the cell membrane potential becoming less negative and closer to the threshold potential for depolarisation. Arrhythmias are therefore more readily initiated.

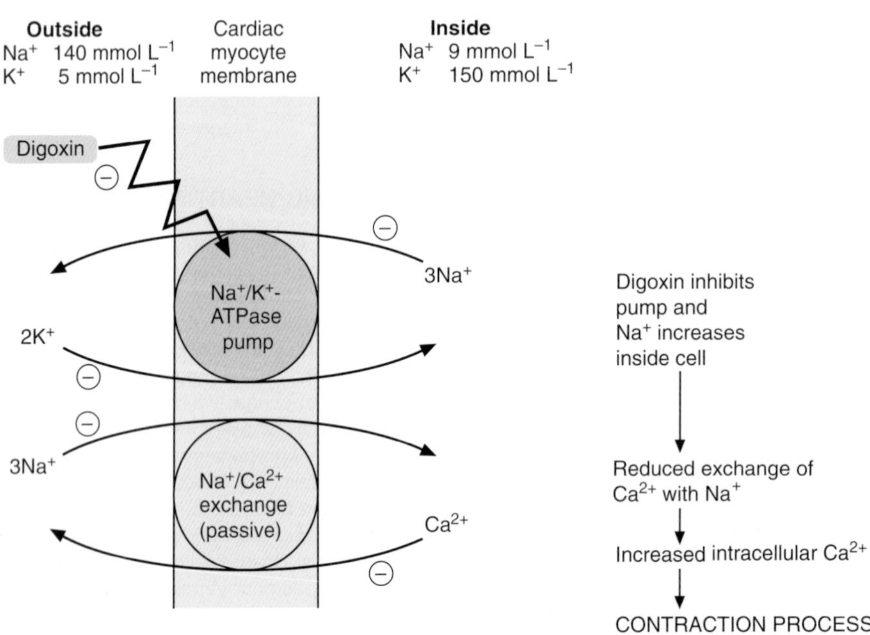

Fig. 7.4 **The action of digoxin on the cardiac myocyte.**

- **Triggering of spontaneous release of Ca^{2+} from the sarcoplasmic reticulum**: this leads to transient depolarisation of the cell immediately following an action potential ('after potentials'), which can initiate arrhythmias (Ch. 8).

Digitalis glycosides also have clinically useful indirect actions on the heart that arise from stimulation of the central vagal nucleus, and that enable them to be used for treating arrhythmias (Ch. 8). The vagal effects on the heart are as follows.

- **Decreased automaticity of the sinoatrial node**: this slightly slows heart rate in sinus rhythm.
- **Increased refractory period of the atrioventricular node**: this slows impulse transmission to the ventricles. This is useful in the management of the fast ventricular rates that result from atrial flutter and fibrillation (Ch. 8).

Pharmacokinetics

Digoxin is the most widely used of the digitalis glycosides. It is well absorbed from the gut, and the kidney is the main route of elimination, partially by active tubular secretion. The half-life of digoxin is very long (about 1.5 days) and is increased if renal function is impaired. The dose must be reduced in the presence of renal impairment, to avoid toxicity (see below). To achieve an early onset of action, loading doses should be given over the first 24 or 36 h (Ch. 2). If a rapid response is essential, digoxin can be given by slow intravenous injection.

Digitoxin is occasionally given when there is renal impairment, since it is extensively metabolised and mainly excreted via the gut. However, it has the disadvantage of an even longer half-life (approximately 8 days).

Unwanted effects

Digitalis glycosides have a narrow therapeutic index, and toxicity is mostly dose-related.

- *Consequences of intracellular Ca^{2+} overload*: increased automaticity of the atrioventricular node and Purkinje fibres produces junctional escape beats, junctional tachycardia, ventricular ectopic beats (including bigeminy: coupling of an ectopic beat after each normal beat) or (less commonly) ventricular tachycardia.
- *Distinctive changes on the ECG*: this includes non-specific T-wave changes and sagging of the S–T segment with an upright T-wave ('reverse tick'). These ECG effects can be mistaken for myocardial ischaemia.
- *Consequences of increased vagal activity*: excessive atrioventricular nodal block can occur; when associated with increased atrial automaticity, this produces atrial tachycardia with 2:1 atrioventricular nodal block, a rhythm characteristic of digitalis toxicity.
- *Gastrointestinal disturbances*: anorexia, nausea and vomiting (largely a central effect at the chemoreceptor trigger zone; Ch. 32), and diarrhoea.
- *Neurological disturbances*: fatigue, malaise, confusion, vertigo, coloured vision (especially yellow halos around lights, possibly from inhibition of Na^+/K^+-ATPase in the cones of the retina).
- *Gynaecomastia*: the steroid structure allows digitalis glycosides to bind to oestrogen receptors in breast tissue.

Exacerbating factors for digitalis glycoside toxicity

- *Hypokalaemia*: reduced extracellular K^+ concentration increases the effects of digitalis glycosides on the Na^+/K^+-ATPase pump. Care must be taken if potassium-losing diuretics, such as furosemide (Ch. 14), are used with digitalis glycosides.
- *Renal impairment reduces the excretion of digoxin*. This is not always obvious in the elderly, who may have a normal plasma creatinine concentration even when renal function is markedly reduced (see Ch. 56).
- *Hypoxaemia*: this sensitises the heart to digitalis glycoside-induced arrhythmias.
- *Hypothyroidism*: the renal elimination of digoxin is decreased because of a reduced glomerular filtration rate.
- *Drugs that displace digoxin from tissue binding sites and interfere with its renal excretion*: these include verapamil (Ch. 5) and quinidine (Ch. 8), which can double the plasma concentration of digoxin; amiodarone (Ch. 8) produces a less marked effect.

Treatment of digitalis toxicity

Digitalis glycoside toxicity can be treated by:

- withholding further doses of digitalis glycoside
- using K^+ supplementation (Ch. 14) for hypokalaemia; this is usually given orally, but should be given by slow intravenous infusion if there are dangerous arrhythmias
- atropine (Ch. 8) for sinus bradycardia or atrioventricular block; temporary transvenous pacing is used for marked bradycardia unresponsive to atropine
- digoxin-specific antibody fragments for serious digoxin toxicity (Ch. 53).

SYMPATHOMIMETIC INOTROPES

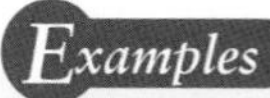

selective β_1-adrenoceptor agonist: dobutamine
selective β_2-adrenoceptor agonist and dopamine receptor agonist: dopexamine
non-selective β-adrenoceptor, α-adrenoceptor and dopamine receptor agonist: dopamine

Mechanisms of action and effects

The mechanisms of action of the sympathomimetic inotropes are also considered in Chapter 4.

Isoprenaline is a non-selective β-adrenoceptor agonist that is now only available in the UK on special order.

Dobutamine, a synthetic dopamine analogue, is a selective β_1-adrenoceptor agonist that produces a powerful inotropic response, with relatively less increase in heart rate and little direct effect on vascular tone, even at high concentrations.

Dopexamine acts on β_2-adrenoceptors to increase heart rate and to vasodilate, and, to a lesser extent, on

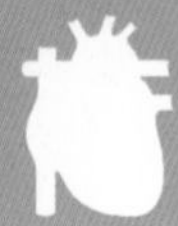

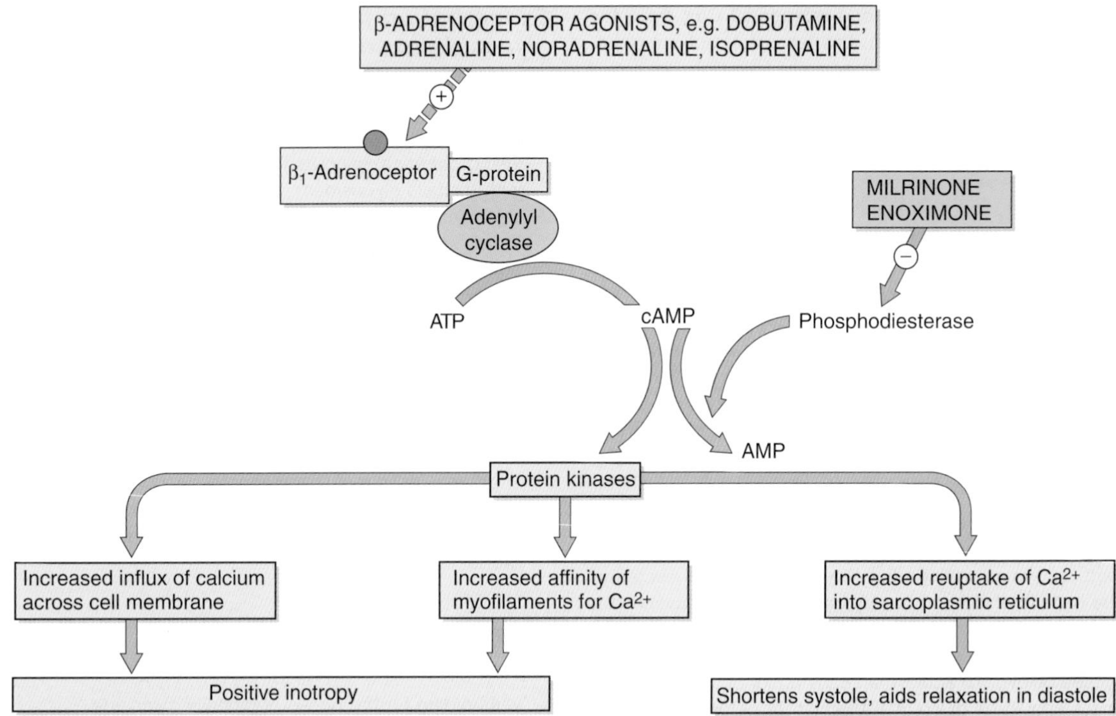

Fig. 7.5 **Mechanisms by which sympathomimetics and phosphodiesterase inhibitors exert their positive inotropic effects.**

β_1-adrenoceptors, giving a weak direct positive inotropic effect. It also acts on peripheral dopamine receptors and produces some increase in renal blood flow, but, unlike dopamine, it does not cause peripheral vasoconstriction with high doses.

Dopamine has dose-related actions at several receptors.

- At low doses, it selectively stimulates peripheral dopamine receptors, which are structurally distinct from those in the central nervous system. This produces renal arterial vasodilation and diuresis (D_1 receptors) and peripheral arterial vasodilation (D_2 presynaptic receptors, which inhibit noradrenaline release from sympathetic nerves).
- At moderate doses, non-selective β-adrenoceptor stimulation produces a positive inotropic response (Fig. 7.5). Tachycardia is more marked than with dobutamine, because of stimulation of both cardiac β_1- and β_2-adrenoceptors and the reflex response to β_2-adrenoceptor-mediated peripheral arterial dilation.
- At high doses, α_1-adrenoceptor stimulation produces peripheral vasoconstriction, which also affects the renal arteries and overcomes D_1-receptor-mediated renal vasodilation.

The doses that produce these different effects differ widely among individuals. Unfortunately, there is no dose that can be relied upon to act selectively at dopamine receptors without stimulating adrenoceptors.

Pharmacokinetics

All sympathomimetic inotropes are administered by intravenous infusion because of their very short half-lives of about 2–10 min. Metabolic inactivation is by the same pathways as for noradrenaline (Ch. 4). Desensitisation and downregulation of β-adrenoceptors (Ch. 1) rapidly reduce the response to sustained infusions over 48–72 h. Because of its unpredictable vasoconstrictor actions, dopamine is usually given into a large central vein.

Unwanted effects

Unwanted effects can be predicted from agonist actions at adrenoceptors (Ch. 4) and mainly relate to excessive cardiac stimulation, with tachycardia, palpitations and arrhythmias.

PHOSPHODIESTERASE INHIBITORS

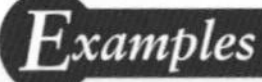

enoximone, milrinone

Mechanism of action and effects

Milrinone and enoximone are specific inhibitors of the isoenzyme of phosphodiesterase (type 3) found in cardiac and smooth muscle. Their inotropic action on the heart results from an increase in intracellular cAMP with increased mobilisation of intracellular Ca^{2+} (Fig. 7.5). Unlike β-adrenoceptor agonists, the activity of phosphodiesterase inhibitors is not limited by desensitisation of cell surface receptors, because they act at a site beyond the receptor. Since they have complementary sites of action, phosphodiesterase inhibitors and β-adrenoceptor agonists will have additive effects on the heart. Phosphodiesterase inhibition in vascular smooth muscle produces peripheral arterial vasodilation.

Pharmacokinetics

Phosphodiesterase inhibitors are only given for short-term treatment by intravenous infusion. Milrinone is eliminated by the kidney and enoximone by hepatic metabolism. They have elimination half-lives of about 1 h.

Unwanted effects

- These are mainly a consequence of excessive cardiac stimulation, and include especially tachycardia, palpitation and potentially serious arrhythmias.
- Long-term oral use increases mortality in heart failure. Oral use has therefore been abandoned.

MANAGEMENT OF HEART FAILURE

ACUTE LEFT VENTRICULAR FAILURE

The immediate aim of pharmacological treatment in acute left ventricular failure is to reduce the excessive venous return. Treatment includes:

- Oxygen in high concentration via a facemask.
- Intravenous opioid analgesic such as morphine (Ch. 19), often given to relieve distress and breathlessness.
- Intravenous injection of a loop diuretic such as furosemide (Ch. 14). This initially produces venodilation, which increases peripheral venous pooling. Symptoms are therefore improved even before the onset of a diuresis that reduces plasma volume and further decreases preload.
- Sublingual glyceryl trinitrate (Ch. 5). This dilates venous capacitance vessels and is a useful alternative or additional emergency treatment to diuretics.

Whenever possible, a precipitating or exacerbating cause should be treated – for example, arrhythmias, anaemia, thyrotoxicosis, acute mitral regurgitation or critical aortic stenosis. However, if there is underlying left ventricular systolic impairment, then management as for chronic heart failure is subsequently necessary.

CARDIOGENIC SHOCK

The immediate aim of treatment is resuscitation, while looking for a remediable cause. If appropriate, early coronary revascularisation is crucial to increase the probability of survival. Supportive measures include the following:

- Oxygen in high concentration via a facemask.
- Correct any acid–base imbalance (especially acidosis) and electrolyte abnormalities (particularly hypokalaemia).
- Relieve pain, usually with an opioid analgesic such as morphine (Ch. 19).
- Correct any cardiac rhythm disturbance (Ch. 8).
- Ensure an adequate left ventricular filling pressure. This can be low after right ventricular infarction, despite a high central venous pressure (right ventricular filling pressure). If intravenous volume is adequate but tissue perfusion remains impaired, dobutamine is the inotropic drug of choice. Dobutamine is often given in combination with low-dose dopamine, with the intention that the dopamine will improve renal perfusion; however, there is little evidence that the addition of dopamine is beneficial.
- Phosphodiesterase inhibitors are sometimes given to improve myocardial contractility and to produce peripheral vasodilation. They are usually reserved for those who fail to improve with maximum tolerated doses of dobutamine.
- When there is profound hypotension, noradrenaline (norepinephrine) (Ch. 4) can be infused intravenously to produce α_1-adrenoceptor-mediated peripheral vasoconstriction and maintain vital organ perfusion. The potential disadvantage is that the increase in peripheral resistance will further impair cardiac output. Vasopressin (Ch. 43) is sometimes given to raise blood pressure, as vascular sensitivity to noradrenaline is impaired in shock. Vasopressin is a vasoconstrictor that also increases vascular sensitivity to noradrenaline.
- Vasodilators can be given to 'offload' the heart once an adequate blood pressure has been established. This strategy is particularly helpful if there is significant mitral regurgitation, since reduced resistance to left ventricular emptying will diminish the regurgitant volume. Either glyceryl trinitrate (Ch. 5) or nitroprusside (Ch. 6) is used.

CHRONIC SYSTOLIC HEART FAILURE

Much of the treatment of chronic heart failure is directed towards counteracting the compensatory mechanisms for the reduced cardiac output and low blood pressure generated by a failing heart, i.e. arterial and venous vasoconstriction and fluid retention. A further desirable action is to reduce or reverse the shape change (remodelling) that occurs in the failing ventricle and makes contraction less efficient. Treatment has two main aims: symptom relief and improved prognosis.

Non-pharmacological treatment

A number of lifestyle changes can be helpful.

- Weight reduction should be encouraged for an obese person; this improves exercise tolerance.
- Bed rest may be appropriate to rest the heart during acute episodes of fluid retention.
- Modest salt restriction is desirable (severe salt restriction is unpleasant and unnecessary).
- Fluid restriction is rarely required unless profound hyponatraemia accompanies severe oedema. In this situation, diuretics may be ineffective until the plasma Na^+ concentration is corrected.
- If possible, drugs that exacerbate heart failure by producing myocardial depression (e.g. most calcium

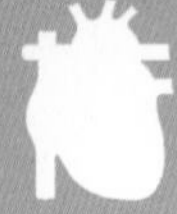

channel blockers) or by promoting fluid retention (e.g. non-steroidal anti-inflammatory drugs [NSAIDs]) should be withdrawn. Beta-adrenoceptor antagonists can cause myocardial depression, but should not be stopped, although a high dose may need to be reduced. Alcohol intake should be moderate at most, since alcohol depresses myocardial contractility and can be arrhythmogenic.
- A graded exercise programme for people with stable heart failure can improve symptoms.

Diuretics

Diuretics remain the mainstay of treatment for chronic heart failure with fluid retention, and are very effective for relief of symptoms (Ch. 14). They are usually taken once daily, in the morning. A thiazide diuretic, such as bendroflumethiazide, when used alone is only useful to relieve mild symptoms, and a loop diuretic (usually furosemide) is used for moderate or severe fluid retention. There is no evidence that the use of a loop or thiazide diuretic alters prognosis. Hypokalaemia is unusual when loop diuretics are used in chronic heart failure, especially as an angiotensin-converting enzyme (ACE) inhibitor or angiotensin receptor antagonist is usually taken concurrently (see below). Nevertheless, the use of a potassium-sparing diuretic is advisable if the plasma K^+ falls below 3.5 mmol L^{-1}, especially if digoxin or antiarrhythmic therapy is given concurrently (because of an increased risk of generating cardiac rhythm disturbances). Spironolactone is preferred in this situation since it improves symptoms and prognosis (at least in severe heart failure) if a low dose is added to maximal therapy with other drugs. Strategies for the management of diuretic-resistant fluid retention are considered in Chapter 14.

Angiotensin-converting enzyme inhibitors and angiotensin receptor antagonists

An ACE inhibitor (Ch. 6) is now considered to be essential in the treatment of systolic heart failure, and is usually started at the same time as a diuretic. ACE inhibitors produce arterial and venous dilation, which improves cardiac function by decreasing ventricular end-diastolic volume and increasing cardiac output (Figs 7.1 and 7.2). An ACE inhibitor usually improves breathlessness and fatigue, and exercise tolerance increases. The full symptomatic response is often delayed for 4 to 6 weeks after the start of treatment, despite early haemodynamic changes. A further benefit of ACE inhibitors is improved survival, which may be due to a reversal of the remodelling of the left ventricle. High doses of an ACE inhibitor are more effective than low doses, and reduce mortality by 20–25% in systolic heart failure.

There is a small risk of symptomatic hypotension after administration of the first dose of an ACE inhibitor; use of a small initial dose of ACE inhibitor reduces the duration of any hypotension. ACE inhibitors promote K^+ retention by the kidney; the combination of an ACE inhibitor with spironolactone in severe heart failure is advantageous in terms of prognosis, although the combination carries a small added risk of serious hyperkalaemia.

If an ACE inhibitor is not tolerated, usually because of cough, an angiotensin receptor antagonist (Ch. 6) can be substituted. These agents have similar efficacy to ACE inhibitors.

Beta-adrenoceptor antagonists

Contrary to traditional teaching, β-adrenoceptor antagonists (Ch. 5) are highly effective for the treatment of heart failure, usually after stabilising the condition with an ACE inhibitor (or an angiotensin receptor antagonist) and diuretic. β-adrenoceptor antagonists were once considered to be contraindicated in heart failure because of their negative inotropic properties. However, if introduced very gradually, starting with low doses, they improve both symptoms and survival. The survival advantage is additive to that produced by an ACE inhibitor, with a further reduction of 30–35% in mortality at all classes of severity of heart failure. Possible explanations for the benefit of β-adrenoceptor antagonists are numerous (Box 7.2), but a reduction in cardiac remodelling is probably important. Unless there are contraindications, all people with heart failure should now be treated with a β-adrenoceptor antagonist once they are clinically stable. The only compounds licensed for this use in the UK are bisoprolol, carvedilol and nebivolol, although there are also data to show the efficacy of a modified-release formulation of metoprolol.

Digoxin

Digitalis glycosides are widely used to control heart rate when heart failure is associated with atrial fibrillation and a rapid ventricular rate. The use of digoxin for heart failure associated with sinus rhythm has been more controversial, but there is now conclusive evidence that its positive inotropic effect can be useful as a supplement to diuretic and ACE inhibitor therapy when there is severe left ventricular systolic dysfunction and persisting symptoms. Digoxin improves symptoms and the need for hospitalisation, and survival may be improved if the serum digoxin concentration is kept low. Importantly, the effective dose of digoxin in sinus rhythm is smaller than that required for control of atrial fibrillation.

Other vasodilators

Treatment with a combination of hydralazine (Ch. 6) and isosorbide dinitrate or mononitrate (Ch. 5), in addition to a

Box 7.2 Possible beneficial effects of β-adrenoceptor antagonists in heart failure

Reduced workload of ischaemic myocardium
Restoration of cardiac excitation–contraction coupling and improved intracellular Ca^{2+} handling
Reduced cardiac hypertrophy and fibrosis
Reduced myocyte apoptosis
Antiarrhythmic effects

diuretic and digoxin, provides balanced arterial and venous dilation. This combination improves exercise tolerance in heart failure but produces only a modest reduction in mortality, although there may be greater benefits in people of Afro-Caribbean origin. The combination can be tried for people who cannot tolerate an ACE inhibitor or angiotensin receptor antagonist (Ch. 6).

Cardiac pacing and defibrillation

Cardiac resynchronisation therapy (CRT; biventricular electrical pacing) is helpful in severe heart failure when the ECG shows left bundle branch block and the ventricles display marked dyssynchronous contraction on echocardiography. About half of all people with heart failure die suddenly of ventricular arrhythmias, and an implantable cardioverter ventricular defibrillator (ICD) can improve prognosis when there is severe left ventricular impairment and a propensity to ventricular arrhythmias. Combined cardiac resynchronisation–defibrillator devices (CRT-D) are also available. Antiarrhythmic drugs do not improve survival in heart failure.

DIASTOLIC HEART FAILURE

The optimal management of diastolic heart failure is not well established. Most of the interventions that improve prognosis in systolic heart failure have shown little impact on survival in diastolic heart failure, and therefore treatment is mainly directed at symptom-relief using the drugs discussed above (with the exception of positive inotropic agents such as digoxin).

FURTHER READING

Ahmed A, Rich MW, Love TE et al (2006) Digoxin and reduction in mortality and hospitalization in heart failure: a comprehensive *post hoc* analysis of the DIG trial. *Eur Heart J* 27, 178–186

Amabile CM, Spencer AP (2004) Keeping your patient with heart failure safe. A review of potentially dangerous medications. *Arch Intern Med* 164, 709–720

Cleland JGF, Coletta A, Witte K (2006) Practical applications of intravenous diuretic therapy in decompensated heart failure. *Am J Med* 119(12A), S26–S36

DiBianco R (2003) Update on therapy for heart failure. *Am J Med* 115, 480–488

Dimopoulos K, Salukhe TV, Coats AJS et al (2004) Meta-analyses of mortality and morbidity effects of an angiotensin receptor blocker in patients with chronic heart failure already receiving an ACE inhibitor (alone or with a β-adrenoceptor antagonist). *Int J Cardiol* 93, 105–111

Eichhorn EJ, Gheorghiade M (2002) Digoxin. *Prog Cardiovasc Dis* 44, 251–266

Farrell MH, Foody JM, Krumholz HM (2002) β-adrenoceptor antagonists in heart failure. Clinical applications. *JAMA* 287, 890–897

Flather MD, Yuisuf S, Kober L et al (2000) Long-term ACE-inhibitor therapy in patients with heart failure or left ventricular dysfunction: a systematic overview of data from individual patients. *Lancet* 355, 1578–1581

Foody JM, Farrell MH, Krumholz HM (2002) β-adrenoceptor antagonist therapy in heart failure. Scientific review. *JAMA* 287, 883–889

Friedrich JO, Adhikari N, Herridge MS et al (2005) Meta-analysis: low-dose dopamine increases urine output but does not prevent renal dysfunction or death. *Ann Intern Med* 142, 510–521

Funck-Brentano C (2006) Beta-blockade in CHF: from contraindication to indication. *Eur Heart J* 8(suppl C), C19–C27

Gowda RM, Fox JT, Khan IA (2008) Cardiogenic shock: basics and clinical considerations. *Int J Cardiol* 123, 221–228

Koerner MM, Loebe M, Lisman KA et al (2001) New strategies for the management of acute decompensated heart failure. *Curr Opin Cardiol* 16, 164–173

McMurray JJV, Pfeffer MA (2006) Heart failure. *Lancet* 365, 1877–1889

Molenaar P, Parsonage WA (2005) Fundamental considerations of β-adrenoceptor subtypes in human heart failure. *Trends Pharmacol Sci* 26, 368–374

Nieminen MS, Böhm M, Cowie MR et al (2005) Executive summary of the guidelines on the diagnosis and treatment of acute heart failure: The Task Force on Acute Heart Failure of the European Society of Cardiology. *Eur Heart J* 26, 384–416

Rathore SS, Curtis JP, Jeptha P et al (2003) Association of serum digoxin concentration and outcomes in patients with heart failure. *JAMA* 289, 871–878

Shammas RL, Khan NUA, Nekkanti R et al (2007) Diastolic heart failure and left ventricular dysfunction: what we know and what we don't know! *Int J Cardiol* 115, 284–292

Silke B (2006) Beta-blockade in CHF: pathophysiological considerations. *Eur Heart J* 8(suppl C), C13–C18

Struthers AD (2006) Angiotensin blockade or aldosterone blockade as the third neuroendocrine-blocking drug in mild but symptomatic heart failure. *Heart* 92, 1728–1731

SELF-ASSESSMENT

1. In the following questions, the first statement, in italics, is true. Is the accompanying statement also true?
   a. *One of the determinants of cardiac output is afterload.* In healthy hearts, myocardial contractility increases following a rise in afterload.
   b. *A major symptom of pulmonary oedema is breathlessness.* Oedema occurs when the pressure in the pulmonary veins is less than the plasma osmotic pressure.
   c. *Detrimental changes in body function in heart failure occur as a result of attempts by the body to compensate for the cardiac dysfunction.* In heart failure, sympathetic outflow increases because of an increase in the sensory input from the baroreceptors in the carotid sinus.
   d. *Treatment of chronic heart failure is directed towards the compensatory mechanisms, i.e. vasoconstriction and fluid retention.* Digoxin is the mainstay of treatment of the vasoconstriction and fluid retention.

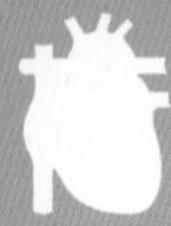

e. *The positive inotropic action of digoxin on the cardiac myocyte is a result of inhibition of the Na^+/K^+-ATPase pump on the myocyte membranes, ultimately increasing intracellular Ca^{2+} concentration.* Potassium ions and digoxin enhance the actions of each other at the Na^+/K^+-ATPase pump.
f. *Digoxin has both direct and indirect effects on the electrical properties of the heart.* Digoxin inhibits the vagus, decreasing the refractory period of the atrioventricular node.
g. *In cardiogenic shock, to improve tissue perfusion in the short term, dobutamine or the phosphodiesterase inhibitor milrinone can be given intravenously; their half-lives are very short.* Desensitisation of the response to dobutamine but not to milrinone can occur with sustained infusion.
h. *Dobutamine increases cardiac output and decreases ventricular filling pressure in heart failure.* Dobutamine produces peripheral vasodilation by its effect on β_2-adrenoceptors.
i. *Digoxin has a half-life of about 1.5 days.* The toxicity of digoxin increases in renal failure.
j. *In heart failure, drugs that do not have a direct action on the heart are very useful.* ACE inhibitors improve survival in chronic heart failure and have added benefit if given together with K^+-sparing diuretics such as spironolactone.

2. Toxicity related to digoxin is common. Which one of the following events is **unlikely** to increase the chance of toxicity occurring?
   A. A decline in renal function
   B. Moderately raised extracellular potassium concentrations
   C. Administration of bendroflumethiazide
   D. Administration of furosemide
   E. Administration of verapamil
3. Case history questions

Mr DY is 78 years of age and had a large anterior myocardial infarction 3 years ago. Echocardiography revealed marked left ventricular systolic dysfunction with a reduced ejection fraction. He presented with several symptoms, including fatigue and decreased exercise ability, shortness of breath and peripheral oedema. Examination demonstrated cardiomegaly, a raised jugular venous pressure and crackles in the lungs. An ECG showed that he is in sinus rhythm.

a. Could long-term oral administration of the phosphodiesterase inhibitor milrinone be used as part of the treatment for Mr DY?
b. Could long-term oral administration of digoxin or a β-adrenoceptor antagonist be used as part of the treatment for Mr DY?
c. What are the choices of diuretic open to you in treating Mr DY?
d. Potassium loss produced by diuretics may lead to hypokalaemia, which should be avoided in people with heart failure, particularly those taking digoxin. What is an effective way of reducing urinary K^+ loss?
e. Mr DY was then started on an ACE inhibitor. What precautionary measures should be taken in starting this new medication and how would its effectiveness be assessed?
f. After 4 weeks of treatment with the ACE inhibitor and a diuretic, Mr DY's symptoms of breathlessness, fatigue and exercise tolerance were much improved. However, he developed a cough while taking the ACE inhibitor, which became unbearable. What is thought to be the reason for the cough and what alternative therapy could be given to avoid this?

ANSWERS

1. a. **True**. In the healthy heart, contractility rises when there is an increase in afterload, thereby maintaining stoke volume. In the failing heart, contractility increases less so, therefore stroke volume falls (Fig. 7.2).
   b. **False**. The plasma osmotic pressure works to move fluid from the interstitium into the vessel, and the hydrostatic pressure in the other direction. Therefore, oedema occurs when the hydrostatic pressure is greater than the plasma osmotic pressure.
   c. **False**. In cardiac failure, the baroreceptor reflex sensory input to the vasomotor centre is reduced, resulting in increased sympathetic outflow.
   d. **False**. Although digoxin may be of benefit, the mainstay of treatment is a diuretic such as furosemide. If diuretics are given concurrently with digoxin, K^+-sparing diuretics may also be required, as hypokalaemia resulting from urinary K^+ loss can increase the risk of digoxin-induced rhythm disturbances.
   e. **False**. Potassium ions and digoxin compete for the pump; therefore, high extracellular K^+ inhibits the effect of digoxin, and low K^+ can increase the arrhythmic potential of digoxin.
   f. **False**. The effect of low therapeutic doses of digoxin is to stimulate the vagus, sensitise baroreceptor outflow and thereby increase vagal outflow from the vasomotor centre; overall, this increases the refractory period of the atrioventricular node. This is the reason that digoxin is useful in some arrhythmias, such as atrial fibrillation.
   g. **True**. Dobutamine acts through stimulation of β_1-adrenoceptors, which results in an increase in cAMP and thereby increases cardiac contractility. Desensitisation occurs because of downregulation of the receptors in response to prolonged stimulation by the drug. Desensitisation to milrinone does not occur, because it 'bypasses' the receptor and increases cAMP by preventing its breakdown. Milrinone is a phosphodiesterase type 3 inhibitor.
   h. **False**. Dobutamine is a selective β_1-adrenoceptor agonist and does not produce vasodilation.
   i. **True**. Digoxin is eliminated unchanged by the kidney. Its half-life can be increased markedly in renal failure.
   j. **True**. ACE inhibitors decrease angiotensin II formation and decrease aldosterone release. This results in less reabsorption of Na^+ in the collecting ducts in exchange for K^+ efflux into the tubules, resulting in increased K^+ retention. Spironolactone can produce additional clinical benefit but care must be taken to

avoid dangerous hyperkalaemia, with regular monitoring of the plasma K^+ concentration.

2. Answer **B**.
   - A. Digoxin is excreted virtually unchanged in the kidney. A decline in renal function, especially in the elderly, increases plasma concentrations.
   - B,C,D. Moderately raised plasma K^+ will not increase the toxicity of digoxin. The inotropic effect of digoxin is a consequence of the inhibition of the cardiac myocyte Na^+/K^+-ATPase (Fig. 7.4). *Reduced* extracellular K^+, for example during use of bendroflumethiazide or furosemide, also inhibits the ATPase, exacerbating toxicity.
   - E. Digoxin and verapamil both delay AV conduction, and an increased chance of AV block may occur when both are administered. Verapamil also increases plasma concentrations of digoxin.
3. Case history answers
   - a. This would not be recommended, as long-term therapy has been shown to increase mortality.
   - b. The place of digoxin is well established in heart failure associated with atrial fibrillation and a rapid ventricular rate, but its benefit in heart failure in sinus rhythm remained controversial until recently. However, evidence is now available for the use of a small dose of digoxin combined with a diuretic and an ACE inhibitor when there is severe left ventricular systolic dysfunction and sinus rhythm. Beta-adrenoceptor antagonists used injudiciously may worsen heart failure by reducing cardiac output. Administration of low doses of β-adrenoceptor antagonists have, however, been shown to be beneficial, but only when the person's condition has been stabilised with diuretics and an ACE inhibitor.
   - c. The treatment of first choice for fluid retention in chronic heart failure is a diuretic. For mild symptoms, a thiazide diuretic may be adequate, but in most people a loop diuretic such as furosemide is used. The loss of renal function in the elderly and renal underperfusion in heart failure means that thiazide diuretics are less effective in older people with this condition.
   - d. The addition of K^+-sparing diuretics such as amiloride to furosemide or thiazide diuretics can reduce hypokalaemia. However, studies have shown that in severe heart failure the K^+-sparing diuretic spironolactone improves symptoms and prognosis (at least in severe heart failure) if a low dose is added to maximal therapy with other drugs; this may therefore be a better option.
   - e. ACE inhibitors slow the progression of heart failure and improve survival. There is a small risk of severe hypotension following the first dose, and omission of the diuretic immediately prior to this may be helpful.
   - f. The cough is thought to be caused by increased concentrations of bradykinin. ACE inhibitors prevent the breakdown of bradykinin by kininase II, which is the same enzyme that converts angiotensin I to angiotensin II. An alternative strategy is to use an angiotensin receptor antagonist such as losartan. These drugs are well tolerated, improve symptoms, and they reduce morbidity and mortality.

Drugs used to treat heart failure

Drug	Half-life and kinetics	Comments
Digitalis glycosides		
Used in heart failure and for supraventricular arrhythmias (particularly atrial fibrillation)		
Digitoxin	8 days (3–16 days) [M + R + B]	Once-daily oral dosage, or even alternate-day dosage
Digoxin	40 h (20–50 h) [R] Eliminated by glomerular filtration; increased half-life in renal impairment	Given once daily orally; a loading dose may be given orally in divided dose over 24 h or by intravenous infusion in an emergency (see Ch. 2)
Phosphodiesterase inhibitors		
Given intravenously		
Enoximone	1.3 h [M] Half-life increased in chronic heart failure; metabolised to a sulphoxide, which is eliminated in urine	Used for congestive heart failure where cardiac output is reduced and filling pressure increased; given by intravenous infusion
Milrinone	0.8–0.9 h [R] Short half-life due to rapid renal tubular secretion and a low volume of distribution	Used for short-term treatment of severe congestive heart failure, and acute heart failure; given by intravenous injection followed by infusion (usually for up to 12 h)

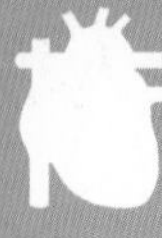

Drugs used to treat heart failure

Drug	Half-life and kinetics	Comments
Sympathomimetic inotropes		
Very short half-lives and negligible oral bioavailability since they are rapidly metabolised by the pathways of noradrenaline metabolism; all given by intravenous infusion		
Dobutamine	2 min [M]	Used for inotropic effect after myocardial infarction, cardiac surgery, cardiomyopathies, septic shock and cardiogenic shock; acts on β_1-adrenoceptors in heart muscle to increase cardiac contractility with little effect on heart rate
Dopamine	7–12 min [M]	Used for cardiogenic shock in exacerbations of chronic heart failure and in heart failure associated with cardiac surgery; acts on β_1-adrenoceptors in heart muscle to increase cardiac contractility with little effect on heart rate, and on peripheral dopamine receptors to increase renal perfusion, but this is offset by α-adrenoceptor-mediated vasoconstriction
Dopexamine	7 min [M]	Used for inotropic effect after myocardial infarction, cardiac surgery, cardiomyopathies, septic shock and cardiogenic shock; acts on β_2-adrenoceptors in heart muscle to increase cardiac contractility and on peripheral dopamine receptors to increase renal perfusion

[B], biliary excretion; [M], metabolism; [R], renal excretion.

8 Cardiac arrhythmias

BASIC CARDIAC ELECTROPHYSIOLOGY

Action potentials in myocardial cells and the associated highly regulated cardiac contractions are a product of transmembrane ion currents generated by the movement of ions through membrane channels (Ch. 1). A variety of specific channels exist for Na^+, Ca^{2+} and K^+ transport in the myocardium (Figs 8.1 and 8.2). These channels cycle through three states: resting, open or closed (inactive and refractory) (Ch. 1). Whether the ion channels are open to allow ion flow or are closed is determined by the membrane potential across the cell membrane; hence they are called voltage-gated ion channels. The direction in which ions move is dependent upon the type of channel, the concentration gradient of the ions, and the transmembrane electrical potential (Figs 8.1 and 8.2). As a result of activity in these channels, the resting potential inside a cardiac cell is approximately –70 to –80 mV compared with the extracellular environment, although this will vary between different regions of the heart.

Cells with pacemaker activity

The action potentials of the sinoatrial (SA) and atrioventricular (AV) nodes, Purkinje fibres and ventricular cells vary substantially in their characteristics (Figs 8.1, 8.2 and 8.5). Action potentials in cardiac cells can be divided into four phases (Figs 8.1a and 8.2); phases 1 and 2 are not clearly evident in the SA and AV nodes because of the different ion channels that are activated (Fig. 8.1a).

The SA node, AV node, bundle of His and Purkinje system are part of the *specialised conducting system* of the heart and all have the intrinsic ability to spontaneously depolarise in phase 4 and to independently generate impulses. These specialised cells are therefore termed *pacemaker cells*. Other populations of myocytes in the heart do not show phase 4 spontaneous depolarisation. The primary pacemaker that drives normal repetitive cardiac impulses is the SA node (producing normal sinus rhythm of 60–100 impulses per minute at rest). The secondary pacemaker, the AV node, depolarises more slowly and can generate 50–60 impulses per minute, while the tertiary pacemakers (the bundle of His, its branches and the Purkinje fibres) can fire 30–60 times per minute. The secondary and tertiary pacemakers will only be utilised if there is a failure of pacemakers which have a faster rate of spontaneous depolarisation.

Control of cell depolarisation in pacemaker and non-pacemaker cells

Pacemaker cells are mainly distinguished from non-pacemaker cells by slow spontaneous repetitive depolarisation during phase 4 of the action potential (compare Fig. 8.1 panels a and c). The intrinsic rate of firing of a pacemaker cell depends on three factors:

- the resting potential
- the threshold potential for initiating an impulse
- the rate of spontaneous depolarisation.

Slow spontaneous depolarisation in phase 4 in all pacemaker cells results from influx of several positive ions into the cell, through a variety of cell membrane ion channels. These include Ca^{2+}, mainly through T-type Ca^{2+} channels, and both Na^+ and K^+ through channels that generate the strangely termed cardiac pacemaker 'funny' current (I_f) (Figs 8.1a and 8.2). The I_f is unusual in being generated by mixed ion transport, being activated by diastolic hyperpolarisation, and having very slow activation and deactivation rates. The rate of activation of the I_f is modulated by the autonomic nervous system; stimulation of β_1-adrenoceptors enhances the rate of activation and vagal stimulation decreases the rate of activation.

Intrinsic depolarisation of pacemaker cells occurs when the membrane reaches a potential that opens Na^+ or Ca^{2+} channels and ion influx occurs (phase 0). The reason that the SA node pacemaker is dominant is that activation of the I_f current in the SA node occurs at more depolarised transmembrane voltages and has a faster activation rate than in the AV node or Purkinje fibres. Therefore, spontaneous diastolic depolarisation in the SA node is initiated earlier and they are the dominant pacemaker cells.

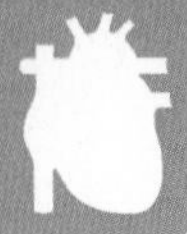

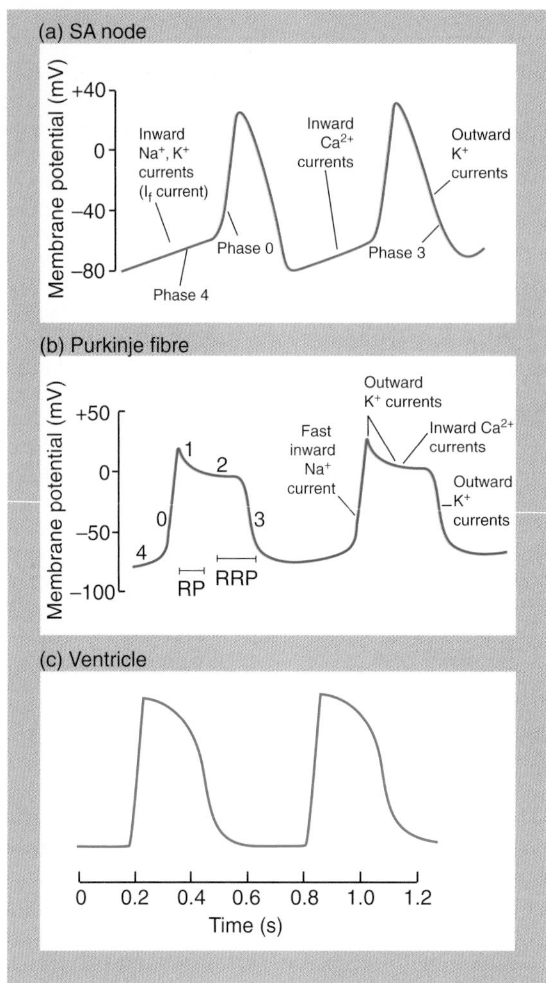

Fig. 8.1 **Action potentials show variations in patterns among different populations of myocytes in different regions of the heart.** This figure should be studied in conjunction with Figure 8.2.

The patterns are determined by the opening and closing of selective gates for Na^+, Ca^{2+} and K^+. The overall stability of the resting transmembrane ionic balance is maintained by active pumps such as the Na^+/K^+-ATPase pump (it is these pumps that maintains the substantial concentration gradients of 140 mmol L^{-1} Na^+ outside and 10–15 mmol L^{-1} Na^+ inside the cell, and 140 mmol L^{-1} K^+ inside and 4 mmol L^{-1} K^+ outside the cell). This results in an electrical gradient at rest of approximately −70 to −80 mV inside the cell, relative to 0 mV outside the cell. Large ion fluxes at rest are prevented by specific pumps and closure of voltage-operated gates. The cardiac action potential is closely ordered. Action potentials in the atrioventricular (AV) node, bundle of His and ventricle are controlled by the sinoatrial (SA) node in the heart when it is in sinus rhythm. The rate of spontaneous depolarisation of the SA node determines its primacy as a pacemaker in the healthy heart.

Phase 0 (Fig. 8.1b,c) occurs when the membrane potential reaches a defined threshold (threshold potential) and an 'all or none' influx of Na^+ through voltage-dependent fast Na^+ channels occurs. This is transient and the gates close after a few milliseconds. Phase 0 is much slower in the SA node and AV node than in ventricular cells, and depends mainly upon Ca^{2+} influx (Fig. 8.1a). This causes the conduction velocity in the SA node to be considerably less than that in the Purkinje fibres, and the refractory period is longer in proportion to the total duration of the action potential. Phase 1, called the early repolarisation and notch, results from K^+ efflux (the transient outward [I_{TO}] current) and reduced Na^+ influx (Fig. 8.2). The phase 2 plateau is primarily a result of Ca^{2+} influx (slow inward, SI current) which is balanced by K^+ efflux over a slow time course. Phase 3 repolarisation results from inactivation of Ca^{2+} influx and increasing K^+ efflux via a number of currents (see text, Table 8.1 and Fig. 8.2). Part of the overall importance of the K^+ currents is to maintain a stable resting membrane potential. Phase 4 (Fig. 8.1 a,b) is termed the diastolic or pacemaker depolarisation generated on hyperpolarisation. The phase 4 inward 'funny' current (I_f) involves Na^+ and K^+ and is gated by both changes in voltage and by cAMP. I_f controls in part the rate of spontaneous beating of the heart and the control of rate by the sympathetic and parasympathetic nervous systems. Ca^{2+} currents may also be involved in pacemaker activity in Phase 4. RP: absolute refractory period, RRP: relative refractory period.

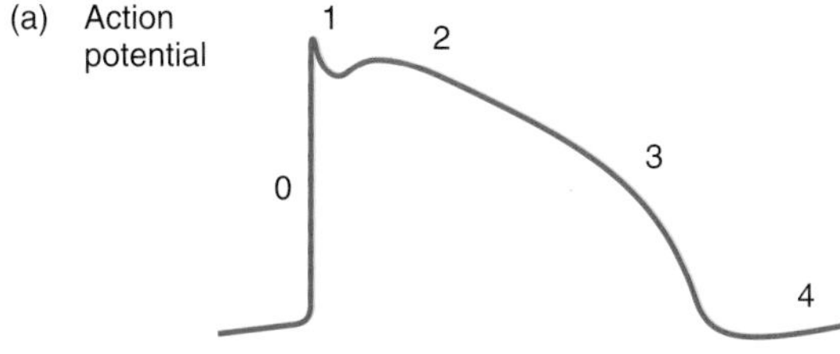

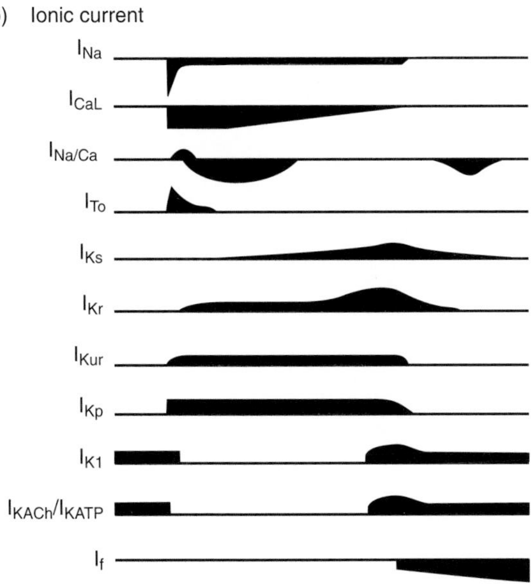

Fig. 8.2 **A schematic representation of the influx and efflux of Na^+, Ca^{2+} and K^+ in Purkinje fibres**. This figure should be read in conjunction with Table 8.1. A downward inflection represents influx of the ion, and upward represents efflux. (Modified and reproduced with permission from Tamargo et al 2004.)

In the SA and AV node, depolarisation in phase 0 arises from the slow influx of Ca^{2+} through voltage-gated L-type channels (Fig. 8.1a; I_{CaL} in Fig. 8.2). This results in slower conduction of the impulse through the AV node. In contrast, in ventricular cells, phase 0 of the action potential is initiated by a rapid influx of Na^+ through specific voltage-gated Na^+ ion channels (fast Na^+ channels) (Fig. 8.1b; I_{Na} in Fig. 8.2). Phase 0 (depolarisation) is triggered when the cell reaches its threshold potential, and sufficient voltage-gated Ca^{2+} or Na^+ channels have been opened to allow a rapid influx of positive ions into the cell.

At the end of phase 0 , the intracellular voltage potential briefly becomes positive, at which point a voltage-triggered 'gate' closes and inactivates the Na^+ or Ca^{2+} channels, preventing further inward ion flow and further depolarisation (Fig. 8.1a,b).

Control of cell repolarisation in pacemaker and non-pacemaker cells

Cells then undergo a process of repolarisation to return the membrane potential to its resting level. This creates the conditions for the next action potential to be initiated (Figs 8.1 and 8.2). In both pacemaker and non-pacemaker cells, repolarisation (phase 3) is initiated by the opening of several types of K^+ channels and transport of K^+ out of the cell (Fig. 8.2). These channels are known as rectifiers (see Table 8.1 for explanation). The opening of most K^+ channels varies according to the membrane potential. The process of repolarisation is, however, temporarily delayed in the Purkinje system and non-pacemaker cardiac cells by influx of Ca^{2+} through L-type channels (phase 2, the plateau phase, I_{CaL} in Fig. 8.2), which balances continued K^+ efflux and prolongs and slows the process of depolarisation. (Fig. 8.1b phase 2).

In the resting phase between action potentials, Na^+ and K^+ transmembrane concentration gradients are restored by a separate exchange pump (Na^+/ K^+-ATPase; see Fig. 7.4). The negative internal resting membrane potential is maintained by high K^+ permeability of resting cell membranes through inward rectifying voltage- and ligand-gated K^+ channels which close when the cell depolarises (see also Ch. 1).

During the period between phase 0 and the end of phase 2 of the action potential, the myocardial cell is refractory to further depolarisation (*the absolute refractory period*, RP). This is because the depolarising channels are inactivated until a sufficiently negative potential is restored inside the cell. During phase 3, a large depolarising stimulus can open sufficient Na^+ channels (many of which will have recovered to the resting state) to overcome the K^+ efflux and initiate a further action potential. This part of the action potential is the *relative refractory period* (RRP, Fig. 8.1b)

The sum of the individual electrical currents that pass from one cell to another through the heart can be recorded as the surface electrocardiogram (ECG) (Fig. 8.3).

MECHANISMS OF ARRHYTHMOGENESIS

Arrhythmias are disorders of rate and rhythm of the heart, which can arise as the result of either abnormal impulse generation or abnormal impulse conduction. There are three principal mechanisms of arrhythmogenesis.

- **Increased automaticity.** Ectopic pacemakers (pacemakers other than the SA node) can arise when pacemaker cells in the specialised conducting tissue develop a more rapid phase 4 depolarisation than the SA node. They can also occur when rapid spontaneous phase 4 depolarisation develops in myocardial cells that usually have a stable phase 4. Ischaemia, or other changes in the microcellular environment, can create conditions that allow a non-specialised myocardial cell to become a pacemaker.
- **Re-entry.** This is the cause of most clinically important arrhythmias. It can occur when an impulse travelling through the heart arrives at a part of the myocardium that is refractory to the stimulus. These conditions are created as a result of abnormally slow repolarisation in a part of the myocardium (Fig. 8.4b). The impulse will bypass the refractory tissue, but if it subsequently arrives at the distal part of the refractory tissue when this tissue has had sufficient time to repolarise, the impulse

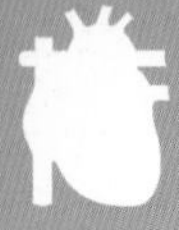

Table 8.1 Selected examples of some K^+ channels and associated currents (this should be studied in conjunction with Fig. 8.2)

Type of gating	Examples of distribution[a]	Comment
K_V voltage-gated channel family		
K_v channels carrying delayed inward rectifying currents	Widely distributed, including brain, heart, pancreas	Multiple subtypes of K^+ channels are involved in delayed inward rectification and are responsible for slow (I_{Ks}), rapid (I_{Kr}) and ultrarapid (I_{Kur}) K currents involved in repolarisation in phases 2 and 3 in the heart. Inhibited by some class I and class III antiarrhythmics, e.g. amiodarone and sotalol
K_v channel carrying transient outward rectifying (I_{KTO}) current		A genetically distinct member of the K_v family of channels. Responsible for the I_{TO} transient current in phase 1. Activated by adenosine; inhibited by quinidine, amiodarone
K_{ir} family		
Inward rectifying	Heart, muscle, brain, pancreas	Inward rectifying, rapidly inactivates cardiac Na^+ channels; sets resting membrane potential (I_{K1}, I_{Kr}). Inhibited by amiodarone
Ligand-gated channels		
ATP-sensitive channels (K_{ATP})	Heart, muscle, pancreas, mitochondria	Comprised of coexpressed K_{ir} and sulphonylurea subunits with varied configurations in different tissues. This provides a weak inward rectifying current. Opened by ischaemia, minoxidil and nicorandil; inhibited by ATP and sulphonylureas
Acetylcholine-sensitive channel (K_{ACh})	SA node, AV node and atria	This is G-protein-linked in SA node, atria and AV node and is a member of the K_{ir} family resulting in an inward rectifying (K_{ir}) current. Opened by adenosine; inhibited by atropine and disopyramide
Two-pore channel (K_{2P})	Heart, brain pancreas	Opened by arachidonic acid; weak inward rectifying current; modulates resting membrane potential
Calcium-activated (K_{Ca} family)		Members of K_{ir} family of channels
Large conductance channel (B_{Kca})	Heart, brain, pancreas	Being investigated for roles in neuroprotection, erectile dysfunction and other disorders
Intermediate conductance channel (I_{Kca})	T-lymphocytes, smooth muscle, brain, heart	Opened by hydralazine

Potassium channels are diverse in structure and behaviour. Each channel consists of a variable number of membrane-spanning subunits. Each subunit consists of a variable number of linked membrane segments (maximum six) which make up the water-filled pore. Some channels can be made up of just two subunits and some four. This diversity results in the possibility of dozens of genetically determined different configurations of K^+ channels, many of which may have particular physiological roles. The genes encoding the channel proteins have in many cases been cloned. Channels with subunit variations are associated with different types of current which are involved in repolarisation at different phases of the cardiac action potential. The channels can be open or closed depending upon the voltage across the cell or the presence of a selective ligand.
Rectifying current: an inward rectifying current means that under conditions of equivalent but opposing electrochemical potentials these channels pass more current inwards than outwards. An outward rectifying current is similar but in an outward direction.
[a]Selected examples only are given.

will then be conducted retrogradely through this tissue (Fig. 8.4c). If there has been sufficient time for the healthy myocardium proximal to the block to repolarise, a self-perpetuating circuit of electrical activity will be initiated (a re-entry circuit) that acts as a pacemaker. Such functional re-entry circuits can be localised within a small area of myocardium that has been damaged by scarring, fibrosis or ischaemia (micro re-entry). The myocardium can also support large anatomical re-entry circuits. These can arise in congenital pathways that bypass the AV node, and conduct electrical activity between the atria and ventricles. Re-entry circuits between the atria and ventricles can also include the AV node (such as occurs in the Wolff–Parkinson–White syndrome).

- **Triggered activity.** A cell can develop transient depolarisations during or following repolarisation ('afterdepolarisations'), which will initiate an action potential if they reach the threshold potential of the cell. Afterdepolarisations are said to be 'early' if they occur during repolarisation (relative refractory period in Fig. 8.1b), or 'delayed' if they occur in phase 4. In many cases, opening of L-type Ca^{2+} channels or the Na^+/Ca^{2+} exchange current during prolonged repolarisation probably initiates afterdepolarisation. Triggered rhythms are an uncommon mechanism of arrhythmogenesis but may be responsible for the proarrhythmic activity of class Ia and III antiarrhythmic agents and digitalis glycosides (see below).

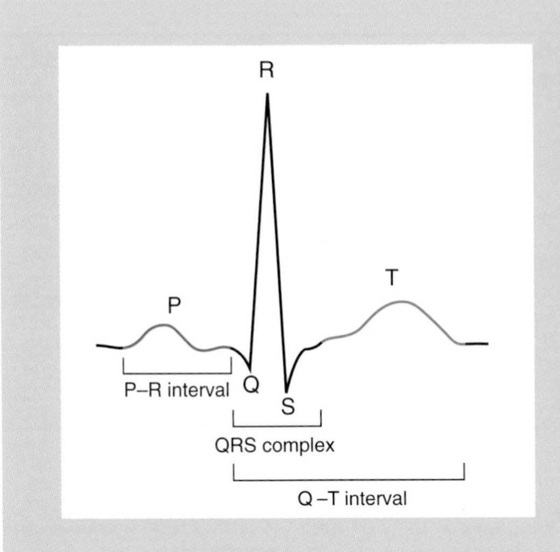

Fig. 8.3 **The waveform for cardiac events seen on a surface electrocardiogram**. The P wave represents the spread of depolarisation through the atria, and the QRS complex is the spread through the ventricles. The T wave represents repolarisation of the ventricle. The P–R interval is the time of conductance from atrium to ventricles, and the QRS time is the time the ventricles are activated. The duration of the ventricle action potential is given by the Q–T interval.

CLASSIFICATION OF ANTIARRHYTHMIC DRUGS

A widely used classification of antiarrhythmic drugs (the Vaughan Williams classification) is based on their effects on the action potential (Fig. 8.5). This classification has many flaws and does not take account of the multiple actions possessed by some drugs, or the fact that the effects of drugs on diseased myocardium may be different from that on healthy myocardium. However, there is no widely accepted alternative classification.

The Vaughan Williams classification recognises four classes of drug (Table 8.2).

Class I

All class I drugs inhibit fast Na^+ channels with variable potency, slow the rate of rise of phase 0, and reduce the excitability of the myocardial cell. They are often called membrane stabilisers. They readily penetrate the phospholipid bilayers of the cell membrane, where they concentrate in the hydrophobic core and bind to hydrophobic amino acids in the Na^+ channel. Class I drugs are subdivided according to their effects on the duration of the action potential.

- *Class Ia*, such as disopyramide, produce moderate Na^+ channel blockade and slow impulse conduction. In addition, they block some K^+ channels (Table 8.1, Figs 8.1 and 8.5a), which prolongs repolarisation and therefore the duration of the action potential. *They are*

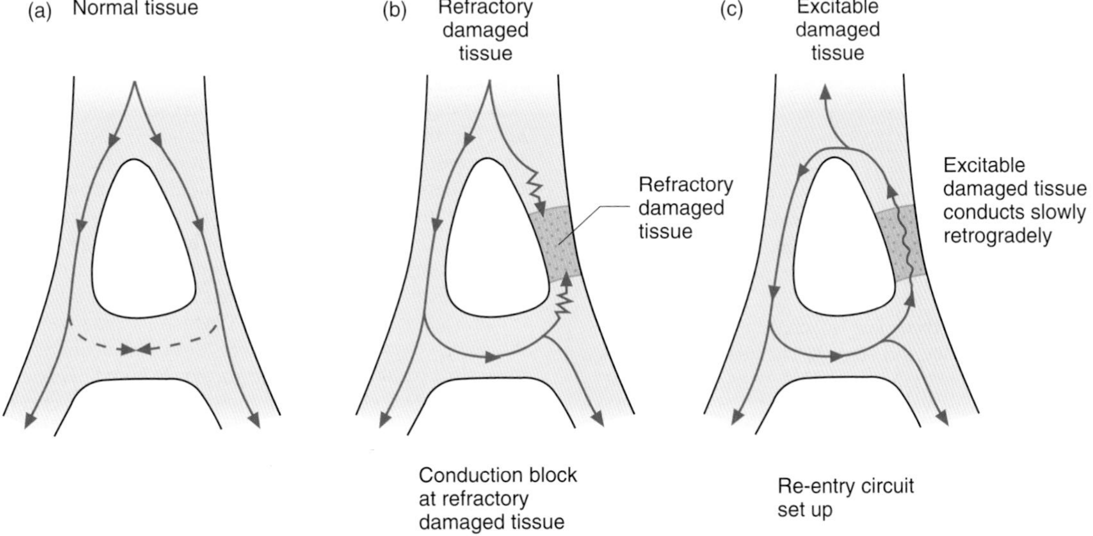

Fig. 8.4 **Conduction in normal and damaged cardiac tissue**. (a) In normal tissue, conduction is carefully ordered. When an action potential has been generated, the cells cannot be immediately reactivated because of refractoriness of the myocardial cells. If conducted impulses meet, they die out. (b) If an area of damage or dysfunction is present, impulses are conducted abnormally. If an action potential arrives at the area of damaged tissue and it is fully refractory, the impulse is blocked and an arrhythmia will not develop. (c) If an action potential arrives at a damaged area and it is capable of being excited and conducting in a retrograde direction, a perpetuating abnormal re-entry circuit may be set up.

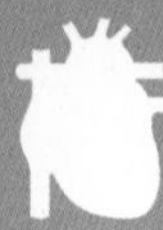

Table 8.2 Principal indications for antiarrhythmic drugs

Class	Examples	Supraventricular arrhythmias	Ventricular arrhythmias
Ia	Disopyramide, procainamide, quinidine	+	+
Ib	Lidocaine	–	+ (especially after myocardial infarction)
Ic	Flecainide, propafenone	+	+
II	β-Adrenoceptor antagonists	+	+ (especially after myocardial infarction)
III	Amiodarone, sotalol	+	+
IV	Calcium channel blockers	+	–

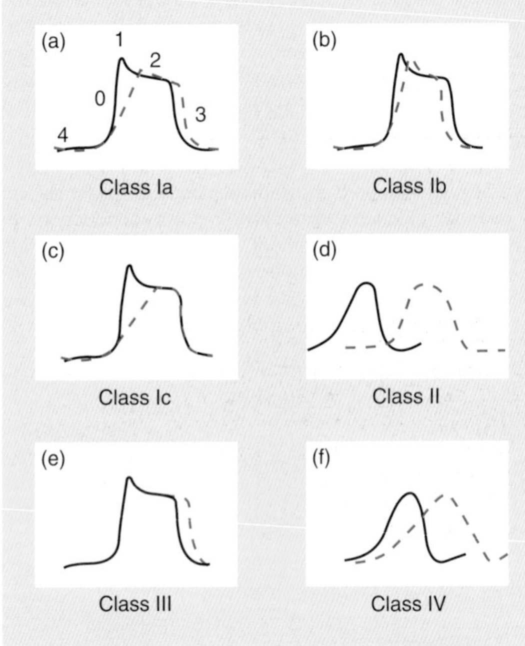

Fig. 8.5 **Effects of different classes of antiarrhythmic drug on the cardiac action potential.** Panels a, b, c and e show drug effects on ventricular cells; panels d and f, effects on the AV node.

a. *Class 1a drugs.* Block fast Na^+ channels in phase 0 with moderate potency and some K^+ channels. Repolarisation is prolonged.
b. *Class 1b drugs.* Weakly block fast Na^+ channels in phase 0 only in abnormal tissue; little effect on K^+ channels.
c. *Class 1c drugs.* Potently block fast Na^+ channels and weakly block Ca^{2+} channels and some K^+ channels.
d. *Class II drugs*. Reduce phase 4 and phase 0 depolarisation in AV and SA nodes. Repolarisation in the AV node is prolonged.
e. *Class III drugs.* Block some K^+ channels, inhibiting repolarisation and prolonging the action potential.
f. *Class IV drugs.* Block L-type Ca^{2+} channels, slowing phase 0 and phase 4 depolarisation, particularly in the AV node, with less effect in the SA node. Repolarisation is prolonged.

effective for the treatment of both supraventricular and ventricular arrhythmias (Table 8.2).

- *Class Ib*, such as lidocaine, produce weak Na^+ channel blockade and slow impulse conduction, but only in abnormal tissue (such as ischaemic myocardium) with no effect in healthy tissue. They do not block K^+ channels and have either no effect on repolarisation or may shorten it (Fig. 8.5b). *They are only effective for the treatment of ventricular arrhythmias.*
- *Class Ic*, such as flecainide, produce marked Na^+ channel blockade and slow impulse conduction. They produce weak blockade of some K^+ channels (Table 8.1), and also block inward Ca^{2+} channels. There is minimal effect on repolarisation (Fig. 8.5c). *They are effective for the treatment of both atrial and ventricular arrhythmias.*

The different effects of the class I subgroups result from their diverse ion-channel binding characteristics. During the time course of the action potential, the access of the drug to its binding site is intermittent and dependent on the state of the channel. Class Ib drugs show marked use-dependency, i.e. the action increases with the frequency of opening of the channel. They associate more rapidly with Na^+ channels during depolarisation and they rapidly dissociate from the channel when it returns to the resting state. Therefore they are more effective when there are repetitive depolarisations, and they will block premature impulses. Depolarised membranes are frequently found in ischaemic myocardium or cells affected by digitalis toxicity. This explains the selectivity of class Ib drugs for ventricular arrhythmias in ischaemic heart disease (ischaemia mainly affects the ventricles). Class Ic drugs also show use-dependent binding, but dissociate slowly from their binding sites in the Na^+ channel and therefore produce prolonged blockade. This results in a widespread reduction in cellular excitability. Class Ia drugs have binding characteristics between those of the other two subgroups.

Class II

The class II drugs are the β-adrenoceptor antagonists which block the actions of catecholamines on the heart. They reduce the rate of spontaneous depolarisation of SA and AV nodal tissue and reduce conduction through the AV node. They also reduce spontaneous depolarisation in phase 4 of some ectopic foci by indirect blockade of adrenoceptor-activated Ca^{2+} channels (Fig. 8.5d). *They are effective for the treatment of both supraventricular and ventricular arrhythmias, particularly if they are catecholamine-dependent.*

Class III

Class III drugs prolong the duration of the action potential, thus increasing the absolute refractory period. This is achieved by inhibition of some K^+ channels involved in repolarisation (Table 8.1, Fig. 8.5e). *They are effective for the treatment of both supraventricular and ventricular arrhythmias.*

Class IV

There are two types of calcium channel in the heart but the class IV drugs selectively block the L-type Ca^{2+} channel. They stabilise phase 4 of the action potential, particularly in the AV node, and slow the rate of spontaneous depolarisation. They do not greatly affect the rate of depolarisation at the SA node since this depends largely on T-type Ca^{2+} channels and the funny current (I_f). The L-type Ca^{2+} channels are also responsible for depolarisation in phase 0 of the action potential in the AV node, and blocking these channels will slow the rate of impulse conduction through the AV node (Fig. 8.5f). *They are only effective for the treatment of supraventricular arrhythmias.*

Unclassified drugs

Four drugs used in the treatment of rhythm disturbances do not fit into the Vaughan Williams classification: digitalis glycosides, adenosine, magnesium sulphate and atropine.

PROARRHYTHMIC ACTIVITY OF ANTIARRHYTHMIC DRUGS

Many antiarrhythmic drugs have the potential to precipitate serious arrhythmias, such as incessant ventricular tachycardia. Several of them (particularly class Ia agents and sotalol) prolong the Q–T interval on the ECG (Fig. 8.3). This predisposes to a polymorphic ventricular tachycardia known as torsades de pointes, which has a characteristic twisting QRS axis on the ECG and can degenerate into ventricular fibrillation. Drug-induced ventricular rhythm disturbances are particularly refractory to treatment.

There are probably multiple mechanisms of drug-induced arrhythmogenesis. Several risk factors have been identified, including the following.

- *Excessive slowing of cardiac impulse conduction*, such as occurs with marked blockade of Na^+ channels.
- *Excessive prolongation of the action potential*, especially if due to blockade of the I_{Kr} current (Table 8.1, Fig. 8.2). Prolonged repolarisation may cause early afterdepolarisations (see above), and variability of the effects of the drugs on cells in the myocardium can lead to differential rates of repolarisation that predisposes to re-entry circuits.
- *Mutations in genes* coding for channels that regulate Na^+, K^+ and Ca^{2+} transmembrane ion flows: these may exist in 5–10% of people, and are probably subclinical variants of the congenital long QT syndrome. These individuals are more susceptible to torsades de pointes when exposed to a drug that prolongs the Q–T interval.
- *Structural heart disease*, especially ischaemic heart disease, with greater slowing of conduction in diseased myocardium.
- *Hypokalaemia*.
- *Female gender*: about 70% of those who develop torsades de pointes are women.

CLASS IA DRUGS

These drugs are no longer widely used in the UK because of their unwanted effects.

Disopyramide

Pharmacokinetics

Oral absorption of disopyramide is almost complete, but an intravenous formulation is available for rapid onset of action. Metabolism in the liver generates a compound with less antiarrhythmic activity but with greater antimuscarinic activity. About half the drug is eliminated unchanged in the urine. Disopyramide has a half-life of 4–10 h.

Unwanted effects

- Gastrointestinal disturbances
- Powerful negative inotropic effect; disopyramide should be avoided in people with left ventricular dysfunction
- Proarrhythmic effects
- Antimuscarinic effects (see Ch. 4), especially urinary retention, dry mouth and blurred vision.

Procainamide

Pharmacokinetics

Procainamide is well absorbed from the gut but is usually used intravenously. Much is excreted unchanged by the kidney, but about 40% is acetylated in the liver to an active metabolite with a longer half-life than procainamide. The rate of acetylation is subject to genetic polymorphism and is slow in some individuals (Ch. 2). The plasma half-life is about 3 h in fast acetylators but increased twofold in slow acetylators.

Unwanted effects

- Gastrointestinal disturbances: nausea, vomiting, anorexia, diarrhoea.
- Negative inotropic effect.
- Systemic lupus erythematosus (SLE)-like syndrome with fever, arthralgia, rashes and pleurisy. The syndrome is more common in slow acetylators; it usually appears after at least 2 months of treatment and is common after 6 months. Consequently, long-term treatment is usually avoided and procainamide is rarely used in the UK.
- Proarrhythmic effects.

Quinidine

Pharmacokinetics

Oral absorption of quinidine is almost complete and about 30% undergoes first-pass metabolism. Metabolism in the liver is extensive and the drug has a half-life of 7 h. Modified-release formulations are used to reduce the peak

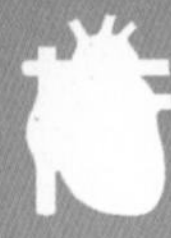

plasma concentration and to minimise unwanted effects. Quinidine is little used in the UK.

Unwanted effects

- Gastrointestinal disturbances: nausea, vomiting, abdominal pain, diarrhoea
- Cinchonism: tinnitus, visual disturbance, flushing, abdominal pain, confusion, headache
- Negative inotropic effect
- Proarrhythmic effects.

CLASS IB DRUGS

Lidocaine

Pharmacokinetics

Extensive first-pass metabolism to a potentially toxic metabolite means that oral administration of lidocaine is not practicable. It is usually given intravenously, initially as a loading dose by bolus injection followed by an infusion. Lidocaine is extensively metabolised in the liver, largely by CYP3A4, to compounds with little antiarrhythmic activity, but one can cause seizures. The half-life of lidocaine is 2 h.

Unwanted effects

- Gastrointestinal disturbances: nausea and vomiting
- Central nervous system (CNS) toxicity: muscle twitching, seizures, dizziness, drowsiness
- Negative inotropic effect
- Bradycardia, proarrhythmic effects.

CLASS IC DRUGS

Flecainide

Pharmacokinetics

Oral absorption of flecainide is complete. An intravenous formulation is also available for rapid onset of action. Flecainide is eliminated both by the kidneys and by hepatic metabolism, and the half-life is long (14 h).

Unwanted effects

- Gastrointestinal disturbances: nausea, vomiting
- CNS toxicity: blurred vision, hallucinations, depression, convulsions, paraesthesiae, ataxia
- Negative inotropic effect
- Proarrhythmic effects, possibly more marked after recent myocardial infarction, when it may increase mortality.

Propafenone

Propafenone has weak β-adrenoceptor antagonist activity in addition to its class Ic action.

Pharmacokinetics

Oral absorption of propafenone is almost complete, but dose-dependent first-pass metabolism can be extensive. Elimination is by cytochrome P450-mediated oxidation, which is saturable and shows genetic polymorphism (Ch. 2). The half-life is therefore dose-dependent and much longer in slow metabolisers of CYP2D6 substrates.

Unwanted effects

- Gastrointestinal disturbances: nausea, vomiting, diarrhoea, bitter taste
- CNS toxicity (as for flecainide)
- Negative inotropic effect, producing hypotension
- Weak β-adrenoceptor antagonist activity can cause bronchoconstriction in individuals with asthma
- Antimuscarinic effects (see Ch. 4): especially urinary retention, dry mouth and blurred vision
- Proarrhythmic effects.

CLASS II DRUGS

Beta-adrenoceptor antagonists (β-blockers)

The β_1-adrenoceptor antagonist activity is responsible for the therapeutic effects of this class. The most widely used agents for treatment of rhythm disturbances are atenolol and propranolol, but any drug in this class will have antiarrhythmic activity. Beta-adrenoceptor antagonists are discussed in more detail in Chapter 5.

Esmolol is an ultra-short-acting β_1-adrenoceptor-selective (cardioselective) agent that is used by bolus intravenous injection exclusively for the treatment of arrhythmias. It is most often used when arrhythmias arise during anaesthesia.

Pharmacokinetics

After bolus intravenous injection, the half-life of esmolol is very short (about 9 min). Its action is terminated by esterases after uptake by erythrocytes.

CLASS III DRUGS

Amiodarone

Amiodarone is a drug with multiple antiarrhythmic actions. It has class III actions by blocking several K^+ channels and shows use-dependence (see above). However, amiodarone also has a class Ib-like action on Na^+ channels, as well as non-competitive β-adrenoceptor antagonist (class II) activity and calcium channel blocking (class IV) actions. The antiarrhythmic effects produced early after intravenous infusion are believed to be due to β-adrenoceptor antagonist activity, while the class III effect is delayed.

Pharmacokinetics

Amiodarone is incompletely absorbed orally and has a large volume of distribution as a result of extensive uptake into adipose tissue. Metabolism in the liver produces an active metabolite, desethylamiodarone, and both amiodarone and its major metabolite have extremely long half-lives, averaging 50–60 days. An intravenous formulation is available. Because of the very long half-life, a prolonged loading dose regimen is used for both routes of administration.

Unwanted effects

- Gastrointestinal disturbances, for example constipation and nausea, most often occur during the loading period.
- Reversible corneal microdeposits develop in almost all people, and can cause dazzling by lights when driving at night.
- Amiodarone has a high iodine content and a structural relationship to thyroid hormone. Particularly in iodine-deficient parts of the world, it can produce a destructive thyroiditis with release of preformed thyroid hormone leading to thyrotoxicosis in up to 10% of those taking it. Thyrotoxicosis is often refractory to treatment, and at least temporary withdrawal of amiodarone may be necessary. In iodine-sufficient areas (such as the UK), inhibition of intracellular thyroxine (T_4) transport and 5′-deiodinase reduces the conversion of T_4 to active triiodothyronine (T_3) (Ch. 41), producing hypothyroidism in about 10% of those treated. Hypothyroidism can be treated by thyroxine replacement without stopping amiodarone (Ch. 41). Amiodarone can also exacerbate underlying asymptomatic autoimmune thyroid disease. Thyroid function should be checked every 6 months during treatment.
- Photosensitive skin rashes are common. Wide-spectrum sunscreen is recommended. Slate-grey skin discoloration can also occur.
- Peripheral neuropathy or myopathy.
- Hepatitis and cirrhosis occur rarely.
- Progressive pneumonitis and lung fibrosis are rare but serious effects of long-term treatment.
- Proarrhythmic effects.
- Drug interactions: the plasma concentrations of warfarin (Ch. 11) and digoxin (Ch. 7) are increased by amiodarone, with consequent potentiation of their effects. Amiodarone inhibits the metabolism of warfarin. It also displaces digoxin from tissue stores and inhibits the renal excretion of digoxin, both actions which increase the risk of digoxin toxicity.

Unlike most antiarrhythmic drugs, amiodarone does not have negative inotropic effects and is safe to use in heart failure.

Sotalol

Sotalol is a non-selective β-adrenoceptor antagonist (Ch. 5) with additional class III properties. It selectively blocks the I_{Kr} current (which is particularly involved in phase 2 and 3 repolarisation), and shows reverse use-dependency (higher receptor binding when the channel is closed) so that it is most effective at slow rates of cell depolarisation (bradycardia). Sotalol is a racemic mixture; the L-isomer has both β-adrenoceptor-blocking and class III activity, while the D-isomer has only class III activity. The class III activity gives sotalol a greater proarrhythmic potential than other β-adrenoceptor antagonists (see above). Sotalol is now reserved for treatment of significant cardiac rhythm disturbances and is not used for the other indications for β-adrenoceptor antagonists.

Pharmacokinetics

Sotalol is almost completely absorbed from the gut and excreted unchanged in the urine. Its half-life varies between 7 and 18 h in different individuals.

Unwanted effects

These are discussed in Chapter 5. The additional proarrhythmic activity of sotalol is discussed above.

CLASS IV DRUGS

Calcium channel blockers (calcium antagonists)

Verapamil and diltiazem (Ch. 5), but not the dihydropyridine derivatives such as nifedipine, have antiarrhythmic activity. Verapamil can be given intravenously for a rapid effect, but this should not be given together with a β-adrenoceptor antagonist, because of summation of myocardial depression and AV nodal conduction block. Details of calcium channel blockers can be found in Chapter 5.

OTHER DRUGS FOR CARDIAC RHYTHM DISTURBANCES

Those drugs used for the management of rhythm disturbances that do not fit into the Vaughan Williams classification are considered here.

Digitalis glycosides

Digitalis glycosides (such as digoxin) are not strictly antiarrhythmic, but they are useful for controlling ventricular rate in atrial flutter and atrial fibrillation by reducing conduction through the AV node. Digitalis glycosides are discussed in Chapter 7.

Adenosine

Mechanism of action and effects

Adenosine is a purine nucleoside that has potent effects on the SA node, producing sinus bradycardia. It also slows impulse conduction through the AV node, but has no effect on conduction in the ventricles. Consequently, it is useful only for the management of supraventricular arrhythmias, particularly those caused by AV nodal re-entry mechanisms. Its electrophysiological actions are mediated by the A_1 subtype of specific G-protein-coupled adenosine receptors, which activate inward rectifier K_{ACh} channels. This enhances the flow of K^+ out of myocardial cells and produces hyperpolarisation of the cell membrane (see Table 8.1). In addition, adenosine antagonises the stimulatory effects of noradrenaline on Ca^{2+} currents. These actions combine to stabilise the myocardial cell membrane.

The A_2 type adenosine receptor reduces Ca^{2+} uptake in vascular smooth muscle, and produces vasodilation. This receptor action enables adenosine to be used as a pharmacological stress to induce ischaemia in people with coronary artery disease so that it can be assessed by radionuclide scanning or echocardiography. Preferential dilation of healthy coronary arteries produces coronary blood flow 'steal' that reduces flow in the stenosed arteries.

Pharmacokinetics

Adenosine is given by rapid bolus intravenous injection. The effect is terminated by uptake into erythrocytes and

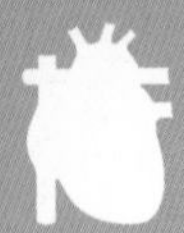

endothelial cells, followed by metabolism to inosine and hypoxanthine. Adenosine has a half-life of less than 10 s, and its duration of action is less than 1 min.

Unwanted effects

Unwanted effects are common and occur in about 25% of those treated with adenosine, but last less than 1 min:

- Bradycardia and AV block
- Malaise, facial flushing, headache, chest pain or tightness, bronchospasm; adenosine should be avoided in people with asthma
- Drug interactions: dipyridamole (Ch. 11) potentiates the effects of adenosine, while methylxanthines such as aminophylline (Ch. 12) inhibit its action.

Atropine

Atropine (see Ch. 4) is given by intravenous bolus injection and reduces the inhibitory effect of the vagus nerve on the heart. Blockade of muscarinic M_2 receptors increases the rate of firing of the SA node and increases conduction through the AV node. This is the result of inhibition of inward rectifying K_{ACh} channels, and prevention of hyperpolarisation of the cell membrane (Table 8.1). Atropine is used specifically for the treatment of sinus bradycardia and AV block. It is metabolised in the liver and has a half-life of 2–5 h.

Magnesium sulphate

Intravenous magnesium sulphate is used to control the ventricular arrhythmia torsades de pointes, and digitalis-induced ventricular arrhythmias. The mechanism is not well understood, but may involve blockade of transmembrane Ca^{2+} currents. Flushing is the main unwanted effect.

DRUG TREATMENT OF ARRHYTHMIAS

Arrhythmias can be asymptomatic, or they can produce a variety of consequences that range from mild symptoms to life-threatening effects on cardiac output. The probability of developing symptoms depends on several factors, the most important of which are the nature of the rhythm disturbance, the rate of an abnormal rhythm and the presence of underlying heart disease. The range of consequences of rhythm disturbances includes:

- awareness of palpitation
- dizziness
- syncope
- precipitation of angina or heart failure
- sudden death.

Treatment may not be necessary for benign or self-terminating arrhythmias; reassurance may be all that is required, but it is important to remove or treat any underlying cause. Vagotonic procedures such as the Valsalva manoeuvre or carotid sinus massage delay conduction through the AV node, and can terminate re-entrant tachycardias involving nodal tissue (but not atrial fibrillation or flutter).

The choice of treatment depends on the situation. With most tachyarrhythmias, sinus rhythm should be restored if possible. Direct current (DC) cardioversion is used to achieve this in severe, life-threatening or drug-resistant arrhythmias; drug therapy is used if there is less need for an immediate effect or to control the ventricular rate if the abnormal rhythm cannot be terminated. Radiofrequency ablation of an arrhythmogenic focus or pathway is increasingly used to prevent arrhythmia. This is carried out after intracardiac electrophysiological studies, using a cardiac catheter. Long-term drug treatment for bradyarrhythmias is not possible and an implanted pacemaker may be necessary.

SUPRAVENTRICULAR TACHYARRHYTHMIAS

Atrial premature beats

Atrial premature beats are very common and usually benign. However, sometimes they are a consequence of digoxin toxicity, and frequent multifocal atrial ectopics can result from organic heart disease. Other than treatment of an underlying cause, specific drug therapy is rarely needed. Some individuals are disturbed by a post-ectopic pause followed by a more forceful beat when sinus rhythm recommences. If treatment is required, then a β-adrenoceptor antagonist, or a calcium channel blocker such as verapamil or diltiazem, can be used to suppress the ectopics.

Atrial tachycardia

Atrial tachycardia is an infrequent rhythm disturbance usually arising from an automatic focus that produces an atrial rate of 150–250 beats min^{-1}. There is usually AV conduction block that results in a slower ventricular rate. Atrial tachycardia is not usually associated with significant cardiac disease, but can be a manifestation of digitalis toxicity. If drug therapy is necessary, an AV nodal blocking agent such as a β-adrenoceptor antagonist or a calcium channel blocker (verapamil or diltiazem) will control the ventricular rate but rarely restores sinus rhythm. Sinus rhythm can be achieved with a class Ic antiarrhythmic agent such as flecainide, given with an AV nodal blocking drug (flecainide alone increases the risk of 1:1 AV nodal conduction if the atrial rate slows sufficiently but sinus rhythm is not restored). Sotalol or amiodarone can also be used to suppress the rhythm disturbance. Ablation of the initiating focus may also be considered.

A less common form of atrial tachycardia is multifocal atrial tachycardia arising from several ectopic foci, usually in individuals with severe pulmonary disease. Calcium channel blockers are usually used for ventricular rate control if treatment is needed.

Atrial flutter

In atrial flutter, the atrial rate is usually 250–350 beats min^{-1}, which is conducted to the ventricles with 2:1 or greater degrees of AV block. Flutter waves may be obvious on the ECG, or appear if the ventricular rate is slowed by vagal manoeuvres or the administration of adenosine. Atrial flutter

Box 8.1 Causes of atrial fibrillation

Structural heart disease
Hypertension
Coronary heart disease
Valvular heart disease (especially mitral)
Cardiomyopathies
Cardiac surgery
Congenital heart disease (especially atrial septal defect)

Other causes
Major infections
Thyrotoxicosis, myxoedema
Alcohol intoxication
Systemic illness (e.g. amyloid, sarcoidosis)

Box 8.2 Factors predicting a high probability of successful restoration of sinus rhythm in people with atrial fibrillation

Short duration of atrial fibrillation (less than 1 year)
Younger age (<50 years)
Absence of underlying heart disease
Normal left ventricular function
Little or no enlargement of the left atrium
Withdrawal or treatment of a precipitating factor, e.g. thyrotoxicosis, alcohol

usually arises from a macro re-entrant circuit in the right atrium. Underlying causes include cardiac surgery, cor pulmonale and congenital heart disease, but it can arise for no obvious reason. It may be paroxysmal, and it can degenerate into atrial fibrillation.

Drug therapy is relatively unsuccessful for restoring sinus rhythm, and DC cardioversion (synchronised to discharge on the R wave of the ECG) or rapid 'overdrive' electrical pacing to capture the ventricle followed by a gradual reduction in the paced rate may be required. Class Ia, Ic and III antiarrhythmic agents can prevent recurrence of paroxysmal atrial flutter. Disopyramide should be avoided as its antimuscarinic action can increase AV conduction and speed up the ventricular response. If a class Ic agent such as flecainide is used, then an AV nodal blocking drug should be given concurrently, since the atrial rate could slow and lead to 1 : 1 AV conduction, with an unacceptably high ventricular rate.

Control of the ventricular rate in atrial flutter can be achieved in a similar manner to that in atrial fibrillation (see below), but treatment is often less successful. For this reason, radiofrequency ablation of the re-entrant pathway via a cardiac catheter is becoming increasingly popular. Prophylaxis against thromboembolism should be given, similar to that for atrial fibrillation.

Atrial fibrillation

Atrial fibrillation is the most common rhythm disturbance in clinical practice. It has a variety of underlying causes (Box 8.1), some of which may be treatable. In younger people, atrial fibrillation often occurs without any obvious underlying cause, when it is called 'lone' atrial fibrillation. The arrhythmia usually arises from multiple re-entry circuits in the atria, although a rapid ectopic focus in a pulmonary vein may be responsible for triggering paroxysmal atrial fibrillation. The ventricular rate will depend on AV nodal function, and when the AV node conducts well, atrial fibrillation produces a rapid ventricular rate. Atrial fibrillation predisposes to atrial thrombus formation and subsequent systemic emboli, which most commonly cause stroke. Clinically, three forms of atrial fibrillation are recognised: paroxysmal, persistent (present for more than 7 days but less than 1 year) and permanent (present for more than 1 year after unsuccessful attempts to maintain sinus rhythm, or if a decision has been made not to attempt this). Management has four underlying aims.

- **To identify and treat the underlying cause.**
- **To restore or maintain sinus rhythm in paroxysmal or persistent atrial fibrillation** (Box 8.2). It is desirable to attempt to restore sinus rhythm in younger people or those who tolerate the rhythm disturbance poorly. In these individuals, symptoms and exercise tolerance are usually improved by restoring sinus rhythm, but the risk of stroke is not removed (see below). However, the case for restoring sinus rhythm is less clear-cut for older people who tolerate the rhythm well, because there is no reduction in the risk of thromboembolic events (probably due to the high rate of recurrence of the arrhythmia), and their quality of life may not improve. Restoration of sinus rhythm is usually possible in lone atrial fibrillation or when there is a treatable underlying cause. It can be achieved with drugs (pharmacological or chemical cardioversion), especially if the rhythm disturbance is of recent onset (40–80% success rate if the arrhythmia is of less than 7 days' duration), but often requires QRS-synchronised DC cardioversion. Pharmacological cardioversion is most rapidly achieved by using a single oral dose of a class Ic drug such as flecainide or propafenone. Intravenous amiodarone is also effective, but takes longer to restore sinus rhythm. Recurrence of atrial fibrillation is most frequent during the first 3–6 months after restoration of sinus rhythm. Drugs are not always recommended for prophylaxis to maintain sinus rhythm after a first cardioversion, because of their proarrhythmic effects. However, if there is a high risk of recurrence, then sinus rhythm can be maintained with the same drugs used for chemical cardioversion, or with sotalol. Amiodarone is the most successful single drug for long-term prevention of recurrence; although it maintains sinus rhythm in only about 75% of people at 1 year, this is superior to sotalol or class 1c drugs (40%). The addition of a second drug such as propafenone or verapamil to amiodarone, or the combination of propafenone and verapamil, can be more effective than amiodarone alone for reducing recurrence. Other drugs can be added to antiarrhythmic therapy to increase the probability of maintaining sinus rhythm. These include angiotensin-converting enzyme (ACE) inhibitors (Ch. 6) and angiotensin receptor blockers (Ch. 6), or β-adrenoceptor antagonists in people with ischaemic heart disease. The mechanisms of action of these drugs in preventing atrial fibrillation are unknown. Digitalis glycosides are

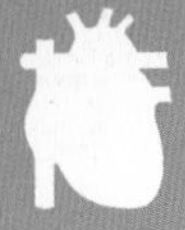

Table 8.3 Risk of stroke in 'non-rheumatic' atrial fibrillation: $CHADS_2$ scoring system[a]

Overall score[a]	Annual risk of stroke (%)	Recommended thromboprophylaxis
0	0.5–2	Aspirin
1	1.5–3	Aspirin or warfarin
2	2.5–4	Warfarin
3	5–6	Warfarin
4	6–8	Warfarin
5	9–12	Warfarin
6	18	Warfarin

[a]The overall score is a summation of the following individual scores: **C**ongestive heart failure, 1; **H**ypertension, 1; **A**ge >75 years, 1 ; **D**iabetes mellitus, 1; prior **S**troke, 2.

ineffective for restoring or maintaining sinus rhythm in paroxysmal atrial fibrillation and should be avoided. Radiofrequency isolation via a cardiac catheter of a pulmonary vein trigger area is becoming increasingly used for younger people with paroxysmal atrial fibrillation. Other curative procedures are infrequently used.

- **To control a rapid ventricular response in persistent or permanent atrial fibrillation.** For rate control both at rest and on exercise, a β-adrenoceptor antagonist, or a ventricular rate-controlling calcium channel blocker, such as verapamil or diltiazem, are the drugs of choice. Rate control at rest can be achieved with digoxin, but a rapid heart rate often still occurs during exercise, so it is only used alone for sedentary people. A β-adrenoceptor antagonist, verapamil, diltiazem or amiodarone can be used together with digoxin if rate control is difficult to achieve. Sotalol has no particular value in sustained atrial fibrillation and should be avoided because of its greater proarrhythmic activity compared with that of other β-adrenoceptor antagonists. If drug combinations do not provide satisfactory rate control, then AV nodal ablation with insertion of a pacemaker can be considered
- **To reduce thromboembolism by long-term anticoagulation** (Ch. 11). Warfarin is the anticoagulant of choice in atrial fibrillation associated with rheumatic heart disease or thyrotoxicosis, and for 1 month before and at least 1 month after DC cardioversion. In non-rheumatic atrial fibrillation, the risk of emboli is greatest in the elderly (over 75 years of age) and if there is coexisting hypertension, diabetes mellitus or recent heart failure (Table 8.3). Almost all those with atrial fibrillation, whether sustained or paroxysmal, should take either aspirin or warfarin. Warfarin (maintaining the international normalised ratio [INR] between 2 and 3; see Ch. 11) reduces the risk of thromboembolism by about two-thirds, and low-dose aspirin reduces the risk of thromboembolism by one-quarter. Warfarin is therefore preferred for people at high risk of embolism, but has little advantage in those at low risk, when the increased risk of bleeding outweighs the benefit. Even after restoration of sinus rhythm in paroxysmal or persistent atrial fibrillation, people at high risk of thromboembolic events should continue to take warfarin, since the risk of stroke does not decrease. This may reflect the high risk of recurrence (often asymptomatic) of atrial fibrillation.

Junctional (nodal) tachycardias

Junctional tachycardias usually arise from a re-entry circuit, and are often initiated by an ectopic beat. The circuit can be within the AV node when there are two functional intranodal pathways (AV nodal re-entry). Such circuits account for 60% of supraventricular tachycardias other than atrial fibrillation/flutter, and are not usually associated with structural cardiac disease. Alternatively, the circuit may involve an accessory AV pathway such as in Wolff–Parkinson–White syndrome (30% of supraventricular tachycardias). Termination of an acute attack can often be achieved with vagotonic manoeuvres such as carotid sinus massage or by adenosine. Beta-adrenoceptor antagonists, diltiazem or verapamil can be used to treat acute episodes or for prophylaxis. Diltiazem, verapamil and digoxin should be avoided if there is an accessory AV pathway, because selective blockade of the AV node by these drugs can predispose to rapid conduction of atrial arrhythmias through the accessory pathway. Junctional tachycardias involving an accessory pathway often respond well to flecainide, sotalol or amiodarone. Radiofrequency ablation of the re-entry circuit, via a cardiac catheter, is being employed increasingly for troublesome junctional tachycardias.

Immediate management of narrow complex tachycardia of uncertain origin

If the rhythm is regular, it is often not possible to determine from the ECG whether the arrhythmia has an atrial or nodal origin. If vagotonic manoeuvres are unsuccessful, and the person is haemodynamically stable, intravenous adenosine should be given. This often converts a junctional tachycardia to sinus rhythm or can slow the ventricular rate sufficiently to identify the origin of the rhythm. If there is a history of severe asthma, intravenous verapamil may be preferred. DC cardioversion is preferred if there is haemodynamic instability.

VENTRICULAR TACHYARRHYTHMIAS

Ventricular ectopic beats

Ventricular ectopic beats can occur in healthy individuals or in association with a variety of cardiac disorders such as ischaemic heart disease and heart failure. Frequent ventricular ectopic beats after myocardial infarction predict a poorer long-term outcome; however, suppressing such ectopics with class I antiarrhythmic agents increases mortality and should be avoided. In contrast, β-adrenoceptor antagonists after myocardial infarction reduce the risk of sudden death (Ch. 5). A β-adrenoceptor antagonist can also suppress ventricular ectopic beats induced by stress or anxiety. In other situations, symptomatic ventricular ectopic beats can be suppressed by a class I drug such as flecainide or disopyramide.

Ventricular tachycardia

Ventricular tachycardia presents with broad QRS complexes on the ECG (broad-complex tachycardia). Although broad complexes can arise with supraventricular tachycardias (when there is bundle branch block), broad-complex tachycardia is usually treated on the assumption that it is ventricular tachycardia. Ventricular tachycardia is often associated with serious underlying heart disease, such as ischaemic heart disease or heart failure, and is more common following myocardial infarction. It can be either sustained or non-sustained. Sustained ventricular tachycardia can be associated with a minimal or absent cardiac output ('pulseless' ventricular tachycardia), when it is treated in the same way as ventricular fibrillation (see below). Polymorphic or incessant ventricular tachycardias can occur as a complication of antiarrhythmic drug therapy (see above) and with other drugs that prolong the Q–T interval on the ECG.

For sustained ventricular tachycardias, drug options include class Ib antiarrhythmic agents such as lidocaine (especially after myocardial infarction), and amiodarone. Sustained ventricular tachycardia is often associated with a poor long-term outlook in ischaemic heart disease, and coronary revascularisation or an automatic implantable cardiac defibrillator may be beneficial. During and after the acute phase of myocardial infarction, a β-adrenoceptor antagonist is the treatment of choice to suppress non-sustained ventricular tachycardias.

Polymorphic or incessant ventricular tachycardias do not respond well to conventional treatments. Withdrawal of a precipitant drug, correction of electrolyte imbalance, and intravenous magnesium sulphate are the therapies of choice. Temporary transvenous overpacing at a rate of 90–110 beats min^{-1} may prevent recurrence. In the congenital form of long QT syndrome, a β-adrenoceptor antagonist is the mainstay of treatment.

Ventricular fibrillation

Ventricular fibrillation is a potentially lethal arrhythmia that constitutes one form of 'cardiac arrest'. An algorithm for the management of cardiac arrest is regularly updated by the European Resuscitation Working Party, and is shown in Figure 8.6. The important principles of resuscitation are the maintenance of adequate cardiac output by external chest compression, and oxygenation by artificial inflation of the lungs, while attempting to restore sinus rhythm. Ventricular fibrillation is the commonest arrhythmia in acute cardiac arrest and it should be assumed to be present at the onset of a cardiac arrest. It should be treated with immediate DC cardioversion if a good ECG monitor read-out is not available. Adrenaline (epinephrine; Ch. 4) may be given to vasoconstrict the peripheries and thus maintain pressure in the central arteries perfusing the heart and brain. For recurrent ventricular fibrillation, suppression may be achieved by long-term use of antiarrhythmic drugs such as sotalol or amiodarone (often combined with a β-adrenoceptor antagonist), but frequently requires an automatic implantable cardiac defibrillator.

BRADYCARDIAS

Sinus bradycardia

Treatment with atropine may be necessary if sinus bradycardia is causing symptoms (e.g. after myocardial infarction). Hypotension precipitated by drugs such as streptokinase (Ch. 11) or the first dose of an ACE inhibitor (Ch. 6) is often associated with vagally mediated bradycardia, which will respond to atropine.

Atrioventricular block ('heart block')

If AV block arises suddenly, then loss of consciousness (Stokes–Adams attack) or death can occur. AV block can be congenital or may accompany a variety of heart diseases. If it occurs after myocardial infarction, it is usually temporary if the infarct is inferior but is often permanent after anterior infarction. First-degree heart block (prolongation of the P–R interval on the ECG) or Wenckebach (Mobitz type 1) second-degree heart block (progressive P–R prolongation until there is a non-conducted P wave) rarely requires treatment, but higher degrees of block (second-degree [Mobitz type 2] and third-degree heart block with non-conducted P waves) should be treated. If the onset is acute, atropine should be given intravenously to increase AV conduction, but external or temporary transvenous electrical cardiac pacing is usually required. Although it is rarely used, the β-adrenoceptor agonist isoprenaline can be given by intravenous infusion if there is likely to be a delay in pacing. However, this usually produces excessive numbers of ectopic beats and rarely improves nodal conduction. If the AV block is permanent, the implantation of a permanent electrical cardiac pacemaker is usually necessary.

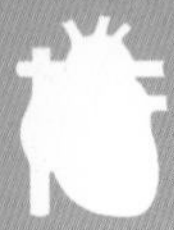

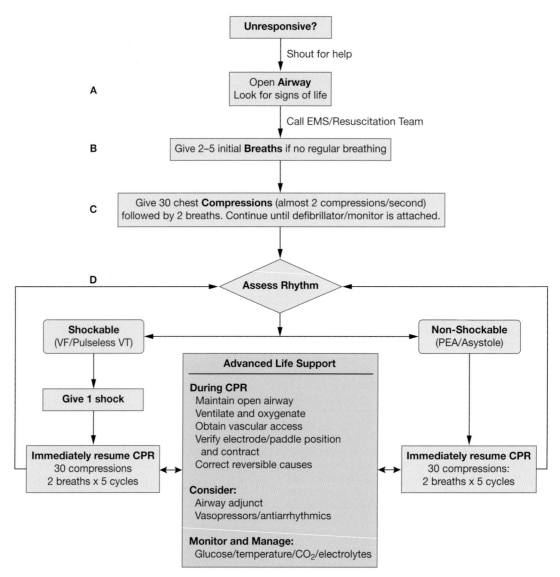

Fig. 8.6 **An algorithm for the management of cardiac arrest.** CPR, cardiopulmonary resuscitation; EMS, emergency medical services; PEA, pulseless electrical activity; VF, ventricular fibrillation; VT, ventricular tachycardia.

FURTHER READING

Blomström-Lundqvist C, Scheinman MM, Aliot EM et al (2003) ACC/AHA/ESC guidelines for the management of patients with supraventricular arrhythmias – executive summary. *Eur Heart J* 24, 1857–1897

Calò L, Sciarra L, Lamberti F et al (2003) Electropharmacological effects of antiarrhythmic drugs on atrial fibrillation termination. Part 1: molecular and ionic fundamentals of antiarrhythmic drug actions. *Ital Heart J* 4, 430–441

Crystal E, Connolly SJ (2004) Role of anticoagulation in management of atrial fibrillation. *Heart* 90, 813–817

Delacrétaz E (2006) Supraventricular tachycardias. *N Engl J Med* 354, 1039–1051

Goette A, Lendeckel U (2004) Nonchannel drug targets in atrial fibrillation. *Pharmacol Ther* 102, 17–36

Grant AO (2001) Molecular biology of sodium channels and their role in cardiac arrhythmias. *Am J Med* 110, 296–305

Gupta A, Lawrence AT, Krishnan K et al (2007) Current concepts in the mechanisms and management of drug-induced QT prolongation and torsade de pointes. *Am Heart J* 153, 891–899

Hancox JC, Patel KCR, Jones JV (2000) Antiarrhythmics – from cell to clinic: past, present, and future. *Heart* 84, 14–24

Hart RG, Pearce LA, Aguilar MI (2007) Meta-analysis: antithrombotic therapy to prevent stroke in patients who have nonvalvular atrial fibrillation. *Ann Intern Med* 146, 857–867

International Liaison Committee on Resuscitation (2005) 2005 International Consensus on Cardiopulmonary Resuscitation and Emergency Cardiovascular Care Science with Treatment Recommendations, Part 1: Introduction. *Resuscitation* 67, 181–186

Iqbal MB, Taneja AK, Lip GYH et al (2005) Recent developments in atrial fibrillation. *BMJ* 330, 238–243

Katz AM (1998) Selectivity and toxicity of antiarrhythmic drugs: molecular interactions with ion channels. *Am J Med* 104, 179–195

Korantzopoulos P, Kolettis TM, Goudevenos JA et al (2005) Errors and pitfalls in the non-invasive management of atrial fibrillation. *Int J Cardiol* 104, 125–130

Lafuente-Lafuente C, Mouly S, Longás-Tejero MA et al (2006) Antiarrhythmic drugs for maintaining sinus rhythm after cardioversion of atrial fibrillation. *Arch Intern Med* 166, 719–728

Lau W, Newman D, Dorian P (2000) Can antiarrhythmic agents be selected based on mechanism of action? *Drugs* 60, 1315–1328

Lip GYH, Tse H-F (2007) Management of atrial fibrillation. *Lancet* 370, 604–618

Markides V, Schilling RJ (2003) Atrial fibrillation: classification, pathophysiology, mechanisms and drug treatment. *Heart* 89, 939–943

Nattel S, Opie LH (2006) Controversies in atrial fibrillation. *Lancet* 367, 262–272

Page RL (2004) Newly diagnosed atrial fibrillation. *N Engl J Med* 351, 2408–2416

Reiffel JA, Reiter MJ, Blitzer M (1998) Antiarrhythmic drugs and devices for the management of ventricular tachyarrhythmias in ischemic heart disease. *Am J Cardiol* 82, 31I–40I

Reiter MJ, Reiffel JA (1998) Importance of beta blockade in the therapy of serious ventricular arrhythmias. *Am J Cardiol* 82, 9I–19I

Roden DM, Balser JR, George AL Jr, Anderson ME (2002) Cardiac ion channels. *Annu Rev Physiol* 64, 431–475

Shorofsky SR, Balke CW (2001) Calcium currents and arrhythmias: insights from molecular biology. *Am J Med* 110, 127–140

Tamargo J, Caballero, R, Gomez, R et al (2004) Pharmacology of cardiac potassium channels. *Cardiovasc Res* 62, 9–33

Wyse DG (2006) Pharmacologic approaches to rhythm versus rate control in atrial fibrillation – where are we now? *Int J Cardiol* 110, 301–312

SELF-ASSESSMENT

1. In the following questions, the first statement, in italics, is true. Is the accompanying statement also true?
   a. *Pacemaker cells in the SA node initiate cardiac rhythm and discharge at a higher frequency than those in other parts of the heart.* Spontaneous or pacemaker depolarisation occurring during diastole results from the inflow of a single cation, Na^+.
   b. *The influx of Na^+ during phase 0 lasts only for milliseconds and the fast Na^+ channels for influx close at the end of phase 1.* Cells are unable to generate further action potentials during phases 0, 1 and 2 of the action potential.
   c. *Reducing the rate of rise in the slope of phase 4 will slow the normal pacemaker rate.* Sympathetic and vagal stimulation reduce the slope of phase 4 depolarisation and, therefore, reduce pacemaker rate.
   d. *The SA node and the AV node have pacemaker activity.* Healthy non-pacemaker cells remain quiescent if not excited by an impulse arising from other regions in the heart.
   e. *Sympathetic stimulation of the AV node increases pacemaker depolarisation rate and conduction through the node.* Beta-adrenoceptor antagonist drugs are useful in stress-induced tachycardias.
   f. *Verapamil has little benefit in ventricular arrhythmias.* Verapamil will affect both the plateau phase 2 and phase 4 of the action potential cycle.
   g. *Adenosine is currently the drug of choice for prompt conversion of AV nodal re-entrant tachycardia to sinus rhythm.* Adenosine is effective in the treatment of ventricular arrhythmias.
2. Considering the flow of ions into cardiac myocytes (inward flow) and out of myocytes (outward flow), identify which one statement **most correctly** describes a situation that would prevent arrhythmias.
   A. Increased inward flow of Na^+ during phase 0 of the action potential
   B. Increased inflow of Ca^{2+} during phase 4 of the action potential
   C. Decreased inflow of Na^+ during phase 0 of the action potential
   D. Increased inflow of Ca^{2+} during phase 2 of the action potential
   E. Decreased outflow of K^+ in phase 3 of the action potential
3. Case history questions

Mr GH, aged 48 years, consulted his GP complaining of palpitations and was found to have an irregular pulse with a pulse rate of 120 beats min^{-1}. He had been suffering from shortness of breath and faintness for the previous 6 h. The symptoms had started after a drinking binge 36 h previously. Examination, blood tests (including thyroid function tests), ECG and chest radiograph revealed no coexisting heart disease, diabetes or hypertension. The ECG confirmed atrial fibrillation.

a. What were the options available for treating Mr GH?

Before any treatment could be instituted, Mr GH spontaneously reverted to sinus rhythm. He was well for a year but then returned to his GP with a 3-day history of palpitations, breathlessness, chest pain and dizziness. Examination and an ECG again revealed atrial fibrillation. He was referred to a cardiologist and echocardiography showed no evidence of structural cardiac disease. Electrical DC cardioversion was carried out and the rhythm reverted to sinus rhythm.

Over the next 5 years, episodes of atrial fibrillation occurred with increasing frequency, and, eventually, sinus rhythm could not be restored with a variety of antiarrhythmic drugs or by DC conversion.

b. What prophylactic treatment should be considered at the time of DC cardioversion? What drug treatments may be useful after DC cardioversion?

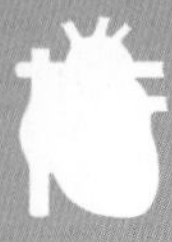

ANSWERS

1. a. **False**. Slow pacemaker depolarisation in pacemaker cells results from an inward flow of Na^+, Ca^{2+} and K^+ (funny I_f current).
   b. **True**. However, during phase 3, the cells are only relatively refractory to further depolarising stimuli and a sufficient stimulus could fire an action potential during this phase.
   c. **False**. Reducing the phase 4 slow depolarisation slope diminishes the pacemaker rate of firing, as it takes longer to reach the threshold potential. However, although vagal stimulation reduces the slope of phase 4, β-adrenoceptor agonists and adrenergic stimulation increase the slope and the firing rate.
   d. **True**. Normally this is true, however if the intracellular Ca^{2+} concentration rises abnormally (e.g. under the influence of cardiac glycosides or noradrenaline [norepinephrine]), this can exchange with Na^+ passing inwards, causing membrane depolarisations. These are called afterdepolarisations or 'triggered activity'.
   e. **True**. Beta-adrenoceptor antagonists reduce pacemaker depolarisation rate by inhibiting the sympathetic stimulation of the cAMP-dependent funny current (I_f) in the SA and AV nodes.
   f. **True**. Although the type of Ca^{2+} channels utilised in the plateau phase 2 is different from those utilised in the pacemaker depolarisation during phase 4 (funny current I_f) of the action potential cycle, verapamil will act both to slow the rate of rise of the pacemaker depolarisation and to reduce the plateau phase, thus shortening the action potential. With these effects, verapamil is useful in supraventricular tachycardias but not in ventricular arrhythmias.
   g. **False**. Adenosine has no beneficial effect on ventricular arrhythmias. Its main effect involves enhancing K^+ conductance and inhibition of Ca^{2+} influx. The result is reduced AV nodal conduction and an increase in the AV nodal refractory period. Adenosine is useful because it has a high efficacy and a short duration of action.
2. Answer **C**.
   A, B. Each of these would increase both depolarisation rate in phase 4 and the rate of firing of the SA and AV nodes.
   C. This would slow the rate of depolarisation in phase 0 and is one of the mechanisms by which class I antiarrhythmics exert their therapeutic actions.
   D, E. Each of these would shorten action potential duration, increasing the likelihood of arrhythmias.
3. Case history answers
   a. The aim at this stage is to restore and maintain sinus rhythm in this man, who appears to have no structural heart disease. Since the arrhythmia is of short duration, pharmacological cardioversion may be successful. This could be achieved by flecainide, propafenone, sotalol or amiodarone. Amiodarone is usually reserved for people with significant cardiac dysfunction or those refractory to other agents. Flecainide and propafenone should be avoided in those with significant cardiac dysfunction or concomitant ischaemic heart disease. However, they are probably suitable for this man. Digoxin, calcium channel blockers and β-adrenoceptor antagonists are ineffective for *terminating* atrial fibrillation. Synchronised DC cardioversion is successful in up to 90% of people with atrial fibrillation who have no structural heart disease or heart failure, who are aged less than 50 years and whose duration of atrial fibrillation is less than 1 year. It could be considered if drugs are unsuccessful. About 50% of the time, recent-onset atrial fibrillation (less than 48 h duration) spontaneously converts to sinus rhythm. In this man, the atrial fibrillation could have been brought on by excess alcohol (so-called 'holiday heart'). If he moderates his alcohol intake, then prophylaxis would not be necessary after a single attack.
   b. Anticoagulation with warfarin is essential for at least 3–4 weeks before and 4 weeks after a DC cardioversion, to minimise the risk of a systemic embolus. For prophylaxis against recurrence, antifibrillatory drugs are usually given for 3–6 months following DC cardioversion, since this is the period of highest risk of recurrence. Digoxin, verapamil and β-adrenoceptor antagonists are not effective for prophylaxis. After 5 years of recurrence of atrial fibrillation, sinus rhythm could not be restored. Therefore, the aim in this man is to control ventricular rate. Digoxin suppresses AV nodal conduction and can reduce the ventricular response rate. This is mediated through potentiation of vagal effects on the heart and is less effective during exercise; therefore, the addition of a β-adrenoceptor antagonist or calcium channel blocker (such as verapamil or diltiazem) may be necessary. However, β-adrenoceptor antagonists (in high doses), verapamil and diltiazem are negatively inotropic and if there is significant cardiac dysfunction or heart failure they are contraindicated. The positive inotropic action of digoxin might be helpful if there is coexisting left ventricular impairment. The major long-term consequence of atrial fibrillation is the risk of thromboembolism and this is greatest in those over 75 years of age. For Mr GH, aspirin is sufficient as he is at a relatively low risk of stroke because of his age and lack of any coexisting hypertension, diabetes or significant left ventricular impairment.

Drugs used to treat cardiac arrhythmias

Drug	Half-life (h) and kinetics	Comments[a]
Class I drugs		
Disopyramide	4–10 [R + M] Oral bioavailability is 90%; main metabolite is less antiarrhythmic but more antimuscarinic	Used for SVT, VF, VT; given orally, or by slow intravenous injection (over at least 5 min) or intravenous infusion
Flecainide	12–30 [R + M] Oral bioavailability is >90%; metabolised by CYP2D6 and conjugation; also excreted in urine	Used for AF, N; treatment should be initiated in hospital; given orally, or by slow intravenous injection (over 10–30 min) or intravenous infusion (for ventricular tachyarrhythmias resistant to other treatments)
Lidocaine	2 [M] Low oral bioavailability; metabolised by CYP3A4; metabolites retain some activity	Used for VA (especially post-MI); given by intravenous injection or intravenous infusion
Moracizine (moricizine)	3 [M] Oral bioavailability is about 30–40% owing to first-pass metabolism; induces its own metabolism by induction of cytochrome P450 (autoinduction)	Used for severe life-threatening VA on a named patient basis only; given orally
Procainamide	3 [R + M] Metabolised by N-acetylation; N-acetyl metabolite is as active as the parent drug and has a longer half-life (6–9 h)	Used for AT, VA; given by slow intravenous injection or by intravenous infusion
Propafenone	4 [M] Low oral bioavailability (10%), which is increased at higher doses and by food; metabolised by oxidation by CYP2D6 + CYP3A4: longer half-life (17 h) in poor metabolisers of CYP2D6 substrates	Used for SVT, N, VA; some β-adrenoceptor antagonist activity; given orally
Quinidine	7 [M + R] Good oral bioavailability (70–80%); metabolised by oxidation; potent inhibitor of CYP2D6	SVT, VA; specialist use only; given orally
Class II drugs: β-adrenoceptor antagonists		
β-Adrenoceptor antagonists are used in a wide variety of indications; they are listed alphabetically in the compendium in Ch. 5		
Class III drugs		
Amiodarone	50–60 days [M] Oral bioavailability is 20–100%; active metabolite, which also has a long half-life (50 days); accumulation occurs, with steady state reached after about 6 months of treatment	Used for all arrhythmias, with treatment usually initiated in hospital or under specialist supervision; given orally or by intravenous infusion; given by intravenous injection (over 3 min) for ventricular fibrillation
Sotalol	7–18 [R] Oral bioavailability is >90%; eliminated largely by glomerular filtration	Also class II β-adrenoceptor antagonist; used for VT (life-threatening); β-adrenoceptor-non-selective; class III antiarrhythmic activity; greater proarrhythmic risk than other β-adrenoceptor antagonists; given orally or by intravenous injection (over 10 min)
Class IV drugs: calcium channel blockers		
For calcium channel blockers, see Ch. 5. Diltiazem has antiarrhythmic properties but is not licensed in the UK for this indication		
Verapamil	2–7 [M] Low oral bioavailability (about 20%); S-isomer is more active form; metabolised by CYP3A4 or CYP1A2	Used for SVT; given orally or by intravenous injection
Other drugs		
Adenosine	2 s [M all cells] Cleared extremely rapidly by metabolism	Used as the treatment of choice for terminating paroxysmal SVT; given intravenously
Atropine	2–5 [M + R] Metabolised in the liver to a number of metabolites	Used for bradycardia, especially if complicated by hypotension; given intravenously
Digoxin	40 (20–50) [R]	Used for AF; may need loading dose; oral or intravenous dosage (see Ch. 7)

[a]The types of arrhythmias commonly treated with different drugs are: AF, atrial fibrillation; AT, atrial tachycardia; N, nodal; SVT, supraventricular tachycardia; VA, ventricular arrhythmias; VF, ventricular fibrillation; VT, ventricular tachycardia.
Other abbreviations: MI, myocardial infarction; [M], metabolism; [R], renal excretion.

9 Cerebrovascular disease and dementia

STROKE

AETIOLOGY

Strokes are a major cause of morbidity and mortality, particularly in older people. They present as a transient or permanent neurological disturbance caused by ischaemic infarction or haemorrhagic disruption of neuronal pathways in the brain.

Ischaemic strokes

These account for about 85% of events. Cerebral infarction can result from intracerebral arterial thrombosis or from emboli travelling to the cerebral arteries, typically from the internal carotid arteries or from the heart. The extent and duration of the resulting functional deficit following a stroke is very variable.

Transient cerebral ischaemic attacks (TIAs) arise from small cerebral arterial emboli which rapidly disperse. They produce short-lived neurological signs and symptoms but leave no functional deficit 24 h later. A completed stroke results from more severe cerebral ischaemia which produces cerebral infarction. The neurological disturbance persists for more than 24 h, and frequently there is some permanent loss of function. Following a TIA there is an increased risk of a subsequent completed stroke. The overall risk is 30% in the 5 years after the initial TIA; however, if there is a significant carotid artery stenosis at the time of the TIA, the risk is 30% in the first month.

Haemorrhagic strokes

Primary intracerebral haemorrhage is responsible for up to15% of events. It often arises from rupture of microaneurysms on intracerebral arteries, usually in association with hypertension. Haemorrhagic strokes commonly leave a permanent functional deficit.

PREVENTION AND TREATMENT

Current treatments produce only a modest limitation of the neurological deficit in acute completed stroke. Most management is directed to:

- primary prevention of a first event (ischaemic or haemorrhagic stroke)
- prevention of recurrence of stroke or of other cardiovascular events
- rehabilitation after the stroke.

About one-third of strokes are recurrent. The recurrence rate for ischaemic stroke is about 3–7% per year for individuals who are in sinus rhythm and about 12% per year for those in atrial fibrillation.

Primary prevention of ischaemic stroke

- **Blood pressure lowering**. Hypertension is the single most powerful predictor of stroke. Pooled trial results indicate that a reduction in diastolic blood pressure by 5–6 mmHg reduces the risk of stroke by about 40% (Ch. 6). For isolated systolic hypertension, a similar reduction in risk has been shown after an average 11 mmHg reduction in systolic blood pressure.
- **Smoking cessation**. The risk of ischaemic stroke is reduced by up to 40% by 2–5 years after smoking cessation. This is probably due to slower progression of arterial atherothrombotic disease.
- **Reduced platelet aggregation**. Aspirin has *not* been shown to prevent a first stroke when taken by healthy individuals who are in sinus rhythm. In contrast, when given to people with atrial fibrillation, aspirin can reduce the risk of a first ischaemic stroke by almost one-third. However, aspirin is less effective than warfarin in this situation and the choice between them will depend on the balance of stroke risk in the individual and the risk of serious bleeding from the antithrombotic therapy (Ch. 11).
- **Inhibition of blood clotting**. Anticoagulation with warfarin (Chs 8 and 11) in people with atrial fibrillation reduces the risk of a first ischaemic stroke by 70–80%. Warfarin, at a dosage giving an INR (international normalised ratio) of 2–3, is superior to aspirin for stroke prevention, but at the expense of more major bleeds

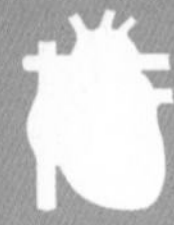

(including a small risk of haemorrhagic stroke). If there are no additional risk factors for cerebral embolic disease other than atrial fibrillation, then the risk–benefit analysis may favour the use of aspirin (see Ch. 11). There is no advantage for warfarin over aspirin for people in sinus rhythm. Warfarin reduces the risk of stroke following myocardial infarction if there is intracardiac clot associated with an akinetic area of the left ventricular wall.

- **Lowering cholesterol**. Reduction of a raised plasma cholesterol with a statin (Ch. 48) produces a 25% reduction in the risk of a first stroke, although much of the evidence for this effect derives from trials in subjects who already have clinical evidence of vascular disease or have diabetes.
- **Carotid endarterectomy**. This is sometimes recommended for asymptomatic carotid artery disease, but the annual risk of an ischaemic stroke is low in this situation, and there is little evidence to support carotid endarterectomy for primary prevention.

Primary prevention of intracerebral haemorrhage

- **Blood pressure lowering**. Lowering a raised blood pressure is the only means of reducing the risk of cerebral haemorrhage.

Treatment of acute ischaemic stroke

Fibrinolytic therapy with recombinant tissue plasminogen activator (rt-PA, alteplase; Ch. 11) can reduce the long-term neurological deficit after an ischaemic stroke. If treatment is started within 3 h of the onset of symptoms, thrombolysis reduces the risk of death or dependency at 3 months, with greater benefit the earlier that treatment is given. However, there is an increased risk of intracerebral haemorrhage, particularly in those with a blood pressure above 185/110 mmHg. If used after 3 h, there may be an adverse effect on outcome because the risk of intracerebral haemorrhage outweighs the benefit from neuronal salvage. Nevertheless, a meta-analysis of several studies suggests that alteplase may be effective until about 4.5 h and possibly 6 h after the event. Further studies will be necessary to confirm the effective treatment window.

Secondary prevention of recurrent ischaemic stroke

Many treatments are similar to those used for primary prevention of ischaemic stroke (see above).

- **Blood pressure lowering**. Lowering blood pressure after a stroke will reduce the risk of recurrence by 30–40%. There is considerable reluctance to reduce blood pressure in the first few days after a stroke, because of concern that cerebral perfusion pressure may fall too much if the normal cerebral artery autoregulation has been disturbed by the stroke. However, there is some evidence that early treatment (after the first 24 h) may be advantageous.
- **Reduced platelet aggregation**. Low-dose aspirin should be given to individuals who are in sinus rhythm following a TIA or a first ischaemic stroke. It reduces the risk of a further non-fatal stroke by about 20–30%. Combining aspirin with dipyridamole is more effective than low-dose aspirin given alone. This combination is recommended for up to 2 years after an ischaemic stroke, when the risk of recurrent stroke is highest, after which aspirin is often used alone. Clopidogrel alone (Ch. 11) is an alternative if aspirin is not tolerated, whereas dipyridamole alone is less effective than aspirin. By contrast, the combination of aspirin and clopidogrel is no more effective than aspirin alone (unlike in acute coronary syndromes – see Ch. 5), and increases the risk of serious bleeds. Warfarin has no role for preventing recurrent stroke in people who are in sinus rhythm. It is no better than aspirin, and carries a greater risk of major bleeds.
- **Inhibition of blood clotting**. After a first stroke in people with atrial fibrillation, warfarin reduces the risk of a further stroke by two-thirds. In contrast, aspirin has no protective effect in this situation (see Ch. 11).
- **Lowering cholesterol**. Cholesterol reduction with a statin is effective in secondary prevention of ischaemic stroke. However, the greatest advantage of cholesterol reduction in this situation is in the prevention of ischaemic cardiac events, since coronary artery disease often coexists with atheromatous cerebrovascular disease.
- **Carotid endarterectomy**. This reduces the risk of recurrent stroke if there have already been transient focal neurological symptoms in the cerebral territory served by a diseased carotid artery. If the stenosis is ≥70% of the vessel diameter (but without near total occlusion), then endarterectomy reduces the risk of recurrent stroke by about 16% over the subsequent 5 years (despite a perioperative risk of stroke or death of 3–5%). There is no benefit if the occlusion is less than 50%, and only marginal benefit if the occlusion is between 50% and 69%, unless the surgery is carried out soon after the event, when the risk of recurrence is highest.

Secondary prevention of recurrent haemorrhagic stroke

- **Blood pressure lowering**. Lowering blood pressure after a haemorrhagic stroke will reduce the risk of recurrence by up to 40%. The reduction in risk is greater than for ischaemic stroke, and even lowering a 'normal' blood pressure may be effective.

SUBARACHNOID HAEMORRHAGE

Most subarachnoid haemorrhages are caused by rupture of a saccular (or berry) aneurysm on an intracranial artery, usually on or close to the circle of Willis. These aneurysms are acquired during life and the cause is unknown, although there is an association with hypertension and conditions that increase cerebral blood flow such as arteriovenous malformations. About 5% of all strokes are caused by subarachnoid haemorrhage. Sudden onset of severe occipital headache is the most common presenting feature, but focal neurological signs or progressive confusion and impaired consciousness can occur. Rebleeding is a significant cause of disability and death, but early surgical intervention in survivors of the initial bleed reduces this risk. A more common cause of permanent neurological disability or later death is delayed cerebral ischaemia. This is produced by cerebral vasospasm, which develops in about 25% of cases, usually at least 3 days after the haemorrhage. The mechanism is poorly understood, but involves activation of voltage-dependent Ca^{2+} channels in intracranial arteries. It presents with confusion, decreased consciousness and new focal neurological deficit.

DRUGS FOR SUBARACHNOID HAEMORRHAGE

Nimodipine

Nimodipine is a dihydropyridine L-type calcium channel blocker (for mechanism of action, see Ch. 5) that is an arterial vasodilator with some selectivity for cerebral arteries. It reduces the risk of vasospasm following subarachnoid haemorrhage, but probably produces most of its benefits by protecting ischaemic neurons from Ca^{2+} overload. There is a theoretical risk that cerebral vasodilation may actually facilitate bleeding, but this does not appear to be a problem in practice. It is usually given intravenously immediately after the event, followed by oral dosing for a total of 5–10 days.

Pharmacokinetics

Nimodipine is well absorbed from the gut and undergoes extensive first-pass metabolism in the liver and gut wall. It has a half-life of 8–9 h, and is eliminated by metabolism in the liver.

Unwanted effects

These are mainly caused by arterial dilation:

- Hypotension, which can have a detrimental effect on cerebral perfusion
- Headache, flushing.

MANAGEMENT OF SUBARACHNOID HAEMORRHAGE

The definitive management of subarachnoid haemorrhage is surgical, with endovascular coil occlusion of the aneurysm or clipping of the neck of the aneurysm that produced the bleeding. Ischaemic cerebral damage can be reduced by using nimodipine in the first few days after the event. Although there is a lack of controlled clinical evidence, most neurosurgical units also use 'triple-H' therapy, a regimen of intravenous fluid replacement to create **H**ypervolaemia, avoidance of **H**ypotension, and **H**aemodilution to reduce ischaemic complications. This is achieved by a combination of intravenous crystalloid (typically isotonic saline) and colloid such as dextrans. Dexamethasone (Ch. 44) is often used to reduce cerebral oedema. The optimum blood pressure in the early period after the haemorrhage is not known, but hypotension should be avoided and blood pressure lowered modestly in those who present with significant hypertension. In the last 20 years, early surgical intervention, combined with medical therapy, has reduced mortality from 20% to about 5–10%.

Box 9.1 Causes of dementia

Treatable causes of dementia	Irreversible and partially treatable causes of dementia
Hypothyroidism	Vascular dementia
Neurosyphilis	Alzheimer's disease
Vitamin B_1 deficiency	Lewy body-type dementia
Normal pressure hydrocephalus	Parkinson's disease dementia
Frontal lobe tumours	Progressive supranuclear palsy
Cerebral vasculitis	Multiple systems atrophy
Cerebral hypoperfusion	

DEMENTIA

Dementia usually begins with forgetfulness and is characterised by disorientation in unfamiliar surroundings, variable mood, restlessness and poor sleep. Deterioration in social behaviour with self-neglect often follows, and may be accompanied by personality change with loss of inhibition. Most dementia results from Alzheimer's disease or from cerebrovascular disease (multi-infarct dementia), but there are other causes (Box 9.1). Memory impairment in dementia tends to be associated with bilateral hippocampal damage.

ALZHEIMER'S DISEASE

Alzheimer's disease is the commonest cause of dementia in people over the age of 65 years. About 10% of people over the age of 65 and about 30% of those over the age of 85 have some signs of Alzheimer's disease. The onset of symptoms is gradual, with progressive deterioration, unlike vascular dementia. It is a neurodegenerative disorder that begins pathologically 20–30 years before the clinical onset.

The cause of Alzheimer's disease is unknown, but there are several distinct factors associated with the disease.

- **Amyloid protein**. Amyloid β is deposited in the medial temporal lobe and cerebral cortex of people with Alzheimer's disease as senile plaques, which also contain typical neurofibrillary tangles. The fundamental defect may be an imbalance between the production and clearance of amyloid β in the brain.
- **Genetic predisposition**. Possession of the apolipoprotein E ε4 allele (APOE ε4) confers a higher risk, while mutations in genes coding for amyloid precursor protein and presenilin 1 and 2 explain much familial disease. APOE ε4 is essential for amyloid β deposition.
- **Inflammatory factors**. Activated microglia and reactive astrocytes surround the plaques, and there is local increase in proinflammatory mediators.
- **Glutamate involvement**. Amyloid deposits may promote neuronal damage by increasing neuronal release of

glutamate. This acts at NMDA (N-methyl-D-aspartate) receptors to generate glutamate-induced excitotoxicity of cholinergic neurons. Hyperactivity of glutamatergic neurons is a common finding in Alzheimer's disease.

- **Free radicals**. There is evidence for excessive free radical production in Alzheimer's disease. Increased oxidative stress may contribute to the condition by producing vascular damage, reducing amyloid β clearance and promoting metabolic derangement in neurons.
- **Loss of cholinergic (nicotinic) function**. There is a marked loss of acetylcholine neurotransmitter synthesis in the cerebral cortex and the hippocampus, particularly affecting the areas involved in cognition and in memory that are impaired in Alzheimer's disease. The defect may be in both cholinergic neurotransmission and neural growth. Muscarinic receptor density appears to be normal but the number of nicotinic receptors is reduced. Depletion of other neurotransmitters is a late and inconsistent finding.

DRUGS FOR ALZHEIMER'S DISEASE

Anticholinesterases

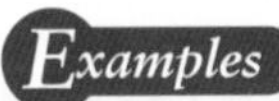

donepezil, galantamine, rivastigmine

Mechanisms of action and effects

The basis of the cholinergic hypothesis of Alzheimer's disease is that loss of cholinergic neurons in the basal forebrain nuclei results in abnormal function at cholinergic terminals in the hippocampus and neocortex, which are involved in memory and cognition. Anticholinesterases increase cholinergic transmission in the brain by inhibition of the enzyme acetylcholinesterase in the synaptic cleft (Ch. 4).

- Donepezil is a reversible inhibitor of acetylcholinesterase with a high degree of selectivity for the central nervous system (CNS).
- Galantamine is a reversible competitive inhibitor of acetylcholinesterase that also has agonist activity at presynaptic nicotinic receptors by allosterically enhancing the receptor response to acetylcholine.
- Rivastigmine is a slowly reversible inhibitor of acetylcholinesterase with selectivity for the CNS, and also inhibits pseudocholinesterase (butyrylcholinesterase) that is present in plasma.

Pharmacokinetics

Donepezil, galantamine and rivastigmine are well absorbed from the gut; donepezil and galantamine are metabolised in the liver, whereas rivastigmine is rapidly inactivated by cholinesterase-mediated hydrolysis. Rivastigmine has a short half-life of 1–2 h, while that of galantamine is longer, at 5–7 h, and that of donepezil is very long, at 70–80 h.

Unwanted effects

- Anorexia, nausea, vomiting, diarrhoea, abdominal pain
- Insomnia, confusion, agitation, dizziness, headache.

NMDA receptor antagonist

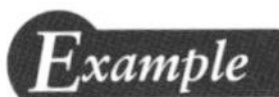

memantine

Mechanism of action and effects

Memantine is a derivative of the antiviral drug amantadine (Ch. 24 and Ch. 51), and is a non-competitive antagonist at glutamate NMDA receptors. Blockade of the NMDA receptor may prevent glutamate-induced excitotoxicity (by limiting long-lasting influx of Ca^{2+} into neurons), but without interfering with the actions of glutamate that are involved in memory and learning. Memantine is also a $5HT_3$ receptor antagonist and a non-competitive nicotinic receptor antagonist, but the significance of these actions for the treatment of dementia is unknown. It can be taken together with an anticholinesterase.

Pharmacokinetics

Memantine is well absorbed from the gut and is partly metabolised in the liver but is largely excreted unchanged by the kidney. It has a very long half-life of 60–80 h.

Unwanted effects

- Constipation
- Insomnia, dizziness, headache, hallucinations.

TREATMENT OF ALZHEIMER'S DISEASE

In the UK, drug treatment for Alzheimer's disease is started only for people who have a Mini-Mental State Examination (MMSE) score of 10–20 points (moderate dementia). The diagnosis of Alzheimer's disease should be first confirmed in a specialist clinic.

Cholinesterase inhibitors produce modest improvement in symptoms, and a delay in the decline of cognitive function and memory, in up to 40% of sufferers. Efficacy should be assessed after 2–4 months of treatment at a suitable dose. Treatment should be continued only if the 'global, functional and behavioural condition remains at a level where the drug is considered to be having a worthwhile effect'. Treatment should be stopped in non-responders. The decline in mental function is delayed by about 3–6 months but not arrested. Rapid progression resumes when the drugs are stopped, but there may be limited benefit from restarting treatment more than a month after withdrawal. Anticholinesterases produce some improvement in other functional measures and behaviour that also affect the quality of life.

Memantine produces moderate improvement in cognition and reduction in functional decline, and is usually well tolerated. However, the evidence for its cost-effectiveness is inconclusive.

Current treatments for Alzheimer's disease do not alter the progression of the underlying disease. New treatment strategies are being developed that are directed either at enhancing the various neurotrophic proteins which protect neuronal systems, or at altering the production or clearance of amyloid protein or Tau protein found in neurofibrillary tangles. Such strategies may offer a more fundamental approach to retarding the progress of Alzheimer's disease. Early studies which suggested that treatment with non-steroidal anti-inflammatory drugs (NSAIDs) retards the progression of Alzheimer's disease have not been supported by recent evidence, but there is some suggestion that NSAIDs may reduce the risk of developing the disease.

VASCULAR DEMENTIA

Cerebrovascular disease is a particularly common cause of dementia over the age of 85 years, and overall is the second most frequent cause of dementia. The deterioration in mental function is produced by multiple cerebral infarcts (multi-infarct dementia), particularly if they affect the white matter. The risk of dementia is increased ninefold in people with stroke. In some of these, dementia may be produced by specific strategically located infarcts, especially in the angular gyrus of the inferior parietal lobule. In contrast to Alzheimer's disease, the initial presentation is usually more acute, and cognitive decline has a stepwise course arising from recurrent cerebrovascular events.

TREATMENT

- Prophylaxis against cerebral emboli with aspirin or warfarin (see prevention of stroke, above). However, the Cochrane database finds that there is no evidence, as yet, that aspirin is of benefit in vascular dementia.
- Control of hypertension (Ch. 6). Trials have shown that calcium channel blockers are effective for reducing the risk of vascular dementia, but it is likely to be an effect related to blood pressure reduction rather than to a more specific effect of this class of drug.
- Anticholinesterases or memantine may produce some improvement in vascular dementia.
- Immunosuppressant drugs (Ch. 38) can be used in the rare cases caused by cerebral vasculitis.

FURTHER READING

Stroke

Amarenco P, Bogousslavsky J, Callahan A et al (2006) High-dose atorvastatin after stroke or transient ischemic attack. *N Engl J Med* 355, 549–559

Bedi A, Flaker GC (2002) How do HMG-CoA reductase inhibitors prevent stroke? *Am J Cardiovasc Drugs* 2, 7–14

Bentley P, Sharma P (2005) Pharmacological treatment of ischaemic stroke. *Pharmacol Ther* 108, 334–352

Briel M, Studer M, Glass TR et al (2004) Effects of statins on stroke prevention in patients with and without coronary heart disease: a meta-analysis of randomized controlled trials. *Am J Med* 117, 596–606

Claiborne JS (2002) Transient ischemic attack. *N Engl J Med* 347, 1687–1692

Donnan GA, Fisher M, MacLeod M et al (2008) Stroke. *Lancet* 371, 1612–1623

ESPRIT Study Group, Halkes PH, van Gijn J, Kappelle LJ, Koudstaall PJ, Algra A (2006) Aspirin plus dipyridamole versus aspirin alone after cerebral ischaemia of arterial origin (ESPRIT): randomised controlled trial. *Lancet* 367, 1665–1773

Fotherby MD, Panayiotou B (1999) Antihypertensive therapy in the prevention of stroke. *Drugs* 58, 663–674

Hacke W, Donnan G, Fieschi C et al (2004) Association of outcome with early stroke treatment: pooled analysis of ATLANTIS, ECASS, and NINDs rt-PA stroke trials. *Lancet* 363, 768–774

Laws PE, Spark JI, Cowled PA, Fitridge RA (2004) The role of statins in vascular disease. *Eur J Vasc Endovasc Surg* 27, 6–16

Muir KW (2004) Secondary prevention for stroke and transient ischaemic attacks. *BMJ* 328, 297–298

Powers WJ (2001) Oral anticoagulant therapy for the prevention of stroke. *N Engl J Med* 345, 1493–1495

Rashid P, Leonardi-Bee J, Bath P (2003) Blood pressure reduction and secondary prevention of stroke and other vascular events: a systematic review. *Stroke* 34, 2741–2748

Rothwell PM, Eliasziw M, Gutnikov SA et al (2003) Analysis of pooled data from the randomised controlled trials of endarterectomy for symptomatic carotid artery stenosis. *Lancet* 361, 107–116

Schellinger PD, Kaste M, Hacke W (2004) An update on thrombolytic therapy for acute stroke. *Curr Opin Neurol* 17, 69–77

Straus SE, Majumdar SR, McAlister FA (2002) New evidence for stroke prevention. Scientific review. *JAMA* 288, 1388–1395

van der Worp HB, van Gijn J (2007) Acute ischemic stroke. *N Engl J Med* 357, 572–579

Wahlgren N, Ahmed N, Davalos A et al (2007) Thrombolysis with alteplase for ischaemic stroke in the Safe Implementation of Thrombolysis in Stroke-Monitoring Study (SITS-MOST): an observational study. *Lancet* 369, 275–282

Waldo AL (2003) Stroke prevention in atrial fibrillation. *JAMA* 290, 1093–1095

Subarachnoid haemorrhage

Al-Shahi R, White PM, Davenport RJ et al (2006) Subarachnoid haemorrhage. *BMJ* 333, 235–240

Sen J, Belli A, Albon H et al (2003) Triple-H therapy in the management of aneurysmal subarachnoid haemorrhage. *Lancet Neurol* 2, 614–621

van Gijn J, Kerr RS, Rinkel GJ (2007) Subarachnoid haemorrhage. *Lancet* 369, 306–318

Dementia

The Cochrane database *http://www.cochrane.org/reviews* allows access to the trials that have been performed using aspirin, nimodipine and *Ginkgo biloba* in dementias and is worth referring to

Blennow K, de Leon MJ, Zetterberg H (2006) Alzheimer's disease. *Lancet* 368, 387–403

Cummings JL (2004) Alzheimer's disease. *N Engl J Med* 351, 56–67

Doraiswamy PM (2002) Non-cholinergic strategies for treating and preventing Alzheimer's disease. *CNS Drugs* 16, 811–824

Doraiswamy PM (2003) Alzheimer's disease and the glutamate NMDA receptor. *Psychopharmacol Bull* 37, 41–49

Farlowe MR (2006) Use of antidementia agents in vascular dementia: beyond Alzheimer disease. *Mayo Clin Proc* 81, 1350–1358

Farlowe MR, Cummings JL (2007) Effective pharmacologic management of Alzheimer's disease. *Am J Med* 120, 388–397

Forette F, Seux M-L, Staessen JA et al (2002) The prevention of dementia with antihypertensive treatment. New evidence from the Systolic Hypertension in Europe (Syst-Eur) study. *Arch Intern Med* 162, 2046–2052

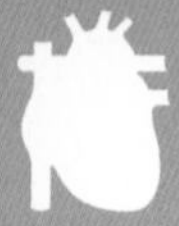

Grutzendler J, Morris JC (2001) Cholinesterase inhibitors for Alzheimer's disease. *Drugs* 61, 41–52

Kawas CH (2003) Early Alzheimer's disease. *N Engl J Med* 349, 1056–1063

O'Brien, Erkinjuntti T, Roman G et al (2003) Vascular cognitive impairment. *Lancet Neurol* 2, 89–98

Raina P, Santaguida P, Ismalia A et al (2008) Effectiveness of cholinesterase inhibitors and mementine for treating dementia: evidence review for a clinical practice guideline. *Ann Intern Med* 148, 379–397

Ritchie K, Lovestone S (2002) The dementias. *Lancet* 360, 1759–1766

Scarpini E, Scheltens P, Feldman H (2003) Treatment of Alzheimer's disease: current status and new perspectives. *Lancet Neurol* 2, 539–547

SELF-ASSESSMENT

1. In the following questions, the first statement, in italics, is true. Is the accompanying statement also true?
   a. *Aspirin has not been shown to prevent a first stroke when given to people in sinus rhythm.* Aspirin cannot prevent a first event in people with persistent atrial fibrillation.
   b. *Approximately 85% of all strokes have an ischaemic aetiology and most of the remaining 15% have a haemorrhagic basis.* If thrombolysis with recombinant tissue-type plasminogen activator (rt-PA; alteplase) is given in acute stroke, antiplatelet and anticoagulant therapies should not be given concurrently.
   c. *Glutamate receptor antagonists lower the neurotoxicity of the neuroexcitatory transmitter glutamate.* Cerebral ischaemia depolarises neurons and causes the release of large amounts of glutamate.
   d. *Cerebral emboli arising from the heart can be caused by atrial fibrillation, infected or damaged prosthetic valves or arise following damage to parts of the myocardium.* Anticoagulation with warfarin or antiplatelet therapy with aspirin are equal first-choice drugs for secondary prevention of recurrent ischaemic strokes in the presence of sinus rhythm.
2. Choose the one **correct** statement from the following:
   A. Alzheimer's disease is associated with a relative lack of cholinergic and glutamatergic neurotransmission.
   B. It is recommended that rivastigmine is prescribed irrespective of the Mini-Mental State Examination (MMSE) score of a person with Alzheimer's disease.
   C. Memantine acts by stimulation of glutamate receptors.
   D. Anticholinesterases should not be co-prescribed with memantine.
   E. Rivastigmine treatment results in stimulation of both muscarinic and nicotinic receptors.
3. Case history questions

A 70-year-old man had a blood pressure of 190/110 mmHg despite intensive antihypertensive drug treatment. He was admitted to hospital 6 h after the acute onset of unilateral weakness and sensory loss. At the time of admission to hospital, most of the neurological signs had resolved. He had no headache or vomiting and remained conscious. He was in sinus rhythm. Following clinical examination and a CT brain scan, this episode was diagnosed as a TIA.

   a. Should thrombolysis be given?
   b. What other therapies should be instituted immediately?
   c. What secondary prevention strategy should be employed?

ANSWERS

1. a. **False**. Aspirin has been shown to reduce the risk of a first embolic stroke in atrial fibrillation.
   b. **True**. The immediate risk of intracranial haemorrhage with alteplase is high and could be compounded by simultaneous administration of antiplatelet or anticoagulant agents. These should be considered later, when the effect of the thrombolytic has waned.
   c. **True**. The excitatory amino acid glutamate can cause a substantial rise in intracellular Ca^{2+}, causing Ca^{2+} overload. This causes cell death by generation of free radicals. However, trials of drugs that interfere with glutamate synthesis or effect have been disappointing.
   d. **False**. In people in sinus rhythm, aspirin alone or possibly together with dipyridamole reduces the risk of stroke; warfarin is no more effective but there is a greater risk of major bleeding.
2. Answer **E**.
   A. Incorrect. Alzheimer's disease is associated with a lack of cholinergic transmission and an overactivity of glutamatergic transmission.
   B. Incorrect. In the UK, it is advised that the anticholinesterases should not be prescribed if the MMSE is below 12.
   C. Incorrect. Memantine inhibits the glutamate NMDA receptor.
   D. Incorrect. They can be useful co-prescribed.
   E. Correct.
3. Case history answers
   a. Thrombolysis is inappropriate in this situation. His blood pressure is high and it is a considerable time since the onset of symptoms. Thrombolysis has been approved for use within 3 h of the onset of symptoms. The rapid resolution of signs indicates a TIA, for which thrombolysis is not given. (Although thrombolysis has been shown in some trials to be useful in the treatment of stroke, safe and effective use is determined by a rigid set of criteria as there is a significant risk of intracranial haemorrhage.)
   b. His blood pressure must be brought under control. Reduction in blood pressure has a major effect on

the prevention of a recurrent stroke. He should be started on a low dose of aspirin.

c. Antiplatelet therapy should be continued. The antiplatelet drug dipyridamole has additional benefit when given together with aspirin. Cholesterol reduction with a statin is effective in secondary prevention of ischaemic stroke. It may be worth treating this man with a statin even if his cholesterol is not raised. An important reason for cholesterol reduction is prevention of ischaemic cardiac events, since coronary artery disease often coexists with atheromatous cerebrovascular disease.

Drugs used to treat cerebrovascular disease and dementia (given orally[a])

Drug	Half-life (h) and kinetics	Comment
Anticholinesterase drugs		
Donepezil	70–80 [M + R] Oral bioavailability is high; metabolised by CYP2D6 (polymorphic) and CYP3A4, and excreted in urine as both parent drug and metabolites	Used for mild to moderate dementia in Alzheimer's disease; given once daily at night
Galantamine	5–7 [R + some M] Almost complete oral bioavailability (>90%); metabolised by CYP2D6 and CYP3A4, and excreted in urine as parent drug and metabolites	Used for mild to moderate dementia in Alzheimer's disease
Rivastigmine	1–2 [M] Oral bioavailability is 30–70% (depending on dose); it is a carbamate inhibitor of cholinesterases which is metabolised by hydrolysis; duration of effect is about 10 h	Used for mild to moderate dementia in Alzheimer's disease
Other drugs		
Clopidogrel and prasugrel		see Ch. 11
Dipyridamole	12 [M] Variable absorption (30–90%); metabolised by glucuronidation	A vasodilator (Ch. 11)
Memantine	60–80 [R] Complete oral bioavailability (100%); renal excretion exceeds glomerular filtration rate (GFR) but is pH-dependent and markedly reduced at high urine pH	NMDA receptor antagonist; used for moderate to severe dementia in Alzheimer's disease
Nimodipine	8–9 [M] Oral bioavailability is 5–10%; metabolised by hepatic cytochrome P450	Calcium channel blocker (Ch. 5); selective for cerebral arteries; use is confined to the prevention and treatment of ischaemic neurological deficits following aneurysmal subarachnoid haemorrhage; given orally or by intravenous infusion

[a]Except nimodipine, which can be given intravenously.
[M], metabolism; [R], renal excretion.

10 Peripheral vascular disease

ATHEROMATOUS PERIPHERAL VASCULAR DISEASE

Atherosclerotic disease in peripheral arteries principally affects the aorta, renal and lower limb arteries. The risk factors for its development are similar to those for coronary artery and cerebrovascular disease (Chs 5 and 9). The strongest associations are with smoking and a raised systolic blood pressure, and to a lesser extent with diabetes mellitus, a raised plasma low-density lipoprotein (LDL) cholesterol and lack of exercise. Not surprisingly, ischaemic heart disease and cerebrovascular disease frequently coexist in people with peripheral vascular disease and are responsible for about 70% of their excess mortality. Only about 50% of people with peripheral vascular disease are alive 10 years after diagnosis; this is three times the mortality of those without peripheral vascular disease.

INTERMITTENT CLAUDICATION

Intermittent claudication is pain in the muscles of the lower limb which is precipitated by walking and is relieved by rest. The symptoms usually arise as a consequence of atherosclerotic stenosis of a lower limb artery. Hypoxia of skeletal muscle occurs when blood flow through the diseased artery fails to increase sufficiently to meet the increased metabolic demand of the muscle during exercise. The metabolic changes that accompany the switch to anaerobic metabolism in the muscle trigger the pain. Depending on the site of the vascular narrowing, pain can be experienced in the calf, thigh or buttock. The development of a collateral arterial circulation (see also Ch. 5) will reduce the severity of the symptoms and influence the long-term outcome. In three-quarters of those with peripheral vascular disease, the symptoms stabilise within a few months of presentation. The remainder experience steady progression, but only 1% per year will develop critical ischaemia which causes pain at rest and distal gangrene (see below).

DRUGS FOR PERIPHERAL VASCULAR DISEASE

Cilostazol

Mechanism of action

Cilostazol appears to have several actions. It is a reversible inhibitor of the enzyme phosphodiesterase type 3 (PDE3), and therefore reduces breakdown of cyclic adenosine monophosphate (cAMP) (Table 1.1). PDE3 is present in vascular smooth muscle cells and platelets, and cilostazol causes vasodilation, inhibits platelet activation and aggregation, and prevents release of prothrombotic inflammatory substances. Cilostazol also inhibits adenosine reuptake, which promotes vasodilation, has favourable effects on plasma lipids by increasing high-density lipoprotein (HDL) cholesterol, and inhibits cell proliferation in vascular smooth muscle. The vasodilatory actions of cilostazol are greater on femoral arteries than on vertebral, carotid or superior mesenteric arteries, and renal arteries do not dilate in response to cilostazol. This may reflect the differences in PDE3 abundance in these tissues.

Pharmacokinetics

Cilostazol is well absorbed orally, and undergoes hepatic metabolism via cytochrome P450 to two metabolites with antiplatelet activity, one of which is more active than cilostazol. Cilostazol has a half-life of about 12 h.

Unwanted effects

- Diarrhoea
- Headache
- Palpitation and tachycardia
- Other phosphodiesterase inhibitors such as milrinone have been shown to decrease survival in people with heart failure (Ch. 7); cilostazol does not appear to increase the risk of life-threatening arrhythmias, but at present its use is contraindicated in people with heart failure or cardiac arrhythmias
- Drug interactions: the pharmacokinetics of cilostazol will be altered by drugs that influence the liver cytochrome P450 CYP3A4 isoenzyme (Ch. 2).

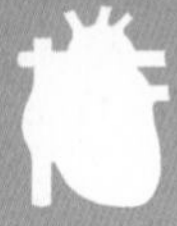

Naftidrofuryl oxalate

Mechanism of action and effects

Naftidrofuryl oxalate promotes the production of high-energy phosphates in ischaemic tissue by activating the enzyme succinic dehydrogenase. It is also a 5-hydroxytryptamine type 2 ($5HT_2$) receptor antagonist, an action which leads to vasodilation in the periphery and reduced platelet aggregation. All these actions could improve blood flow to ischaemic tissues and tissue nutrition, but the effect on walking distance is modest.

Pharmacokinetics

Naftidrofuryl is well absorbed from the gut and metabolised in the liver. It has a half-life of 3–4 h.

Unwanted effects

- Nausea, epigastric pain
- Rash
- Hepatitis is a rare, but potentially serious, complication.

MANAGEMENT OF INTERMITTENT CLAUDICATION

Non-pharmacological treatment

- Stopping smoking slows the progression of peripheral atherosclerosis and may improve walking distance by improving blood oxygen transport.
- Regular exercise, up to the point of claudication, can improve walking distance by 150% over 3–12 months.

Pharmacological treatment

- Low-dose aspirin inhibits platelet aggregation and reduces cardiac and cerebrovascular events (Chs 11 and 29).
- Intensive management of hypertension reduces progression of atheroma. Conventional antihypertensive therapy is used (Ch. 6). Although β-adrenoceptor antagonists could theoretically exacerbate intermittent claudication by reducing cardiac output and impairing vasodilation of arteries supplying skeletal muscle (Ch. 5), there is little evidence that they are disadvantageous unless there is critical limb ischaemia.
- Lowering serum LDL cholesterol (Ch. 48) can stabilise or regress atherosclerotic plaques. It is not known whether this improves limb survival or reduces the need for subsequent surgery. A greater benefit from cholesterol lowering may be reduced morbidity and mortality from coexistent ischaemic heart disease (Ch. 5).
- Cilostazol can improve walking distance by up to 50% over 3–6 months of treatment, but the impact of this on quality of life is often minimal. It is not known whether cilostazol has any effect on long-term outcome or on the subsequent need for surgery.
- Naftidrofuryl oxalate has only a modest effect on walking distance. It should not be used routinely, but a trial of treatment may be justified for those who remain restricted by the disease after 6–12 months of conservative treatment. Withdrawal is advised after 3–6 months of treatment, to assess whether spontaneous improvement has occurred.
- Pentoxifylline, nicotinic acid derivatives, and cinnarizine are licensed for treatment of peripheral vascular disease, but are relatively ineffective and are not recommended.

Surgical treatment

Surgical treatment is usually considered if quality of life is significantly impaired by claudication or if tissue integrity is at risk. Percutaneous transluminal angioplasty, often with insertion of a stent, is used particularly for stenoses above the inguinal ligament, while bypass surgery is used for most other disease.

ACUTE AND CRITICAL LIMB ISCHAEMIA

Acute and critical limb ischaemia in peripheral vascular disease is usually caused by thrombosis superimposed on a pre-existing atheromatous plaque. Acute limb ischaemia is caused by an arterial embolus from an intracardiac site, usually associated with atrial fibrillation (Ch. 8) or following a myocardial infarction (Ch. 5), or aortic thrombus. Emboli can occlude previously healthy vessels. The clinical presentation is with acute onset of severe pain at rest, associated with signs of critically impaired tissue perfusion. Critical limb ischaemia results from chronic, severe, subtotal occlusion of an artery. The symptoms include rest pain, often worse at night and relieved by hanging the leg out of the bed.

MANAGEMENT

Unless treatment of acute or acute-on-chronic critical limb ischaemia is rapid, the person may be left with a chronically ischaemic limb, or occasionally the limb may be lost through gangrene.

If the limb is still viable, then a peripheral arterial angiogram should be carried out. For acute embolic arterial occlusion, embolectomy is the treatment of choice. Intra-arterial thrombolysis, either with streptokinase or tissue plasminogen activator (rt-PA, alteplase) (Ch. 11), is used to dissolve an acute thrombus occluding a previously diseased vessel. Alteplase produces more rapid lysis, but there is no evidence that limb salvage is any better than with streptokinase. The thrombolytic agent can be infused via a catheter for up to 24 h or given as repeated boluses. Reperfusion takes several hours, and in about 25% of acute vascular occlusions lysis is not achieved, especially if there is embolic occlusion. The risk of intracerebral haemorrhage is also a concern. A surgical bypass may be considered if there is no time for thrombolysis.

Secondary prevention measures to reduce other cardiovascular events (see above) should also be started.

RAYNAUD'S PHENOMENON

Raynaud's phenomenon is a profound and exaggerated vasospastic response of blood vessels in the extremities on exposure to cold or during emotional upset. This leads to episodes of ischaemia which can be provoked by even small changes of temperature and most commonly affect the fingers (occasionally also in the toes, ear lobes or the nipples). A typical attack initially produces pallor of the affected part, followed by cyanosis then redness as flow returns. About two-thirds of cases occur in women (typically presenting under the age of 40 years), in whom the overall prevalence is about 15%. Common symptoms include discomfort, numbness and tingling, with loss of function and pain if the condition is severe. Rarely, digital ulceration can occur.

The majority of cases of Raynaud's phenomenon are idiopathic (primary Raynaud's phenomenon; also called Raynaud's disease), when the cause of the excessive vascular reactivity is unknown. Vascular function in other tissues is often abnormal in primary Raynaud's phenomenon: for example, in the cerebral vessels (giving an association with migraine), the coronary circulation (producing variant angina) or, more rarely, in the pulmonary circulation (leading to pulmonary hypertension).

In about 10% of cases, Raynaud's phenomenon is secondary to another disorder. This is most commonly scleroderma, but there are many other associated conditions (Box 10.1). Structural damage to arteries is common in secondary Raynaud's phenomenon, and digital ulceration is much more common than in the primary type.

Other disorders of the peripheral circulation should also be considered in the differential diagnosis of Raynaud's phenomenon.

- Acrocyanosis usually affects the hands and produces persistently cold, bluish fingers which are often sweaty or oedematous. The management of this condition is similar to that of Raynaud's phenomenon.
- Chilblains are an inflammatory disorder with erythematous lesions on the feet, or less commonly the hands or face, that are precipitated by cold and humidity followed by rapid rewarming. The lesions are often painful or itchy. Treatments used for Raynaud's phenomenon may help, with the addition of topical non-steroidal anti-inflammatory agents (Ch. 29).
- Erythromelalgia is a painful, burning condition often affecting the hands and feet that, unlike Raynaud's phenomenon, is usually provoked by heat. It sometimes responds to treatment with a calcium channel blocker (Ch. 5) or gabapentin (Ch. 23).
- Vibration white finger is a patchy digital vasospasm associated with prolonged use of vibrating tools. If drug treatment is necessary, it is similar to that for Raynaud's phenomenon.

Box 10.1 Conditions associated with Raynaud's phenomenon

Connective tissue disorders
Systemic sclerosis
Systemic lupus erythematosus
Rheumatoid arthritis
Dermatomyositis and polymyositis

Obstructive arterial disorders
Carpal tunnel syndrome
Thoracic outlet syndrome
Atherosclerosis
Thromboangiitis obliterans

Drugs and chemicals
Ergotamine
Beta-adrenoceptor antagonists
Bleomycin, vinblastine, cisplatin
Oral contraceptives
Vinyl chloride

Occupational
Vibrating tools
Cold environment

Blood disorders
Polycythaemia
Cold agglutinin disease
Monoclonal gammopathies
Thrombocytosis

MANAGEMENT

Many people with Raynaud's phenomenon are only mildly inconvenienced by their symptoms and respond to simple measures. Drug treatment is usually reserved for those suffering from more intense vasospasm with pain, impairment of function or trophic changes. Responses to individual treatments are unpredictable, and are less satisfactory in secondary Raynaud's phenomenon because of structural changes to the vessel wall.

Non-pharmacological treatment

- Often, minimising changes in ambient temperature with insulating clothing is enough to reduce the numbers of attacks, although electrically heated gloves or socks may be useful for more severely affected people.
- Smoking should be strongly discouraged. Nicotine promotes vasospasm and may also reduce the threshold for other provoking factors.
- Aggravating factors should be withdrawn or corrected whenever possible (see Box 10.1). Beta-adrenoceptor antagonists (Ch. 5) produce peripheral circulatory problems sufficient to necessitate stopping treatment in about 3–5% of people with hypertension.
- Surgical sympathectomy is occasionally used for advanced disease.

Pharmacological treatment

Arterial vasodilators

- Calcium channel blockers (Ch. 5): modified-release nifedipine is the drug of first choice for Raynaud's phenomenon, and reduces the frequency, duration and intensity of vasospastic episodes. Several other dihydropyridines are probably equally effective, but diltiazem

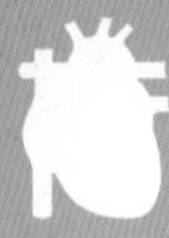

is less effective and verapamil ineffective in this condition.

- Naftidrofuryl oxalate may produce a modest reduction in the severity of attacks.
- Alpha$_1$-adrenoceptor antagonists (Ch. 6): moxisylyte may be effective and does not lower blood pressure, unlike other α-adrenoceptor antagonists; prazosin has also been shown to be helpful.
- Angiotensin receptor antagonists (Ch. 6): losartan has shown some benefit.
- Sildenafil (Ch. 16) has been used successfully in secondary Raynaud's phenomenon that is resistant to other vasodilators.
- Bosentan, an endothelin receptor antagonist (Ch. 6), has shown promise in severe Raynaud's phenomenon.
- Fluoxetine (Ch. 22), a selective serotonin reuptake inhibitor (SSRI) antidepressant, is effective in some people.
- Calcitonin gene-related peptide (CGRP) is effective for prolonged periods when given by short intravenous infusions over 5 or more consecutive days. It is a neurotransmitter at vasodilator cutaneous sensorimotor nerves in the fingers and toes. CGRP is usually reserved for failure to respond to epoprostenol (see below).

Drugs acting primarily on blood components

- Prostaglandins: short intravenous infusions of epoprostenol (prostacyclin, PGI_2, Ch. 11) over at least 5 consecutive days produces immediate vasodilation, but long-term improvement in symptoms and healing of ulcers over a period of 10–16 weeks. These effects are believed to be caused by actions on the flow properties of blood, i.e. reduced platelet aggregation, increased red cell deformability and reduced neutrophil adhesiveness. Epoprostenol is rapidly inactivated in plasma by hydrolysis, and has a very short half-life of about 3 min. Unwanted effects are due to vasodilation, and include flushing, headache and hypotension.
- Inositol nicotinate (a nicotinic acid derivative) produces a gradual onset of clinical response and only modest improvement. Its action may result more from fibrinolysis (reducing plasma viscosity) and reduction in platelet aggregation than from vasodilation.

FURTHER READING

Boin F, Wigley FM (2005) Understanding, assessing and treating Raynaud's phenomenon. *Curr Opin Rheumatol* 17, 752–760

Bowling JCR, Dowd PM (2003) Raynaud's disease. *Lancet* 361, 2078–2080

Hankey GJ, Norman PE, Eikelboom JW (2006) Medical treatment of peripheral arterial disease. *JAMA* 295, 547–553

Herrick AL (2003) Treatment of Raynaud's phenomenon: new insights and developments. *Curr Rheumatol Rep* 5, 168–174

Levien TL (2006) Phosphodiesterase inhibitors in Raynaud's phenomenon. *Ann Pharmacother* 40, 1388–1393

Mannava K, Money SR (2007) Current management of peripheral arterial occlusive disease: a review of pharmacologic agents and other interventions. *Am J Cardiovasc Drugs* 7, 59–66

Regensteiner JG, Hiatt WR (2002) Current medical therapies for patients with peripheral arterial disease: a critical review. *Am J Med* 112, 49–57

Tilley DG, Maurice DH (2002) Vascular smooth muscle cell phosphodiesterase (PDE) 3 and PDE4 activities and levels are regulated by cyclic AMP in vivo. *Mol Pharmacol* 63, 497–506

Warfarin Antiplatelet Vascular Evaluation Trial Investigators (2007) Oral anticoagulant and antiplatelet therapy and peripheral arterial disease. *N Engl J Med* 357, 217–227

Wright C (2007) Intermittent claudication. *N Engl J Med* 356, 1241–1250

SELF-ASSESSMENT

1. In the following questions, the first statement, in italics, is true. Is the accompanying statement also true?
   a. *There is an additive effect of diabetes mellitus, hypertension and smoking on the risk of developing peripheral vascular disease.* People with intermittent claudication do not have an increased risk of developing coronary disease.
   b. *'Statins' are indicated in people with symptomatic atherosclerotic peripheral vascular disease.* Simvastatin increases the expression of hepatic low-density lipoprotein (LDL) receptors.
   c. *Drugs such as ergotamine, used in migraine treatment, can precipitate Raynaud's phenomenon*. Verapamil is the calcium channel blocker of choice in the treatment of Raynaud's phenomenon.
2. Choose the one **correct** statement from the following:
   A. Cilostazol inhibits phosphodiesterase type 3 in vascular tissues.
   B. Cilostazol is useful in the treatment of congestive heart failure.
   C. Cilostazol is mainly excreted unchanged in the urine.
   D. Cilostazol has little effect on platelet aggregation.
   E. Cilostazol decreases plasma HDL cholesterol.

3. Case history questions

> Mr TH, aged 67 years, was an insulin-dependent diabetic and smoked 20 cigarettes a day. His plasma cholesterol level was raised at 7 mmol L^{-1} and his blood pressure was 160/110 mmHg. After walking 50 m, he developed pain in his left calf muscle, which was relieved by rest. He occasionally, but rarely, had rest pain at night. On examination, both popliteal and posterior tibial pulses were absent and femoropopliteal obstruction was diagnosed.

a. Comment on the usefulness and drawbacks of the following drugs to treat this patient with peripheral vascular disease.
   A. Propranolol
   B. Atenolol
   C. Nifedipine
   D. A statin
   E. Low-dose aspirin
   F. Cilostazol
b. What other therapy could be of benefit?
c. Should the use of an electric blanket be discouraged?

ANSWERS

1. a. **False**. There is a two- to fourfold increase in risk of developing coronary disease, stroke or heart failure compared with age-matched subjects who do not have intermittent claudication.
   b. **True**. By reducing cholesterol synthesis, simvastatin increases hepatic LDL receptors, which results in reduced LDL cholesterol in blood and a small accompanying increase in high-density lipoprotein (HDL) cholesterol (Ch. 48). The main potential benefit of lowered LDL cholesterol in these patients is a reduction in coronary artery disease events.
   c. **False**. Verapamil is ineffective in the treatment of Raynaud's phenomenon, and the agent of choice is nifedipine.
2. Answer **A**.
   A. Correct. Cilostazol inhibits phosphodiesterase type 3 in vascular smooth muscle cells and in platelets, increasing the levels of cAMP.
   B. Incorrect. Unlike the other phosphodiesterase-3 inhibitors such as milrinone, cilostazol does not increase the incidence of arrhythmias. However, it is not recommended that cilostazol is used in patients with congestive heart failure and cardiac arrhythmia.
   C. Incorrect. Cilostazol is extensively metabolised by CYP3A4 and CYP2C19 isoenzymes in the liver.
   D. Incorrect. Cilostazol inhibits platelet aggregation.
   E. Incorrect. Cilostazol increases plasma HDL cholesterol.
3. Case history answers
   a. A. A β-adrenoceptor antagonist should probably be avoided in this man. Firstly it would not be the drug of choice in the initial treatment of his high blood pressure (Ch. 6). Secondly, by reducing cardiac output and inhibiting vasodilation, it could reduce blood flow further in critical limb ischaemia.
      B. Cardioselective β-adrenoceptor antagonists such as atenolol do not cause deterioration in walking distance when used alone.
      C. Vasodilators will lower blood pressure but do not improve walking distance. In some people, they may redirect blood from the maximally dilated ischaemic tissues to healthy tissues (vascular steal). This can be particularly troublesome in critical limb ischaemia, or when the cardiac output is also reduced by concurrent use of a β-adrenoceptor antagonist.
      D. Lowering LDL cholesterol can stabilise atherosclerotic plaques, perhaps reducing the consequences of coexistent heart disease; it is not known if walking distance or limb survival is improved.
      E. Low-dose aspirin inhibits platelet aggregation and reduces future cardiac events, which are common in this group of patients.
      F. Cilostazol can increase walking distance by up to 35%.
   b. Intensive management of blood pressure, control of diabetes and antiplatelet therapy will reduce the risk of cardiac events. An exercise programme can improve walking distance. Smoking is a major contributory factor to impaired walking distance and cardiac events.
   c. Yes. Excessive warming of limbs may dilate normal arteries, 'stealing' blood from diseased arteries.

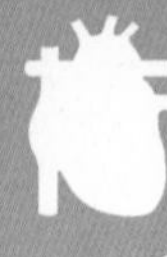

Drugs used to treat peripheral vascular disease (all, except epoprostenol, given orally)

Drug	Half-life (h) and kinetics	Comment
Cilostazol	12 [M] Absorption increased by food; metabolised by CYP3A4 and CYP2C19 to active metabolites	Reversibly reduces platelet aggregation by inhibition of phosphodiesterase (PDE) type 3
Cinnarizine	24 [M] Slow oral absorption; eliminated largely by CYP2D6 (polymorphic) metabolism	Antihistamine; used primarily for vestibular disorders
Epoprostenol	3 min [M] Eliminated very rapidly by hydrolysis	Prostaglandin that opposes the actions of thromboxane A_2; given by intravenous infusion
Inositol nicotinate	Few data available; probably eliminated by hydrolysis	Also used for hyperlipidaemias
Moxisylyte	1 (DAM) [M] Good oral bioavailability; a prodrug which is rapidly deacetylated in plasma to an active metabolite (DAM)	Used for the short-term treatment of primary Raynaud's phenomenon
Naftidrofuryl oxalate	3–4 [M + some R] Good oral bioavailability; metabolised by oxidation and hydrolysis	Activates succinic dehydrogenase and is a 5-hydroxytryptamine type 2 ($5HT_2$) receptor antagonist
Pentoxifylline	1 [M] Metabolised in liver and blood (clearance greatly exceeds liver blood flow)	Increases erythrocyte flexibility and decreases blood viscosity, possibly by increasing erythrocyte cAMP by inhibition of phosphodiesterase

[M], metabolism; [R], renal excretion.

11 Haemostasis

Haemostasis is a complex process involving vasoconstriction, platelet aggregation, blood coagulation and the interactions between them. The descriptions of the processes of platelet aggregation and coagulation pathways in this chapter are restricted to essential knowledge required for understanding the actions of pharmacological agents.

PLATELETS AND PLATELET AGGREGATION

Platelets are critical components of the blood for initiating thrombus formation, and have a lifespan in the circulation of 7–10 days. Platelets aggregate following adhesion to an injured blood vessel and subsequent activation. When the integrity of vascular endothelium is breached, subendothelial proteins such as von Willebrand factor and collagen come into contact with blood. These proteins interact with a family of platelet-surface glycoprotein (GP) receptors (integrin receptors) such as GPIb/IX and GPIa/IIa, resulting in platelets adhering at the site of injury and formation of a platelet plug (Fig. 11.1).

Extension of the platelet plug requires activation of further platelets and their subsequent aggregation together. Platelets are activated by exposure to soluble agonists such as thrombin, ADP, collagen and thromboxane A_2, with an increase in intracellular Ca^{2+} and phosphorylation of myosin light chains in the platelet. These processes produce a rearrangement of the platelet cytoskeleton and a change in cell shape, followed by a critical upregulation and activation of GPIIb/IIIa receptors on the surface of the platelets (Figs 11.1 and 11.2). The increase in platelet intracellular Ca^{2+} also activates phospholipase A_2, which releases arachidonic acid (AA) that is then converted in the platelet to thromboxane A_2. This is the most potent naturally occurring pro-aggregating agent. Platelet aggregation occurs when upregulated GPIIb/IIIa receptors are cross-linked with circulating fibrinogen in the blood.

Platelet activation also enhances exocytosis of platelet storage granules, releasing substances such as platelet factor 4, β-thromboglobulin, ADP and serotonin (5-HT). These initiate or enhance the coagulation cascade by:

- reducing prostacyclin (prostaglandin I_2) synthesis by vascular endothelium; prostacyclin is a vasodilator and a potent inhibitor of platelet aggregation
- inhibiting the action of heparin sulphate produced by vascular endothelium; this enhances activity of the coagulation cascade.

Thrombin produced during the process of coagulation leads to further platelet activation.

Expression of platelet GPIIb/IIIa surface receptors can be inhibited by an increase in the concentration of cyclic adenosine monophosphate (cAMP) in the platelet; this is the mechanism by which prostacyclin (PGI_2) inhibits platelet aggregation (Figs 11.1 and 11.2).

Polyunsaturated (omega-3) fatty acids in fish oils are precursors for thromboxane A_3, which causes less platelet aggregation than thromboxane A_2; they also increase production of a modified form of prostacyclin (PGI_3) by vascular endothelium which has equal anti-aggregatory activity to PGI_2. A high intake of fish oils, therefore, creates a state in which platelets are less able to aggregate.

BLOOD COAGULATION AND THE COAGULATION CASCADE

Both coagulant and anticoagulant factors regulate haemostasis. Activation of the coagulation cascade is divided into extrinsic and intrinsic pathways (Fig. 11.3). The factors involved in these cascades amplify the coagulation response and work together to produce a thrombus. The extrinsic pathway accounts for most of the coagulation in vivo.

The extrinsic system is initiated by the release of tissue factors (TF) from many cell types in damaged tissue and is activated rapidly within minutes of endothelial disruption.

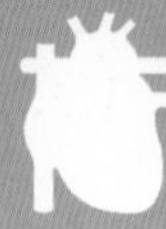

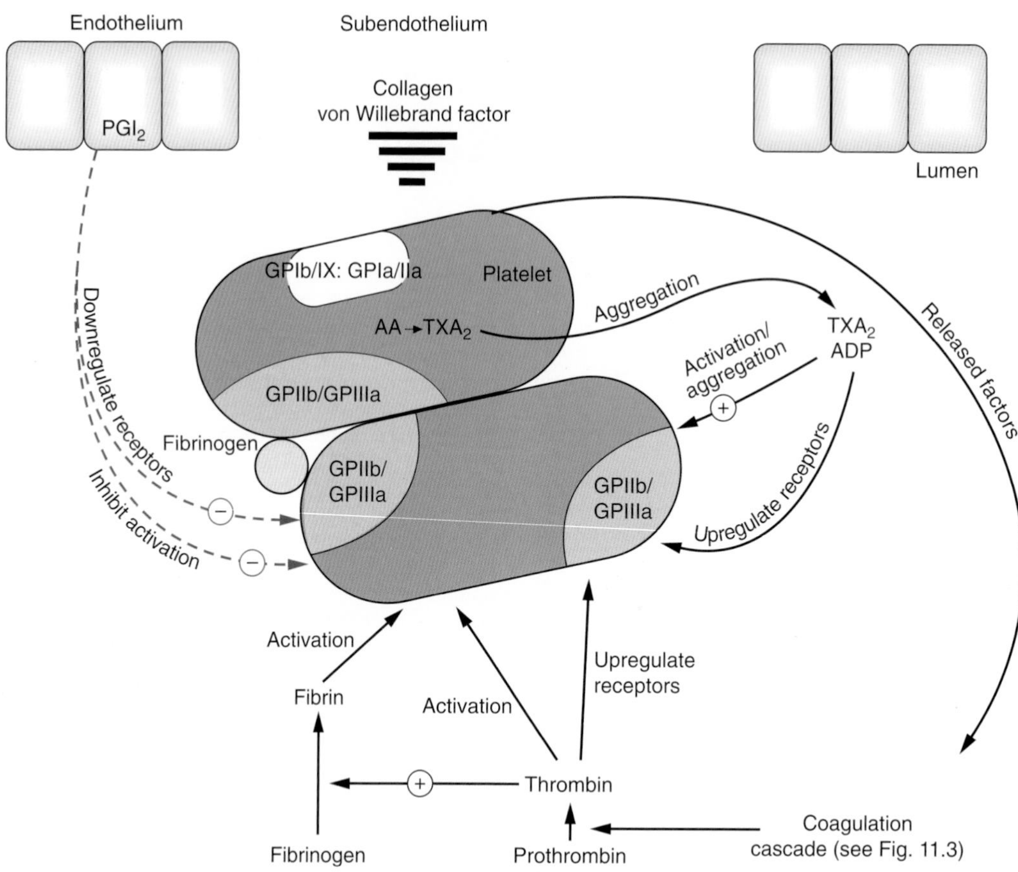

Fig. 11.1 **Platelets and platelet aggregation.** Subendothelial macromolecules such as von Willebrand factor and collagen interact with glycoprotein receptors (GPIb/IX and GPIa/IIa) on platelets, causing activation of platelets and upregulation of GPIIb/IIIa receptors, which are cross-linked by fibrinogen, resulting in aggregation. During the initial processes of aggregation, stimulation of the synthesis and release of a number of platelet-derived substances, such as thromboxane A_2 (TXA_2), ADP and other factors (see text), further promote aggregation by upregulation of GPIIb/IIIa receptors. Conversely, prostacyclin (PGI_2) from endothelial cells inhibits activation and upregulation of GPIIb/IIIa receptors. Thrombin is generated by the action of factor Xa on prothrombin (see Fig. 11.3). AA, arachidonic acid.

Formation of complexes of TF with factor VIIa, and the presence of phospholipids and Ca^{2+} triggers the cascade. The intrinsic system is triggered by contact of blood with a negatively charged surface such as subendothelial collagen, and its activation is delayed by more than 10 min after tissue disruption. Both coagulation pathways respond to breaches in endothelial integrity much more slowly than platelet aggregation.

The intrinsic coagulation cascade comprises a series of enzyme-mediated reactions involving activation of clotting factors (e.g. conversion of inactive factor X to active Xa), which ultimately leads to generation of thrombin. Thrombin is responsible for activation of the final common step in the pathways of coagulation (Fig. 11.3). The actions of active thrombin (factor IIa) and several other activated coagulation factors (Fig 11.3) are inhibited by circulating antithrombin. Antithrombin inhibits coagulation factors after forming complexes with heparin-like molecules that are produced by intact endothelial cells, and with heparin from mast cells. Once sufficient thrombin has been produced to overcome the effect of circulating antithrombin, the soluble protein fibrinogen is converted to an insoluble fibrin gel. The fibrin then forms a meshwork in a mature thrombus that traps and stabilises circulating platelets leucocytes and red blood cells. Each activated clotting factor is inactivated extremely rapidly so that the coagulation process remains localised at the site of the initiating event. In some circumstances, aggregates of platelets combined with fibrin thrombi can embolise and occlude more distal parts of the circulation.

Arterial and venous thrombosis

There are differences in the composition of an arterial or venous thrombus. Arterial thrombosis occurs in the setting of high flow and high shear stress, and platelets play a prominent role in the initiation and growth of the thrombus. In contrast, venous thrombi form in a low flow, low shear stress environment. Venous thrombus usually forms initially in the valve pockets of deep veins, and consists mainly of fibrin and red cells with few platelets.

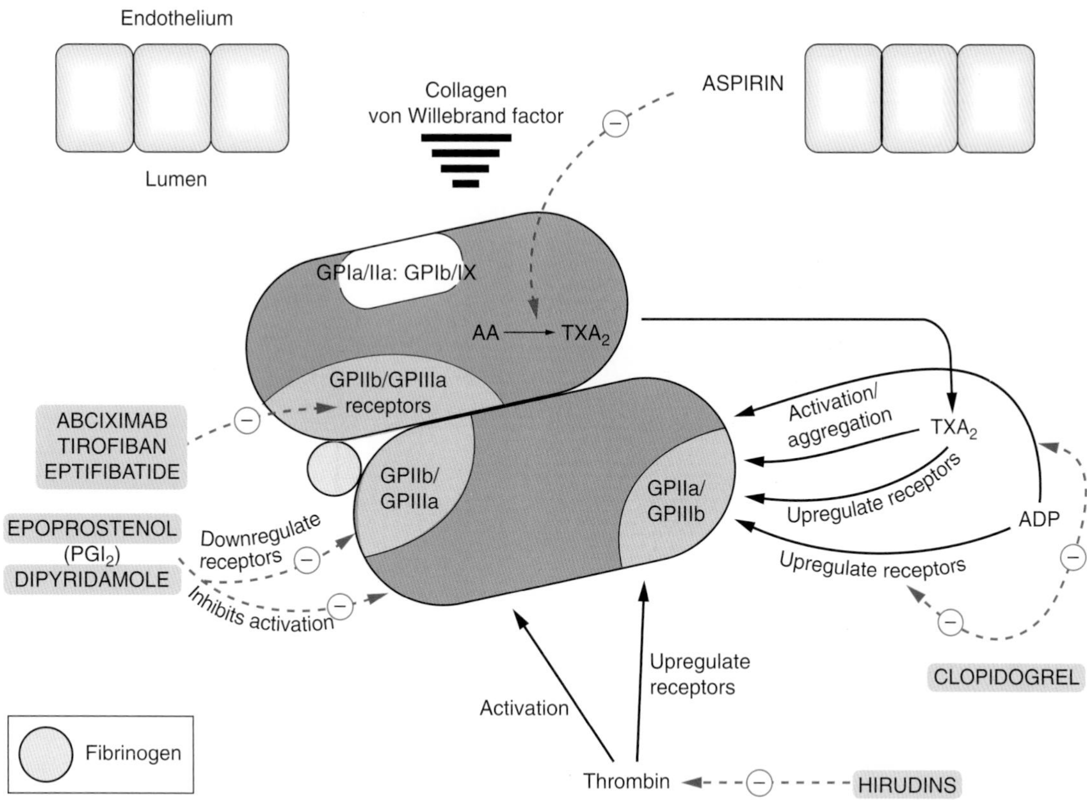

Fig. 11.2 **Sites of action of major drugs used in haemostasis.** Drugs act directly or indirectly to inhibit activation of platelets or to block or reduce upregulation of the glycoprotein GPIIb/IIIa receptors (integrin receptor family), which are necessary for aggregation of platelets. Abciximab is an antibody, tirofiban a non-peptide inhibitor, and eptifibatide a peptide inhibitor of these glycoprotein receptors. Epoprostenol and dipyridamole inhibit activation of platelets and downregulate the glycoprotein receptors via generation of cAMP. Clopidogrel inhibits ADP receptors and prevents ADP-induced upregulation of the glycoprotein GPIIb/IIIa receptors and platelet aggregation. Hirudin prevents the effects of thrombin. Aspirin inhibits the generation of thromboxane A_2 (TXA_2), which causes activation of platelets and upregulation of GPIIb/IIIa receptors. AA, arachidonic acid. For effects of heparin and hirudins on thrombin, see Fig. 11.3.

ANTIPLATELET DRUGS

CYCLO-OXYGENASE INHIBITORS

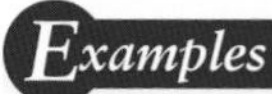

aspirin

Mechanism of action on platelets

The highly potent platelet-aggregating agent thromboxane A_2 is formed in platelets from arachidonic acid by the enzyme cyclo-oxygenase type 1 (COX-1). Aspirin irreversibly inhibits COX-1 and inhibits platelet aggregation (Ch. 29). Because of the irreversible nature of inhibition by aspirin, COX-1 cannot be reactivated and the platelet will have reduced ability to aggregate throughout its lifespan. Aspirin reduces expression of cell surface GPIIb/IIIa receptors and inhibits platelet aggregation, but does not eliminate it completely, because other pathways for platelet activation still function (Figs 11.1 and 11.2). The antiplatelet action of aspirin occurs at very low doses that have little analgesic or anti-inflammatory actions. Details of the pharmacology of aspirin can be found in Chapter 29.

PHOSPHODIESTERASE INHIBITORS

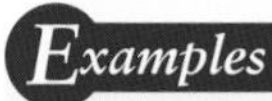

dipyridamole

Mechanism of action

Dipyridamole inhibits the enzyme phosphodiesterase type 5, which degrades cyclic nucleotides. In the platelets, this increases intracellular concentrations of cAMP and reduces activation and expression of cell surface GPIIb/IIIa receptors, leading to inhibition of platelet aggregation (Fig. 11.2).

Pharmacokinetics

Dipyridamole is incompletely absorbed from the gut and is metabolised in the liver. It has a half-life of 12 h. A modified-release formulation is better tolerated than the standard formulation.

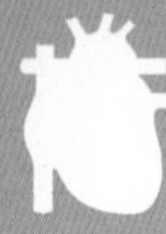

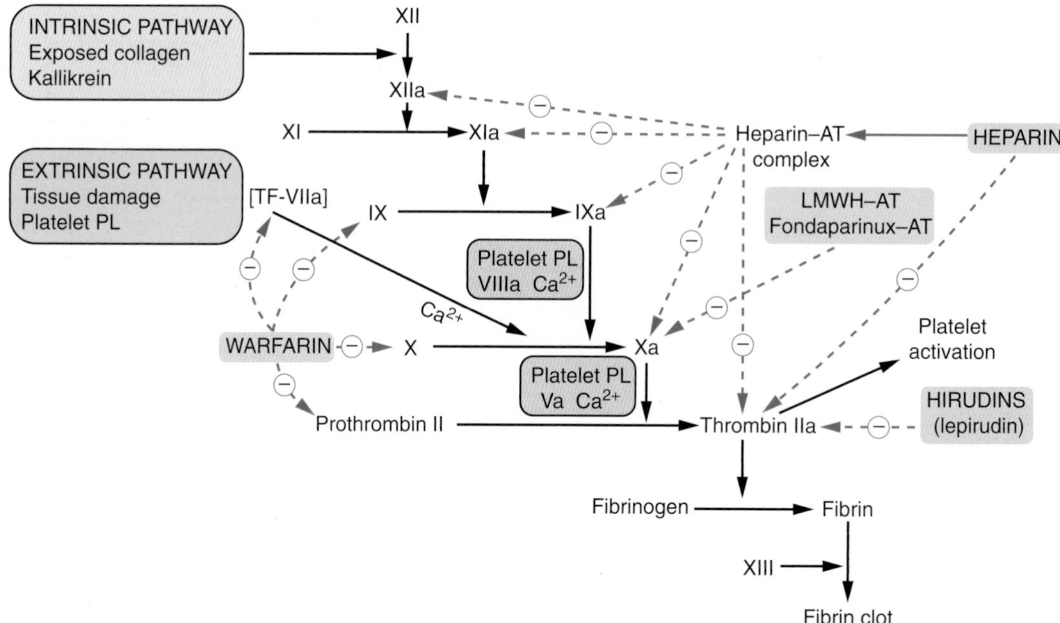

Fig. 11.3 **The coagulation cascade and action of anticoagulants.** The complex cascade of clotting factor synthesis is initiated extrinsically by tissue damage. Activation of the clotting factors after damage depends upon platelet factors, tissue factor, phospholipids, Ca^{2+} and vitamin K. The provision of platelet products is further enhanced by the formation of thrombin, which then activates further platelets as well as causing fibrin formation. Heparin acts at various sites in the cascade by complexing with the anticlotting factor antithrombin III (AT) and inhibiting the activated clotting factors shown. Low-molecular-weight heparin (LMWH) complexes with AT but in a different manner to unfractionated heparin and inhibits only factor Xa. Hirudins inhibit thrombin (IIa) action and formation. Warfarin inhibits the synthesis of the vitamin K-dependent clotting factors VII, IX, X and II (prothrombin). Roman numerals indicate the individual clotting factors; PL, phospholipid; TF tissue factor.

Unwanted effects

- Gastrointestinal effects
- Myalgia
- Dizziness, headache
- Flushing, hypotension, tachycardia
- Hypersensitivity reactions, including rash, urticaria, bronchospasm and angioedema.

ADP RECEPTOR ANTAGONISTS

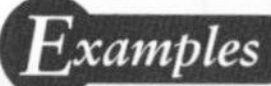

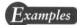

clopidogrel, prasugrel

Mechanism of action

Clopidogrel and prasugrel inhibit platelet aggregation by irreversibly binding to the purinergic P_2 receptors for ADP on the platelet surface (Fig. 11.2). This reduces the mobilisation of Ca^{2+} from intracellular platelet stores, and reduces expression of GPIIb/IIIa receptors. Prasugrel has a similar mechanism of action to clopidogrel. It is an inactive prodrug that is well absorbed from the gut and metabolised rapidly in the liver to an active metabolite which has a half life of 8 days; its effect is more predictable than that of clopidogrel.

Pharmacokinetics

Clopidogrel is a prodrug. It is well absorbed from the gut, and is activated by metabolism in the liver. It undergoes further metabolism to inactive derivatives in the liver, and has a half-life of 7 h.

Unwanted effects

- Bleeding, although the risk is low
- Gastrointestinal upset, especially with dyspepsia, abdominal pain and diarrhoea
- Headache, dizziness, paraesthesia
- Rashes.

Glycoprotein IIb/IIIa receptor antagonists

abciximab, tirofiban

Mechanism of action

Abciximab is a murine monoclonal antibody to the GPIIb/IIIa receptors with the Fc fragment removed to prevent immunogenicity. The Fab fragment is then joined to a human Fc region to form a chimeric molecule. Abciximab binds irreversibly to the GPIIb/IIIa receptors and blocks the binding of fibrinogen (Fig. 11.2). Abciximab can reduce platelet aggregation by more than 90%.

Tirofiban binds reversibly to and blocks the GPIIb/IIIa receptor.

Pharmacokinetics

Abciximab must be given intravenously, usually as an initial bolus followed by continuous infusion. Platelet inhibition occurs rapidly with a bolus injection and largely recovers by 48 h after cessation of the infusion as new platelets are synthesised. The duration of receptor blockade is longer than predicted from its very short half-life of 30 min.

Tirofiban also requires continuous infusion, has a short half-life of about 2 h, and is eliminated by the kidney. Platelet aggregation recovers more rapidly than with abciximab.

Unwanted effects

- Bleeding, especially in the elderly and those of low body weight; the risk is reduced if the dose is adjusted for body weight
- Thrombocytopenia
- Abciximab can cause nausea, vomiting, hypotension, bradycardia, headache, and, occasionally, hypersensitivity reactions.

Epoprostenol

Mechanism of action

Epoprostenol (PGI_2) increases platelet cAMP, which at low concentrations inhibits platelet aggregation and at higher concentrations reduces platelet adhesion. Epoprostenol is also a peripheral arterial vasodilator.

Pharmacokinetics

Epoprostenol is given by intravenous infusion. Unlike most other prostaglandins, it is not significantly metabolised in the lung, as it is rapidly metabolised by hydrolysis in plasma and peripheral tissues, giving a very short half-life of about 3 min.

Unwanted effects

These can be reduced by starting with a low dose and include:

- Facial flushing
- Headache
- Hypotension
- Gastrointestinal disturbances.

CLINICAL USES OF ANTIPLATELET DRUGS

Aspirin and clopidogrel used alone show similar efficacy in most conditions that can be treated with oral antiplatelet drugs, but dipyridamole is less effective for treating coronary heart disease. When a single antiplatelet drug is used, aspirin is usually the drug of choice. Combinations of two antiplatelet drugs may be advantageous in selected circumstances. Main uses of antiplatelet drugs are:

- **Prevention of embolic stroke and transient cerebral ischaemic attacks** (aspirin, clopidogrel or dipyridamole). Dipyridamole combined with aspirin has an additive effect in prevention of stroke (Ch. 9).
- **Secondary prevention after myocardial infarction** (aspirin or clopidogrel). The combination of aspirin and clopidogrel is better than either alone (Ch. 5). The GPIIb/IIIa inhibitor tirofiban further reduces events in non-ST-elevation myocardial infarction when added to aspirin and heparin, but is not widely used (see Ch. 5).
- **Prevention of myocardial infarction in stable angina or peripheral vascular disease** (aspirin or clopidogrel alone; the combination has no advantage) (Chs 5 and 10).
- **Primary prevention of ischaemic heart disease in people with hypertension who have a 10-year predicted risk of cardiovascular disease greater than 20%** (aspirin). Below this level of risk, the potential for serious haemorrhage offsets much of the potential benefit.
- **Anticoagulation in extracorporeal circulations** – for example, cardiopulmonary bypass and renal haemodialysis (epoprostenol).
- **Symptom relief in Raynaud's phenomenon** (epoprostenol) (Ch. 10).
- **Reduction of ischaemic complications produced by sudden vessel closure following percutaneous coronary interventional procedures with stent insertion**; these complications include myocardial infarction, the need for emergency surgical revascularisation and death (aspirin with clopidogrel or prasugrel; abciximab).
- **Dipyridamole is used as a pharmacological stress for the coronary circulation, in order to detect myocardial ischaemia in people who are unable to exercise.** This is related to its ability to block the cellular uptake of adenosine. In the heart, adenosine acts on specific receptors in the small resistance coronary arteries to produce vasodilation. Dipyridamole can divert blood away from myocardium supplied by stenosed coronary arteries by preferentially dilating healthy vascular beds (vascular steal).

ANTICOAGULANT DRUGS

Anticoagulation can be achieved with either injectable or oral drug therapy. A comparison of some of the properties of heparins and warfarin are shown in Table 11.1.

INJECTABLE ANTICOAGULANTS

Heparins

Heparins are a family of highly sulphated acidic mucopolysaccharides (glycosaminoglycans) that are found in mast cells, basophils and endothelium. Heparins have a variable molecular weight between 3000 and 30 000 Da with variable numbers of polysaccharide subunits.

Mechanism of action and effects

Heparin is available as an unfractionated preparation, or as low-molecular-weight heparins (LMWHs), which consist of the heparin subfractions that have molecular weights less than 7000 Da.

Unfractionated heparin forms a complex with and conformationally alters antithrombin III; the complex can then inactivate thrombin and several other clotting factors (Fig. 11.3). LMWH interacts with antithrombin III in a different manner to unfractionated heparin; the LMWH–antithrombin

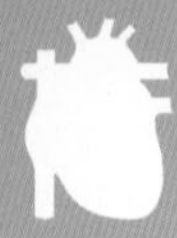

Table 11.1 Comparison of some properties of heparins and warfarin

	Heparins	Warfarin
Route of administration	Intravenous, subcutaneous	Oral
Onset	Immediate	1–3 days
Site of action	Free thrombin and clotting factors in blood	Clotting factors II, VII, IX, X in liver
Duration of action	3–6 h	3–6 days
Antagonist	Protamine but this is less effective against LMWH	Vitamin K_1
Monitoring	APTT	PT, INR
Fate	Partially degraded in liver	Inactivated in liver
Variability in individual response	Little	Great, because of genetic differences particularly in CYP2C9 isoenzyme
Potential for drug interactions	Few	Many
Placental transfer to fetus	Does not cross placenta	Crosses placenta; teratogenic

APTT, activated partial thromboplastin time; INR, international normalised ratio; LMWH, low-molecular-weight heparin; PT, prothrombin time.

complexes have a more selective anticoagulant action (Fig. 11.3).

Actions of the heparins are as follows:

- LMWH–antithrombin complexes mainly inactivate factor Xa; they are four times more active in this respect than unfractionated heparin.
- High-molecular-weight heparin–antithrombin complexes inactivate thrombin and factors IXa, Xa, XIa and XIIa.
- Promotion of tissue factor pathway inhibitor (TFPI) release from the vascular wall contributes to the antithrombotic effects of heparin. TFPI inhibits formation of factor Xa.
- Inhibition of platelet aggregation through binding to platelet factor 4 (mainly unfractionated heparin).
- Activation of lipoprotein lipase, which in addition to promoting lipolysis also reduces platelet adhesiveness.

Danaparoid is a heparinoid, related to heparin and derived from porcine gut mucosa. It contains the anticoagulant glycosaminoglycans heparan sulphate, dermatan sulphate and chondroitin sulphate. Its mechanism of action is similar to that of LMWHs.

Pharmacokinetics

Heparins are inactive orally and are given intravenously or by subcutaneous injection. They have a rapid onset of action. Heparins do not cross the placenta or enter breast milk. The two principal forms of heparin have different pharmacokinetic properties.

Unfractionated heparin

This is extracted from porcine intestinal mucosa or bovine lung, and consists of a mean of 45 polysaccharide units. It has dose-dependent pharmacokinetics: the half-life is very short (about 30 min) at low doses, increasing some fivefold at higher doses. Variable binding to plasma proteins contributes to inter-individual variation in the dose required to achieve target levels of anticoagulation. Most heparin is metabolised in endothelial cells after binding to surface receptors, but some is metabolised in the liver, with a small amount excreted unchanged by the kidney. Unfractionated heparin can be given by repeated intravenous bolus injections or more often by continuous intravenous infusion for full anticoagulation. Low-dose subcutaneous injections are used for prophylaxis against venous thrombosis, although bioavailability by this route is only about 30%.

Low-molecular-weight heparins

LMWHs have a mean of 15 polysaccharide units. They are almost completely absorbed after subcutaneous administration and only need to be given once or twice daily by subcutaneous injection for full anticoagulation. LMWHs have a low affinity for plasma protein binding sites and for endothelial cell heparin receptors. They have two routes of elimination: a rapid, saturable liver uptake and slower renal excretion. The different LMWHs have half-lives in the range 2–6 h. The dose of a LMWH is based on body weight, and they produce a more predictable anticoagulant effect compared with unfractionated heparin.

Danaparoid

Danaparoid has a very long half-life (17–28 h), is given subcutaneously, has high bioavailability, and is eliminated predominantly by renal excretion.

Control of heparin therapy

The therapeutic index for heparin is low. The degree of anticoagulation with unfractionated heparin is usually monitored with the activated partial thromboplastin time (APTT, a global test of the intrinsic coagulation pathway), which should be prolonged by 1.5–2.0 times the control value for full anticoagulation. Monitoring is *not required* when low-dose subcutaneous unfractionated heparin is used (see below). The anticoagulant effect of LMWHs can be monitored by the degree of factor Xa inhibition, but this is not carried out routinely since their effect is much more predictable than that of unfractionated heparin.

Unwanted effects

- *Haemorrhage* is the most common problem. The risk is greater in the elderly, especially if there is a history of heavy alcohol intake. The effect of unfractionated heparin can be rapidly reversed by intravenous injection of protamine sulphate, a basic peptide which binds strongly to the acidic heparin components. Protamine binds poorly to LMWHs and only partially reverses their action.
- *Osteoporosis* is a rare complication which can occur when heparin is given for several weeks; heparin binds to osteoblasts, and inhibits their activity. The risk is less with LMWH.

- *Thrombocytopenia* can occur 5–15 days after starting intravenous heparin in about 2% of people, and arises from the development of antibodies to the heparin–platelet factor 4 complex. This causes platelet activation, aggregation and thrombosis. Danaparoid or lepirudin (see below) are used if continued anticoagulation is necessary. LMWHs have much less effect on platelet aggregation and their lower binding to endothelium also reduces interference with platelet–vessel wall interaction.
- *Hyperkalaemia* by inhibition of aldosterone secretion. This is most likely to occur after 7 days of treatment.
- *Hypersensitivity reactions*.

Fondaparinux

Mechanism of action

Fondaparinux is a synthetic pentasaccharide almost identical to the natural pentasaccharide sequence of heparin that binds to antithrombin. Like LMWH, it enhances the innate ability of antithrombin to inhibit factor Xa.

Pharmacokinetics

Fondaparinux is given by subcutaneous injection. It is predictably absorbed from the injection site, eliminated unchanged by the kidney, and has a long half-life (18 h).

Unwanted effects

- Haemorrhage
- Thrombocytopenia
- Oedema
- Gastrointestinal upset.

Hirudins

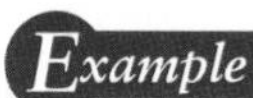

lepirudin

Mechanism of action and use

Hirudin is a naturally occurring substance produced by the salivary gland of the leech. Lepirudin is a recombinant hirudin that binds directly to thrombin and inhibits its action (Fig. 11.3). Lepirudin binds to both the substrate binding site and the catalytic site on the thrombin molecule and therefore inactivates both free and clot-bound thrombin. Its effect is monitored by measurement of the APTT. Lepirudin is used for anticoagulation in place of heparin when there has been heparin-induced thrombocytopenia.

Pharmacokinetics

Lepirudin is given intravenously, and is largely eliminated in urine and possibly also by hydrolysis; it has a short half-life (1.5 h).

Unwanted effects

- Bleeding
- Fever
- Hypersensitivity reactions.

ORAL ANTICOAGULANTS

Vitamin K antagonists

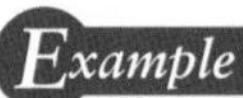

warfarin

Mechanism of action

These drugs are antagonists of vitamin K by inhibiting hepatic vitamin K epoxide reductase, which is the enzyme that converts vitamin K to its active (hydroquinone) form. As a result, the hepatic synthesis of vitamin K-dependent clotting factors (II [prothrombin], VII, IX and X) is impaired (Fig. 11.3). There is a delay in the onset of the anticoagulant effect, owing to the presence of previously synthesised and circulating clotting factors.

Pharmacokinetics

Warfarin is the most widely used oral anticoagulant. It is almost completely absorbed from the gut and is highly bound to plasma albumin. It is eliminated by cytochrome P450-mediated hepatic metabolism (CYP2C9) and has a very long half-life of 1–2 days. Functional consequences of CYP2C9 polymorphisms contribute to considerable inter-individual variability in warfarin sensitivity. The plasma concentration of warfarin does not correlate directly with the clinical effect of the drug, which is determined by the balance between the rates of synthesis and degradation of clotting factors. The maximum effect of an individual dose of warfarin is reflected in the blood coagulation time some 24–36 h later. On stopping treatment, the duration of anticoagulant action is determined largely by the time required to synthesise new clotting factors.

Control of oral anticoagulant therapy

Factor VII is the clotting factor that is most sensitive to vitamin K deficiency, since it has the shortest half-life of the vitamin K-sensitive clotting factors. Therefore, a test of the extrinsic coagulation pathway – the prothrombin time – is used as a measure of effectiveness. The degree of prolongation of the prothrombin time is standardised by comparison with control plasma from a single source, and referred to as the INR (international normalised ratio). Therapeutic INR ranges differ according to the condition being treated:

- 2–2.5 for prophylaxis of deep vein thrombosis
- 2–3 for thromboprophylaxis in hip surgery and fractured femur operations, for treatment of deep vein thrombosis and pulmonary embolism, and for prevention of thromboembolism in atrial fibrillation
- 3–4.5 for prevention of recurrent deep vein thrombosis and for preventing thrombosis on mechanical prosthetic heart valves.

Unwanted effects

Warfarin is an important example of a drug that has a narrow therapeutic index.

- Haemorrhage. The most effective antidote to warfarin is phytomenadione (vitamin K_1). For major bleeding, this is

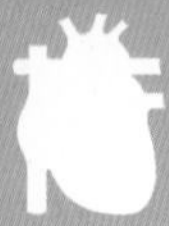

given intravenously and controls bleeding within 6 h. An immediate coagulant effect is achieved by also giving an intravenous injection of prothrombin complex concentrate (vitamin K-dependent clotting factors) or an infusion of fresh frozen plasma. After giving a large dose of phytomenadione, it can be difficult to restore therapeutic anticoagulation with warfarin for up to 3 weeks. If the INR is >8.0 but there is no bleeding or only minor bleeding, then a smaller dose of phytomenadione is given intravenously or orally.

- Alopecia, skin necrosis and hypersensitivity reactions occur rarely.
- Warfarin crosses the placenta and can have undesirable effects on the fetus. It is teratogenic and should be avoided in the first trimester of pregnancy, except when essential; furthermore, it should not be used in the last trimester, as it increases the risk of intracranial haemorrhage in the baby during delivery.
- Drug interactions. These are particularly important. The anticoagulant effect of warfarin can be increased by broad-spectrum antibacterial agents that suppress the production of vitamin K by gut bacteria. Drugs such as amiodarone (Ch. 8) and the histamine H_2 receptor antagonist cimetidine (Ch. 33) which inhibit CYP2C9-mediated metabolism of warfarin enhance its effects. Drugs that induce CYP2C9 – for example, phenytoin, phenobarbital (Ch. 23) and alcohol (Ch. 54) – reduce the effect of warfarin by increasing its elimination.

DIRECT FACTOR XA INHIBITOR

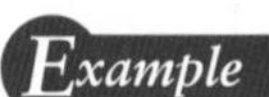

rivaroxaban

Mechanism of action

Rivaroxaban is an orally active factor Xa inhibitor with a predictable anticoagulant action, unlike warfarin. It is currently licensed for prophylaxis of venous thromboembolism after orthopaedic surgery.

Pharmacokinetics

Rivaroxaban is well absorbed from the gut. It is partially metabolised in the liver and partially excreted by the kidneys. Its half life is 9–12 h.

Unwanted effects

- nausea, and less often other gastrointestinal upset
- haemorrhage

Direct thrombin inhibitors

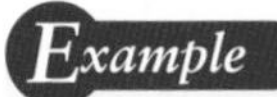

dabigatran etexilate

Mechanism of action

Dabigatran is a selective, competitive thrombin inhibitor that binds to and inhibits both free circulating and thrombus-bound thrombin (factor IIa). This is distinct from heparin, which only affects free thrombin, mainly via activation of antithrombin. Unlike heparin, it does not bind to plasma proteins, so the dosing is more predictable. There is no known antagonist.

Pharmacokinetics

Dabigatran etexilate is a prodrug that has a low oral bioavailability and undergoes first-pass metabolism to its active derivative dabigatran. The active metabolite is excreted unchanged by the kidneys, and has a short half-life of about 40 min.

Unwanted effects

- Bleeding, with a similar risk to warfarin.

CLINICAL USES OF ANTICOAGULANTS

Venous thromboembolism

Pulmonary embolism remains a major cause of morbidity and death and has been estimated to be responsible for 10% of all deaths in hospital. Most serious pulmonary emboli arise from deep vein thrombosis of the lower limb, particularly if this extends to the larger veins above the calf. Following a deep vein thrombosis, chronic post-phlebitic syndrome can develop, with pain, swelling and ulceration of the affected leg.

Factors predisposing to venous thromboembolism (Table 11.2) include prolonged immobility, a variety of coexisting medical conditions such as cancer, and various inherited or acquired disorders of the coagulation system. Use

Table 11.2 Risk of thromboembolism in people admitted to hospital

Risk	Procedure
Low	Minor surgery, no other risk factor Major surgery, age <40 years, no other risk factors Minor trauma or illness
Moderate	Major surgery; age ≥40 years or other risk factor Heart failure, recent myocardial infarction, malignancy, inflammatory bowel disease Major trauma or burns Minor surgery, trauma or illness in patient with previous deep vein thrombosis or pulmonary embolism
High	Fracture or major orthopaedic surgery of pelvis, hips or lower limb Major pelvic or abdominal surgery for cancer Major surgery, trauma or illness in patient with previous deep vein thrombosis or pulmonary embolism Lower limb paralysis Major lower limb amputation

of the oral contraceptive pill by older women who smoke (see Ch. 45) is also a factor. Many episodes of deep vein thrombosis occur in hospital, particularly in people over 40 years of age following major illness, trauma or surgery. After an initial spontaneous deep vein thrombosis, the risk of recurrence is about 25% after 4 years, but is much lower after postoperative thrombosis.

Prevention of deep vein thrombosis

In hospitalised people, the most appropriate method to prevent deep vein thrombosis will depend on the degree of risk.

Mechanical methods

These are used for those at moderate risk and include graduated elastic compression stockings and intermittent pneumatic compression devices to improve venous flow and limit stasis in venous valve pockets. They can also be used to supplement pharmacological prophylaxis in high-risk people.

Low-dose subcutaneous heparin

This is the treatment of choice in those at high risk and in many people at moderate risk. Heparin reduces both initiation and extension of fibrin-rich thrombi at doses which have little effect on other measurements of blood coagulation and, therefore, laboratory monitoring is unnecessary. Low-dose unfractionated heparin reduces deep venous thrombosis and fatal pulmonary emboli by about two-thirds, with minimal risk of serious bleeding, although minor bleeding is increased. LMWHs or fondaparinux are more effective than unfractionated heparin for those at highest risk, particularly during orthopaedic surgery and both dabigatran and rivaroxaban are as effective as LMWHs. Prophylaxis should be started before surgery.

Low-dose aspirin or warfarin

Warfarin may be more effective than heparin for prophylaxis in people at highest risk. Although a meta-analysis of several studies suggests that low-dose aspirin reduces deep venous thrombosis, it is less effective than heparin.

Treatment of established venous thromboembolism

The goals of treatment for deep vein thrombosis are to prevent pulmonary emboli and to restore patency of the occluded vessel, with preservation of the function of venous valves. In about 50% of people with deep venous thrombosis, the vessel will recanalise within 3 months if appropriately treated.

Full anticoagulation

This is the treatment of choice for deep vein thrombosis and for most pulmonary emboli; it substantially reduces mortality. Heparin is given initially for its rapid onset of effect. Unfractionated heparin given by intravenous infusion is now being replaced by LMWH given subcutaneously as a convenient and effective alternative. Heparin is usually given for 3–5 days, with concurrent initiation of treatment with warfarin. Heparin can be stopped once warfarin has produced adequate anticoagulation (i.e. the INR is within the therapeutic range; see above). When deep vein thrombosis occurs in someone with cancer, there is a high risk of both bleeding and recurrence during treatment with warfarin. In this situation, prolonged treatment with LMWH (6 months, or lifelong if remission is not achieved) is usually advocated. The optimal duration of anticoagulant therapy is not well defined, but suggested periods are shown in Table 11.3.

Table 11.3 Suggested duration of anticoagulant therapy for venous thromboembolism

Risk of recurrence	Clinical setting	Duration
Low	Temporary risk factors for thromboembolism	3 months
Intermediate	Continuing medical risk factors for thromboembolism	3–6 months
High	Recurrent thromboembolism; inherited thrombophilic tendency	Indefinite

Surgical venous thrombectomy

This may be required for massive iliofemoral thrombosis if it threatens the viability of the limb. Pulmonary embolectomy is occasionally carried out for large pulmonary emboli.

Fibrinolytic treatment with streptokinase

This treatment (see below) has no advantage over warfarin in uncomplicated deep venous thrombosis, but is sometimes used to disintegrate massive pulmonary emboli.

Other treatments

For pulmonary emboli that continue to occur despite adequate anticoagulation, or when anticoagulation is contraindicated, inferior vena caval plication or insertion of a 'filter' device to trap emboli in the inferior vena cava can be considered.

Arterial thromboembolism

Warfarin is used long term for the prevention of thrombosis on prosthetic heart valves. Atrial fibrillation (Ch. 8) and mural thrombus in the left ventricle following a myocardial infarction predispose to arterial embolism and are indications for anticoagulation with warfarin. Dabigatran is effective for prevention of thromboembolism in atrial fibrillation and may provide an alternative to warfarin.

THE FIBRINOLYTIC SYSTEM

Fibrinolysis is the physiological mechanism for dissolving the fibrin meshwork in a thrombus. The process is initiated by activation of plasminogen, a circulating α_2-globulin (Fig. 11.4). Tissue plasminogen activator (t-PA) is released from damaged vessels and cleaves plasminogen to the active enzyme plasmin. In the circulation, plasminogen activator inhibitors 1 and 2 rapidly inactivate t-PA. However, t-PA

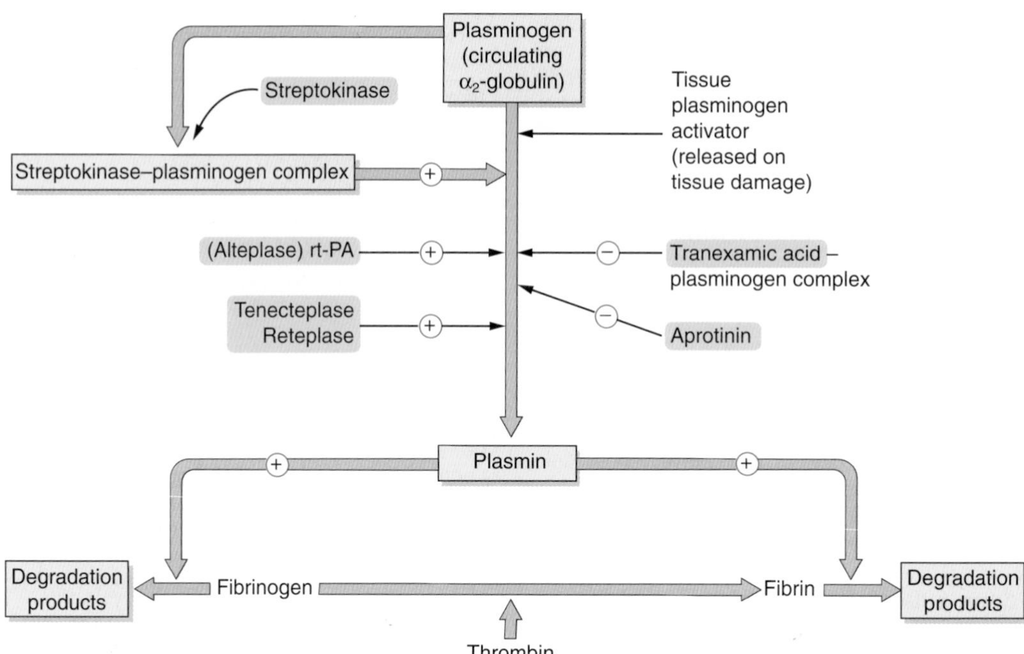

Fig. 11.4 **The fibrinolytic system.** The fibrinolytic system is linked intimately with the coagulation cascade and platelet function. When a clot is formed via the prothrombotic system, activation of plasminogen to the fibrinolytically active plasmin is initiated by several tissue plasminogen activators, thus lysing the clot. The drugs promoting this act as plasminogen activators (alteplase and derivatives) or bind to plasminogen (streptokinase), promoting plasmin activity. The antifibrinolytic drugs tranexamic acid and aprotinin (recently withdrawn) inhibit plasminogen activation. Aprotinin also has other actions to inhibit the fibrinolytic cascade.

binds locally at the site of release to fibrin, and converts fibrin-bound plasminogen to plasmin. Plasmin splits both fibrinogen and fibrin into degradation products; if this occurs at the site of a thrombus, it produces lysis of the clot matrix. Fibrinolytic therapy (also called thrombolytic therapy) is achieved by using a plasminogen activator in such large quantities that the inhibitory controls are overwhelmed.

FIBRINOLYTIC (THROMBOLYTIC) AGENTS

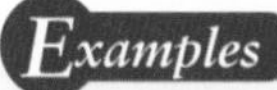

alteplase (recombinant tissue-type plasminogen activator, rt-PA), reteplase, streptokinase, tenecteplase

Mechanism of action

All fibrinolytic drugs enhance fibrinolysis by activating plasminogen, which enables them to enhance the degradation of thrombi and act as fibrinolytic agents. Alteplase is a genetically engineered copy of the naturally occurring t-PA which binds to fibrinogen and fibrin. Reteplase is a recombinant deletion-modified form of t-PA that binds less strongly to both fibrinogen and fibrin, has similar sensitivity to plasminogen activator inhibitors but has a longer duration of action. Tenecteplase is a genetically engineered multiply-modified form of t-PA with increased fibrin specificity, less sensitivity to plasminogen activator inhibitors, and a longer duration of action than t-PA.

Streptokinase is obtained from haemolytic streptococci. Unlike alteplase and related compounds, streptokinase is inactive until it forms a complex with circulating plasminogen; the resultant streptokinase–plasminogen activator complex substitutes for t-PA in the fibrinolytic cascade, causing plasminogen activation.

The effectiveness of any fibrinolytic agent depends on the age of the thrombus (most effective with new thrombus) and the surface area of thrombus exposed to it.

Pharmacokinetics

All fibrinolytic agents are given intravenously or intra-arterially. Alteplase and related compounds are metabolised in the liver. The streptokinase–plasminogen activator complex is degraded enzymatically in the circulation. Some streptokinase is cleared from the plasma before it forms an active complex, by combining with circulating neutralising antibody formed during previous exposure to streptokinase. After the use of streptokinase, or following a streptococcal infection, neutralising antibodies can persist in high titre for several years and substantially reduce the effectiveness of subsequent therapy with streptokinase.

Streptokinase has a slower onset of action than alteplase or its derivatives owing to slow combination with plasminogen. Consequently, the reperfusion of occluded vessels is slower. The half-life of streptokinase (1 h) is longer than that of alteplase or reteplase (0.5 h) but similar to that of tenecteplase. Streptokinase is usually given as a short (1 h) infusion for the treatment of coronary artery occlusion, although longer infusions are usual for peripheral arterial occlusions or pulmonary embolism. Infusions of alteplase are given over longer periods, usually for between 3 and 24 h, depending on the condition being treated. Reteplase is given as two bolus injections separated by 90 min, and tenecteplase as a single bolus. Because of its short duration of action, when alteplase has been used to lyse coronary artery thrombus, subsequent anticoagulation with heparin for 48 h is necessary to reduce the risk of reocclusion. Heparin is also given after reteplase and tenecteplase.

Unwanted effects

- *Haemorrhage* is usually minor but can occasionally be serious – for example, intracerebral haemorrhage, which occurs in about 1% of those treated (and is slightly more frequent with alteplase and related drugs than with streptokinase). Bleeding can be stopped by antifibrinolytic drugs (see below) or by transfusion of fresh frozen plasma.
- *Hypotension*: this is dose-related and more common with streptokinase. It may be caused by enzymatic release of the vasodilator bradykinin from its circulating precursor. If the infusion of the thrombolytic is stopped for a brief period, the blood pressure usually recovers rapidly and treatment can be continued.
- *Allergic reactions*: these are rare but can occur with streptokinase, as a consequence of its bacterial origin.

CLINICAL USES OF FIBRINOLYTIC AGENTS

Fibrinolytic agents are used to treat the following:

- acute myocardial infarction (Ch. 5)
- ischaemic stroke (Ch. 9)
- pulmonary embolism or deep venous thrombosis, in a minority of cases (see above)
- peripheral arterial thromboembolism (Ch. 10)
- intravenous catheters occluded by clot: this is particularly useful to restore patency of 'long lines' inserted for intravenous nutrition or administration of cytotoxic drugs.

ANTIFIBRINOLYTIC AND HAEMOSTATIC AGENTS

Antifibrinolytic agents

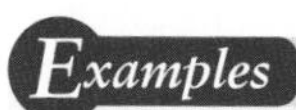

tranexamic acid

Mechanisms of action

Tranexamic acid competitively inhibits the activation of plasminogen, so fibrinolysis is inhibited.

Pharmacokinetics

Tranexamic acid is a synthetic amino acid that is incompletely absorbed from the gut and can also be given intravenously. It is excreted unchanged by the kidney and has a short half-life (1–2 h).

Unwanted effects

- Nausea, vomiting, diarrhoea, and disturbances of colour vision.
- The theoretical risk of a creating a thrombotic tendency does not appear to be a clinical problem.

Desmopressin

Desmopressin (Ch. 43) briefly increases the plasma concentration of clotting factor VIII and von Willebrand factor, an adhesion protein in blood vessel walls. Factor VIII accelerates the process of fibrin formation and von Willebrand factor enhances platelet adhesion to subendothelial tissue.

CLINICAL USES OF ANTIFIBRINOLYTIC AND HAEMOSTATIC AGENTS

Haemostatic agents have a number of clinical uses.

- Tranexamic acid is used to prevent bleeding after surgery, especially of the prostate, or after dental extraction in individuals with haemophilia.
- Desmopressin is used in mild congenital bleeding disorders such as haemophilia A or von Willebrand's disease; it is given to reduce spontaneous or traumatic bleeding, or as a prophylactic before surgery.
- Tranexamic acid is used for the treatment of menorrhagia, epistaxis or bleeding following overdose of a fibrinolytic drug.
- Tranexamic acid is mainly used prophylactically for reduction of bleeding during cardiovascular surgery with extracorporeal circulation.
- Tranexamic acid is used for treatment of hereditary angioedema.

FURTHER READING

Antiplatelet agents

Antiplatelet Trialist's Collaboration (2002) Collaborative meta-analysis of randomised trials of antiplatelet therapy for prevention of death, myocardial infarction and stroke in high risk patients. *BMJ* 324, 71–86

Behan MW, Storey RF (2004) Antiplatelet therapy in cardiovascular disease. *Postgrad Med J* 80, 155–164

Bhatt DL, Fox KAA, Hacke W et al (2006) Clopidogrel and aspirin versus aspirin alone for the prevention of atherothrombotic events. *N Engl J Med* 354, 1706–1717

Cryer B (2005) Reducing the risks of gastrointestinal bleeding with antiplatelet therapies. *N Engl J Med* 352, 287–289

Gladding P, Webster M, Ormiston J et al (2008) Antiplatelet drug unresponsiveness. *Am Heart J* 155, 591–599

Kong DF, Hasselblad V, Harrington RA et al (2003) Meta-analysis of survival with platelet glycoprotein IIb/IIIa antagonists for

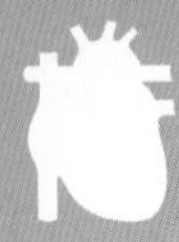

percutaneous coronary interventions. *Am J Cardiol* 92, 651–655

McQuaid KR, Laine L (2006) Systematic review and meta-analysis of adverse events of low-dose aspirin and clopidogrel in randomised controlled trials. *Am J Med* 119, 624–638

Micelli G, Cavallini A (2004) New therapeutic strategies with antiplatelet agents. *Neurol Sci* 25(suppl 1), S13–S15

Vorchheimer DA, Badimon JJ, Fuster VV (1999) Platelet glycoprotein IIb/IIIa receptor antagonists in cardiovascular disease. *JAMA* 281, 1407–1414

Anticoagulants

Agnelli G, Becattini C, Kirschstein T (2002) Thrombolysis versus heparin in the treatment of pulmonary embolism. A clinical outcome-based meta-analysis. *Arch Intern Med* 162, 2537–2541

Blann AD, Lip YH (2006) Venous thromboembolism. *BMJ* 332, 215–219

Cayley WE (2007) Preventing deep vein thrombosis in hospital inpatients. *BMJ* 335, 147–151

DeZee KJ, Shimeall WT, Douglas et al (2006) Treatment of excessive anticoagulation with phytonadione (vitamin K). A meta-analysis. *Arch Intern Med* 166, 391–397

Ginsberg JS, Greer I, Hirsch J (2001) Use of antithrombotic agents during pregnancy. *Chest* 119, s122–s131

Goldhaber SZ (2004) Pulmonary embolism. *Lancet* 363, 1295–1305

Haemostasis and Thrombosis Task Force of the British Society for Haematology (1998) Guidelines on anticoagulation: third edition. *Br J Haematol* 101, 374–387

Hamm CW (2003) Anti-integrin therapy *Annu Rev Med* 54, 425–435

Hodl R, Klein W (2003) The role of low-molecular-weight heparins in cardiovascular medicine. *J Clin Pharm Ther* 28, 371–378

Konstantinides S (2008) Acute pulmonary embolism. *N Engl J Med* 359, 2804–2813

Kyrle PA, Eichinger S (2005) Deep vein thrombosis. *Lancet* 365, 1163–1174

Schulman S (2003) Unresolved issues in anticoagulant therapy. *J Thromb Haemost* 1, 1464–1470

Tapson VF (2008) Acute pulmonary embolism. *N Engl J Med* 358, 1037–1052

Fibrinolytic drugs

Khan IJ, Gowda RM (2003) Clinical perspectives and therapeutics of thrombolysis. *Int J Cardiol* 91, 115–127

Nordt TK, Bode C (2003) Thrombolysis: newer thrombolytic agents and their role in clinical medicine. *Heart* 89, 1358–1362

Haemostatic drugs

Mannucci PM, Levi M (2007) Prevention and treatment of major blood loss. *N Engl J Med* 356, 2301–2311

Wellington K, Wagstaff AJ (2003) Tranexamic acid. A review of its use in the management of menorrhagia. *Drugs* 63, 1417–1433

SELF-ASSESSMENT

1. In the following questions, the first statement, in italics, is true. Is the accompanying statement also true?
   a. *Tenecteplase is a modified form of tissue-type plasminogen activator (t-PA) with a longer half-life than t-PA.* Fibrinolytic infusions of recombinant tissue-type plasminogen activator (rt-PA; alteplase) for myocardial infarction are usually given for a duration of 1 h whereas streptokinase is given for 3–24 h.
   b. *Warfarin has a long half-life (36 h) in plasma.* Warfarin readily crosses the placenta.
   c. *Clopidogrel, dipyridamole and aspirin inhibit platelet aggregation.* Clopidogrel has its antithrombotic action by enhancing the action of ADP on platelets.
   d. *Abciximab in conjunction with heparin and aspirin is used before coronary angioplasty with stenting for high-risk procedures.* Abciximab is an antibody directed against the glycoprotein GPIIb/IIIa receptor on platelets.
   e. *Aspirin irreversibly inhibits cyclo-oxygenase enzymes.* Aspirin inhibits platelet aggregation at doses below those needed for an anti-inflammatory effect.
   f. *Warfarin inhibits the activation of clotting factors II, VII, IX and X, which depend upon vitamin K for their synthesis.* Anticoagulant activity of warfarin is inhibited by broad-spectrum antibacterial agents.
   g. *Tranexamic acid is an antifibrinolytic agent used in the treatment of menorrhagia.* Tranexamic acid enhances plasminogen activation.
   h. *LMWHs have longer half-lives than unfractionated heparin.* Once administered, the action of heparin cannot be reversed.
2. Comparing heparin, warfarin and lepirudin, choose the one **correct** statement.
   A. In people treated with heparin or lepirudin, their INR would need to be regularly monitored.
   B. If a predictable oral anticoagulant is required for rapid anticoagulant activity before surgery, heparin is the drug of choice.
   C. Dosage adjustment of warfarin but not heparin would be required if a person was prescribed concomitant treatment with the H_2 receptor antagonist cimetidine.
   D. In overdose, the effects of heparin but not of warfarin can be reversed with appropriate antagonists.
   E. During treatment with a broad-spectrum antibacterial, the anticoagulant effects of warfarin and lepirudin can be inhibited.
3. Case history questions

A 51-year-old obese female was treated with oestrogen replacement therapy for 18 months because of peri-menopausal symptoms. She was scheduled for a hip replacement.

   a. Was anticoagulant therapy necessary for this woman?
   b. Should thromboprophylaxis have been started before surgery?
   c. Should heparin or warfarin have been chosen for prophylaxis and what routes of administration were appropriate?

The hip replacement was carried out successfully and the woman was discharged from hospital after 5 days, although heparin therapy was continued for a further 5 days.

d. Why was therapy continued for this extended period and what out-of-hospital therapeutic prophylaxis could be considered?

ANSWERS

1. a. **False**. Streptokinase is usually infused for 1 h and alteplase for 3 h. Streptokinase has a longer half-life (1 h, alteplase 0.5 h), permitting a shorter infusion time.
   b. **True**. Warfarin can cause fetal abnormalities and, unless essential, should not be given in early or late pregnancy.
   c. **False**. Clopidogrel prevents the platelet aggregatory action of ADP. Clopidogrel also inhibits thrombin-induced platelet aggregation.
   d. **True**. The increased expression of GPIIb/IIIa receptors on platelets is essential for aggregation as fibrinogen links adjacent platelets by binding to GPIIb/IIIa receptors, thereby initiating aggregation.
   e. **True**. Thromboxane A_2 (TXA_2) required for platelet aggregation is synthesised by the cyclo-oxygenase type 1 (COX-1) enzyme, whereas prostaglandins synthesised during inflammation are synthesised predominantly, but not exclusively, by cyclo-oxygenase type 2 (COX-2) enzymes. Aspirin is 160 times more active at inhibiting COX-1 than COX-2. Therefore, at the low doses required to inhibit TXA_2 synthesis, it has no anti-inflammatory effect.
   f. **False**. Vitamin K is produced by gut bacteria. Alteration of gut flora by broad-spectrum antibacterials will reduce vitamin K formation and hence reduce vitamin K-dependent clotting factors. This will enhance the activity of warfarin.
   g. **False**. Tranexamic acid inhibits plasminogen activation, reducing fibrin degradation and the risk of bleeding.
   h. **False**. The action of unfractionated heparin but not LMWH can be reversed by the strongly basic protein protamine, which rapidly binds to it, forming an inactive complex.
2. Answer **C**.
   A. Incorrect. Regular INR monitoring is required in people taking warfarin but not heparin or lepirudin, when the activated partial thromboplastin time (APTT) is used.
   B. Incorrect. Heparin is inactive orally and must be given by intravenous or subcutaneous routes.
   C. Correct. Warfarin is metabolised by the liver cytochrome P450 metabolising isoenzyme CYP2C9. Cimetidine inhibits this isoenzyme.
   D. Incorrect. The effects of heparin can be reversed with the drug protamine and those of warfarin can be reversed with vitamin K_1.
   E. Incorrect. Broad-spectrum antibacterials may suppress the production of vitamin K by gut bacteria and increase the activity of warfarin. It would not affect the actions of lepirudin.
3. Case history answers
   a. Anticoagulant therapy is necessary. Postoperative venous thromboembolism occurs in 40–50% of people who undergo hip replacement, and fatal pulmonary embolism in 1–5%, if prophylactic anticoagulant therapy is not given. This woman is also at increased risk because of obesity.
   b. This is controversial. Initiating prophylaxis postoperatively allows more effective haemostatic control during and immediately after surgery and does not reduce the effectiveness of treatment.
   c. Heparin is active given intravenously or subcutaneously and the onset of action of heparin is rapid, whereas warfarin takes several days for full effectiveness but can be given orally. Heparin would therefore be chosen if started pre- or postoperatively.
   d. The woman was obese, a risk factor for postoperative venous thrombosis. Daily self-administered subcutaneous prophylaxis with LMWH could be used. LMWH has a better bioavailability, a longer half-life and a lower risk of producing thrombocytopenia. Unlike unfractionated heparin, its effect is predictable.

Drugs used to affect haemostasis

Drug	Half-life (h) and kinetics	Comments
Antiplatelet drugs		
Abciximab	0.5 [M] Mechanism of elimination not defined (probably tissue uptake and proteolysis)	Used as an adjunct to heparin and aspirin in high-risk individuals (specialist use only); antibody fragment to glycoprotein IIb/IIIa receptor on platelets; produces long-lasting blockade of receptors; given intravenously
Aspirin	0.25–0.35 [M] The half-life of active salicylic acid metabolite is 3–20 h	Low dose used for the secondary prevention of thrombotic cerebrovascular or cardiovascular disease; given orally
Clopidogrel	5–8 (inactive metabolite) [M] Prodrug requiring hepatic bioactivation in two steps, one by CYP3A4; acts via an active thiol metabolite that is unstable and has not been identified; the half-life is for an inactive metabolite (and may not relate to the duration of clinical effect)	Used for the prevention of ischaemic events in people with a history of symptomatic ischaemic disease; given orally

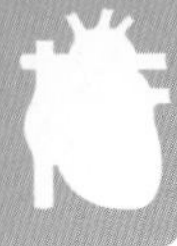

Drugs used to affect haemostasis

Drug	Half-life (h) and kinetics	Comments
Dipyridamole	12 [M] Metabolised largely to glucuronic acid conjugates which are excreted in bile with some enterohepatic circulation	Used as an adjunct to oral anticoagulants in people with prosthetic heart valves and for the secondary prevention of ischaemic stroke; given orally or by intravenous injection (for diagnostic purposes)
Epoprostenol	3 min [M] Eliminated very rapidly by hydrolysis	Used intravenously in combination with heparin during renal dialysis and in combination with oral anticoagulants for primary pulmonary hypertension resistant to other treatments; potent vasodilator
Prasugrel	8 days (active metabolite) [M] A prodrug activated rapidly by esterases and then several CYPs	Used for the prevention of ischaemic events in people with a history of symptomatic ischaemic disease; compared with clopidogrel it has more rapid onset and inhibits platelet aggregation more completely. Greater incidence of bleeding; given orally
Eptifibatide	1.5–2 [R + M] Eliminated unchanged in urine and as a deaminated product	A cyclic hexapeptide given as an adjunct to heparin and aspirin in high-risk people with unstable angina (specialist use only); glycoprotein IIb/IIIa receptor inhibitor; given intravenously
Tirofiban	2 [R + B] Limited metabolism; eliminated in urine and bile	A non-peptide glycoprotein IIb/IIIa receptor inhibitor; used as an adjunct to heparin and aspirin in high-risk people with unstable angina (specialist use only); given intravenously
Anticoagulants (heparin-like)		
All drugs are macromolecules and given by injection; they are eliminated by tissue uptake and degradation; LMWHs are as effective as unfractionated heparin; the longer half-life allows treatment by once-daily subcutaneous injection		
Bemiparin	4–5[a]	LMWH
Dalteparin sodium	2–4[a] [R] Unlike heparin, elimination is not dose-dependent	LMWH
Danaparoid sodium	17–28[a] [R] Unlike heparin, elimination is not dose-dependent	A heparinoid substance; useful in prophylaxis of deep vein thrombosis on a named patient basis only
Enoxaparin	3–6[a] [M + R] Eliminated by hepatic degradation and limited renal excretion	LMWH
Fondaparinux	18 [R] Excreted in the urine unchanged	A synthetic pentasaccharide which, like heparin, enhances the ability of antithrombin to inhibit factor Xa; used for prophylaxis in people undergoing major orthopaedic surgery of the legs
Heparin (also known as unfractionated heparin)	0.4–2.5[a] Eliminated by tissue uptake and metabolism; half-life is dose-dependent	Used as the initial treatment for deep vein thrombosis and pulmonary embolism, as an intravenous loading dose followed by an intravenous infusion or intermittent subcutaneous injection; also given by subcutaneous injection for deep vein thrombosis prophylaxis in general surgery
Tinzaparin	3–4[a] [R + M] Eliminated largely by renal excretion with some hepatic degradation	LMWH
Direct thrombin inhibitors		
Either peptides that are related to hirudin and are given intravenously (lepirudin and bivalirudin) or non-peptides that can be given orally (dabigatran etexilate)		
Bivalirudin	0.5 [R + M] Eliminated by a combination of glomerular filtration and metabolism (peptide cleavage)	Used for people undergoing percutaneous coronary intervention

Drugs used to affect haemostasis

Drug	Half-life (h) and kinetics	Comments
Dabigatran etexilate	40 min [R – metabolite] A prodrug; low oral bioavailability; metabolised to active derivative dabigatran which is excreted unchanged by the kidneys	Selective, competitive thrombin inhibitor acting on both free and clot-bound thrombin (factor IIa); administered orally
Lepirudin	1.5 [R + M?] Eliminated by glomerular filtration; very prolonged half-life in renal failure; possibly some metabolism	Used for people with heparin-associated thrombocytopenia type II who require parenteral anticoagulation; a recombinant hirudin (not related to heparins); given by slow intravenous injection or intravenous infusion
Anticoagulants (oral)		
Warfarin is the drug of choice and the others are seldom required		
Acenocoumarol	7 (R-isomer) 1 (S-isomer) [M] R- and S-enantiomers show different kinetics; the more potent S-isomer is metabolised by CYP2C9; genetic variants of CYP2C9 affect pharmacodynamic response and the risk of bleeding	Uses are as given for warfarin
Phenindione	5–6 [M + R] Urinary metabolites give a reddish colour to alkalinised urine	Uses are as given for warfarin
Rivaroxaban	9–12 [M + R]	Anticoagulant action by inhibiting factor Xa. Used for prophylaxis after hip and knee replacement surgery; given orally
Warfarin	18–35 (S-isomer) 20–60 (R-isomer) [M] Activated by oxidation; S-enantiomer more active and oxidised by CYP2C9; R-enantiomer is reduced	Used mainly for deep vein thrombosis; also used for pulmonary embolism, and for prophylaxis of embolism in rheumatic heart disease, atrial fibrillation and after insertion of prosthetic heart valves
Thrombolytic agents (also known as fibrinolytic agents)		
Activate plasminogen to plasmin; used in the treatment of myocardial infarction; macromolecules that are given intravenously		
Alteplase (rt-PA)	0.5 [M] Hepatic uptake and degradation	Tissue-type plasminogen activator; given by intravenous injection (when the action may be limited by distribution, which has a half-life of only 3–11 min) or by intravenous infusion
Reteplase	0.4–0.5 [M] Cleared by liver and kidney	Given by intravenous injection over not more than 2 min
Streptokinase	1 [M] Binding to plasminogen	Also used for life-threatening venous thrombosis and pulmonary embolism; given by intravenous infusion; rapid initial decrease in concentrations when there is a high antibody titre
Tenecteplase	1.5–2 [M] Eliminated by hepatic metabolism	A modified tissue-type plasminogen activator produced by recombinant DNA technology; higher selectivity than alteplase for fibrin; given by intravenous injection over 10 s
Antifibrinolytic drugs and haemostatic agents		
Etamsylate	No published kinetic data available	Reduces capillary bleeding, probably by affecting platelet adhesion; given orally
Tranexamic acid	1.4 [R] Eliminated by glomerular filtration	Used in hereditary angioedema, epistaxis and after excessive thrombolytic dosage; given orally or by slow intravenous injection

[a]Value depends on the clotting factor measured to reflect drug presence and activity, rather than chemical analysis of the drug.
[B], biliary excretion; [M], metabolism; [R], renal excretion; LMWH, low-molecular-weight heparin.

3

The respiratory system

12 Asthma and chronic obstructive pulmonary disease

Asthma and chronic obstructive pulmonary disease (COPD) show several similarities in their clinical features but have some distinct pathophysiological – including immunological – differences. Both are inflammatory disorders of the bronchi. Clinically, they are characterised by airflow obstruction (a forced expiratory volume in 1 second [FEV_1] below 80% of predicted and a ratio of FEV_1 to forced vital capacity of less than 70%).

ASTHMA

The characteristic feature of asthma is reversible airflow obstruction. Asthma is often associated with an atopic disposition, and exposure to allergens or other environmental air pollutants may then result in expression of the condition. More severe and adult-onset asthma is often non-allergic and accounts for 10–30% of cases; the pathological findings are similar.

The most common symptoms of asthma are wheeze and breathlessness, although cough may be the only symptom in younger people, especially at night. Airflow obstruction in asthma typically shows marked variability over time and greater than 15% improvement in response to any inhaled bronchodilator (see below).

The pathogenesis of asthma involves several processes but our knowledge is incomplete (Figs 12.1 and 12.2). Immune dysfunction in asthma may result from impaired regulation and imbalance between different T-regulatory and T-helper lymphocyte subsets and also epithelial and airway dendritic cells. Chronic inflammation of the bronchial mucosa is prominent, with infiltration of activated T-lymphocytes and granulocytes. This leads to the release of several powerful chemical mediators that can damage the epithelial lining of the airways and produce symptoms (Figs 12.1 and 12.2).

Figure 12.1 shows that exposure to a relevant allergen (such as pollen or the faeces of house-dust mite) cross-links IgE that is over-expressed on mast cells as a result of the immune response in atopic individuals; this causes mast cell degranulation. Degranulation and the subsequent pathological processes can also sometimes occur in non-atopic asthmatics with normal levels of IgE. Degranulation produces immediate bronchoconstriction (early phase) due to the release of a number of spasmogens (Fig. 12.1). Other released mediators act as chemotactic agents promoting an influx of inflammatory cells which 4–6 h later results in a late-phase bronchoconstrictor response and the commencement of a cascade of other pathological events in the airways. The persistent release of spasmogens and inflammatory mediators by these infiltrating cells can leave the bronchi hyperreactive to various irritants for several weeks. Mediators also produce mucosal oedema, which narrows the airways and stimulates smooth muscle contraction, leading to bronchoconstriction. Excessive production of mucus can cause further airways obstruction by plugging the bronchiolar lumen. Viral upper respiratory tract infections can exacerbate the mucosal inflammatory process. In hypersensitive individuals this sequence of events can occur in the absence of atopy.

In *mild to moderate* asthma, there is an increase in the number and activation of eosinophils (accompanied by some neutrophils and macrophages) in the airway and hyperresponsiveness to irritants and spasmogens. Airway smooth muscle cells undergo hypertrophy, and there is proliferation of blood vessels, transformation of epithelial cells into mucus-secreting cells, and increased deposition of matrix. Although all airways are involved in the inflammatory process in mild to moderate asthma, the degree of submucosal fibrosis and mucus secretion is modest, with no parenchymal destruction. In mild to moderate asthma there is a persistent and excessive $CD4^+$ T-helper cell type 2 (Th2)-dominated immune response; the cytokines produced by Th2 cells include interleukin-4 (IL-4), IL-5, IL-9, IL-13 and other cytokines producing a range of biological responses (Fig. 12.2).

In *severe asthma* there is evidence of additional, greater infiltration of neutrophils, tissue destruction and airways remodelling, with progressive thickening and loss of elastic recoil, especially in the peripheral airways. In addition to the changes seen in mild to moderate asthma, in severe disease there is increased expression of T-helper cell type 1 (Th1) derived cytokines (such as tumour necrosis factor alpha [TNFα] and IL-8). Disturbances in other immune regulatory functions are also present.

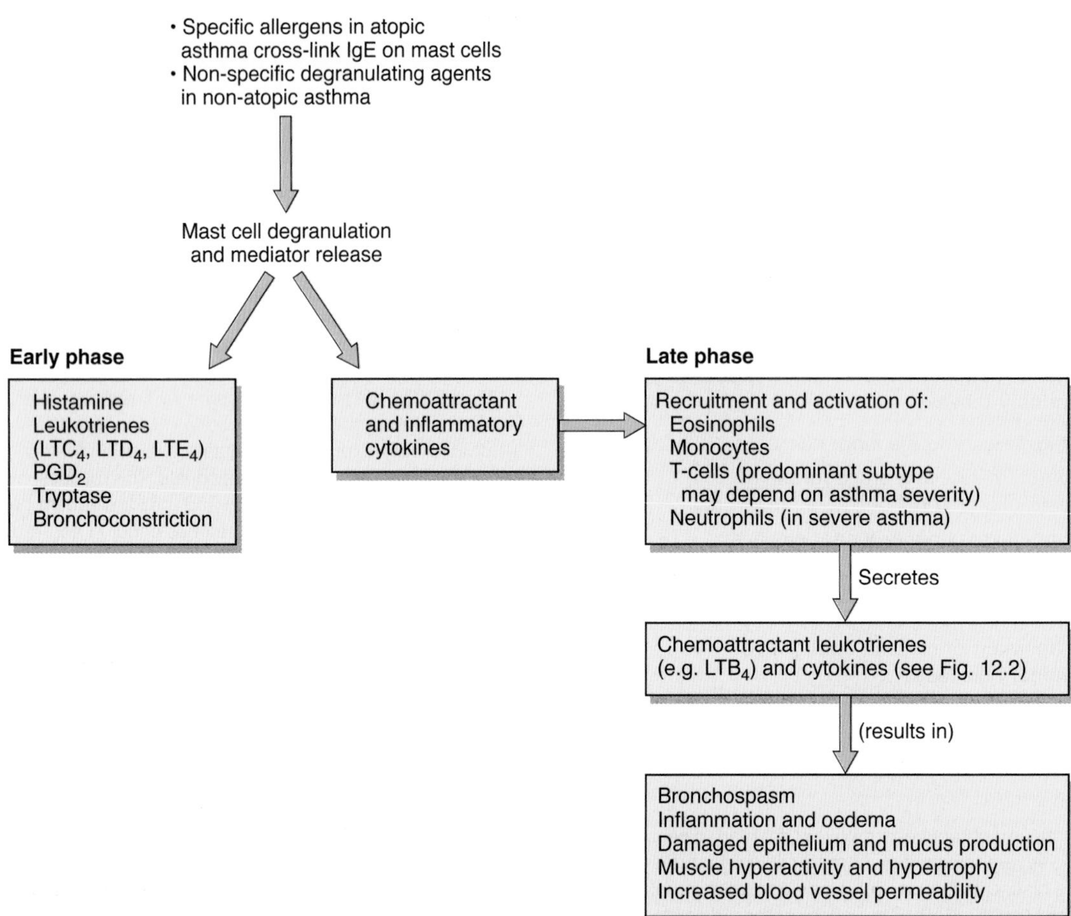

Fig. 12.1 **Some aspects of the early- and late-phase responses in asthma.** Cross-linking of the over-expressed IgE on mast cells of atopic individuals and non-immunogenic stimulants in more severe non-atopic asthma can degranulate mast cells, resulting in secretion of mediators that contribute to the pathogenesis of asthma. These mediators can directly produce bronchoconstriction and can both initiate the acute inflammatory response and attract and activate cells responsible for further inflammatory mediator production and persistent chronic inflammation. The roles of other agents, e.g. adenosine, nitric oxide, platelet activating factor, are uncertain despite the fact that they can have significant biological actions. LT, leukotriene; PG, prostaglandin.

Overall dysregulation in a vast number of inflammatory mediators appears to be involved in asthma, including leukotrienes, histamine, and a variety of cytokines including those termed chemokines (chemoattractant cytokines), but, unlike COPD, there is relatively little evidence of an increase in reactive oxygen species.

CHRONIC OBSTRUCTIVE PULMONARY DISEASE

About 95% of people with COPD are, or have been, cigarette smokers. There is wide variability in the rate of decline in pulmonary function in persistent smokers, with about 10–20% showing an accelerated decline that may reflect a genetic susceptibility. The other causes of COPD are exposure to air pollution and inherited α_1-antiprotease deficiency.

COPD is a symptom complex that is characterised by persistent airflow obstruction, with most people showing limited reversibility in response to a bronchodilator; however, about 10% of people with COPD do show considerable bronchodilator-induced reversibility of the airflow obstruction, and have a mixed inflammatory pattern in the airways, which probably represents an overlap between asthma and COPD (wheezy bronchitis). The airflow obstruction in COPD is usually slowly progressive. It is often accompanied by chronic bronchitis (production of mucoid sputum for all or part of the year) and emphysema (see below).

The most frequent symptoms of COPD are gradually progressive breathlessness and cough. The cough is often productive and usually worse in the morning; its severity is

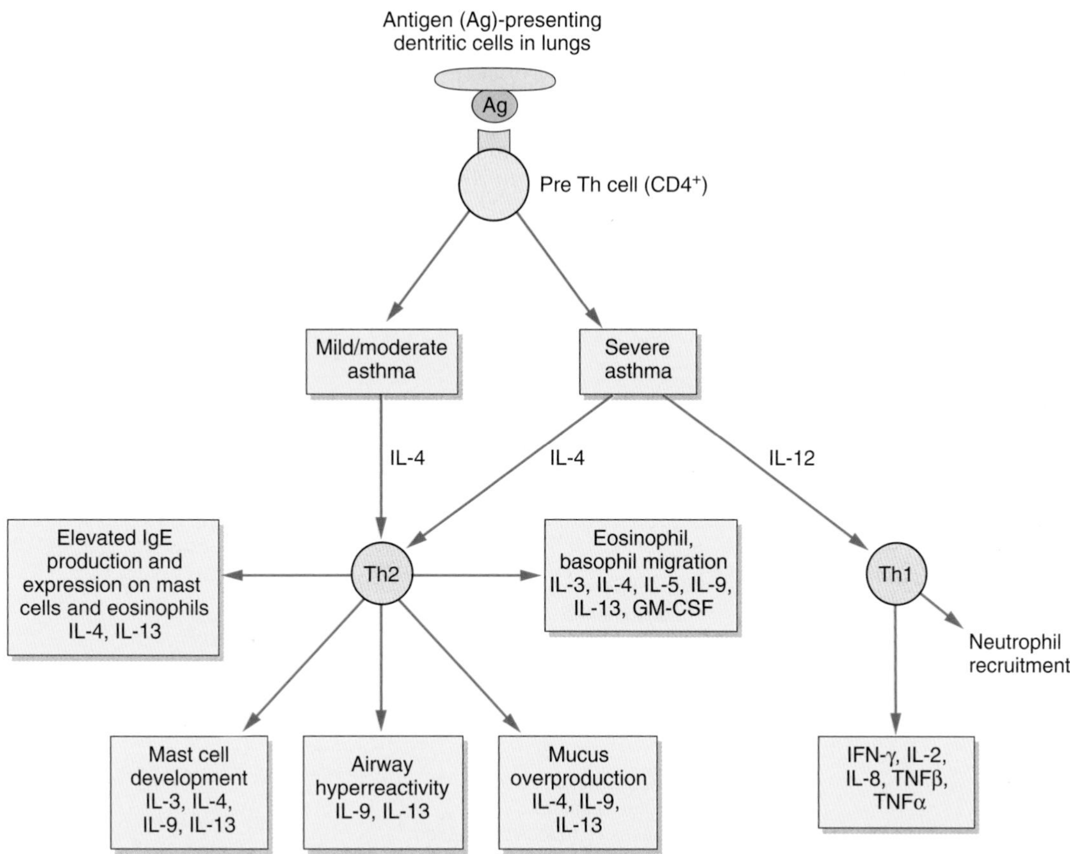

Fig. 12.2 **T-cells and asthma.** In allergic asthma there are complex and still poorly understood imbalances in the immune system. This includes alterations in functioning of several T-cell subsets and additional dysregulation in epithelial cells and airway dendritic cells. In allergic asthma, the T-helper type 2 (Th2) response is amplified, and Th2 cytokines contribute to many of the pathophysiological features of asthma. In severe asthma there is a greater pathological role for T-helper type 1 (Th1) cytokines and neutrophils compared with mild asthma, where Th2 cytokines and eosinophils predominate. IL, interleukin; GM-CSF, granulocyte–macrophage colony-stimulating factor; IFN, interferon; TNF, tissue necrosis factor.

unrelated to the degree of airflow obstruction. Repeated respiratory infections are common, and are often associated with exacerbations of the airflow obstruction and symptomatic deterioration.

In COPD there is an inflammatory process that predominantly affects the peripheral airways. The predominant infiltrating cells are neutrophils, macrophages and cytotoxic $CD8^+$ T-lymphocytes (Fig. 12.3). The major inflammatory mediators are leukotriene B_4 (LTB_4), TNFα and IL-8; an increase in growth-related oncogenes is also seen. There is increased oxidative stress due to reactive oxygen species, derived from cigarette smoke and other pollutants and released from neutrophils and inflammatory macrophages. There is a marked fibrotic reaction, parenchymal destruction and excessive bronchial mucus secretion.

The airflow obstruction in COPD results from a combination of decreased bronchial luminal diameter (produced by wall thickening, intraluminal mucus and changes in the fluid lining the small airways) and dynamic airways collapse due to emphysema (defined below). Corresponding histological changes include an increase in goblet cells in the bronchial mucosa and an increase in muscle mass in the bronchial wall, with interstitial fibrosis. Inflammation of the wall of the airway, particularly involving mononuclear cells, is common, especially in the early phases.

Emphysema is a pathological description, and is defined as enlargement of airways distal to the terminal bronchioles owing to destructive changes that may involve the entire acinus (panacinar) or the central part of the acinus (centriacinar). Lung parenchymal destruction is largely mediated by tissue proteases such as the matrix metalloproteinase gelatinase B (MMP-9) and cathepsins that are released by neutrophils and macrophages. Generation of excessive amounts of reactive oxygen species inhibits the antiproteases that normally protect the lung against such attack. Tissue destruction leads to a loss of lung recoil on expiration. Emphysema is probably the dominant factor in severe COPD.

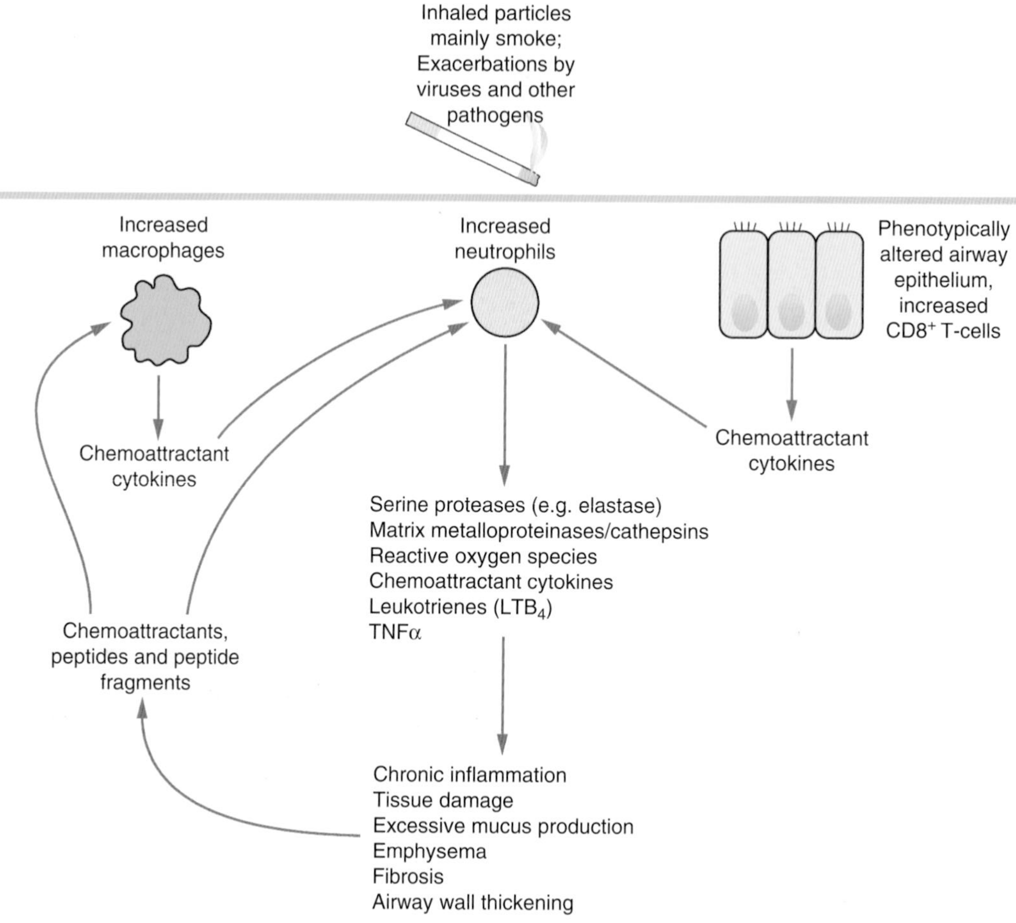

Fig 12.3 **Some pathophysiological factors in COPD**. A small percentage of smokers are particularly susceptible to the development of COPD; susceptibility may be determined by variability in inflammatory or protective genes. Chronic alterations in the recruitment, activation and control in function of neutrophils, macrophages and subsets of T-cells results in chronic parenchymal damage. Increased expression of chemoattractant cytokines (chemokines), growth-related oncogenes and expression of receptors for chemokines such as CXCR2 on macrophages, neutrophils and T-cells are involved. The precise roles and interplay of individual $CD4^+$ (helper) and $CD8^+$ (cytotoxic) T-cells with other cell types are still being characterised.

DRUGS FOR ASTHMA AND CHRONIC OBSTRUCTIVE PULMONARY DISEASE

DRUG DELIVERY TO THE LUNG

For the treatment of airways disease, direct delivery of drug to the lung by inhalation allows the use of smaller doses and therefore reduces the incidence of unwanted systemic effects (see Table 12.1). Drug is usually delivered in an aerosol; the size of the aerosol particle that is inhaled determines whether or not it will reach the airways and where in the airways it will be deposited. The optimal particle size for treatment is 2–5 μm. Particles larger than 10 μm impact on the upper airways and will be swallowed. Particles smaller than 1 μm will not deposit in the lower respiratory tract and are either absorbed into the blood from the alveoli or are exhaled. There are several methods for delivery of inhaled drug.

Pressurised metered-dose inhaler (pMDI)

This is the most common device for delivery of bronchodilator and anti-inflammatory drugs used in the treatment of asthma and COPD. Manually activated inhalers are widely used since they are convenient and inexpensive, but they require coordination of simultaneous device activation and inhalation. The delivery and uptake of the drug is suboptimal if inspiratory flow is low, if inspiration is not full and is not preceded by full expiration, or if inspiration is followed by a breath hold of less than 6 s. About one-third of users find coordination difficult, and, even if it is optimal, around 70–90% of the aerosol is deposited in the oropharynx, and swallowed. Chlorofluorocarbon (CFC) propellants in these inhalers are being phased out and replaced by hydrofluoroalkanes (HFAs) because of concerns over

Table 12.1 Comparison of aerosol and oral therapy for asthma

	Aerosol	Oral
Ideal pharmacokinetics	Slow absorption from the lung surface and rapid systemic clearance	Good oral absorption and long systemic action
Dose	Low dose delivered direct to target	High systemic dose necessary to achieve an appropriate concentration in the lung
Systemic drug concentration	Low	High
Incidence of unwanted effects	Low	High
Distribution in the lung	Reduced in severe disease	Unaffected by disease
Compliance	Good with bronchodilators, poor with anti-inflammatory drugs	Good
Ease of administration	Difficult for small children and infirm people[a]	Good
Effectiveness	Good in mild to moderate disease	Good even in severe disease

[a]May be improved by breath-activated inhalers or spacing devices. Nebulisers can be used for severe exacerbations.

atmospheric ozone depletion. The inhaler should be shaken before use.

pMDI with a large-volume spacer

The use of spacers is recommended for children and adults with mild to moderate asthma, to remove the need to coordinate aerosol activation and inspiration. For an adult, a plastic reservoir of about 750 mL volume can be attached to a metered-dose inhaler. The inhaler is activated into the spacer, and the person breathes normally through the mouthpiece. For young children, a small-volume (350 mL) spacer is used (attached to a facemask for very young children). Inhalation of the contents should be completed within 10 s. The spacer allows evaporation of propellant and may create more droplets of the correct size to deposit in the airways. It also reduces drug deposition in the oropharynx. When the device is washed, it should not be wiped dry, since this creates an electrostatic charge which attracts particles and reduces drug delivery. Addition of a spacer makes a metered-dose inhaler system less portable. To overcome this, one manufacturer has incorporated a collapsible spacer into its inhaler device.

Breath-actuated inhaler (BAI)

There are several types, delivering either an aerosol or dry powder. The aerosol type is a modified metered-dose inhaler that is activated by inspiration. Activation requires air to be drawn through the mouthpiece at a flow rate of about 30 L min^{-1}. BAIs are therefore less useful than pMDIs for those with severe airflow obstruction. Dry-powder inhalers contain particles of drug of optimal size for deposition. Inspiration through the device generates turbulence, which disperses the particles in the inspired air.

Nebulisers

These are devices that are used with a facemask or mouthpiece to deliver drug from a reservoir solution. There are two types. Jet nebulisers use air or oxygen passing through a narrow orifice to suck drug solution from a reservoir into a feed tube with fine ligaments. The impact of the solution on these ligaments generates droplets (Venturi principle). Ultrasonic nebulisers use a piezoelectric crystal vibrating at high frequency. The vibrations are transmitted through a buffer to the drug solution and form a fountain of liquid in the nebulisation chamber. Ultrasonic nebulisers produce a more uniform particle size than do jet nebulisers. Up to 10 times the amount of drug is required in a nebuliser to produce the same degree of bronchodilation achieved by a metered-dose inhaler. Delivery is more efficient via a mouthpiece than via a mask.

SYMPTOM-RELIEVING DRUGS FOR AIRFLOW OBSTRUCTION (BRONCHODILATORS; 'RELIEVERS')

Beta$_2$-adrenoceptor agonists

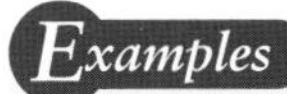

short-acting: salbutamol, terbutaline
long-acting: formoterol, salmeterol

Mechanism of action and effects

Beta$_2$-adrenoceptors are widely distributed in the lung; the receptor density is higher in bronchial smooth muscle than in other cell types such as epithelial and endothelial cells and mast cells. Receptor stimulation causes stabilisation of the receptor in its active rather than inactive configuration; this results in increased generation of cyclic adenosine monophosphate (cAMP) and activation of protein kinase A (PKA), which phosphorylates proteins that are central to the regulation of smooth muscle tone. Major actions are:

- bronchodilation due to reduced Ca^{2+} release from intracellular stores, and reduced Ca^{2+} entry into smooth muscle cells
- inhibition of mediator release from mast cells and monocytes
- enhanced mucociliary clearance.

Recent studies have suggested that the bronchodilation may in part be due to direct interaction of G proteins with K^+ channels in smooth muscle rather than through cAMP-activated pathways.

Pharmacokinetics

The selectivity of β_2-adrenoceptor agonists is dose-dependent. Inhalation of drug aids selectivity since it delivers small

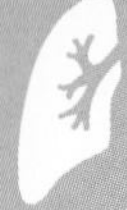

but effective doses to the airways and minimises systemic exposure and hence the stimulation of β_1-adrenoceptors (Table 12.1). The dose–response relationship for bronchodilation is log-linear and a 10-fold increase in dose is required to double the effect.

Agents such as salbutamol are short-acting because they are hydrophilic and are therefore rapidly metabolised and eliminated. The onset of drug action is rapid, often within 5 min. and they produce bronchodilation for up to about 6 h. Their duration of action is far longer than the natural adrenoceptor agonists such as adrenaline, because they are not substrates for uptake into the presynaptic neuron (uptake 1, Ch. 4) or for catechol-O-methyl transferase, the enzyme which metabolises catecholamines outside adrenergic neurons (Ch. 4).

Salmeterol and formoterol are longer-acting because they are more lipophilic than short-acting agents. Salmeterol has a lipophilic side-chain that binds to the membrane adjacent to the receptor. Formoterol enters the lipid bilayer of the cell membrane and is then gradually released. They act for up to 12 h and have a slower onset of action than short-acting agents.

Salbutamol and terbutaline can also be given orally (as conventional or modified-release formulations), by subcutaneous or intramuscular injections, or by intravenous infusion. Much larger doses are required to deliver an adequate amount of drug to the lungs by any of these routes. This reduces the selectivity for β_2-adrenoceptors, and systemic unwanted effects can be troublesome.

Unwanted effects

- Fine skeletal muscle tremor from stimulation of β_2-adrenoceptors.
- Tachycardia and arrhythmias result from both β_1- and β_2-adrenoceptor stimulation when high doses of inhaled drug are used, or after oral or parenteral administration.
- Hypokalaemia, due to promotion of cellular uptake of K^+ by a cAMP-dependent action on the Na^+/K^+ pump, can be an acute metabolic response to a high dose of β_2-adrenoceptor agonist. Hypomagnesaemia and hyperglycaemia can also occur. These effects do not persist during long-term use.
- Paradoxical bronchospasm has been reported with inhalation, usually when given for the first time or with a new canister.
- Headache.
- Tolerance to the bronchodilator effects can occur with prolonged use of β_2-adrenoceptor agonists, probably as a result of desensitisation and downregulation of the adrenoceptor. The process of receptor desensitisation appears to be more rapid for mast cells than for bronchial smooth muscle. Corticosteroids may reduce desensitisation by increasing β_2-adrenoceptor gene transcription and enhancing coupling of the receptor to adenylyl cyclase.

Regular use of high doses of short-acting or inhaled long-acting β_2-adrenoceptor agonists has been linked with asthma deaths. One possibility is that they precipitate serious cardiac arrhythmias during severe asthma exacerbations. It is also possible that their use might allow people to tolerate initial exposure to larger doses of allergens or irritants, which then produce an enhanced late asthmatic response. The excess mortality, although of concern, is extremely low. Recent investigation has raised the possibility that β_2-adrenoceptor polymorphism may modify the response to these drugs in some individuals, but it is not known whether this explains the risk of adverse events.

Antimuscarinic agents

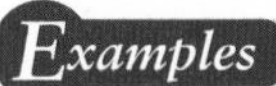

ipratropium, tiotropium

Mechanism of action and effects

Many cell types in the respiratory system, including both neuronal and non-neuronal cells, have nicotinic and muscarinic surface receptors. These mediate a multitude of actions in response to parasympathetic nervous system stimulation. There are three main types of muscarinic receptors in the airways, of which the M_3 receptor subtype appears to be the most important in the pathophysiology and treatment of asthma and COPD. M_1 and M_2 receptor stimulation results in actions that would be expected to benefit asthma; therefore blockade of all subtypes by the use of non-selective muscarinic antagonists in asthma may result in less benefit than might be expected.

- M_3 receptors are postsynaptic and may be involved in asthma in the following ways: they mediate airways smooth muscle contraction (and thus bronchoconstriction), mucus secretion and ciliary beating. M_3 receptor stimulation activates phospholipase C with subsequent formation of IP_3 and DAG (key events in the signalling pathway that increases intracellular Ca^{2+}, Ch. 1; Fig. 1.5). M_3 receptors are also involved in the regulation of smooth muscle proliferation in response to peptide growth factors (which are increased in allergic airway inflammation), but it is not known whether inhibition of airway remodelling contributes to the clinical effects of antimuscarinic drugs.
- M_1 receptors may facilitate cholinergic neurotransmission at parasympathetic ganglia, although this effect is small. They are also involved in inhibition of histamine release from mast cells and therefore their blockade in this context would not help relieve asthma.
- M_2 receptors are presynaptic autoreceptors on cholinergic neurons and provide negative feedback that modulates acetylcholine release, thereby potentially limiting bronchoconstriction. This effect is increased by glucocorticoid treatment.

Parasympathetic stimulation has also been shown to affect the functioning of mast cells, macrophages and epithelial cells, but in the clinical situation it remains uncertain whether the effect of therapeutic doses of antimuscarinic drugs on these cells is of relevance.

The antimuscarinic drugs used for bronchodilation are non-selective, and bind to all three types of muscarinic receptors in the lung. Their main benefit is in COPD; they are of less value for bronchodilation in acute mild to moderate asthma, but may have a place when added to β_2-adrenoceptor agonists in severe exacerbations of asthma.

Pharmacokinetics

The antimuscarinic drugs used for bronchodilation are N-quaternary congeners of the tertiary-structured atropine; they are poorly absorbed orally and do not cross the blood–brain barrier. They are given exclusively by inhalation (as a powder or aerosol) or via a nebuliser. They have a slower onset of action (30–60 min) than salbutamol (5–10 min), probably due to slow absorption from the surface of the airways. The duration of action is related to the rate of removal locally from the airways, and not the half-life of elimination from the circulation.

Unwanted effects

Similarly to inhaled β_2-adrenoceptor agonists, direct delivery of antimuscarinic drugs to the lung is the main reason for the relative lack of unwanted systemic effects.

- Dry mouth is the most common effect
- Nausea, constipation
- Headache
- Tiotropium can cause urinary retention in men with prostatism
- Exacerbation of angle-closure glaucoma (Ch. 50).

Methylxanthines

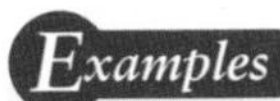

aminophylline, theophylline

Mechanism of action and effects

Methylxanthines are a group of naturally occurring substances found in coffee, tea, chocolate and related foodstuffs. Naturally occurring theophylline (1,3-dimethylxanthine), and its ester derivative aminophylline, are the only compounds in clinical use. They are chemically similar to caffeine. Methylxanthines have vasodilator, anti-inflammatory and immunomodulatory actions. The mechanisms of action of methylxanthines are multiple, controversial and uncertain.

- Inhibition of the enzyme phosphodiesterase (PDE), which degrades cyclic nucleotide second messengers, may partly explain the actions of methylxanthines. Theophylline preferentially inhibits PDE3 and PDE4 isoenzymes, which are found in bronchial smooth muscle and several inflammatory cells, including mast cells, and are responsible for degradation of cAMP. Theophylline also inhibits PDE5 and reduces the breakdown of cGMP. The rise in intracellular cAMP in bronchial smooth muscle stimulates large conductance voltage-gated Ca^{2+}-activated K^+ channels (BK_{Ca}) in the cell membrane, leading to cell hyperpolarisation and muscle relaxation. However, theophylline only produces bronchodilation at relatively high plasma concentrations (10–20 mg L^{-1}) and drugs that are more effective PDE inhibitors (such as dipyridamole) do not bronchodilate. Prolonging the duration of action of cyclic nucleotides may potentiate the action of β_2-adrenoceptor agonists and produce a synergistic dilator effect on bronchial smooth muscle. PDE inhibition also stimulates ciliary beat frequency in the airways and enhances water transport across the airway epithelium, which increase mucociliary clearance. In contrast, theophylline increases the force and rate of contraction of cardiac muscle (Ch. 7).
- Increased diaphragmatic contractility and reduced fatigue have been reported at lower plasma theophylline concentrations than those required for bronchodilation. This may improve lung ventilation.
- Adenosine receptor antagonism may be relevant to some of the clinical effects of methylxanthines (see also adenosine; Ch. 8). Adenosine releases histamine and leukotrienes from mast cells, which results in the constriction of hyperresponsive airways in individuals with asthma. Theophylline is a potent antagonist at adenosine A_1 and A_2 receptors (Ch. 1) and may reduce bronchoconstriction by this mechanism. Adenosine receptor antagonism is responsible for central nervous system (CNS) stimulation, which improves mental performance and alertness, and in the kidney reduces tubular Na^+ reabsorption and leads to natriuresis and diuresis.
- Activation of histone deacetylases (see corticosteroids below). Acetylation of core histones, which form part of the structure of DNA, activates pro-inflammatory transcription factors, such as nuclear factor-κB and activator protein-1. If histone acetylation is reversed by increasing the activity of histone deacetylases, then the inflammatory genes will be suppressed. Theophylline produces its anti-inflammatory effects at drug plasma concentrations of 5–10 mg L^{-1}, similar to those that produce clinical benefit. This action may potentiate the anti-inflammatory effects of corticosteroids (see Ch. 44), since histone deacetylases only become effective at the site of inflammation when glucocorticoid receptors are activated.

Pharmacokinetics

The extent of absorption of theophylline from the gut is unpredictable, with considerable inter-individual variation. This, and the short but highly variable plasma half-life, has resulted in the widespread use of modified-release formulations. Theophylline has a narrow therapeutic index, and since different formulations vary in their release characteristics, they are not readily interchangeable. Theophylline is metabolised in the liver by cytochrome P450 (CYP1A2 and, to a lesser extent, by CYP3A4), giving the potential for drug interactions. Aminophylline is a more water-soluble ester prodrug, which is hydrolysed rapidly after absorption from the gut to theophylline and ethylenediamine. Aminophylline can also be given by intravenous infusion. Measurement of blood theophylline concentrations is valuable as a guide to effective dosing.

Unwanted effects

Most are dose-related and can arise within the accepted therapeutic plasma concentration range.

- Gastrointestinal upset, including nausea, vomiting (from PDE4 inhibition in the vomiting centre) and diarrhoea.
- CNS stimulation, including insomnia, irritability, occasionally seizures at high plasma concentrations (from adenosine receptor antagonism) and headache (from PDE3 inhibition).
- Hypotension from peripheral vasodilation (from PDE3 inhibition in the smooth muscle cells of many blood

vessels). In contrast, cerebral arteries are constricted by methylxanthines (adenosine is a vasodilator of cranial blood vessels and methylxanthines may act as adenosine receptor antagonists in this vascular bed).

- Cardiac stimulation produces various arrhythmias.
- Hypokalaemia can occur acutely, especially after intravenous injection, which also promotes cardiac arrhythmias.
- Tolerance to the beneficial effects of methylxanthines can occur.
- Drug interactions can be troublesome, due to the narrow therapeutic index of theophylline. Hepatic CYP1A2 enzyme inhibitors such as ciprofloxacin, erythromycin, clarithromycin, fluconazole and ketoconazole (Ch. 51, Table 2.9). can precipitate theophylline toxicity.

ANTI-INFLAMMATORY DRUGS FOR AIRWAYS OBSTRUCTION ('PREVENTERS')

Corticosteroids

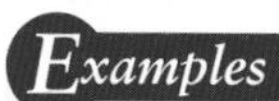

beclometasone dipropionate, budesonide, fluticasone propionate, hydrocortisone, mometasone, prednisolone

Mechanism of action and effects

Glucocorticoids are the most effective class of drug in the treatment of chronic asthma but are relatively ineffective in COPD. They act to suppress inflammation and the immune response but are not bronchodilators and are therefore ineffective in the initial stages of an acute attack of asthma. Powerful glucocorticoids, devoid of significant mineralocorticoid activity, are usually used.

Intracellular events involved in the anti-inflammatory action of corticosteroids are described in Chapters 38 and 44. A major effect in asthma is probably activation of glucocorticoid receptors that inhibit transcription of genes coding for the cytokines involved in inflammation. Glucocorticoid receptors recruit histone deacetylases to the transcription complex of activated inflammatory genes. The deacetylation of core histones at the transcription complex silences genes that have been activated by inflammatory stimuli. Used long term, corticosteroids reduce airway responsiveness to several bronchoconstrictor mediators and block both the early and late reactions to allergen. Following a delay of 6–12 h, several anti-inflammatory actions occur which may be important in asthma.

Short-term anti-inflammatory effects include:

- reduced inflammatory cell activation (including macrophages, T-lymphocytes, eosinophils and airway epithelial cells)
- decreased IgE synthesis
- reduced mucosal oedema and decreased local generation of inflammatory prostaglandins and leukotrienes by inhibition of phospholipase A_2 (see also Ch. 29)
- β_2-adrenoceptor upregulation and better coupling to adenylyl cyclase, which restores responsiveness to β_2-adrenoceptor agonists
- enhanced activity of the M_2 autoreceptors on acetylcholine nerve endings inhibits acetylcholine release and relieves bronchoconstriction.

Long-term anti-inflammatory effects include:

- reduced T-cell cytokine production (Ch. 38) and reduced dendritic cell signalling to T-cells
- reduced eosinophil deposition in bronchial mucosa (by removing cytokine stimulation, reducing expression of epithelial adhesion molecules and enhancing apoptosis)
- reduced mast cell deposition in bronchial mucosa (although the release of mediators from these cells is unaffected)
- suppression of the excess epithelial cell shedding and goblet cell hyperplasia found in the bronchial epithelium in asthma.

Inhaled corticosteroids produce some improvement in asthmatic symptoms after 24 h and a maximum response after 1–2 weeks. Reduction in airway responsiveness to allergens and irritants occurs gradually over several months: many of the chronic structural changes in the airways in asthma are not affected by corticosteroids.

Pharmacokinetics

Whenever possible, corticosteroids are given by inhalation of an aerosol or dry powder in order to minimise systemic unwanted effects, but they can be used intravenously or orally in severe asthma. Desirable properties of an inhaled corticosteroid include a low rate of absorption across mucosal surfaces (such as the lung, but also the gut for swallowed drug) and rapid inactivation once absorbed. Beclometasone dipropionate fulfils the former criterion, but it is only slowly inactivated once it reaches the systemic circulation. Inhaled budesonide (which is inactivated by extensive first-pass metabolism in the liver following oral absorption) or fluticasone (which is very poorly absorbed from the gut) may be preferred if high doses of inhaled drug are needed, or for the treatment of children, in whom the systemic effects can be more problematic.

Unwanted effects

The unwanted effects of oral and parenteral corticosteroids are described in Chapter 44. Inhaled corticosteroids only have systemic actions when given in high doses. The amount of swallowed drug can be minimised by using a large-volume spacer (see above); large aerosol particles, which would otherwise be deposited on the oropharyngeal mucosa, are trapped in the spacer and only the smaller particles are inhaled.

There are some specific problems with inhaled corticosteroids:

- Dysphonia (hoarseness), caused by deposition on vocal cords and myopathy of laryngeal muscles, occurs in up to one-third of those using inhaled corticosteroids. This may be less troublesome with breath-actuated delivery, since the method of inspiration leads to protection of the vocal cords by the false cords.
- Oral candidiasis can occur but can be prevented by using a spacer device or by gargling after use of the inhaler.

Cromones

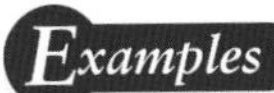

sodium cromoglicate, nedocromil sodium

The cromones are used to prevent asthma attacks; because they have no bronchodilator activity, they are of no use in acute attacks of asthma. Prophylaxis with these agents is usually less effective than with inhaled corticosteroids, and only about one-third of people benefit from treatment with cromones. Currently, their major use is as a prophylactic agent in the treatment of mild to moderate antigen-, pollutant- and exercise-induced asthma. They are also used as a nasal inhalant to treat seasonal allergic rhinitis (Ch. 39) and as an ophthalmic solution to treat allergic conjunctivitis (Ch. 50).

Mechanisms of action and effects

- Mast cell stabilisation. Sodium cromoglicate was originally introduced as a mast cell stabiliser. It enhances phosphorylation of a protein that normally forms a substrate for the intracellular enzyme protein kinase C, and interferes with the signal transduction for inflammatory mediator release. This action may protect against immediate bronchoconstriction induced by allergens, exercise or cold air.
- Inhibition of sensory C-fibre neurons by antagonism of the effects of the tachykinins, substance P and neurokinin B, which are involved in generation of sensory stimuli. This is probably responsible for protection against bronchoconstriction produced by irritants such as sulphur dioxide.
- Inhibition of accumulation of eosinophils in the lungs and reduced activation of eosinophils, neutrophils and macrophages in inflamed lung tissue. These actions may be important in preventing the 'late-phase' response to allergen and the development of bronchial hyperreactivity.
- Reduced IgE production. Inhibition of B-cell switching to IgE production probably also contributes to the long-term effects of these drugs.

A single dose of either nedocromil sodium or sodium cromoglicate will prevent the early-phase bronchoconstrictor response to allergen, but treatment for 1–2 months may be necessary to block the late-phase reaction.

Pharmacokinetics

Both sodium cromoglicate and nedocromil sodium are highly ionised and poorly absorbed across biological membranes. They are therefore largely retained at the site of action on bronchial mucosa after inhalation as a powder or from a metered-dose aerosol inhaler. Swallowed drug is unabsorbed and voided in the faeces.

Unwanted effects

Cough, wheeze and throat irritation may be provoked transiently following inhalation.

Leukotriene receptor antagonists

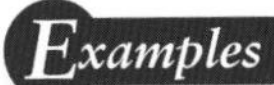

montelukast, zafirlukast

These are oral agents for the prevention of chronic asthma and have an additive effect with corticosteroid treatment.

Mechanisms of action and effects

The leukotriene receptor antagonists are given orally and inhibit the bronchoconstriction induced by leukotrienes (Ch. 29), by blocking the receptors for the cysteinyl leukotrienes (LTC_4, LTD_4 and LTE_4). Cysteinyl leukotrienes are released from various cells, including activated mast cells and eosinophils, in response to several airway insults, and their synthesis is increased by many mediators, such as cytokines. Cysteinyl leukotrienes can contribute to airway oedema, smooth muscle contraction and enhanced secretion of mucus (Fig. 12.1).

Leukotriene receptor antagonists prevent both the early and late bronchoconstrictor responses to allergen, and may be most useful in mild and moderate asthma, exercise-induced asthma, and asthma provoked by non-steroidal anti-inflammatory drugs (NSAIDs; Ch. 29).

Unwanted effects

- Headache, irritability
- Gastrointestinal upset
- Dry mouth, thirst
- Oedema
- Hypersensitivity reactions, including anaphylaxis, angioedema and skin rashes.

Magnesium sulphate

Mechanism of action and effects

Intravenous magnesium sulphate can be given for the treatment of severe asthma in adults if life-threatening features are present. Magnesium bronchodilates by blocking Ca^{2+} channels in smooth muscle cell membranes, therefore reducing Ca^{2+} influx into the cell.

Pharmacokinetics

Magnesium sulphate is given intravenously and is widely distributed. It crosses the placenta and passes into breast milk. The Mg^{2+} is excreted by the kidney, with a half-life of 4 h.

Unwanted effects

- Atrioventricular block
- Enhancement of neuromuscular blockade by neuromuscular blocking agents
- Potentiates the hypotensive effects of calcium channel blockers
- Diarrhoea.

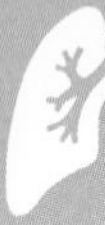

Antibody to immunoglobulin E (IgE)

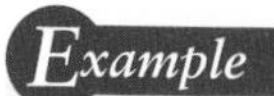

omalizumab

Mechanism of action

Omalizumab is licensed for the treatment of persistent severe allergic asthma that cannot be controlled with corticosteroids and long-acting β_2-adrenoceptor agonists. It is a recombinant DNA-derived humanised IgG1κ monoclonal antibody that binds selectively to IgE and removes both circulating and tissue IgE. This leads to a reduction in the high-affinity IgE receptors on mast cells, basophils and dendritic cells. Treatment with omalizumab gradually reduces airway inflammation in asthma, with a peak response after 12–16 weeks.

Pharmacokinetics

Omalizumab is given subcutaneously, in a dose that is determined by the recipient's plasma IgE concentration and body weight. It forms complexes with IgE that are removed by the reticuloendothelial system and endothelial cells. The half-life is very long, at about 26 days.

Unwanted effects

- Headache
- Injection site reactions.

MANAGEMENT OF ASTHMA

Treatment of asthma has two aims:

- relief of symptoms
- reduction of airways inflammation.

The acute attack

Mild infrequent attacks of asthma can often be controlled by occasional use of an inhaled β_2-adrenoceptor agonist. Antimuscarinic agents are most effective when asthma coexists with chronic obstructive airways disease. More severe attacks require intensive treatment with bronchodilators and systemic corticosteroids. The signs of severe and life-threatening asthma are shown in Table 12.2.

Treatment of acute severe asthma should include:

- ensuring adequate hydration
- 40–60% oxygen via a facemask
- nebulised β_2-adrenoceptor agonist such as salbutamol (preferably nebulised by oxygen)
- intravenous hydrocortisone and/or high-dose oral prednisolone.

If there are life-threatening features, additional treatment should be given:

- nebulised ipratropium
- intravenous aminophylline or β_2-adrenoceptor agonist such as salbutamol
- intravenous magnesium sulphate
- assisted ventilation if there is not rapid clinical improvement.

Table 12.2 Signs of severe and life-threatening asthma

Severe	Life-threatening
Inability to complete a sentence	A silent chest
Pulse ≥110 beats min^{-1}	Bradycardia or hypotension
Peak expiratory flow rate ≤50% of predicted or previous best	Peak expiratory flow rate ≤33% of predicted or previous best
	Exhaustion, confusion or coma
Arterial blood gas markers of severe asthma Normal (5–6 kPa) or high arterial carbon dioxide ($Pa\text{CO}_2$) Severe hypoxaemia ($Pa\text{O}_2$ < 8 kPa) Low or high plasma pH	

After recovery from a severe asthma attack, an oral corticosteroid should be continued until there are no residual symptoms, especially at night, and the peak expiratory flow rate is at least 80% of the person's previous best. High doses of these drugs can be stopped abruptly if used for 3 weeks or less, or tapered off if they have been used for a longer period (Ch. 44).

Prophylaxis of recurrent attacks

An initial attempt should be made to identify and exclude precipitating factors – for example, allergens, occupational precipitants, NSAIDs (see below) and β-adrenoceptor antagonists (including eye-drops) (Ch. 5). After initially gaining control of asthma symptoms, long-term treatment is guided by a stepwise treatment plan recommended by the British Thoracic Society and Scottish Intercollegiate Guidelines Network (for last version *http://www.sign.ac.uk/guidelines/fulltext/101/index.html*).

The recommendations for adults and schoolchildren are:

Step 1. Mild intermittent asthma. Inhaled short-acting β_2-adrenoceptor agonist, such as salbutamol, taken as required. For those who are intolerant to this treatment, inhaled ipratropium and oral theophylline are alternative options but there is a higher risk of unwanted effects with the latter. Additional treatment should be considered if more than one dose of short-acting β_2-adrenoceptor agonist is required each day.

Step 2. Regular inhaled preventer therapy. For adults, a corticosteroid such as beclometasone is most often used. In children and some adults, initial treatment with cromoglicate or nedocromil or a leukotriene receptor antagonist could be tried. These agents are generally less effective than inhaled corticosteroid.

Step 3. Inhaled corticosteroid plus long-acting inhaled β_2-adrenoceptor agonist. If the symptoms are not controlled by standard doses of inhaled corticosteroid, a long-acting β_2-adrenoceptor agonist such as salmeterol is usually more effective than increasing the dose of corticosteroid. If there is no response to the long-acting β_2-adrenoceptor agonist, it should be stopped and the corticosteroid dose increased. For persistent poor control, sequential add-on therapy with a leukotriene receptor antagonist, a modified-release theophylline formulation or a modified-release oral β_2-adrenoceptor agonist should be tried.

Step 4. High-dose inhaled corticosteroid plus regular bronchodilators. High-dose inhaled corticosteroid with a short-acting β_2-adrenoceptor agonist as required, and usually an inhaled long-acting β_2-adrenoceptor agonist plus a sequential trial of one or more of the following:

- leukotriene receptor antagonist
- oral modified-release theophylline formulation
- oral modified-release β_2-adrenoceptor agonist.

Step 5. Regular oral corticosteroid. Oral prednisolone is taken in addition to other measures outlined above.

Aspirin-induced asthma

About 5% of people with asthma experience exacerbations when they take aspirin or other NSAIDs (Ch. 29), and have an eosinophilic rhinosinusitis and nasal polyposis in addition to asthma. The condition may be initiated by priming of the respiratory mucosa by an immune reaction to a viral infection or other insult which upregulates cysteinyl leukotriene receptors. However, bronchoconstriction is prevented since lipoxygenase activity (and therefore production of bronchoconstrictor leukotrienes) remains under partial inhibitory control by PGE_2. Aspirin is an irreversible cyclooxygenase type 1 (COX-1) and COX-2 inhibitor with greater effect on COX-1 inhibition. COX inhibition reduces PGE_2 synthesis, which releases the inhibition of leukotriene synthesis, provoking bronchospasm (see Fig. 29.1).

Symptoms begin within 3 h of ingesting aspirin, accompanied by profuse rhinorrhoea, conjunctival injection and, sometimes, flushing or urticaria. Airways inflammation can persist for many weeks after an aspirin challenge. Only NSAIDs that inhibit COX-1 induce bronchoconstriction; the newer selective COX-2 inhibitors do not provoke asthma. Leukotriene receptor antagonists produce symptom relief in some people with aspirin-induced asthma. Treatment of the asthmatic attack is the same as for any other episode. Sometimes, long-term use of an oral corticosteroid is the only way to control persistent symptoms; in which case desensitisation to aspirin should be attempted. Nasal polypectomy may be necessary to control rhinosinusitis.

Asthma resistant to standard treatment

For people with resistant disease, especially those who require maintenance treatment with oral corticosteroids, the use of immunosuppressive drugs such as ciclosporin or methotrexate (Ch. 38) has been advocated. Omalizumab can reduce the frequency of asthma attacks in severe persistent allergic asthma, but only about two-thirds of people given the drug show any response. More recently, small studies have shown benefit from the anti-TNFα fusion protein etanercept (Ch. 30) in severe asthma.

MANAGEMENT OF CHRONIC OBSTRUCTIVE PULMONARY DISEASE

There are two goals in the treatment of COPD: to minimise symptoms (including a reduction in acute exacerbations) and to preserve lung function.

- **Cessation of smoking**. Stopping smoking (see Ch. 54) is the only effective way to alter the natural history of COPD. Smoking cessation slows the rate of decline in lung function to that naturally seen with ageing, although any loss of lung function due to smoking cannot be restored. Occupational exposure to inhaled pollutants should also be minimised.
- **Pneumococcal and influenza vaccination**. These can reduce infectious exacerbations in people with COPD.
- **Bronchodilators.** The principles are similar to those for asthma, although the limited reversibility of the airway obstruction means that the benefit is less marked, except during an acute exacerbation of symptoms. Some improvement in symptoms and functional capacity can occur without changes in standard lung function tests and the main benefit is improved lung emptying during expiration, with reduced hyperinflation at rest. Inhaled bronchodilators reduce the frequency of exacerbations of COPD. Beta$_2$-adrenoceptor agonists and antimuscarinic agents are equally effective, and produce additive improvements in lung function when taken together. Recent studies suggest that either a long-acting β_2-adrenoceptor agonist or tiotropium can slow the rate of decline in lung function in COPD, but there is no evidence to show additional benefit on decline in lung function from combining these treatments. Theophylline is usually reserved for advanced COPD when symptoms persist despite use of inhaled long-acting bronchodilators. Nebulised bronchodilators can be useful for severe exacerbations.
- **Corticosteroids**. Many of the inflammatory changes in COPD do not respond to corticosteroids; nevertheless, an oral corticosteroid should be used for 7–14 days when treating an acute exacerbation of symptoms. Long-term use of an inhaled corticosteroid can reduce the number and severity of exacerbations, and should be considered if there are two or more exacerbations in a 12-month period. An inhaled corticosteroid can also produce some symptomatic benefit for people who remain breathless despite the use of a long-acting bronchodilator. About 10% of people with COPD will have an improvement in their forced expiratory flow rate with an inhaled corticosteroid, and when combined with a long-acting bronchodilator, there may be an additive effect on reducing the rate of decline in lung function.
- **Antibacterial drugs**. One-third of infective exacerbations are due to viral infection, but antibacterial drugs (Ch. 51) produce earlier symptomatic improvement if there is moderate-to-severe acute exacerbation of symptoms with purulent sputum.

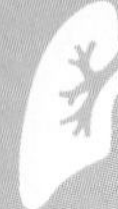

- **Mucolytic agents**. Mecysteine hydrochloride or carbocisteine (Ch. 13) may reduce the frequency of exacerbations. An initial 1-month trial should be considered if COPD is accompanied by a chronic productive cough or if there are prolonged severe exacerbations. Treatment should only be continued if there is a perceived benefit.
- **Oxygen therapy**. This is extremely important to treat hypoxaemia during acute exacerbations. Care must be taken to raise the arterial oxygen saturation (if possible to ≥90%) without increasing the arterial carbon dioxide tension. To avoid suppressing hypoxic drive in type 2 respiratory failure (hypoxaemia with a raised arterial carbon dioxide concentration), low-dose supplementary oxygen may be necessary (e.g. 24% via Venturi mask or 1–2 L min^{-1} via nasal cannulae). Long-term domiciliary oxygen treatment, usually from an oxygen concentrator which removes nitrogen from air and delivers via nasal cannulae, improves symptoms and survival in COPD with respiratory failure (with an arterial oxygen tension less than 7.3 kPa). It should only be considered if respiratory failure persists for 3–4 weeks despite optimal drug therapy and without a clinical exacerbation, and if the person does not smoke (because of the fire risk). To improve survival, oxygen must be used for at least 15 h per day.
- **Ventilatory support.** This may be required during exacerbations. Intubation and mechanical ventilation may be necessary, but non-invasive assisted ventilation is preferable. Nasal intermittent positive pressure ventilation (NIPPV) is being increasingly used during exacerbations for people who fail to respond to maximal medical therapy, especially if there is carbon dioxide retention. The respiratory stimulant doxapram (Ch. 13) is occasionally used to produce short-term improvement in blood gas tensions while awaiting initiation of non-invasive ventilation.
- **Pulmonary rehabilitation**. This improves exercise capacity, reduces the sensation of breathlessness, and can substantially improve morale.

FURTHER READING

Asthma

Adcock IM, Caramori G, Chung KF (2008) New targets for drug development in asthma. *Lancet* 372, 1073–1087

Barnes PJ (2000) Molecular basis for corticosteroid action in asthma. *Chem Immunol* 78, 72–80

Bloebaum RM, Grant JA, Sur S (2004) Immunomodulation: the future of allergy and asthma treatment. *Curr Opin Allergy Clin Immunol* 4, 63–67

British Thoracic Society, Scottish Intercollegiate Guidelines Network (SIGN) (2005) British guideline on the management of asthma. http://www.brit-thoracic.org.uk (accessed December 2007)

Corry DB (2002) Emerging immune targets for the therapy of allergic asthma. *Nat Rev Drug Discov* 1, 55–64

Foresi A, Paggiaro P (2003) Inhaled corticosteroids and leukotriene modifiers in the acute treatment of asthma exacerbations. *Curr Opin Pulm Med* 9, 52–56

Hamid Q, Tulic MK, Liu MC, Moqbel R (2003) Inflammatory cells in asthma: mechanisms and implications for therapy. *J Allergy Clin Immunol* 111(suppl), S5–S12; discussion S12–S17

Holgate ST, Polosa R (2006) The mechanisms, diagnosis and management of severe asthma in adults. *Lancet* 368, 780–793

Johnson M (2006) Molecular mechanisms of β_2 adrenergic receptor function, response and regulation. *J Allergy Clin Immunol* 117, 18–24

Kaiser HB (2004) Risk factors in allergy/asthma. *Allergy Asthma Proc* 25, 7–10

Lin H, Casale TB (2002) Treatment of allergic asthma. *Am J Med* 113(9A), 8s–16s

Lipworth BJ, Jackson CM (2002) Second-line controller therapy for persistent asthma uncontrolled on inhaled corticosteroids. *Drugs* 62, 2315–2332

Livingston M, Heaney LG, Ennis M (2004) Adenosine, inflammation and asthma – a review. *Inflamm Res* 53, 171–178

Luft C, Hausding M, Finotto S (2004) Regulation of T cells in asthma: implications for genetic manipulation. *Curr Opin Allergy Clin Immunol* 4, 69–74

Nayak A (2004) A review of montelukast in the treatment of asthma and allergic rhinitis. *Expert Opin Pharmacother* 3, 679–686

O'Byrne PM, Parameswaran K (2006) Pharmacological management of mild or moderate persistent asthma. *Lancet* 368, 794–803

Ormiston TM, Salpeter EE (2004) Respiratory tolerance to regular β_2-agonist use in patients with asthma. *Ann Intern Med* 140, 802–814

Prescott SL Dunstan JA (2005) Immune dysregulation in allergic respiratory disease: the role of T regulatory cells. *Pulm Pharmacol Ther* 18 217–228

Racke K, Juergens UR, Matthiesen S (2006) Control by cholinergic mechanisms. *Eur J Pharmacol* 533, 57–68

Rees J (2006) Asthma control in adults. *BMJ* 332, 767–771

Rodrigo GJ (2003) Inhaled therapy for acute adult asthma. *Curr Opin Allergy Clin Immunol* 32, 169–175

Rodrigo GJ, Rodrigo C (2002) The role of anticholinergics in acute asthma treatment: an evidence-based evaluation. *Chest* 121, 1977–1988

Rowe BH, Bretzlaff JA, Bourdon C, Bota GW, Camargo CA Jr (2000) Intravenous magnesium sulfate treatment for acute asthma in the emergency department: a systematic review of the literature. *Ann Emerg Med* 3, 6181–6190

Salpeter SR, Buckley NS, Ormiston TM, Salpeter EE (2006) Meta-analysis: effect of long-acting β-agonists on severe exacerbations and asthma-related deaths. *Ann Intern Med* 144, 904–912

Spina D (2003) Theophylline and PDE4 inhibitors in asthma. *Curr Opin Pulm Med* 9, 57–64

Szczeklik A, Stevenson DD (2003) Aspirin-induced asthma: advances in pathogenesis, diagnosis, and management. *J Allergy Clin Immunol* 111, 913–921

Szczeklik A, Sanak M, Nizankowska-Mogilnicka E, Kielbasa B (2004) Aspirin intolerance and the cyclooxygenase-leukotriene pathways. *Curr Opin Pulm Med* 10, 51–56

Vancheri C, Mastruzzo C, Sortino MA, Crimi N (2004) The lung as a privileged site for the beneficial actions of PGE2. *Trends Immunol* 25, 40–46

Vignola AM (2003) Effects of inhaled corticosteroids, leukotriene receptor antagonists, or both, plus long-acting beta2-agonists on asthma pathophysiology: a review of the evidence. *Drugs* 63(suppl 2), 35–51

Chronic obstructive pulmonary disease

Anzueto A (2006) Clinical course of chronic obstructive pulmonary disease: review of therapeutic interventions. *Am J Med* 119, S46–S53

Barcelo B, Pons J, Fuster A et al (2006) Intracellular cytokine profile of T lymphocytes in patients with chronic obstructive pulmonary disease. *Clin Exp Immunol* 145, 474–479

Barnes PJ (2002) Theophylline. New perspectives for an old drug. *Am J Respir Crit Care Med* 167, 813–818

Barnes PJ, Ito K, Adcock IM (2004) Corticosteroid resistance in chronic obstructive pulmonary disease: inactivation of histone deacetylase. *Lancet* 363, 731–733

Calverly PMA, Walker P (2003) Chronic obstructive pulmonary disease. *Lancet* 362, 1053–1061

Criner GJ (2007) Optimal treatment of chronic obstructive pulmonary disease: the search for the magic combination of inhaled bronchodilators and corticosteroids. *Ann Intern Med* 146, 606–608

Disse B (2001) Antimuscarinic treatment for lung diseases. From research to clinical practice. *Life Sci* 68, 2557–2564

Hansel T, Barnes P (2009) New drugs for exacerbations of chronic obstructive pulmonary disease. *Lancet* 374, 744–755

Knight DA, Holgate ST (2003) The airway epithelium: structural and functional properties in health and disease. *Respirology* 4, 432–446

Lipworth BJ (2005) Phosphodiesterase-4 inhibitors for asthma and chronic obstructive pulmonary disease. *Lancet*, 365, 167–175

MacNee W, Calverley PMA (2003) Chronic obstructive pulmonary disease 7: management of COPD. *Thorax* 58, 261–265

Man SPF, McAlister FA, Anthonisen NR et al (2003) Contemporary management of chronic obstructive pulmonary disease: clinical applications. *JAMA* 290, 2313–2316

Plant PK, Elliot MW (2003) Chronic obstructive pulmonary disease 9: management of ventilatory failure in COPD. *Thorax* 58, 537–542

Sin DD, McAlister FA, Man SPF et al (2003) Contemporary management of chronic obstructive pulmonary disease: scientific review. *JAMA* 290, 2301–2312

Singh JM, Palda VA, Stanbrook MB et al (2002) Corticosteroid therapy for patients with acute exacerbations of chronic obstructive pulmonary disease. *Arch Intern Med* 162, 2527–2536

Smit JJ Lukacs, NW (2006) The missing link: chemokine receptors and tissue matrix breakdown in COPD. *Trends Pharmcol Sci* 27, 555–557

Stoller JK (2002) Acute exacerbations of chronic obstructive pulmonary disease. *N Engl J Med* 346, 988–994

Sutherland ER, Cherniak RM (2004) Management of chronic obstructive pulmonary disease. *N Engl J Med* 350, 2689–2697

Wilt J, Niewoehner D, MacDonald R et al (2007) Management of stable chronic obstructive pulmonary disease: a systematic review for a clinical practice guideline. *Ann Intern Med* 147, 639–653

Wilt J, Weinberger S, Shekelle P et al (2007) Diagnosis and management of stable chronic obstructive pulmonary disease: a clinical practice guideline from the American College of Physicians. *Ann Intern Med* 147, 633–638

SELF-ASSESSMENT

In the questions 1–8, the first statement, in italics, is correct. Are the accompanying statements also true?

1. *In people with asthma, an inherited tendency to develop allergy or airway hyperresponsiveness is exacerbated by allergens, irritants, infection and smoking.*
   a. An influx of Th2 lymphocytes occurs in the late phase of response following an asthmatic attack.
   b. Leukotriene C_4 is an important bronchodilator released from eosinophils.
2. *Exercise-induced asthma appears to involve only the immediate (early)-phase response.* The β_2-adrenoceptor agonists are effective in preventing exercise-induced asthma.
3. *After recovery from the bronchospasm that follows an acute attack of asthma, increased hyperreactivity and inflammation can last for weeks.* The late-phase response is characterised by bronchial muscle hyperresponsiveness but normal epithelial cell morphology.
4. *In addition to their bronchodilator action, β_2-adrenoceptor agonists enhance mucus clearance by acting on cilia.* Tolerance to β_2-adrenoceptor agonists can occur.
5. *The mechanism of the bronchodilator action of the methylxanthines is unclear but may include inhibition of phosphodiesterases and antagonism at adenosine receptors.*
   a. The plasma concentration of theophylline is increased by simultaneous administration of erythromycin or ciprofloxacin.
   b. Methylxanthines cause drowsiness.
   c. An unwanted effect of theophylline is stimulation of the heart.
6. *The muscarinic receptor antagonist ipratropium can be given in combination with a β_2-adrenoceptor agonist and a corticosteroid.*
   a. Ipratropium is more effective than salbutamol for preventing bronchospasm following challenge with an allergen.
   b. Ipratropium causes bradycardia.
   c. Ipratropium is poorly absorbed from the bronchi into the systemic circulation.
7. *Leukotriene C_4 may be important in the precipitation of asthma in people who are intolerant to aspirin.*
   a. Montelukast inhibits the lipoxygenase enzymes that convert arachidonic acid to leukotrienes.
   b. The leukotriene antagonists are only effective if given prophylactically.
8. *Glucocorticoids are ineffective in the treatment of the early-phase response in an asthmatic attack.* Glucocorticoids reduce dendritic cell signalling to T-cells, T-cell cytokine production and eosinophil deposition in bronchial mucosa.
9. Extended-matching questions
   Which is the **most appropriate** option A–H for add-on treatment to the current medication that is being prescribed in each case scenario (9.1–9.5)?
   A. Ipratropium
   B. Ciprofloxacin
   C. Salmeterol
   D. A spacer
   E. Modified-release theophylline
   F. Intravenous magnesium sulphate
   G. Oral prednisolone
   H. Modified-release theophylline.

9.1. A 25-year-old woman was admitted to A&E with an acute exacerbation of her asthma. Her peak expiratory flow rate was 150 L min^{-1}. Her pulse rate was 145 beats min^{-1}, her respiratory rate was 30 min^{-1}, respiration was shallow and she was confused. She was treated with 60% oxygen, nebulised salbutamol, nebulised ipratropium, intravenous aminophylline and intravenous hydrocortisone. Arterial blood gases on admission, breathing air, showed a $P\text{O}_2$ of 8.4 kPa, $P\text{CO}_2$ 7.2 kPa and pH 7.29. There was little clinical improvement and she was transferred to the intensive care unit.

9.2. A 64-year-old man had mild asthma that was well controlled taking salbutamol two to three times a week and inhaled beclometasone twice daily. He complained of soreness of the mouth and hoarseness and was advised about oral hygiene.

9.3. A 67-year-old man had COPD with a chronic cough producing clear sputum. The cough and sputum production had not recently changed. He had stopped smoking 3 months ago because of his dyspnoea. Prior to that time, he had smoked 20 cigarettes a day for 50 years. He denied alcohol use. He had no other significant medical illnesses. His FEV_1 was 1.34 (about 45% of that predicted). He was taking salbutamol four times daily. A trial of inhaled beclometasone 3 months previously had provided no benefit and had been stopped.

9.4. A 60-year-old woman attended the A&E department with increasing shortness of breath, increased production of green–yellow sputum and fever over the previous 4 days. She was known to have COPD. She was taking daily salbutamol and ipratropium by breath-activated inhalers.

9.5. A 30-year-old man had mild asthma and allergic rhinitis. He was taking inhaled salbutamol and beclometasone, both twice daily. Recently he had been waking most nights with a persistent cough. He was a non-smoker and had no other medical history.

10. Extended-matching questions

Which is the **most appropriate** option A–G that relates to the statements 10.1–10.5? The choice of options A–G must be used once only.

A. Theophylline
B. Celecoxib
C. Prostaglandin $F_{2\alpha}$
D. Salbutamol
E. Montelukast
F. Aspirin
G. Leukotriene B_4

10.1. Increases the synthesis of cAMP
10.2. Decreases the breakdown of cAMP
10.3. Results in an increase in the synthesis of leukotriene C_4/D_4 in sensitive asthmatics
10.4. Inhibits NSAID-induced bronchoconstriction
10.5. Causes bronchoconstriction

11. Which one of the following is the **most appropriate** description of an unwanted effect of high-dose salbutamol?

A. Bradycardia
B. Hypokalaemia
C. Hypoglycaemia
D. Mydriasis
E. Constipation

ANSWERS

1. a. **True**. This is particularly important and the Th2 cells are involved in the generation of cytokines that promote activation of eosinophils and expression of IgE receptors on mast cells and eosinophils. The Th2 cells also express endothelial adhesion molecules that attract eosinophils.
   b. **False**. Leukotriene C_4 is a bronchoconstrictor, increasing mucus secretion and oedema.
2. **True**. Salbutamol is effective taken before exercise but the longer-acting β_2-adrenoceptor agonists are slower in onset. Cromoglicate taken prophylactically may also be effective.
3. **False**. Hyperreactivity of airways is seen but epithelial cells show variable damage.
4. **True**. There is evidence of tolerance to β_2-adrenoceptor agonists; the development of tolerance can be reduced by administration of corticosteroids.
5. a. **True**. Erythromycin and ciprofloxacin inhibit liver cytochrome P450 enzymes, which metabolise theophylline.
   b. **False**. The methylxanthines (present in coffee) increase alertness and can cause irritability and headache.
   c. **True**. All methylxanthines have positive inotropic and chronotropic activity and a narrow therapeutic index.
6. a. **False**. Ipratropium is less effective against allergen challenge but can be useful as an adjunct and in the management of COPD.
   b. **False**. Ipratropium can cause a modest tachycardia owing to blockade of muscarinic receptors in the heart.
   c. **True**. Ipratropium has a quaternary structure and, therefore, is poorly absorbed.
7. a. **False**. Montelukast inhibits receptors for the cysteinyl leukotrienes (C_4, D_4, E_4).
   b. **True**. The leukotriene antagonists need to be administered orally on a regular prophylactic basis to reduce asthma attacks. They are much less effective once an attack has started.
8. **True**. Glucocorticoids affect several steps in the inflammatory pathways involved in the genesis of asthma.
9. Extended-matching answers

   9.1. Answer **F**. This woman is being treated according to the British Thoracic Society Guidelines. An appropriate add-on medication that has been added to the guidelines recently for use in life-threatening situations is intravenous magnesium sulphate.

   9.2. Answer **D**. This man should additionally be advised to use a spacer with all inhaled drugs. This improves the effectiveness of the medication and will reduce deposition of corticosteroids in the mouth and oropharynx, reducing the occurrence of fungal growth and hoarseness.

9.3. Answer **A**. The antimuscarinic drug ipratropium provides equal or greater benefit to β_2-adrenoceptor agonists in COPD and will reduce the volume of sputum produced. Corticosteroids are of modest benefit in only a small percentage of patients with COPD.

9.4. Answer **B**. This woman has an infection-related exacerbation of her COPD and should be treated with an appropriate antibiotic. Nebulised salbutamol and ipratropium should also be started.

9.5. Answer **C**. Approximately 80% of severe asthmatic attacks occur between midnight and 8 a.m. Salbutamol is a short-acting β_2-adrenoceptor agonist, providing relief for 2–6 h. A trial of salmeterol or formoterol, which provide bronchodilation for 12 h or longer, should be considered. The long-acting drugs should not be used for relief of acute asthma episodes.

10. Extended-matching answers

10.1. Answer **D**. Salbutamol acts selectively on the β_2-adrenoceptors in airways, which are coupled to G-protein-linked receptors, and its bronchodilator action results from the cellular events following the increase in cAMP.

10.2. Answer **A**. Theophylline inhibits the breakdown of cAMP by phosphodiesterases.

10.3. Answer **F**. Aspirin can induce bronchoconstriction in a subset of sensitive asthmatics (as many as one in five). This results from inhibition of COX-1-generated prostaglandin E_2, which normally inhibits the formation of the bronchoconstrictor leukotriene C_4/D_4. Celecoxib, which is a selective COX-2-inhibiting NSAID, does not have this effect, but should still be used with care in asthmatics.

10.4. Answer **E**. Montelukast selectively inhibits receptors for the bronchoconstrictor cysteinyl leukotrienes $C_4/D_4/E_4$.

10.5. Answer **C**. Prostaglandin $F_{2\alpha}$ is a bronchoconstrictor and asthmatics are more sensitive to its action.

11. Answer **B**. Salbutamol is a β_2-adrenoceptor agonist and produces hypokalaemia and also, at higher doses, tachycardia, hypomagnesaemia and hyperglycaemia.

Drugs used to treat asthma or chronic obstructive pulmonary disease (COPD)

Drug	Half-life[a] (h) and kinetics	Comment
β-Adrenoceptor agonists		
Bambuterol	8–22 [M] Long-acting prodrug hydrolysed by pseudocholinesterase (butyrylcholinesterase, plasma cholinesterase) to terbutaline, which has a half-life of 14–18 h	Not recommended for children; given orally
Ephedrine	6 [R + M] High oral bioavailability; eliminated largely by renal excretion; metabolised to norephedrine, which has central stimulant effects	Direct- + indirect-acting sympathomimetic; given orally
Fenoterol	6–7 [M + R] Eliminated by conjugation with sulphate	Given by inhalation in combination with ipratropium
Formoterol	2–3 [M] Eliminated largely by glucuronidation	Given by dry-powder inhalation; duration of action in airways exceeds the elimination half-life
Orciprenaline	6 [M] Has a low oral bioavailability (about 10%); eliminated by conjugation with glucuronic acid	The 3,4-dihydroxy isomer of the old, non-selective drug isoprenaline; given orally
Salbutamol	4–6 [R+ M] Eliminated by conjugation with sulphate	Given by inhalation, orally, intravenously or subcutaneously
Salmeterol	3–5 [M] Extensively oxidised; metabolite retains some activity	Given by inhalation; long-acting
Terbutaline	14–18 [R + M] Eliminated by glomerular filtration and by conjugation with sulphate	Given by inhalation, orally, intravenously or subcutaneously
Antimuscarinics		
Ipratropium	4 [R + M] Little drug enters the circulation after inhalation and most is swallowed and not absorbed from the gut; the absorbed fraction is eliminated by the kidneys and hydrolysis	Given by inhalation for short-term relief in asthma and for COPD

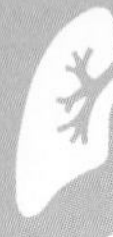

Drugs used to treat asthma or chronic obstructive pulmonary disease (COPD)

Drug	Half-life[a] (h) and kinetics	Comment
Tiotropium	5–6 days [R] The small amounts of drug that enter the circulation after inhalation are eliminated in the urine	Given by inhalation for COPD; not recommended for children
Methylxanthines		
Aminophylline	Minutes [M] Very rapidly broken down by hydrolysis to constituents	Water-soluble mixture of theophylline and ethylenediamine; given orally or by injection
Theophylline	1–13 [M + some R] Metabolised by CYP1A2, which is induced by smoking; half-life is shorter in children than in adults	Given orally
Corticosteroids		
Given by inhalation (see Ch. 44 for corticosteroids such as prednisolone and hydrocortisone which are given orally or by intravenous injection in the treatment of asthma); high-dose preparations are not recommended for children		
Beclometasone dipropionate	15 [M] Hydrolysed rapidly by esterases to the 17-monopropionate, which is almost 30 times more potent, or 21-monopropionate, which is inactive	Inhaled using aerosol or powder formulation; standard- and high-dose preparations available
Budesonide	2 [M] Metabolites are inactive; oral bioavailability is about 10%	Inhaled using aerosol or powder formulation
Ciclesonide	0.7 [M] Metabolised in lung to active metabolite which is metabolised by hepatic CYP3A4 and has a half-life of 7 h	Prodrug; inhaled using powder formulation
Fluticasone propionate	3 [M] Oxidised by liver to inactive acid metabolite, which is excreted in bile; any swallowed dose undergoes 100% first-pass inactivation	Inhaled using aerosol or powder formulation
Mometasone furoate	5 [M] Metabolised by CYP3A4-mediated oxidation to multiple metabolites that are eliminated in bile	Originally used as a topical corticosteroid in dermatology; inhaled using powder formulation; not recommended for children
Cromones		
Highly polar molecules that are slowly absorbed from sites of deposition in the airways		
Nedocromil sodium	2 [R] High polarity gives slow absorption from lung; negligible absorption from gut, and oral half-life is 23 h because of absorption rate-limited kinetics	Similar to cromoglicate
Sodium cromoglicate	1–1.5 [R] High polarity gives slow absorption from lung; negligible absorption from gut	Given by inhalation
Leukotriene activity modulators		
Montelukast	3–5 [M] Good oral bioavailability (about 70%); oxidised by hepatic CYP3A4 and CYP2C9	Antagonist of LTD_4 at the cysteinyl leukotriene receptor found in the human airway; given orally at bedtime
Zafirlukast	10 [M] Believed to undergo extensive first-pass metabolism; metabolised by CYP2C9; inhibits CYP3A4 and CYP2C9	Inhibits the binding of LTD_4 and LTE_4, at the cysteinyl leukotriene receptor; given orally; not recommended for children under 12 years
Anti-IgE antibody		
Omalizumab	22 days [M] Eliminated by very slow turnover/recycling of immunoglobulins	Binds to the high-affinity Fc receptor of human IgE and prevents the binding of IgE to cells associated with the allergic response; given by subcutaneous injection
Other agents		
Ketotifen	22 [M] Oral bioavailability is about 50%; eliminated by oxidation and also by conjugation with glucuronic acid	An antihistamine with actions similar to cromoglicate, and which has proved to be of limited value in asthma

[a]The half-life refers to the systemic elimination half-life from the general circulation, which may not correlate with the duration of action following inhalation, when this is dependent on very slow uptake from the airways.
[M], metabolism; [R], renal excretion.

13 Respiratory disorders: cough, respiratory stimulants, cystic fibrosis and neonatal respiratory distress syndrome

COUGH

Cough is a protective mechanism for the airways that removes excessive mucus, abnormal substances such as fluid or pus, or inhaled foreign material from the upper airways. Cough is under both voluntary and involuntary control.

The cough reflex is initiated by irritant receptors located at the epithelial surface of the airway mucosa, which can be activated by either chemical or mechanical stimuli. These receptors have been identified at and below the oropharynx in the large airways, and are probably present in the external auditory canals and tympanic membrane in the ear, as well as in other sites such as the oesophagus and stomach. Rapidly adapting receptors that respond mainly to mechanical stimuli may be of primary importance in eliciting the cough reflex. Neuropeptides are produced by the mechanosensitive neurons following viral infection or allergen challenge, and probably sensitise the cough reflex.

Afferent fibres from these receptors in the airways travel in the vagus and superior laryngeal nerves to the medullary 'cough network' in the region of the nucleus tractus solitarius. Neuronal pathways connect the network to the respiratory pattern generator, from where efferent fibres travel in somatic nerves to respiratory muscles. Projections from the cerebral cortex to the medulla can also initiate cough or modulate the cough reflex.

Several mediators are involved in the cough reflex pathways in the medulla. One proposed model is that the afferent input to the cough centre is via glutamatergic neurons that stimulate NMDA (N-methyl-D-aspartate) receptors. These neurons can be inhibited by presynaptic serotonergic nerve synapses via serotonin type 1 (5-HT_1) receptors. Opioids facilitate the inhibitory action of the serotonergic neurons through further interneuronal connections. The complexity of these pathways is illustrated by the number of mediators and antagonists that can experimentally initiate or inhibit cough. Selective opioids such as κ- and δ-opioid receptor agonists, tachykinin receptor antagonists, bradykinin receptor antagonists, and vanilloid receptor (TRPV1) antagonists all have potential as future antitussives.

A cough is initiated by a rapid inspiration followed by brief closure of the glottis. Forced expiration against the closed glottis raises intrathoracic pressure, and sudden opening of the glottis expels air together with secretions and debris. Flow rates can approach the speed of sound, producing vibration of upper airway structures and the typical sound of cough.

Cough has several diverse causes (Box 13.1). In some situations, a cough is unproductive and has no useful function. An ineffective cough may result from respiratory muscle weakness, or when the mucus on the airway wall is thick and more adhesive. In other situations, a cough can be considered useful, clearing excess secretions or inhaled foreign matter. An effective cough that can clear the airway depends on the ability to generate high airflow.

There are two clinical categories of cough: acute, lasting less than 3 weeks, and chronic. Acute cough is most often caused by the common cold. Chronic productive cough is usually related to smoking or bronchiectasis, while the most common causes of a non-productive cough in non-smokers are upper airway cough syndrome (also called post-nasal drip syndrome), asthma and gastro-oesophageal reflux disease.

DRUGS FOR TREATMENT OF COUGH

Antitussives (cough suppressants)

Cough suppressants fall into three classes.

Centrally acting drugs (opioids)

These increase the threshold for stimulation of neurons in the medullary cough centre, and are thought to modulate a gating mechanism in the brain, analogous to that identified for pain reception. They are most effective for cough arising from the lower airways. Weak opioid analgesics (Ch. 19) are most commonly used, especially codeine and pholcodine; they are less addictive than morphine, which should be reserved for terminal conditions. Dextromethorphan is structurally related to opioids, but is a glutamate NMDA receptor antagonist that has no analgesic or sedative activity but does have antitussive properties.

Peripherally acting drugs

Local anaesthetics such as lidocaine (Ch. 18) are used as an oropharyngeal spray to reduce cough during bronchoscopy. Antihistamines (Ch. 39) reduce post-nasal drip from allergic rhinitis, which can stimulate cough, but probably

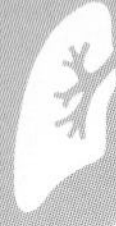

Box 13.1 Common causes of cough

Acute respiratory infection
- Upper respiratory tract infection
- Pneumonia, including aspiration

Chronic respiratory infection
- Cystic fibrosis
- Bronchiectasis
- Post-nasal drip (upper airway cough syndrome)

Airway disease
- Asthma
- Chronic obstructive pulmonary disease

Parenchymal lung disease
- Interstitial fibrosis

Irritant
- Cigarette smoke
- Inhaled foreign body

Bronchopulmonary malignancy

Drug-induced
- Angiotensin-converting enzyme inhibitors
- Inhaled drugs

have little direct antitussive activity. Sedative antihistamines (Ch. 39), such as diphenhydramine, are commonly used in compound cough preparations on sale to the public.

Locally acting drugs

Demulcents line the surface of the airway above the larynx, reducing local irritation. The syrup in simple linctus acts by this mechanism.

Expectorants and mucolytics

Expectorants such as guaifenesin and squill are often included in compound cough preparations on sale to the public, with the intention of improving clearance of mucus from the airways. There is no evidence of clinical value.

Mucolytics such as mecysteine hydrochloride, erdosteine and carbocisteine can be given orally to reduce the viscosity of bronchial secretions by breaking disulphide cross-linking between molecules. Mucolytics are occasionally useful in chronic obstructive pulmonary disease (Ch. 12) and bronchiectasis.

MANAGEMENT OF COUGH

An acute cough should be treated only if it is unproductive or excessive. A self-limiting non-productive acute cough, such as that caused by a viral illness, can be suppressed by simple linctus or a weak opioid. Any cough of unknown origin that is still present after 14 days should be investigated further to identify an underlying cause.

For chronic cough, non-specific therapy has a limited role, since it should be possible to identify and treat the cause. Specific treatment for left ventricular failure, asthma, upper airway cough syndrome (with an antihistamine and a decongestant) or gastro-oesophageal reflux disease should eliminate the cough associated with those conditions. Cough is a common unwanted effect of angiotensin-converting enzyme (ACE) inhibitors (Ch. 6) and occurs in up to 15% of people who take them. It sometimes appears soon after starting treatment, but can arise after several months. The cough may improve with a reduction in drug dosage, but changing to another class of drug is usually necessary to eliminate the cough.

When symptomatic therapy is required for cough, there are few options. Opioids are most useful for chronic non-productive cough in terminal lung cancer. Mucolytics may make clearance of mucus easier, but are probably no more effective than hydration from inhaling steam or nebulised hypertonic saline. The value of mucolytics in chronic bronchitis is uncertain, but they may be useful in chronic obstructive pulmonary disease (Ch. 12). Mucolytics do not improve lung function in cystic fibrosis.

RESPIRATORY STIMULANTS (ANALEPTIC DRUGS)

Doxapram has a limited place in the short-term treatment of ventilatory failure, particularly in hypercapnoeic respiratory failure due to chronic obstructive pulmonary disease which is causing drowsiness. It increases respiratory drive and arousal, and improves both rate and depth of ventilation. When combined with physiotherapy, doxapram may encourage coughing and clearance of excessive secretions. However, its use has largely been superseded by non-invasive ventilatory support, such as with nasal intermittent positive pressure ventilation. There is also a minor role for doxapram to reverse postoperative respiratory depression. Doxapram stimulates the medullary respiratory centre both by a direct action and by peripheral stimulation of the carotid body. Given by intravenous injection, its action is very brief, owing to rapid metabolism by the liver, and a continuous infusion is often used. Restlessness, muscle twitching and vomiting are common unwanted effects, and seizures can occur due to generalised stimulation of the central nervous system.

Acetazolamide (Ch. 14) is an inhibitor of carbonic anhydrase that stimulates the respiratory centre by creating a mild metabolic acidosis. This action may contribute to its ability to reduce the headache, nausea, vomiting and lethargy of acute mountain sickness by decreasing periodic nocturnal apnoea and maintaining arterial oxygen saturation. Use of acetazolamide is not a substitute for gradual acclimatisation to altitude.

CYSTIC FIBROSIS

Cystic fibrosis is an autosomal recessive disorder caused by a single gene mutation on the long arm of chromosome 7. This gene encodes the cystic fibrosis transmembrane conductance regulator (CFTR), a Cl^- and HCO_3^- channel in epithelial cell membranes. The negative ions are accompanied by paracellular diffusion of Na^+ and water, creating a fluid secretion from the cell. If the *CFTR* gene is faulty, then the function of the transporter is impaired or absent and Cl^- transport is defective in epithelial cells in many organs, including the respiratory, hepatobiliary, gastrointestinal and reproductive tracts and the pancreas. As a result of the defective electrolyte flows, secretions become thicker. This causes obstruction in (and destruction of) exocrine glandular ducts, and clogs respiratory cilia with mucus. Over 1500 *CFTR* gene mutations have already been identified (although about 15 of these account for more than 75% of clinical cases), but even a single type of mutation produces different severities of disease, suggesting that there is involvement of other genes and/or environmental factors.

In cystic fibrosis there is a sustained and exaggerated inflammatory response to infection in the lung, the reasons for which are not fully understood. The lung becomes colonised with bacteria that are impossible to eradicate. A chronic inflammatory response is established in the airway both in response to, and independently of, the infection.

The most common clinical consequences in cystic fibrosis are lung disease (bronchiectasis and chronic airflow obstruction) and pancreatic exocrine insufficiency leading to malabsorption. These problems affect about 90% of those with the gene defect. About 20% develop pancreatic endocrine insufficiency with insulin-dependent diabetes and a smaller number develop meconium ileus in infancy or obstructive biliary tract disease. Death in 90% of people with cystic fibrosis is due to progressive lung disease, but median survival is now over 30 years due to improved treatment.

Drug treatment of cystic fibrosis

Much of the treatment for cystic fibrosis is supportive, including physiotherapy and regular inhaled antibacterial drugs to reduce exacerbations of lung disease, and intensive antibacterial therapy for exacerbations of lung disease. Nebulised hypertonic saline improves mucociliary clearance, and reduces the frequency of infective exacerbations: it can sometimes produce bronchospasm, which can be prevented by prior use of an inhaled β_2-adrenoceptor agonist such as salbutamol (Ch. 12). Nutritional supplements are important because of the frequency of fat malabsorption.

Prevention of infection (and cross-infection), particularly during hospital admission, is important, and improved treatment of infection is the main reason for the prolongation of life expectancy in recent years. *Staphylococcus aureus* and *Haemophilus influenzae* are common pathogens in the very young person with cystic fibrosis, while *Burkholderia cepacia* and *Burkholderia dolosa* are particularly virulent pathogens. In the early years of life, anti-staphylococcal therapy is usually appropriate for exacerbations of lung disease (Ch. 51). By adolescence, *Pseudomonas aeruginosa* becomes the predominant pathogen, and is treated with intravenous or nebulised antibacterials. Nebulised tobramycin or colistimethate sodium, perhaps combined with oral ciprofloxacin, are increasingly used in this age group and subsequently (Ch. 51). It is almost impossible to eradicate *P. aeruginosa* from sputum, but rapid and intensive treatment of clinical infection slows the decline in lung function.

Since inflammation is a major component of the airway disease, several anti-inflammatory therapies have been studied. Oral corticosteroids (Ch. 44) reduce the rate of decline in lung function and reduce the frequency of infections, but unwanted effects preclude their long-term use. Inhaled corticosteroid does not improve lung function unless there is associated airway hyperreactivity. There are several pharmacological interventions under investigation for improving the conductance of the defective Cl^- channel in cystic fibrosis, but none has yet been shown to improve the long-term outcome of the lung disease.

In addition to antibacterial treatment of respiratory infection, current therapies for respiratory and gastrointestinal symptoms of cystic fibrosis include the following.

Dornase alfa (recombinant human deoxyribonuclease I; rhDNase I)

This enzyme can digest extracellular DNA. DNA released from dying polymorphonuclear neutrophils in the airways contributes to the increased sputum viscosity in cystic fibrosis. Dornase alfa is given by inhalation using a jet nebuliser (see Ch. 12), and is probably most effective when given on alternate days. It reduces sputum viscoelasticity, improves lung function in the short- to medium-term (although long-term benefits are much less certain), and results in fewer exacerbations of lung disease. Unwanted effects include transient pharyngitis and hoarseness. Currently, use of dornase alfa is usually confined to those with reduced lung function (but forced vital capacity preserved at greater than 40% of predicted) and chronic sputum production who require regular courses of intravenous antibacterials for recurrent chest infections, but there is also benefit in people with more severe lung disease. Improved lung function should be measurable after 2 weeks in responders.

Pancreatic enzyme supplements (pancreatin)

Pancreatin consists of protease, lipase and amylase, which are inactivated by gastric acid and by heat. Supplements, therefore, must be taken with food (but not mixed with very hot food), and either concurrently with gastric acid suppression therapy (e.g. with cimetidine; Ch. 33) or as enteric-coated formulations. Pancreatin preparations in clinical use are of porcine origin. Dosage is adjusted according to the size, number and consistency of stools. Unwanted effects include irritation of the mouth and perianal skin, nausea, vomiting and abdominal discomfort. Some higher-strength formulations should be avoided in children under 15 years of age with cystic fibrosis, since they have been associated with the formation of large bowel strictures.

Ursodeoxycholic acid

This synthetic bile acid (see Ch. 36) improves abnormal liver function tests in those with cystic fibrosis by improving bile acid flow, and by increasing the bicarbonate content of bile. It is not known whether this prevents progressive liver disease in the small group for whom this is a significant problem.

NEONATAL RESPIRATORY DISTRESS SYNDROME

Pulmonary surfactant is responsible for reducing surface tension at the air–liquid interface in the alveoli, preventing lung collapse at resting lung pressures. Surfactant is a macromolecular complex largely composed of phospholipids, mainly phosphatidylcholine (of which dipalmitoylphosphatidylcholine is the major surface-active component),

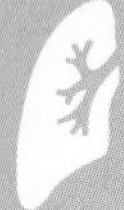

neutral lipids and surfactant-specific proteins. The phospholipid monolayer stabilises the lungs and prevents end-expiratory alveolar collapse by reducing the deflating force in the alveolus. The hydrophobic surfactant proteins B and C are critical for adsorption and spreading of the surfactant layer at the air–liquid interface. The hydrophilic surfactant proteins A and D are involved in surfactant metabolism and host defence.

Surfactant is synthesised by epithelial cells lining the alveoli and is normally present in substantial amounts at full term delivery. However, preterm infants may produce too little surfactant, leading to neonatal respiratory distress syndrome.

Mortality is high in neonatal respiratory distress syndrome, but it can be reduced by administration of surfactant via an endotracheal tube into the lung. There are two natural agents: beractant (bovine lung extract) and poractant alfa (porcine lung phospholipid fraction), which do not however retain the surfactant proteins A and D. New synthetic compounds with peptides that mimic the natural surfactant proteins are under clinical development. The potential advantages of a synthetic compound include easier production and elimination of the infection risk associated with animal products.

The use of a surfactant in neonatal respiratory distress syndrome reduces the risk of death by 40%, whether the treatment is given prophylactically or as a rescue treatment. There is also a reduced risk of pneumothorax and of subsequent chronic lung disease. Surfactant is given as soon as possible after delivery to infants with neonatal respiratory distress syndrome, or to those considered to be at risk of developing it.

In women at risk of preterm delivery, a corticosteroid such as dexamethasone will increase the production of surfactant in the fetal lung, which may prevent neonatal respiratory distress syndrome (Ch. 45).

FURTHER READING

Cough

Bolser DC (2006) Current and future centrally acting antitussives. *Resp Physiol Neurobiol* 152, 349–355

Chang AB (2006) The physiology of cough. *Paediatr Resp Rev* 7, 2–8

Chung KF (2003) Current and future prospects for drugs to suppress cough. *Drugs* 6, 781–786

Dicpinigaitis PV (2006) Current and future peripherally-acting antitussives. *Respir Physiol Neurobiol* 152, 356–362

Fox AJ (1996) Modulation of cough and airway sensory fibres. *Pulm Pharmacol* 9, 335–342

Irwin RS, Baumann MH, Bolser DC et al (2006) Diagnosis and management of cough. *Chest* 129, 1S–23S

Irwin RS, Madison JM (2000) Primary care: the diagnosis and treatment of cough. *N Engl J Med* 343, 1715–1721

Reynolds SM, Mackenzie AJ, Spina D, Page CP (2004) The pharmacology of cough. *Trends Pharmacol Sci* 25, 569–576

Cystic fibrosis

Boyle MP (2007) Adult cystic fibrosis. *JAMA* 298, 1787–1793

Davies JC, Alton EWFW, Bush A (2007) Cystic fibrosis. *BMJ* 335, 1255–1259

Elborn JS (2006) Practical management of cystic fibrosis. *Chron Resp Dis* 3, 161–165

Lukacs GL, Durie PR (2003) Pharmacological approaches to correcting the basic defect in cystic fibrosis. *N Engl J Med* 349, 1401–1404

Ratjen F, Döring G (2003) Cystic fibrosis. *Lancet* 361, 681–689

Rowe SM, Clancy JP (2006) Advance in cystic fibrosis therapies. *Curr Opin Pediatr* 18, 604–613

Neonatal respiratory distress syndrome

Curstedt T, Johansson J (2005) New synthetic surfactants – basic science. *Biol Neonate* 87, 332–337

Pfister RH, Soll RF (2005) New synthetic surfactants: the next generation? *Biol Neonate* 87, 338–344

Whitsett JA, Weaver TE (2002) Mechanisms of disease: hydrophobic surfactant proteins in lung function and disease. *N Engl J Med* 347, 2142–2148

SELF-ASSESSMENT

In questions 1 and 2, the first statements, in italics, are correct. Are the accompanying statements also true?

1. *Postviral cough can last for 3–6 weeks. Treatment should include increased humidity of inspired air and cough suppressants. Other drugs are of little value.*
   a. Many compound cough preparations sold over the counter contain sedating antihistamines.
   b. Dextromethorphan is a synthetic opioid used as a cough suppressant, but has no analgesic action.
2. *There is little evidence that any preparation can specifically facilitate expectoration; they may serve a useful placebo function.*
   a. Pulmonary surfactant increases surface tension in the alveoli.
   b. Doxapram should not be used in postoperative respiratory failure.
   c. The mucolytic mecysteine acts by inhibiting the production of mucus.
3. Choose the one **correct** statement from the following, concerning cough.
   A. Angiotensin receptor antagonists cause coughs.
   B. Guaifenesin inhibits cough-reflex sensitivity.
   C. All opioids are equally effective as cough suppressants.
   D. Dextromethorphan has similar unwanted effects to the opioid codeine.

E. Antitussives are effective in the treatment of acute cough.

ANSWERS

1. a. **True**. Diphenhydramine and chlorpheniramine are common constituents of compound cough mixtures.
   b. **True**. Dextromethorphan has the same cough suppressant potency as codeine but is not analgesic.
2. a. **False**. Surfactant acts like a detergent and lowers the surface tension, enabling the alveoli to expand and retain an expanded shape.
   b. **False**. Doxapram is used in hospitals for postoperative respiratory failure. It stimulates the respiratory centre and the carotid chemoreceptors, but its precise mode of action is unknown.
   c. **False**. Mecysteine breaks the disulphide cross-bridges that maintain the polymeric gel-like structure of mucus.
3. Answer **B**.
   A. Incorrect. Angiotensin receptor antagonists do not cause cough. Inhibition of angiotensin-converting enzyme (ACE), which reduces the formation of angiotensin II, also prevents the breakdown of bradykinin and this increases coughing. ACE inhibitors may also increase substance P and thromboxane, which are implicated in cough.
   B. Correct. Guaifenesin is included in many cough remedies and is particularly useful in the treatment of dry cough.
   C. Incorrect. Opioids vary widely in their abilities to suppress cough.
   D. Incorrect. Dextromethorphan has none of the analgesic, sedative, or respiratory depressive properties associated with the opioids.
   E. Incorrect. The Cochrane database states that there is no good evidence that antitussives are useful in acute cough.

Drugs used to treat respiratory disorders

Drug	Half-life (h) and kinetics	Comment
Cough suppressants		
All drugs given below are opioid derivatives (see Ch. 19 and its compendium for details); usually given orally as a linctus. Sedating antihistamines (Ch. 39) are also sometimes given for their cough suppressant actions		
Codeine	3–4 [M]	Use is associated with constipation
Dextromethorphan	3 [M + R] Extensive first-pass metabolism; metabolised by oxidation to dextrorphan, which is a non-opioid cough suppressant, and by glucuronidation	Fewer unwanted effects than codeine; not used as an analgesic
Methadone	6–8 [M + R]	Used mainly in palliative care for the distressing cough of terminal lung cancer (used less than other opioids)
Morphine	1–5 [M + R]	Used in palliative care for the distressing cough of terminal lung cancer
Pholcodine	32–43 [M + R] Slowly eliminated owing to very high apparent volume of distribution (50 L kg^{-1}) rather than low clearance, which is largely due to hepatic metabolism	Fewer unwanted effects than codeine
Mucolytics		
Given orally		
Carbocisteine	? [M + R] Good oral absorption; eliminated unchanged and as metabolites in urine	
Dornase alfa	Few data available Measurable concentrations have not been found in the blood after inhalation administration; activity in sputum is measurable for at least 6 h	Recombinant human deoxyribonuclease preparation used for cystic fibrosis; given by inhalation of a nebulised solution
Erdosteine	? [M] Undergoes first-pass metabolism to an active metabolite(s) containing a thiol (-SH) group	
Mecysteine	? [M + R] Few kinetic data available	

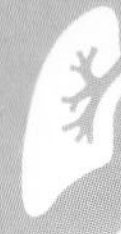

Drugs used to treat respiratory disorders

Drug	Half-life (h) and kinetics	Comment
Pulmonary surfactants		
Used for respiratory distress in preterm infants		
Beractant	No human kinetic data available; the apparent half-life of the natural surfactant (phosphatidylglycerol) is about 30 h	Given by endotracheal tube; activity occurs at the alveolar surface without systemic absorption; respiratory distress syndrome may enhance permeability and uptake
Poractant alfa	See beractant	See beractant
Respiratory stimulants		
Given only under expert supervision		
Doxapram	2–4 [M] Metabolised by oxidation in the liver; the keto metabolite is less active than the parent drug but is eliminated more slowly	Given by intravenous injection (over 30 s) or by continuous intravenous infusion

[M], metabolism; [R], renal excretion.

4

The renal system

14 Diuretics

FUNCTIONS OF THE KIDNEY

The kidney has several important functions:

- regulation of plasma electrolyte concentrations and fluid balance
- regulation of acid–base balance
- elimination of waste products
- conservation of essential nutrients.

Of these, a basic knowledge of the mechanisms of electrolyte and fluid handling by the kidney is essential for understanding the uses and the unwanted effects of diuretics.

Diuretics are drugs that act on the kidney to increase the tubular concentration and elimination of Na^+ ions. This can be useful in the management of a wide range of conditions that produce oedema (e.g. heart failure, cirrhosis of the liver and nephrotic syndrome) and for the treatment of hypertension.

The kidney and maintenance of salt and water balance

Each day the renal glomeruli of a healthy adult filter about 180 L of fluid, together with its content of ions such as Na^+, K^+ and Cl^-. Since the urine output is only 1–2 L in 24 h, it is clear that most of the filtered fluid and solutes is absorbed back from the tubule into the blood. Different regions of the tubule and collecting duct vary in their capacity to reabsorb water and solutes (Figs 14.1 and 14.2).

The proximal tubule

In the proximal tubule, about 60–70% of the filtered Na^+ is reabsorbed together with equivalent amounts of water. Therefore, on leaving the proximal tubule, the tubular fluid still has the same osmolarity as plasma. The proximal tubule has many transport mechanisms for the secretion of organic anions into the tubular lumen (the organic anion transport mechanism Fig. 14.1, site 1; see also Ch. 2), and the reabsorption of water-soluble essential nutrients, such as glucose and amino acids, from the lumen. The organic anion transport mechanism is important for the transport of many drugs and their metabolites from the blood into the tubule (e.g. see acetazolamide and loop diuretics below). Reabsorption of ions from the proximal tubule into the renal tubular cells is passive (Fig. 14.1, site 1). The activity of the Na^+/K^+-ATPase pump on the basolateral surface of the tubular cell (transporting 3 Na^+ out of the tubular cell in exchange for 2 K^+) helps to establish the electrochemical gradient for passive Na^+ reabsorption from the tubular lumen into the tubule cell. This inward Na^+ gradient provides the drive for several other carriers, such as that for glucose. Bicarbonate is also reabsorbed from the proximal tubule by a mechanism dependent on the enzyme carbonic anhydrase (Fig. 14.1, site 2). Water reabsorption by the proximal renal tubule is driven by the osmotic gradient across the tubular cells, which is created by the active transport of Na^+ out of the cell across the basolateral membrane. The extent of the proximal tubular reabsorption of Na^+ and water is determined by two regulatory mechanisms: glomerulotubular feedback (enhanced tubular Na^+ reabsorption when the glomerular filtration rate rises), and various neural and hormonal influences such as the sympathetic nervous system, angiotensin II, endothelin, dopamine and parathyroid hormone.

The loop of Henle

The descending limb of the loop of Henle is permeable to water but not to Na^+. Water passes from the tubule into the interstitium of the renal medulla, where the fluid is hypertonic as a result of ion transport in the ascending limb of the loop of Henle (see below). The thick ascending limb of the loop of Henle is impermeable to water but has an active $Na^+/K^+/2Cl^-$ cotransporter complex in the luminal (apical) membrane (Fig. 14.1, site 3). Active extrusion of Na^+ from the tubular cells by the Na^+/K^+-ATPase pump in the basolateral membrane creates a low intracellular Na^+ concentration and therefore a Na^+ ion gradient that drives this cotransporter. The ascending limb of the loop of Henle can reabsorb up to 30% of the Na^+ filtered at the glomerulus. K^+ that is carried from the tubule into the cells of the loop by the cotransporter is recycled back into the tubular lumen, which ensures that there is always enough tubular K^+ to continue to favour Na^+ reabsorption. K^+ recycling also creates a lumen-positive transepithelial voltage gradient. This, in turn, drives a paracellular ionic current which is responsible for half the total Na^+ reabsorbed by this region of the kidney, along with Ca^{2+} and Mg^{2+}.

The reabsorption of Na^+ but not water by the thick ascending limb of the loop of Henle establishes the hypertonicity of the medullary interstitium (the corticomedullary concentration gradient). This interstitial hypertonicity is responsible for an osmotic gradient across the collecting ducts, which permits the formation of hypertonic urine (see below). There are various hormonal regulators of Na^+ reabsorption in the ascending limb of the loop of Henle, including calcitonin, parathyroid hormone and prostaglandin E_2.

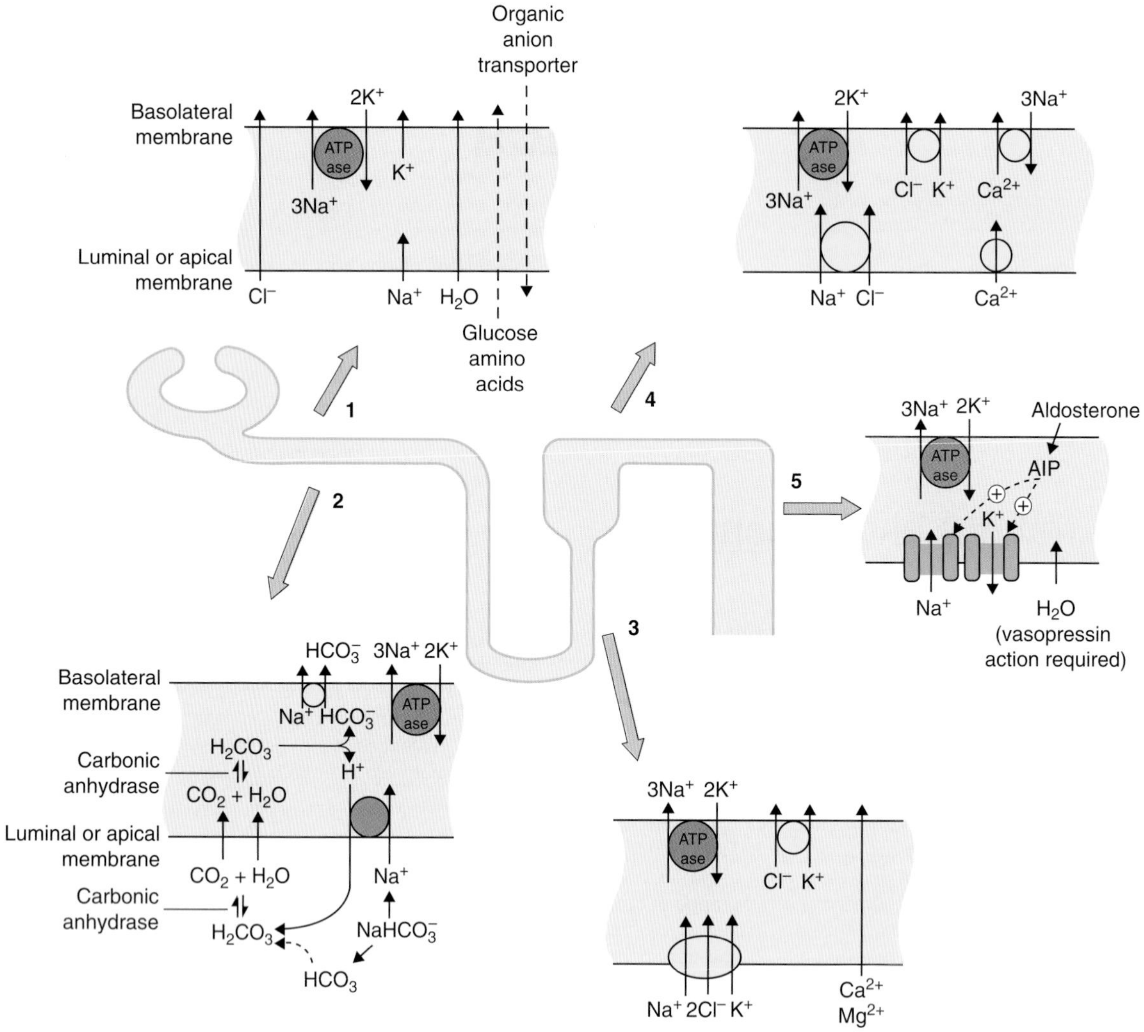

Fig. 14.1 **Transport mechanisms for solutes in the kidney.** In all segments of the renal tubule there is active transport of Na^+ out of and K^+ into the cell, across the basolateral membrane, using Na^+/K^+-ATPase proton pumps. This sets up electrochemical gradients for the transport of other ions. In the proximal tubule (sites 1 and 2), considerable amounts of Na^+, glucose and amino acids are taken up from the lumen along with water. The principal function of the organic anion transporter (site 1) (Ch. 2) is the elimination of metabolites of ingested foreign substances (xenobiotics). It is also the route that drugs such as furosemide use to gain access to the ion transporters that they inhibit on apical membranes in the tubule. Hydrogen ions are excreted in exchange for Na^+ uptake and this, in part, depends upon the activity of carbonic anhydrase. In the ascending limb of the loop of Henle (site 3), the luminal membrane has a cotransport mechanism for $Na^+/Cl^-/K^+$ but is impermeable to water. In the proximal part of the distal tubule (cortical diluting segment; site 4), Na^+ and Cl^- are co-absorbed but not water. Ca^{2+} also exchanges with 3 Na^+ at the basolateral border at this site. In the distal part of the distal tubule and collecting duct (site 5), Na^+ is reabsorbed from the lumen in exchange for K^+ through selective channels. The channels transporting these ions are regulated by aldosterone. Water is reabsorbed in the collecting duct under the influence of antidiuretic hormone (vasopressin) acting through receptors in the basolateral membrane. AIP, aldosterone-induced protein.

The proximal (cortical) diluting segment of the distal tubule

The filtrate leaving the loop of Henle is hypotonic and passes to the proximal part of the distal tubule (also known as the cortical diluting segment of the distal tubule). This part of the renal tubule is impermeable to water but has a luminal Na^+/Cl^- cotransporter (Fig 14.1, site 4). The driving force for this cotransporter is again generated by the Na^+/K^+-ATPase pump in the basolateral membrane. About 5% of the filtered Na^+ load can be reabsorbed at this site. The rich blood supply to this region allows rapid diffusion of the reabsorbed ions into the plasma and prevents the interstitium from becoming hypertonic. Reabsorption of Ca^{2+} is also regulated at this site, under the influence of parathyroid hormone and calcitriol (Ch. 42). The rate of Ca^{2+} transport

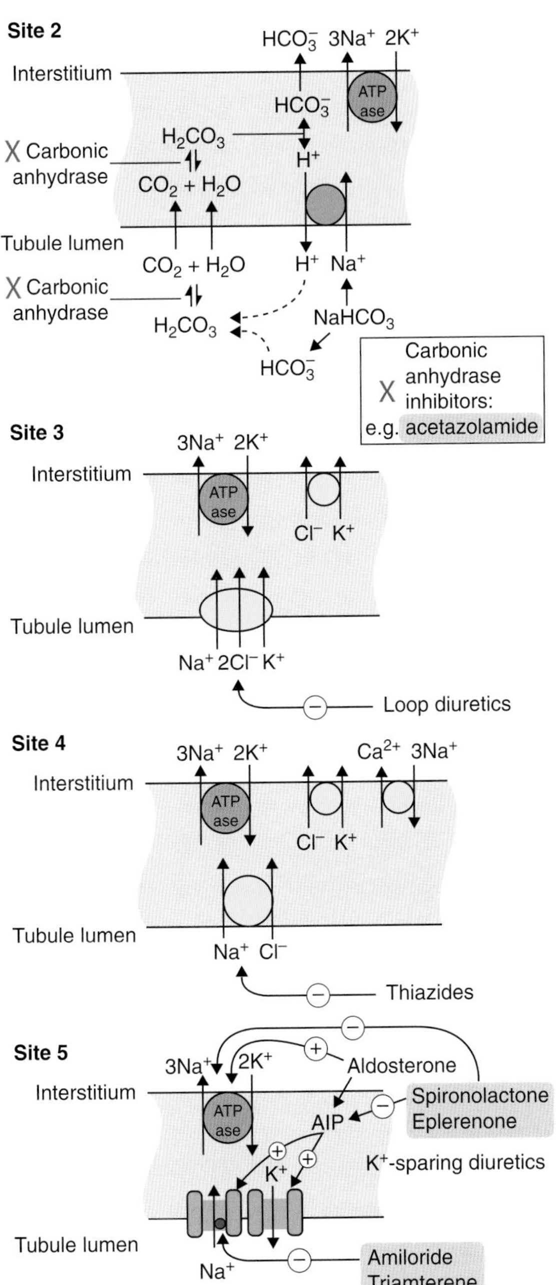

Fig. 14.2 **Sites of action of diuretics.** For location of these sites, see Fig. 14.1. Drugs gain access to the membrane transporters after secretion into the tubule by the organic anion transporter in the proximal tubule. Acetazolamide inhibits carbonic anhydrase and is a weak self-limiting diuretic, now largely used for other conditions such as glaucoma. Osmotic diuretics increase osmotic pressure through the tubule, reducing electrolyte reabsorption across the luminal membrane. Loop diuretics can inhibit the cotransporter for $Na^+/Cl^-/K^+$ and inhibit up to 30% of filtered Na^+ reabsorption. Thiazide diuretics and potassium-sparing diuretics inhibit the reuptake of a maximum of about 5% of filtered Na^+. The potassium-sparing diuretic spironolactone acts by inhibiting Na^+/K^+ exchange mechanisms in the basolateral membrane and inhibiting AIP synthesis which participates in the formation and Na^+ and K^+ channels in the apical membrane. Amiloride and triamterene act directly to block the activity of the Na^+ transporter. AIP, aldosterone-induced protein.

is inversely related to that of Na^+ transport; this is because Na^+ inside the tubular cell either inhibits luminal voltage-gated Ca^{2+} channels or reduces the activity of the basolateral Na^+/Ca^{2+} exchanger.

In this region of the kidney, the increased luminal concentration of Na^+ or Cl^- initiates two responses that limit Na^+ loss. The first is tubuloglomerular feedback, a mechanism (possibly mediated by adenosine) that constricts the afferent glomerular arteriole to that nephron. The second is secretion of renin, which, through activation of the renin–angiotensin system, eventually increases the release of aldosterone from the adrenal cortex and increases Na^+ reabsorption at the distal part of the distal convoluted tubule (Chs 6 and 44, and below).

The distal part of the distal tubule and the collecting duct

The tubular fluid that has become yet more hypotonic in the cortical diluting segment of the distal tubule is delivered to the distal part of the distal tubule and then to the collecting duct. There are two cell types in this region.

In the principal cell, Na^+ is reabsorbed through a highly specific amiloride-sensitive epithelial Na^+ channel (Fig. 14.2). This depolarises the luminal membrane, and activates inwardly rectifying K^+_{ATP} channels, which secrete K^+ into the tubule. Therefore, Na^+ reabsorption from the distal part of the distal tubule is accompanied by obligatory K^+ loss into the urine. Aldosterone enhances Na^+ reabsorption at this site by generating aldosterone-induced proteins (AIPs). One of these, serum- and glucocorticoid-regulated kinase (SGK 1), phosphorylates and activates the epithelial Na^+ channel. Another, channel-inducing factor, regulates the Na^+/K^+-ATPase in the basolateral membrane, which provides the driving force for Na^+ reabsorption from the tubule. There are other less important hormonal regulators of Na^+ reabsorption in the distal part of the distal tubule and the collecting duct, including calcitonin, bradykinin and the family of natriuretic peptides. Overall, only about 3–5% of filtered Na^+ is reabsorbed at the distal part of the distal tubule. However, the distal renal tubule is the primary site in the kidney responsible for maintenance of K^+ homeostasis. Relatively small changes in extracellular K^+ concentration can affect cardiac muscle, skeletal muscle and brain function.

The principal cell is also the site of action of antidiuretic hormone (ADH, vasopressin; Ch. 43). This hormone is secreted by the posterior pituitary gland and binds to receptors in the basolateral membrane, where it increases the permeability of the cell to water by upregulating aquaporin 2 channels. In the presence of ADH, water reabsorption into the hypertonic medullary interstitium is increased, which concentrates the urine as it passes through the collecting duct.

Intercalated cells are the second cell type (not illustrated in Figs 14.1 and 14.2). These cells actively secrete H^+ into the lumen and conserve HCO_3^-. They are upregulated in systemic acidosis, and stimulated by aldosterone.

DIURETIC DRUGS

Proximal tubular diuretics: carbonic anhydrase inhibitors

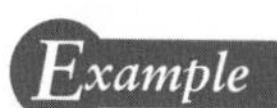

acetazolamide

Mechanism of action

Acetazolamide interferes with the small proportion of Na^+ that is actively reabsorbed in the proximal tubule in exchange for H^+ (Fig. 14.2, site 2), a process dependent on the enzyme carbonic anhydrase. Acetazolamide inhibits carbonic anhydrase, and therefore increases HCO_3^-, Na^+ and K^+ secretion, causing alkaline urine. H^+ retention produces a mild acidosis in the blood, but the fall in plasma HCO_3^- concentration stimulates carbonic anhydrase activity, which rapidly leads to tolerance to the diuretic action of acetazolamide. In consequence, acetazolamide does not have a clinically useful diuretic action. It is used for treatment of mountain sickness and glaucoma.

Pharmacokinetics

Acetazolamide is well absorbed from the gut and is eliminated unchanged by the kidney. It is secreted into the proximal renal tubule via the organic acid transport mechanism, and works at the luminal surface of the proximal tubule. It has a half-life of 6–9 h.

Unwanted effects

- Nausea and vomiting, anorexia
- Paraesthesia, dizziness, fatigue
- Hypokalaemia (see loop diuretics)
- Drowsiness.

Osmotic diuretics

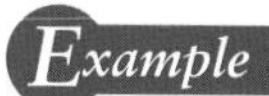

mannitol

Mechanism of action

Mannitol is filtered at the glomerulus but not reabsorbed from the renal tubule. It exerts osmotic activity within the proximal renal tubule and particularly the descending limb of the loop of Henle, and limits passive tubular reabsorption of water. Water loss produced by mannitol is accompanied by a variable natriuresis (up to 25% of filtered Na^+). Unlike other diuretics, the osmotic action of mannitol produces an initial expansion of plasma and extracellular fluid volume, which limits its clinical uses.

Mannitol does not readily cross the blood–brain barrier. It is used to treat some forms of acute brain injury, when the main mechanism of action may be through haemodilution and reduced blood viscosity which may limit ischaemic damage, rather than a dehydrating action on cerebral tissues.

Pharmacokinetics

Mannitol is given by intravenous infusion and is excreted unchanged at the glomerulus. It has a half-life of 2 h, which is substantially increased in renal impairment.

Unwanted effects

- Expansion of plasma volume can precipitate heart failure.
- Urinary K^+ loss can lead to hypokalaemia (see loop diuretics).

Loop diuretics

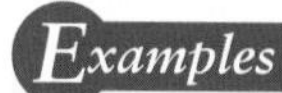

bumetanide, furosemide

Mechanism of action and effects

Loop diuretics, such as furosemide, must be secreted into the proximal kidney tubule by the tubular anion transport mechanism to access their site of action. The extent of the natriuresis and diuresis is dependent on the rate of delivery of the drug to the renal tubule via this secretory mechanism. Once the renal transporter sites are saturated, no increase in diuresis or natriuresis can be achieved by increasing the dose of the diuretic. Loop diuretics bind to the $Na^+/K^+/2Cl^-$ cotransporter complex at the luminal border of the thick ascending limb of the loop of Henle, and inhibit Cl^- reabsorption. This diminishes the electrochemical gradient across the cell, and reduces Na^+ reabsorption from the tubular fluid. Loop diuretics therefore reduce the ability of the kidney to generate the medullary ionic concentration gradient, and inhibit generation of concentrated urine in the collecting duct. Loop diuretics also inhibit the tubuloglomerular feedback mechanism and the afferent artery vasoconstriction in response to the increased tubular concentrations of Na^+ and Cl^-. They are powerful, 'high ceiling' diuretics which can inhibit reabsorption of up to 20–25% of the Na^+ that appears in the glomerular filtrate.

The dose–response curves of loop diuretics are steep, but the doses required to achieve maximal inhibition of Na^+ reabsorption show wide inter-individual variation. Their short duration of action results in partial compensation for the natriuresis by subsequent rebound Na^+ uptake from the tubular fluid after their action has finished. Loop diuretics remain effective even in advanced renal failure, but larger doses are necessary to deliver an effective concentration of drug to the remaining renal tubules, since the reduced proximal tubular secretion of the drug results in greater drug metabolism in the liver.

When injected intravenously, furosemide releases vasodilator prostaglandins, such as prostacyclin, from the kidney and produces a short-lived venodilation. Pooling of blood in the capacitance vessels reduces central blood volume, which can be useful in the treatment of acute left ventricular failure (Ch. 7). Loop diuretics also produce arterial vasodilation (see thiazide diuretics), but because of their short duration of action they are not widely used to treat hypertension, except in renal failure.

Pharmacokinetics

Furosemide is incompletely and erratically absorbed from the gut, with considerable inter-individual variation. Bumetanide is more completely absorbed, with less variation. Both are partially metabolised in the liver. They can also be given intravenously by slow bolus injection or by infusion. Loop diuretics are highly protein bound in plasma, and little drug is filtered at the glomerulus. Unmetabolised drug is actively secreted into the proximal tubular lumen via the organic anion transporter, and the rate of urinary Na^+ excretion is directly related to the urinary excretion rate of the diuretic. Renal failure impairs the delivery of drug to the tubular fluid, since the ability of the kidney to secrete organic anions is reduced and other metabolic substrates compete with the diuretic for tubular secretion. If renal function is normal, then the plasma half-life of a loop diuretic is short, at about 1–4 h. Natriuresis and diuresis begin about 30 min after an oral dose and last up to 6 h, by which time the urinary concentration of drug has fallen below the diuretic threshold. Intravenous injection produces a more rapid effect, with an onset of diuresis within minutes, lasting about 2–3 h.

Unwanted effects

- *Excessive salt and water depletion* can cause intravascular volume depletion, hypotension and renal impairment.
- *Dilutional hyponatraemia* can arise from excessive Na^+ loss that exceeds water loss. Hyponatraemia is far less common than with thiazide diuretics, since the prolonged block of Na^+/K^+ cotransport in the distal tubule by thiazides (where water cannot be reabsorbed) impairs free water clearance. Stimulation of ADH secretion in response to plasma volume contraction also contributes to hyponatraemia by promoting reabsorption of water from the collecting duct. Hyponatraemia can present with lethargy, impaired consciousness, and eventually coma and seizures.
- *Hypokalaemia,* which is dose-related but less severe than with longer-acting diuretics such as thiazides (see below). It arises from increased urinary K^+ loss from the distal part of the distal renal tubule.
  - Since diuretics increase the delivery of Na^+ to the distal tubule, there is enhanced Na^+ reabsorption at this site. This creates a negative luminal gradient that promotes K^+ diffusion into the tubular lumen.
  - The reduced K^+ concentration in the dilute urine increases the K^+ gradient across the tubular membrane, which also favours K^+ diffusion into the tubular lumen.
  - In addition, diuretic-induced hypovolaemia stimulates renin release, causing secondary hyperaldosteronism. Aldosterone further enhances Na^+ reabsorption in the distal tubule at the expense of increased K^+ excretion.
  - Obligatory urinary Cl^- loss with the K^+ creates a mild metabolic alkalosis in the plasma. To counteract the alkalosis, H^+ is shifted out of cells in exchange for intracellular accumulation of K^+, which exacerbates the hypokalaemia.

  The consequences and treatment of hypokalaemia are discussed below.
- Hypomagnesaemia can accompany hypokalaemia and makes the correction of hypokalaemia more difficult. About 70% of filtered Mg^{2+} is reabsorbed by paracellular diffusion in the loop of Henle, and this is impaired by loop diuretics, which inhibit the electrical gradient necessary for Mg^{2+} reabsorption. Hypomagnesaemia predisposes to cardiac arrhythmias.
- Increased urinary Ca^{2+} excretion from inhibition of paracellular reabsorption of Ca^{2+} at the loop of Henle. Hypocalcaemia does not occur, but this action can be helpful in the management of hypercalcaemia (Ch. 42).
- Hyperuricaemia arises from reduced glomerular filtration of uric acid following reduction of plasma volume. There may be an additional reduction of proximal tubular urate secretion as a result of competition between uric acid and the diuretic for the organic anion transporter. Clinical gout is unusual (Ch. 31), and less common with loop than with thiazide diuretics.
- Incontinence can result from the rapid increase in urine volume. In older males with prostatic hypertrophy, retention of urine can occur.

- Ototoxicity with deafness can result from cochlear damage, especially when renal failure reduces the rate of drug excretion or when very large doses of a loop diuretic are used. Vertigo may result from vestibular damage. Both are more common with furosemide than bumetanide and are usually reversible.

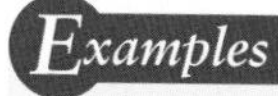

bendroflumethiazide, chlortalidone, metolazone

Thiazide and thiazide-like diuretics

Mechanisms of action and effects

The thiazides are structurally related to sulphonamides. They act at the luminal surface of the cortical (proximal) diluting segment of the distal convoluted tubule by inhibition of the Na^+/Cl^- cotransporter. This prevents Na^+, Cl^- and therefore water from entering the tubular cell. Several structurally different 'thiazide-like' drugs, such as chlortalidone and metolazone, share this site of action. Thiazides have a lower efficacy than loop diuretics, achieving a maximum natriuresis of about 5–8% of the filtered Na^+ load, and have a shallow dose–response curve. The onset of diuresis is slow, and they also have a longer duration of action than loop diuretics. However, this varies among the drugs; for example, bendroflumethiazide produces a natriuresis for up to 6–12 h and chlortalidone for 48–72 h. Most thiazide diuretics are less effective in renal failure (especially when the glomerular filtration rate is below 20 mL min^{-1}). Metolazone differs from other thiazide diuretics in that it works in advanced renal failure. Thiazide diuretics, unlike the loop diuretics, reduce urinary Ca^{2+} loss by inhibiting Ca^{2+} transport in the proximal and distal tubules.

Thiazides produce arterial vasodilation during long-term use, which is the basis of their hypotensive effect (Ch. 6). The mechanism of vasodilation is incompletely understood. It may involve inhibition of agonist-induced vasoconstriction by Ca^{2+} desensitization in smooth muscle cells linked to the Rho-Rho kinase pathway (a key regulator of force and velocity of actomyosin cross-bridging). This vascular action is maximal at lower dosages than are required for diuresis.

Pharmacokinetics

The thiazides and related drugs are fairly well absorbed from the gut and most are extensively metabolised in the liver. They are highly protein bound and little is filtered at the glomerulus. Thiazides act from within the renal tubular lumen after secretion of the parent drug via the proximal tubule organic anion transport mechanism (see also loop diuretics). The half-lives of thiazides and related drugs are between 4 and 90 h, and this contributes to their more prolonged duration of action compared with loop diuretics.

Unwanted effects

- *Hypokalaemia* (see loop diuretics). Clinically this is more important with thiazides than with loop diuretics. The greatest reduction in plasma K^+ usually occurs within 2 weeks of starting treatment.
- *Salt and water depletion.* The combination of a thiazide with amiloride (see below) is particularly associated with dilutional hyponatraemia (see loop diuretics).
- *Hyperuricaemia* (see loop diuretics). Gout occurs infrequently and is less common in women.
- *Decreased urinary Ca^{2+} excretion.* This is in contrast to loop diuretics and the mechanism is not well understood. Hypercalcaemia is unusual unless there is another underlying disturbance of Ca^{2+} metabolism, such as hyperparathyroidism.
- *Glucose intolerance.* This is dose-related, with a progressive increase in plasma glucose over many months. The major cause is prolonged hypokalaemia and the consequent reduced intracellular K^+ concentration. This inhibits insulin release and impairs tissue uptake of glucose in response to insulin. The glucose intolerance usually reverses over several months if the thiazide is stopped (see Ch. 40).
- *Hyperlipidaemia.* There is a dose-related increase in low-density lipoprotein cholesterol and triglycerides. The long-term effects (>1 year) are small, but may increase atherogenic risk if high doses are used (Ch. 48).
- *Impotence.* This is reported by up to 10% of middle-aged hypertensive men treated with high doses of thiazides (Ch. 16).
- *Nocturia* and urinary frequency can result from prolonged diuresis.

Potassium-sparing diuretics

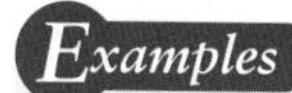

amiloride, eplerenone, spironolactone, triamterene

Mechanism of action and effects

Drugs in this class produce a mild diuresis while limiting urinary K^+ loss. All potassium-sparing diuretics act at the late distal convoluted tubule and cortical collecting duct. Spironolactone and eplerenone are the only diuretics that do not act at the luminal membrane of the tubular cells, but bind to the cytoplasmic aldosterone receptor. They only work in the presence of aldosterone and therefore their effect is enhanced in hyperaldosteronism. Aldosterone binds to a cytoplasmic mineralocorticoid receptor, a DNA transcription factor, which migrates to the nucleus and increases the synthesis of aldosterone-induced proteins (AIP) that induce Na^+ channel activity (Fig. 14.2, site 5; and see above). Spironolactone, its active metabolite canrenone, and eplerenone compete with aldosterone for its cytoplasmic receptors. Receptors occupied by these molecules do not attach to DNA, and AIP synthesis is reduced.

Amiloride and triamterene have a different mechanism of action, and block the epithelial Na^+ channel at the luminal surface of the renal tubule (Fig. 14.2). This action is independent of the presence of aldosterone.

The maximum natriuresis achieved by potassium-sparing diuretics is small (less than 2–3% of filtered Na^+) unless there is marked secondary hyperaldosteronism, when spironolactone and eplerenone are more effective. With this group of drugs, Na^+ and water loss is accompanied by preservation of plasma K^+, because of reduced Na^+/K^+ exchange. When used together with thiazide or loop diuretics, potassium-sparing diuretics reduce or eliminate the excess urinary K^+ loss.

Pharmacokinetics

All potassium-sparing diuretics are given orally. Spironolactone is metabolised in the wall of the gut and the liver to canrenone, which is probably responsible for most of the diuretic effect. The half-life of spironolactone (1 h) is much shorter than that of canrenone (17–22 h). The onset of action is slow, starting after 1 day and becoming maximal by 3–4 days; this slow effect is largely a consequence of its mechanism of action rather than its pharmacokinetics. Eplerenone has a half-life of 4–6 h, and is partially metabolised to inactive derivatives in the liver. It also has a slow onset of action.

Triamterene is extensively metabolised in the liver, and tubular secretion of the sulphate ester metabolite is responsible for the diuretic action. Triamterene has a short half-life (2 h). Amiloride is secreted unchanged into the proximal renal tubule and has a half-life of 6–9 h. The onset of action of amiloride and triamterene is rapid.

Unwanted effects

- Hyperkalaemia. This is more common in the presence of pre-existing renal disease, in the elderly and during combination treatment with angiotensin-converting enzyme (ACE) inhibitors or angiotensin receptor antagonists (Ch. 6). Retention of Mg^{2+} also occurs, in contrast to the loss with the thiazides and loop diuretics.
- Hyponatraemia. This is more common with thiazide–amiloride combinations.
- Spironolactone has an anti-androgenic effect, a consequence of its ability to bind to androgen receptors and prevent their interaction with dihydrotestosterone. This causes gynaecomastia and impotence in males, and menstrual irregularities in women. The anti-androgenic effect is sometimes used to treat hirsutism, male-pattern hair loss and acne in females. Eplerenone has greater aldosterone receptor selectivity and does not cause these problems.
- Gastrointestinal disturbances.
- Spironolactone is carcinogenic at high doses in rats but there is no evidence of a problem in humans.

MANAGEMENT OF DIURETIC-INDUCED HYPOKALAEMIA

A modest reduction in plasma K^+ concentration is common during treatment with loop or thiazide diuretics. Marked hypokalaemia (below 3.0 mmol L^{-1}) predisposes to cardiac rhythm disturbances, particularly in the presence of acute myocardial ischaemia, during treatment with digitalis glycosides (Ch. 7) or with antiarrhythmic agents that prolong the Q–T interval on the electrocardiogram (Ch. 8). It may also precipitate encephalopathy in people with liver failure. The risk of hypokalaemia is greatest with:

- thiazide rather than loop diuretics, because of their longer duration of action
- low oral intake of K^+
- high doses of diuretic
- hyperaldosteronism, for example in hepatic cirrhosis and nephrotic syndrome.

Both treatment and prevention of diuretic-induced hypokalaemia can be achieved by using either oral K^+ supplements or a potassium-sparing diuretic. Potassium supplements are less effective unless used in large quantities, which often cause gastric irritation. Modified-release tablets and effervescent formulations of K^+ are available, and supplements of greater than 30 mmol daily are usually needed. Intravenous K^+ treatment is rarely needed unless there is severe K^+ depletion. Rapid intravenous injection of K^+ can produce potentially lethal hyperkalaemia (provoking asystole), and a maximum infusion rate of 10 mmol h^{-1} is recommended, with hourly monitoring of the plasma K^+ concentration if such a high infusion rate is necessary.

It is unnecessary to routinely prescribe a potassium-sparing diuretic with a thiazide or loop diuretic, but they are widely used, often as fixed-dose combination tablets. A pragmatic approach would be to reserve their use for those at high risk from hypokalaemia, or those who develop significant hypokalaemia during regular diuretic treatment.

MAJOR USES OF DIURETICS

Diuretics can be used to treat a number of conditions.

Oedema in heart failure (Ch. 7), nephrotic syndrome and hepatic cirrhosis

Mild oedema can sometimes be controlled by a thiazide diuretic, but more marked oedema usually requires the use of a loop diuretic. Modest doses of a loop diuretic provide a near-maximal response if renal function is normal, but large doses are sometimes necessary if there is renal failure (see above). Long-term use of a loop diuretic can occasionally produce tolerance, due to hypertrophy of epithelial cells of the cortical diluting segment of the distal convoluted tubule, which results in increased Na^+ reabsorption at this site. There are various strategies that can be tried if fluid retention is resistant to oral furosemide:

- Salt restriction and avoidance of salt-retaining drugs, such as non-steroidal anti-inflammatory drugs (Ch. 29).
- Divided oral doses of a loop diuretic can be used to give more prolonged drug delivery to the kidney. This also reduces post-diuretic rebound Na^+ retention.
- Oral bumetanide can be used rather than furosemide, because of its more consistent oral absorption.
- A loop diuretic can be given by intravenous infusion to prolong the duration of action. Slow intravenous infusion of higher drug doses will help to avoid ototoxicity.
- The addition of a thiazide diuretic or metolazone to a loop diuretic. Sequential inhibition of tubular Na^+ reabsorption can produce a dramatic diuresis and natriuresis. However, hyponatraemia, hypokalaemia, hypovolaemia and renal impairment can be troublesome with such combinations.
- If there is marked secondary hyperaldosteronism (e.g. in ascites associated with cirrhosis of the liver), spironolactone can be particularly useful. Eplerenone is currently reserved for people who are intolerant of spironolactone.

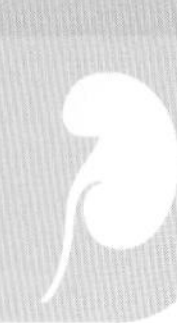

Hypertension (Ch. 6)

Low doses of a thiazide diuretic are usually used. A loop diuretic or spironolactone can be useful for resistant hypertension or when there is renal impairment.

Acute renal failure

A loop diuretic has been advocated for incipient acute renal failure to prevent it from becoming established. Recent analyses do not show any evidence that this strategy alters the need for subsequent renal replacement therapy, and it is not recommended.

Hypercalciuria with renal stone formation

Thiazides can be used to reduce urinary Ca^{2+} excretion.

Glaucoma

Acetazolamide can be used to reduce intraocular pressure (Ch. 50). Tolerance does not occur to this effect, unlike the diuretic action.

Mountain sickness

An unlicensed use for acetazolamide is the prevention and treatment of mountain sickness (Ch. 13). It should be taken for several days before ascending to altitude, and continued until descent. The mechanism is unknown.

Hypoventilation in chronic obstructive pulmonary disease

Acetazolamide creates a mild metabolic acidosis. This can stimulate respiration in the short term, and reduce carbon dioxide retention (Ch. 12).

Acute brain injury

Mannitol is occasionally used to reduce ischaemic cerebral damage, for example after neurosurgery or in acute traumatic brain injury. Fluid loss via the kidney should be replaced with intravenous crystalloid to avoid dehydration.

FURTHER READING

Brater DC (2000) Pharmacology of diuretics. *Am J Med Sci* 319, 38–50

De Bruyne LKM (2003) Mechanisms and management of diuretic resistance in congestive heart failure. *Postgrad Med J* 79, 268–271

Greenberg A (2000) Diuretic complications. *Am J Med Sci* 319, 10–24

Herbert SC (1999) Molecular mechanisms. *Semin Nephrol* 19, 504–523

Krämer BK, Schweda F, Riegger GAJ (1999) Diuretic treatment and diuretic resistance in heart failure. *Am J Med* 106, 90–96

Shankar SS, Brater DC (2003) Loop diuretics: from the Na-K-2Cl transporter to clinical use. *Am J Physiol Renal Physiol* 284, F11–F21

Wright SH, Dantzler WH (2004) Molecular and cellular physiology of renal organic cation and anion transport. *Physiol Rev* 84, 987–1049

SELF-ASSESSMENT

In questions 1–11, the first statement, in italics, is correct. Are the accompanying statements true or false?

1. *A fall in plasma K^+ concentration can affect cardiac muscle and brain function.* The main renal site of K^+ loss in the urine is from the proximal tubule.
2. *Electrogenic gradients are set up in many segments of the tubule by the Na^+/K^+-ATPase pump on the basolateral membrane.* The thick ascending limb of the loop of Henle is impermeable to water.
3. *Osmotic diuretics are poorly reabsorbed from the renal tubule.* Osmotic diuretics exert their activity on the proximal tubule, descending limb of the loop of Henle and the collecting ducts.
4. *Osmotic diuretics cause expansion of the extracellular fluid volume.* Osmotic diuretics should not be given in heart failure.
5. *The carbonic anhydrase inhibitor acetazolamide is used to inhibit the formation of aqueous humour in glaucoma.* Tolerance to the diuretic effect of acetazolamide develops.
6. *Approximately 20–30% of filtered Na^+ is reabsorbed in the thick ascending limb of the loop of Henle.* Loop diuretics increase the hypertonicity of the interstitium in the medullary region.
7. *In addition to its diuretic properties, furosemide has a venodilator action possibly as a result of the release of prostaglandins.*
   a. Loop diuretics are useful in the treatment of acute pulmonary oedema.
   b. Loop diuretics and thiazide diuretics should not be administered together.
   c. Loop diuretics do not produce hypokalaemia.
   d. There is no upper limit to the diuretic or natriuretic activity of a loop diuretic.
   e. Loop diuretics can produce ototoxicity.
8. *Unlike loop diuretics, which are short-acting, some thiazide diuretics such as chlortalidone can produce a diuresis for up to 48–72 h.*
   a. Thiazide diuretics act by inhibiting the Na^+ and Cl^- cotransport in the basolateral membrane.
   b. Like the loop diuretics, the thiazides increase urinary Ca^{2+} excretion.
   c. The diuretic effect of metolazone is greater than that of other thiazide diuretics.
   d. Thiazide diuretics can produce glucose intolerance.

9. *Spironolactone and amiloride reduce K^+ loss by inhibiting the uptake of Na^+ which exchange for K^+ in the late distal convoluted tubule and the cortical collecting duct.*
   a. Spironolactone and amiloride act by identical mechanisms to reduce K^+ loss.
   b. Potassium-sparing diuretics can cause a potentially harmful interaction if given with ACE inhibitors.
10. *Thiazide or loop diuretics are often given together with potassium-sparing diuretics.*
   a. The combination of amiloride and bendroflumethiazide produces no greater natriuresis than bendroflumethiazide given alone.
   b. Spironolactone is metabolised to the inactive metabolite canrenone.
11. *Non-steroidal anti-inflammatory drugs (NSAIDs) reduce the diuretic response to thiazide and loop diuretics.* Prostaglandins synthesised within the kidney increase renal blood flow and cause natriuresis.
12. Extended-matching questions
   Choose the **most likely** option (A–G) that would relate to the case scenarios (12.1–12.4).
   A. Raised serum K^+ concentration
   B. Lowered serum K^+ concentration
   C. Reduced natriuresis
   D. Increased natriuresis
   E. Raised plasma glucose
   F. Lowered plasma glucose
   G. Lowered plasma Ca^{2+}
   12.1. A 58-year-old woman was taken to the A&E department with dyspnoea and bradycardia of 40 beats min^{-1}. She had previously had a myocardial infarction and coronary angioplasty. She was taking the ACE inhibitor lisinopril, and the diuretics bendroflumethiazide and amiloride, and had recently had the dose of lisinopril increased.
   12.2. A 68-year-old woman with hypertension was taking bendroflumethiazide. Her blood pressure had been controlled at 136/88 mmHg. She had recently started taking naproxen for the aches and pains of osteoarthritis. Her blood pressure was found to be elevated (146/100 mmHg).
   12.3. A 40-year-old man with type 1 diabetes and hypertension was being treated with insulin. He had started on chlortalidone 2 months previously for his hypertension and was seeking medical advice about his increased tiredness and lethargy.
   12.4. A 55-year-old man with congestive heart failure was treated with digoxin and lisinopril. Furosemide was added because of oedema and he subsequently complained of palpitation. He was admitted to hospital and the electrocardiogram showed atrial tachycardia.

ANSWERS

1. **False**. Much of the K^+ filtered at the glomerulus is reabsorbed in the proximal tubule and in the loop of Henle. Secretory loss into the urine is mainly in exchange for Na^+, occurring through specialised K^+ channels in the collecting ducts.
2. **True**. Impermeability to water and an active $Na^+/Cl^-/K^+$ cotransporter that transports these ions from the lumen into the tubular cell in the thick ascending limb are pertinent to the generation of the hyperosmotic interstitium and the counter-current mechanisms for concentrating urine in the collecting duct.
3. **True**. These regions are permeable to water, where an osmotic effect can be exerted.
4. **True**. As a result of extracting water from intracellular compartments and expanding extracellular and intravascular fluid volume, they can precipitate pulmonary oedema.
5. **True**. Acetazolamide results in a mild metabolic acidosis and a reduced plasma HCO_3^- concentration, which limits the H^+/Na^+ exchange at the luminal membrane.
6. **False**. By inhibiting the $Na^+/K^+/Cl^-$ cotransporter, the medullary interstitial hypertonicity falls. Because the interstitial hypertonicity provides the osmotic force for the reabsorption of water in the collecting ducts (in the presence of antidiuretic hormone [vasopressin]), the lower osmotic pressure results in reduced water reabsorption. Loop diuretics are highly protein bound and little is filtered at the glomerulus. The drugs reach the luminal membrane cotransporter by secretion into the proximal tubule via the organic acid transport mechanism.
7. a. **True**. Loop diuretics are widely used in the control of oedema in heart failure for the elimination of the excessive salt and water load. The direct venodilator activity of furosemide reduces central blood volume.
   b. **False**. A thiazide diuretic or metolazone can be added to a loop diuretic to act sequentially at different sites in the nephron, thus producing a marked diuresis and natriuresis.
   c. **False**. Delivery of greater concentrations of Na^+ to the collecting ducts increases the exchange for K^+ at that site, thus increasing K^+ loss.
   d. **False**. Once the cotransporter mechanism is maximally inhibited, no further water or salt excretion can occur.
   e. **True**. When high doses are used, especially in the presence of renal impairment, or when taken with another ototoxic drug such as an aminoglycoside antibacterial, ototoxicity can occur.
8. a. **False**. Like the loop diuretics, the thiazides have to act from the renal tubular lumen on the cotransporter that is on the luminal (apical) membrane. The thiazides are secreted by the proximal tubule transport mechanism into the lumen.
   b. **False**. The thiazide diuretics do not increase Ca^{2+} excretion, unlike the loop diuretics.
   c. **True**. Metolazone is more effective than other thiazide diuretics and when given together with furosemide in advanced renal impairment.
   d. **True**. Thiazide diuretics could exacerbate diabetes mellitus. The mechanism may be through inhibition of insulin synthesis.
9. a. **False**. Although both drugs ultimately reduce activity of the Na^+ reuptake channel, amiloride blocks the channel directly, whereas spironolactone prevents the actions of aldosterone-induced proteins, which enhance the Na^+ channel numbers and activity.
   b. **True**. ACE inhibitors, by inhibiting aldosterone secretion, will increase K^+ concentration in the inter-

stitium and blood by reducing K^+ excretion. Hyperkalaemia may result

10. a. **False**. Because the diuretics act at different sites, an additional natriuresis is produced.
    b. **False**. Canrenone is an active diuretic, responsible for most of the effects of spironolactone.
11. **True**. Some diuretics may act partly by the generation of prostaglandins. In addition, prostaglandins help to maintain renal blood flow. Therefore, NSAIDs can reduce diuretic activity.
12. Extended-matching answers
    12.1. Answer **A**. Amiloride is a potassium-sparing diuretic. Lisinopril can also increase plasma K^+ concentrations by increasing the levels of aldosterone. The raised K^+ levels may have been the cause of the profound bradycardia.
    12.2. Answer **C**. One component of the antihypertensive action of bendroflumethiazide is via prostaglandins, which promote sodium excretion by the kidney and cause vasodilation. Because NSAIDs such as naproxen will prevent prostaglandin formation by inhibiting cyclo-oxygenase, their administration will diminish the antihypertensive actions of bendroflumethiazide at the vascular and renal levels.
    12.3. Answer **E**. Thiazide-like diuretics can worsen insulin resistance, resulting in an increased plasma glucose concentration.
    12.4. Answer **B**. The loop diuretic may cause hypokalaemia. This enhances the toxicity of digoxin, resulting in arrhythmias.

Diuretic drugs (all given orally unless otherwise stated)

Drug	Half-life (h) and kinetics	Comment
Carbonic anhydrase inhibitors		
Acetazolamide	6–9 [R] 100% is eliminated unchanged within 24 h	Of little clinical value as a diuretic, because of the rapid development of tolerance. Used in glaucoma (Ch. 50)
Osmotic diuretics		
Mannitol	2–36 [R] Half-life is 2 h in healthy people but very prolonged in cardiac or renal failure	Given by rapid intravenous infusion; used in cerebral oedema but not used in heart failure as it may expand plasma volume
Loop diuretics		
Used for heart failure, oedema and oliguria due to renal failure		
Bumetanide	1–2 [R + M] Well absorbed from the gut; about 50% is conjugated with glucuronic acid and excreted in urine and bile	Given orally or by intravenous or intramuscular injection
Furosemide	1 [R + M] Incomplete and erratic absorption from gut; limited metabolism (15%) by glucuronidation	Given orally or by intravenous or intramuscular injection
Torasemide	2–4 [M + R] Good oral absorption; about 25% cleared by kidney and remainder by metabolism; half-life unchanged in renal failure	Compared with bumetanide and furosemide, the diuretic action of torasemide is less affected by renal failure, but it should still be used with caution in renal impairment
Thiazide diuretics		
Weak acids, therefore renal clearance affected by urine pH; given orally; used for heart failure, oedema and hypertension		
Bendroflumethiazide	3–9 [M + R] Complete absorption from gut; 30% excreted in urine unchanged; metabolites not characterised	
Chlortalidone	50–90 [R] Incomplete oral absorption; long half-life because of its large volume of distribution and high plasma protein binding which reduces glomerular filtration	
Cyclopenthiazide	? [R]	Offers no advantages over other thiazides and is now little used in the UK
Hydrochlorothiazide	8–12 [R]	Offers no advantages over other thiazides and is now little used in the UK

Diuretic drugs (all given orally unless otherwise stated)

Drug	Half-life (h) and kinetics	Comment
Indapamide	10–22 [M + R] Rapidly and extensively absorbed from the gut; extensive hepatic metabolism; only 5% of dose is excreted unchanged	
Metolazone	4–5 [R] Good oral absorption; urine is main route of elimination (80% as parent drug)	
Xipamide	5 [M + R] Rapidly and extensively absorbed from the gut; about a half is excreted unchanged in the urine and a third as a glucuronide conjugate	
Potassium-sparing diuretics		
Prevention of diuretic-induced hypokalemia, hyperaldosteronism, ascites associated with liver cirrhosis		
Amiloride	6–9 [R + F] Absorbed drug is excreted unchanged in urine	Used in combination with thiazides and loop diuretics to conserve K^+
Eplerenone	4–6 [M] Metabolised by CYP3A4 to inactive products	More selective than spironolactone for aldosterone receptor
Spironolactone	1 [M] Variable absorption from gut, enhanced if taken with food; metabolised to an active metabolite (canrenone), which has a half-life of 17–22 h and is eliminated in urine as an ester glucuronide	
Triamterene	2 [M] Variable absorption owing to first-pass metabolism; metabolised by oxidation to a hydroxy metabolite and conjugated with sulphate; the conjugate retains activity	Used in combination with thiazides and loop diuretics to conserve K^+

[F], faecal excretion; [M], metabolism; [R], renal excretion.

15 Disorders of micturition

PATHOPHYSIOLOGY OF MICTURITION

The urinary bladder is a smooth muscle organ composed chiefly of the detrusor muscle, which relaxes to allow bladder filling up to 500–600 mL. A smaller muscle, the trigone, is found between the ureteric orifices and bladder neck. Internal and external distal sphincter mechanisms are normally constricted to prevent bladder emptying and maintain continence (Fig. 15.1). Coordination of these components of the lower urinary tract and the coordination of bladder filling, continence and emptying are brought about by an area in the frontal lobe, the pontine micturition centre. Conscious sensations of bladder fullness are processed by the cerebral cortex, which then sends signals to the micturition centre.

During *bladder filling*, sympathetic nervous system stimulation via the hypogastric nerve relaxes the bladder smooth muscle (via β_2-adrenoceptors in the detrusor and generation of intracellular cyclic adenosine monophosphate [cAMP]). At the same time, sympathetic stimulation of a subtype of α_1-adrenoceptors (α_{1A}- and to a lesser extent α_{1B}-adrenoceptors), via the vesical nerve, contracts the smooth muscle of the internal urethral sphincter. Somatic stimulation of the striated muscle of the voluntary external urethral sphincter via the pudendal nerve, aided by pelvic muscle control in women, contributes to maintenance of sphincter tone and continence. The sensation of urge to micturate occurs in adults at a bladder volume of 200–300 mL.

Bladder emptying is initiated by myogenic stretch receptor activity produced by distention of the detrusor, and by sensory signals from the urothelium (the epithelial cell lining of the bladder). Release of ATP from the urothelium stimulates P2X purinoreceptors on the sensory afferent neurons, and other local transmitters also modulate the sensitivity of this system (see Ch. 1). The afferent nerves project to the pontine micturition centre which initiates activity in efferent pathways. Bladder contraction and thus voiding results from stimulation of the pelvic nerve and parasympathetic muscarinic M_3 receptors in the detrusor muscle by acetylcholine, leading to generation of intracellular inositol 1,4,5-triphosphate (IP_3) and diacylglycerol (DAG). At the same time, stimulation of muscarinic M_2 receptors on presynaptic nerve terminals inhibits intracellular cAMP production, and therefore opposes the effects of sympathetic activity. Non-cholinergic-mediated contractions (mediated by ATP acting via P2X purinoreceptors) also contributes to bladder contraction, and this component becomes more prominent in unstable bladders. Contraction of the detrusor is coordinated with inhibition of the tonic control of distal sphincter mechanisms and the bladder neck, thus relaxing the bladder outflow tract. Bladder emptying may be augmented by contraction of the diaphragm and abdominal muscles. M_3 and M_2 receptors are present in detrusor muscle but the M_3 subtype appears to be more important for detrusor contraction.

Disorders of micturition

Disorders of micturition can arise from a disturbance of bladder function or from abnormalities affecting bladder outflow. Although there are distinct clinical syndromes, many people have mixed incontinence, e.g. both stress and urge incontinence (see below). Management of disorders of micturition should also consider possible contributory factors, such as diuretics, α_1-adrenoceptor antagonists used for treatment of hypertension, and stool impaction which inhibits sacral parasympathetic neurotransmission.

OVERACTIVE BLADDER (DETRUSOR INSTABILITY)

Detrusor instability produces uncontrolled bladder contractions during normal filling. Symptoms from this include urinary frequency, nocturia and urgency (overactive bladder syndrome), often accompanied by urge incontinence (a sudden compelling desire to urinate). Most cases in women are idiopathic, but in men, bladder outflow obstruction is the commonest cause. Upper motor neuron lesions, such as those produced by stroke, spinal cord injuries or multiple sclerosis, can also produce an overactive bladder. Fluid management, with reduction in excessive intake, and behavioural training that includes pelvic muscle training and suppression of urge are first-line approaches to management.

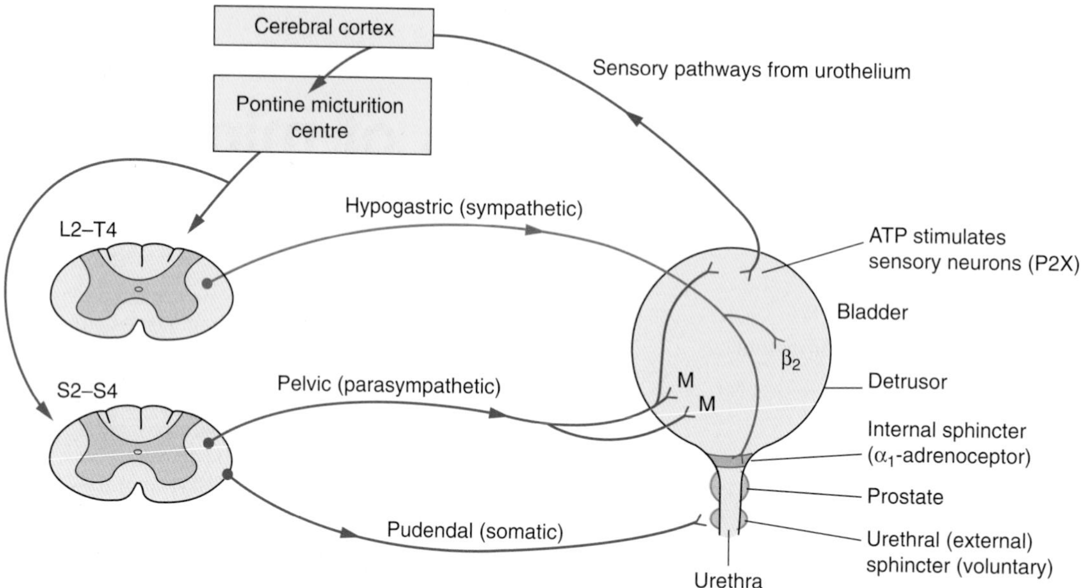

Fig. 15.1 **Aspects of the bladder/prostate structures and the innervation involved in the micturition reflex.** Bladder filling provides neuronal signals to the micturition centre via sensory input from purinoceptors on neurons in the urothelium. To accommodate filling and continence, sympathetic stimulation both relaxes the smooth muscle of the bladder via β-adrenoceptors (β_2) and stimulates sphincter mechanisms through α_1-adrenoceptor subtypes. Somatic control of the external sphincter also aids continence. Voluntary urination involves parasympathetic stimulation of bladder smooth muscle through M_3 and M_2 muscarinic receptor subtypes (M) and inhibition of the sympathetic and somatic outflow. Aspects of bladder control may involve other less understood transmitter substances. For example, gamma-aminobutyric acid (GABA) interneurons inhibit bladder contraction. M: M_2 and M_3 muscarinic receptors. β_2, β_2-adrenoceptors. P2X, purinergic receptors.

DRUG TREATMENT OF OVERACTIVE BLADDER

Increased understanding of the neural pathways involved in initiating micturition is opening up new avenues for drug therapy to augment the relatively ineffective treatments currently available. Drugs used at present to treat overactive bladder act at peripheral muscarinic receptors to decrease bladder activity.

Muscarinic receptor antagonists

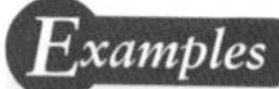

Examples

darifenacin, oxybutynin, propiverine, solifenacin, tolterodine, trospium

These drugs act with various degrees of selectivity at muscarinic receptor subtypes. Antimuscarinic unwanted effects (Ch. 4) are most troublesome with oxybutynin, particularly central nervous system effects (from M_1 receptor blockade) and dry mouth (from M_3 receptor blockade in salivary glands). The need for continued use of these drugs should be reviewed after 6 months.

- *Oxybutynin* is selective for M_1 and M_3 receptors and has additional weak muscle relaxant properties through calcium channel blocking actions and local anaesthetic activity. Oxybutynin is rapidly absorbed from the gut and metabolised in the liver; an active metabolite may contribute many of the unwanted effects of this drug. Modified-release and transdermal formulations are available because oxybutynin has a short half-life (1–3 h) and use of standard formulations can result in large fluctuations in plasma drug concentrations and increase the severity of unwanted effects.
- *Tolterodine* and *trospium* are non-selective muscarinic receptor blockers with no additional properties and less lipophilicity than oxybutynin. Both tolterodine and trospium have short half-lives (2 h in most people – but see compendium for tolterodine). Tolterodine is better tolerated in a modified-release formulation.
- *Darifenacin* and *solifenacin* are more selective for M_3 receptors.
- *Propiverine* is a non-selective muscarinic receptor blocker, with additional calcium channel blocking actions. It is an option for overactive bladder syndrome, but less effective for urge incontinence.
- *Tricyclic antidepressants*, for example imipramine and amitriptyline (Ch. 22), have antimuscarinic actions but are now little used for detrusor instability, because of their troublesome unwanted effects.

Other drugs

- *Topical vaginal oestrogen* replacement therapy (Ch. 45) reverses atrophic changes in the lower genital tract in postmenopausal women and may be helpful for overactive bladder syndrome.

- *Desmopressin,* a synthetic antidiuretic hormone analogue (Ch. 43), is sometimes helpful to reduce nocturia in unstable bladder syndrome. It is taken orally; the nasal spray is no longer licensed for this indication because of the risk of water intoxication in children.

HYPOTONIC BLADDER

Hypotonic bladder is often a result of lower motor neuron lesions, or can arise from bladder distension following chronic urinary retention. Drugs with antimuscarinic properties (tricyclic antidepressants and see above) can make the symptoms worse. Hypotonic bladder leads to incomplete bladder emptying, with urinary retention and overflow incontinence. Treatment depends on the cause.

- Chronic urinary retention is often caused by bladder outlet obstruction. If renal function is impaired, it should be managed by bladder catheterisation and correction of the underlying cause.
- Neurogenic problems are sometimes treated with muscarinic agonists which increase the force of detrusor contraction (Ch. 4), although they are probably ineffective. They should not be used in the presence of urinary outflow obstruction. The most frequently used drug is the anticholinesterase distigmine; the direct-acting agonist bethanechol is no longer recommended.

URETHRAL SPHINCTER INCOMPETENCE

Urethral sphincter incompetence produces stress incontinence in women (urine leakage with effort, exertion, sneezing or coughing) or sphincter weakness incontinence in men. The most common cause in women is loss of collagenous support in the pelvic floor or perineum; it also arises from trauma to the membranous urethra (sphincter mechanism), such as may occur from pelvic trauma or following prostatectomy in males. Drugs such as α_1-adrenoceptor antagonists (see below) can make the symptoms worse. Pelvic floor muscle training may be helpful, while minimal access surgical sling procedures or colposuspension to provide urethral support are among the surgical options. Drug therapy is limited, and only recommended if surgical treatment is not suitable.

Duloxetine is a selective serotonin and noradrenaline reuptake inhibitor (see Ch. 22). It is believed to augment sympathetic activity which relaxes the detrusor, and to enhance external urethral sphincter activity by increasing efferent impulses in the motor neurons of the pudendal nerve when the bladder is placed under stress. It reduces the frequency of incontinence episodes significantly in about half of those treated.

BENIGN PROSTATIC HYPERTROPHY

Benign prostatic hypertrophy (BPH) produces symptoms in more than 25% of men above the age of 60 years, and up to 70% of men over the age of 70 years. The spectrum of symptoms is often called prostatism (Box 15.1). Left untreated, spontaneous improvement occurs or symptoms remain stable in up to half of all those with prostatism. Acute urinary retention occurs at a rate of 1–2% per year. Scoring systems can reliably quantify the extent to which symptoms affect the quality of life.

Box 15.1 Symptoms of benign prostatic hypertrophy

Obstructive	Irritative
Hesitancy	Urgency
Poor stream	Frequency
Straining to pass urine	Nocturia
Prolonged micturition	Urge incontinence
Feeling of incomplete bladder emptying	
Urinary retention	

DRUG TREATMENT OF PROSTATISM

Many symptomatic individuals do not require or want treatment, and a policy of 'watchful waiting' will be appropriate. The aim of drug treatment is either to reduce prostatic size or to relax the smooth muscle that restricts urine outflow. There is no evidence that medical treatment avoids the need for surgery in the long term.

Alpha$_1$-adrenoceptor antagonists

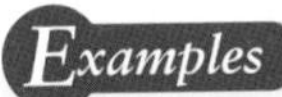

alfuzosin, doxazosin, prazosin, tamsulosin

Selective α_1-adrenoceptor antagonists inhibit contraction in prostatic and bladder neck smooth muscle, without affecting the detrusor. Relaxation of these muscles improves urine flow rate and symptoms of BPH. Alfuzosin and tamsulosin are claimed to be more selective antagonists at the α_{1A}-adrenoceptor subtype in the smooth muscle of the urinary tract and may produce fewer vasodilatory unwanted effects compared with other less selective α_1-adrenoceptor antagonists that also block α_{1B}- and α_{1D}-adrenoceptors in blood vessels; however, the clinical advantages of the α_{1A}-adrenoceptor selective drugs are equivocal. Symptomatic improvement usually occurs within 1 month, and is seen in about two-thirds of those treated. Selective α_1-adrenoceptor antagonists are the first-choice drugs for improving symptoms and urinary flow rates.

5α-Reductase inhibitors

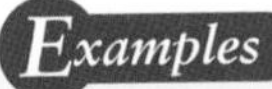

dutasteride, finasteride

Inhibition of the enzyme 5α-reductase reduces the conversion of testosterone to dihydrotestosterone (DHT) within prostatic cells, but does not affect circulating testosterone levels. DHT is involved in prostate growth, and inhibition of its production can reduce prostate volume by up to 30%. There are two isoenzymes of 5α-reductase, both found in the prostate. Finasteride only inhibits the type 2 isoenzyme, while dutasteride inhibits both the type 1 and 2 isoenzymes, but it is not yet known whether this confers any clinical advantage. 5α-Reductase inhibitors usually take 3–6 months to improve symptoms of prostatism, but the improvements are maintained. The drugs may be more effective with larger-volume prostates. Additional symptomatic benefit can be obtained from combining finasteride with an α_1-adrenoceptor antagonist.

Pharmacokinetics

Both finasteride and dutasteride are well absorbed after oral administration and eliminated by hepatic metabolism. Finasteride has a half-life of about 6 h, whereas that of dutasteride is extremely long at about 4 weeks.

Unwanted effects

These occur in up to 10% of people taking the drugs, and include:

- Reduced libido
- Erectile impotence or decreased ejaculation
- Reduction of the plasma concentration of prostate-specific antigen by an average of 50%, which should be considered when screening for prostate cancer.

Plant extracts

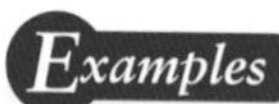

saw palmetto plant extracts, β-sitosterol plant extract

These products are available direct to consumers, but their composition varies between suppliers. Very limited trial evidence suggests that they produce modest short-term improvements in symptoms of prostatism, but a more rigorous study found no benefit for a preparation of saw palmetto extract compared to placebo. The mechanism of action, if any, is uncertain, but these extracts may reduce the synthesis of DHT or inhibit expression of prostatic growth factors. They are well tolerated, with unwanted effects mainly confined to gastrointestinal upset.

SURGICAL TREATMENT

Surgical treatment is usually required for severe symptoms or complications of BPH (Box 15.2). Transurethral resection of the prostate improves symptoms in 70–90% of those with prostatism. Long-term sequelae include impotence (5–10%), retrograde ejaculation (80–90%) and incontinence (<5%). Several less invasive procedures are now available, but they may be less successful for relieving symptoms, and do not reduce the risk of long-term consequences, although they produce fewer immediate postoperative complications.

Box 15.2 Indications for surgery in patients with benign prostatic hypertrophy (BPH)

Acute retention of urine
Chronic retention of urine
Recurrent urinary tract infection
Bladder stones
Renal insufficiency owing to BPH
Large bladder diverticula
Severe symptoms

FURTHER READING

Appel RA (2006) Pharmacotherapy for overactive bladder. *Drugs* 66, 1361–1370

Barendrecht MM, Oelke M, Laguna MP et al (2007) Is the use of parasympathetics for treating an underactive urinary bladder evidence-based? *BJU Int* 99, 749–752

Chapple RC, Yamanishi T, Chess-Williams R (2002) Muscarinic receptor subtypes and management of the overactive bladder. *Urology* 60(suppl 5A), 82–89

Connolly SS, Fitzpatrick JM (2007) Medical treatment of benign prostatic hyperplasia. *Postgrad Med J* 83, 73–78

Foley CL, Kirby RS (2003) 5-alpha-reductase inhibitors: what's new? *Curr Opin Urol* 13, 31–37

Gerber GS (2002) Phytotherapy for benign prostatic hyperplasia. *Curr Urol Rep* 3, 285–291

Hashim H, Abrams P (2006) Pharmacological management of women with mixed incontinence. *Drugs* 66, 591–606

Norton P, Brubaker L (2006) Urinary incontinence in women. *Lancet* 367, 57–67

Rogers RG (2008) Urinary stress incontinence in women. *N Engl J Med* 358, 1029–1036

Shamliyan TA, Kane RL, Wyman J et al (2008) Randomised, controlled trials of non-surgical treatments for urinary incontinence in women. *Ann Intern Med* 148, 459–473

Shefchyk SJ (2001) Sacral spinal interneurones and the control of urinary bladder and urethral striated sphincter muscle function. *J Physiol* 533, 57–63

Thorpe A, Neal D (2003) Benign prostatic hyperplasia. *Lancet* 361, 1359–1367

Wilt TJ, Dow JN (2008) Benign prostatic hyperplasia. Part 2 – Management. *BMJ* 336, 206–210

SELF-ASSESSMENT

1. In this question, the first statement, in italics, is correct. Are the accompanying statements also true?
   Urinary bladder function is controlled by involuntary parasympathetic and sympathetic innervation of the detrusor and sphincter muscles and voluntary control via the somatic nervous system.
   a. Darifenacin causes urinary frequency and urge incontinence.
   b. The antidepressant drug duloxetine can be used to treat stress incontinence.
   c. The anticholinesterase distigmine can be given safely if there is urinary outflow obstruction.
2. Case history questions

A 65-year-old man developed progressive urinary problems over a 5-year period. He had difficulty passing urine and was getting up three times in the night to pass urine. A rectal examination by his GP showed an enlarged prostate. Ultrasound, flow tests and prostate-specific antigen measurements suggested benign prostatic hypertrophy (BPH).

   a. What pharmacological approaches to the treatment of BPH could be considered?
   b. What are the unwanted effects of these treatments?
   c. What are the possible outcomes of not giving treating?
3. Extended-matching questions
   Choose the **most appropriate** pharmacological option A–F to fit the case scenarios described in 3.1–3.3.
   A. Tamsulosin
   B. Finasteride
   C. Duloxetine
   D. Amitriptyline
   E. Bethanecol
   F. Oxybutynin
   3.1. A 50-year-old man with a 2-year history of difficulty in urinating and hesitancy was diagnosed with BPH and an enlarged prostate. He was given a 1-month trial of an α_1-adrenoceptor antagonist, which did not improve his symptoms. He did not at this stage want to undergo surgery. What pharmacological treatment might be of benefit?
   3.2. A 30-year-old woman with normal bladder function complained of difficulty in urination after being prescribed new medication for her depression. She was found to have urinary retention. What class of antidepressant could cause this effect?
   3.3. A 60-year-old woman had severe urge incontinence. She urinated 16–20 times a day and had leakage two to three times a day and at night. What treatment could she be given?

ANSWERS

1. a. **False**. Darifenacin blocks muscarinic receptors with some selectivity for the M_3 subtype, inhibiting the parasympathetic effects on the detrusor muscle. It is used for treatment of overactive bladder.
   b. **True**. Duloxetine inhibits the reuptake of amines and increases the contractility of the urethral sphincters.
   c. **False**. Distigmine contracts detrusor muscle, which is undesirable in the presence of urinary outflow obstruction.
2. Case history answers
   a. Drugs may be used in mild disease and while awaiting a transurethral resection of the prostate. Selective α_1-adrenoceptor antagonists increase urine flow to a limited extent but also decrease urgency, frequency and hesitancy. Antagonists selective for α_{1A}-adrenoceptors, such as tamsulosin, are claimed to have fewer unwanted effects. Finasteride, which inhibits conversion of testosterone to dihydrotestosterone, reduces prostate size slowly.
   b. Alpha$_1$-adrenoceptor antagonists can cause postural hypotension, especially with the first dose. They cause dizziness and can interact with other drugs to lower blood pressure. Finasteride can reduce libido and cause impotence.
   c. The outcome is variable; symptoms may not worsen appreciably for many years, but moderate symptoms can lead to a poor quality of life. Complications include urinary retention, incontinence and renal insufficiency owing to hydronephrosis.
3. Extended-matching answers
   3.1. Answer **B**. Finasteride inhibits the conversion of testosterone to dihydrotestosterone, which is a promoter of prostatic cell growth. A reduction of up to 30% in prostate size can be obtained. Benefit may be increased if finasteride and an α_1-adrenoceptor antagonist are given together
   3.2. Answer **D**. Amitriptyline is an inhibitor of muscarinic receptors and inhibits the micturition reflex.
   3.3. Answer **C**. Duloxetine could be tried if the condition were caused by sphincter incompetence. Duloxetine increases the levels of noradrenaline and serotonin in the synapse and the activity of the motor neurons in the pudendal nerve. Pelvic floor exercises should also be suggested. Drug therapy is of limited benefit.

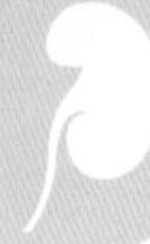

Drugs used to treat disorders of micturition

Drug	Half-life (h) and kinetics	Comment
Drugs for urinary retention		
All drugs taken orally		
α_1-Adrenoceptor antagonists		
Alfuzosin	4–10 [M + R] Oral bioavailability is about 50% when given with food; metabolised in the liver by CYP3A4 to inactive metabolites; about 11% is excreted by the kidneys	Relative selectivity for α_{1A}-adrenoceptors in the genitourinary tract
Doxazosin	10–20 [M + R] Oral bioavailability is 65%; longer half-lives (20 h) found after treatment to steady state; eliminated largely by oxidative metabolism to a number of products, one of which is a potent α_1-adrenoceptor antagonist	
Indoramin	5 (2–10) [M + R] Undergoes extensive hepatic first-pass metabolism; oral bioavailability is about 10–20% (but 70% in people with hepatic cirrhosis); longer half-life and much higher blood levels (fivefold) in the elderly	
Prazosin	2–4 [M + R] Oral bioavailability is about 60%; metabolised in the liver by dealkylation and conjugation	
Tamsulosin	15 [M + R] Food reduces bioavailability to about 60%; eliminated by hepatic oxidation followed by conjugation with glucuronic acid and sulphate	Relative selectivity for α_{1A}-adrenoceptors in the genitourinary tract; normally taken with food (to reduce unwanted effects)
Terazosin	10–12 [M + R] High oral bioavailability (90%); metabolised in liver; eliminated in faeces and urine as parent drug and metabolites	
Parasympathomimetics		
Bethanechol	? Few data available; poorly absorbed; not hydrolysed by cholinesterases	
Distigmine	70 [R + hydrolysis] Very poor oral bioavailability (5%), especially if taken with food; hydrolysed by plasma esterases	
5α-Reductase inhibitors		
Dutasteride	4–5 weeks [M] Oral bioavailability is about 60%; eliminated by CYP3A4 metabolism; the very long half-life results from low clearance (0.5 L h^{-1}) and a large apparent volume of distribution (500 L); it takes about 6 months to reach steady state	Safety profile similar to that of finasteride
Finasteride	6 (3–16) [M] Oral bioavailability is about 60–80%; eliminated as metabolites in faeces and in urine	

Drugs used to treat disorders of micturition

Drug	Half-life (h) and kinetics	Comment
Drugs for urinary frequency and incontinence		
All drugs taken orally		
Inhibitors of muscarinic receptors		
Darifenacin	13–19 [M] Low oral bioavailability; metabolised by CYP2D6 and CYP3A4; higher plasma levels in CYP2D6 poor metabolisers	Selective M_3 receptor antagonist (about nine-fold difference compared with M_1)
Flavoxate	? [R + M] Metabolised to a carboxylic acid derivative; also eliminated unchanged in urine; few other kinetic data are available (high oral bioavailability in rats)	
Oxybutynin	1–3 [M] Very low oral bioavailability (6%) owing to extensive first-pass metabolism; cholinergic antagonism in vivo probably results from the desethyl metabolite, which is formed in the liver during first-pass metabolism and is as active as the parent compound	
Propantheline	1–2 [M] Oral bioavailability is about 10–25% and variable; undergoes first-pass metabolism; metabolites are inactive	Quaternary amino compound
Propiverine	4 [M] Oral bioavailability is about 50%; metabolised mainly by N-oxidation	
Solifenacin	55 [M + R] High oral bioavailability; eliminated by CYP3A4 metabolism; <15% excreted in urine unchanged	Selective M_3 receptor antagonist
Tolterodine	2 (EM); 10 (PM): [M] High oral bioavailability (about 75%); metabolised by CYP2D6 to an active metabolite responsible for part of the therapeutic effect; subjects with low CYP2D6 activity (poor metabolisers; PM) metabolise the drug by CYP3A4; PM have higher levels of parent drug and lower levels of the metabolite, but, as both compounds are active, they show similar responses to extensive metabolisers (EM); the drug shows dose-dependent kinetics in the therapeutic range	
Trospium	1–2 [R + M] Very low oral bioavailability (<10%); about 40% of that absorbed undergoes metabolism; about one-half is excreted unchanged	A quaternary amino compound
Inhibitor of noradrenaline and serotonin reuptake		
Duloxetine	9–19 [M] Good oral absorption; undergoes extensive hepatic oxidation by CYP2D6 and CYP1A2 to numerous inactive metabolites	

[M], metabolism; [R], renal excretion.

16 Erectile dysfunction

PHYSIOLOGY OF ERECTION

Achieving and maintaining an erection is a spinal reflex that involves a complex series of interactions between the central nervous system, the autonomic nervous system and local mediators; psychological, visual, olfactory and tactile stimuli are also important. The primary erectile innervation is the parasympathetic nervous system. There are four phases in the processes of penile erection.

Phase 1. Parasympathetic stimulation relaxes both arterial smooth muscle and the smooth muscle that forms bands (trabeculae) with connective tissue in the highly vascular erectile tissues of the penis (corpus cavernosa and corpus spongiosum). This increases the influx of blood into the sinusoidal spaces of the corpus cavernosa, which engorge with blood (Fig. 16.1). Conversely, sympathetic stimulation inhibits erection by increasing vascular smooth muscle tone.

Phase 2. Within the corpus cavernosum, pressure rises and the sinusoids expand. The penis elongates and widens.

Phase 3. The rise in pressure in the sinusoids compresses the venous plexus and reduces venous outflow, thus maintaining the erection (the corporeal veno-occlusive mechanism).

Phase 4. The pudendal nerve (part of the parasympathetic innervation) stimulates the ischiocavernous muscle. This squeezes the crura at the base of the penis and stops both arterial inflow and venous outflow, maintaining full erection. Muscle fatigue eventually allows return of perfusion.

There are also many locally produced mediators that appear to be involved in achieving and maintaining an erection. Nitric oxide synthesised by blood vessel endothelial cells and released from non-adrenergic non-cholinergic (NANC) nerves in the corpora appears to be crucial for cavernosal smooth muscle relaxation via generation of cyclic guanosine monophosphate (cGMP) and activation of protein kinase G. Cyclic GMP is degraded by phosphodiesterase type 5 (PDE5) (see Table 1.1) to GMP, terminating its effects; inhibition of PDE5 is a primary target for the pharmacological treatment of erectile dysfunction (see below). The precise role of other vasodilators that seem to be involved in modulating penile vascular smooth muscle relaxation and blood flow, such as vasoactive intestinal peptide (VIP), calcitonin gene-related peptide (CGRP) and prostaglandin E_1, are less well understood. Numerous central facilitatory mediators have been identified, including dopamine, acetylcholine and a variety of peptides. These are involved in the psychological preparedness that is essential for an erection to occur.

Erectile dysfunction

Erectile dysfunction is defined as the consistent inability to achieve or sustain an erection of sufficient rigidity for sexual intercourse. It is a common problem, affecting up to 20% of adult men, with up to 10% over the age of 40 years having complete erectile dysfunction. Any disease process that affects penile neural supply, arterial inflow or venous outflow can produce erectile dysfunction. There is a physical cause in about 80% of cases (Box 16.1) but a psychological component often coexists. Psychogenic erectile dysfunction is more common in younger men. Drugs are an important cause of erectile dysfunction, particularly antihypertensive, psychotropic and 'recreational' drugs, and account for up to 25% of cases (Table 16.1).

MANAGEMENT OF ERECTILE DYSFUNCTION

A number of strategies can be used in the management of erectile dysfunction. Initially there should be an assessment and treatment of any underlying psychological cause or physical disease or withdrawal of a causative drug. Treatment options for persistent dysfunction include:

- pharmacological, using the drugs described below
- mechanical aids, such as the vacuum constriction device: these are usually advised for older people who do not respond to pharmacological treatment and do not wish to have surgery
- penile implants using a malleable or inflatable prosthesis
- testosterone replacement therapy for hypogonadism (Ch. 46), an uncommon cause of impotence
- hyperprolactinaemia impairs erection; it is most commonly caused by drug therapy (e.g. with phenothiazines) and can be improved by oral bromocriptine (Ch. 43) if the cause cannot be treated.

Oral phosphodiesterase inhibitors

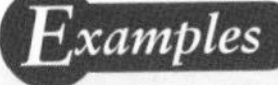

sildenafil, tadalafil, vardenafil

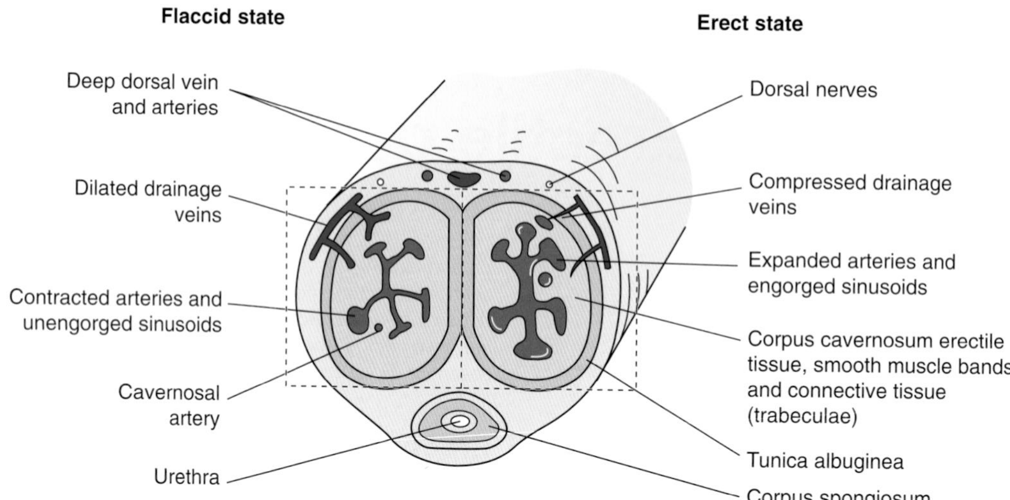

Fig. 16.1 **Cross-section of the penis, showing structures involved in erection.** This diagram shows only part of the rich nervous and vascular filling and drainage system in the penis. The left-hand area shows the situation in the flaccid penis and the right-hand area the erect penis. The rising pressure during erection limits the venous outflow, thus maintaining the erection. The penis contains three cylinders of erectile tissue: two corpora cavernosa and the corpus spongiosum. The corpus spongiosum contains the urethra. The cylinders of erectile tissue are divided into spaces known as sinusoids or lacunae, which are lined by vascular epithelium. The walls of these spaces are made up of thick bundles of smooth muscle cells within a framework of fibroblasts, collagen and elastin (trabeculae). The erectile tissues are supplied with blood from the cavernosal and helicine arteries, which drain into the sinusoidal spaces. Blood is drained from the sinusoidal spaces through emissary veins. The venules join together to form larger veins that drain into the deep dorsal vein or other veins at different parts of the penis. Arterial and sinusoid dilation is important for erection, while swelling is limited by the inelastic tunica albuginea.

Box 16.1 Common causes of erectile dysfunction

Diabetes
Vascular disease
Surgery
Drugs (Table 16.1)
Substance abuse, e.g. nicotine, alcohol, recreational drugs
Hormonal imbalance
Neurological disease, e.g. multiple sclerosis, Alzheimer's disease, epilepsy
Spinal cord injury
Psychological (20% as a primary cause, more commonly secondary to physical problems)

Endothelial-derived nitric oxide increases the synthesis of cGMP that acts via protein kinases to cause blood vessel dilation (see Ch. 5, Fig. 5.3). Cyclic GMP is broken down in penile tissue by PDE5. Sildenafil, tadalafil and vardenafil are orally active analogues of cGMP that selectively inhibit the enzyme. PDE5 is also found in lower concentrations in other vascular and visceral smooth muscles, and in skeletal muscle and platelets. Prolonging the vasodilator effect of nitric oxide on penile vascular smooth muscle results in erection; sexual stimulation resulting in the release of nitric oxide is a prerequisite for these drugs to produce an erection. If an appropriate dose of the drug is used, about 60% of men with erectile dysfunction will achieve erections sufficient to permit intercourse. The response is often better if precipitating factors are also treated, such as depression or excess alcohol consumption.

Sildenafil is also used to treat pulmonary hypertension (Ch. 6).

Pharmacokinetics

Sildenafil is relatively well absorbed orally, but vardenafil and tadalafil are less well absorbed. The median time to onset of action for all is about 30 min. The absorption of sildenafil and vardenafil are delayed by a fatty meal, whereas the absorption of tadalafil is rapid and is unaffected by food. All are eliminated by hepatic metabolism mediated primarily by CYP3A4. Sildenafil and vardenafil have half-lives of less than 6 h, and should be taken 30–60 min before sexual activity for maximum benefit. The half-life of tadalafil is longer (17 h), and its duration of action is up to about 24–36 h; therefore, planning of sexual activity (and its timing in relation to drug dosage) is less relevant with this drug. Sildenafil and vardenafil both have active metabolites, but tadalafil does not.

Unwanted effects

- Dyspepsia, nausea, vomiting.
- Hypotension, dizziness, flushing, headache and nasal congestion from systemic vasodilation.
- PDE6 (involved in phototransduction in the eye) is inhibited by high doses of sildenafil, but less so by tadalafil or vardenafil. This can cause visual disturbance (enhanced perception of bright lights, or a 'blue halo' effect) and raised intraocular pressure.
- Priapism, a painful and sustained erection, can occur rarely.

Table 16.1 Drugs that commonly cause male sexual dysfunction

	Ejaculatory dysfunction	Erectile dysfunction	Loss of libido
Antihypertensives			
β-Adrenoceptor antagonists		+	
α-Adrenoceptor antagonists	+		
Methyldopa	+	+	+
Thiazide diuretics		+	
Psychotropic drugs			
Phenothiazines	+	+	+
Benzodiazepines	+	+	+
Tricyclic antidepressants		+	+
Selective serotonin reuptake inhibitors (SSRIs)		+	+
Other			
Spironolactone			+
Digoxin		+	
Cimetidine/ranitidine		+	+
Metoclopramide		+	+
Carbamazepine		+	+
Recreational drugs			
Alcohol	+	+	
Marijuana		+	
Cocaine		+	+
Amphetamines	+	+	+
Anabolic steroids		+	+

- Drug interactions: oral PDE5 inhibitors should not be used together with nitrates or nicorandil (see Ch. 5), because of a synergistic effect on vascular nitric oxide with exaggerated vasodilator effects. Several antiviral drugs, such as saquinavir (Table 2.9 and Ch. 51), inhibit the CYP3A4 isoenzyme that metabolises oral PDE5 inhibitors, and can potentiate their effects.

Other vasodilators

Sublingual apomorphine

Apomorphine is a dopamine D_2 receptor agonist used in Parkinson's disease (Ch. 24); its mechanism of action in erectile dysfunction is uncertain and probably involves hypothalamic stimulation in the brain. Until recently it was only available in a formulation for subcutaneous administration, but sublingual preparations have been developed. Limited absorption through the buccal mucosa reduces the nausea and hypotension that are troublesome following subcutaneous injection. It is effective about 10–20 min after administration, and gives most benefit in psychogenic impotence.

Intracavernosal injection of vasodilators

These are more effective if arterial flow is normal, such as with neurogenic and psychogenic impotence. Bleeding tendencies preclude this form of treatment, as does poor manual dexterity or morbid obesity. The injection is made into the side of the penis, directly into the corpus cavernosum.

- **Alprostadil.** This is a synthetic prostaglandin E_1 analogue. It vasodilates by acting on smooth muscle cell surface receptors to increase intracellular cAMP, which in turn reduces the intracellular Ca^{2+} concentration. Local pain after injection is a common unwanted effect, reported by one-third of users, and can be reduced by the addition of a local anaesthetic such as procaine (Ch. 18). Rapid local metabolism of alprostadil minimises unwanted systemic effects. High doses of *intraurethral alprostadil* can be given as a pellet using a plastic applicator, but are less effective than the injection. In responders, an erection develops within 15 min and lasts for 30–60 min. Because of the uterine stimulant activity of alprostadil, a sheath is recommended if the partner is pregnant.

- **Phentolamine.** This is a non-selective α-adrenoceptor antagonist (Ch. 6). It is relatively ineffective when used alone, because it does not reduce venous outflow, and is used in combination with papaverine.
- **Papaverine.** This is a non-selective phosphodiesterase inhibitor that increases intracellular cAMP and cGMP, reduces intracellular Ca^{2+} in vascular smooth muscle, and produces relaxation. Papaverine is not licensed in the UK. The success rate in impotence is about 50%, but there is a high incidence of prolonged erection (lasting more than 4 h) or priapism, so this drug is rarely used except in combination with alprostadil and phentolamine for non-responders to alprostadil given alone. Fibrosis within the penis can result from the acidity of the solution.

Combinations of drugs, e.g. sildenafil with apomorphine, can be effective when monotherapy fails.

FURTHER READING

Andersson K-E (2001) Pharmacology of penile erection. *Pharmacol Rev* 53, 417–450

Corbin JD, Francis SH (2002) Pharmacology of phosphodiesterase-5 inhibitors. *Int J Clin Pract* 56, 453–459

Fink HA, MacDonald R, Rutks I et al (2002) Sildenafil for male erectile dysfunction. *Arch Intern Med* 162, 1349–1360

McVary KT (2007) Erectile dysfunction. *N Engl J Med* 357, 2472–2481

Morgentaler A (1999) Male impotence. *Lancet* 354, 1713–1718

Sivalingam S, Hashim H, Schwaibold H (2006) An overview of the diagnosis and treatment of erectile dysfunction. *Drugs* 66, 2339–2355

SELF-ASSESSMENT

1. Are the following statements true or false?
   a. Sildenafil should not be taken by men already taking nitrates.
   b. Sildenafil can cause an increase in blood pressure if taken with nitrates.
   c. Phosphodiesterase type 5 is only found in the vasculature in the penis.
   d. Increased parasympathetic outflow to the penis causes a failure of erection.
   e. Erections caused by injected drugs such as papaverine or alprostadil are not easy to control.
   f. Impotence caused by hypogonadism can be treated with oestrogen.
   g. Diabetes can cause impotence.
   h. The duration of biological actions of sildenafil and tadalafil are similar.
   i. Sildenafil inhibits the breakdown of cAMP.
2. Which one of the following statements concerning drug action and erectile dysfunction is **false?**
   A. Alcohol can cause erectile difficulties.
   B. Cimetidine can exacerbate the potential for sildenafil to cause headache.
   C. Nicorandil is safe when taken together with tadalafil.
   D. Amitriptyline can cause impotence.
   E. Sildenafil prevents the breakdown of cGMP.
3. Case history questions

Mr JA, aged 56 years, presented with erectile dysfunction of gradual onset over the last 2–3 years. He was hypertensive, with a blood pressure of 160/96 mmHg, and was being treated with atenolol and bendroflumethiazide. There was a family history of coronary artery disease. He smokes 30 cigarettes a day and drinks 4 pints of beer a night. Examination revealed that he was hypercholesterolaemic and there were signs of coronary artery disease. Tests for liver function and testosterone were normal and no organic reason for the dysfunction was found. Mr JA also suffers from recurrent heartburn, for which he is taking cimetidine on most days.

It was decided not to prescribe a pharmacological agent for his erectile dysfunction at this stage, but a number of suggestions and recommendations were made.

After 3 months, during which time Mr JA followed the advice he was given, his blood pressure was within normal limits and his cholesterol was lower. He was regularly taking cimetidine. However, his erectile dysfunction persisted.

Following discussions, it was decided that Mr JA should try sildenafil.

a. Which of the above factors could contribute to his erectile dysfunction and what recommendations would you suggest?
b. From his history, what precautions should be taken in prescribing sildenafil and what advice should Mr JA be given?

ANSWERS

1. a. **True**. Nitrates result in increased nitric oxide production and elevate cGMP. Sildenafil has a similar effect by preventing cGMP breakdown. This can lead to additive unwanted effects, particularly hypotension.
   b. **False**. These two drugs can act together to cause hypotension.
   c. **False**. Phosphodiesterase type 5 is found in other blood vessels and tissues, which can result in unwanted effects when sildenafil is given.
   d. **False**. Parasympathetic stimulation enhances erection. Drugs known to inhibit the parasympathetic outflow, e.g. tricyclic antidepressants, can cause erectile failure.
   e. **True**. Painful priapism with erections lasting many hours can occur.
   f. **False**. Testosterone can be useful if the impotence is due to hypogonadism.
   g. **True**. Probably through vascular dysfunction.
   h. **False**. Although both are mainly metabolised in the liver, tadalafil has a much longer biological half-life than sildenafil.
   i. **False**. Sildenafil inhibits the breakdown of cGMP.
2. Answer **C**.
   A. True
   B. True. Cimetidine inhibits the isoenzyme CYP3A4 that metabolises sildenafil, enhancing its vasodilator action
   C. False. Nicorandil is a K^+ channel opener (Ch. 5) which also has a nitrate structure; this increases cGMP formation and would add to the effects of tadalafil with the potential for increased unwanted effects
   D. True. Amitriptyline has antimuscarinic actions that could decrease blood vessel dilation in the penis, thereby inhibiting erection.
   E. True. This is the main mechanism of action of sildenafil. Cyclic GMP decreases Ca^{2+} availability, resulting in vasodilation.
3. Case history answers
   a. The following points should be noted.
      - The contribution of psychological factors in his erectile dysfunction needs to be assessed and dealt with if they are present.
      - Vascular disease, smoking and his level of alcohol consumption may all contribute to the erectile dysfunction, and Mr JA should be helped to manage these.
      - Because of the evidence of coronary artery disease, it would be advisable to be more aggressive in treating his blood pressure and reducing his cholesterol levels. Although lowering his blood pressure and cholesterol alone are unlikely to restore the erectile function, they may improve the patient's well-being and have a psychological benefit. Coronary artery disease is known to be associated with erectile dysfunction.
      - Beta-adrenoceptor antagonist drugs and thiazide diuretics can contribute to erectile problems, and Mr JA could be changed to enalapril, which has not been shown to contribute to impotence.
   b. Cimetidine is an inhibitor of hepatic CYP3A4 (Table 2.9) that metabolises sildenafil. The initial dose of sildenafil should be reduced. Alternatively, Mr JA could use ranitidine, which does not inhibit the P450 enzymes. Studies of sildenafil in patients with a history of cardiovascular disease have shown that sildenafil is safe but the simultaneous use of nitrates is an absolute contraindication. Mr JA should be told about the dangers of drug interactions and possible unwanted effects.

Drugs used to treat erectile dysfunction (all should be used with caution in people with cardiovascular disease)

Drug	Half-life (h) and kinetics	Comments
Phosphodiesterase type 5 inhibitors		
All drugs given orally		
Sildenafil	2 [M] Incomplete oral bioavailability (about 40%) due to first-pass metabolism; absorption delayed by fatty food; oxidised by hepatic CYP3A4 and CYP2C9; one metabolite retains some activity and contributes to the clinical effect; metabolites are eliminated mainly in the faeces (80%)	Taken between 0.5 and 4 h before sexual activity; also used for pulmonary hypertension
Tadalafil	17 [M] Bioavailability has not been defined, but absorption is rapid and not affected by food; eliminated by CYP3A4-catalysed oxidation in the liver	Due to the long half-life and duration of action, it can be taken between 30 min and 12 h before sexual activity
Vardenafil	4–5 [M] Incomplete oral bioavailability (about 15%); absorption delayed by fatty food; eliminated by oxidation catalysed by CYP3A4; the major metabolite retains some activity; metabolites are eliminated mainly in the faeces (80%)	Usually taken about 1 h before sexual activity

Drugs used to treat erectile dysfunction (all should be used with caution in people with cardiovascular disease)

Drug	Half-life (h) and kinetics	Comments
Other drugs used for erectile dysfunction		
Alprostadil	30 s [M] Pathways of metabolism undefined	Prostaglandin E_1 analogue; given by intracavernosal injection or urethral application; care needed if partner is pregnant; can cause priapism; can be given with papaverine (see below)
Apomorphine	0.5 [M] Sublingual bioavailability is 10–20%; metabolised by hepatic oxidation and conjugation with sulphate and glucuronic acid	Increases erections via agonist activity on dopamine receptors in the hypothalamus and limbic system; stimulation of the chemoreceptor trigger zone (CTZ) produces potent emetic actions; taken sublingually 20 min before sexual activity; not licensed for this indication in the BNF
Papaverine	2 [M] Eliminated by oxidation in the liver; the 4-hydroxy metabolite is a phosphodiesterase inhibitor	Smooth muscle relaxant; given by intracavernosal injection; not licensed in the UK
Phentolamine	1.5 [M + R] Eliminated in urine largely as oxidised metabolites plus some unchanged drug	Given by intracavernosal injection

[M], metabolism; [R], renal excretion.

5

The nervous system

17 General anaesthetics

General anaesthetics work in the brain to induce unconsciousness. This allows surgical or other painful procedures to be undertaken without the person being aware. General anaesthesia was introduced into clinical practice in the 19th century, with the inhalation of vapours such as diethyl ether and chloroform. Major drawbacks with such compounds included the time taken to cause loss of consciousness, slow recovery, unpleasant taste, irritant properties and their potential to explode. Cardiac and hepatic toxicity also limited the usefulness of chloroform. The perfect general anaesthetic would possess the properties shown in Box 17.1. Because no single anaesthetic agent possesses all of these, it is normal practice to use a combination of general anaesthetics, analgesics and muscle relaxants to produce balanced general anaesthesia (see below and Table 17.2). This maximises the advantages of each agent, and minimises the disadvantages. General anaesthesia for surgical procedures involves several steps:

- premedication
- induction
- muscle relaxation and intubation
- maintenance of anaesthesia
- analgesia
- reversal.

Premedication in adults is given to reduce anxiety and produce amnesia, usually with a benzodiazepine such as diazepam, midazolam, temazepam or lorazepam (Ch. 20). In addition, an antiemetic such as metoclopramide (Ch. 32) may be used.

Anaesthesia was originally induced and maintained solely by inhalation of a volatile agent. If this method is used, several stages of general anaesthesia are experienced during induction and recovery (Table 17.1), some of which are undesirable. In adults, use of only an inhalational anaesthetic for induction of anaesthesia is usually associated with troublesome excitation and struggling; this can be overcome by using a bolus of intravenous anaesthetic for rapid induction, followed by an inhalational anaesthetic for maintenance. In children, this is less of a problem, and anaesthesia is often both induced and maintained with an inhalational anaesthetic agent. For some short surgical procedures in adults, total intravenous anaesthesia can be used.

For abdominal and thoracic surgery, and for long operations, adjunctive neuromuscular-blocking drugs (Ch. 27) are used, in which case endotracheal intubation and mechanical ventilation are necessary. Analgesia can be provided by an intravenous opioid for systemic analgesia, or by a local anaesthetic (Ch. 18) to provide regional analgesia, such as into the epidural space (epidural analgesia) or on peripheral nerves.

At the end of an operation, resumption of consciousness (reversal of anaesthesia) occurs when intravenous anaesthetics are redistributed or metabolised, or when inhalational anaesthetics are redistributed or exhaled. Residual neuromuscular blockade by competitive blocking agents may need reversal with an anticholinesterase such as neostigmine (Ch. 27). Attentiveness, and therefore the ability to drive safely, may be impaired for up to 24 h after general anaesthesia.

The management of a person undergoing general anaesthesia requires the administration of several drugs having different desirable and unwanted effects. The appropriate combination of these agents produces a 'balanced anaesthesia' with a suitable degree of sedation, analgesia and muscle relaxation (Table 17.2).

MECHANISMS OF ACTION OF GENERAL ANAESTHETICS

General anaesthesia can be produced by compounds of widely differing chemical structure: simple gases such as nitrous oxide; volatile liquids such as isoflurane; and non-volatile solids such as propofol (Fig. 17.1). Anaesthetic potency of the volatile anaesthetics is measured as the minimum alveolar concentration (MAC) of an agent necessary to immobilise 50% of subjects exposed to a noxious stimulus (which in humans is a surgical skin incision). Therefore, MAC is the equivalent of the ED_{50} (the 50% effective dose) for other drugs (Ch. 1). The MAC for inhaled anaesthetics correlates *inversely* with the oil : gas partition coefficient, which is a measure of the anaesthetic's lipid solubility (see Table 17.3); the more potent anaesthetics (e.g. halothane compared with nitrous oxide) therefore have higher lipid solubility and a lower MAC.

In contrast, the time to induction and recovery correlates *directly* with the blood : gas partition coefficient (see Table 17.3). For an anaesthetic such as nitrous oxide which has a low blood : gas partition coefficient, the partial pressure of the nitrous oxide in the blood and the brain reaches the partial pressure of the nitrous oxide in the inspired air more rapidly than for a drug such as halothane which has a higher

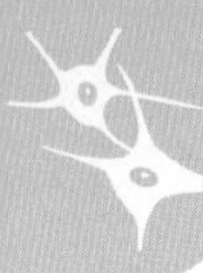

Box 17.1 Properties of an ideal inhalational anaesthetic

Inherently stable
Non-flammable and non-explosive when mixed with air, oxygen or nitrous oxide
Potent, allowing the use of a high inspired oxygen concentration
Low blood solubility, allowing rapid induction (with minimal excitation stage); rapid emergence from anaesthesia, with no hangover; and rapid adjustment of the depth of anaesthesia
Non-irritant to the airways
Non-toxic
Lack of sensitisation of the heart to catecholamines
Analgesic
Easily reversible
Minimal interactions with other drugs
Inexpensive

Table 17.1 The stages of anaesthesia

Stage	Description	Effects produced
I	Analgesia	Analgesia without amnesia or loss of touch sensation; consciousness retained
II	Excitation	Excitation and delirium with struggling: respiration rapid and irregular; frequent eye movements with increased pupil diameter; amnesia
III	Surgical anaesthesia	Loss of consciousness; subdivided into four levels or planes of increasing depth; plane I shows a decrease in eye movements and some pupillary constriction; plane II shows loss of corneal reflex; planes III and IV show increasing loss of pharyngeal reflex, and a progressive decrease in thoracic breathing and general muscle tone
IV	Medullary depression	Loss of spontaneous respiration and progressive depression of cardiovascular reflexes, no eye movements; should be considered as an overdose requiring respiratory and circulatory support

blood : gas partition coefficient. Therefore, induction and recovery times for nitrous oxide are faster than for halothane.

General anaesthetics act at cell membranes, and the relationship between lipid solubility and potency led to the hypothesis that their incorporation into lipids altered the properties of the cell membrane, perhaps resulting in the increased membrane fluidity and neural volume expansion. However, this does not account for many of the properties of general anaesthetics. Although it is not known precisely how general anaesthetics work, there is increasing evidence that implicates actions at ligand-gated ion channels in the production of general anaesthesia (Table 17.4). Individual intravenous or inhalational anaesthetic agents have diverse abilities to inhibit or enhance the functions of a number of ion channels or receptors, thus explaining the differences in their capacities to produce hypnosis, amnesia, analgesia and muscle relaxation. In general terms, their actions are to *inhibit* the functions of excitatory receptors for acetylcholine (nicotinic) and for glutamate (NMDA [N-methyl-D-aspartate] and AMPA [α-amino-3-hydroxy-5-methyl-4-isoxazole propionic acid] receptors). In contrast, they might *enhance* the functioning of inhibitory receptors for gamma-aminobutyric acid ($GABA_A$) and glycine, or

(a) Nitrous oxide: gas

N_2O

(b) Isoflurane: organic liquid

F–C(F)(F)–C(H)(Cl)–O–C(F)(F)–H

(c) Propofol: oil in water emulsion

2,6-$(CH(CH_3)_2)_2$ phenol: OH, $(CH_3)_2HC$, $CH(CH_3)_2$

Fig. 17.1 **Examples of general anaesthetics of different chemical natures.**

Table 17.2 The concept of 'balanced anaesthesia'– drugs are used in combination to produce the appropriate balance of sedation, analgesia and muscle relaxation while minimising unwanted effects; at particular doses and concentrations, each contributes minor or major effects to achieve this balance. Excessive or inadequate doses of any one agent could disturb the balance

	Sedation	Analgesia	Muscle relaxation
Drugs exerting a major effect	Inhalational anaesthetics Propofol Premedicant benzodiazepines	Fentanyl Alfentanil Local anaesthetics	Neuromuscular blocking drugs (Ch. 27)
Drugs exerting a minor effect	Fentanyl Alfentanil Nitrous oxide	Nitrous oxide	Inhalational anaesthetics

Table 17.3 Inhalational anaesthetics[a]

Compound	Blood:gas partition coefficient	Induction time[b]	Oil:gas partition coefficient	MAC (%)[c]	Metabolism (%)[d]
Nitrous oxide	0.5	Fast	1.4	>100[e]	0
Isoflurane	1.4	Medium	91	1.12	0.2
Enflurane	1.9	Medium	96	1.7	2.10
Halothane[f]	2.3	Medium	224	0.8	15
Sevoflurane	0.6	Fast	53	2.1	≈5
Diethyl ether[g]	12.1	Slow	65	2	5–10

[a]Most cause cardiac and respiratory depression and muscle relaxation. They have varying effects on cerebral blood flow.
[b]Time for induction if used as the sole anaesthetic; correlates with blood:gas partition coefficient.
[c]MAC is the minimum alveolar concentration necessary for surgical anaesthesia (inversely proportional to potency); correlates inversely with oil:gas coefficient.
[d]Percentage eliminated as urinary metabolites; most of the remainder is eliminated in the expired air; influenced by volatility and blood:gas coefficient.
[e]Theoretical value.
[f]No longer available in the UK.
[g]Not used clinically, included for comparative purposes.
The blood:gas partition coefficient correlates more closely with the time to induction, and the oil:gas partition correlates with the potency of the anaesthetic.

Table 17.4 Possible sites of action of inhalation and intravenous general anaesthetics[a]

Drug group	Properties of group	Receptor and channel targets
Etodimate, propofol, thiopental	Potent amnesics Potent hypnotics Weak muscle relaxants	Enhance activity at $GABA_A$ receptors
Nitrous oxide, ketamine	Potent analgesics Weak hypnotics Weak muscle relaxants	Inhibit NMDA, AMPA (glutamate) receptors Inhibit ACh nicotinic receptors Open two-pore K^+ channels
Sevoflurane, isoflurane, desflurane	Potent amnesics Potent hypnotics Potent muscle relaxants	Enhance activity at $GABA_A$ receptors Enhance glycine receptor activity Inhibit NMDA, AMPA (glutamate) receptors Inhibit ACh nicotinic receptors Open two-pore K^+ channels

[a]Information for this table is derived mainly from Solt and Forman (2007) and is based on data from in vitro studies and in vivo studies in transgenic animals.

activate two-pore K^+ channels that are widely expressed in GABA interneurons. Receptor binding sites for general anaesthetics have not yet been identified, but are probably on excitable membrane proteins. Binding of the drug to these proteins occurs preferentially when the ion channels are in their open state, and general anaesthetics may compete with endogenous ligands that are essential for the activity of these proteins. The interaction of a general anaesthetic with the various ion channels alters postsynaptic receptor activity and inhibits both local and long-range (such as thalamocortical) cortical neural circuits. The amnesic and immobilising actions of an anaesthetic may result from effects on the hippocampus and spinal cord.

The various stages of anaesthesia (Table 17.1) probably arise as a result of the different sizes of neurons affected by anaesthetics and their accessibility to the anaesthetic agent. A rapid action on small neurons in the dorsal horn of the spinal cord (nociceptive impulses; Ch. 19) and inhibitory cells in the brain (see effects of alcohol; Ch. 54) explain the early analgesic and excitation phases. By contrast, neurons of the medullary centres are less insensitive.

DRUGS USED IN ANAESTHESIA

General anaesthetics can be grouped according to their route of administration, which is either intravenous or inhalational.

INTRAVENOUS ANAESTHETICS

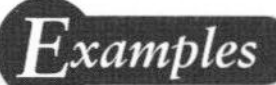

etomidate, ketamine, propofol, thiopental

Intravenous anaesthetics can be administered over a short time period for rapid induction of anaesthesia and then replaced by inhalational anaesthetics for longer-term maintenance of anaesthesia. However, the intravenous anaesthetics propofol and ketamine (but not etomidate or thiopental) can be given continuously without inhalational anaesthesia for short operations (total intravenous anaesthesia). Ketamine is analgesic, unlike all other available intravenous anaesthetics, but it does not reliably suppress

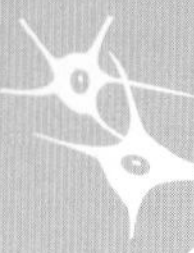

Table 17.5 Some properties of common intravenous anaesthetics

Drug	Type	Speed of induction	Recovery	Hangover effect	Analgesic	Comment
Thiopental	Barbiturate	Rapid	Slow, owing to redistribution. Slow liver metabolism	Yes	No	Widely used; sloughing of tissue if extravasation occurs from the blood vessel or the site of injection; cannot be given by long-term continuous infusion; can cause bradycardia
Propofol	Phenol	Rapid	Rapid. Liver metabolism	Low	No	Does not accumulate during infusion; continuous infusion can be used in intensive care; occasional bradycardia
Etomidate	Imidazole	Rapid	Fairly rapid. Liver metabolism	Low	No	Not infused continuously; cardiac depressant; enhances GABA activity; repeated doses suppress adrenocortical function
Ketamine	Cyclohexanone	Slower	Slower	No	Yes	Hallucinations on recovery; cardiac stimulant, raises blood pressure; can be given continuously; analgesia that outlasts anaesthesia; bronchodilator

laryngeal reflexes, which can make endotracheal intubation more difficult. It is now rarely used, except for paediatric anaesthesia. Some properties of commonly used intravenous anaesthetics are shown in Table 17.5.

Pharmacokinetics

Thiobarbiturates, such as thiopental, have a very rapid onset of action (within 30 s) owing to their high lipid solubility and ease of passage across the blood–brain barrier. The duration of action after a bolus dose is very short (about 2–5 min); blood concentrations fall rapidly, initially because of redistribution into tissues with greatest blood flow; redistribution then occurs more slowly into the major muscle groups and into the blood flow-poor but lipid-rich fat (Fig. 17.2; see also Ch. 2). With thiopental, total intravenous anaesthesia is not practicable, as during a lengthy procedure the brain and blood and slowly equilibrating tissues would reach equilibrium. Recovery from anaesthesia on cessation of anaesthetic administration would then depend on the elimination half-life (3–8 h for thiopental, related to hepatic metabolism) not the distribution half-life (about 3 min). Therefore, following induction of anaesthesia with thiopental, an inhaled agent is used for maintenance of anaesthesia.

Propofol has a slightly slower onset of action (about 30 s) compared with thiopental, but its duration of action is also limited by redistribution after a bolus dose. It can be given as an infusion for total intravenous anaesthesia (and for sedation in intensive care), but under these circumstances its duration of action is determined by a slower tissue redistribution phase (half-life 0.5–1 h), whereas after prolonged use its duration of action is determined by hepatic clearance (half-life about 6 h). Propofol is particularly useful for day surgery, because of its rapid elimination

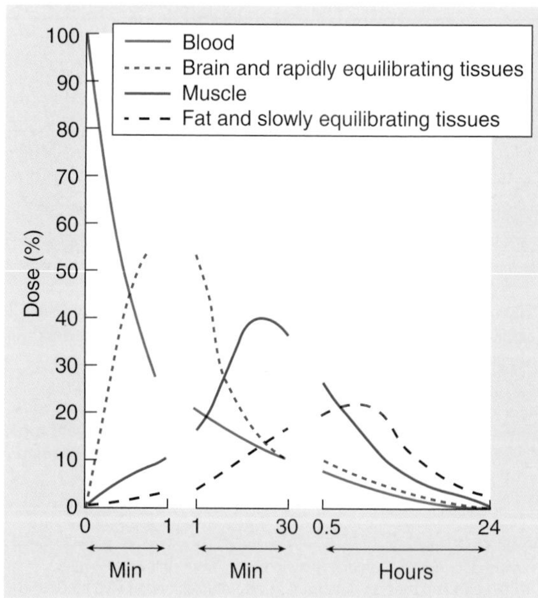

Fig. 17.2 **The amounts of thiopental in blood, brain (and other rapidly equilibrating tissues), muscle, adipose tissue and other slowly equilibrating tissues after an intravenous infusion over 10 s.** NB: the time axis is not linear: the continued uptake into muscle between 1 and 30 min lowers the concentration in the blood and in all rapidly equilibrating tissues (including the brain); the terminal elimination slopes are parallel for all tissues; metabolism removes about 15% of the body load per hour.

and absence of hangover effects. It also has an antiemetic action. Propofol can also be used by intravenous infusion for up to 3 days for sedation in conscious people requiring controlled ventilation in an intensive care unit.

Ketamine can be given by intramuscular injection or intravenously by bolus injection or infusion. The anaesthetic action is terminated largely by redistribution (half-life about 15 min).

Etomidate has a rapid onset of action after intravenous injection, and its action is terminated by rapid metabolism in plasma and the liver, so that the duration of action is about 6–10 min with minimal hangover. It is not used to maintain anaesthesia because prolonged infusion can suppress adrenocortical function.

Unwanted effects

- On the central nervous system (CNS): general depression of the CNS can also produce respiratory and cardiovascular depression. Slow release of thiopental distributed into tissues may result in some sedation for up to 24 h after use. Hallucinations and vivid dreams are common during recovery from ketamine (emergence reactions), but are less frequent in children.
- On muscles: extraneous muscle movement is common with etomidate, and to a lesser degree with propofol. They can be reduced by a benzodiazepine or opioid analgesic given before induction. Ketamine increases muscle tone.
- On the heart: thiopental, propofol and to a lesser extent etomidate depress the heart, producing bradycardia and reducing blood pressure. In contrast, ketamine produces tachycardia and an increase in blood pressure.
- Nausea and vomiting during recovery is experienced by up to 40% of people but rarely persists for more than 24 h. Propofol has an antiemetic action.
- Convulsions have been reported after propofol. These can be delayed, indicating the need for special caution after day surgery.
- Pain on injection: propofol, being lipid-soluble, is given in a complex vehicle, which may cause pain during intravenous injection. Thiopental is an alkaline solution that is irritant if injected outside the vein.

INTRAVENOUS OPIOIDS

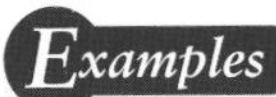

alfentanil, fentanyl, remifentanil

Intravenous opioids are given at induction for intraoperative analgesia and to reduce the dose requirement of anaesthetic agents. In high doses, they stimulate the vagus and produce bradycardia; this can be helpful to reduce the tachycardia and hypertension produced by sympathetic nervous system activation during surgery. Attenuation of surgical stress can be particularly useful, for example during cardiac surgery. Details of the mechanism of action of opioids can be found in Chapter 19.

Pharmacokinetics

After intravenous injection, fentanyl has a rapid onset of action, within 1–2 min. After a single dose, the action of fentanyl is short, owing to rapid redistribution. The effect is maintained by repeated injections or infusion. With prolonged use, fentanyl has a long duration of action determined by its hepatic elimination (half-life about 4 h), so that prolonged ventilatory support may be necessary after surgery.

Remifentanil is an opioid ester that has a similar rapid onset to fentanyl but a very short half-life of about 5 min, due to metabolism by tissue and plasma esterases. After an initial bolus dose of remifentanil, continuous intravenous infusion is used to maintain its effects.

Alfentanil has a redistribution half-life of 5 min and an elimination half-life of 1.5 h.

Unwanted effects

- **Muscle rigidity**: this can be controlled during surgery with muscle relaxants, but myoclonus and rigidity can persist after recovery, and require reversal with the opioid antagonist naloxone (Ch. 19)
- **Respiratory depression**: this may be profound and means that assisted ventilation is usually necessary during surgery when large doses have been used.

INHALATIONAL ANAESTHETICS

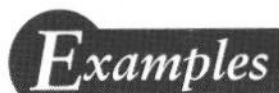

desflurane, halothane, isoflurane, nitrous oxide, sevoflurane

Inhalational anaesthetics are given with oxygen to avoid hypoxia during anaesthesia. Following induction with an intravenous anaesthetic, a single inhalational agent can be used to maintain anaesthesia. Nitrous oxide is not sufficiently potent to be used alone (Table 17.3), but it has the advantage of producing analgesia (unlike the other inhalational anaesthetics) and is often used in combination with other anaesthetics, thus reducing the required dose of the other agent. Nitrous oxide can only be used as the sole inhalational agent when combined with an intravenous opioid and a neuromuscular junction blocking drug (Ch. 27), but there is a risk of awareness during surgery. Sevoflurane is widely used for children as it has a pleasant odour, an advantage when using it for induction. Recovery is rapid after sevoflurane, since it is eliminated more quickly than halothane or isoflurane, and therefore early postoperative analgesia may be necessary.

Pharmacokinetics

In order to produce general anaesthesia, the concentration of anaesthetic used in the inhaled gas and the duration of inhalation necessary to give sufficient concentration of drug in the CNS will depend on the relationships shown in Figure 17.3 and Table 17.3. There are four factors that are important.

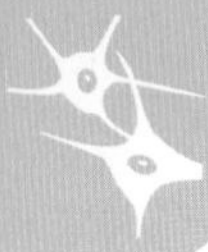

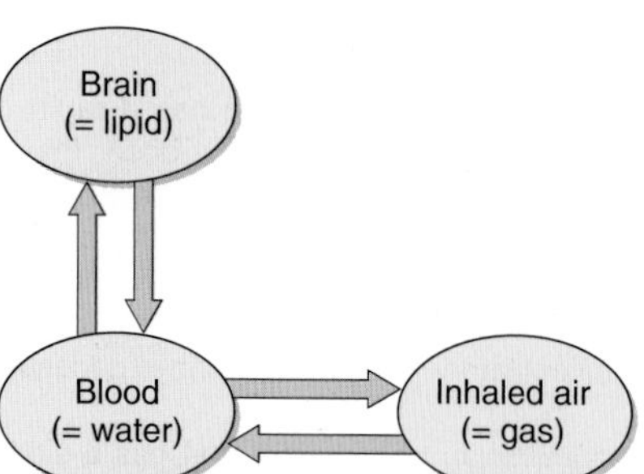

Fig. 17.3 **Equilibration of inhalational general anaesthetics between air, blood and brain.** The concentration ratio between blood and air at equilibrium is estimated from in vivo studies of the blood : gas partition coefficient and correlates with the induction time of the drug (Table 17.3). The concentrations in brain and blood at equilibrium reflect the different affinities of the two body compartments for general anaesthetics. The brain : blood ratio is 1–3 : 1 for all commonly used anaesthetics. The concentration in the inspired air required to give the necessary concentration in brain membranes (minimum alveolar concentration; MAC) correlates inversely with the blood : gas partition coefficient which is an indication of the potency of the compound.

- The rate of absorption across the alveolar membranes. This depends on both the concentration of drug in the inspired air and the rate of drug delivery, i.e. the rate and depth of inspiration. These factors are important if an inhaled agent is used for induction, but less significant once equilibrium has been established between the inhaled concentration and that in the brain. Lung conditions such as emphysema, which result in poor alveolar ventilation, will slow the induction of anaesthesia and also slow the recovery from agents eliminated by exhalation.
- The rate at which the concentration of drug in the blood reaches equilibrium with that in the inspired air. An important factor in this context is the solubility of the anaesthetic in blood and rapidly equilibrating tissues such as the brain. A high relative solubility in blood compared with the brain will be associated with a slow attainment of equilibrium.
- The cardiac output, which will determine circulation time and drug delivery to the brain. This is not usually a limiting factor.
- The relative concentrations of the drug in the brain and blood at equilibrium. The rate of entry of drug into the brain is not limiting for lipid-soluble drugs such as anaesthetics. The rate-limiting step is the rate of delivery via the inhaled gas compared with the total amount in the body at equilibrium.

There are two physicochemical properties that affect the action of an inhaled anaesthetic agent.

- The blood : gas partition coefficient or blood/gas ratio. This indicates the relative solubilities of the drug in blood and air. A high solubility in blood, and therefore in all rapidly equilibrating body tissues, means that a greater amount of the agent will need to be administered before the partial pressure of the agent in the blood is in equilibrium with that in the inspired air. Diethyl ether, although not used clinically, has been included in Table 17.3 since this illustrates well the relationship between a high blood : air partition coefficient and a long induction period. (Note: the data in Table 17.3 conform to the basic pharmacokinetic principle explained in Chapter 2, that compounds with a large apparent volume of distribution take longer to reach steady state during a constant rate of drug input.)
- The oil : gas partition coefficient or oil/gas ratio. This reflects the ratio between the concentration in the lipid membranes of brain cells (oil) and the inhaled concentration. The higher the partition coefficient, then the lower will be the inhaled concentration of gas required to maintain anaesthesia. This is well illustrated by the data in Table 17.3. Nitrous oxide has a low oil : gas partition coefficient, and, if given alone, surgical anaesthesia could only be achieved with an inspired concentration of drug that would not allow an adequate inspired oxygen concentration.

The major route of elimination of inhalational anaesthetics is via the airways. Factors that influence the duration of the induction phase, such as ventilation rate and the blood : gas partition coefficient, will also affect the time taken to eliminate the anaesthetic and thus the recovery time. The recovery time may also depend on the duration of inhalation, which can affect the extent to which the drug has entered slowly equilibrating tissues. Elimination from these tissues is slow, which can maintain the plasma concentration of the drug and delay recovery. During recovery, the depth of anaesthesia reverses through the stages discussed above to consciousness; a rapid recovery which minimises stage II (Table 17.1) is beneficial. Comparing the data in Table 17.3, it is hardly surprising that diethyl ether is no longer used.

General anaesthetics are also partly eliminated by metabolism, the extent of which depends on the time that the agent is retained in the body and is available to the metabolising enzymes. Thus, exhalation and metabolism can be regarded as alternative pathways of elimination, the proportions of which are determined largely by the volatility of the agent and its blood : gas partition coefficient (see Table 17.3).

Unwanted effects

A number of unwanted effects are common to most clinically useful inhalational anaesthetics; however, each agent also has a unique profile of additional unwanted effects.

- Cardiovascular system. Most agents depress myocardial contractility and produce bradycardia by interfering with transmembrane Ca^{2+} flux. This decreases cardiac output and blood pressure. Isoflurane is less cardiodepressant, but may reduce blood pressure by arterial vasodilation. Nitrous oxide also has less depressant effect on the heart and circulation and its use in combination with other agents may permit reduction in their dosage and, therefore, reduce their depressant effect on the heart. Inhalational anaesthetics often increase cerebral blood flow, which can exacerbate an elevated intracranial pressure.

- Respiratory system. All agents depress the response of the respiratory centre in the medulla to carbon dioxide and hypoxia. They also decrease tidal volume and increase respiratory rate. Desflurane and isoflurane are irritant and can cause coughing and laryngospasm if used for induction.
- Liver. Most agents decrease liver blood flow. Mild hepatic dysfunction, because of specific hepatic toxicity, is common after treatment with halothane. However, about 1 in 30 000 people will develop severe hepatic necrosis following the use of halothane, especially after repeat exposure within a short time interval. For this reason, halothane is only used after a careful anaesthetic history (especially in the preceding 3 months) and is avoided in those with a history of unexplained jaundice or pyrexia following exposure to halothane. Halothane is only available in the UK on special order. Hepatotoxicity is rare with other halogenated anaesthetics.
- Kidney. Both renal blood flow and renal vascular resistance decrease, resulting in a reduced glomerular filtration rate.
- Uterus. There is relaxation of the uterus, which may increase the risk of haemorrhage when anaesthesia is used in labour. Nitrous oxide has less effect on uterine muscle compared with the other agents.
- Skeletal muscle. Most agents produce some muscle relaxation, which enhances the activity of neuromuscular-blocking drugs (Ch. 27). With sevoflurane, this may be sufficient to enable tracheal intubation without the use of a neuromuscular blocker.
- Chemoreceptor trigger zone. Inhalational anaesthetics trigger postoperative nausea and vomiting. This may be most pronounced with nitrous oxide.
- Postoperative shivering. This occurs in up to 65% of those recovering from general anaesthesia. The aetiology is unclear.
- Malignant hyperthermia. This is a rare but potentially fatal complication of inhalational anaesthesia. It is genetically determined, and results from a defect in the ryanodine receptor (RYR1) that regulates release of Ca^{2+} from the sarcoplasmic reticulum in muscle cells (Ch. 5, Fig. 5.4). A sudden increase in intracellular Ca^{2+} produces tachycardia, unstable blood pressure, hypercapnoea, fever and hyperventilation, followed by hyperkalaemia and metabolic acidosis. Muscle rigidity may occur. Treatment is with dantrolene, which is an RYR1 antagonist (Ch. 24).

FURTHER READING

Campagna JA, Miller KW, Forman SA (2003) Mechanisms of actions of inhaled anaesthetics. *N Engl J Med* 348, 2110–2124

Dodds C (1999) General anaesthesia: practical recommendations and recent advances. *Drugs* 58, 453–467

Fox AJ, Rowbottam DJ (1999) Anaesthesia. *BMJ* 319, 557–560

Litman RS, Rosenberg H (2005) Malignant hyperthermia. Update on susceptibility testing. *JAMA* 293, 2918–2924

Millar KW (2002) The nature and sites of general anaesthetic action. *Br J Anaesth* 89, 17–31

Nathan N, Odin I (2007) Induction of anaesthesia. A guide to drug choice. *Drugs* 67, 701–723

Solt K, Forman SA (2007) Correlating the clinical actions and molecular mechanisms of general anesthetics. *Curr Opin Anaesthesiol* 20, 300–306

Wiklund RA, Rosenbaum SH (1997) Anaesthesiology Parts I and II. *N Engl J Med* 337, 1132–1141, 1215–1219

SELF-ASSESSMENT

In questions 1–6, the initial statement, in italics, is true. Are the accompanying statements also true?

1. *The minimum alveolar concentration (MAC) of an inhalational anaesthetic required to produce surgical anaesthesia correlates inversely with the oil:gas partition coefficient of drug.*
   a. Inhalational anaesthetics may have their effect by interacting with specific receptors.
   b. Inhalational anaesthetics are all gases.
   c. Most inhalational anaesthetics are sulphur-containing compounds.
2. *Properties of an ideal inhalational anaesthetic are that it is stable, non-inflammable, potent, low lipid solubility, non-irritant, non-toxic, analgesic and does not sensitise the heart to catecholamines.*
   a. Halothane closely approaches the properties of an ideal inhalational anaesthetic.
   b. The risk of hangover effects with inhalational anaesthetics increases if the operation is long.
   c. Nitrous oxide, when administered alone, reaches the MAC necessary for surgical anaesthesia if its concentration in inspired air is 50%.
   d. Nitrous oxide is frequently given with oxygen and a fluorinated anaesthetic agent to produce effective surgical anaesthesia.
3. *Isoflurane is a widely used volatile anaesthetic.* Isoflurane is metabolised as extensively as halothane.
4. *The short duration of action of thiopental is due to its redistribution into richly perfused tissues such as muscles.*
   a. The elimination half-life of thiopental is similar to the distribution half-life.
   b. Propofol cannot be given alone by continuous intravenous infusion to maintain anaesthesia.
   c. Accidental injection of thiopental into an artery can have serious consequences.
   d. Ketamine is a sedative but is without analgesic action.
5. *Fentanyl is a lipid-soluble opioid analgesic.* Fentanyl should not be administered concurrently with inhalational anaesthetics.

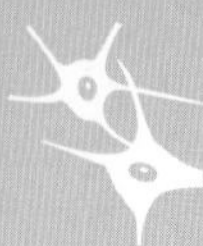

6. *Because of the rapid activity of modern anaesthetics, the individual well-defined stages of anaesthesia are not clearly seen.*
   a. When administering an inhalational anaesthetic, the excitement stage of anaesthesia is prolonged if an intravenous anaesthetic is not given beforehand.
   b. Most inhalational anaesthetics have a depressant effect on the cardiovascular system.
   c. Inhalational anaesthetics reduce the sensitivity of the respiratory centre to carbon dioxide and hypoxia.
   d. Sevoflurane has the advantage of a fast onset of action and rapid elimination.
7. Considering the pharmacology of agents used in anaesthesia, choose the one **most appropriate** statement.
   A. The minimum percentage concentration of nitrous oxide in alveolar air (MAC) for surgical anaesthesia is 50%.
   B. The major route of elimination of most inhalational anaesthetics is via the liver.
   C. Ketamine is an intravenous anaesthetic and also has analgesic properties.
   D. The intravenous opioid fentanyl should not be administered together with sevoflurane.
   E. Atropine is a commonly administered pre-operative agent.
8. Case history question (this should be attempted in conjunction with information from Ch. 27)

> A 40-year-old woman is scheduled for a laparotomy because of an abdominal swelling. She has not had a previous operation and is otherwise healthy, with normal cardiovascular and respiratory function. She was premedicated with pethidine (meperidine) and atropine. The operation lasted 40 minutes.

   a. Why is atropine little used in adults as pre-anaesthetic medication nowadays?
   b. Do the muscarinic receptor antagonists atropine and hyoscine have the same properties?

> The woman was intubated after the administration of thiopental, fentanyl and suxamethonium (succinylcholine).

   c. Why has the routine use of suxamethonium to facilitate endotracheal intubation been reduced?

> Following intubation, pancuronium and fentanyl were given and she was ventilated with nitrous oxide, enflurane and oxygen. An ovarian cyst was removed and the operation took 40 min.

   d. Is pancuronium the most suitable choice of muscle relaxant? What alternatives are available?

> After the operation, she did not breathe spontaneously, despite the administration of neostigmine and glycopyrronium.

   e. What are the possible reasons for the apnoea and how could they be treated?
   f. Would mivacurium (a short-duration muscle relaxant) have been a preferable muscle relaxant to use in this patient?
   g. What is the reason for administering glycopyrronium with neostigmine at the end of the operation?

ANSWERS

1. a. **True**. It was thought for many years that there are not distinctive receptors at which general anaesthetics act, but rather they produce more general effects on constituents of the cell membrane such as lipids or proteins. However, it is now considered that they have actions at a number of excitatory and inhibitory receptors (Table 17.4).
   b. **False**. Many inhalational anaesthetics are volatile liquids.
   c. **False**. The main inhalational anaesthetics are halogenated compounds.
2. a. **False**. It causes cardiac arrhythmias, hepatotoxicity with repeated use, and hypotension. It also sensitises the heart to catecholamines. It is, however, a potent anaesthetic.
   b. **True**. This is particularly true with highly lipid-soluble agents, which will accumulate in body fat stores and be slowly released after the operation.
   c. **False**. Even at concentrations higher than 50%, nitrous oxide is not potent enough to produce effective surgical anaesthesia on its own.
   d. **True**. Nitrous oxide and oxygen are used concurrently with fluorinated anaesthetics. The other attribute of nitrous oxide is that, unlike fluorinated compounds, it has analgesic activity.
3. **False**. Halothane undergoes substantial metabolism, but the other halogenated anaesthetics do not.
4. a. **False**. The half-life of the rapid distribution phase of thiopental is only about 3 min, hence its short duration of action. However, the elimination of thiopental from the body is much slower and the half-life is 3–8 h. This partially accounts for the hangover effect seen with this drug.
   b. **False**. Propofol is useful for short operations, where it has rapid elimination and little hangover effect. The hepatic clearance of propofol has a half-life of 1–2 h. It can also be given by continuous infusion in intensive care units.
   c. **True**. Either extravascular injections of thiopental or intra-arterial injections can have damaging consequences, because its pH is approximately 9–10.
   d. **False**. Ketamine does have analgesic action, unlike other available intravenous anaesthetics. It can be useful when pain is difficult to control.
5. **False**. Fentanyl is increasingly given for intraoperative analgesia. It is short-acting and with rapid recovery; consequently, it has a low incidence of hangover effects.
6. a. **True**. This was true when slow-acting anaesthetics were given, but it is less problematic because of the rapid onset of action of modern anaesthetics.

b. **True**. Most are negatively inotropic and they depress myocardial function by interfering with Ca^{2+} fluxes. Halothane also sensitises the heart to catecholamines and can lead to arrhythmias.
c. **True**. Inhalational anaesthetics reduce the ventilatory response to carbon dioxide and hypoxia and increase the arterial partial pressure of carbon dioxide.
d. **True**. Sevoflurane is rapid in onset and also is more rapidly eliminated than halothane or isoflurane.

7. Answer **C**.
   A. The MAC of nitrous oxide required for anaesthesia if given alone would be greater than 100%!
   B. The major route of elimination is via the airways.
   C. Unlike other intravenous anaesthetics, ketamine is analgesic.
   D. Fentanyl is often used as an analgesic given together with many inhalational anaesthetics.
   E. With modern anaesthetic practice, atropine is seldom given to dry bronchial and salivary secretions.
8. Case history answers
   a. Atropine (and hyoscine) blocks muscarinic receptors, blocking bronchial and salivary secretions. Modern anaesthetics have less irritant effect, thus reducing this problem. Muscarinic antagonists can reduce the bradycardia caused by some inhalation anaesthetics and suxamethonium.
   b. Atropine can cause CNS excitation, whereas hyoscine causes sedation and has antiemetic properties.
   c. Relatively minor but frequent complications occur with suxamethonium, including bradycardia, postoperative myalgia, transient elevation of the plasma K^+ concentration and raised intraocular, intracranial and intragastric pressures. A rare, but potentially fatal, complication is malignant hyperthermia, which is genetically determined. The short-acting nondepolarising blocking drug rocuronium has a short duration of action and does not cause these problems.
   d. Pancuronium is probably not the ideal muscle relaxant to use. It does not cause histamine release, but it can cause tachycardia and hypertension and is long-acting (Ch. 27). An alternative would be vecuronium, which has an intermediate duration of action, does not release histamine, and lacks cardiovascular effects. The short-acting rocuronium is more expensive but has a rapid onset and short duration of action and a low risk of cardiovascular effects.
   e. There are at least three possible reasons for the postoperative apnoea. (A) Opioid-induced apnoea. The use of pethidine followed by fentanyl may be generous for a short operation, resulting in respiratory depression. The effect could be reversed by the administration of naloxone. (B) The dose of neostigmine given may have been insufficient to reverse the competitive blocking effect of the long-acting pancuronium. (C) The woman could have a genetically determined deficiency of pseudocholinesterase (plasma cholinesterase, butyrylcholinesterase), which metabolises suxamethonium. This is present in about 1 in 2000 individuals. If respiratory depression is caused by suxamethonium, administration of neostigmine would make it worse. Fresh frozen plasma containing pseudocholinesterase could be administered.
   f. Although mivacurium is a short-acting muscle relaxant, it is metabolised by pseudocholinesterase and its effect would be prolonged if there is a reduced level of this metabolising enzyme.
   g. Neostigmine inhibits acetylcholinesterase. It partially or fully reverses the actions of competitive neuromuscular-blocking drugs acting at N_2 receptors at skeletal muscle but also enhances the activity of acetylcholine at muscarinic receptors, causing bradycardia and respiratory bronchoconstriction. Glycopyrronium selectivity blocks muscarinic receptors, thus reducing excess muscarinic stimulation.

General anaesthetics

Drug	Half-life (h) and kinetics	Comments
Intravenous anaesthetics		
Following a bolus dose, the duration of action depends on the rate of redistribution and not the elimination half-life given below		
Etomidate	1–2 [M] Hydrolysed and oxidised in liver to inactive products	Used for induction without hangover; suppresses adrenocortical function on continuous dosage and should not be used for maintenance anaesthesia
Ketamine	2–4 [M] Redistribution half-life from well-perfused to poorly perfused tissues is about 15 min; hepatic metabolism produces numerous oxidation products, one of which retains activity	Can also be given by intramuscular injection for short procedures
Propofol	3–12 [M] Redistribution half-life of 0.5–1 h; rapid glucuronidation in the liver and other tissues contributes to recovery; drug that has entered poorly perfused tissues (during prolonged administration) is eliminated more slowly, with a half-life of about 3–12 h	Duration of action partly determined by redistribution

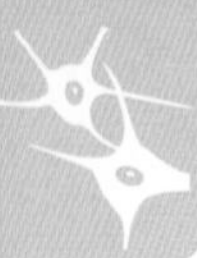

General anaesthetics

Drug	Half-life (h) and kinetics	Comments
Thiopental	3–8 [M] Slow oxidation to an inactive product; repeated doses have a cumulative and prolonged effect as the blood and poorly perfused tissues reach equilibrium	Reconstituted solution is highly alkaline; duration of action determined by redistribution
Intravenous opioids		
Provide analgesia and enhance anaesthesia		
Alfentanil	0.7–2 [M] Oxidised in liver by CYP3A4, and conjugated with glucuronic acid	Used especially during short procedures and for outpatient surgery; respiratory depression may persist after the end of the procedure if repeated doses are given
Fentanyl	1–6 [M] Rapid initial uptake from the blood into lungs, followed by redistribution and elimination; metabolised in the liver largely by CYP3A4	Respiratory depression may persist after the end of the procedure if repeated doses are given
Remifentanil	0.1 [M] Very rapid clearance by blood and tissue esterases (clearance is 3 L min^{-1}, which exceeds liver blood flow); metabolite inactive	Given as an intravenous infusion
Inhalational anaesthetics		
Desflurane	[E] <0.1% is metabolised by CYP2E1; brain : blood ratio is 1.3 : 1	Not recommended for induction in children because of cough, laryngospasm and increased secretions; rapid recovery (minutes) but present in exhaled air for days
Enflurane	[E + M] About 8% is metabolised by CYP2E1; brain : blood ratio is 1.4 : 1; rapid recovery; multiple phases are present in the elimination curve, with half-lives ranging from 2 min to 34 h owing to uptake and release from tissues	Powerful cardiorespiratory depressant
Halothane	[E + M] About 20% is metabolised by CYP2E1 to fluorine derivatives; metabolism produces a reactive metabolite, possibly trifluoroacetyl chloride, which reacts with cellular proteins	Use is limited by the risk of hepatotoxicity (see text); now available in the UK on special order only
Isoflurane	[E] <0.2% metabolism by CYP2E1; brain : blood ratio is 2.6 : 1; multiple half-lives reported, <1 min to 40 h, requires a five-compartmental mathematical model; rapid recovery during redistribution phases	An isomer of enflurane
Nitrous oxide	[E] Eliminated by exhalation, without metabolism; brain : blood ratio is 1.0 : 1; may reduce cerebrovascular effects of halothane when used in combination	Low potency compared with other inhaled agents; rapid recovery owing to low potency and low tissue affinity
Sevoflurane	[E + M] About 5% metabolism by CYP2E1; brain : blood ratio is 1.7 : 1; complex elimination kinetics; recovery may be particularly rapid after short procedures	

Comment – various other drugs, such as anxiolytics and analgesics, are used in the perioperative period.
[E], exhalation; [M], metabolism.

18 Local anaesthetics

Local anaesthetics are drugs that reversibly block the transmission of pain stimuli locally at their site of administration.

Examples

benzocaine, bupivacaine, cocaine, lidocaine, prilocaine, ropivacaine, tetracaine

PHARMACOLOGY

MECHANISM OF ACTION

At rest, the neuronal cell membrane has only limited permeability to Na^+ but about 50–70 times greater permeability to K^+ because of the greater number of channels open for passive transport of K^+ out of the cell. The maintenance of a negative resting membrane electrical potential is largely determined by the K^+ gradient across the cell membrane, with a smaller contribution from the active Na^+/K^+-ATPase pump, which pumps out 3 Na^+ ions for every 2 K^+ ions it transports in. Conduction of a nerve action potential results from opening of voltage-dependent Na^+ channels, and rapid influx of Na^+ to depolarise the cell (see Fig. 18.2). Na^+ channels cycle between three states:

- *resting*, when the channel is closed but able to open in response to a change in transmembrane potential
- *open*, when the channel opens in response to an action potential and allows the rapid influx of Na^+ ions through to the cytoplasm
- *inactivated* due to a very rapid change in conformation at the cytoplasmic end of the channel occurring very soon after the action potential has passed; during this stage the channel is resistant to depolarising influences, but sensitivity returns when the membrane potential returns to resting level.

There is considerable redundancy in the membrane Na^+ channels; as a consequence, nerve conduction can continue even when 90% of the channels are blocked.

Local anaesthetics produce reversible nerve conduction blockade and prevent impulse transmission in nerve fibres by blocking the voltage-dependent Na^+ channels that depolarise the cell. They bind to the Na^+ channel at a site on the inner surface of the membrane, and progressively interrupt Na^+ channel-mediated depolarisation until conduction fails. Because they act by such a ubiquitous mechanism, local anaesthetics have a wide spectrum of action and will block conduction in all nerve fibres (Table 18.1).

The probability that propagation of a nerve impulse will fail at a particular segment of the nerve is related to:

- the local concentration of the anaesthetic drug
- the size of the nerve fibre
- if the nerve is myelinated
- the length of the nerve exposed to the drug.

In general, nerve transmission is blocked in smaller-diameter fibres before that in larger fibres. Thus, the myelinated Aδ and small non-myelinated C fibres that are pain-transmitting (nociceptive) fibres are blocked before larger touch and pressure and motor fibres. Therefore, pain pathways are most rapidly and intensely blocked by local anaesthetics (Table 18.1), and also show the longest duration of local anaesthetic effect. In myelinated nerves, the drug penetrates at the nodes of Ranvier and must block at least three consecutive nodes to produce conduction block. Unmyelinated nerves must be blocked over sufficient length, and around the full circumference of the nerve.

Structural requirements of local anaesthetics

The action of local anaesthetics results mainly from binding of the ionic form of the anaesthetic to a site on the inside (axoplasmic opening) of the Na^+ channel. Membrane penetration, however, is better with the un-ionised (lipid-soluble) form. The structural requirements for local anaesthetic activity appear to involve a minimum of a hydrophobic aromatic ring structure connected to a hydrophilic amine group by a short ester or amide linkage (Fig. 18.1). Clinically used potent local anaesthetics are secondary or tertiary amines with a central amide or ester structure. The length of the intermediate bonding chain is critical to local anaesthetic activity and is optimal between 3 and 7 carbon equivalents. The lipophilic aromatic group enables the molecule to cross the nerve membrane, and the potency of the drug is directly related to its lipid solubility. Many local anaesthetics are structurally closely related. Bupivacaine is a racemic mixture of the *S*(–)- and *R*(+)-isomers, while levobupivacaine is the *S*(–)-isomer of bupivacaine; ropivacaine is an *S*(–)-isomer of an analogue of bupivacaine in which a butyl group is replaced by a propyl group (see compendium).

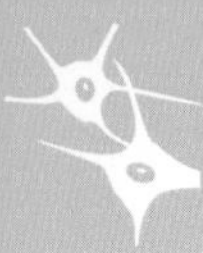

Table 18.1 Nerve fibres and their responsiveness to local anaesthetics

Fibre type	Site or function	Myelination	Diameter (μm)	Sensitivity to anaesthesia[a]
A				
Alpha	Motor	Yes	12–20	+
Beta	Touch, pressure	Yes	5–12	+
Gamma	Muscle spindle	Yes	3–6	++
Delta	Thermal, chemical, mechanical	Yes	2–5	+++
B	Preganglionic autonomic	Yes	1–3	+++
C	Thermal, chemical, mechanical	No	0.4–1.2	+++
	Postganglionic	No	0.3–1.3	+++

[a]Increasing number of + indicates increasing sensitivity to local anaesthesia.

Lidocaine

Lipid-soluble (aromatic) centre — Amide bond — Hydrophilic (polar) centre

Tetracaine

$CH_3CH_2CH_2CH_2NH$–(benzene ring)–$C(=O)$-O-$CH_2CH_2N(CH_3)_2$

Lipid-soluble centre — Ester bond — Hydrophilic centre

Fig. 18.1 **General structure of local anaesthetics.** Differences in structure alter the speed of onset, duration of action and the metabolism of the drugs (see the drug compendium table).

Specific intraneuronal binding

Local anaesthetics bind to a receptor protein within the axoplasmic opening of the Na^+ channel. Therefore, compounds with high binding affinity stay at the site of action for longer and have a long duration of action. Thus, procaine, which has a low binding affinity and a weak association with the Na^+ channel, has a short duration of action, whereas bupivacaine has a high binding affinity and has a long duration of action.

The pK_a of the drug determines the extent of ionisation at physiological pH and the speed of onset of the conduction block. All local anaesthetics are weak bases and will be relatively more ionised at a pH below the pK_a (which for most local anaesthetics is between 7.7 and 9.1). Because the water solubility of a local anaesthetic is greatest in the ionised form, injectable preparations are formulated as the hydrochloride salts with a pH of 5.0–6.0. However, the base (un-ionised) form is more lipid-soluble and more readily penetrates lipid membranes; therefore, after injection, the drug solution (pH 5.0–6.0) must be buffered to physiological pH (7.4) before a significant amount of un-ionised local anaesthetic is available to penetrate the nerve and reach its site of action. The higher the pK_a of the drug, the greater the percentage that is in the cationic form at physiological pH, and the speed of onset of anaesthesia will be slower. Alkalinisation of the injected solution by adding bicarbonate will increase the proportion of the drug in its un-ionised lipid-soluble form and therefore increase the rate of absorption of the anaesthetic into the nerve and accelerate the onset of action.

In contrast, it is the ionised form of the drug that binds to the receptor within the axoplasmic opening of the Na^+ channel. Therefore, drugs with a higher pK_a will re-ionise to a greater extent within the cell (pH 7.4) and produce more effective blockade. Although some un-ionised anaesthetic may reach the binding site by diffusion within the cell membrane and become ionised within the Na^+ channel, the majority passes across the cell membrane, enters the cytosol, where it becomes ionised, and then reaches the receptor via the cytoplasm. The binding site is most accessible when the channel is in its open (activated) state (Fig. 18.2). For this reason, the effectiveness of most local anaesthetics is dependent on the frequency of firing of the neuron (use-dependency), and a faster onset of local anaesthesia occurs in rapidly firing neurons. Once the local anaesthetic has bound to the channel, the influx of Na^+ is blocked and the channel remains in the *inactivated* state and resistant to further depolarisation. The local anaesthetic does not dissociate from the channel when it is in the *inactivated* state as it has a high affinity for the channel in this state. The local anaesthetic moves off the binding site when the membrane potential returns to its resting level, and the channel is in the *resting* state. This is further facilitated when the cytoplasmic concentration of the drug decreases as it diffuses away from the site of administration.

Local anaesthetics also bind to other ion channels and cell receptors, including presynaptic Ca^{2+} channels, tachy-

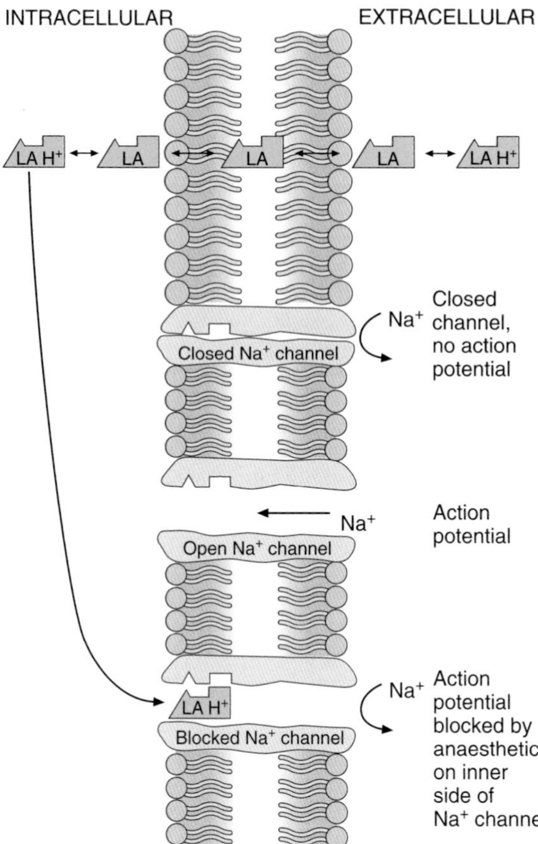

Fig. 18.2 **Site and mechanism of action of local anaesthetics.** Weakly basic local anaesthetics exist in an equilibrium between ionised (LA H^+) and un-ionised (LA) forms. The ionised form binds to the intracellular receptor, and the un-ionised form is lipid-soluble and crosses the axonal membrane. Some un-ionised anaesthetic may reach the ion channel by diffusion within the cell membrane, become ionised within the Na^+ channel, and then bind to the receptor site.

kinin type 1 receptors, glutamate, bradykinin B_2 and acetylcholine receptors. These actions may be involved in reducing nociceptive neurotransmission and in the production of spinal anaesthesia.

PHARMACOKINETICS

The speed of onset of local anaesthetic action is largely determined by the physicochemical properties of the drug molecule. The duration of action of local anaesthetics is dependent on the degree of receptor binding (see above) and on their rate of removal from the site of administration, rather than their systemic elimination by metabolism. Most local anaesthetics cause vasodilation at the site of injection, which will enhance their removal. In contrast, cocaine, which blocks noradrenaline reuptake by noradrenergic neurons (uptake 1; Ch. 4), produces intense vasoconstriction and has a long duration of action. Because of this, cocaine is never given by injection, and its medical use is restricted to topical anaesthesia in otolaryngology. The duration of action of any local anaesthetic can be extended considerably by co-administration with a vasoconstrictor such as an α_1-adrenoceptor agonist, for example adrenaline (epinephrine). However, the pH of the solution must be 2.0–3.0 to prevent decomposition of the adrenaline (epinephrine). Local anaesthetic preparations with other vasoconstrictors such as phenylephrine or felypressin are also available.

Once the local anaesthetic has diffused away from the site of administration, it enters the general circulation and undergoes elimination from the body. Most local anaesthetics have a central amide bond, and are eliminated at least in part by hepatic hydrolysis of the amide bond. The half-life of amide local anaesthetics within the circulation is generally short (between 1 and 3 h). In contrast, the plasma half-lives of the ester drugs procaine and tetracaine are 3 min or less, since ester bonds are very rapidly hydrolysed by plasma esterases.

UNWANTED EFFECTS

Local effects

These occur at the site of administration and include irritation and inflammation. Local ischaemia can occur if local anaesthetics are co-administered with a vasoconstrictor; therefore this should be avoided in the extremities such as the digits. Tissue damage/necrosis can follow inappropriate administration (e.g. accidental intra-arterial administration or spinal administration of an epidural dose).

Systemic effects

These are related to the anaesthetic action, and usually result from excessive plasma concentrations that affect other excitable membranes such as the heart (see antiarrhythmic action of lidocaine; Ch. 8). After regional anaesthesia, the maximum plasma drug concentration occurs within 30 min.

- High plasma concentrations (especially after accidental intravenous injection, or rapid absorption from inflamed tissues) can cause cardiovascular collapse from systemic vasodilation and a negative inotropic effect. Cardiotoxicity with serious arrhythmias is a particular problem with bupivacaine and is caused by its avid tissue binding in the heart. As a result of its high lipid solubility and high protein binding, it has a fast-in, slow-out kinetic pattern at the Na^+ channel. Bupivacaine (particularly the *R*(+)-isomer) blocks the normal cardiac conducting system and predisposes to ventricular re-entrant pathways and intractable ventricular arrhythmias (see Ch. 8). Levobupivacaine and ropivacaine have about the same local anaesthetic potency but less potential to produce cardiac effects, having less effect on cardiac Na^+ channels.
- In the central nervous system (CNS), local anaesthetics can produce light-headedness, then sedation and loss of consciousness. Severe reactions can be accompanied by convulsions. Metabolites of lidocaine can cause generalised excitation and seizures.

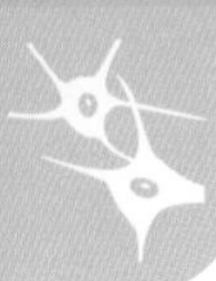

- True allergy is rare, but can occur with ester agents, related to their metabolism to *p*-amino benzoic acid.

TECHNIQUES OF ADMINISTRATION

The extent of local anaesthesia depends largely on the technique of administration.

Surface administration

High concentrations (up to 10%) of drug in an oily vehicle can slowly penetrate the skin or mucous membranes to give a small localised area of anaesthesia. Lidocaine can be applied as a cream to an area before a minor skin procedure or venepuncture. Benzocaine is a relatively non-polar weak non-amino local anaesthetic that is included in some throat pastilles to produce anaesthesia of mucous membranes. Cocaine is restricted to topical use in otolaryngeal procedures, to produce vasoconstriction and reduce mucosal bleeding.

Infiltration anaesthesia

A localised injection of an aqueous solution of local anaesthetic, sometimes with a vasoconstrictor, produces a local field of anaesthesia. The anaesthetic effect produced is more efficient than surface anaesthesia, but requires a relatively large amount of drug. Smaller volumes can be used for field block anaesthesia, involving subcutaneous injection close to nerves around the area to be anaesthetised. This technique is used extensively in dentistry.

Peripheral nerve block anaesthesia

Injection of an aqueous solution around a nerve trunk produces a field of anaesthesia distal to the site of injection. This can be used for temporary sympathetic nerve block, such as the stellate ganglion, or for lumbar sympathectomy.

Epidural anaesthesia

Injection or slow infusion via a cannula of an aqueous solution adjacent to the spinal column, but outside the dura mater, produces anaesthesia both above and below the site of injection. The extent of anaesthesia depends on the volume of drug administered. This technique is used extensively in obstetrics and some surgical procedures. The concentration of drug used is the same as that for spinal anaesthesia, but the volume, and therefore the dose, is greater. For this reason, systemic unwanted effects are more frequent than with spinal anaesthesia. Sympathetic fibres are particularly sensitive to local anaesthetics (Table 18.1); this can result in hypotension and may be particularly exaggerated during pregnancy (probably related to the concurrent effects of high progesterone concentrations). Backache is a frequent postoperative complication with epidural and spinal anaesthesia.

Spinal anaesthesia

This involves injection of an aqueous solution into the lumbar subarachnoid space, usually between the third and fourth lumbar vertebrae. The spread of anaesthetic within the subarachnoid space depends on the density of the solution (a solution in 10% glucose is more dense than cerebrospinal fluid) and the posture of the person during the first 10–15 min while the solution flows up or down the subarachnoid space. Spinal and epidural anaesthesia can be used together, often using an opioid (Ch. 17) alone or in combination with a local anaesthetic.

Intravenous regional anaesthesia

This involves injection of a dilute solution of local anaesthetic into a limb after application of a tourniquet (Bier's block). It is used for manipulation of fractures and minor surgical procedures. Arterial blood flow must not be occluded for more than 20 min.

FURTHER READING

French RJ, Zamponi GW, Sierralta IE (1998) Molecular and kinetic determinants of local anaesthetic action on sodium channels. *Toxicol Lett* 100/101, 247–254

Heavner SE (2007) Local anaesthetics. *Curr Opin Anaesthesiol* 20, 336–342

Tetzlaff JE (2000) The pharmacology of local anesthetics. *Anesth Clin North Am* 18, 217–233

Veering BT (2003) Complications and local anaesthetic toxicity in regional anaesthesia. *Curr Opin Anaesthesiol* 16, 455–459

Wiklund RA, Rosenbaum SH (1997) Anesthesiology. Part II. *N Engl J Med* 337, 1215–1219

Yanagidate F, Strichartz GR (2007) Local anesthetics. *Handb Exp Pharmacol* 177, 95–127

SELF-ASSESSMENT

In questions 1 and 2, the first statements, in italics, are true. Are the accompanying statements true or false?

1. *Most anaesthetics exhibit use-dependence. The block is more rapid and complete when the nerve is actively firing. This is because most local anaesthetics gain better access to binding sites in Na^+ channels that are in the open state.*
   a. Local anaesthetics have no systemic unwanted effects.
   b. The main mechanism by which the effect of local anaesthesia wears off is through liver metabolism of the anaesthetic.
   c. Local anaesthetics block smaller myelinated axons more effectively than large myelinated axons.
   d. The α_1-adrenoceptor antagonist prazosin is added to local anaesthetics to extend their duration of activity.

2. *Local anaesthetics that are in their lipid-soluble form penetrate the axon more readily than their ionised (water-soluble) form and reach the innerside of the Na^+ channel before blocking it. However, it is the ionised component which blocks the Na^+ channel.* Ropivacaine is a long-acting local anaesthetic.
3. Choose the one **most appropriate** statement from the following options.
   A. Raising the pH of a local anaesthetic solution will increase its speed of onset.
   B. Liver metabolism is the primary mechanism in terminating local anaesthetic action.
   C. The effectiveness of a local anaesthetic is not altered by local tissue pH.
   D. Direct effects on blood vessel diameter of most commonly used local anaesthetics prolong their duration of action.
   E. Adrenaline (epinephrine) is given with a local anaesthetic injection in digits and appendages to increase the duration of anaesthesia.
4. Extended-matching questions
   Choose the **most appropriate** option A–F that could be used in the situations 4.1–4.4 below.
   A. Cocaine
   B. Adrenaline (epinephrine)
   C. Salbutamol
   D. Tetracaine
   E. Lidocaine
   F. Benzocaine
   4.1. A child needed a minor surgical procedure on her nasopharynx and you chose to use a single agent that could be administered topically which would reduce mucous membrane bleeding.
   4.2. An agent that would extend the duration and potency of a local anaesthetic.
   4.3. An agent that could be applied topically to produce anaesthesia of the conjunctiva which would not cause vasoconstriction.
   4.4. An agent that could be administered intravenously in the treatment of ventricular arrhythmias.

ANSWERS

1. a. **False**. If absorbed, systemic high doses of local anaesthetics can produce cardiovascular collapse and CNS depression.
   b. **False**. Initial decline in local activity is due to removal into the systemic circulation. The anaesthetic is then metabolised by liver enzyme metabolism or plasma cholinesterases.
   c. **True**. For example Aδ axons (2–5 μm diameter) are blocked more readily than motor fibres (12–20 μm diameter).
   d. **False**. Prazosin is a vasodilator and would increase the removal of the local anaesthetic from its injection site: adrenaline (epinephrine) or other local vasoconstrictors are necessary.
2. **True**. It is a long-acting local anaesthetic (2–4 h) similar to bupivacaine but may be less arrhythmogenic.
3. Answer **A**.
   A. Most local anaesthetics are weak bases, pK_a 7–9. Raising the pH will increase the relative amount of the non-ionised species and will therefore enhance lipid solubility and membrane penetration. (Increased pH may, however, reduce the water solubility of the drug in solution.)
   B. Uptake into the systemic circulation is the most important primary determinant in terminating the local action and also producing toxicity. Following most regional anaesthetic procedures, maximum arterial plasma concentrations of anaesthetic develop within about 10 to 25 min. Avoidance of intravascular administration is essential.
   C. Altered local pH could change the ratio of cationic to non-ionised species of the local anaesthetic, affecting its potential to penetrate membranes (non-ionised species) and block Na^+ channels (cationic species).
   D. With the exception of cocaine, local anaesthetics dilate blood vessels, hastening their removal from the site of injection.
   E. Adrenaline (epinephrine) should not be given with a local anaesthetic for injection in digits and appendages, because of the risk of ischaemic necrosis.
4. Extended-matching answers
   4.1. Answer **A**. Cocaine can be administered topically and, unlike other local anaesthetics, inhibits the neuronal reuptake of released noradrenaline, resulting in vasoconstriction.
   4.2. Answer **B**. Adrenaline (epinephrine) causes vasoconstriction and the administered local anaesthetic resides at its site of injection for a longer period.
   4.3. Answer **D**. Tetracaine is poorly absorbed and is used topically for conjunctival anaesthesia.
   4.4. Answer **E**. Lidocaine can be given intravenously for the treatment of ventricular arrhythmias.

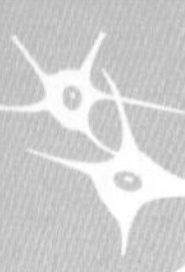

Local anaesthetics (all given by injection [see text], except for benzocaine)

Drug	Half-life (h) and kinetics	Comments
Articaine	1 [M] Half-life data are from subjects treated to produce regional anaesthesia; hydrolysed to inactive articainic acid by plasma esterases	Used in dentistry; concentrations in tooth alveolus are 100 times those in circulation
Benzocaine	<1 min [M] Minimal oral absorption; metabolised in liver	Differs from other drugs by not having a secondary amino group; used in throat lozenges
Bupivacaine	2–4 [M] Metabolised mainly by N-dealkylation and hydroxylation; less than 10% is excreted in urine	Bupivacaine is a racemic mixture of *S*(–)- and *R*(+)-isomers of 1-butyl-N-(2,6-dimethyl phenyl)-piperidine-2-carboxamide; used for local infiltration anaesthesia, peripheral nerve block, epidural block and sympathetic block; onset of action 1–10 min; duration of action 3–9 h
Cocaine	1–2 [M] Rapidly and extensively metabolised to products that are excreted in urine; half-life may be longer after topical dosage	Very rapid onset of action; used topically on mucosal surfaces (the only legal route!); profound CNS effects limit clinical usefulness
Levobupivacaine	1.3 [M] Metabolised by hepatic CYP3A4; less cardiotoxic than bupivacaine	The *S*(–)-isomer of the drug bupivacaine
Lidocaine	1–2 [M] Metabolised by dealkylation, catalysed by CYP3A4, followed by hydrolysis	Used for local infiltration anaesthesia, intravenous regional anaesthesia, nerve blocks and dental anaesthesia; also used topically
Mepivacaine	2–3 [M] Metabolised in liver by N-dealkylation and hydroxylation; metabolites excreted in bile and subject to enterohepatic circulation	Used in dentistry
Prilocaine	1–2 [M] Metabolised mainly by amide hydrolysis in the liver	Used for local infiltration anaesthesia, intravenous anaesthesia, nerve blocks and dental anaesthesia; may cause methaemoglobinaemia (especially in infants)
Procaine	Not relevant [0.5][M] Very rapid ester hydrolysis at site of injection; any which escaped into the blood would be rapidly hydrolysed by plasma esterases, with a half-life of less than 1 min	Seldom used now; local infiltration anaesthesia
Ropivacaine	2–4 [M] Oxidised by hepatic CYP1A2 and to some extent by CYP3A4	Ropivacaine is the *S*(–)-isomer of 1-propyl-N-(2,6-dimethylphenyl)-piperidine-2-carboxamide; used for epidural, major nerve block and field block
Tetracaine	3 min [M] Poorly absorbed; hydrolysed to metabolites by pseudocholinesterase (butyrylcholinesterase, plasma cholinesterase)	Mostly used topically

[M], metabolism.

19 Opioid analgesics and the management of pain

PAIN AND PAIN PERCEPTION

Pain is a complex phenomenon that involves the person's awareness and response to a noxious stimulation. Pain is highly subjective to the individual, and psychological factors will determine to what extent the individual experiences suffering or distress (Fig. 19.1). Pain can be **acute**, lasting only until the initiating trauma resolves, which is sometimes described as **nociceptive pain**. Pain can also become protracted and **chronic**, outlasting the original trauma, and can in some cases become intractable as a result of persistent pathological change in the way that the nociceptive (pain-carrying) neuronal pathways function (**neuropathic pain**).

Nociceptive pain is a defensive response to a variety stimuli (e.g. mechanical, thermal or chemical) that activates nociceptor sensory units on nerve endings. It is defensive as it induces behaviour that may aid healing and avoid exacerbation of the pain. Painful stimuli are transmitted to the central nervous system (CNS) by fast fibres in the neospinothalamic pathways and slow fibres in the paleospinothalamic pathways (Fig. 19.2).

Neuropathic pain may result from abnormal neuronal activity that persists beyond the time expected for healing of the injury. For example, phantom limb pain of amputation, and shingles may cause pain well beyond the time expected. There are multiple pathophysiological mechanisms underlying neuropathic pain.

Neuropathic pain can be spontaneous (stimulus-independent), when it is usually described by the sufferer as shooting or lancinating sensations, electric-shock-like pain or an abnormal unpleasant sensation (dysaesthesia). Alternatively, it can be an exaggerated response to a painful stimulus (hyperalgesia) or a painful response to a trivial stimulus (allodynia).

Some pain states have mixed nociceptive and neuropathic elements, for example mechanical spinal pain with local nerve damage such as radiculopathy or myelopathy.

The pathophysiological and molecular explanations for nociceptive and neuropathic pain and the endogenous responses that modulate pain are complex and incompletely understood. In brief, the genesis of pain results from initial stimulation of afferent sensory neurons (nociceptors) by thermal, mechanical or chemical stimuli sufficient to stimulate the nociceptors (free nerve endings responsive to high-threshold noxious stimuli) in Aδ and C axons (Fig. 19.3). The particular type of painful stimulus may determine which receptors or channels are activated. The many mediators, receptors and channels involved in painful nerve impulses include bradykinin, ATP, vanilloid type receptors (*transient receptor potential vanilloid receptor TRPV*$_1$) and mechanosensitive channels (ion channels responsive to touch, pressure etc.). Activation of the channels or receptors results in an influx of Na^+/Ca^{2+} sufficient to generate action potentials in the nerve (Fig. 19.3). When tissue damage occurs, nociceptors which were not normally active (described as silent or sleeping) can be recruited and fire persistently. Chemical transmission of the afferent impulse across synapses in the dorsal horn of the spinal cord results from the release of transmitters such as glutamate, substance P and calcitonin gene-related peptide (CGRP) from vesicles in the presynaptic membrane. These depolarise the postsynaptic neuron by acting on a variety of receptors and channels in the postsynaptic membrane. Synaptic transmission responsible for nociceptive pain can be reduced by local inhibitory neurons and by stimulation of the multifaceted descending modulatory pathways. Endogenous opioids, GABA, glycine, noradrenaline (acting on α_2-adrenoceptors) and other amines are all involved in pain modulation. Activation of these systems produces hyperpolarisation of neurons in the pain pathways (by inhibiting Na^+/Ca^{2+} influx and enhancing K^+ efflux) and prevents nociceptive action potential generation (Figs 19.4 and 19.5). The endogenous cannabinoids anandamide and 2-arachidonyl glycerol are also being investigated for their modulatory functions.

Neuropathic pain persisting beyond the time when the original pathology has resolved may result from chronic hypersensitisation and phenotypic change in neurons. These changes can occur both peripherally and centrally, probably as a result of repetitive stimulation of synaptic transmission. In neuropathic and other chronic pain states, the following possibilities may exist:

- **Sensitisation of afferent inputs**: this may include recruitment of silent nociceptors, lower threshold for generation of action potentials, and enhanced and spontaneous release of increased amounts of substance P, glutamate and CGRP from afferent terminals, leading to enhanced action potential generation (Figs 19.3 and 19.5).

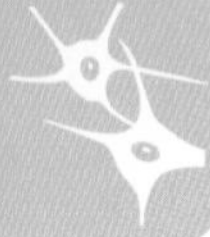

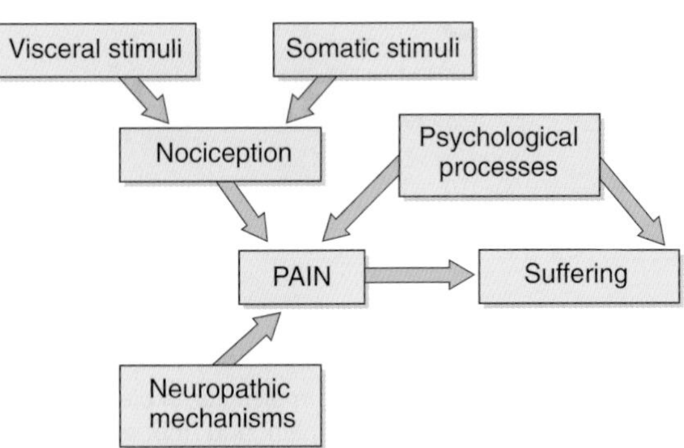

Fig. 19.1 **The origin of pain and suffering.**

- **Dysfunctional descending pain modulatory and facilitatory pathways**: the functioning of the descending modulatory pathway (Fig. 19.4) may become inadequate as a result of persistent nociceptive pain and this may be related to the overactivity of endogenous pain facilitatory pathways that exist in tracts from the medulla to the spinal dorsal horn, which then maintain neuropathic pain states.
- **Loss of inhibitory neurons and generation of new synapses that act as nociceptive neurons (neuronal plasticity)**: in neuropathic pain, Aβ nerve fibres which normally transmit tactile stimuli can sometimes phenotypically alter and take on the properties of a nociceptive neuron.

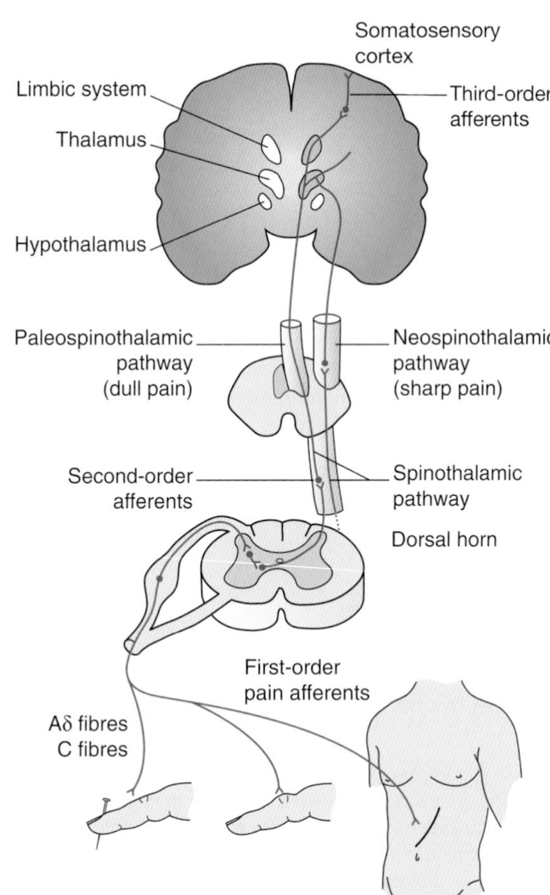

Fig. 19.2 **Ascending pathways of pain perception.** Ascending pathways are activated following stimulation of afferent sensory nociceptive nerve terminals. Many mediators and neurotransmitters are involved during afferent stimulation of the nociceptive pathway. Mediator release (bradykinin, serotonin, prostaglandins) and thermal and mechanical influences can stimulate and sensitise the sensory nerve terminals of pain fibres, resulting in increased cation influx, depolarisation and generation of action potentials (see Fig 19.3). Onward afferent transmission of ascending nerve impulses at the synapses in the dorsal horn involves transmitters such as substance P, glutamate and calcitonin gene-related peptide (CGRP) (Fig. 19.5). Hyperexcitability of pain fibres can also be promoted by other mediators. Prolonged activation of the nociceptive pathways can produce pathophysiological and phenotypic changes resulting in neuropathic pain that persists when the original pathological cause of the pain has resolved, and generation of nociceptive signals can occur at low levels of axonal stimulation.

ANALGESIC DRUGS

Non-steroidal anti-inflammatory drugs (NSAIDs; Ch. 29) and opioids are the major classes of pain-relieving (analgesic) drugs. They act at different levels in the pain-transmitting pathways to influence the production and recognition of pain as indicated in Figures 19.3 and 19.4.

Non-steroidal anti-inflammatory drugs

These act mainly by blocking the peripheral generation of the nociceptive impulses. Prostaglandins enhance nociceptive impulses in peripheral afferent neurons by increasing the ability of thermal, mechanical or chemical stimuli to increase Na^+/Ca^{2+} influx and thereby to generate action potentials in nociceptive afferent neurons. NSAIDs inhibit the production of prostaglandins by the cyclo-oxygenase type 1 and type 2 (COX-1, COX-2) isoenzymes and reduce the sensitivity of sensory nociceptive nerve endings to agents released by injured tissue that initiate pain, such as bradykinin and substance P. These drugs are considered fully in Chapter 29.

Opioids

These act on the spinal cord and limbic system, and stimulate the long descending inhibitory pathways from the midbrain to the dorsal horn. They produce their effects via specific receptors that are closely associated with the neuronal pathways which transmit pain from the periphery to the CNS.

Non-opioid, non-NSAID analgesics

A variety of drugs which are used more widely for other purposes are being used increasingly for their analgesic actions when NSAIDs and opioids are less effective, for example in neuropathic pain (see Table 19.2).

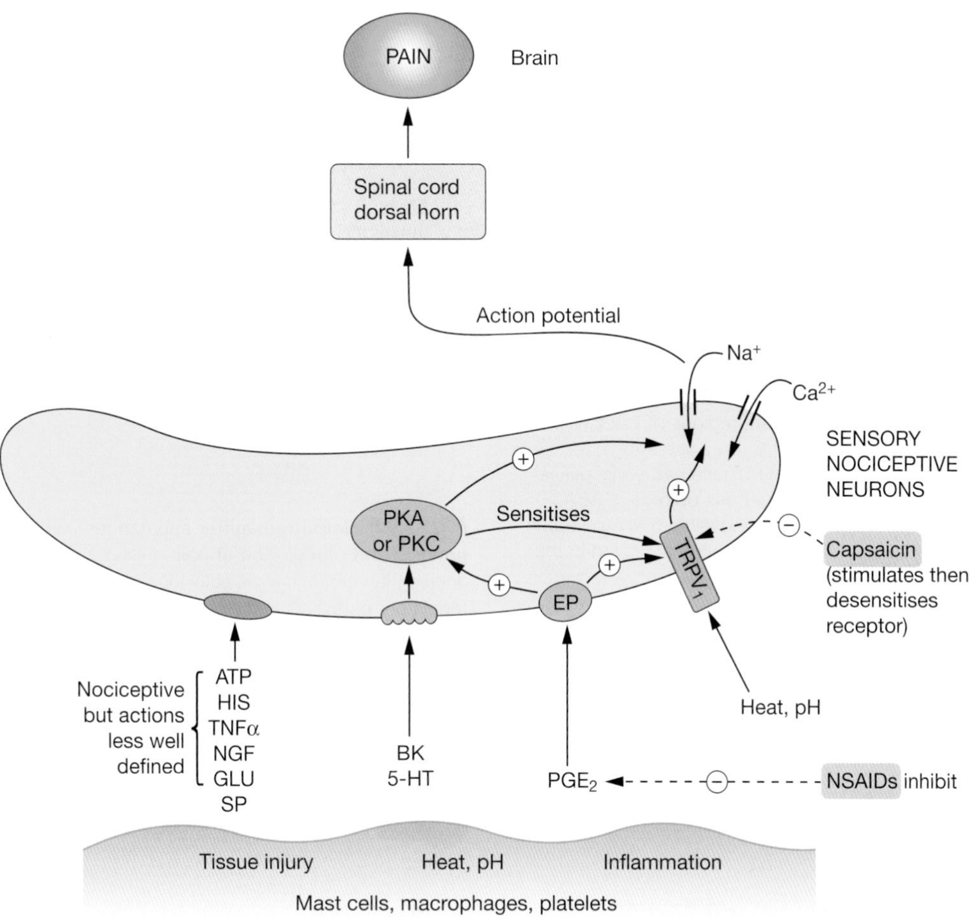

Fig 19.3 **Mediators involved in the genesis and modulation of pain.** Numerous mediators are able to stimulate or sensitise primary sensory neurons (nociceptors), leading to activation of nociceptive fibres. Tissue injury and other noxious stimuli such as heat or extremes of pH can stimulate the release of substances that act to promote pain, such as bradykinin (BK) and serotonin (5-HT). PGE_2 acting at prostaglandin E receptors (EP) sensitises the nerve endings to the actions of nociceptive mediators such as BK and 5-HT. Adenosine triphosphate (ATP) and histamine (HIS) also have nociceptive actions, acting in, as yet, less well-defined ways. Heat and H^+ stimulate the $TRPV_1$ receptor, producing pain. The $TRPV_1$ channel receptor is also sensitised by many other mediators. Capsaicin and other $TRPV_1$ receptor stimulants desensitise the receptor on persistent stimulation, resulting in an analgesic effect. Non-steroidal anti-inflammatory drugs (NSAIDs) inhibit the production of PGE_2. Overall the effect of nociceptive stimuli is to depolarise the neuron, setting up action potentials in the fibres to the dorsal horn and pain-perceiving areas of the brain. Substance P and calcitonin gene-related peptide (CGRP) may also be involved in nociception. GLU, glutamate; NGF, nerve growth factor; PKA, protein kinase A; PKC, protein kinase C; TNFα, tumour necrosis factor alpha; $TRPV_1$, transient receptor potential vanilloid receptor.

OPIOID ANALGESICS

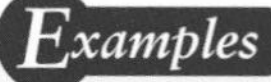

buprenorphine, codeine, diamorphine (heroin), dihydrocodeine, fentanyl, meptazinol, methadone, morphine, oxycodone, pentazocine, pethidine (known as meperidine in the USA), tramadol

Opioid is a term used for both naturally occurring and synthetic molecules that produce their effects by an agonist action at opioid receptors. The terms opiate analgesics (specifically, drugs derived from the juice of the opium poppy, *Papaver somniferum*) and narcotic analgesic (which literally means a 'stupor-inducing pain killer') are no longer used.

Mechanism of action

The brain produces several endogenous opioid peptides, which are neurotransmitters that act via specific opioid receptors. Among these are the two pentapeptide enkephalins. These each contain the amino acid sequence Tyr-Gly-Gly-Phe as the message domain, linked to either leucine or methionine, and are called leu-enkephalin and

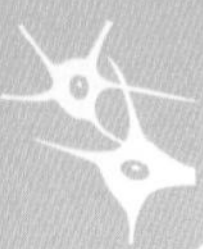

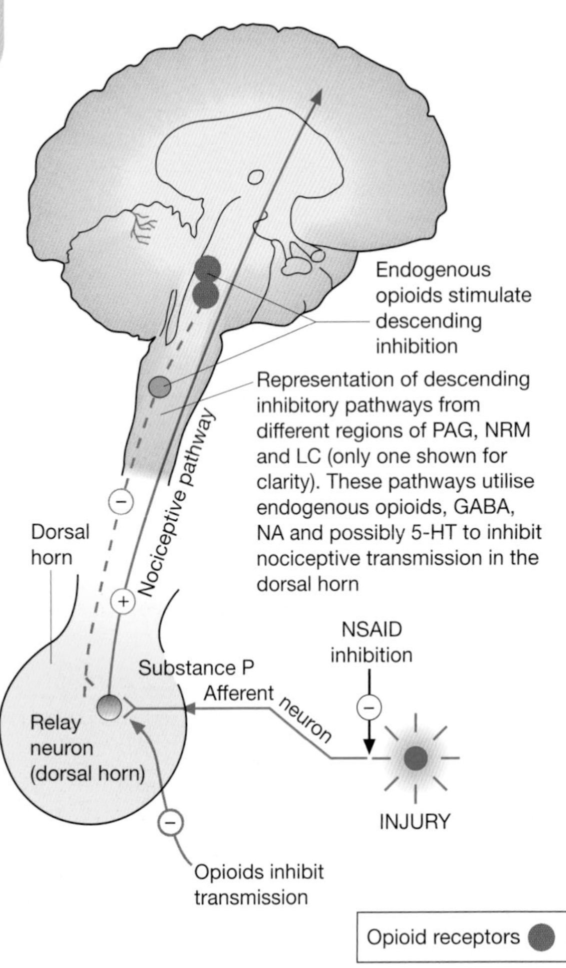

Fig. 19.4 **Transmitters and receptors for pain perception and control.** The afferent nociceptive pathways are subject to inhibitory control. Opioids act at opioid receptor-rich sites in the periaqueductal grey matter (PAG), the nucleus raphe magnus (NRM) and other spinal sites to stimulate descending inhibitory fibres that inhibit nociceptive transmission in the dorsal horn. Descending pathways from the locus ceruleus (LC) that are noradrenergic are also involved. Opioids also act at a local level in the dorsal horn (Fig. 19.5). Inhibitory modulation of nociceptive transmission via local nerve networks also results from actions of other agents (Fig. 19.5). 5-HT, 5-hydroxytryptamine (serotonin); GABA, gamma-aminobutyric acid; NA, noradrenaline; NSAID, non-steroidal anti-inflammatory drug.

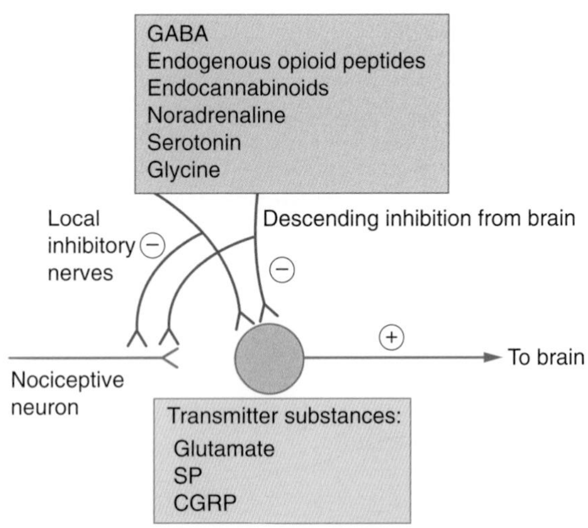

Fig. 19.5 **Neurotransmitter substances involved in the genesis and modulation of pain.** Inhibitory modulation of nociception can occur via activation of the descending regulatory pathways and also by actions of local interneurons. Inhibitory transmitters are shown in the blue box and excitatory transmitters in the pink box. 5-HT, 5-hydroxytryptamine (serotonin); CGRP, calcitonin gene-related peptide; GABA, gamma-aminobutyric acid; SP, substance P.

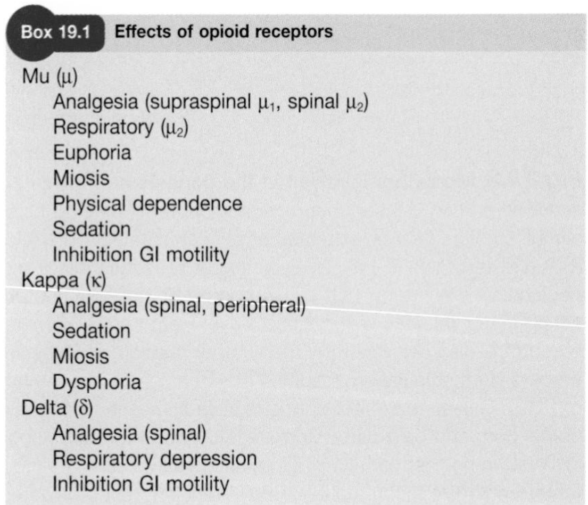

Box 19.1 Effects of opioid receptors

Mu (μ)
- Analgesia (supraspinal μ_1, spinal μ_2)
- Respiratory (μ_2)
- Euphoria
- Miosis
- Physical dependence
- Sedation
- Inhibition GI motility

Kappa (κ)
- Analgesia (spinal, peripheral)
- Sedation
- Miosis
- Dysphoria

Delta (δ)
- Analgesia (spinal)
- Respiratory depression
- Inhibition GI motility

met-enkephalin. Other agonists incorporating the same amino acid sequence are dynorphins A and B and the most potent agonist β-endorphin, a 31-amino-acid peptide with met-enkephalin at its carboxyl end. Two further peptides, endomorphins 1 and 2, have been identified that have a Tyr-Pro-Phe/Trp message domain sequence. All opioid peptides are derived by selective cleavage of larger precursor molecules.

Opioid receptors are found on the presynaptic and postsynaptic membranes of neurons in the pain pathways of the CNS, and have also been identified in the peripheral nervous system. Three major classes of opioid receptor have been identified, which mediate distinct effects: the μ (mu), κ (kappa), and δ (delta) receptors (Box 19.1). There is a distinctive regional distribution of opioid peptides and their receptors in the CNS, with high concentrations in the limbic system and spinal cord. These regions also contain high concentrations of a neutral endopeptidase (enkephalinase), which rapidly hydrolyses the pentapeptides into fragments. The various endogenous opioid peptides show preferential receptor binding affinities: β-endorphin binds equally to μ- and δ-receptors; endomorphins bind mainly to μ-receptors; dynorphins bind preferentially to κ-receptors; and the enkephalins bind preferentially to δ-receptors. The different physiological effects produced by these receptors are due to their specific neuronal distributions. An 'orphan' opioid receptor has been identified, which is principally found in the medulla and facilitates descending enkephalinergic pathways in the spinal cord. This receptor has been named NOP (nociceptin/orphanin peptide receptor), after its specific endogenous agonist known as nociceptin or orphanin FQ.

All opioid receptors are coupled to inhibitory G-proteins (G_i/G_0). Receptor activation has many consequences, including inhibition of adenylyl cyclase with reduced intracellular generation of cyclic adenosine monophosphate (cAMP), and other second messengers. The G-proteins are also directly coupled to inwardly rectifying K^+ channels and voltage-operated Ca^{2+} channels. Opioids increase K^+ conductance and hyperpolarise the target cells, making them less responsive to depolarising impulses, and also inhibit Ca^{2+} influx. These actions reduce neurotransmitter release from the neurons and reduce postsynaptic impulse generation. Opioids have a complementary analgesic effect with NSAIDs, as they act by different mechanisms to relieve pain (Ch. 29).

Morphine and synthetic opioid analgesics produce their effects largely by acting as agonists at specific opioid receptors in the CNS. The analgesic action of opioids is the end result of a complex series of neuronal interactions. In the nucleus raphe magnus of the brain, μ-receptor stimulation decreases activity in inhibitory gamma-aminobutyric acid (GABA) neurons that project to descending inhibitory serotonergic neurons in the brainstem. These neurons in turn connect presynaptically with afferent nociceptive fibres in the dorsal horn of the spinal cord. Inhibition of the GABA neurons permits increased firing of these descending inhibitory serotonergic neurons. Analgesia is produced by inhibition of the release of the pain pathway mediators, substance P, glutamate and nitric oxide, from the afferent nociceptive neurons (Fig. 19.5). Activation of κ-receptors antagonises the analgesia produced by μ-receptor stimulation, by inhibiting the descending (pain-modulating) serotonergic neurons in the pain pathway. However, there is a paradoxical spinal analgesic effect from unopposed κ-receptor activation.

Opioid receptors are also present on peripheral nerves in the pain pathways, and a μ-receptor agonist reduces the sensitivity of peripheral nociceptive neurons to pain stimuli, particularly in inflamed tissues. Non-neuronal κ-receptors are involved in the inflammatory response, and are found on endothelial cells, T-lymphocytes and macrophages; κ-receptor agonists are being developed to modulate the inflammatory response orchestrated by these cells.

Opioid drugs show receptor selectivity and can have agonist, partial agonist or antagonist properties at various opioid receptor types (Table 19.1).

- **Full agonists**: these act principally at μ-receptors and include morphine, diamorphine, fentanyl, pethidine, codeine and dihydrocodeine. They also have weak agonist activity at δ- and κ-receptors.
- **Mixed agonist–antagonist**: pentazocine has agonist effects at the κ-receptor (and, to a lesser extent, the δ-receptor) and is a weak μ-receptor antagonist.
- **Mixed partial agonist–antagonist**: buprenorphine is a potent partial agonist at the μ-receptor and has antagonist activity at κ-receptors. The latter action will enhance the analgesic action produced via the μ-receptors.

Some opioids have additional properties: meptazinol is a μ-receptor agonist with muscarinic receptor agonist activity; tramadol and methadone are μ-receptor agonists that also inhibit neuronal noradrenaline and serotonin (5-hydroxytryptamine, 5-HT) reuptake. These supplementary actions of tramadol and methadone contribute to their analgesic actions, since enhanced amine-mediated neurotransmission potentiates descending inhibitory pain pathways (Fig. 19.4). Methadone is also an antagonist at glutamate NMDA (N-methyl-D-aspartate) receptors, an action which can also inhibit pain transmission (Fig. 19.5).

Opioid receptor antagonists, such as naloxone without analgesic actions and are used in the treatment of opioid overdose (Ch. 53).

Effects and clinical uses

Effects on the central nervous system

Analgesia

The analgesia produced by morphine is most effective for chronic visceral pain, but can still be helpful for some types of neuropathic pain. In addition to its antinociceptive effect, morphine alters the perception of pain, making it less unpleasant. This supraspinal effect, possibly at the limbic system, is less marked with some opioids such as pentazocine. Opioid analgesics have no anti-inflammatory effect. In fact, morphine can release the inflammatory mediator histamine locally at the site of an injection. Full μ-receptor agonists are the most powerful opioid analgesics (see Table 19.1 for list of full and partial agonists). However, some full μ-receptor agonists, for example codeine, are weak agonists and their ceiling analgesic effect in clinical use is low. There is growing evidence that the antagonist action of methadone at NMDA receptors can produce effective analgesia in people who have become tolerant to high doses of morphine (see below).

The ceiling analgesic effect of a μ-receptor partial agonist is lower than that of a full agonist. If a person receiving high doses of a potent full μ-receptor agonist is given a μ-receptor partial agonist (e.g. buprenorphine) or a μ-receptor antagonist (e.g. pentazocine), then some of the full agonist molecules will be displaced from receptor sites by the less effective molecules. The degree of analgesia may then be reduced, and in dependent individuals withdrawal symptoms can be produced (see below and Table 19.1).

Short-acting opioids such as alfentanil, fentanyl and remifentanil are used for analgesia during anaesthesia (Ch. 17).

Euphoria

The use of morphine is often associated with an elevated sense of well-being (euphoria, mediated by μ-receptors), an action that contributes considerably to its analgesic efficacy. The opposite effect (dysphoria, mediated by agonist activity at κ-receptors) counteracts the euphoric action, and the degree of euphoria produced will depend on the receptor binding characteristics of the drug.

Respiratory depression

The sensitivity of the respiratory centre to stimulation by carbon dioxide is reduced by morphine at doses that

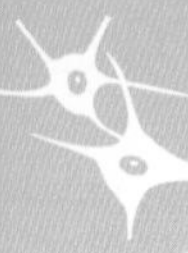

Table 19.1 Opioid analgesics

Compound	Analgesic potency	Tolerance and dependence	Clinical uses and comments
Alfentanil	+++	–	Used by injection for intraoperative analgesia; not used for management of chronic pain and therefore tolerance and dependence not relevant
Buprenorphine	++++	++	Used as an alternative to morphine for analgesia, but nausea may limit its tolerability; a partial agonist at μ opioid receptors
Codeine	+	+	See text; also used when the non-analgesic effects such as antitussive or antidiarrhoeal actions are needed; produces little respiratory depression
Dextropropoxyphene	(+)	+	Withdrawn in the UK in 2005; reports of fatalities with overdose, especially when taken with alcohol
Diamorphine (heroin)	++++	++++	Clinical uses restricted because of high abuse potential; given orally or by infusion for the pain of terminal cancer; given for acute severe pain, e.g. myocardial infarction
Dihydrocodeine	+	+	Used largely as an alternative to codeine for moderate pain
Dipipanone	++	++	Less sedating than morphine, but the only available formulation in the UK contains cyclizine (an antiemetic), which makes it unsuitable for palliative care
Fentanyl	+++	+	Increasingly used by transdermal patch for intractable pain; intravenous adjunct in anaesthesia
Hydromorphone	+++	+++	Similar to morphine in most properties; shorter duration of action may limit usefulness in chronic pain compared with morphine
Meptazinol	+	–	Behaves as a mixed agonist/antagonist and lacks withdrawal and dependence symptoms
Methadone	+++	++	Major use is for withdrawal from morphine/heroin dependence
Morphine	+++	+++	See text
Nalbuphine	+++	+	Fewer side-effects than morphine and a lower abuse potential; may produce opiate withdrawal if administered to opioid-dependent people, due to its mixed opioid agonist and antagonist activity
Oxycodone	+++	++	Similar profile to morphine; used primarily to control pain in palliative care as an alternative in people who cannot tolerate morphine
Pentazocine	+++	++	See text; will provoke a withdrawal syndrome in a morphine-dependent person because of weak antagonist or partial agonist action on μ-receptors (but not cross-tolerance to morphine)
Pethidine (meperidine)	++	+	Not useful for antitussive or antidiarrhoeal effects
Remifentanil	+++	–	Used by injection for intraoperative analgesia; not used for management of chronic pain and therefore tolerance and dependence not relevant
Tramadol	+	+	Obstetric analgesia; less potential for respiratory depression; WHO-classified step II agent; it is also a monoamine reuptake blocker

produce analgesia. Respiratory depression is a common cause of death in opioid overdose. Occasionally, the effect on respiratory rate can be of clinical benefit; for example, intravenous morphine relieves the dyspnoea associated with acute pulmonary oedema, and morphine is used orally or by subcutaneous infusion for the treatment of breathlessness in palliative care. Meptazinol and tramadol are claimed to cause less respiratory depression than other opioids; meptazinol is used for obstetric analgesia, to reduce the risk of respiratory depression in the neonate.

Suppression of the cough centre

Opioids possess an antitussive action. Compounds such as codeine and dextromethorphan are highly effective for cough suppression (Ch. 13), despite having relatively weak analgesic effects.

Vomiting

Opioids stimulate the chemoreceptor trigger zone, and cause vomiting in up to 30% of people. Tolerance to the nausea and vomiting can occur with repeated doses. Powerful opioids such as morphine are usually given with an antiemetic (Ch. 32), particularly when used for acute pain.

Miosis

Stimulation of the third-nerve nucleus results in pupillary constriction. Pinpoint pupils, together with coma and slow respiration, are signs of opioid overdose (Ch. 53).

Endocrine effects

Opioids inhibit the hypothalamic–pituitary–adrenal axis, leading to a progressive decline in plasma cortisol levels (Ch. 44). They also increase prolactin and decrease luteinising hormone release, which leads to testosterone deficiency in men and a reduction in oestrogen in women (Chs 45 and 46). Men usually benefit from testosterone replacement during long-term opioid use (Ch. 46).

Peripheral effects

Gastrointestinal tract

There is a general increase in resting tone of the gut wall and sphincters. These effects arise from stimulation of μ- and κ-receptors on neuronal plexuses in the gut wall. An increase in biliary pressure caused by opioid-induced spasm at the sphincter of Oddi can exacerbate biliary colic. In the stomach, a decrease in motility and pyloric tone can produce anorexia, nausea and vomiting. In the small and large intestines there is increased segmenting activity and decreased propulsive activity. Thus, opioid administration is associated with constipation, and up to 80% of people who take opioids long term will need a laxative. Methylnaltrexone, a specific antagonist of peripheral opioid receptors, is used to treat opioid-induced constipation during palliative care when laxatives are inadequate. The effects of opioids on gastrointestinal motility make them useful in the treatment of diarrhoea (Ch. 35). Pethidine and tramadol have less effect on the gastrointestinal tract than do equianalgesic doses of morphine.

Cardiovascular system

Opioids have little effect on the heart or circulation except at high doses that can depress the medullary vasomotor centre. Hypotension can occur with parenteral use of morphine, possibly because of histamine release.

Other systems

Opioids have minor effects on other systems. For example, there is an increase in tone of the bladder wall and sphincter, which can lead to urinary retention. There is increasing evidence that long-term use of opioids suppresses immune function by inhibiting the development and differentiation of many types of immune cells. The clinical relevance of this is not known.

Tolerance and dependence

Tolerance and dependence result from changes in the functioning of opioid receptors during continuous opioid administration. As a consequence of adaptive changes, more of the drug is necessary to produce the same effect (tolerance) and withdrawal of the drug produces adverse physiological effects until the compensatory changes are reset (dependence).

Tolerance to opioids occurs in two ways. Associative (learned) tolerance has a major psychological component. Non-associative (adaptive) tolerance involves downregulation or desensitisation of opioid receptors. This arises in response to increased firing of neurons in the noradrenergic pathways of the locus ceruleus, which is rich in inhibitory opioid receptors, and activation of the reward pathway in the brain (see Ch. 54). It may also involve increased activity at NMDA receptors for excitatory glutamate-mediated neurotransmission in spinal and supraspinal circuits. Tolerance to the analgesia, euphoria, respiratory depression and emesis develops rapidly during long-term opioid administration, but much less to the constipation or miosis. A high degree of cross-tolerance is shown by many opioids; consequently, individuals who develop tolerance to one opioid are often (but not invariably) tolerant to another. Opioid-induced NMDA receptor activation can also produce abnormal pain sensitivity at spinal cord dorsal horn cells. This sensitisation process can be confused with tolerance and lead to opioid dose escalation. Methadone may be useful in this situation (see above).

Dependence manifests itself as a withdrawal syndrome, which can be precipitated when individuals who have taken the drug for a long period of time have their intake stopped or are given an opioid antagonist or partial agonist (Ch. 54). This is most often a problem for people who abuse the drug, but can occur from long-term intake of a prescribed opioid.

During the first 12 h after opioid withdrawal, effects such as nervousness, sweating and craving are largely psychological, because they can be alleviated by the administration of a placebo. Following this period, the effects of physiological dependence manifest themselves – for example, dilated pupils, anorexia, weakness, depression, insomnia, gastrointestinal and skeletal muscle cramps, increased respiratory rate, pyrexia, piloerection with goose-pimples, and diarrhoea. The time course for the development and resolution of these symptoms varies among the opioids. In the case of morphine, the maximum withdrawal effects occur quickly (after about 1–2 days) and subside rapidly (about 5–10 days), but the intensity of the symptoms may be intolerable. In contrast, withdrawal from methadone is a slow process because of its very long half-life, but the effects are far less intense (peak effect at almost 1 week and symptoms persist for about 3 weeks). Therefore, morphine- or heroin-dependent individuals who have been abusing the drug are often transferred from their drug of abuse to methadone prior to withdrawal. Methadone also produces less euphoria than morphine or heroin. After a period of treatment with methadone, the methadone dosage is gradually reduced and the person undergoes a more tolerable withdrawal.

More recently, buprenorphine has been used as an alternative to methadone, due to the low severity of withdrawal symptoms. It can be given for 6 days in a rapid detoxification programme. Long-term maintenance with buprenorphine has also shown promise for reducing relapse in people who are addicted to opioids, since its partial agonist activity blocks the 'high' from illicit opioid use.

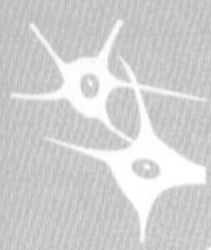

Rapid in-hospital tapering of opioids over 2 weeks has an 80% success rate. On an outpatient basis, slow tapering over 6 months is more successful than rapid withdrawal, but still leads to only a 40% success rate. Long-term buprenorphine therapy, combined with high-intensity psychosocial group therapy treatment, has achieved up to 75% withdrawal rates after 1 year. Detoxification from opioids can also be helped by the presynaptic α_2-adrenoceptor agonists clonidine or lofexidine (a clonidine analogue with fewer unwanted effects). These inhibit the excessive sympathetic nervous system activity associated with opioid withdrawal, such as lacrimation, rhinorrhoea, muscle pain, joint pain and gastrointestinal symptoms. However, the lethargy, insomnia and restlessness persist.

Pharmacokinetics

The pharmacokinetic properties of individual opioid analgesics are summarised in the drug compendium at the end of this chapter. Most opioids are available for oral use. Buprenorphine is formulated for sublingual absorption, and fentanyl is available as lozenges for rapid pain relief. Some opioids, such as morphine, buprenorphine, meptazinol, methadone, oxycodone and tramadol, can be given by intravenous or intramuscular injection. Morphine and oxycodone can also be given by subcutaneous infusion in palliative care. Diamorphine is more water-soluble than morphine and can be given by subcutaneous infusion in smaller volumes, which can be useful for emaciated people. Morphine and pentazocine are available as a suppository. Fentanyl and buprenorphine can be delivered transdermally via self-adhesive patches for prolonged analgesia.

Some opioids, such as morphine, have a low and variable absorption across the gut wall, and the dose should be reduced when they are given parenterally to achieve equivalent analgesia and avoid unwanted effects. Others, such as dihydrocodeine, have a low oral bioavailability due to extensive first-pass metabolism. Opioids are eliminated by hepatic metabolism. A metabolite of morphine, morphine 6-glucuronide, has more analgesic activity than the parent compound and is excreted by the kidney. The dose of morphine must therefore be reduced in renal failure. Diamorphine is an acetylated morphine derivative that is converted to morphine by hydrolysis in plasma and in most tissues, including the brain. Codeine is a prodrug that is metabolised by CYP2D6, which shows genetic polymorphism, to several active metabolites. Codeine 6-glucuronide is responsible for most of the analgesic activity, while about 5% is converted to morphine. About 10% of people have low CYP2D6 activity, and have a reduced analgesic response to codeine.

Most opioid analgesics have half-lives in the range 1–6 h. For long-term pain control, morphine is often given as a modified-release formulation to prolong the duration of action. Fentanyl has a short half-life (1–6 h), but can be given as a transdermal delivery patch, when pain relief lasts 12–24 h due to slow drug delivery (Ch. 2). In addition, the effect persists for several hours after removing the patch owing to build-up of a subcutaneous drug reservoir at the site of application. Care is necessary both to maintain analgesia and to avoid unwanted opioid effects if analgesia is changed between different doses of fentanyl patches or between fentanyl patches and another opioid.

Table 19.2 The mechanisms of action of some non-opioid non-NSAID analgesics[a]

Drug	Mechanism (see also Fig. 19.3)
Gabapentin, pregabalin	GABA concentrations increased
Carbamazepine, lamotrigine	Membrane stabilisation. Na^+ channel blockade. Attenuation of glutamate-related synaptic transmission
Baclofen	$GABA_B$ receptor agonist. Attenuation of glutamate-related synaptic transmission
Clonidine	α_2-Adrenoceptor agonist
Tricyclic antidepressants; imipramine, amitriptyline	Increase noradrenaline availability
Ketamine, dextromethorphan	NMDA (glutamate) receptor antagonists
Local anaesthetics	Neuronal transmission (Na^+ channel block)
Capsaicin	SP depletion, stimulation of vanilloid ($TRPV_1$) receptor followed by desensitisation
Cannabinoids	Stimulation of cannabinoid receptors

[a]The mechanisms of pain control by these classes of drugs are imperfectly understood. Some are selective in their actions. For example, pain related to diabetic neuropathy and postherpetic neuralgia (shingles), but not lower back pain, responds to tricyclic antidepressants.

GABA, gamma-aminobutyric acid; SP, substance P; $TRPV_1$, transient receptor potential vanilloid receptor.

Unwanted effects

The unwanted effects of opioids are caused by their actions on those opioid receptors that are not the primary site for therapeutic benefit (see above). For example, respiratory depression and constipation are unwanted effects when an opioid is used as an analgesic, but the same effects are therapeutically beneficial in the treatment of breathlessness or diarrhoea. Tolerance and dependence can also be regarded as unwanted problems associated with long term use.

NON-OPIOID, NON-NSAID AGENTS USED FOR ANALGESIA

A diverse group of drugs are now being used for pain control in circumstances where opioids and NSAIDs are inadequate (Table 19.2). These are dealt with individually in the next section and the detailed pharmacology of the drugs is given in the chapters describing their main clinical uses.

PAIN MANAGEMENT

Appropriate management of pain depends on its origin and severity. The 'analgesic ladder' developed by the World

Box 19.2 The 'analgesic ladder'

Step 1: non-opioid analgesics, e.g. paracetamol, NSAIDs
Step 2: opioid suitable for moderate pain ± simple analgesics
Step 3: opioid suitable for severe pain ± simple analgesics

Adjuvant analgesics (non-opioid, non-NSAID) may be required at any step (see text)

Health Organisation (WHO) is useful for choosing drug therapy appropriate to the level of pain (Box 19.2).

Step 1 drugs

Paracetamol (Ch. 29) is suitable for mild pain. However, an NSAID (Ch. 29) may be more appropriate if there is local inflammation. The choice will be determined by the balance of benefits and risks of NSAIDs. Examples of pain that respond better to an NSAID are soft-tissue injury, tissue compression, visceral pain caused by pleural or peritoneal irritation, and bone pain caused by metastatic deposits. Bone metastases cause local secretion of prostaglandins, and NSAIDs can be particularly effective. Individual responses to an NSAID vary; about 60% of people will respond to an alternative drug even if the first was ineffective.

Step 2 drugs

A weak opioid should be added to a step 1 drug for moderate pain, or when the response to a step 1 drug is inadequate. Opioids suitable for moderate pain include codeine and dihydrocodeine. These are often used in combination with paracetamol, such as co-codamol (codeine and paracetamol), although the dose of opioid in some combinations is too low to produce useful additional analgesia. Tramadol has been advocated at this stage, but it is no more effective than co-codamol, and claims that it has less effect on respiration and gastrointestinal motility are of uncertain clinical importance.

Step 3 drugs

The drug of choice for moderate to severe pain is morphine. It is usually effective orally, using a rapid-onset formulation for initial pain control. Doctors are often unwilling to give adequate doses of strong opioid because of concern about addiction. In severe chronic pain with terminal illness, this is not an issue, and it should not be used as a reason for avoiding the use of morphine in non-cancer pain. Opioid addiction is not a problem when opioids are given appropriately for relief of pain.

Acute pain

Acute pain usually has an obvious cause and is often accompanied by anxiety. For rapid pain relief in a self-limiting condition, for example migraine, a readily absorbed, short-acting drug will be appropriate. For more protracted conditions, for example sprains, a long-acting drug may be helpful to improve adherence by reducing the frequency of administration.

The principles of the WHO analgesic ladder should be followed. Very severe acute pain, for example with myocardial infarction, will require a powerful opioid such as morphine given intravenously for rapid effect. Intramuscular injection should be avoided if possible, since severe pain is often accompanied by sympathetic nervous system stimulation which produces peripheral vasoconstriction and thereby delays drug absorption. Some acute severe pain, such as that arising postoperatively or from trauma, cholecystitis, pancreatitis or sickle cell crisis, should be treated initially with a powerful analgesic, then using less powerful analgesics as the condition resolves. This involves applying the principles of the WHO analgesic ladder in reverse.

Chronic pain

Chronic pain (usually defined as pain lasting for at least 3–6 months) can be a result of chronic nociceptive stimulation or can have a neuropathic origin. Effective management of much chronic pain is facilitated by multidisciplinary pain teams. Drug therapy is not the only solution for chronic pain, and, depending on the cause, non-pharmacological or local treatments are often appropriate. Examples include:

- surgery for neoplastic, structural or ischaemic disorders
- physical methods such as acupuncture, transcutaneous electrical nerve stimulation (TENS – which activates spinal inhibitory neurons by acting as a counter-irritant) and local anaesthetic nerve block (Ch. 18)
- behavioural modification, e.g. biofeedback, relaxation techniques, hypnosis
- a corticosteroid (Ch. 44) for raised intracranial pressure or spinal cord compression, or to reduce inflammation which can be associated with a cancer.

The principles of escalation of analgesia described in the WHO analgesic ladder should be followed. For most severe chronic nociceptive pain, morphine is the treatment of choice. If pain remains severe with a low initial dosage of morphine, the dosage should be increased by 50–100% every 24 h; once the pain is moderate in intensity, increments of 25–50% daily are usually sufficient to achieve control without excessive unwanted effects. A modified-release formulation of morphine can be substituted once a stable dosage has been determined, although a rapid-acting formulation may still be required to treat breakthrough pain. Oral administration may not be possible if there is vomiting, dysphagia or intestinal obstruction. In these circumstances, rectal administration of morphine or subcutaneous infusion of morphine using a syringe driver can be used. Diamorphine can also be given by epidural or intrathecal injection for intractable pain. Transdermal delivery of an opioid such as fentanyl from an adhesive patch is an alternative to modified-release oral morphine. There is increasing evidence that if a person is unable to tolerate a particular opioid, an alternative opioid may be better tolerated. The factors that predict intolerance to a particular agent are poorly understood, although it is now recognised that intolerance to morphine may be associated with a mutation in the multidrug resistance 1 transporter protein (Chs 2 and 52).

Neuropathic pain

Neuropathic pain, such as trigeminal neuralgia, postherpetic neuralgia and phantom limb pain after an amputation,

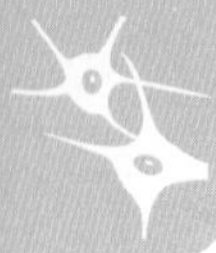

often responds poorly to conventional analgesia. However, mechanisms of neuropathic pain are now beginning to be better understood, allowing a more rational approach to treatment.

Stimulus-independent pain usually arises from spontaneous ectopic impulses arising in afferent nociceptive fibres. Stimulus-evoked pain can also be due to this mechanism, especially following nerve injury, but is more likely to result from peripheral nociceptor sensitisation or loss of inhibitory controls at a spinal level (increased glutamate activity at excitatory NMDA receptors or decreased GABA-mediated inhibition). The afferent fibres involved in hyperalgesia are usually the lightly myelinated Aδ fibres or unmyelinated C fibres (Ch. 18) that transmit nociceptive stimuli. By contrast, allodynia usually involves aberrant transmission in larger myelinated Aβ fibres that normally transmit tactile stimuli.

Stimulus-independent symptoms respond best to membrane-stabilising agents, such as carbamazepine and phenytoin (Ch. 23). Burning pain can be treated with tricyclic antidepressants (Ch. 22) that increase synaptic noradrenaline and serotonin concentrations in the descending spinal inhibitory pathways (Figs 19.4 and 19.5). The importance of noradrenaline is shown by the lack of efficacy of selective serotonin reuptake inhibitor (SSRI) antidepressants for neuropathic pain. Opioids are useful in some cases of stimulus-independent pain.

Of the *stimulus-evoked pains*, hyperalgesia may respond to topical treatment. Lidocaine cream may work, through its local anaesthetic actions (Ch. 18). Alternatively, capsaicin, a derivative of red chilli peppers that stimulates C fibres in the afferent nociceptive pathway, can be applied topically as a counter-irritant. This releases substance P and stimulates the vanilloid receptor TRPV$_1$ and initially provokes hyperalgesia by promoting depolarisation and action potential generation. Subsequent depletion of substance P and even nerve terminal degeneration then blocks nerve function (Fig. 19.3).

If local treatment is inappropriate or ineffective, a membrane-stabilising drug can be used. For allodynia, gabapentin (Ch. 23) is particularly effective for increasing inhibitory pathway activity. Alternatives include tricyclic antidepressants, the α_2-adrenoceptor agonist clonidine (Ch. 6), baclofen (Ch. 24) and the NMDA receptor antagonist ketamine (Ch. 17), all of which modulate spinal transmission of the pain signal. Opioids can be helpful in some cases of allodynia (Table 19.1).

The use of cannabinoids (the active components of cannabis; Ch. 54) for relief of hyperalgesia in conditions such as multiple sclerosis is receiving considerable attention. Stimulation of cannabinoid receptors produces an antinociceptive action and inhibits pain transmission in the spinal cord.

FURTHER READING

Ballantyne JC, Mao J (2003) Opioid therapy for chronic pain. *N Engl J Med* 349, 1943–1953

Berde CB, Sethna NF (2002) Analgesics for the treatment of pain in children. *N Engl J Med* 347, 1094–1103

Bennetto L, Patel NK, Fuller G (2007) Trigeminal neuralgia and its management. *BMJ* 334, 201–205

Carr DB, Goudas LC (1999) Acute pain. *Lancet* 353, 2051–2058

Croxford JL (2003) Therapeutic potential of cannabinoids in CNS disease. *CNS Drugs* 17, 179–202

Eisenberg E, McNichol ED, Carr DB (2005) Efficacy and safety of opioid agonists in the treatment of neuropathic pain of nonmalignant origin. *JAMA* 293, 3043–3052

Gonzalez G, Oliveto A, Kosten TR (2002) Treatment of heroin (diamorphine) addiction. *Drugs* 62, 1331–1343

Holdcroft A, Power I (2003) Management of pain. *BMJ* 326, 635–639

Jensen TS (2002) Anticonvulsants in neuropathic pain: rationale and clinical evidence. *Eur J Pain* 6(suppl A), 61–68

Johnson RW, Dworkin RH (2003) Treatment of herpes zoster and postherpetic neuralgia. *BMJ* 326, 748–750

McMahon SB, Koltzenburg M (eds) (2006) Wall and Melzack's Textbook of Pain. Elsevier

McQuay H (1999) Opioids in pain management. *Lancet* 353, 2229–2232

Mendell JR, Sahenk Z (2003) Painful sensory neuropathy. *N Engl J Med* 348, 1243–1255

O'Connor AB, Dworkin RH (2009) Treatment of neuropathic pain: an overview of recent guidelines. *Am J Med* 122 (Suppl 1), S22–S32

Quigley C (2005) The role of opioids in cancer pain. *BMJ* 331, 825–829

Rea K, Roche M, Finn DP (2007) Supraspinal modulation of pain by cannabinoids: the role of GABA and glutamate. *Br J Pharmacol* 152, 633–648

Ripamonti C, Dickerson ED (2001) Strategies for the treatment of cancer pain in the new millennium. *Drugs* 61, 955–977

Szalliasi A, Cruz F, Geppetti P (2006) TRPV1: a therapeutic target for novel analgesic drugs. *Trends Mol Med* 12, 545–554

Somogyi AA, Barratt DT, Coller JK (2007) Pharmacogenetics of opioids. *Clin Pharm Ther* 81, 429–444

Vadalouca A, Siafaka I, Argyra E et al (2007) Therapeutic management of chronic neuropathic pain: an examination of pharmacologic treatment. *Ann NY Acad Sci* 1088, 164–186

Vanderah TW (2007) Pathophysiology of pain. *Med Clin North Am* 91, 1–12

Ward J, Hall W, Mattick RP (1999) Role of maintenance treatment in opioid dependence. *Lancet* 353, 221–226

Westaway SM (2007) The potential of the transient receptor potential vanilloid type 1 receptor channel modulators for the treatment of pain. *J Med Chem* 50, 2589–2596

Woolf CJ, Mannion RJ (1999) Neuropathic pain: aetiology, symptoms, mechanisms and management. *Lancet* 353, 1959–1964

SELF-ASSESSMENT

In questions 1–4, the initial statements, in italics, are true. Are the accompanying statements also true?

1. *Opioids are analgesic by acting at the level of the dorsal horn to inhibit transmission in the ascending nociceptive pathway. They also act at the level of the periaqueductal grey matter to stimulate descending inhibitory pathways that further inhibit dorsal horn synaptic transmission.*
   a. Opioids can cause euphoria or dysphoria.
   b. Tolerance develops uniformly to all of the biological effects of the opioids.
   c. Methadone has a rapid onset of action and a short half-life.

2. *Concerns about dependence potential should not inhibit the administration of adequate doses of opioids to treat severe chronic pain.*
   a. Meptazinol is a pure μ-receptor agonist.
   b. Naloxone is a short-acting opioid agonist.
3. *Chronic neuropathic pain may be more difficult to manage with opioids than acute pain, and may require treatment with non-opioid, non-NSAID drugs.*
   a. Drugs that inhibit the reuptake of noradrenaline can be effective analgesics in some cases of neuropathic pain.
   b. Anticonvulsants are ineffective in treatment of neuropathic pain.
4. *Pentazocine and buprenorphine are partial agonists at opioid receptors and have less abuse liability than morphine.* Pentazocine can precipitate withdrawal symptoms in morphine addicts.
5. Choose the **most appropriate** statement from the following options.
   A. In the elderly, tolerance rapidly develops to the constipatory effects of morphine.
   B. An opioid analgesic is the drug of choice for chronic limb pain following a below-knee amputation after a road traffic accident.
   C. Naloxone is an agonist at μ-opioid receptors.
   D. Tolerance does not develop to the miotic effect of opioids.
   E. Fentanyl can be used for opioid withdrawal and maintenance of the chronically relapsing heroin addict.
6. Case history questions – pain control in terminal cancer. The case notes highlight the pharmacology of analgesic usage and the necessary involvement of other drugs given concomitantly to manage unwanted effects.

A 60-year-old man was admitted to a hospice. He had previously had a left nephrectomy for renal cell carcinoma and now had intense metastatic bone pain in his ankles, right iliac crest and left upper arm. He was also having periods of dyspnoea. Prior to admission, his medication was the compound analgesic co-codamol and diclofenac (150 mg) at night. He was also taking cimetidine (400 mg) twice daily. His pain was not well controlled on admission. After a week of assessment and optimisation of drug therapy, his treatment comprised the following drugs:

morphine, slow release	260 mg	twice daily (MST)
morphine, oral solution	50 mg	when required
diclofenac, slow release	150 mg	at night
dexamethasone	2 mg	three times daily
metoclopramide	10 mg	three times daily (antiemetic)
cimetidine	400 mg	twice daily
docusate sodium	100 mg	three times daily (laxative)
temazepam	20 mg	at night

Morphine is the optimum drug of choice for pain control in the majority of people with cancer.

   a. How does morphine exert its pharmacological action as an analgesic?
   b. Why was morphine oral solution (which is an immediate-release form) also made available in addition to the modified-release formulation?
   c. Was the addictive potential of morphine likely to present a problem in this man?
   d. What alternative opioids as an immediate replacement for morphine might you consider?
   e. How does diclofenac control inflammation and inflammatory pain?
   f. Why was diclofenac useful in this man?
   g. What was the rationale for the use of dexamethasone in this man?
   h. Metoclopramide is an antiemetic. Why do you think that this man was likely to suffer from nausea and possibly vomiting?
   i. How does metoclopramide act to alleviate nausea?
   j. What other drugs could be used to alleviate nausea?
   k. Why might gastric or duodenal ulceration be a problem in this man?
   l. How might cimetidine reduce the problem of gastric or duodenal ulceration?
   m. Why was constipation likely to be a problem in this man?
   n. What is the mechanism of action of docusate sodium?
   o. What alternative laxative agents to docusate sodium could have been used?
   p. Why was temazepam given?

ANSWERS

1. a. **True**. In people who have pain, analgesia is often associated with well-being (μ-receptors), whereas in pain-free people, dysphoria can occur (κ-receptors).
   b. **False**. Tolerance to miosis and the constipatory effects of opioids develops much less than that to the other biological effects, including analgesia and respiratory depression. Cross-tolerance to opioids is common but not uniform between opioids.
   c. **False**. Because of its long half-life and less potential to cause euphoria, it is used in controlled withdrawal in people with opioid dependence. It is orally well absorbed and has a slow onset of action. Withdrawal symptoms occur more gradually and are less intense with methadone.
2. a. **True**. Because the μ-opioid receptors produce analgesia and the κ-receptors are involved in respiratory depression, it is claimed that meptazinol has less respiratory depressant action. However, this is of limited significance in clinical practice.
   b. **False**. Naloxone is short-acting opioid antagonist acting at μ-, κ- and δ-receptors. It is used in opioid overdosage. Severe withdrawal symptoms can occur in addicts following naloxone administration.
3. a. **True**. Tricyclic antidepressants can be effective for the treatment of pain of neuropathic origin. They may act by enhancing amine levels in the descending inhibitory pathways that control the pain gate mechanism.
   b. **False**. Phenytoin, carbamazepine and sodium valproate can be of use in the treatment of neuropathic

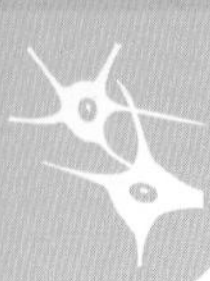

pain, probably by stabilising neuronal membranes and inhibiting neurotransmitter release.

4. **True**. Because it is a partial agonist, it can actually reduce the effects of morphine.
5. Answer **D**.
   A. Constipation continues to be a problem with long-term morphine treatment, and laxatives are often required
   B. Chronic pain is usually less responsive to opioids, and non-opioid treatments (e.g. anticonvulsants) may be required.
   C. Naloxone is an antagonist used to treat opioid overdosage.
   D. This is correct. Miosis is one of the signs of opioid abuse.
   E. Fentanyl is not suitable. Methadone can be used as a substitute in the detoxification process.
6. Case history answers
   a. Morphine acts at specific opioid receptors at spinal and supraspinal sites to produce analgesia and also at other sites to produce unwanted effects. Morphine is a strong agonist at μ-opioid receptors that produce analgesia, euphoria, sedation, respiratory depression, dependence and inhibition of gastrointestinal motility.
   b. Morphine oral solution is used to control short-term breakthrough exacerbations of pain on a patient-initiated basis. Repeated use of this form of morphine should signal a reassessment of the dose of the long-acting morphine. When the person is unable to take oral medication because of weakness or vomiting, rectal or continuous subcutaneous infusion may be required (see d). Normally, 80% of people require less than 200 mg morphine per day to control severe pain. With terminally ill people having persistent severe pain, the dose is gradually increased over a period of 1–2 weeks until an appropriate level of control is achieved. The maximum level may be as high as 2–3 g per day. Unwanted effects can occur; therefore, close monitoring is needed when treatment is first initiated or dosage altered.
   c. For reasons that are not easily explained from a theoretical viewpoint, addiction seldom occurs in people with a high degree of pain. Possible reasons may be a high natural opioid level or high catecholamine levels.
   d. Diamorphine can be used instead of morphine. It is more potent, but is no more efficacious. Its major advantage in practice is its high solubility, which reduces the volume of intramuscular injections or continuous subcutaneous infusion if these are required. Infrequently, an unusual response to morphine may require its replacement by other opioids. Fentanyl is a suitable replacement delivered via a transdermal patch and having fewer unwanted effects.
   e. Diclofenac is an aspirin-like NSAID often used in the treatment of arthritic conditions. Unlike opioids, it has both analgesic and anti-inflammatory actions. NSAIDs appear to have only a small central component to their actions.
   f. The pain from metastases is compounded by local inflammation: in this case, the bone metastases cause 'inflammatory pain', which may be reduced by diclofenac, thereby reducing the requirement for morphine.
   g. Inflammation increases local pressure (and hence pain) within the bone; dexamethasone is a potent corticosteroid, reducing inflammation and swelling.
   h. Nausea is an unwanted effect caused by morphine, occurring particularly during the first week of administration, but may also be a consequence of the cancer itself or related complications such as hypercalcaemia. Tolerance to the nausea induced by morphine occurs.
   i. Metoclopramide is a dopamine antagonist that acts on the chemoreceptor trigger zone (CTZ) to reduce chemical and radiation-induced nausea.
   j. A centrally acting antiemetic such as prochlorperazine can be used. They have the same mechanism of action as metoclopramide.
   k. Gastric and/or duodenal inflammation (which may cause considerable discomfort) or even ulceration may occur with prolonged use of diclofenac and a corticosteroid. Cimetidine in this person relieved the gastric discomfort associated with oral administration of diclofenac.
   l. Cimetidine is a histamine H_2 receptor antagonist reducing histamine-related acid secretion by the parietal gland. Note: cimetidine inhibits the enzymes that convert codeine into morphine and may reduce its analgesic effect. (Diclofenac is also available in a combined formulation with the prostaglandin analogue misoprostol, which has gastroprotective activity.)
   m. Constipation is a feature of morphine therapy. Tolerance does not develop to opioid-induced constipation. Peristalsis is reduced, while the tone of the intestinal muscle is increased.
   n. Docusate sodium has some faecal-softening properties and is a stimulant of intestinal smooth muscle, which restores peristalsis.
   o. In practice, terminally ill people are often given danthron, in combination with either docusate sodium (co-danthrusate) or poloxamer (co-danthramer). Danthron is a stimulant drug and stool softener and is particularly useful when 'bowel movements must be by strain'. The irritant properties of danthron and its carcinogenic potential restrict its general use. The alternatives in use include senna preparations (stimulants) and magnesium sulphate (a bulk purgative). Most recently, the peripheral opioid receptor antagonist methylnaltrexone is available to treat constipation which has not fully responded to laxatives.
   p. Temazepam is a short-acting benzodiazepine used to aid sleeping.

   Note. Pain control must also take note of the psychological, social and spiritual condition of the patient. At all times, if pain control is inadequate, adjuvant treatments such as radiotherapy or transcutaneous electrical nerve stimulation should be considered. Where neuropathic pain is evident, tricyclic antidepressants or anticonvulsants should also be considered.

Opioids and related drugs

Drug	Half-life (h) and kinetics	Comments
Opioids used primarily for analgesia		
Alfentanil	1–2 [M] Oxidised in liver by CYP3A4, and conjugated with glucuronic acid	Used at surgery (Ch. 17); given by intravenous injection; respiratory depression may persist after the end of the procedure if repeated doses are given
Buprenorphine	1–7 [M] Bioavailability sublingual > oral; metabolised by CYP3A4 to an active metabolite and by conjugation	Has both agonist and antagonist properties and can precipitate withdrawal in individuals dependent on other opioids; action only partly reversed by naloxone; given sublingually, by slow intravenous or intramuscular injection, or as transdermal patches
Codeine	3–4 [M + R] Eliminated by metabolism by CYP3A4 and CYP2D6 and excreted unchanged (10%); demethylated to morphine (5–15%) by the polymorphic enzyme CYP2D6; variability in response linked to CYP2D6 polymorphism	Given orally for mild to moderate pain or by intramuscular injection
Diamorphine	2–5 min [Hydrolysis] Readily crosses the blood–brain barrier and is rapidly hydrolysed to morphine	Acetylated prodrug which is more lipid-soluble and more potent than morphine; given by intramuscular or subcutaneous injection
Dihydrocodeine	3–5 [M] Undergoes extensive first-pass metabolism; role of metabolites in activity is unknown	Similar potency to codeine; given orally or by intramuscular or subcutaneous injection
Dipipanone	3–4 [M] Clinical effects suggest good oral absorption but very few data are available	Given orally
Fentanyl	1–6 [M] Rapid initial uptake from the blood into lungs, followed by redistribution and elimination; metabolised in the liver largely by CYP3A4; not metabolised in the skin (transdermal)	Usually given by injection, or by transdermal or buccal routes; also used at surgery (Ch. 17); respiratory depression may persist after the end of the procedure if repeated doses are given
Hydromorphone	2–3 [M] Oral bioavailability of 60%; eliminated largely by conjugation with glucuronic acid and by reduction	A potent μ-receptor agonist with a duration of action of about 3–4 h; given orally
Meptazinol	1–3 [M + R] Rapid absorption but low oral bioavailability (5–20%); eliminated by conjugation with sulphate and glucuronic acid	Less potent than morphine with possibly a reduced risk of respiratory depression; given orally or by intramuscular or slow intravenous injection
Methadone	6–8 [M + R] Good oral bioavailability (40–100%); substrate for P-glycoprotein, which may inhibit its absorption across the gut wall; eliminated by hepatic oxidation by a number of CYP isoenzymes which may undergo autoinduction on repeated dosage	Potent μ-receptor agonist but less sedating than morphine; longer action with reduced excitation leads to its use in managing opioid withdrawal; given orally or by subcutaneous or intramuscular injection
Morphine	1–5 [M] Oral bioavailability is low (10–50%); eliminated by conjugation with glucuronic acid to morphine-3-glucuronide (inactive major metabolite) and morphine-6-glucuronide (active minor metabolite which crosses blood–brain barrier despite polarity)	Can be given orally, rectally as suppositories, or by subcutaneous, intramuscular or slow intravenous injection
Nalbuphine	2–4 (i.v.) 3–8 (oral) [M + R] Extensive first-pass metabolism (bioavailability 10–20%)	Similar potency and efficacy to morphine but with fewer unwanted effects and a lower abuse potential; given by subcutaneous, intramuscular or intravenous injection
Oxycodone	3–5 [M + R] Bioavailability is about 50–90%; eliminated mostly by hepatic metabolism	A potent μ-receptor agonist with similar efficacy and adverse effect profile to morphine; used largely in palliative care; given orally (normal or modified-release tablets) or by subcutaneous or slow intravenous injection

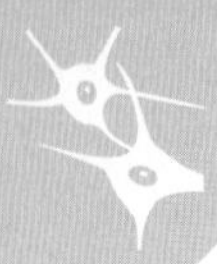

Opioids and related drugs

Drug	Half-life (h) and kinetics	Comments
Pentazocine	2–3 [M + R] Oral bioavailability is 11–32%; eliminated by hepatic oxidation and conjugation	Is a racemate and the L-isomer has both agonist and antagonist properties; it can precipitate withdrawal in people dependent on other opioids; given orally, rectally, or by subcutaneous or slow intravenous injection
Pethidine (meperidine)	3–8 [M + R] Oral bioavailability about 50%; metabolised by hydrolysis and demethylation to normeperidine (norpethidine), which is about 50% as potent as the parent compound but has a long half-life (15–30 h) and may accumulate on repeated dosage	Produces rapid but short-lasting analgesia; frequently used in labour; given orally or by subcutaneous or slow intravenous injection
Remifentanil	0.1 [M] Very rapid clearance by blood and tissue esterases (clearance is 3 L min^{-1}, which exceeds liver blood flow); metabolite inactive	Used at surgery (Ch. 17); given as an infusion
Tramadol	5–6 [M + R] Oral bioavailability about 60–70%; undergoes CYP2D6-mediated O-demethylation to a metabolite which is a more potent agonist at μ-receptors, also has a half-life of about 6 h and is responsible for most of the activity of the drug	Has a dual mechanism of action; a μ-opioid receptor agonist and a weak inhibitor of norepinephrine and serotonin reuptake; acts as an opioid agonist and also produces analgesia via enhancement of serotonergic and noradrenergic pathways, with the different optical isomers of tramadol showing a different spectrum of affinities; given orally or by intramuscular or intravenous injection
Opioid antagonists		
Methylnaltrexone	2–3 [R + M] Quarternary ammonium compound (N-methylnaltrexone), oral absorption 40–50%; does not cross the blood–brain barrier; undergoes limited demethylation; the majority is excreted unchanged in urine	Peripheral μ–opioid receptor antagonist; reduces opioid-induced constipation without affecting central actions including analgesia or inducing withdrawal symptoms; used in combination with laxatives in palliative care when laxatives alone have failed and also used to reduce postoperative paralytic ileus; unwanted effects include abdominal pain, flatulence nausea, dizziness; given by subcutaneous injection
Naloxone	1–1.5 [M] Half-life is shorter than that of morphine and repeated doses may be necessary; eliminated by conjugation with glucuronic acid	Opioid antagonist used to treat opioid overdose (Chs 53 and 54); administered by injection, giving a rapid onset of action (1–2 min)
Naltrexone	4 [M] Complete oral bioavailability; metabolised in the liver and possibly other tissues; an active metabolite has a half-life of 14 h; much longer absorption rate-limited half-lives (5–10 days) after intramuscular injection	Oral opioid receptor antagonist; longer duration of action than naloxone; oral, subcutaneous or intravenous administration
Opioids used primarily for non-analgesic effects		
Dextromethorphan	11 [M] Rapidly absorbed orally; metabolised primarily by the polymorphic enzyme CYP2D6	Methyl ether of the *d*-isomer of levorphanol (a codeine analogue); the antitussive action is the only opioid activity shown; antagonist to NMDA receptors; given orally
Diphenoxylate	2–3 [M] Oral bioavailability may be limited due to incomplete dissolution in gut; undergoes extensive hepatic metabolism to an active metabolite, diphenoxylic acid, which has a half-life of 3–14 h, and to inactive metabolites	Opioid agonist; used in acute diarrhoea (Ch. 35); may exert its effects locally on smooth muscle rather than via opioid receptors; given orally
Loperamide	11 [M + F] Oral bioavailability is 40%; undergoes hepatic metabolism mainly by CYP2C8 and CYP3A4; 30% excreted unchanged in faeces	Chemically related to the opioids but does not show any characteristics other than an anti-diarrhoeal action; tolerance does not develop; given orally
Related drugs or actions		
Lofexidine	? [M + F] Few data available; mainly metabolised, with 12% excreted unchanged in urine	α_2-Adrenoceptor antagonist; useful in opioid withdrawal; given orally

[F], faecal excretion; [M], metabolism; [R], renal excretion.

20 Anxiolytics, sedatives and hypnotics

There is considerable overlap in the pharmacology of drugs that have anxiolytic (anxiety-relieving) and hypnotic (sleep-inducing) properties. Compounds with sedative properties (moderating excitement and calming) at low doses often have hypnotic effects at higher doses. In addition, sedative drugs may have anxiolytic properties when used at doses that are too low to produce sedation. More recently, compounds such as buspirone have been developed that have anxiolytic properties but do not sedate.

ANXIETY DISORDERS

BIOLOGICAL BASIS OF ANXIETY DISORDERS

Anxiety disorders are among the most common psychiatric syndromes, and affect 15% of the general population at some time during their life. The clinical manifestations of anxiety are both psychological and physical. Anxiety is only pathological when it is inappropriate to the degree of stress to which the individual is exposed. A variety of anxiety disorders are recognised (Box 20.1). Of these, mixed anxiety and depressive disorder is the most common, followed by generalised anxiety disorder.

The symptoms vary among the anxiety disorders, but usually include apprehension, worry, fear and nervousness. Increased sympathetic nervous system activity frequently accompanies these feelings, causing sweating, tachycardia and epigastric discomfort. Sleep is often disturbed, with difficulty getting to sleep being a common feature. Many anxiety syndromes present early in life, and tend to become chronic if untreated. They are often associated with substance abuse.

Dysfunction of neurotransmission in the limbic region of the brain underlies the genesis of anxiety. The amygdala is a central part of the system that processes a fear stimulus and selects a response based on previous experience. Implementation of the response is through the locus ceruleus (autonomic and neuroendocrine responses) and nucleus paragigantocellularis (autonomic responses) in the brainstem, and the hypothalamus. There are many neurobiological theories that attempt to explain the origin of anxiety disorders. These try to integrate our understanding of the neurochemical disturbances with genetic predisposition and environmental triggers. It is now thought that generalised anxiety disorder and major depression may share a genetic basis, and that expression of the clinical syndrome is determined by environmental factors.

Excessive serotonergic (5-HT) and, to a lesser extent, noradrenergic excitatory neurotransmission in the limbic system has been implicated in many anxiety syndromes. In particular, overactivity at pre- and postsynaptic 5-hydroxytryptamine type 1A ($5HT_{1A}$) receptors, and postsynaptic $5HT_{2A}$ and $5HT_{1C}$ receptors may be important, associated with upregulation of presynaptic α_2-adrenoceptors. Deficient inhibition of limbic neurotransmission by gamma-aminobutyric acid (GABA) interneurons is found in many anxiety disorders, with subsensitivity of postsynaptic $GABA_A$ receptors. Excessive activity in excitatory glutamatergic neurons at NMDA (N-methyl-D-aspartate) receptors in the amygdala has also been implicated, and may be responsible for fear conditioning. Supersensitivity of receptors for peptide neurotransmitters such as cholecystokinin and neuropeptide Y may also occur. There is increasing evidence for the central role of brain-derived neurotrophic factor (BDNF) in modulating neural plasticity in anxiety states (see Fig. 22.2). BDNF is regulated by most of the neurotransmitters implicated in the genesis of anxiety states, and a decrease in BDNF correlates with anxiety and memory deficits.

In some anxiety syndromes, there is excess secretion of corticotrophin-releasing factor (CRF), but a low plasma cortisol concentration and upregulation of corticosteroid receptors. CRF is a neurotransmitter in the limbic system, and upregulation may occur from early adverse experiences, leading to conditioning of those with a genetic predisposition to anxiety disorder in later life.

DRUG THERAPY FOR ANXIETY

Drugs used to treat anxiety are called anxiolytics.

Benzodiazepines

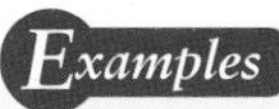

chlordiazepoxide, diazepam, lorazepam, midazolam, temazepam

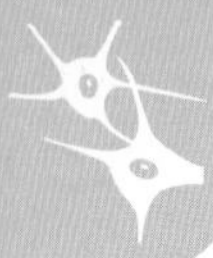

In addition to their anxiolytic effect, benzodiazepines have several other properties that are clinically useful. This section also considers drugs that are not used primarily for treatment of anxiety.

Mechanism of action and effects

Benzodiazepines act by potentiating the actions of GABA, the primary inhibitory neurotransmitter in the central nervous system (CNS). They act at a regulatory site closely linked to the $GABA_A$ receptor which mediates fast inhibitory synaptic neurotransmission (Fig. 20.1). The $GABA_A$ receptor is also the binding site for some volatile anaesthetics and alcohol, propofol, etomidate and barbiturates. Binding of a benzodiazepine to subunits of the receptor induces a conformational change in the GABA receptor that enhances its affinity for the neurotransmitter (Fig. 20.1). GABA increases the influx of Cl^- into the neuron, hyperpolarises the cell membrane and decreases cell excitability. Benzodiazepines act only in the presence of GABA to enhance GABA-mediated opening of the ion channel; they have no direct action on the channel (Fig. 20.1). The $GABA_A$ receptor has thus far been shown to be composed of different combinations of 5 subunits from the 19 subunits that have been identified (Fig. 20.1 and legend). The presence of an α_1-subunit is responsible for the sedative, amnesic and anticonvulsant properties of benzodiazepines, while both α_2 and α_3 appear to be involved in the anxiolytic and muscle relaxant effects. The many receptor configurations also show differences in their regional distributions in the brain. Benzodiazepines are relatively non-selective in their binding to the different configurations but some non-benzodiazepines do show a degree of selectivity (Fig. 20.1). The increase in inhibitory neurotransmission produced by benzodiazepines has the following potentially useful effects:

- sedation from reduced sensory input to the reticular activating system
- sleep induction at high drug concentrations
- anterograde amnesia
- anxiolysis from actions on the limbic system and hypothalamus
- anticonvulsant activity (Ch. 23)
- reduction of muscle tone (Ch. 24).

Box 20.1 Simplified classification of anxiety disorders

Phobic anxiety disorder
Other anxiety disorder (including panic disorder and mixed anxiety and depressive disorder)
Obsessive compulsive disorder
Reaction to severe stress (including post-traumatic stress disorder)
Conversion disorders
Somatoform disorders
Other neurotic disorders (including neurasthenia)

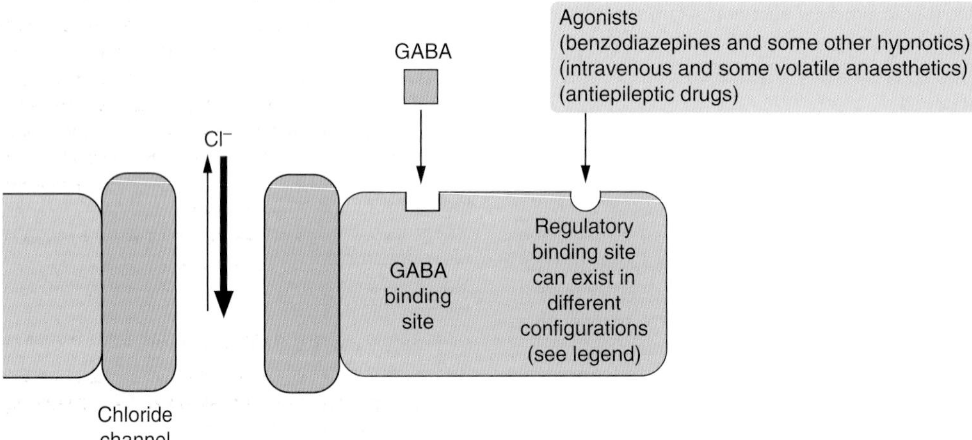

Fig. 20.1 **The $GABA_A$ (benzodiazepine) receptor.** The $GABA_A$ receptor has a GABA binding site and an allosteric regulatory binding site; the receptor can exist in many possible configurations. Binding of GABA to its receptor mediates opening of the Cl^- channel; this action is enhanced by drugs stimulating the regulatory allosteric binding site on the GABA receptor, which is distinct from the GABA binding site. Influx of Cl^- ions hyperpolarises the cell. The GABA receptor consists of five transmembrane subunits configured from the 19 possible subunits that have been identified; thus, a multitude of configurations in the GABA receptor could possibly exist. These subunits are known as α_{1-6}, β_{1-4}, γ_{1-3}, δ, ε, π and ρ_{1-3}. The most abundant configurations contain either $\alpha_1\beta_2\gamma_2$- or $\alpha_2\beta_3\gamma_2$-subunits plus two other subunits. The α_1-subtype-containing configurations are preferentially found in the cortex and thalamus, and α_2-subtypes in the hippocampus, amygdala and striatum. The presence of certain subunits in the receptor confers particular properties. For example, receptors with α_1-subunits have greater sedative, amnesic and anticonvulsant properties, while those with α_2-subunits have greater anxiolytic and muscle relaxant properties. Diazepam and lorazepam and other 'classic' benzodiazepines are non-selective and act on all subunit configurations so far identified; their biological action also requires that a γ_2-subunit is present. Compounds such as zolpidem have a higher affinity for α_1-subunits. The intravenous anaesthetics propofol and etomidate bind to β_2- and β_3-subunits.

Pharmacokinetics

Benzodiazepines are well absorbed from the gut, and their lipid solubility ensures ready penetration into the brain. Many, including diazepam, are subsequently metabolised in the liver to active compounds (see Fig. 2.12) that contribute to a prolonged duration of action through relatively slow elimination from the body. Metabolism of some benzodiazepines, for example temazepam (used as a hypnotic – see below), produces inactive derivatives. The pharmacokinetics of individual benzodiazepines determines their major clinical uses.

Benzodiazepines that are useful for inducing sleep (e.g. temazepam) are rapidly absorbed from the gut. This produces a fast onset of sedation, then sleep. A brief duration of action is desirable, to avoid hangover sedation in the morning; this is more likely if the drug is inactivated by its metabolism in the liver (e.g. temazepam). Repeated dosing, particularly with long-acting compounds such as diazepam, increases the risk of accumulation, producing a prolonged sedative effect.

The anxiolytic properties of benzodiazepines are best exploited by using a compound with a long duration of action. Smaller doses can then be used, to minimise sedation, and the rebound in anxiety symptoms that can occur between doses of a short-acting drug is avoided.

Diazepam, lorazepam and midazolam can also be given by intravenous injection to provide rapid sedation preoperatively or before procedures such as endoscopy. Intravenous lorazepam and diazepam can be useful for treatment of status epilepticus (Ch. 23). Long-acting benzodiazepines, such as clobazam, clonazepam, diazepam and lorazepam, are used in the treatment of epilepsy (see Ch. 23).

Unwanted effects

- Drowsiness, which may cause problems with driving or operating machinery.
- Lightheadedness.
- Confusion, especially in the elderly.
- Paradoxical increase in aggression.
- Impaired memory.
- Ataxia.
- Muscle weakness.
- Potentiation of the sedative effects of other CNS depressant drugs such as alcohol. In overdose, such combinations can lead to severe respiratory depression. Flumazenil is a competitive antagonist of benzodiazepines and can be used in acute overdose to reverse respiratory depression (Ch. 53).
- Tolerance and dependence:
  - **Tolerance** to the therapeutic effects of benzodiazepines is common. Hypnotic effects are lost quite early, and the rebound insomnia on withdrawal can perpetuate benzodiazepine use.
  - **Dependence** with physical and psychological withdrawal symptoms occurs during long-term treatment. The risk is highest in people with personality disorders, or a previous history of dependence on alcohol or drugs, and is more likely to occur if high doses of benzodiazepines are used. Restricting their use to a maximum of 4 weeks will minimise the risk of dependence. With long-acting drugs, withdrawal symptoms may be delayed by up to 3 weeks. Anxiety is the most frequent symptom, while insomnia, depression, and abnormalities of perception, such as altered sensitivity to noise, light or touch, also occur. More severe reactions such as psychosis or convulsions arise occasionally. Some withdrawal symptoms may resemble those for which the drug was originally prescribed, encouraging continued use. Gradual withdrawal of a benzodiazepine over 4–8 weeks is desirable after long-term use, although complete withdrawal may take up to a year. Lorazepam is a potent benzodiazepine with a relatively short duration of action that proves particularly difficult to stop because of the intensity of withdrawal symptoms that begin a few hours after cessation of treatment. Substitution with the longer-acting drug diazepam may be helpful before withdrawal is attempted. There are no proven treatments for reducing symptoms associated with withdrawal. Beta-adrenoceptor antagonists (Ch. 5) are sometimes helpful, or an antidepressant (Ch. 22) if there are depressive symptoms or panic attacks.

Azapirones

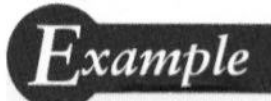

buspirone

Mechanism of action and effects

Buspirone is a partial agonist at presynaptic $5HT_{1A}$ receptors, producing negative feedback to inhibit serotonin release. It has no effect on GABA receptors. Initial exacerbation of anxiety may occur, possibly caused by postsynaptic $5HT_{1A}$ receptor stimulation. The onset of the anxiolytic action of buspirone is slow, reaching a maximum effect at approximately 4 weeks, so the mechanism of action may involve gradual changes in neural plasticity (enhancement of neural performance or changes in neural connections; Ch. 22). It has no sedative action, and is ineffective for panic attacks.

Pharmacokinetics

Buspirone is well absorbed from the gut and undergoes extensive first-pass metabolism in the liver. The half-life is short (2–4 h).

Unwanted effects

- Nausea
- Dizziness, lightheadedness and headache
- Nervousness.

Neither tolerance nor dependence has been reported.

MANAGEMENT OF ANXIETY

Symptoms of anxiety, if mild, may respond to counselling and psychotherapy, such as relaxation training. For more severe or persistent symptoms, benzodiazepines are the most effective drugs, with a rapid onset of action over 15–60 min. Problems of dependence should limit their use

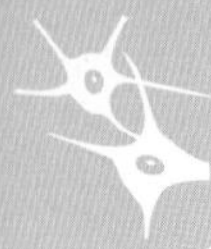

to a maximum of 4 weeks, and the dose should be gradually reduced after the first 2 weeks. Buspirone has similar efficacy to benzodiazepines, but the slow onset of action (3 days) makes it less versatile for managing short-term anxiety. In addition, anxiety that responds well to benzodiazepines often responds less well to buspirone, possibly due to a relative lack of effect on somatic symptoms. Somatic symptoms of anxiety (e.g. tremor, palpitations) are often helped by a β-adrenoceptor antagonist (Ch. 5).

Generalised anxiety disorder often requires long-term treatment, and there is now considerable evidence that antidepressants (Ch. 22) are useful in this situation. Tricyclic antidepressants and selective serotonin reuptake inhibitors (SSRIs) appear to be equally effective. Antidepressants can initially exacerbate anxiety, and a benzodiazepine may be necessary for the first 2–3 weeks of treatment to prevent this. The optimal duration of antidepressant treatment in this situation is uncertain, but similar treatment periods as for depression (Ch. 22) are usually recommended.

Social anxiety disorder responds to monoamine oxidase inhibitors (MAOIs; Ch. 22) better than to most other agents. Moclobemide is the treatment of choice, but phenelzine is also used. Phobic disorders usually need a different approach, and cognitive behavioural therapy is often most effective. Panic disorder is usually treated with tricyclic antidepressants or SSRIs; MAOIs are used for people who do not respond.

INSOMNIA

Defining insomnia is complicated by the considerable variability in the normal pattern of sleep. Most healthy adults sleep between 7 and 9 hours per night, but much shorter or even longer periods can be normal. Insomnia is considered to be present if there is ‘inability to initiate or maintain sleep’. There are three major categories of insomnia (Table 20.1). Symptoms include sleep-onset insomnia (difficulty falling asleep, more common in younger people), frequent nocturnal awakening (difficulty maintaining sleep, more common in older people), early morning awakening (with difficulty getting back to sleep) and difficulty functioning in the daytime due to perceived poor sleep.

The reticular formation in the midbrain, medulla and pons is responsible for maintaining wakefulness. Activity in the reticular formation is dependent on sensory input via collateral connections from the main sensory pathways. Neurotransmitter systems involved in the regulation of sleep are complex. Cortical arousal is regulated by noradrenergic pathways from the locus ceruleus, cholinergic ascending tracts from brainstem nuclei, histaminergic neurons from the tuberomammillary nucleus, and serotonergic neurons from the raphe nuclei. Orexins (hypocretins) are important neuropeptide transmitters found in the lateral hypothalamus which, through connections with other hypothalamic and brainstem nuclei, promote wakefulness (see also narcolepsy Ch. 22). Sleep is induced by GABA and galanin (a predominantly inhibitory neuropeptide) neurotransmission from the anterior hypothalamus, which inhibits these arousal neurons.

Table 20.1 Types of insomnia

Type of insomnia	Duration	Likely causes
Transient	2–3 days	Acute situational or environmental stress (e.g. jet lag, shift work)
Short-term	<3 weeks	Ongoing personal stress
Long-term	>3 weeks	Psychiatric illness, behavioural reasons, medical reasons

SLEEP PATTERNS

The two main types of sleep pattern are non-rapid eye movement (non-REM) sleep and rapid eye movement (REM) sleep. These sleep patterns occur in cycles (Fig. 20.2), with non-REM sleep varying between light sleep (stages 1 and 2) and slow-wave sleep (stages 3 and 4). Two-thirds of sleep is usually spent in stages 2–4, characterised by continuous or intermittent delta waves (slow waves) on the electroencephalogram. These deeper stages of sleep are the recuperative phase, while most dreaming occurs during the REM-sleep periods. Increasing age is associated with more nocturnal awakening and longer periods of REM sleep.

DRUGS FOR TREATING INSOMNIA (HYPNOTICS)

Benzodiazepines

Benzodiazepines have dose-related hypnotic effects. See above for details.

Non-benzodiazepine drugs that modulate the $GABA_A$/chloride channel

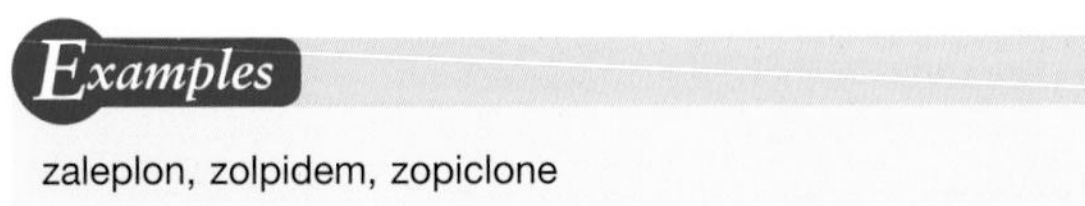

zaleplon, zolpidem, zopiclone

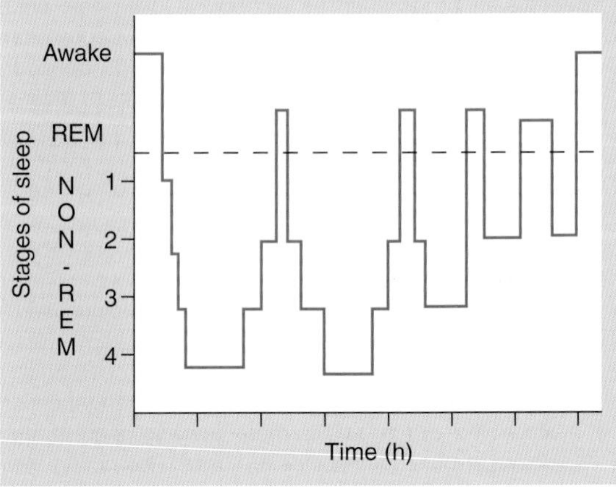

Fig. 20.2 **Typical sleep pattern in a young adult.** REM, rapid eye movement.

Mechanism of action and effects

Zaleplon, zolpidem and zopiclone (the 'Z' drugs) belong to different chemical classes but interact in a similar manner with the postsynaptic $GABA_A$ receptor on neuronal membranes. They bind to regulatory binding sites on the receptor that are close to, but distinct from, the benzodiazepine binding site (Fig. 20.1) Like the benzodiazepines, they increase GABA-mediated Cl^- influx into the cell, which inhibits neurotransmission. Zolpidem and zaleplon are selective for the α_1-subunit on the GABA receptor. Zopiclone also acts on the α_2-subunit of the GABA receptor. Although zopiclone also possesses anxiolytic and anticonvulsant activity, its short duration of action makes it unsuitable for these indications.

Pharmacokinetics

The 'Z' drugs are rapidly absorbed from the gut and have short half-lives (1–6 h), which makes them well suited to their use as hypnotics. Metabolism in the liver is responsible for elimination.

Unwanted effects

- Bitter metallic taste (zopiclone)
- Gastrointestinal disturbances, including nausea and vomiting
- Incoordination
- Drowsiness, dizziness, headache and fatigue
- Depression, confusion, amnesia
- There is only anecdotal evidence for tolerance, but dependence with withdrawal symptoms has been reported.

Clomethiazole

Mechanism of action, effects and clinical uses

It probably enhances GABA receptor activity by interaction with a site similar to that of the barbiturates (Fig. 20.1 and Ch. 23). Clomethiazole has sedative, hypnotic and anticonvulsant properties, but is now rarely used as a hypnotic. Clinical uses are limited, but it is sometimes used in the management of alcohol withdrawal (Ch. 54).

Pharmacokinetics

Clomethiazole is readily absorbed from the gut but undergoes extensive first-pass metabolism in the liver. The half-life is 4–6 h.

Unwanted effects

- Nasal congestion and conjunctival irritation early in use
- Headache
- Hangover effects
- Respiratory depression in overdose, especially if taken with alcohol
- Dependence is common, which restricts the drug's usefulness. To minimise the risk of dependence, clomethiazole should not be given for more than 9 days.

Chloral derivatives

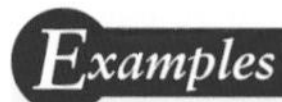

chloral hydrate, triclofos sodium

Mechanism of action and effects

The alcohol metabolite trichloroethanol is mainly responsible for the hypnotic effects of chloral derivatives. It may act in part by modulating GABAergic inhibitory neurotransmission, although it has effects on several other receptors and ligand-activated ion channels. Chloral derivatives have a narrow therapeutic index and therefore are not ideal hypnotic drugs. They are considered less suitable than other hypnotics and are only recommended for short-term use.

Pharmacokinetics

Chloral hydrate is a prodrug that is well absorbed from the gut, then rapidly metabolised to trichloroethanol by alcohol dehydrogenase. The drug competes with ethanol for metabolism. Trichloroethanol has a half-life of 8–12 h.

Unwanted effects

- Unpleasant taste and gastric irritation
- Ataxia and nightmares
- Hangover effects
- Tolerance and dependence are frequent, as with benzodiazepines
- Respiratory and myocardial depression can occur in overdose.

MANAGEMENT OF INSOMNIA

Drugs play only a small part in the treatment of insomnia. Explanation of the normal variations in sleep patterns and avoidance of diuretics or of drinks containing caffeine or alcohol in the hours before retiring can help. Eliminating excessive noise or heat in the bedroom, encouraging regular exercise in the day and minimising daytime napping may also be useful.

Hypnotic drugs are reserved for times when abnormal sleep markedly affects quality of life. The ideal hypnotic would induce good-quality prolonged sleep without disturbance of the normal sleep pattern. It should have a rapid onset of action, with no 'hangover' sedation in the morning, and should not produce tolerance or dependence. Few drugs come close to this ideal profile. Benzodiazepines reduce sleep latency (the time between settling down and falling asleep) and prolong sleep duration. However, they reduce the time spent in REM sleep, with more time spent in stage 2 sleep. Short-acting benzodiazepines may permit wakefulness early in the morning but longer-acting drugs carry the risk of hangover effects the following day. The 'Z' drugs produce less disturbance of sleep 'architecture', having less effect on the amount of REM sleep while increasing the duration of deeper (slow-wave) sleep.

Hypnotic drugs should be used only for short periods and intermittently if possible; tolerance to hypnotics frequently occurs after 2 weeks. If a benzodiazepine is used continuously for 4–6 weeks, rebound insomnia, caused by

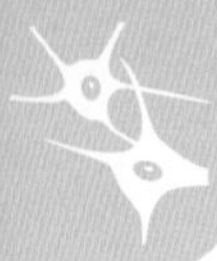

mild dependence, is common when the drug is stopped. Nevertheless, benzodiazepines are still widely used since they are safe in overdose. The 'Z' drugs carry a similar risk of dependence.

Of the other hypnotics, chloral derivatives and clomethiazole should usually be avoided. Other compounds with sedative actions as a part of their therapeutic profile can be useful to aid sleep. For example, a sedative antihistamine such as promazine (Ch. 39) can be helpful for children suffering from somnambulism (sleep walking) or night terrors. Sedative tricyclic antidepressants (Ch. 22), such as amitriptyline, should be considered if there is an underlying depressive illness. If less sedative antidepressants are used, short-term concurrent use of a benzodiazepine may be necessary while awaiting the onset of the antidepressant effect.

FURTHER READING

Abramowitz JS, Taylor S, McKay D (2009) Obsessive compulsive disorder. *Lancet* 374, 491–499

Aranda M, Hanson CW (2000) Anesthetics, sedatives and paralytics. Understanding their use in the intensive care unit. *Surg Clin North Am* 80, 933–947

Doble A (1999) New insights into the mechanism of action of hypnotics. *J Psychopharmacol* 13, S11–S20

Ebert B, Wafford KA, Deacon S (2006) Treating insomnia: current and investigational pharmacological approaches. *Pharmacol Ther* 112, 612–629

Fricehione G (2004) Generalized anxiety disorder. *N Engl J Med* 351, 675–682

Gale C, Davidson O (2007) Generalized anxiety disorder. *BMJ* 334, 579–581

Gottesmann C (2002) GABA mechanisms and sleep. *Neuroscience* 111, 231–239

Lader MH (1999) Limitations on the use of benzodiazepines in anxiety and insomnia: are they justified? *Eur Neuropsychopharmacol* 9(suppl 6), S399–S405

Lerch C, Park GR (1999) Sedation and analgesia. *Br Med Bull* 55, 76–95

Longo LP, Johnson B (2000) Addiction: Part I. Benzodiazepines – side effects, abuse risk and alternatives. *Am Fam Physician* 61, 2121–2128

Lydiard RB (2003) The role of GABA in anxiety. *J Clin Psychiatry* 64(suppl 3), 21–27

Michels G, Moss SJ (2007) $GABA_A$ receptors: properties and trafficking. *Crit Rev Biochem Mol Biol* 42, 3–14

Mohler H, Fritschy JM, Rudolph U (2002) A new benzodiazepine pharmacology. *J Pharmacol Exp Ther* 300, 2–8

Roy-Byrne PP, Craske MG, Stein MB (2006) Panic disorder. *Lancet* 368, 1023–1032

Schenk CH, Mahowald MW, Sack RL (2003) Assessment and management of insomnia. *JAMA* 289, 2475–2479

Schneier FR (2006) Social anxiety disorder. *N Engl J Med* 355, 1029–1036

Szabadi E (2006) Drugs for sleep disorders: mechanisms and therapeutic prospects. *Br J Clin Pharmacol* 61, 761–766

Tyrer P, Baldwin D (2006) Generalised anxiety disorder. *Lancet* 368, 2156–2166

Whiting PJ (2003) GABA receptor subtypes in the brain: a paradigm for CNS drug discovery. *Drug Discovery Today* 8, 445–450

Young C, Knudsen N, Hilton A, Reves JG (2000) Sedation in the intensive care unit. *Crit Care Med* 28, 853–866

SELF-ASSESSMENT

In questions 1–3, the first statement, in italics, is true. Are the accompanying statements also true?

1. *Benzodiazepines with a medium to long duration of action are useful for treating anxiety states.*
   a. Long-term use of benzodiazepines is recommended in anxiety states.
   b. Potentiation of CNS effects of benzodiazepines occurs with concurrent alcohol administration.
2. *CNS depressant effects of benzodiazepines can be reversed with the antagonist flumazenil.*
   a. Lower doses of benzodiazepines should be used in the elderly.
   b. Buspirone is more sedative than temazepam.
3. *Benzodiazepines used to treat anxiety should be administered for as short a time as possible and in the lowest dose possible.* Benzodiazepines have no effect on sleep patterns as measured by the duration of REM sleep.
4. You are considering options for the treatment of a patient with insomnia and anxiety who has been taking diazepam for several months without clear benefit. Choose the one **most appropriate** statement from the following.
   A. If there is no response to one hypnotic, it is advisable to switch to another.
   B. Withdrawal symptoms abate within 3 weeks of abruptly stopping diazepam.
   C. Barbiturates are the drugs of choice in patients with insomnia and anxiety.
   D. Buspirone decreases anxiety by acting at the GABA receptor site.
   E. Benzodiazepines act to potentiate the inhibitory actions of GABA at its receptor.
5. Case history questions

Mrs FL was a 46-year-old mother of three who was finding it very hard to cope following the sudden death of her husband 3 months previously. She had returned to work but did not sleep properly, experienced occasional periods of anxiety during the day, and felt that she was at risk of losing her job because tiredness and anxiety about her financial difficulties prevented her concentrating on her work.

   a. What drug might you prescribe to help Mrs FL's insomnia? What factors may determine your choice of this drug?
   b. How does your chosen drug work to reduce insomnia and anxiety? What potential unwanted effects

and drug interactions should you warn Mrs FL about?

c. Mrs FL returned 2 weeks later, saying that she regularly woke at 4 a.m. and could not get back to sleep. Consider the 'pros' and 'cons' of changing her to a longer-acting drug or to another 'newer' hypnotic.
d. What are the problems associated with long-term use of benzodiazepines? What other options should be considered to help to manage Mrs FL's problems in the long-term?

6. Extended-matching questions
Choose the **most appropriate** statement A–E for the next course of action in the case scenarios described in 6.1 and 6.2. These are not 'complete' case studies. Only the pharmacological aspects of cases are dealt with; the equally important roles of psychological and psychiatric help must always be considered.
   A. Gradual tapering of the medication over many months.
   B. Gradual tapering of the medication over several days.
   C. Prescribe another course of the same benzodiazepine.
   D. Consider giving paroxetine.
   6.1. A 54-year-old woman had a history of anxiety. Seven years earlier, she had received a prescription of lorazepam, the first of a series of prescriptions. For the last 3 years, her doctor had been refilling prescription requests without reassessing the clinical need. There is no indication of depressive illness. The woman now wishes to stop her medication.
   6.2. You have been treating a woman aged 25 for a year. She has been having up to 10 intense panic attacks a month. At any time of day, she suddenly developed a peculiar and very strong feeling of being lightheaded, jumpy and being smothered. Her heart rate increased dramatically. It came on so quickly and was so severe that she felt she might be dying. Then she felt very shaky, sweaty, and unsteady. This whole experience reached peak intensity within 2 min but she was often unable to continue work and needed to go home. She had been treated with intermittent courses of diazepam for a year without improvement.

ANSWERS

1. a. **False**. Dependence, tolerance and withdrawal symptoms occur with long-term continuous usage.
   b. **True**. Additional CNS depression can occur.
2. a. **True**. Benzodiazepines are metabolised largely by the liver and rate of metabolism is reduced in the elderly; the elderly are also more sensitive to the effects of the drugs.
   b. **False**. Buspirone is not a benzodiazepine and has less sedative action than temazepam.
3. **False**. Benzodiazepines affect the structure of sleep, with loss of REM sleep. Zolpidem has less effect on sleep architecture than benzodiazepines.
4. Answer **E**.
   A. An alternative hypnotic is unlikely to work and switching between hypnotics is not good practice.
   B. With long-acting benzodiazepines, withdrawal symptoms may take more than 3 weeks to appear.
   C. Barbiturates are contraindicated as hypnotics because of unwanted effects, tolerance and dependence liability.
   D. Buspirone acts at the $5HT_{1A}$ receptor. It is used in general anxiety disorders and is not sedative.
   E. Benzodiazepines potentiate the entry of Cl^- through the receptor-operated channel which is part of the $GABA_A$ receptor.
5. Case history answers
   a. Mrs FL's insomnia and anxiety are a response to bereavement and might present fewer long-term problems than chronic 'endogenous' anxiety. Benzodiazepines and the newer hypnotics are barbiturates. Nevertheless, the central concept in benzodiazepine therapy is to use the minimal effective dose for the shortest possible period. A short-acting benzodiazepine (e.g. temazepam) taken at night should help to restore her sleep pattern and may improve her daytime tiredness. The relatively short half-life of temazepam (5–12 h) should minimise risk of sedation during the working day. However, if the daytime anxiety also warrants treatment, a long-acting benzodiazepine (e.g. diazepam) given at night may be the drug to choose. The anxiolytic buspirone is not sedative, but it is ineffective against panic attacks. Only short or intermittent courses of treatment should be given.
   b. Benzodiazepines are $GABA_A$ agonists that enhance $GABA_A$-mediated inhibition of neuronal activity in the brain and spinal cord. Benzodiazepines bind to $GABA_A$ receptors at a site separate from GABA itself and increase the frequency of GABA-induced channel opening, enhancing Cl^- entry into the cell and neuronal hyperpolarisation. Benzodiazepines are relatively free of serious unwanted effects if used correctly and are safe in overdose, but sedation and psychomotor impairment may interfere markedly with driving and operating machinery (worsened by interaction with alcohol, barbiturates, and older sedative antihistamines). Other unwanted effects include headache, dry mouth, hypotension, anterograde amnesia, skin rashes and blood dyscrasias. Psychotic reactions (hallucinations) have been reported with triazolam.
   c. Rebound wakefulness may indicate a need for a longer-acting benzodiazepine such as nitrazepam or diazepam, which may also help to reduce Mrs FL's daytime anxiety and panic attacks. Conversely, daytime sedation may interfere with driving and work, exacerbated by long-acting metabolites of these drugs. An alternative may be to prescribe buspirone; however, this requires 1–2 weeks for a response. Switching to a newer hypnotic such as zolpidem is unlikely to make a difference.
   d. Long-term use of a benzodiazepine is associated with dependence, manifested mainly as a

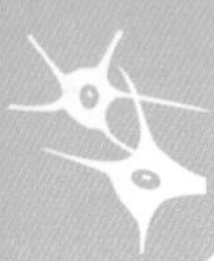

withdrawal reaction, which may include rebound anxiety, tremor, nausea, irritability, anorexia and dysphoria. Together with rapid development of tolerance (especially to hypnotic action), these contraindicate benzodiazepine treatment for more than 3 weeks. In the longer term, a course of antidepressants may be indicated. Mrs FL's recovery from bereavement may be aided by psychological counselling and support from family and employer.

6. Extended-matching answers
   6.1. Answer **A**. Withdrawal from long courses of benzodiazepines is difficult. She is liable to show withdrawal symptoms or return of the original complaints that determined the original prescription. Psychological and other forms of counselling may be advisable. Withdrawal should include gradual dosage reduction and anxiety management. Long-term psychological support is equally important for successful outcome, particularly for reducing the incidence and severity of post-withdrawal syndromes.
   6.2. Answer **D**. Continuing with a benzodiazepine is unlikely to improve matters after a year of treatment. The use of anxiolytics may be masking depression. An option might be to assess for depression and to use an SSRI such as paroxetine. Some of the SSRIs are licensed for the treatment of anxiety and panic disorders. General assessment is also recommended, to rule out other disorders, and non-pharmacological treatments should be considered.

Anxiolytics, sedatives and hypnotics

Drug	Half-life (h) and kinetics	Comments
Anxiolytics		
Short-term use; given orally unless other otherwise indicated		
Alprazolam	6–16 [M] Almost complete oral bioavailability; eliminated largely by oxidation by CYP3A4 to inactive metabolites which are conjugated with glucuronic acid	
Buspirone	2–4 [M] Rapid absorption but extensive first-pass metabolism, so that the bioavailability is only about 4%, but increased if taken with food; metabolised by CYP3A4-mediated oxidative dealkylation and hydroxylation	
Chlordiazepoxide	5–30 [M] Complete oral bioavailability; slowly eliminated by hepatic metabolism; a number of the metabolites retain activity, have very long half-lives (15–100 h) and contribute significantly to the effect	Also used as an adjunct in alcohol withdrawal
Diazepam	20–100 [M] Complete oral bioavailability; metabolised to N-desmethyl metabolite, which has a longer half-life (30–200 h), and to temazepam; N-desmethyldiazepam is oxidised to oxazepam	May be given orally, rectally or by intramuscular or slow intravenous injection; also used for insomnia, status epilepticus and muscle spasm and in surgical premedication
Lorazepam	4–25 [M] High bioavailability; eliminated mainly as the glucuronic acid conjugate	May be given orally or by intramuscular or slow intravenous dosage; also used for insomnia and in surgical premedication
Meprobamate	8–11 [M + R] Good oral absorption; eliminated by hepatic metabolism to inactive metabolites and some renal excretion of the parent drug	Not recommended because of potential toxicity and dependence
Oxazepam	4–25 [M] High bioavailability; eliminated mainly as the glucuronic acid conjugate	
Sedative and hypnotics		
All given orally and recommended for short-term use only (unless otherwise indicated)		
Chloral hydrate	0.1 [M] Extensive first-pass metabolism; rapidly reduced to trichloroethanol (TCE) (half-life 8–12 h) and oxidised to trichloroacetic acid (half-life 60–70 h), the hypnotic effect is believed to be caused by TCE	

Anxiolytics, sedatives and hypnotics

Drug	Half-life (h) and kinetics	Comments
Clomethiazole	4–6 [M] Rapid absorption but extensive (40–95%) first-pass metabolism; metabolised by dechlorination and oxidation	Used only for severe insomnia in the elderly (with little hangover) and for alcohol withdrawal
Flurazepam	2–3 [M] Good oral absorption; oxidised in the liver to active metabolites which have half-lives of 30–100 and 2–4 h	
Loprazolam	7 [M + B] Good oral absorption; metabolised by formation of a more polar N-oxide; metabolite and parent drug are eliminated in bile	
Lormetazepam	8–10 [M] Unlike many benzodiazepines, it is not extensively oxidised but is eliminated as the glucuronic acid conjugate of the parent drug; limited oxidation (about 10%) to lorazepam (the N-desmethyl analogue)	
Midazolam	1–5 [M] Eliminated by hydroxylation in the liver	Used primarily in surgical premedication; given by slow intravenous or intramuscular injection
Nitrazepam	20–48 [M] Rapid absorption but variable bioavailability (50–90%); metabolism is mainly by nitro-reduction, followed by N-acetylation of the resultant amino group; only the parent drug is active	
Promethazine	7–4 [M] Incomplete oral bioavailability (about 20%); metabolised by S-oxidation and N-dealkylation in the liver; the S-oxide (which is the main metabolite) is inactive	Sedative and hypnotic antihistamine that has a prolonged effect
Temazepam	5–12 [M] High oral bioavailability; oxidised by N-demethylation to oxazepam and by conjugation with glucuronic acid; most activity is probably due to the parent compound	Also used in surgical premedication
Triclofos	? [M] Phosphate ester of trichloroethanol that is hydrolysed in vivo; causes fewer gastrointestinal effects than chloral hydrate	Similar to chloral hydrate (see above); few published data available
Zaleplon	1 [M] Rapid absorption with a bioavailability of 30%; metabolised by aldehyde oxidase and CYP3A4 to inactive products	Binds to α_1-subunit of the benzodiazepine receptor; may be used for up to 2 weeks
Zolpidem	2–4 [M] Good oral bioavailability (about 70%); metabolised largely by CYP3A4 to inactive metabolites	Binds to α_1-subunit of the benzodiazepine receptor; may be used for up to 4 weeks
Zopiclone	4–6 [M] Rapid absorption and a high bioavailability (about 80%); metabolised by N-dealkylation, N-oxidation and decarboxylation; the metabolites and about 5% of unchanged parent drug are eliminated in the urine	Hypnotic but also binds to α_2-subunit of the benzodiazepine receptor; may be used for up to 4 weeks
Drugs that reverse sedative effects of benzodiazepines		
Flumazenil	1 [M] Eliminated by hepatic metabolism; half-life 2–3 h in patients with severe hepatic dysfunction	Blocks the benzodiazepine binding site; given by intravenous injection or infusion

[B], biliary excretion; [M], metabolism; [R], renal excretion.

21

The major psychotic disorders: schizophrenia and mania

PSYCHOTIC DISORDERS

The term psychosis indicates that the person affected has lost contact with reality. This is usually experienced as hallucination, delusion or a disruption in thought processes. The two most profound functional psychotic conditions are schizophrenia and mania. These disorders probably represent extremes of a continuum that embraces the so-called schizoaffective disorders (Box 21.1). Organic disease caused by metabolic disturbance, toxic substances or psychoactive drugs can also cause psychosis.

SCHIZOPHRENIA

Schizophrenia is more common in males and usually presents relatively early in life. The onset is usually gradual but can be abrupt. Once established, it can have a relapsing or persistent course. Clinical features are categorised as positive or negative (Table 21.1), although none are pathognomonic of the disorder. The positive features are disordered versions of thinking, perception, formation of ideas, or sense of self. They include hallucinations (false sensory perceptions) and delusions (false beliefs held with absolute certainty and unexplained by the person's socioeconomic background). The negative features are often the most debilitating in the long term.

Biological basis of schizophrenia

There is a strong genetic component to schizophrenia and probably several risk genes; environmental influences probably only affect those with a genetic predisposition. Many neurobiological abnormalities have been described in schizophrenia, including disturbances in neuronal numbers and synaptic connections in the cortical, thalamic and hippocampal areas. These disturbances become more marked as the illness progresses.

Glutamate/dopamine interactions and their possible involvement in schizophrenia

The limbic region and prefrontal cortex are involved in cognition, emotional memory and the initiation of behaviour. Schizophrenia is believed to involve interconnected abnormalities of glutamate and dopamine transmission in these regions of the brain. Whether decreased glutamate or increased dopamine is the primary abnormality is uncertain. The current view is that there is *hypoactivity* in glutamate NMDA (N-methyl-D-aspartate) receptor neurotransmission, which leads to defective modulation of dopaminergic activity in subcortical cell bodies, resulting in *hyperactivity* of the dopaminergic neurons in mesolimbic areas.

The dopaminergic systems in the central nervous system (CNS) arise from the substantia nigra (among the basal ganglia) and ventral tegmental area in the midbrain. One major dopaminergic pathway has its origin in the substantia nigra and projects to gamma-aminobutyric acid (GABA)-ergic inhibitory interneurons in the corpus striatum and globus pallidus through the nigrostriatal pathways (Ch. 24). This pathway modulates motor and behavioural function via ongoing projections to the thalamus and cortex; the striatum receives both positive and negative glutamatergic inputs from the cortex. Other major pathways connect the ventral tegmental area via the mesolimbic projections to the limbic region (especially the hippocampus) and via the mesocortical projections to the prefrontal cortex. The limbic region also receives cortical afferents. Several receptors for the neurotransmitter dopamine are found in the brain (see receptor table at end of Ch. 1). CNS dopamine receptors belong to two families, D_1-like (which includes subtypes D_1 and D_5) and D_2-like (which includes subtypes D_2, D_3 and D_4). Postsynaptic D_1 and D_2 subtypes are found in the striatum, limbic system, thalamus and hypothalamus, all areas that receive dopaminergic innervation. D_2 receptors are also present in the pituitary. Presynaptic D_3 receptors are present on the dopaminergic neuronal terminals in the striatum and limbic system, and stimulation inhibits dopamine release in these areas. D_4 receptors are found in the limbic system and frontal cortex.

There are several pieces of evidence that support the involvement of defective glutamatergic and dopaminergic neurotransmission in the genesis of schizophrenia:

- amfetamine-induced dopamine release is greater in people with schizophrenia.
- striatal dopamine accumulation is higher in people with schizophrenia.
- antipsychotic actions of drugs are achieved by blockade of the D_2 family of receptors.

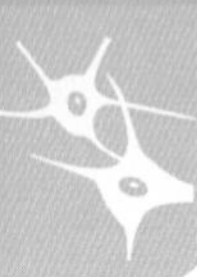

Box 21.1 Classification of major psychotic disorders

Schizophrenia
Persistent delusional disorders (includes paranoid psychosis, paraphrenia)
Acute and transient psychotic disorders
Schizoaffective disorders
Manic episode
Bipolar affective disorder

Table 21.1 Clinical features of schizophrenia

Features	Characteristics
Positive features	
Hallucinations	Third-person auditory hallucinations (voices talking about the person as 'he' or 'she') Second-person commands Olfactory, tactile or visual hallucinations
Delusions	Thought withdrawal (thoughts being taken from your mind) Thought insertion (alien thoughts inserted in your mind) Though broadcast (thoughts are known to others) Actions are caused or controlled from outside Bodily sensations are imposed from outside Delusional perception (a sudden, fully formed delusion, in the wake of a normal perception)
Negative features	
Loss of interest in others, initiative or sense of enjoyment Blunted emotions Limited speech	

- increased stimulation of D_2-like receptors worsens positive symptoms
- glutamate NMDA receptor antagonists (ketamine, phencyclidine) produce positive and negative symptoms, similar to those of schizophrenia
- NMDA receptor agonists such as glycine improve symptoms.

In schizophrenia there is down-regulation of D_3 and D_4 receptors in the frontal cortex and of D_4 receptors in the limbic system. Abnormalities of other neurotransmitter systems may also be important in schizophrenia, but their precise roles are as yet unresolved. Dysfunctions in systems using noradrenaline, serotonin and neuropeptides such as neurotensin, cholecystokinin and somatostatin may also be involved.

MANIA AND BIPOLAR DISORDER

Mania is a disorder of elevated mood that can occur alone (unipolar mania) or more usually interspersed with episodes of depression (bipolar affective disorder or manic-depressive illness). Mild mania is termed hypomania. Sometimes, the fluctuations of mood are less marked, and the disorder is termed cyclothymia.

Mania can occur gradually or suddenly and varies in severity from mild elation, increased drive and sociability, to grandiose ideas, marked overactivity, overspending and socially embarrassing behaviour. Onset is usually early in adult life. Mania and bipolar disorder have (and share) a stronger genetic component than any other grouping of major psychiatric disorders.

Biological basis of bipolar disorder

The biological basis for bipolar disorder is less well understood than that for depression. Susceptibility genes have been identified that are shared with those for schizophrenia, but the environmental stressors that result in expression of the disorder are poorly understood. The dysregulation of neuronal function is probably triggered by altered expression of critical neuronal proteins, determined by the genetic predisposition. In bipolar disorder, there is increased CNS monoamine neurotransmitter activity (particularly serotonin and dopamine) and reduced acetylcholine and GABA neurotransmission. These may all be important in orchestrating changes in neuronal function within the prefrontal cortex, visual association cortex and limbic circuitry.

The changes in neurotransmitter regulation produce functional disruption in the target neurons. Reduced neuronal levels of brain-derived neurotrophic factor (BDNF) may be important in the genesis of bipolar disorder (see also depression, Ch. 22). BDNF regulates several intracellular signal transduction pathways, including myristoylated alanine-rich C kinase substrate (MARKS), protein kinase C and phosphatidylinositol. Dysregulation of these pathways may produce the neuroplastic changes (especially synaptic plasticity) and neuronal cell loss that are features of bipolar disorder.

ANTIPSYCHOTIC DRUGS

Classification

Antipsychotic drugs (also known as neuroleptics or major tranquillisers) have a common mechanism for their beneficial clinical effects, but belong to various chemical classes that differ in their propensity to cause sedation, and antimuscarinic or extrapyramidal effects (Table 21.2). They are commonly considered in two groups that differ in their unwanted effects (although the distinction between these groups is frequently hazy): the conventional and atypical antipsychotics.

Conventional antipsychotic drugs

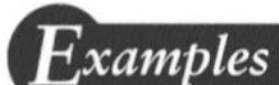

chlorpromazine, flupentixol, haloperidol, sulpiride

Mechanism of action and effects

The antipsychotic action of all these drugs arises primarily from blockade of CNS dopamine receptors in mesolimbic

Table 21.2 Some unwanted effects of antipsychotic drugs

Drug type	Example	Sedative	Antimuscarinic	Extrapyramidal	Hypotension
Conventional antipsychotics					
Phenothiazines					
Group 1 (aliphatic)					
	Chlorpromazine	+++	++	++	+++
	Levomepromazine	+++	++	++	+++
	Promazine	+++	++	++	+++
Group 2 (piperidine)					
	Pericyazine	++	+++	+	++
	Pipotiazine	+	++	++	++
	Thioridazine	++	+++	+	++
Group 3 (piperazine)					
	Fluphenazine	++	+	+++	+
	Perphenazine	++	++	+++	++
	Prochlorperazine	++	++	+++	++
	Trifluoperazine	++	++	+++	+
Thioxanthenes					
	Flupentixol	+	+	+++	+
	Zuclopenthixol	+	+	+++	+
Butyrophenones					
	Benperidol	+	+	+++	+
	Haloperidol	+	+	+++	++
Diphenylbutylpiperidines					
	Pimozide	0	+	+++	+
Substituted benzamides					
	Sulpiride	+	+	+	0
Atypical antipsychotics					
	Amisulpride	+	+	0	+
	Aripiprazole	++	+	+	+
	Clozapine	++	+	0	+
	Olanzapine	++	+	0	+
	Quetiapine	++	0	0	+
	Risperidone	+	0	+	+
	Sertindole	+	0	0	++
	Zotepine	++	0	0	+

+++, high; ++, moderate; +, low; 0, minimal.

pathways. High affinity for the family of D_2 receptors is a common feature of all conventional antipsychotics, and the affinity of the drug for these receptors correlates well with its effective dose. Conventional antipsychotics have a higher affinity than dopamine for D_2 receptors, and dissociate slowly from the receptor. At least 65% D_2 receptor occupancy in the mesolimbic system is required for clinical benefit during long-term treatment of psychotic disorders. However, 80% or more D_2 receptor blockade in the striatum will produce extrapyramidal unwanted effects (see below). Many conventional antipsychotics also block serotonin $5HT_{2A}$ and $5HT_{2C}$ receptors, actions that may contribute to

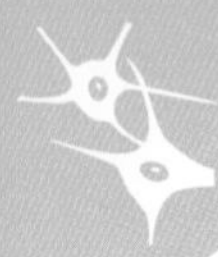

their clinical effects. Antagonist activity at other receptors, including α_1-adrenoceptors and histamine H_1 receptors, does not influence their efficacy in psychotic illness but can produce unwanted effects (in which respect they resemble tricyclic antidepressants; Ch. 22). The severity of these varies considerably among the different drugs.

Clinical improvement with antipsychotic drugs develops slowly, despite an immediate onset of dopamine receptor blockade. There is increasing evidence that these drugs affect neuroplasticity, leading to changes in synaptic connections in areas of the brain known to be involved in psychotic illness, and these changes may be important for their long-term benefit. Clinically useful effects produced by antipsychotic drugs include the following:

- A depressant action on conditioned responses and emotional responsiveness. In psychoses this is particularly helpful for the management of thought disorders, abnormalities of perception and delusional beliefs.
- A sedative action, which is useful for the treatment of restlessness and confusion. Sensory input into the reticular activating system is reduced by blockade of collateral fibres from the lemniscal pathways, but spontaneous activity is preserved; arousal stimuli therefore produce less response.
- An antiemetic effect through dopamine receptor blockade at the chemoreceptor trigger zone (CTZ), which is useful to treat vomiting, such as that associated with drugs (e.g. cytotoxics, opioid analgesics) and uraemia. Some antipsychotic drugs are also effective in motion sickness, through muscarinic receptor blockade (Ch. 32).
- Antihistaminic activity produced by histamine H_1-receptor blockade can be used for treatment of allergic reactions (Ch. 39).

Pharmacokinetics

Antipsychotics are rapidly absorbed from the gut but most undergo extensive first-pass metabolism. For some drugs, the plasma concentrations of active drug (including metabolites) can vary up to 10-fold among individuals, but there is not a close relationship between plasma drug concentration and clinical response. Elimination is by metabolism in the liver. Several antipsychotic drugs, such as chlorpromazine, haloperidol, perphenazine, and zuclopenthixol, are metabolised predominantly by the polymorphic enzyme CYP2D6: significant relationships have been reported between the steady-state plasma concentrations (see Ch. 2) and the CYP2D6 genotype. Sulpiride and amisulpride (an atypical antipsychotic) do not undergo first-pass metabolism and are largely eliminated unchanged by the kidney. The half-lives of the antipsychotics vary widely; for example, that of sulpiride is 6–8 h, while that of pimozide is very long, at 2 days. Some antipsychotics, such as chlorpromazine and haloperidol, can be given by intramuscular injection for more rapid onset of action. Since adherence to treatment is often poor in psychotic disorders, depot formulations of many antipsychotics have been developed. They are given by intramuscular injection as a prodrug – which is the active compound esterified to a long-chain fatty acid and dissolved in a vegetable oil – that slowly releases the drug for between 1 and 12 weeks (depending on the formulation). When given as a depot preparation or by intramuscular injection, the doses used are smaller than those for oral treatment, because of the absence of first-pass metabolism. The half-lives given in the drug table do not reflect the slow absorption rate-limited half-life of the depot form (see Ch. 2). Examples of a depot preparation are flupentixol decanoate and pipotiazine palmitate.

Unwanted effects

The antipsychotic drugs differ mainly in the degree of associated or unwanted effects (Table 21.2).

- Extrapyramidal effects: acute dystonias (tongue protrusion, torticollis, oculogyric crisis) are most common after a few doses in children and young adults. Akathisia (restlessness) usually follows large initial doses, while parkinsonism has a gradual onset usually in adults or the elderly. All arise from D_2 receptor blockade in the nigrostriatal pathways. Extrapyramidal effects (Ch. 24) occur in more than half of those being treated with conventional antipsychotics, but are usually reversible if the drug is stopped. With prolonged use, tardive dyskinesias or dystonias can develop. These consist of choreoathetoid and repetitive orofacial movements that arise after months or years of continued treatment and often do not resolve when the drug is withdrawn. Their aetiology is uncertain: upregulation of D_2 receptors may contribute, but damage to inhibitory GABAergic neurons and/or dysfunction in other neurotransmitter pathways is probably involved. Extrapyramidal effects are most common with piperazine phenothiazines (such as fluphenazine and prochlorperazine) and the butyrophenones (such as haloperidol) (Table 21.2).
- Drowsiness and cognitive impairment can occur as a result of histamine and dopamine receptor blockade.
- Galactorrhoea, with gynaecomastia, amenorrhoea, or impotence: >70% D_2 receptor blockade in hypothalamic pathways produces hyperprolactinaemia and reduced gonadotrophin secretion.
- Antimuscarinic effects: peripheral antimuscarinic actions include dry mouth, constipation, micturition difficulties and blurred vision (Ch. 4). CNS muscarinic receptor blockade predisposes to acute confusional states.
- Postural hypotension, nasal stuffiness and impaired ejaculation, due to α_1-adrenoceptor blockade.
- Hypothermia as a consequence of depressed hypothalamic function. Altered serotonergic neuronal activity may be responsible.
- Reduced seizure threshold with conventional antipsychotics.
- Hypersensitivity reactions include cholestatic jaundice, skin reactions and bone marrow depression.
- Photosensitivity and skin discoloration (especially with chlorpromazine).
- Cognitive impairment.
- Weight gain, with an increased risk of insulin resistance and glucose intolerance.
- Prolongation of the Q–T interval on the electrocardiogram, a particular problem with pimozide, predisposes to ventricular arrhythmias (Ch. 8).
- Neuroleptic malignant syndrome is a rare genetically determined disorder caused by a polymorphism in the D_2 receptor and consequent abnormal dopamine receptor blockade in the corpus striatum and hypothalamus.

In those with a receptor abnormality, antipsychotic drugs produce high fever, muscle rigidity, autonomic instability with hypertension, urinary incontinence and sweating, and altered consciousness. Immediate withdrawal of the antipsychotic and treatment with dantrolene or a dopamine receptor agonist (Ch. 24) may be life-saving. Symptoms can take up to 1 week to subside, or longer after a depot preparation. Cautious reintroduction of an antipsychotic may be possible without recurrence, but at least 2 weeks should be allowed after symptoms of the syndrome have resolved.

- Sudden withdrawal after long-term use can produce nausea, vomiting, anorexia, diarrhoea, sweating, myalgias, paraesthesiae, insomnia and agitation. These usually subside within 2 weeks.

Atypical antipsychotic drugs

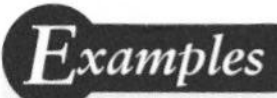

amisulpride, aripiprazole, clozapine, olanzapine, risperidone

Mechanism of action and effects

The antipsychotic action of atypical antipsychotic drugs, like that of conventional antipsychotics, arises primarily from blockade of CNS dopamine D_2 receptors in mesolimbic pathways. Compared with conventional drugs, the atypical antipsychotic drugs have different receptor affinities. In particular, their affinity for D_2 receptors is much lower than that of conventional antipsychotics, and less than that of dopamine, with much more transient receptor occupancy. This may underlie their lower propensity for producing movement disorders (Ch. 24).

- Clozapine is a relatively weak D_2 receptor antagonist with selective cortical receptor occupancy, and shows greater blockade at D_1 and D_4 receptors. It has a much higher affinity for blockade of serotonin $5HT_{2A}$ and $5HT_{2C}$ receptors, and also blocks α_1-adrenoceptors and muscarinic receptors.
- Olanzapine has a similar profile to clozapine, with additional antagonist activity at some other serotonin receptors and histamine H_1 receptors.
- Risperidone has higher-affinity binding to D_2 and D_4 receptors, with dose-dependent limbic selectivity. It also binds to $5HT_{2A}$ receptors, and to α_1- and α_2-adrenoceptors, but not to muscarinic or histamine receptors.
- Aripiprazole has partial agonist activity at the D_2 and D_3 receptor which limits the degree of receptor blockade. It is also a partial agonist at 5-HT_{1A} receptors, but an antagonist at 5-HT_{2A} receptors.
- Amisulpride blocks both pre- and postsynaptic D_2 receptors. Presynaptic receptor blockade increases endogenous dopamine release in the striatum.

Since atypical antipsychotics cause fewer extrapyramidal effects than do conventional drugs, this improves compliance and may explain their apparently greater efficacy when compared with conventional antipsychotics. Clozapine, however, uniquely is clearly superior to all other drugs for refractory schizophrenia.

Pharmacokinetics

Atypical antipsychotics are rapidly absorbed from the gut and most undergo extensive first-pass metabolism to inactive metabolites. The half-lives of the atypical antipsychotics vary widely and are listed in the compendium. Some atypical antipsychotics, such as risperidone, can be given in a depot formulation.

Unwanted effects

The atypical antipsychotic drugs show some differences from conventional antipsychotics in their unwanted effects (Table 21.2).

- *Extrapyramidal effects*: atypical antipsychotics have a lower risk of extrapyramidal effects, except at high dosages, when the risk is similar to conventional antipsychotics.
- *Drowsiness* and cognitive impairment can occur, but is less marked than with conventional antipsychotics. Risperidone can causes insomnia and agitation.
- *Galactorrhoea and sexual dysfunction* are less common with atypical antipsychotics, except risperidone and amisulpride.
- *Antimuscarinic effects* are uncommon with atypical antipsychotics.
- *Postural hypotension*, especially during initial dose titration.
- *Reduced seizure threshold* with clozapine.
- *Agranulocytosis* is a particular problem with clozapine (1–2% risk) and regular blood tests are mandatory during treatment with this drug.
- *Weight gain* with clozapine and olanzapine.
- *Neuroleptic malignant syndrome* occurs rarely.
- *Sudden withdrawal syndrome*.

MOOD-STABILISING DRUGS

Lithium

Mechanism of action

The mechanism of action of lithium is not well understood, but it has multiple effects in the CNS.

- Lithium has complex effects on the generation of intracellular second messengers in cortical neuronal pathways. It attenuates the function of G_s-proteins coupled to adenylyl cyclase but increases basal adenylyl cyclase activity, effects that alter cAMP synthesis. Lithium also inhibits intracellular inositol monophosphatase, and therefore interferes with substrate generation for second messengers involved in phosphoinositide pathway signalling. These actions will affect several monoaminergic and cholinergic systems in the CNS. The overall action of lithium may be to stabilise intracellular signalling by enhancing basal activity but decreasing maximum activity.
- Suppression of the expression of pro-apoptotic genes and increased expression of anti-apoptotic genes, with consequent neuroprotection. Lithium inhibits the multifunctional enzyme glucose synthase kinase-3 (GSK-3), a regulator of many signal transduction pathways that are involved in neuronal apoptosis. Inhibition of the

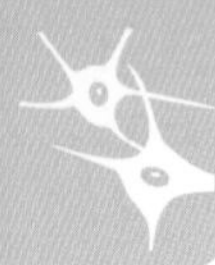

activity of the pro-apoptotic enzyme caspase-3 by lithium also confers neuroprotection.

- Increased neurogenesis has been found in the hippocampus after lithium treatment, which may be one consequence of the complex changes in intracellular signalling.

Pharmacokinetics

Lithium is given as a salt (e.g. carbonate, citrate), which is rapidly absorbed from the gut. To avoid high peak plasma concentrations (which are associated with unwanted effects), modified-release formulations are normally used. Lithium is widely distributed in the body but enters the brain slowly. It is selectively concentrated in bone and the thyroid gland. Excretion is by glomerular filtration, with 80% reabsorbed in the proximal tubule by the same mechanism as Na^+ although, unlike Na^+, lithium is not reabsorbed from more distal parts of the kidney. When the body is depleted of salt and water, for example by vomiting or diarrhoea, then enhanced reabsorption of Na^+ in the proximal tubule is accompanied by enhanced lithium reabsorption, which can produce acute toxicity. Lithium has a long half-life of about 1 day and has a narrow therapeutic index. Regular monitoring of plasma concentrations (which should be measured 12 h after dosing so that the absorption and distribution phases are completed) is mandatory at least every 3 months during long-term treatment.

Unwanted effects

- Nausea and diarrhoea can occur at low plasma concentrations.
- CNS effects, including tremor, giddiness, ataxia and dysarthria.
- Hypothyroidism can be caused by interference with thyroxine synthesis during long-term treatment.
- Reduced responsiveness of the distal renal tubule to antidiuretic hormone (ADH, vasopressin). This occasionally produces a reversible nephrogenic diabetes insipidus with polyuria and consequent polydipsia.
- Severe intoxication produces coma, convulsions, and profound hypotension with oliguria.

Drug interactions

Diuretics can reduce lithium excretion by producing dehydration (see above). This is most marked with thiazides (Ch. 14) because of their prolonged action. Angiotensin-converting enzyme inhibitors (Ch. 6) and some non-steroidal anti-inflammatory drugs (Ch. 29) also reduce the excretion of lithium. The risk of extrapyramidal effects may be increased when lithium is prescribed concurrently with antipsychotic drugs.

Anticonvulsants used in mania

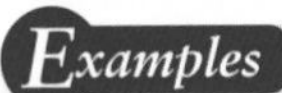

carbamazepine, sodium valproate

Mechanism of action in mania

The mode of action of the anticonvulsants carbamazepine and sodium valproate in mania may be related to facilitation of GABAergic inhibitory neurotransmission, and consequent modulation of excitatory glutamatergic neurons. Like lithium, anticonvulsants modulate cAMP-mediated intracellular events, reduce inositol generation in the phosphoinositide signalling pathway and activate neuroprotective anti-apoptotic genes. They also stimulate hippocampal neurogenesis. Antiepileptic drugs are discussed in Chapter 23.

MANAGEMENT OF PSYCHOTIC DISORDERS

MANAGEMENT OF SCHIZOPHRENIA

Acute psychotic symptoms such as hallucinations and delusions can be controlled relatively rapidly with an antipsychotic drug such as haloperidol or chlorpromazine. The initial sedative actions of these drugs can be particularly helpful. However, reductions in thought disturbance, withdrawal and apathy are delayed and the clinical improvement is gradual over several weeks of treatment.

Treatment for schizophrenia is not curative, and long-term maintenance therapy is usually required to prevent relapse. The duration of this treatment is determined by the number of acute episodes, and is usually at least 2–5 years. Intermittent treatment that is introduced only for relapses is associated with a higher overall relapse rate (50–80%, compared with 25–40% in those taking prophylactic therapy). The relapse rate is lowest with atypical antipsychotics. Adherence to maintenance treatment is often poor in schizophrenia, and can be improved by depot injections given every 1–4 weeks. Continuous antipsychotic treatment provides relief of symptoms for more than 70% of people with schizophrenia. Resistance to conventional antipsychotics is particularly common if negative symptoms predominate.

Atypical antipsychotics should be considered:

- when choosing first-line treatment for newly diagnosed schizophrenia
- if there are unacceptable unwanted effects with a conventional drug
- during an acute schizophrenic episode when discussion with the person is not possible.

Atypical antipsychotic drugs produce greater relief of negative symptoms than the conventional antipsychotic drugs, although this may be due to better adherence to treatment. There is some limited evidence to support the concurrent use of a selective serotonin reuptake inhibitor (SSRI; Ch. 22) with an atypical antipsychotic drug for those whose negative symptoms do not respond to the antipsychotic drug alone. Clozapine is the only antipsychotic drug shown to be effective in treatment resistance (incomplete recovery), but the risk of agranulocytosis has limited its use. It should always be tried if symptoms have failed to respond to two antipsychotic drugs, one of which should be an atypical drug, each given for 6–8 weeks. Between 30% and 50% of those who are resistant to other treatments will respond to clozapine.

Various psychological treatments to improve social skills are important as an adjunct to drug treatment and should be provided along with social support.

MANAGEMENT OF MANIA AND BIPOLAR DISORDER

When symptoms of acute mania are mild or moderate, they can usually be controlled by lithium, although the therapeutic effect may be delayed for at least a week. For this reason, a benzodiazepine (Ch. 20) is usually given as well for the first 7 days. The anticonvulsants carbamazepine and sodium valproate are effective alternatives to lithium for the acute phase. Carbamazepine has a delayed onset of action, and is also used initially with a benzodiazepine. The sedative action of sodium valproate produces a response in 1–4 days when used alone.

If manic symptoms are more severe, it is usually necessary to give an antipsychotic drug in combination with lithium, carbamazepine or sodium valproate. Conventional antipsychotic drugs are only recommended for short-term use, because of their extrapyramidal unwanted effects. Combination therapy with an anticonvulsant, and perhaps use of a benzodiazepine, can reduce the dose of antipsychotic drug needed to control symptoms. The atypical antipsychotic drugs such as olanzapine have antimanic activity, with a lower risk of extrapyramidal unwanted effects.

If a person with bipolar disorder has had at least two episodes of either mania or depression in 5 years, then prophylactic therapy is recommended. Lithium is the conventional treatment of choice for prophylaxis, but carbamazepine is equally effective. There is less evidence to support the use of sodium valproate, which is usually reserved for those who do not tolerate first-line treatments, or for when these are ineffective. Other anticonvulsant drugs, including lamotrigine, gabapentin and topiramate, may be useful as alternatives to carbamazepine for prophylaxis, but the evidence is limited at present. The optimal duration of prophylactic therapy is unknown, but if a decision is made to discontinue treatment, then gradual withdrawal is recommended, to reduce the risk of relapse, especially of mania.

Treatment of depression in bipolar disorder usually requires a combination of lithium and an antidepressant. However, the response to antidepressant therapy is less satisfactory than with unipolar depression, and there is a risk of provoking a manic 'switch'. There is limited evidence that mania is less likely to be provoked by an SSRI than by a tricyclic antidepressant (Ch. 22). As an alternative to combination therapy, lamotrigine has been reported to be effective as sole therapy for bipolar depression.

Electroconvulsive therapy is used for refractory episodes of both mania and depression, and has a much more rapid action than drug therapy. As for schizophrenia, psychological treatments are an important adjunct to drug therapy in bipolar disorder.

FURTHER READING

Altamura AC, Sassella F, Santini A et al (2003) Intramuscular preparations of antipsychotics. *Drugs* 63, 493–512

Belmaker RH (2004) Bipolar disorder. *N Engl J Med* 351, 476–486

Geddes J, Freemantle N, Harrison P, Bebbington P (2000) Atypical antipsychotics in the treatment of schizophrenia: systematic overview and meta-regression analysis. *BMJ* 321, 1371–1376

Harwood AJ, Agam G (2003) Search for a common mechanism of action of mood stabilizers. *Biochem Pharmacol* 66, 179–189

Horacek J, Bubenikov-Valesova V, Kopecek M et al (2006) Mechanism of action of atypical antipsychotic drugs and the neurobiology of schizophrenia. *CNS Drugs* 20, 389–409

Laruelle M, Kegele S, Abi-Darham A (2003) Glutamate dopamine and schizophrenia. From pathology to treatment *Ann NY Acad Sci* 1003, 138–158

Laruelle M, Frankle WG, Narenran R et al (2007) Mechanism of action of antipsychotic drugs: from dopamine D_2 receptor antagonism to glutamate NMDA facilitation. *Clin Ther* 27(suppl A), S16–S24

Li X, Ketter TA, Frye MA (2002) Synaptic, intracellular, and neuroprotective mechanisms of anticonvulsants: are they relevant for the treatment and course of bipolar disorders? *J Affect Disord* 69, 1–14

Miyamoto S, Duncan GE, Marx CE et al (2005) Treatments for schizophrenia: a critical review of pharmacology and mechanisms of action of antipsychotic drugs. *Mol Psychiatry* 10, 79–104

Möller H-J (2003) Management of the negative symptoms of schizophrenia. *CNS Drugs* 17, 793–823

Mueser KT, McGurk SR (2004) Schizophrenia. *Lancet* 363, 2063–2072

Müller-Oerlinghausen B, Berghöfer A, Bauer M (2002) Bipolar disorder. *Lancet* 359, 241–247

Picchioni MM, Murray RM (2007) Schizophrenia. *BMJ* 335, 91–95

Rochon PA, Stukel TA, Sykora A et al (2005) Atypical antipsychotics and parkinsonism. *Arch Intern Med* 165, 1882–1888

van OS J, Kapur S (2009) Schizophrenia. *Lancet* 374, 635–645

SELF-ASSESSMENT

In questions 1–3, the first statement, in italics, is true. Are the accompanying statements also true?

1. *Some antipsychotic drugs such as clozapine have relatively few effects on the extrapyramidal system and have low affinity for the dopamine receptors in the substantia nigra.*
   a. The atypical antipsychotic clozapine has greater antimuscarinic activity than chlorpromazine.
   b. Clozapine causes agranulocytosis.
   c. Chlorpromazine given as the decanoate in a depot preparation has to be injected weekly.
2. *The beneficial effects of antipsychotics take several weeks for their full effect to be seen.*
   a. The 'positive' symptoms of schizophrenia (e.g. delusions) are more readily controlled than negative (withdrawal) symptoms.
   b. There is a close correlation between plasma levels of chlorpromazine and its antipsychotic effect.
3. *Antipsychotics are effective in treating only about 70% of people with schizophrenia.* Clozapine and thioridazine cause relatively few extrapyramidal symptoms.

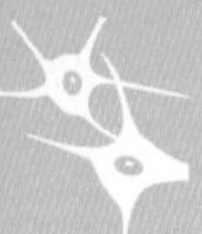

4. From the following statements regarding properties of antipsychotics, choose the one **most appropriate** option.
   A. Clozapine is associated with a high incidence of extrapyramidal side-effects.
   B. Regular blood tests are required in people taking clozapine.
   C. Clozapine causes little sedation.
   D. Haloperidol causes nausea.
   E. Lithium is reabsorbed through the distal convoluted tubule in the kidney.
5. You wish to compare the beneficial and unwanted effect profile of a new antipsychotic. Which one of the following is likely to contribute to its antipsychotic rather than unwanted effect potential?
   A. Its potential to block dopamine receptors in the substantia nigra.
   B. Its potential to block muscarinic receptors.
   C. Its potential to block α_1-adrenoceptors.
   D. Its potential to block serotonin (5-HT) receptors.
   E. Its potential to block histamine receptors.
6. Case history questions

A 25-year-old man (Mr PS) with schizophrenia had been treated with high-dose oral chlorpromazine for 2 years. His main symptoms of auditory hallucinations and delusional thoughts (*'The people in the flat above are broadcasting my thoughts on their radio'*) had improved, but he remained socially withdrawn and apathetic and described a number of new problems, including feeling very tired, faintness on standing up, dry mouth, sexual problems, blurred and darkened vision, occasional difficulty with fine control of movement (writing/typing) and weight gain.

   a. Which neural pathways are thought to be dysfunctional in schizophrenia and what is the evidence for this? How does chlorpromazine exert its antipsychotic action?
   b. Which unwanted effect(s) reported by Mr PS are likely to be caused by chlorpromazine acting at dopamine receptors? Why are movement disorders less frequent with chlorpromazine than with some other antipsychotic drugs?
   c. Which unwanted effects reported by Mr PS are likely to be caused by blockade of histamine receptors, muscarinic receptors and α-adrenoceptors?
   d. Mr PS has had two severe relapses requiring hospitalisation within the last 18 months and is vague on whether he always takes his medication as directed. How might you improve adherence to treatment? Consider alternative antipsychotic drugs that might help Mr PS. What special care is required with the drug(s) you suggest?

ANSWERS

1. a. **False**. The atypical antipsychotics have less antimuscarinic activity than the phenothiazines.
   b. **True**. Regular blood monitoring is required.
   c. **False**. Injections are at 1- to 3-month intervals.
2. a. **True**. Negative symptoms are more difficult to treat; 'atypical' antipsychotics may have greater activity against negative symptoms.
   b. **False**. The plasma levels of chlorpromazine are highly variable and do not correlate with clinical effect.
3. **True**. See Table 21.2. They also have antimuscarinic activity which may also reduce extrapyramidal side-effects (see antimuscarinic drug use in parkinsonism, Ch. 24).
4. Answer **B**.
   A. Clozapine has a very low incidence of extrapyramidal side-effects.
   B. Clozapine can cause agranulocytosis, and blood monitoring is necessary.
   C. Clozapine has a sedative action
   D. Antipsychotics do not cause nausea and some are used in the treatment of nausea and vomiting.
   E. Lithium is reabsorbed through the proximal convoluted tubule in the kidney at the same site that Na^+ is absorbed.
5. Answer **D**.
   A. The ability to block dopamine receptors in the substantia nigra will increase the extrapyramidal unwanted effects.
   B. Blockade of muscarinic receptors will increase unwanted effects such as confusion, although it may reduce parkinsonian-like effects.
   C. Block of α_1-adrenoceptors will cause hypotension.
   D. Serotonin receptor blocking activity could contribute to its antipsychotic potential.
   E. Blockade of histamine receptors will contribute to its sedative effect.
6. Case history answers
   a. Positive symptoms of schizophrenia may be associated with overactivity of dopaminergic pathways in the mesolimbic area and medial temporal lobe, e.g. hippocampus and amygdala; this may be related to reduced glutamatergic modulation of dopamine synthesis in the striatum. Pharmacologically, positive symptoms of schizophrenia may be mimicked by dopamine agonists (e.g. amphetamines) and are improved by dopamine antagonists. Antipsychotic activity correlates most closely with antagonism of dopamine D_2 (and possibly D_3) receptors.
   b. Distinct from their antipsychotic activity, drugs also block dopamine D_2 receptors in nigrostriatal pathways. This upsets the 'balance' between dopaminergic and cholinergic activity, leading to extrapyramidal movement disorders (e.g. tremor, akathisia, tardive dyskinesia). The movement disorders thus mimic those seen in Parkinson's disease, where they are caused by a neurological deficit in dopaminergic activity. As with parkinsonian patients, antimuscarinic drugs are sometimes used in schizophrenia to ameliorate extrapyramidal unwanted effects. Mr PS's movement disorders (problems with writing/typing) appear relatively mild, possibly because chlorpromazine (an early phenothiazine) also has antimuscarinic activity. Paradoxically, newer and more selective phenothiazines (e.g. fluphenazine) often produce worse movement disorders than chlorpromazine. Mr PS's weight gain may

be due to excess corticosteroid release, caused by chlorpromazine antagonising the dopamine-dependent suppression of adrenocorticotrophic hormone (ACTH) release from the hypothalamus.

c. As well as the above caused by dopamine antagonism, many antipsychotic drugs (especially conventional ones) produce unwanted effects due to blockade of histamine receptors (sedation, tiredness), muscarinic receptors (dry mouth, blurred vision, impotence) and α_1-adrenoceptors (vasodilation and postural hypotension). Chlorpromazine may also produce 'yellowing' or darkening of vision because of idiosyncratic deposition in the cornea.

d. Approaches include the possible use of a long-acting depot preparation (decanoates, etc.) and the importance of support from the patient's GP and family in maintaining adherence. A principal cause of poor adherence is unwanted effects of antipsychotic therapy. Since unwanted effects vary widely from drug to drug, the choice of drug may have major impact on adherence.

e. Mr PS may benefit from a different antipsychotic drug, like fluphenazine or flupentixol, which produce less antagonism of histamine receptors (less sedation) and muscarinic receptors (less dry mouth, blurred vision, etc.), even though movement disorders may be worse than with chlorpromazine. Negative symptoms (apathy, withdrawal) are relatively poorly controlled with most antipsychotics compared with 'positive' symptoms (delusions, hallucinations), and both types of symptoms may be particularly resistant in a proportion of people. An 'atypical' antipsychotic drug (clozapine, sulpiride) may help with the apathy and withdrawal reported by Mr PS, with relatively little sedation and movement disorders. Clozapine can cause blood disorders (agranulocytosis and aplastic anaemia), and blood monitoring is mandatory.

Antipsychotic drugs

Drug	**Half-life (h) and kinetics**	**Comments**
Conventional antipsychotics		
Benperidol	5–7 [M] Incomplete oral bioavailability (about 40–50%); metabolites are inactive	Given orally; main indication for control of deviant antisocial sexual behavior (but efficacy uncertain)
Chlorpromazine	8–35 [M] Incomplete oral bioavailability (10–33%); numerous pathways of metabolism, with some metabolites detectable months after cessation of treatment	Oral, suppository and injection formulations available; also used as antiemetic in palliative care
Flupentixol	35 [M] Oral bioavailability is about 40%; the half-life for release from the depot injection is about 17 days; parent drug undergoes enterohepatic circulation following biliary excretion as a glucuronide	Given orally (as hydrochloride) or by depot injection (as the decanoate ester prodrug)
Fluphenazine	16 [M] Oral bioavailability is about 50%; the half-life for release from the depot injection is about 26 days; metabolites of fluphenazine retain activity and may be responsible for about 50% of the total activity	Given orally (as hydrochloride) or by depot injection (as the decanoate ester prodrug)
Haloperidol	20 (9–67) [M] Oral bioavailability is about 60%; the half-life for release from the depot injection is about 21 days; reduced to an active metabolite in liver and extrahepatic tissues; undergoes enterohepatic circulation	Given orally and by injection, or by depot injection (as the decanoate prodrug)
Levomepromazine	15–70 [M] Oral bioavailability is about 50%; numerous metabolites and wide inter-individual variation in kinetics	Given orally or by injection (i.m. or i.v.); also used for pain relief and as antiemetic in palliative care
Pericyazine	? [M?] No data available	Given orally, early drug; few published data available
Perphenazine	9 [M] Variable oral bioavailability due to first-pass metabolism; oxidised by CYP2D6 but also undergoes S-oxidation and glucuronidation; metabolites eliminated over many weeks after cessation of treatment	Given orally; also used as antiemetic

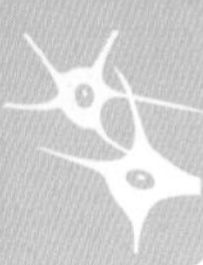

Antipsychotic drugs

Drug	Half-life (h) and kinetics	Comments
Pimozide	55 [M] Oral bioavailability is about 60–80%; metabolised to inactive products by CYP3A4	Given orally
Pipotiazine palmitate	15–16 days [M] Long half-life results from slow release from depot injection; the active drug (pipotiazide) has an elimination half-life of a few hours only	Given only as a depot injection formulation
Prochlorperazine	6–7 [M] Variable absorption of oral doses; undergoes extensive hepatic metabolism	Given orally, rectally or by deep i.m. injection; also used as antiemetic
Promazine	? [M] Metabolised in the liver by N-demethylation and S-oxidation	Given orally; it is a low-potency metabolite of chlorpromazine with little antipsychotic activity; used as sedative
Sulpiride	6–8 [R] Incomplete oral bioavailability (about 30–40%) owing to poor absorption; water-soluble compound eliminated largely unchanged in urine and faeces; clearance approximates to glomerular filtration rate	Given orally
Trifluoperazine	14 (7–18) [M] Oral bioavailability has not been defined (because of the absence of i.v. reference data); numerous metabolites formed	Given orally; also used as antiemetic
Zuclopenthixol	20 (13–23) [M] Oral bioavailability (of zuclopenthixol dihydrochloride) is about 60%; the half-lives of the depot forms (acetate and decanoate) are about 19 days; zuclopenthixol is converted into numerous inactive metabolites	Given orally (as the dihydrochloride) or as deep i.m. depot injection (as the decanoate ester)
Atypical antipsychotics		
Amisulpride	12 [R] Oral bioavailability is about 50%; eliminated largely by the kidneys	D_2/D_3 antagonistic with presynaptic and limbic system selectivity; given orally
Aripiprazole	60 [M] High oral bioavailability; metabolised by CYP3A4 and CYP2D6; undergoes dehydrogenation, hydroxylation, and N-dealkylation; one metabolite retains activity; CYP2D6 poor metabolisers have higher levels of the parent drug but lower levels of the active metabolite	*Partial agonist* at D_2 and $5HT_{1A}$ receptors and an antagonist at $5HT_{2A}$ receptors; given orally
Clozapine	12 (6–33) [M] Oral bioavailability is 30–50%; metabolised by hepatic oxidation (CYP1A2, CYP2D6 and CYP3A4); the desmethyl metabolite is pharmacologically active and its formation may be related to development of neutropenia	High affinity for D_1 and D_4 receptors; given orally
Olanzapine	30 (21–54) [M] Oral bioavailability is 60%; metabolised by CYP1A2 and CYP2D6 to inactive products	Antagonist at D_1, D_2, D_4 and $5HT_2$ receptors; given orally
Quetiapine	6 [M] Good oral absorption; metabolised by hepatic CYP3A4 to an inactive sulphoxide metabolite	Antagonist at $5HT_2$ and D_2 receptors; given orally
Risperidone	2–4 (EM), 17–22 (PM) [M + R] Oral bioavailability is about 70%; antagonist at $5HT_2$ and D_2 receptors; metabolised by hepatic CYP2D6 with extensive metabolisers (EM) eliminating the drug 5–10 times more rapidly than poor metabolisers (PM), who excrete about 30% unchanged in urine	Antagonist at $5HT_2$ and D_2 receptors; given orally or by deep i.m. depot injection

Antipsychotic drugs

Drug	Half-life (h) and kinetics	Comments
Sertindole	60–90 [M] Metabolised by CYP2D6 and CYP3A4; poor metabolisers of CYP2D6 substrates show lower clearance	Selective antagonist at $5HT_2$ receptors and D_2 receptors; given orally
Zotepine	12–24 [M] Low oral bioavailability (7–13%); numerous metabolites formed	Antagonist at $5HT_2$ and D_2 receptors; given orally
Mood-stabilising drugs		
Lithium	8–45 [R] Complete oral absorption; filtered at the glomerulus and reabsorbed (about 80%) in the proximal, but not distal, parts of the renal tubule	Given orally

[M], metabolism; [R], renal; i.m., intramuscular; i.v., intravenous.

22 Depression, attention deficit hyperactivity disorder and narcolepsy

DEPRESSION

Clinical depression is characterised by diverse psychological symptoms such as low mood, loss of interest and enjoyment of activities, and reduced energy. It is often accompanied by a sense of guilt and worthlessness, as well as physical symptoms including sleep disturbance, reduced appetite and loss of libido. Depression can present with only physical rather than psychological symptoms. If depression is severe, there may be marked suicidal tendencies and psychotic symptoms (hallucinations and delusions). The existence of mixed anxiety–depression disorder is now also well accepted.

Depression involves a negative emotional bias that may lead the person to preferentially recall negative events. This negative information is processed in the amygdala, which is hyperactive in people with depression. Both a genetic predisposition and the effects of specific stresses in early life may determine whether a person is susceptible to depressive illness in later life.

BIOLOGICAL BASIS OF DEPRESSION

The cause of depression is unknown and there may not be a single mechanism. The most widely accepted hypothesis is that there is a fundamental abnormality in central nervous system (CNS) monoaminergic neurotransmission. However, dysfunctions in many other signalling pathways have been identified, some in only discrete subsets of depressed individuals.

Serotonergic and noradrenergic pathways in the brain

Most serotonergic neurons are found in the raphe area of the midbrain, from where they project to the hippocampus in the limbic system and the cerebral cortex. Presynaptic α_2-adrenoceptors and $5HT_1$ (not shown in Fig. 22.1) autoreceptors inhibit serotonin release. Somatodendritic $5HT_1$, α_1- and β-adrenoceptor autoreceptors on the neuronal cell bodies of the raphe nuclei also regulate firing in serotonergic neurons. Postsynaptic $5HT_2$ receptors mediate the effects of serotonin, and are widely distributed in the cerebral cortex, but especially the prefrontal cortex. A schematic of these mechanisms is shown in Figure 22.1.

In contrast, most noradrenergic neurons arise in the locus ceruleus and the lateral tegmental areas of the brainstem. The locus ceruleus and the raphe region have many reciprocal neural projections, and therefore the pathways are interdependent. For example, noradrenergic neurotransmission stimulates serotonergic neurons by activating somatodendritic α_1-adrenoceptors, but also inhibits serotonin synthesis and release through presynaptic α_2-adrenoceptors.

Pathways mediated by glutamate, GABA and substance P also modulate monoaminergic neurotransmission.

Monoamine neurotransmitters and depression

Serotonergic pathways in the CNS are believed to be mainly involved in mood, while noradrenergic pathways are involved in stress systems, drive and energy state. These monoaminergic circuits in the brain are closely integrated. Simplistically, it has been hypothesised that the following biological changes in the monoamine system are important in depression:

- low levels of monoamine neurotransmitters
- upregulation of postsynaptic monoamine receptors
- upregulation of the inhibitory presynaptic and somatodendritic autoreceptors that control monoamine release.

There are increased $5HT_2$ receptor numbers in the frontal cortex of depressed suicide victims, while other studies have indicated that serotonin and noradrenaline concentrations in the brain are reduced in depression. Overall, evidence for the 'monoamine' theory as a molecular basis for depression is limited, but the response to drugs that increase monoamine neurotransmission supports the concept.

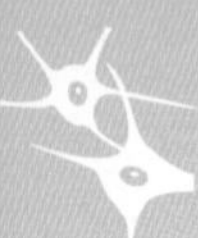

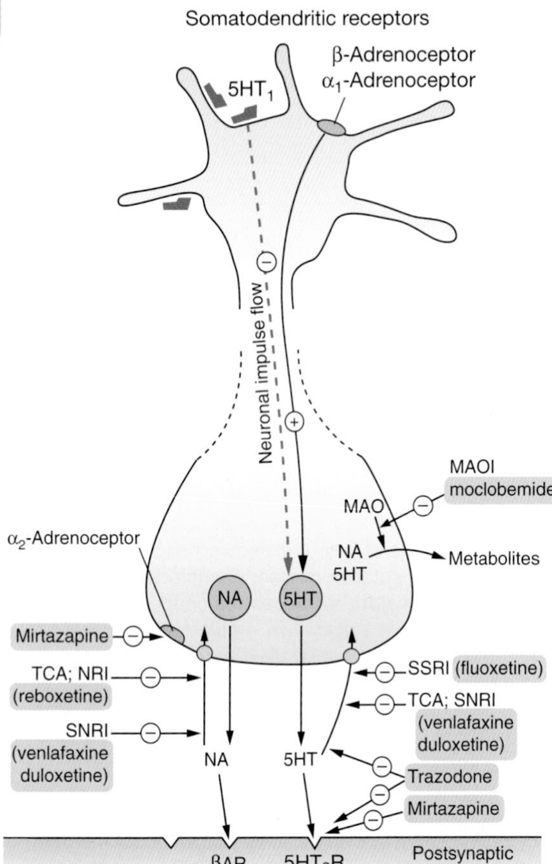

Fig. 22.1 **The effect of drugs used in the treatment of depression on CNS serotonergic and adrenergic functioning.** Some of the bewildering array of adrenergic and (serotonin, 5HT) receptor subtypes are omitted for clarity. The primary action of many drugs in current clinical use is to enhance serotonin and noradrenaline availability. The majority of released serotonin and noradrenaline is rapidly removed from the synapse by reuptake into the neuron (yellow circles). There is a range of antidepressants, which vary in their abilities to inhibit the reuptake of serotonin or noradrenaline, thus enhancing the synapse concentrations of these transmitters. Stimulation of presynaptic α_2-adrenoceptors reduces monoamine release; mirtazapine, by blocking these presynaptic autoreceptors, increases noradrenaline and serotonin release and transmission. Other drugs act by significantly blocking postsynaptic receptors which are upregulated in depression. It is not clear whether the different types of antidepressants have significant advantages in terms of their antidepressant activity, but they differ markedly in their side-effect profiles. MAO, monoamine oxidase; NA, noradrenaline; NRI, (selective) noradrenaline reuptake inhibitor; SNRI, serotonin and noradrenaline reuptake inhibitor; SSRI, selective serotonin reuptake inhibitor; TCA, 'classic' tricyclic antidepressant.

Extending the monoamine theory of depression

The monoamine–cAMP response element binding protein (CREB)–brain-derived neurotrophic factor (BDNF) cascade

Although the mechanisms of action of many current pharmacological treatments for depression support the monoamine theory, it has long been recognised that this explanation is far from complete. Current research is attempting to elucidate how monoamine signalling relates to other signalling systems in the brain that may be dysfunctional in depression. The observation that the clinical benefit of antidepressant therapy is delayed, despite rapid increases in CNS monoamine concentrations, suggests that more gradual adaptive changes occur as a result of increased monoaminergic neurotransmission. These pharmacologically induced changes are incompletely understood, but they may help to normalise the fundamental dysfunction in intracellular signalling pathways and transduction mechanisms that have been described in depression.

There is evidence for the central role of cAMP response element binding protein (CREB) and brain-derived neurotrophic factor (BDNF) in depression. The monoamine–CREB–BDNF cascade is shown in Figure 22.2. Dysfunction in several steps of the cascade have been described in depression (Box 22.1) Decreased expression and activities of CREB and BDNF have adverse effects on neuronal plasticity which may underlie some of the neuronal deficits identified in people with depression. However, it remains unclear whether dysfunction in this cascade is central to all clinical syndromes of depression, or only occurs in subsets of depressed individuals.

Corticotrophin-releasing factor

In depression, there is also hypersecretion of the 'stressor' peptide corticotrophin-releasing factor (CRF; Ch. 43), which has detrimental effects on neural synaptic plasticity and neurogenesis, and promotes neuronal excitotoxicity (Box 22.1). CRF depresses serotonergic neurotransmission, and is also a neurotransmitter that orchestrates the CNS control of many behavioural, endocrine, autonomic and immunological responses. In people who are genetically predisposed to depression, stress can initiate remodelling and elimination of hippocampal circuits involved in regulation of mood, cognition and behaviour. Many of these circuits involve glutamatergic neurotransmission via the excitatory NMDA (N-methyl-D-aspartate) receptor, which provides a potential target for the treatment of depression. CRF also increases cortisol secretion, which also reduces the expression of BDNF in the hippocampus.

ANTIDEPRESSANT DRUG ACTION

Most of the current clinically used antidepressant drugs target the mechanisms involved in the control of neurotransmitter monoamine turnover or monoamine receptor function. There seems to be little difference in efficacy between drugs that act predominantly on serotonergic or on noradrenergic pathways. The ways that major antidepressants work to modify monoamine turnover and function is shown in Figure 22.1.

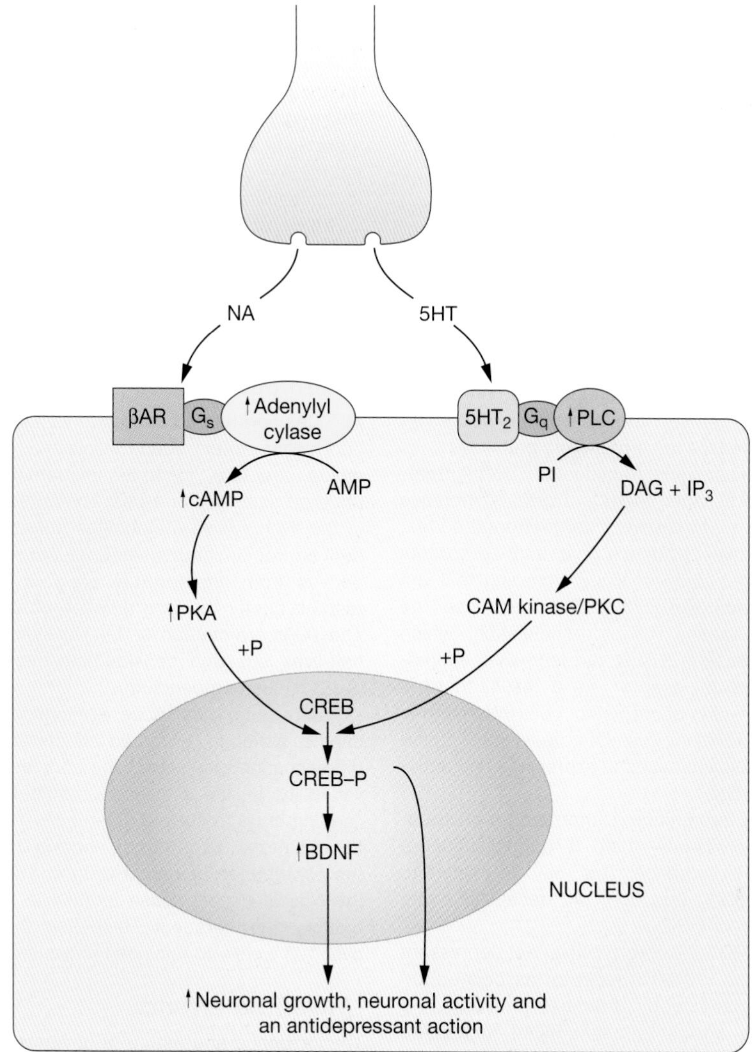

Fig 22.2 **The monoamine–cAMP response element binding protein (CREB)–brain-derived neurotrophic factor (BDNF) cascade.** Only some of the elements involved in this cascade are shown. Adequate levels of CREB-P and BDNF are considered necessary for neuronal growth and plasticity, which may be dysfunctional in depression. These are controlled by amine stimulation. An increase in cAMP can result from noradrenaline acting on β-adrenoceptor subtypes. An increase in DAG can result from serotonin acting on $5HT_2$ type receptors. There is also evidence that serotonin acting on $5HT_4$ and $5HT_7$ receptors can increase cAMP, and noradrenaline acting on α_1-adrenoceptors can increase DAG. Critical points in this cascade may be dysfunctional in subsets of depressed individuals. βAR, β-adrenoceptor; CAM kinase, calmodulin-dependent protein kinase; cAMP, cyclic adenosine monophosphate; DAG, diacylglycerol; IP_3, inositol triphosphate; NA, noradrenaline; PI phosphatidyl inositol; PKA, protein kinase A; PKC, protein kinase C; PLC phospholipase C.

Box 22.1 Some dysfunctional biological processes associated with depression[a]

- Reduced levels of monoamines and altered CNS receptor densities for noradrenaline and serotonin. Decreased CSF levels of serotonin and catecholamine metabolites
- Dysfunction in aspects of the monoamine–CREB–BDNF cascade, including reduced coupling of G_s to adenylyl cyclase, reduced PKA, reduced phosphorylation of CREB (Fig. 22.2)
- Volume loss, neuronal atrophy and cell death in hippocampus and cortex
- Increased cortisol and corticotrophin-releasing factor
- Genetic polymorphisms in $5HT_1$ receptors and tryptophan hydroxylase involved in the synthesis of serotonin

[a]Dysfunction in multiple systems has been identified in depression and only a selection is included here; the dopaminergic, cholinergic, glutamatergic and GABAergic systems also show changes. Research into these dysfunctional aspects has in many cases been carried out in animals and the applicability to humans is not proven. Some of the dysfunctions appear only to apply to particular subsets of people with depression.

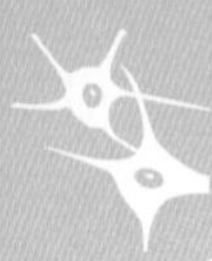

Long-term treatment with antidepressants promotes both the structural and functional integrity of the neural circuits that regulate mood. The mechanisms by which they achieve this are complex.

- Enhanced CNS monoamine levels. The initial action of most drugs used in the treatment of depression is to enhance CNS monoaminergic neurotransmission, and particularly serotonergic neurotransmission. Increased noradrenergic activity enhances serotonergic neurotransmission by stimulating somatodendritic α_1-adrenoceptors on serotonergic neurons. However, although antidepressants rapidly increase synaptic monoamine levels, clinical improvement is delayed. In part, this may be due to slow reduction in the number of upregulated inhibitory somatodendritic and presynaptic $5HT_1$ autoreceptors (see above), which is necessary before activity increases in serotonergic pathways.
- Effects on intracellular signal transduction. During treatment with antidepressants, there is a gradual increase in responsiveness to serotonin in the prefrontal cortex. There is considerable evidence that antidepressants reverse the changes in intracellular signalling that are found in depression (Box 22.1). They enhance the response to monoamine receptor stimulation, which reverses the decrease in CREB and increases expression of BDNF and its receptor. As a result, there is enhanced differentiation of progenitor cells into neurons and increased neuronal survival. Of note, electroconvulsive therapy can also increase the expression and activity of CREB and BDNF.
- Regulation of CRF production. During long-term treatment with antidepressants, there is normalisation of overexpressed CRF secretion. This may be related to upregulation of CNS glucocorticoid receptors, with feedback inhibition of CRF.
- Antagonism of NMDA receptor action. Antidepressant drugs bind to a site in NMDA receptor-associated ion channels in the hippocampus and cerebral cortex, and may protect cells against stress-induced 'glutamate excitotoxicity'.

ANTIDEPRESSANT DRUGS

Tricyclic antidepressant drugs and related compounds

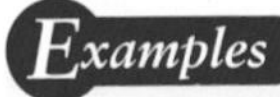

tricyclic compounds: amitriptyline, imipramine, lofepramine
non-tricyclic compounds: amoxapine, maprotiline

Mechanism of action

The first-generation compounds in this class have a triple carbon ring structure (tricyclic antidepressants; TCAs). Many of the newer drugs are structurally unrelated to tricyclic compounds despite having a similar mechanism of action. These include tetracyclic, bicyclic and even non-cyclic structures.

TCAs and related drugs inhibit the reuptake of monoamine neurotransmitters into the presynaptic neuron by competitive inhibition of the ATPase in the membrane monoamine uptake pump (Fig. 22.1). Some drugs show little monoamine selectivity, while other compounds are more selective for one monoamine (Table 22.1). However, the degree of monoamine selectivity has not been shown to influence efficacy.

Many of the unwanted effects of these drugs are a consequence of blockade of other postsynaptic receptors (e.g. muscarinic and histamine H_1 receptors and α_1-adrenoceptors) (Table 22.1), which do not influence their antidepressant action.

Pharmacokinetics

All TCAs and related drugs are well absorbed from the gut and highly protein bound in plasma. Those with a tertiary amine structure, such as imipramine and amitriptyline, undergo extensive first-pass metabolism by demethylation in the liver. Active metabolites (for example, desipramine derived from imipramine and lofepramine, and nortriptyline derived from amitriptyline) are formed and are partially responsible for the long duration of action of these drugs. The TCAs are metabolised in the liver and most have long half-lives but with considerable inter-individual variation (8–90 h; see compendium).

There is no clear dose relationship for the therapeutic effects, although unwanted effects are dose related. This differentiation may reflect the considerable inter-individual variability in the first-pass metabolism of most TCAs (leading to up to 40-fold differences in the plasma concentrations of the parent drug), and the difficulty in quantifying the contribution of parent drug and active metabolites to the clinical effects. Dose titration is usually necessary to optimise the therapeutic response; this should be gradual over 1–2 weeks to minimise unwanted effects.

Unwanted effects

The incidence and nature of unwanted effects vary widely among the different drugs. In general, tertiary amine TCAs have the most α_1-adrenoceptor, histamine H_1 and muscarinic receptor blocking activity, and this is reflected in the frequency of certain unwanted effects with these drugs. See Table 22.1 for the differences among some of the more commonly used drugs.

- Sedation as a result of histamine H_1 and α_1-adrenoceptor blockade (Ch. 39). Some compounds are highly sedative, for example amitriptyline, and others less so, for example amoxapine. Sedation can be useful to help restore sleep patterns in depression (using a larger dose of a sedative drug at night) but can be troublesome or dangerous during the day.
- Antimuscarinic effects (see Ch. 4). Dry mouth is a frequent occurrence, and less commonly constipation, urinary retention, impotence and visual disturbance. Tolerance to these effects can occur, and gradual increases in dose may reduce their incidence.
- Excessive sweating and tremor. The mechanisms behind these effects are uncertain.
- Postural hypotension produced by peripheral α_1-adrenoceptor blockade (Ch. 4) can be particularly troublesome in the elderly, although tolerance can occur.

Table 22.1 Comparative properties of some commonly used antidepressant drugs[a]

	Uptake inhibition	Muscarinic receptor block	$Alpha_1$-adrenoceptor block	Histamine H_1 receptor block	P450-related metabolism[b]	Sedative
TCAs						
Amitriptyline	Serotonin=NA	+++	+++	++++	Inhibition	+++
Imipramine	Serotonin=NA	++	++	+++	Inhibition	++
Amoxapine	Serotonin=NA	+	+++	+++	+	+
Clomipramine	Serotonin>NA	+++	+++	+++	Inhibition	++
Doxepin	Serotonin=NA	++	+++	++++	?	++
Dosulepin	Serotonin=NA	++	+	++	–	++
Lofepramine	NA≫Serotonin	+	+	+	?	+/–
SSRIs						
Citalopram	Serotonin≫NA	0	+	+	Weak inhibition	0
Fluoxetine	Serotonin≫NA	0	0	0	Inhibition	0
Fluvoxamine	Serotonin≫NA	0	0	0	Inhibition	0
Paroxetine	Serotonin>NA	++	+	+	Inhibition	0
Sertraline	Serotonin≫NA	0	++	0	Weak inhibition	0
Other drugs						
Mirtazapine[c]	–	+	+	+++++	Weak inhibition	+
Reboxetine	NA≫Serotonin	Low	Low	Low	–	0
Venlafaxine	Weak NA=Serotonin	0	0	0	Weak inhibition	0
Maprotiline[d]	NA≫Serotonin	+	0	++	+	+
Mianserin[c]	–	+	Low	+++++	+	+
Trazodone[c]	Weak Serotonin	Low	+	+	+	+
Duloxetine	serotonin≥NA	Low	Low	Low	Low	Low

[a]The table is constructed for approximate comparison only and is derived from a number of sources where data are available but mainly from Richelson (2002). The drugs are listed under their major actions or conventional groupings but many of them have mixed actions or their mechanism is uncertain.
[b]Many antidepressants utilise particular isoforms of P450 enzymes for metabolism and this can result in drug interactions. Many are inhibitors of discrete CYP isoforms and this is particularly true for some SSRIs (see Table 2.9). Other antidepressants can be weaker inhibitors of some CYP isoforms. Several are substrates for the CYP2D6 isoform and are subject to polymorphic metabolism.
[c]Serotonin and/or NA pre- or postsynaptic receptor blockade.
[d]Maprotiline has been withdrawn in the UK but is still available in some other countries.
NA, noradrenaline; SSRIs, selective serotonin reuptake inhibitors; TCAs, tricyclic antidepressants.

- Epileptogenic effects. Seizures can be provoked, even when there is no previous clinical history.
- Cardiotoxicity in overdose. Most tricyclic drugs depress myocardial contractility. They can produce tachycardia and severe arrhythmias when taken in overdose, due to both antimuscarinic effects and excessive noradrenergic stimulation. Lofepramine appears to be less cardiotoxic than other drugs in this class.
- Weight gain. Appetite stimulation is common, probably due to histamine H_1 receptor blockade.
- Hyponatraemia from inappropriate antidiuretic hormone (ADH, vasopressin) secretion, leading to drowsiness, confusion and convulsions.
- Sudden withdrawal syndrome. During long-term treatment, doses should be gradually reduced over 4 weeks to avoid agitation, headache, malaise, sweating and gastrointestinal upset, which can accompany sudden withdrawal. These may result from excessive cholinergic activity following prolonged muscarinic receptor blockade.

Drug interactions

Several important drug interactions are recognised. TCAs potentiate the central depressant activity of many drugs, including alcohol. A dangerous interaction can result from giving a monoamine oxidase (MAO) inhibitor (MAOI) (see below) and a TCA together due to prolonged action of the increased serotonin released from the neuron. The interaction can lead to hyperpyrexia, convulsions and coma, and can occur up to 2 weeks after stopping an MAOI due to the long duration of MAO inhibition.

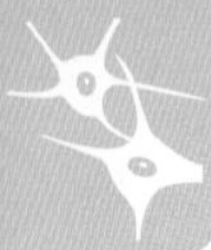

The risk of serious arrhythmias is increased when TCAs are taken with drugs that prolong the Q–T interval on the electrocardiogram (Ch. 8). Such drugs include the class III antiarrhythmic sotalol, and all class I antiarrhythmics.

Selective serotonin reuptake inhibitors and related antidepressants

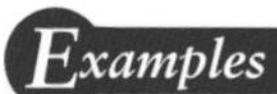

citalopram, fluoxetine, paroxetine, sertraline

Mechanism of action

Unlike the TCAs, the selective serotonin reuptake inhibitors (SSRIs) reduce the neuronal reuptake of serotonin but have less or no effect on noradrenaline reuptake (Table 22.1). They have a more favourable profile of unwanted effects than TCAs because of low affinity for muscarinic and histamine receptors and α_1-adrenoceptors. Paroxetine is unusual in having affinity for muscarinic M_3 receptors, found in the brain, salivary glands and smooth muscle.

The proposed mechanism of action of SSRIs is as follows:

- The increase in synaptic serotonin concentration as a result of reduced neuronal uptake leads to downregulation of the $5HT_1$ somatodendritic and axon terminal presynaptic inhibitory autoreceptors.
- Reduced inhibitory autoreceptor activity increases serotonin release at the axon terminal. The prolonged increase in synaptic serotonin concentration (as a result of both increased release and reduced neuronal uptake) downregulates postsynaptic $5HT_2$ receptors and produces changes in cellular function as described for TCAs.

Pharmacokinetics

SSRIs are well absorbed from the gut and metabolised in the liver. Paroxetine has a long half-life (10–20 h), which is greater in poor metabolisers of CYP2D6 substrates (30–50 h). Citalopram, fluoxetine and sertraline have very long half-lives in the range 23–75 h. Norfluoxetine, the active metabolite of fluoxetine, has a half-life of 6 days, and the resulting very long duration of action can be a disadvantage if an MAOI is used subsequently (see below).

Unwanted effects

In contrast to the TCAs, SSRIs have few antimuscarinic effects (apart from paroxetine), cause little sedation or weight gain, and are not cardiotoxic in overdose. However, they may cause:

- nausea (frequent), dyspepsia, abdominal pain or diarrhoea (less frequent)
- insomnia, anxiety and agitation
- anorexia with weight loss
- rashes
- hyponatraemia due to inappropriate secretion of ADH
- dry mouth and constipation with paroxetine
- sudden withdrawal syndrome after long-term use, which may be most troublesome with paroxetine; it presents in a similar manner to the syndrome after withdrawal of TCAs
- increase in suicidal thoughts in children and adolescents.

Drug interactions

The most serious interaction is with MAOIs (see TCAs above). An interval of 5 weeks is recommended after stopping fluoxetine, or 2 weeks after paroxetine or sertraline, before an MAOI (including selegiline, Ch. 24) is taken. Fluoxetine and other SSRIs inhibit hepatic CYP2D6 (Table 2.9), and this can increase the plasma concentration of drugs metabolised by this enzyme.

Serotonin and noradrenaline reuptake inhibitors (SNRIs)

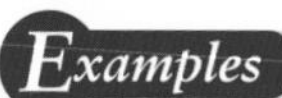

duloxetine, venlafaxine

Mechanism of action and uses

Venlafaxine and duloxetine are classified as a serotonin and noradrenaline reuptake inhibitors (SNRIs) although they have a greater effect on serotonin reuptake at lower doses (Table 22.1). Like the TCAs, they inhibit neuronal reuptake of both serotonin and noradrenaline, but share with SSRIs a low affinity for muscarinic and histamine receptors and α_1-adrenoceptors. Their unwanted-effect profiles are therefore closer to those of the SSRIs than the TCAs. There is limited evidence that clinical improvement with venlafaxine may begin earlier than with other antidepressant drugs.

Duloxetine is also used as an adjunctive treatment for smoking cessation (Ch. 54), and in urinary stress incontinence (Ch. 15).

Pharmacokinetics

Venlafaxine is rapidly absorbed from the gut and undergoes extensive first-pass metabolism in the liver. The main active metabolite has a long half-life (11 h). Duloxetine is well absorbed from the gut and undergoes extensive first-pass metabolism in the liver; its half-life is 9–19 h.

Unwanted effects

- Nausea, vomiting, anorexia, dyspepsia, constipation
- Hypertension, palpitation
- Dry mouth
- Drowsiness, insomnia, dizziness, confusion
- QT-segment prolongation on the ECG which predisposes to ventricular arrhythmias (see Ch. 8); venlafaxine should be avoided in people at high risk of arrhythmias.

Selective noradrenaline reuptake inhibitors (NRIs)

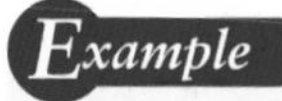

reboxetine

Mechanism of action

Reboxetine is related to fluoxetine but selectively inhibits noradrenaline reuptake. Increased noradrenergic activity at somatodendritic α_1-adrenoceptors enhances serotonergic neurotransmission. Reboxetine, in common with the SSRIs, has little activity at muscarinic and histamine receptors and α_1-adrenoceptors. It therefore has fewer unwanted effects than do TCAs.

Pharmacokinetics

Reboxetine is rapidly absorbed orally. It is eliminated by hepatic metabolism and has a long half-life (15 h).

Unwanted effects

- Nausea, anorexia, constipation
- Palpitation, postural hypotension
- Dry mouth, urinary retention,
- Sweating
- Headache, insomnia, dizziness, paraesthesia.

Presynaptic α_2-adrenoceptor blockers

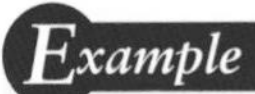

mirtazapine

Mechanism of action

Mirtazapine is a tetracyclic drug unrelated structurally to the TCAs. In addition to potent postsynaptic $5HT_{2C}$ receptor-blocking activity in the cortex (see serotonin receptor blockers below), mirtazapine blocks presynaptic α_2-adrenoceptors (Fig. 22.1). This reduces negative feedback inhibition of serotonin release from raphe nucleus neurons in their terminal projections to regions such as the cortex and hippocampus. Mirtazapine blocks histamine H_1 receptors but has a low affinity for muscarinic receptors and postsynaptic α_1-adrenoceptors. It has minimal effects on monoamine reuptake.

Pharmacokinetics

Mirtazapine is well absorbed from the gut. It is metabolised in the liver and has a very long half-life (20–40 h).

Unwanted effects

- Drowsiness and sedation, especially at lower doses, due to histamine H_1 receptor blockade. At higher doses, increased noradrenergic neurotransmission offsets some of the sedative effects.
- Increased appetite and weight gain.
- Oedema.

Serotonin receptor blockers

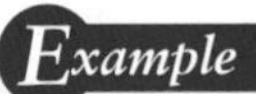

trazodone

Mechanism of action

Trazodone is structurally unrelated to TCAs. The most significant antidepressant action is blockade of postsynaptic $5HT_{2C}$ receptors, which increases activity of dopamine and noradrenaline in the frontal cortex. It also produces weak inhibition of presynaptic serotonin reuptake, but does not inhibit noradrenaline reuptake. Trazodone blocks α_1-adrenoceptors and weakly blocks muscarinic and histamine H_1 receptors.

Pharmacokinetics

Trazodone is well absorbed orally, and metabolised in the liver. The half-life is 7–13 h.

Unwanted effects

- These are similar to those of TCAs, but with fewer antimuscarinic and cardiovascular effects
- Priapism.

Classic (non-selective) monoamine oxidase inhibitors

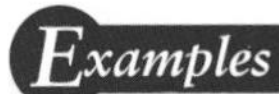

phenelzine, tranylcypromine

Mechanism of action

The mechanism of action of classic (non-selective) MAOIs is complex, but their primary action is to inhibit intracellular MAO, which is the enzyme responsible for degrading free monoamines in the presynaptic nerve terminal. This leads to accumulation of monoamine neurotransmitters in the presynaptic neuron and increased release when the nerve is stimulated (Fig. 22.1). Two MAO isoenzymes have been identified (Fig. 22.3). MAO-B is the predominant enzyme in many parts of the brain, but MAO-A is present in noradrenergic and serotonergic neurons, especially in the locus ceruleus and other cells of the brainstem, as well as being the main enzyme in peripheral tissues. Inhibition of MAO-A in the brain produces the therapeutic effects of these drugs, but classic inhibitors (MAOIs) are not selective for this isoenzyme. Inhibition of both MAO-A and MAO-B in the gut wall and liver also has important consequences (see below). MAOIs also inhibit various drug-metabolising enzymes in the liver, which predisposes to drug interactions but does not contribute to clinical efficacy.

Pharmacokinetics

All drugs in this class are well absorbed from the gut. Structurally, they are either derivatives of hydrazine (e.g. phenelzine) or similar to amfetamine (e.g. tranylcypromine). They are irreversible enzyme inhibitors and therefore their prolonged duration of action is unrelated to the half-life of the drug. Drug withdrawal is followed by gradual restoration of normal MAO activity over about 2 weeks as new enzyme is synthesised.

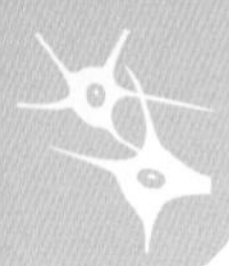

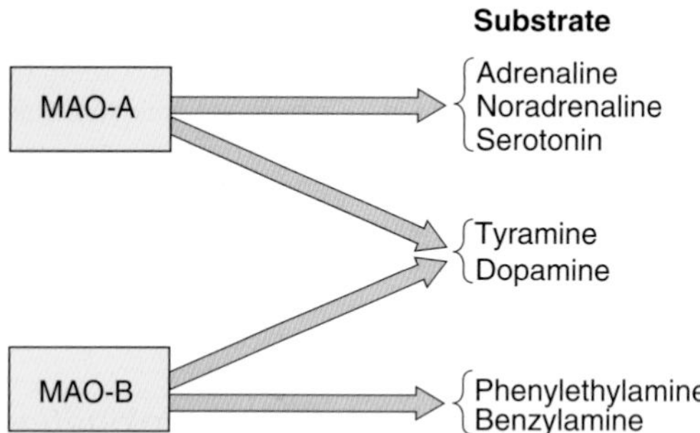

Fig. 22.3 **Actions of monoamine oxidase.** The relative selectivity of the substrates for MAO is shown. MAO-A is the target for drugs useful in treating depression. Non-selective inhibition of both MAO-A and MAO-B blocks the metabolism of tyramine, which is responsible for the food reaction that occurs with these drugs. Reversible inhibition of MAO-A (RIMA) blocks only subtype A. Therefore, tyramine is still metabolised by subtype B and the food reaction is reduced.

Unwanted effects

- Compared with the TCAs, antimuscarinic effects are unusual and there is no predisposition to seizures (except in overdose – see below).
- Dose-related postural hypotension can occur. Unlike with the TCAs, tolerance does not arise. The mechanism may involve conversion of tyramine (normally degraded by MAO) to octopamine, a false neurotransmitter which competes with noradrenaline at sympathetic nerve terminals.
- CNS stimulation with tranylcypromine leads to irritability and insomnia. These are amfetamine-like actions (Ch. 54) and doses should be given early in the day to avoid disturbing sleep.
- Hepatitis is a rare idiosyncratic reaction to the hydrazine derivative phenelzine.
- Acute overdose produces delayed toxic effects after some 12 h. Excessive adrenergic stimulation leads to chest pain, headache and hyperactivity, progressing to confusion and severe hypertension, with eventually profound hypotension and seizures.
- Food interactions can occur because MAO in the gut wall and liver usually prevents the absorption of natural amines, particularly tyramine, which is an indirect-acting sympathomimetic (Ch. 4). If food containing tyramine, for example cheese, yeast extracts (such as Bovril®, Oxo® or Marmite®), pickled herrings, chianti or caviar, or broad bean pods (which contain L-dopa) is eaten, the increased absorption of tyramine and consequently greater release of noradrenaline result in vasoconstriction and severe hypertension. The first indication of this is a throbbing headache. A warning card should be supplied to people who take MAOIs.

Drug interactions

A number of drug interactions can occur. Indirect-acting sympathomimetics (Ch. 4) in cold remedies (e.g. ephedrine, phenylpropanolamine), and L-dopa (treatment of Parkinson's disease, Ch. 24) will be more active, with a risk of hypertensive crisis. The toxicity of the triptans ($5HT_1$ receptor agonists used for treatment of migraine, Ch. 26) and sibutramine (treatment of obesity, Ch. 37) will be potentiated. All these drugs should be avoided for 2 weeks after stopping an MAOI. The combination of MAOIs with TCAs or SSRIs (see above) can be dangerous. Other important interactions occur because MAOIs can impair the hepatic metabolism of certain drugs, especially opioid analgesics.

Reversible inhibitors of monoamine oxidase A (RIMAs)

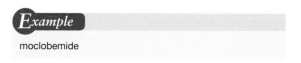

moclobemide

Mechanism of action and effects

Moclobemide is a selective reversible inhibitor of MAO-A (RIMA). This isoenzyme is the target for the antidepressant action of classic MAOIs. If tyramine is absorbed from the gut, MAO-B is able to degrade it, and the food reaction described above for classic MAOIs is very unlikely to occur. Also, since the action of moclobemide on MAO-A is reversible, high concentrations of tyramine will displace the drug from the enzyme, further facilitating degradation of tyramine. If moclobemide is taken after meals, then inhibition of MAO-A in the gut during absorption of tyramine will be minimised, providing further protection. Enzyme inhibition by moclobemide lasts less than 24 h after a single dose.

Pharmacokinetics

Oral absorption is good but there is substantial first-pass metabolism, partially to an active metabolite. Extensive hepatic metabolism gives moclobemide a short half-life (1–2 h).

Unwanted effects

- Sleep disturbance, agitation
- Gastrointestinal upset
- Dizziness, headache
- Dry mouth, visual disturbances
- Oedema.

Drug interactions

Inhibition of cytochrome P450 activity in the liver by cimetidine (Ch. 33) substantially reduces the metabolism of moclobemide, and smaller starting doses are recommended in this situation. Moclobemide should not be given with other antidepressants, and the recommendations for stopping these drugs before prescribing moclobemide are the same as for classic MAOIs.

Melatonin receptor agonist and serotonin receptor antagonist

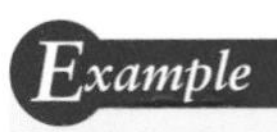

agomelatine

Mechanism of action and effects

Agomelatine is a synthetic agonist of the naturally occurring substance melatonin, which is secreted by the pineal gland and is involved in regulation of circadian rhythms and therefore sleep pattern. Agomelatine is an agonist at both melatonin MT_1 receptors (attenuating alerting signals to the cortex) and MT_2 receptors (producing a phase-shifting action on the circadian rhythm of sleep). Agomelatine significantly improves sleep quality when taken at night to mimic the natural rhythm of melatonin release. It is a weak antagonist at $5HT_{2C}$ receptors (see serotonin receptor blockers above), and has antidepressant efficacy similar to SSRIs.

Pharmacokinetics

Agomelatine is almost completely absorbed from the gut, and undergoes first-pass metabolism. It is metabolised in the liver to derivatives with low affinity for melatonin receptors, and has a short half-life of 1–2 h.

Unwanted effects

- Nausea, bowel disturbances
- Headache dizziness, somnolence

MANAGEMENT OF DEPRESSION

Drugs form only part of the management of depression but are usually necessary for moderate, severe or protracted symptoms. However, in mild to moderate depression, cognitive therapy is as effective as drug treatment and should be tried first. The herbal remedy *Hypericum perforatum* (St John's Wort) is an effective alternative to drug treatment for mild depression, and does not often cause unwanted effects. However, the concentrations of the active constituents vary between different preparations. St John's Wort can induce cytochrome P450, and should not be taken with a prescribed antidepressant. All antidepressant drugs have a delayed onset of action, and people who are severely ill should be considered for electroconvulsive therapy (ECT), which gives a more rapid response.

The TCAs are now less frequently prescribed for depression. They have serious cardiotoxic effects when taken in overdose and should usually be avoided when treating people who are at high risk of attempting suicide. Encouraging adherence to treatment with TCAs may initially be difficult, since antimuscarinic unwanted effects can be troublesome before any benefit is perceived. Starting with a small dose with gradual dose titration is desirable. There is now evidence that large doses of a TCA do not necessarily enhance the treatment response but do increase unwanted effects. The use of low dosages may therefore be preferred.

The newer drugs, for example SSRIs, SNRIs and some drugs related to the TCAs, are no more effective than TCAs and do not work any faster, but they are better tolerated. They are certainly safer than TCAs when there is a high risk of suicide. The use of SSRIs or SNRIs as the first-line treatment for depression is now well established.

Up to 70% of depressed people will respond to drug therapy if the dosage is adequate, compared with about 30% taking placebo. However, only 50% will respond to an individual drug, and up to a further 20% of people with depression will respond if the drug is changed after failure of the initial treatment. Responders show an initial improvement in sleep pattern within a few days. Psychomotor retardation responds more gradually over several days, leading to greater involvement with everyday activities and to enjoyment of life. Improvement in the depressed mood is delayed, beginning up to two or more weeks after commencing treatment with an adequate drug dosage. The response of most symptoms tends to be erratic, with good and bad days.

Initial treatment with an antidepressant should be for 4–6 weeks. If there is no response after this time, and if it is believed that adherence to treatment is not a problem, then either the dose should be increased if unwanted effects permit, or an alternative drug can be substituted. If there is a good response, then the dosage can usually be reduced, but maintenance treatment should be continued for at least 4–6 months after the first episode of depression to minimise the risk of relapse. A longer period of maintenance treatment to prevent recurrence (at least 1 year) is often recommended for the elderly, for others who are at high risk of recurrence, and for people who have experienced two or more depressive episodes. About half of all people who experience depression only have a single episode. In recurrent illness, relapse occurs within a year in up to 65% of those who stop treatment, but only in 15% of people who continue treatment.

Classic MAOIs are usually reserved for atypical depression with hypochondriacal and phobic symptoms, or when TCAs have failed. The therapeutic place of the newer antidepressants such as SNRIs and RIMAs in this situation has yet to be fully established. Small doses of a phenothiazine such as flupentixol (Ch. 21) are sometimes used for treatment of depressed elderly people; evidence for a true antidepressant effect is slight, but some symptoms undoubtedly do improve.

Treatment is most difficult in severe depression, especially if there are psychotic features, or where depression forms part of a bipolar affective disorder (Ch. 21). ECT is used for treatment-resistant depression, and in the elderly who overall are particularly likely to show a response.

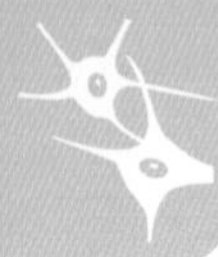

Overall, ECT is probably more effective than drug therapy but does produce some lasting cognitive impairment, especially if given bilaterally rather than unilaterally, or given frequently or with high currents. ECT should be combined with prolonged antidepressant drug treatment. Lithium (Ch. 21) is used for people with severe recurrent depressive episodes and for prophylaxis of bipolar affective disorder. The effect of lithium can take several months to become fully established. The treatment of depression in bipolar disorder is discussed in Chapter 21.

ATTENTION DEFICIT HYPERACTIVITY DISORDER AND NARCOLEPSY

Several drugs with similar mechanisms of action to antidepressants, as well as central stimulant drugs, have limited uses in the management of attention deficit hyperactivity disorder (ADHD) and narcolepsy.

Attention deficit hyperactivity disorder

ADHD is the most common behavioural and cognitive disorder in children of school age, but often remains a problem in adult life. The mechanism is poorly understood, but may involve dopamine deficiency in the prefrontal cortex. There are three subtypes:

- predominantly inattentive subtype: failing to pay attention to details, difficulty with sustained attention, disorganisation and forgetfulness
- predominantly hyperactive-impulsive subtype: excessive fidgeting and squirming, restlessness, frequently interrupting and intruding on others
- predominantly inattentive/hyperactive-impulsive subtype: features of both subtypes in two areas of life and causing dysfunction in at least one area.

Adults with ADHD often present with poor occupational performance, marital instability, poor self-discipline or self-organisation, and restlessness. Sleep disturbances may also be prominent.

Narcolepsy

Narcolepsy usually begins in adolescence and is characterised by overwhelming daytime sleepiness, even if nighttime sleep has been adequate. Sudden daytime naps are frequent and there may be prolonged periods of drowsiness. Hallucinations may be troublesome on falling asleep or awakening. The condition may coexist with cataplexy, characterised by sudden loss of muscle function ranging from weakness to collapse that is often precipitated by laughter. People with narcolepsy have an abnormal sleep pattern, with rapid eye movement sleep at the onset of sleep rather than after a period of non-rapid eye movement sleep (Ch. 20). Narcolepsy has a genetic predisposition and there may be an autoimmune component. There is some evidence for an abnormality of orexin neurotransmission in the hypothalamus. Orexins can regulate wakefulness (see modafinil, mechanism of action below).

DRUGS FOR ATTENTION DEFICIT HYPERACTIVITY DISORDER AND NARCOLEPSY

Atomoxetine

Mechanism of action

Atomoxetine is a selective inhibitor of presynaptic neuronal uptake of noradrenaline. There is a secondary increase in dopaminergic activity in the prefrontal cortex. It has antidepressant activity, but the mechanism of action in ADHD is not known.

Pharmacokinetics

Atomoxetine is well absorbed from the gut. It is metabolised in the liver and has a half-life of 6 h in most individuals (extensive metabolisers), but 19 h in poor metabolisers of CYP2D6 substrates.

Unwanted effects

- Anorexia, dry mouth, nausea, vomiting, abdominal pain, constipation
- Palpitation, hypertension, postural hypotension
- Sleep disturbance, dizziness, headache, fatigue, irritability, depression, tremor
- Urinary retention, sexual dysfunction.

Methylphenidate

Mechanism of action

Methylphenidate activates the brainstem arousal system, but the mechanism is not established. There is evidence that the drug blocks the presynaptic reuptake of noradrenaline and dopamine, and increases dopaminergic neurotransmission in the prefrontal cortex.

Pharmacokinetics

Methylphenidate is well absorbed from the gut. It is metabolised in the liver and has a short half-life (3 h).

Unwanted effects

- Dry mouth, nausea, vomiting, abdominal pain
- Palpitation, hypertension, postural hypotension
- Sleep disturbance, dizziness, headache, fatigue, irritability, depression
- Fever, arthralgia, rash.

Dexamfetamine

The effects of dexamfetamine are discussed in Chapter 54.

Unwanted effects

- Sleep disturbance, dizziness, headache, fatigue, irritability, depression, tremor, seizures, psychosis
- Anorexia, dry mouth, gastrointestinal upset
- Palpitation, hypertension
- Tolerance and dependence.

Modafinil

Mechanism of action

Modafinil blocks the presynaptic reuptake of noradrenaline and dopamine, increasing dopaminergic neurotransmission in the prefrontal cortex. There is also evidence that modafinil activates orexin-releasing neurons in the hypothalamus and may also increase histamine release in the brain. Orexins (also known as hypocretins) are neurotransmitters that regulate wakefulness by releasing dopamine and noradrenaline, which excite histaminergic tuberomammillary neurons.

Pharmacokinetics

Modafinil is well absorbed from the gut. It is metabolised in the liver and has a long half-life of 15 h.

Unwanted effects

- Anorexia, dry mouth, nausea, dyspepsia, abdominal pain, diarrhoea
- Palpitation, chest pain
- Sleep disturbance, dizziness, confusion, agitation, depression.

MANAGEMENT OF ATTENTION DEFICIT HYPERACTIVITY DISORDER

Behaviour management and psychotherapy have a role, but are more effective when combined with drug treatment. However, there is some concern that the benefits of the currently available compounds may be short-lived, with loss of efficacy after about 3 years. Methylphenidate is usually the first choice, while dexamfetamine can be tried if there is no improvement with methylphenidate. Atomoxetine is used when stimulant drugs are ineffective.

MANAGEMENT OF NARCOLEPSY

Planned short naps may avoid the need for drug treatment, but drowsiness may require use of a CNS stimulant. Dexamfetamine or modafinil are usually chosen, but methylphenidate may be helpful. Cataplexy can respond to a tricyclic antidepressant or selective serotonin reuptake inhibitors.

FURTHER READING

Depression

Alexopoulos GS (2005) Depression in the elderly. *Lancet* 365, 1961–1970

Anderson IM, Nutt DJ, Deakin JFW (2000) Evidence-based guidelines for treating depressive disorder with antidepressants: a revision of the 1993 British Association for Psychopharmacology guidelines. *J Psychopharmacol* 14, 3–20

Belmaker RH, Agam G (2008) Major depressive disorder. *N Engl J Med* 358, 55–68

Cryan JF, Leonard BE (2000) $5HT_{1A}$ and beyond: the role of serotonin and its receptors in depression and the antidepressant response. *Hum Psychopharmacol Clin Exp* 15, 113–135

Donati RJ, Rasenick MM (2003) G-protein signaling and the molecular basis of antidepressant action. *Life Sci* 73, 1–17

Duman RS (2004) Role of neurotrophic factors in the etiology and treatment of mood disorders. *Neuromolecular Med* 5, 11–25

Ebmeier, KB, Donaghey C, Steele JD (2006) Recent developments and current controversies in depression. *Lancet* 367, 153–167

Furukawa TA, McGuire H, Barbui C (2002) Meta-analysis of effects and side effects of low dosage tricyclic antidepressants in depression: systematic review. *BMJ* 325, 991–995

Geddes JR, Carney SM, Davies C et al (2003) Relapse prevention with antidepressant drug treatment in depressive disorders: a systematic review. *Lancet* 361, 653–661

Leonard BE (2001) The immune system, depression and the action of antidepressants. *Prog Neuropsychopharmacol Biol Psychiatry* 25, 767–780

Mann JJ (2005) The medical management of depression. *N Engl J Med* 353, 1819–1834

Millan MJ (2006) Multi-target strategies for the improved treatment of depressive states: conceptual foundations and neuronal substrates, drug discovery and therapeutic application. *Pharmacol Ther* 110, 135–370

Nair A, Vaidya VA (2006) Cyclic AMP response element binding protein and brain derived neurotrophic factor: molecules that modulate our mood. *J Biosci* 31, 423–434

Nemeroff CB, Gutman DA (2007) Neurobiology of depression and treatment strategies. *http://www.medscape.com/viewarticle/441626* (accessed April 2008)

Richelson E (2002) The clinical relevance of antidepressant interaction with neurotransmitter transporters and receptors. *Psychopharmacol Bull* 36, 133–150

Rosenzweig-Lipson S, Beyer CE, Hughes ZA et al (2006) Differentiating antidepressants of the future: efficacy and safety. *Pharmacol Ther* 113, 134–153

Shelton RC (2007) The molecular biology of depression. *Psychiatr Clin North Am* 30, 1–11

Skolnick P (2002) Beyond monoamine-based therapies: clues to new approaches. *J Clin Psychiatry* 63(suppl 2), 19–23

Timonen M, LiuKonen T (2008) Management of depression in adults. *BMJ* 336, 435–439

Young LT, Bakish D, Beaulieu S (2002) The neurobiology of treatment response to antidepressants and mood stabilizing medications. *J Psychiatry Neurosci* 27, 260–265

Narcolepsy and ADHD

Jamdar S, Sathyamoorthy BT (2007) Management of attention deficit/hyperactivity disorder. *Br J Hosp Med* 68, 360–366

Keam S, Walker MC (2007) Therapies for narcolepsy with or without cataplexy: evidence-based review. *Curr Opin Neurol* 20, 699–703

Pliszka SR (2007) Pharmacologic treatment of attention-deficit/hyperactivity disorder: efficacy, safety and mechanisms of action. *Neuropsychol Rev* 17, 61–72

Young TJ, Silber MH (2006) Hypersomnias of central origin. *Chest* 130, 913–920

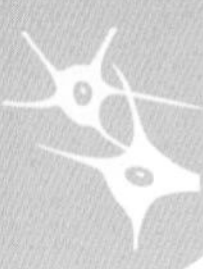

SELF-ASSESSMENT

In questions 1–4, the first statement, in italics, is true. Are the accompanying statements also true?

1. *Despite the fact that the monoamine hypothesis does not adequately explain all the processes of depression, alteration of monoamine transmission remains the mainstay of successful drug treatment.*
   a. Downregulation of $5HT_2$ receptors occurs during antidepressant treatment.
   b. Most TCAs inhibit the reuptake of noradrenaline and serotonin equally.
   c. TCAs have a less satisfactory therapeutic ratio than do SSRIs.
2. *Statistically, inhibitors of noradrenaline or serotonin reuptake are equally effective as antidepressants.*
   a. Lofepramine is more cardiotoxic than amitriptyline.
   b. Co-administration of an SSRI and an MAOI can cause cardiovascular collapse.
3. *Antidepressants include compounds such as trazodone, which act mainly by blocking serotonin receptors.*
   a. Trazodone is an antidepressant that is only a weak inhibitor of monoamine reuptake.
   b. Venlafaxine has marked sedative and antimuscarinic actions.
   c. Venlafaxine has a low incidence of cardiovascular toxicity.
4. *During antidepressant treatment, only 30–40% of people with depression improve as a result of the drug.*
   a. TCAs potentiate the central depressant effects of alcohol.
   b. The half-life of lithium is about 30 min.
   c. Lithium is only used for treatment of bipolar affective disorder.
5. Which one of the following statements concerning antidepressant drugs is the **most appropriate**?
   A. A TCA would be more suitable than an SSRI for a patient with urinary outflow problems due to benign prostate hypertrophy.
   B. A drug that blocks muscarinic receptors would be a more effective antidepressant than one that blocks serotonin receptors.
   C. People taking moclobemide are likely to get an adverse reaction if they eat cheese.
   D. An SSRI would be more suitable than a TCA to treat a person with serious depression and suicidal tendencies.
   E. Increase in brain monoamine levels occurs only after 4–5 weeks treatment with a TCA.
6. Which is the one **most appropriate** statement concerning the antidepressant venlafaxine?
   A. It is a $5HT_2$ receptor antagonist.
   B. It inhibits the neuronal reuptake of noradrenaline and serotonin.
   C. It has potent antimuscarinic activity.
   D. It does not exhibit drug interactions with MAOIs.
   E. It has a low incidence of cardiovascular toxicity.
7. Case history questions

DW, a 30-year-old female financier, was a former Olympic athlete. In 2000 she was appointed manager of the Emerging Countries Fund of a large Unit Trust Company. In early 2005 the company was taken over and DW had a new boss and was moved to assistant manager of the Fund. From 2005 to 2006 she had put on 10 kg in weight, and in January 2006 started a strict diet and worked out at a gym four times a week. In June 2006 she visited her GP with a 6-month history of increasing insomnia, lack of concentration, irritability and anxiety. She had begun to withdraw from a busy social calendar and was becoming indecisive. This was now affecting her work. For the previous 4 weeks she had had recurrent thoughts of suicide. She had also lost 4 kg in weight during that period. The GP diagnosed that she was depressed, arranged a psychiatric consultation for her and started her on a TCA.

   a. What are the risk factors for depression? Was DW at risk prior to the diagnosis?
   b. What neurochemical and receptor changes are associated with depressive illness?
   c. Are TCAs an appropriate first choice of drug for this patient?
   d. What are the unwanted effects of TCAs?
   e. How successful is antidepressant treatment?
   f. After therapy for 3 months and some improvement, DW decided that the side effects of the TCAs were unacceptable. What alternative antidepressant therapies could be given and what are the unwanted effects?

ANSWERS

1. a. **True**. Downregulation of $5HT_2$ receptors parallels the time course of improvement of clinical condition, whereas the time course of the increase in amine transmitters does not.
   b. **False**. Different TCAs vary widely in their abilities to independently affect noradrenaline and serotonin reuptake.
   c. **True**. TCAs have a greater potential to produce serious unwanted effects, e.g. causing cardiac arrhythmias in acute overdose. Lofepramine has a lower incidence of unwanted effects than does most other TCAs.
2. a. **False**. Lofepramine is among the least cardiotoxic of the tricyclic and related antidepressants.
   b. **True**. An MAOI and an SSRI should not be combined. The combination can cause CNS excitation, tremor and hyperthermia. An MAOI should not be started until 1–5 weeks after stopping the SSRI, depending upon which SSRI has been taken.
3. a. **True**. Trazodone blocks $5HT_2$ receptors and is a weak inhibitor of serotonin reuptake.
   b. **False**. Although, like TCAs, venlafaxine inhibits both noradrenaline and serotonin reuptake, it lacks the sedative and antimuscarinic effects of TCAs.

c. **False**. Venlafaxine is associated with an increased incidence of cardiovascular events in high-risk depressed people such as those with uncontrolled blood pressure.

4. a. **True**. Alcohol should not be consumed by people taking TCAs.
   b. **False**. The half-life of lithium is long (about 24 h).
   c. **False**. Although it is most commonly used in bipolar affective disorder, it is also used in those with severe recurrent depressive episodes that do not respond to other treatment.
5. Answer **D**.
   A. Many TCAs have antimuscarinic activity, which could exacerbate urinary retention.
   B. This statement is false, as the antidepressant activity resides in the ability of the drugs to block serotonin receptors and not muscarinic receptors.
   C. Moclobemide is a selective reversible inhibitor of MAO-A, and has relatively little effect on MAO-B. As both MAO-A and MAO-B metabolise tyramine in cheese, which is the source of the hypertension in the 'cheese reaction', tyramine would be effectively metabolised.
   D. Generally, an SSRI is more suitable than most TCAs in this situation because of the lower toxicity in overdose. The effectiveness of the drugs is not different. Some TCAs, however, such as lofepramine, have a low toxicity in overdose despite being a tricyclic structure.
   E. This is false. The increase in brain monoamine levels occurs in hours to days following treatment with a TCA. However, the effect on behaviour, mood and the depression may take 4–6 weeks or longer to come into play.
6. Answer **B**.
   A. **False.** Venlafaxine is predominantly an inhibitor of reuptake of noradrenaline and serotonin. It has little activity in blocking the serotonin receptors.
   B. **True.** Venlafaxine is generally considered to be in the class of the serotonin and noradrenaline reuptake inhibitors, although it does have a greater effect on serotonin reuptake.
   C. **False.** Venlafaxine has relatively little activity in blocking muscarinic receptors.
   D. **False.** Venlafaxine increases monoamines in the synaptic clefts, as does an MAOI. These two drugs can, therefore, exacerbate each other's action on monoamine levels.
   E. **False.** Warnings have been issued to restrict the use of venlafaxine in high-risk groups as increased cardiovascular events have been recorded.
7. Case history answers
   a. Risk factors include gender (more frequent in women), age (peak age 20–40 years), family history of depression, marital status (higher rates in separated and divorced) and stress. It is possible, but we cannot be certain, that any of the circumstances in the clinical history were contributory to her depression.
   b. There is a biological association of depression with reduced CNS monoaminergic neurotransmission, notably noradrenaline and serotonin, but it is still unclear whether this is cause or effect. Drugs that deplete monoamines can induce depression, and when monoamines are replete, symptoms decrease. Probably because of the depletion of monoamines, there is an upregulation of postsynaptic monoamine receptors. These include $5HT_2$ and α_1-adrenoceptors; β_1-adrenoceptors may also be upregulated. Drugs used to treat depression increase CNS serotonin and/or noradrenaline in the synaptic cleft, which eventually results in receptor downregulation and a return to normal in the postsynaptic receptor numbers. There are also dysfunctions in other CNS signalling systems (see text).
   c. TCAs may not be the most appropriate choice if DW was showing suicidal tendencies. Their safety is low and a better choice would be an SSRI.
   d. Unwanted effects include muscarinic receptor blockade (dry mouth, blurred vision, constipation), cardiotoxicity, sedation (variable) and postural hypotension.
   e. The onset of action is delayed for at least 2–4 weeks. Two-thirds of depressed people improve, one-third do not. One-third of people with depression would have got better without drug therapy. Whether TCAs prevent recurrence is unknown.
   f. Alternative treatments include SSRIs such as fluoxetine. This has fewer unwanted effects such as cardiotoxicity and antimuscarinic actions, but causes nausea, insomnia and agitation in some patients. Its antidepressant action is no better than that of TCAs. Other possibilities are MAOIs, which have considerable unwanted effects and require dietary restriction of tyramine (cheese) intake; they are less used now. RIMAs (e.g. moclobemide) are selective for inhibition of the MAO-A isoenzyme, leaving type B unaltered, and this is able to metabolise tyramine. Drugs previously called atypical antidepressants act partially by blocking monoamine receptors. Trazodone blocks postsynaptic $5HT_2$ receptors and has only a small effect on the inhibition of serotonin reuptake.

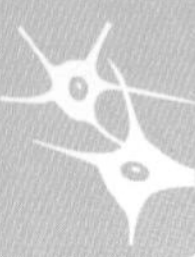

Drugs used to treat depression

Drug	Half-life (h)	Comments
Depression		
Tricyclic antidepressants (TCAs) and related compounds		
Most show high apparent volumes of distribution (Ch. 2) (10–50 L kg^{-1} body weight), which explains the combination of high first-pass metabolism and high clearance but a long elimination half-life; given orally		
Amitriptyline	10–28 [M] Bioavailability is 30–60%; oxidised by hepatic CYP3A4-mediated demethylation to nortriptyline (see below), which has a slightly longer half-life	Particularly useful when sedation is required; also used for nocturnal enuresis in children, for neuropathic pain and for prophylaxis of migraine
Amoxapine	8–14 [M] Bioavailability is 18–54%; metabolised to hydroxy compounds which are eliminated as conjugates; 8-hydroxy-amoxapine is active and has a longer half-life (30 h) and is present at twofold greater concentrations than amoxapine during repeated dosage	
Clomipramine	12–36 [M] Oral bioavailability is about 50%; oxidised by demethylation followed by hydroxylation and conjugation; selective and potent inhibitor of serotonin uptake	Also used for phobic and obsessive states
Dosulepin	11–40 [M] Bioavailability has not been defined; oxidised by demethylation and S-oxidation	Particularly useful when sedation is required
Doxepin	8–25 [M] Bioavailability is about 30%; extensive demethylation in the liver by the polymorphic CYP2D6 to the active desmethyl metabolite, which has a half-life of 30–50 h; subjects who are poor metabolisers are at increased risk of unwanted effects	Particularly useful when sedation is required
Imipramine	8–20 [M] Bioavailability is about 50%; metabolised by demethylation to an active metabolite (desipramine) and by hydroxylation; desipramine is metabolised by CYP2D6	Also used for nocturnal enuresis in children
Lofepramine	5 [M] Undergoes extensive first-pass metabolism but absolute bioavailability is not known; metabolised to desipramine, which is probably responsible for much of the activity	
Maprotiline	30–60 [M] Oral bioavailability is 40–70%; extensively metabolised, with metabolites eliminated in urine and bile; the desmethyl metabolite retains activity	Tetracyclic compound; particularly useful when sedation is required; discontinued in the UK in 2006 but still available in the USA
Mianserin	10–20 [M] Oral bioavailability is 20–30%; major metabolite is desmethyl compound (demethylation product) which has weak α_2-adrenoceptor agonist properties	Tetracyclic compound; also acts by blocking postsynaptic $5HT_2$ receptors; particularly useful when sedation is required; risk of neutropenia and aplastic anaemia in elderly
Nortriptyline	18–90 [M] Bioavailability is 50–60%; oxidised by CYP2D6 to a 10-hydroxy metabolite (which retains some activity) that is conjugated and excreted; CYP2D6 poor metabolisers have higher plasma concentrations of the parent drug but do not show an increased incidence of unwanted effects	Also used for nocturnal enuresis in children and for neuropathic pain
Trazodone	7–13 [M] Complete oral bioavailability (100%); rapidly metabolised by CYP3A4 oxidation to an active metabolite (that has higher plasma concentrations than the parent compound)	Particularly useful when sedation is required; tetracyclic compound
Trimipramine	20–26 [M] Bioavailability is 40%; metabolised by demethylation and hydroxylation catalysed by multiple P450 isoenzymes; the desmethyl metabolite is active but is present only at low concentrations	Particularly useful when sedation is required

Drugs used to treat depression

Drug	Half-life (h)	Comments
Selective serotonin (5-hydroxytryptamine, 5-HT) reuptake inhibitors (SSRIs)		
Given orally		
Citalopram	23–75 [M + R] Oral bioavailability is 80%; oxidised in liver by CYP3A4 and CYP2C19 to a range of metabolites, some of which retain weak activity; weak inhibitor of, but not a substrate for, CYP2D6; about 20% cleared by the kidneys	Also used for panic disorder
Escitalopram	27–32 [M + R] Oxidised in liver mostly by CYP3A4 and CYP2C19; about 8% cleared by the kidneys	Also used for panic disorder; an isomer of citalopram
Fluoxetine	48–72 [M] Essentially complete bioavailability; metabolised by CYP2D6; poor metabolisers have a twofold longer half-life and excrete more of the parent compound in the urine; the major desmethyl metabolite (norfluoxetine) is as active as the parent drug and has a longer half-life (6 days); both parent drug and metabolite are potent inhibitors of CYP2D6 (which metabolises desipramine)	Also used for bulimia nervosa and obsessive-compulsive disorder
Fluvoxamine	7–70 [M] High oral bioavailability (absolute bioavailability is not known); extensively metabolised by oxidation (not by CYP2D6)	Also used for obsessive-compulsive disorder
Paroxetine	10–20 (EM) 30–50 (PM) [M] Good but variable absorption; eliminated by CYP2D6-catalysed oxidation; the half-life in poor metabolisers (PM) is longer than in extensive metabolisers (EM); the metabolites are inactive; during repeated dosage the steady-state plasma concentrations are similar in EM and PM subjects because CYP2D6 is saturated in both groups, and other non-saturated enzymes (e.g. CYP3A4) determine the clearance	Also used for obsessive-compulsive disorder, panic disorder, social phobia, post-traumatic stress disorder and generalised anxiety disorder
Sertraline	26 [M] Oral bioavailability is low and increased if given with food (absolute bioavailability is not known); undergoes hepatic demethylation and oxidation to largely inactive metabolites	Also used for obsessive-compulsive disorder and post-traumatic stress disorder
Serotonin and noradrenaline reuptake inhibitors (SNRIs)		
Given orally		
Duloxetine	9–19 [M] Good oral absorption; high apparent volume of distribution contributes to long half-life; eliminated by hepatic metabolism to a number of inactive metabolites	Also used in diabetic neuropathy and stress urinary incontinence (Ch. 15)
Venlafaxine	5 [M] Low oral bioavailability (about 40%) due to first-pass metabolism; oxidised by hepatic CYP2D6 to the active *O*-desmethyl metabolite which is responsible for much of the therapeutic activity and has a longer half-life (11 h); other minor metabolites, such as the N-desmethyl metabolite, are inactive	Also used for generalised anxiety disorder
Classic (non-selective) monoamine oxidase inhibitors (MAOIs)		
Given orally		
Isocarboxazid	2–3 [M] Essentially complete bioavailability; rapidly hydrolysed by esterases; duration of action is measured in days; slow onset of clinical action (weeks)	
Phenelzine	1 [M] Extensively absorbed; rapidly metabolised by N-acetylation; produces profound and prolonged inhibition of MAO with a slow onset of clinical action (weeks)	

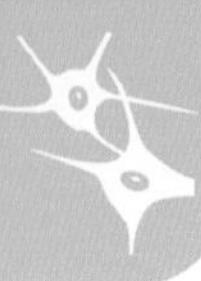

Drugs used to treat depression

Drug	Half-life (h)	Comments
Tranylcypromine	2–3 [M] Extensively absorbed; metabolised by oxidation, N-acetylation and N-glucuronidation (a rare metabolic reaction); onset of action is more rapid than for the other drugs in this group	
Reversible inhibitors of monoamine oxidase A (RIMAs)		
Given orally		
Moclobemide	1–2 [M] Bioavailability is about 50%; numerous metabolites formed; metabolised by polymorphic CYP2C19 (CYP2C19 metabolises mephenytoin); in poor metabolisers of mephenytoin (low CYP2C19) the half-life of moclobemide is 4 h, compared with 2 h in extensive metabolisers of mephenytoin (high CYP2C19)	Also used for social phobia
Other antidepressant drugs		
Agomelatine	1–2 [M] Bioavailability 80%	Agonist at melatonin receptors and a weak antagonist at $5HT_{2C}$ receptors. Also anxiolytic properties. Administered orally
Given orally		
Flupentixol	35 [M] Bioavailability is about 40%; parent drug undergoes enterohepatic circulation following biliary excretion as a glucuronide	Particularly useful for associated psychoses
Lithium	8–45 [R] Complete oral absorption; filtered at the glomerulus and reabsorbed (about 80%) in the proximal, but not distal, parts of the renal tubule	Used for severe recurrent depressive episodes and for prophylaxis of bipolar affective disorder
Mirtazapine	20–40 [M] Bioavailability is about 50%; metabolised by oxidation followed by glucuronidation; metabolised by CYP2D6 and CYP3A4	Principal action is inhibition of central presynaptic α_2-adrenoceptors and blocking of postsynaptic $5HT_2$ receptors
Reboxetine	15 [M + R] Complete oral bioavailability; oxidised by hepatic CYP3A4 plus some renal clearance (10%)	Selective inhibitor of noradrenaline uptake
Tryptophan	2 [M] Actively absorbed from the intestinal tract and transported across the blood–brain barrier (in competition with other amino acids); undergoes decarboxylation and deamination	Very restricted hospital use as an adjunct to conventional treatments
Drugs used to treat attention deficit hyperactivity disorder (ADHD) or ADHD and narcolepsy		
All drugs given orally		
Atomoxetine	6 (EM) 19 (PM) [M] Rapidly absorbed; metabolised by CYP2D6; poor metabolisers (PM) of CYP2D6 substrates (see Ch. 2) have a 50% higher oral bioavailability and 10-fold lower clearance which result in 10-fold higher plasma levels	
Dexamfetamine	6–12 [R + M] Rapidly and completely absorbed; eliminated unchanged in urine (pH-dependent) plus deamination in the liver	Also used for narcolepsy
Methylphenidate	3 [M] Well absorbed orally; metabolised by hepatic de-esterification	Also used for narcolepsy
Modafinil	10–15 [M] Rapid absorption; a racemic compound with the D-isomer eliminated three times faster; metabolised in the liver via deamination, S-oxidation, hydroxylation and glucuronide conjugation	Used primarily for daytime sleepiness
Sodium oxybate	? [M] Rapid but incomplete (25%) absorption probably due to saturable first-pass metabolism	The sodium salt of gamma-hydroxybutyric acid or 'GHB'; given orally

[M], metabolism; [R], renal excretion.

23 Epilepsy

PATHOLOGICAL BASIS OF EPILEPSY

Epilepsy affects 0.1% of the population and is characterised by recurrent epileptic seizures without any immediate provoking cause. Epileptic seizures are sudden, transient and usually unpredictable episodes of motor, sensory, autonomic or psychic disturbance triggered by abnormal neuronal discharges in the brain. The clinical manifestations depend on the site of the discharge.

- In *partial or focal seizures*, the discharge starts in a localised area of the brain and may remain localised or may secondarily spread to affect the whole brain.
- In *generalised seizures*, the abnormal discharge affects the whole of the brain (Table 23.1).

Identification of the type of seizure is important in the selection of the most appropriate therapy.

The origin of epilepsy is complex. For most people with epilepsy, structural damage in the brain, such as that resulting from trauma, tumours, cerebrovascular disease or haemorrhage, may provide the initial focus of abnormal neuronal activity. Seizures may also be caused by metabolic disturbance, such as hypoglycaemia or alcohol abuse. There is a large genetic component in about 30% of cases where there is no identifiable structural or metabolic disorder (idiopathic epilepsy).

NEUROTRANSMITTERS AND EPILEPSY

Coordinated activity among neurons depends on a controlled balance between excitatory and inhibitory influences on the electrical activity across neuronal cell membranes. An epileptic seizure probably arises from a localised imbalance between excitatory neurotransmission, principally mediated by glutamate, and inhibitory neurotransmission, mediated by gamma-aminobutyric acid (GABA), which leads to a focus of neuronal instability. Neuronal networks cooperate by oscillatory electrical activity between different parts of the brain. Generalised epilepsy involves a change from these oscillations to abnormally synchronised activity across large-scale neuronal networks, in particular involving both the cortex and subcortical structures such as the thalamus. Structural changes in neuronal networks in the brain are often found in people with epilepsy and this may provide the basis for generation of the abnormal discharges. These include an increase in excitatory axons; a loss in excitatory neurons whose specific action is to control inhibitory neurons also occurs and a loss of inhibitory neurons.

In healthy neuronal circuits, depolarising inward Na^+ and Ca^{2+} ionic currents (e.g. activated by glutamate receptors) are balanced by repolarising outward K^+ currents (e.g. activated by $GABA_B$ receptors). Influx of Cl^- ions into the neuron, produced by $GABA_A$ receptor activation, hyperpolarises the cell, and inhibits impulse generation. Membrane-bound ATPase pumps also act to maintain the correct resting membrane potential by active transport of ions across the cell membrane (Ch. 8). Any defect in these currents that results in incomplete repolarisation of the cell will leave the neuron closer to its threshold potential for firing, and create a hyperexcitable state. This instability could initiate the burst of firing that produces epileptiform activity. Once an electrical discharge is triggered, spontaneous repetitive firing of the focus is maintained by a feedback mechanism known as post-tetanic potentiation. Several inherited epilepsy syndromes have now been characterised at a cellular level, and arise from mutations of proteins involved in ion channel function. Reduction in the activity of membrane-bound ATPases linked to neuronal transmembrane ion pumps has also been found in the brains of people with primary generalised epilepsy. Ion channel dysfunction may therefore provide the basis for the genesis of many types of generalised seizures. The genesis of partial seizures is less well understood. These arise from focal lesions in the brain that promote formation of abnormal hyperexcitable circuits. These circuits may be enhanced by disruption of glial cell function and changes in the neuronal microenvironment.

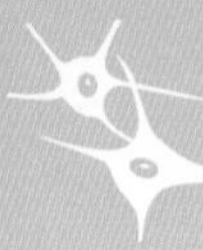

Table 23.1 Simplified classification of epileptic seizures

Seizure type	Characteristics
Partial (focal) seizures	
Simple partial seizures	Motor, somatosensory or psychic symptoms; consciousness is not impaired
Complex partial seizures	Temporal lobe, psychomotor; consciousness is impaired
Secondary generalised seizures	These begin as partial seizures
Generalised seizures	Affect whole brain with loss of consciousness
Clonic, tonic, or tonic–clonic	Initial rigid extensor spasm, respiration stops, defecation, micturition and salivation occur (tonic phase, ~1 min); violent synchronous jerks (clonic phase, 2–4 min)
Myoclonic	Seizures of a muscle or group of muscles
Absence	Abrupt loss of awareness of surroundings, little motor disturbance (occur in children)
Atonic	Loss of muscle tone/strength
Unclassified seizures	

ANTIEPILEPTIC DRUGS

Most antiepileptic drugs act either by blockade of depolarising ion channels, or by enhancing the inhibitory actions of GABA.

Carbamazepine and oxcarbazepine

Mechanism of action and uses

Carbamazepine and oxcarbazepine are effective in most types of epilepsy, *except for myoclonic epilepsy and absences, which they can exacerbate.* Their mechanisms of action are incompletely understood, and may include:

- use-dependent blockade of Na^+ channels which inhibits repetitive neuronal firing; this is probably the principal mechanism
- attenuation of the action of glutamate at NMDA (N-methyl-D-aspartate) receptors, and reduced glutamate release.

Carbamazepine and oxcarbazepine are also used in the management of trigeminal neuralgia (Ch. 19), and carbamazepine in the management of bipolar disorder (Ch. 21).

Pharmacokinetics

Absorption of carbamazepine is slow and incomplete after oral administration. It is metabolised in the liver to an active epoxide metabolite that is present in plasma at lower concentrations than the parent drug. The half-life of carbamazepine is initially very long, at about 1.5 days, but decreases by two-thirds over the first 2 to 3 weeks of treatment because of 'autoinduction' of its own metabolism in the liver. Seizure control may then require an increase in dose. The plasma or salivary concentration of carbamazepine correlates well with its clinical efficacy, but the substantial fluctuations in plasma concentration between doses make interpretation of a single value difficult. Transient unwanted neurological effects, which may occur in association with the peak plasma drug concentration when using the conventional formulation of carbamazepine, are minimised by the use of a modified-release formulation.

Oxcarbazepine is well absorbed orally and is rapidly and extensively converted in the liver to an active metabolite with a half-life of 9 h.

Unwanted effects

The unwanted effects with oxcarbazepine are less severe than with carbamazepine.

- Nausea and vomiting (especially early in treatment), constipation, diarrhea, anorexia.
- Rashes, especially transient generalised erythema, but more severe reactions also occur. If a rash is produced by carbamazepine, oxcarbazepine can often be given without recurrence. Stevens–Johnson syndrome occasionally occurs with carbamazepine, and is more frequent in people with HLA-B*1502, who are most often of Asian origin. Testing for this allele is recommended in people with certain Asian origins before using carbamazepine.
- Central nervous system (CNS) toxicity leads to double vision, dizziness, drowsiness or confusion. Ataxia can occur at high doses.
- Transient leucopenia is common, especially early in treatment, but severe bone marrow depression is rare.
- Hyponatraemia, caused by potentiation of the action of antidiuretic hormone on the kidney, can lead to confusion and decreased control of seizures. This may be more pronounced with oxcarbazepine.
- Teratogenicity in the form of neural tube defects is common (see below).
- Induction of hepatic CYP3A4 (Table 2.9) by carbamazepine can lead to drug interactions. The most common interaction is with the oral combined contraceptive pill (Ch. 45), and the dose of oestrogen should be increased to avoid failure of contraception. The metabolism of warfarin (Ch. 11) and ciclosporin (Ch. 38) are also accelerated. Interactions of carbamazepine with other antiepileptic drugs are discussed below. Oxcarbazepine has little effect on cytochrome P450 and therefore has few drug interactions.

Phenytoin and fosphenytoin

Mechanism of action and uses

Phenytoin and its prodrug fosphenytoin have a broad spectrum of activity and are effective against all forms of epilepsy, *except absences*. They have several actions that may contribute to the anticonvulsant activity:

- use-dependent blockade of Na^+ channels, which reduces cell excitability, is the main mechanism of action
- blockade of voltage-gated L-type Ca^{2+} channels
- potentiation of the action of GABA at $GABA_A$ receptors.

Phenytoin is sometimes used in the management of trigeminal neuralgia (Ch. 19).

Pharmacokinetics

Phenytoin is well, but slowly, absorbed from the gut. Slow intravenous injection can be used if a rapid onset of action is needed. Intramuscular injection of phenytoin should be avoided since absorption by this route is erratic and unpredictable, and muscle damage can occur. Phenytoin is eliminated by hepatic metabolism, but the enzyme is readily saturated and at saturating plasma concentrations the elimination changes from first-order (linear) kinetics to zero-order (non-linear) kinetics (Ch. 2; Fig. 23.1). This occurs in some individuals at plasma drug concentrations below or near the lower end of the therapeutic range. Once the enzyme is saturated, a small change in dose produces a large change in the plasma concentration at steady state (Ch. 2), and the elimination half-life is increased fourfold from about 12 h to almost 2 days. Plasma phenytoin concentrations are closely correlated to the clinical effect, and their measurement is useful as a guide to dosing. Phenytoin is highly protein bound (about 90%) and can be displaced from its binding sites by sodium valproate and salicylates, which briefly enhance the clinical effect of phenytoin to an unpredictable extent. The concentration of phenytoin in saliva reflects the free or unbound drug concentration in plasma, and measurement of the salivary concentration can be useful to guide dose adjustment if protein binding is altered, for example in pregnancy or renal failure. Salivary measurements are also useful for monitoring treatment in children, to avoid blood sampling.

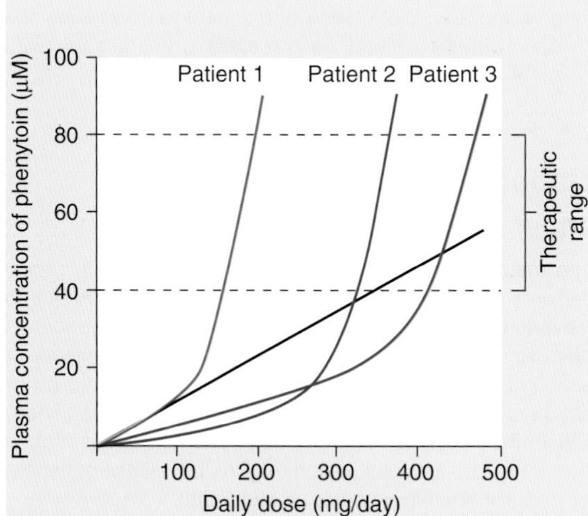

Fig. 23.1 **Inter-individual variation in the plasma concentration of phenytoin at steady state in relation to the daily dose.** The figure illustrates possible relationships between daily dose and plasma concentrations that might be seen in different individuals. The straight line illustrates the increase in plasma concentrations of phenytoin in subject 1 that would occur if the metabolism were not saturated (i.e. first-order kinetics). The relationship of dose and plasma concentration may be non-linear within the desired therapeutic range due to saturation of metabolism in some subjects leads to difficulties in dosage adjustment.

Fosphenytoin is only available for parenteral use, and can be given by intramuscular injection (absorption from this route is good, unlike that of phenytoin) or by intravenous infusion. It is completely metabolised to phenytoin.

Unwanted effects

Most unwanted effects of these drugs are dose-related.

- Nausea, vomiting, constipation, anorexia.
- CNS effects: impaired brainstem and cerebellar function, producing confusion, dizziness, tremor, nervousness or insomnia. Nystagmus, blurred vision, ataxia and dysarthria are signs of overdosage.
- Chronic connective tissue effects: gum hypertrophy, coarsening of facial features, hirsutism and acne. It is therefore usual to avoid phenytoin in young women or adolescents.
- Rashes.
- Folic acid metabolism is increased by phenytoin, producing megaloblastic haemopoiesis, although anaemia with a macrocytic blood picture is rare.
- Increased vitamin D metabolism can produce vitamin D deficiency; in rare cases this results in osteomalacia.
- Teratogenicity with carbamazepine including facial and digital malformations, occur in up to 10% of pregnancies.
- Induction of hepatic cytochrome P450 enzymes (Ch. 2) predisposes to several drug interactions. In particular, the metabolism of warfarin and ciclosporin are increased; interactions with other anticonvulsants are discussed below.

Sodium valproate

Mechanism of action and uses

Valproate has a wide spectrum of antiepileptic activity, and suppresses the initial seizure discharge as well as the spread of seizure activity. It is effective for all forms of epilepsy. Valproate has multiple actions, but their contributions to the clinical effects are incompletely understood. These actions include:

- potentiation of the effect of the inhibitory amino acid GABA, possibly by enhanced synthesis and release, and reduced degradation
- use-dependent blockade of transmembrane Na^+ channels, thus stabilising neuronal membranes; this is probably not the most important action of the drug
- attenuation of the excitatory action of glutamate at NMDA receptors
- inhibition of voltage-gated T-type Ca^{2+} channels
- activation of neuroprotective/neurotrophic intracellular proteins such as brain-derived neurotrophic factor (BDNF) (see Ch. 22).

The immediate anticonvulsant effects may be due to extracellular actions on neuronal ion channels, but slow diffusion into neurons produces delayed intracellular effects. The full benefit of treatment may not be apparent for several weeks. Valproate is also used for the management of bipolar disorder (Ch. 21), prophylaxis of migraine (Ch. 26) and in the management of neuropathic pain (Ch. 19).

Pharmacokinetics

Sodium valproate is well absorbed from the gut. Conventional-formulation tablets should be taken with food in order

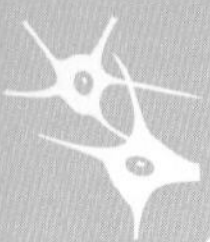

to reduce gastric upset. Plasma protein binding of valproate is high (90–95% at low to moderate plasma concentrations), but the proportion of free (and therefore active) drug rises with increasing blood concentration of the drug. Although valproate is highly ionised at physiological pH, it is rapidly transported across the blood–brain barrier via an anion exchange transporter, then passively and slowly diffuses into neurons. Slow diffusion into and out of neurons may in part explain why the drug concentration in plasma does not correlate well with its therapeutic effect, and the monitoring of blood concentrations is only useful to assess compliance. Valproate is extensively metabolised in the liver and has a long half-life (9–21 h). Valproate is also available in a modified-release formulation (both as sodium valproate and valproic acid), and there is an intravenous preparation of sodium valproate for rapid seizure control.

Unwanted effects

- Gastrointestinal upset: nausea, vomiting, anorexia, abdominal pain and bowel disturbance. These can be minimised by gradual dosage titration. Valproate may rarely cause pancreatitis, and serum amylase should be measured if symptoms such as abdominal pain or nausea and vomiting arise.
- Weight gain caused by appetite stimulation.
- Transient hair loss, with regrowth of curly hair.
- Ataxia, tremor, confusion and, rarely, encephalopathy and coma. These can be minimised by slow dosage titration.
- Thrombocytopenia or impaired platelet activity.
- Severe hepatotoxicity can develop but is rare, and usually occurs in the first 6 months of therapy. This is most frequent in children under 3 years of age or in people with organic brain disorders who are receiving multiple drug therapy for seizures. Transiently raised liver enzymes are common but usually do not progress to more serious liver dysfunction.
- Teratogenicity in the form of neural tube defects (see below).
- Inhibition of hepatic cytochrome P450 enzymes, leading to interactions with other antiepileptic drugs (see below).

Phenobarbital and primidone

Mechanism of action and effects

These drugs have a wide spectrum of activity and are effective in most forms of epilepsy, but unwanted effects limit their use. Phenobarbital is a barbiturate, and its major mechanism of action is activation of postsynaptic neuronal $GABA_A$ receptors (see also Ch. 20). This increases the duration of opening of the transmembrane Cl^- channel associated with the receptor, and the neuronal membrane is therefore hyperpolarised and less likely to fire. The GABA receptors are activated by phenobarbital independently of the presence of the inhibitory amino acid neurotransmitter, but phenobarbital will also potentiate the effect of GABA (Ch. 20). The action of primidone is due in part to its conversion to phenobarbital. Primidone has no advantage over phenobarbital and is generally less well tolerated. People with epilepsy who do not respond to or who are unable to tolerate phenobarbital are unlikely to benefit from primidone.

Pharmacokinetics

Oral absorption of phenobarbital is almost complete. Elimination is by hepatic metabolism and renal excretion, with about 25% excreted unchanged in the urine. The half-life is very long, at about 4 days, but with considerable inter-individual variation.

Primidone is well absorbed orally and is converted in the liver to two active metabolites, one of which is phenobarbital.

The plasma concentrations of phenobarbital and primidone relate poorly to the control of seizures; they are only useful as a guide to adherence to treatment. Control of seizures or unwanted effects should be used to determine dosages.

Unwanted effects

- CNS effects: sedation, fatigue and memory impairment are common in adults; paradoxical excitement, confusion and restlessness can occur in the elderly, and hyperactivity in children.
- Folic acid metabolism is increased by phenobarbital, producing megaloblastic haemopoiesis, although anaemia with a macrocytic blood picture is rare.
- Increased vitamin D metabolism can produce vitamin D deficiency; in rare cases this results in osteomalacia.
- Tolerance to both unwanted and therapeutic effects occurs during long-term treatment.
- Dependence with a physical withdrawal reaction is seen after long-term treatment.
- Teratogenicity (see below).
- Induction of hepatic cytochrome P450 enzymes (Ch. 2) leads to increased metabolism of phenobarbital itself and warfarin, ciclosporin and oestrogen (reducing the effectiveness of oral contraception). Interactions with other antiepileptic drugs are considered below.

Gabapentin and pregabalin

Mechanism of action and uses

The major use of gabapentin and pregabalin is in partial seizures with or without secondary generalisation. Although designed as a structural analogue of GABA, gabapentin does not mimic GABA in the brain. The mechanisms of action of gabapentin and pregabalin are unclear, but probably involve blockade of P/Q-type voltage-gated Ca^{2+} channels in the neocortex and hippocampus. The drugs reduce Ca^{2+} entry into neurons, which may inhibit release of excitatory neurotransmitters such as glutamate.

Gabapentin and pregabalin are also used in the management of neuropathic pain (Ch. 19), and pregabalin for generalised anxiety disorder (Ch. 20).

Pharmacokinetics

Gabapentin is incompletely absorbed from the gut, via a saturable transport mechanism, and is excreted unchanged by the kidney. It has a half-life of 5–7 h. Pregabalin is well absorbed from the gut, and also largely excreted unchanged by the kidney. It has a half-life of 6 h.

Unwanted effects

- Nausea, vomiting, dry mouth, diarrhoea, constipation, abdominal pain
- CNS effects, including drowsiness, dizziness, ataxia, fatigue, headache, tremor, diplopia, confusion and emotional lability
- Weight gain from stimulation of appetite
- Rhinitis, cough, dyspnoea
- Myalgia, arthralgia
- Rashes.

Lamotrigine

Mechanism of action and uses

Lamotrigine has a wide spectrum of efficacy for partial and generalised seizures. It produces use-dependent inhibition of neuronal voltage-gated Na^+ channels. Unlike carbamazepine and phenytoin, it selectively targets dendrites of pyramidal neurons that synthesise glutamate and aspartate and reduces glutamate release. Lamotrigine may further reduce glutamate release through blockade of voltage-gated N- and P/Q-type Ca^{2+} channels.

Lamotrigine is also used for neuropathic pain (Ch. 19).

Pharmacokinetics

Lamotrigine is well absorbed orally and is extensively metabolised in the liver. The half-life is long, at 15–60 h.

Unwanted effects

- Hypersensitivity syndrome with fever, rash, lymphadenopathy and hepatic dysfunction
- Rashes: some disappear despite continued treatment, but severe skin reactions, including Stevens–Johnson syndrome and toxic epidermal necrolysis, occasionally occur, particularly in children, following rapid dose escalation or with concurrent use of sodium valproate
- Nausea, vomiting, diarrhoea
- CNS effects: drowsiness, headache, fatigue, dizziness, double vision and ataxia; tremor can be troublesome at high dosages
- Bone marrow suppression.

Levetiracetam

Mechanism of action and uses

Levetiracetam is used for adjunctive treatment of partial seizures with or without secondary generalisation. Its mechanisms of action remain uncertain. Levetiracetam binds to a protein on the presynaptic neuronal plasma membrane and modulates release of excitatory neurotransmitters, such as glutamate. It also produces blockade of voltage-gated N-type Ca^{2+} channels. The end result is selective inhibition of synchronised epileptiform burst firing and propagation of seizure activity in the hippocampus, without affecting neuronal excitability.

Pharmacokinetics

Levetiracetam is rapidly absorbed after oral administration. It is largely eliminated unchanged by the kidney, but up to one-third undergoes hepatic metabolism. The half-life of levetiracetam is 7 h.

Unwanted effects

- CNS effects: drowsiness, lethargy, dizziness, ataxia, headache, tremor, insomnia, emotional lability, impaired concentration
- Anorexia, nausea, vomiting, dyspepsia, diarrhoea
- Cough.

Tiagabine

Mechanism of action and uses

Tiagabine is used as an adjunctive (add-on) therapy for partial seizures with or without secondary generalisation. It is a potent inhibitor of GABA transporter 1 (GAT-1) and decreases glial and presynaptic neuronal uptake of the inhibitory amino acid GABA. This is the mechanism that normally limits the duration of action of GABA at its receptor. The action of tiagabine is relatively selective for the hippocampus and thalamus.

Pharmacokinetics

Tiagabine is well absorbed from the gut. It is metabolised in the liver and has a half-life of 5–8 h.

Unwanted effects

- CNS effects: dizziness, lethargy, nervousness, impaired concentration, emotional lability, tremor
- Nausea, diarrhoea.

Topiramate

Mechanism of action and uses

Topiramate is used alone or as an add-on treatment for drug-resistant partial or generalised seizures. Various mechanisms of action have been proposed:

- Use-dependent blockade of neuronal Na^+ channels
- Enhancement of the action of GABA at $GABA_A$ receptors, although the mechanism of this interaction is unknown
- Antagonist activity at the AMPA/kainite subtype of receptor for the excitatory amino acid glutamate
- Inhibition of carbonic anhydrase isoenzymes, producing multiple effects on transmembrane ionic fluxes.

Pharmacokinetics

Topiramate is rapidly absorbed orally and up to 70% is eliminated unchanged by the kidney, while the rest is metabolised in the liver. It has a long half-life (20–30 h).

Unwanted effects

- CNS effects, including impaired concentration, cognitive impairment, confusion, dizziness, ataxia, headache agitation, emotional lability or depression
- Gastrointestinal upset, with nausea, abdominal pain, anorexia, dry mouth and weight loss
- Acute angle-closure glaucoma, especially within 1 month of starting treatment.

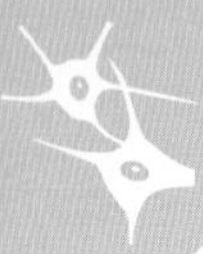

Vigabatrin

Mechanism of action and uses

Vigabatrin is only used in combination with other drugs to treat epilepsy that is resistant to other drug combinations, or when they are poorly tolerated. It is effective in partial epilepsy with or without secondary generalisation, but its use is now restricted because of the unacceptably high risk of visual field defects (see below). It is, however, still useful for infantile spasms. Vigabatrin has a unique mechanism of action. It is a structural analogue of GABA and produces irreversible inhibition of GABA transaminase (GABA-T), the enzyme that inactivates GABA. The generalised increase in CNS concentrations of GABA inhibits the spread of epileptic discharges.

Pharmacokinetics

Vigabatrin is rapidly absorbed from the gut and is excreted unchanged by the kidney. Irreversible drug binding to the target enzyme means that the long duration of action is determined by the time required for enzyme synthesis, rather than the half-life of elimination of the drug (7–8 h). GABA-T activity recovers to about 60% of baseline after 5 days. The efficacy of vigabatrin, therefore, is unrelated to the plasma drug concentration, and blood concentration monitoring is of no value.

Unwanted effects

- CNS effects: sedation and fatigue, dizziness, nervousness, irritability, depression, impaired concentration, ataxia, nystagmus and tremor
- Psychotic reactions, especially if there is a history of psychiatric disorder
- Severe peripheral visual field defects during prolonged use; they can arise from 1 month to several years after starting treatment, and are usually irreversible; regular monitoring of visual fields at 6-month intervals is recommended
- Alopecia, rash
- Weight gain, oedema.

Zonisamide

Mechanism of action and uses

Zonisamide is used for adjunctive treatment of refractory partial seizures with or without secondary generalisation. Its mechanisms of action remain uncertain but may include:

- use-dependent blockade of neuronal Na^+ channels, which stabilises cell membranes
- blockade of voltage-dependent T-type Ca^{2+} channels, also stabilising cell membranes
- enhancement of neuronal uptake of the excitatory amino acid glutamate.

Pharmacokinetics

Zonisamide is well absorbed from the gut and is eliminated by metabolism. It binds selectively to red blood cells and has a very long half-life of about 60 h.

Unwanted effects

- CNS effects: drowsiness, lethargy, dizziness, confusion, ataxia, emotional lability, impaired concentration
- Anorexia, weight loss, nausea, abdominal pain, diarrhoea
- Rash.

Benzodiazepines

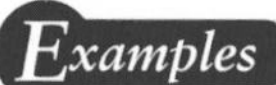

clobazam, clonazepam, diazepam, lorazepam

Mechanism of action and uses

These drugs enhance the action of the inhibitory neurotransmitter GABA (Ch. 20). Clonazepam and clobazam are used orally for prophylaxis, usually as an adjunct to other drugs. Lorazepam, diazepam or clonazepam can be used intravenously to treat individual fits; if intravenous access is not available, then rectal diazepam or buccal or intranasal midazolam can be used. Intravenous diazepam is formulated as an emulsion to reduce the incidence of thrombophlebitis.

Pharmacokinetics

These are long-acting benzodiazepines, discussed in detail in Chapter 20.

Unwanted effects

These are discussed in Chapter 20. Partial or complete tolerance to the antiepileptic action of benzodiazepines often occurs after about 4–6 months of continuous treatment.

Ethosuximide

Mechanism of action and uses

Ethosuximide is a drug of choice in absence seizures, and may be effective for myoclonic seizures, and tonic or atonic seizures. It is ineffective in other types of epilepsy. In absence seizures, T-type Ca^{2+} channels are believed to be responsible for generating excessive activity in thalamocortical relay neurons. Ethosuximide blocks these channels and prevents synchronised neuronal firing.

Pharmacokinetics

Absorption of ethosuximide from the gut is almost complete. Metabolism in the liver is extensive and the half-life is very long, at 2–3 days, although it is shorter in children. Plasma and salivary drug concentrations correlate well with control of seizures and can be used to monitor treatment.

Unwanted effects

- Nausea, vomiting, anorexia (less frequent if the drug is taken with food and if the dose is gradually increased)
- Drowsiness, dizziness, ataxia, dyskinesias, photophobia, headache and depression
- Rashes
- Agranulocytosis and aplastic anaemia are rare complications
- Teratogenicity.

DRUG INTERACTIONS AMONG ANTICONVULSANTS

Many antiepileptics affect hepatic drug-metabolising enzymes, especially cytochrome P450 isoenzymes (see Table 2.9); therefore, drug interactions are frequent. Interactions when two or more antiepileptics are used together can have major clinical implications for seizure control and/or toxicity. Plasma drug concentration monitoring is often advisable when more than one drug is used. Common interactions are listed below.

Carbamazepine. This is an enzyme inducer that can lower the plasma concentrations of clobazam, clonazepam, lamotrigine, tiagabine, topiramate, sodium valproate and an active metabolite of oxcarbazepine.

Phenobarbital and primidone. These are enzyme inducers that lower the plasma concentrations of carbamazepine, clonazepam, lamotrigine, tiagabine, phenytoin, sodium valproate and an active metabolite of oxcarbazepine.

Phenytoin. This is an enzyme inducer and it often lowers the plasma concentrations of carbamazepine, clonazepam, lamotrigine, tiagabine, topiramate, sodium valproate and an active metabolite of oxcarbazepine.

Valproate. Inhibition of hepatic drug metabolism by valproate often increases the plasma concentrations of phenobarbital and lamotrigine, as well as those of an active metabolite of carbamazepine. Sodium valproate can displace phenytoin from plasma protein binding sites but also inhibits the metabolism of phenytoin, and the net result is an increase in the active free component.

Vigabatrin. This drug often reduces plasma phenytoin concentration by an unknown mechanism.

MANAGEMENT OF EPILEPSY

TREATMENT OF INDIVIDUAL SEIZURES

The initial management of a seizure involves positioning the person to avoid injury. Particular attention must also be given to maintaining the airways and ensuring adequate oxygenation. A correctable cause such as hypoglycaemia should be sought and treated, and intravenous thiamine given if alcohol abuse is suspected.

Prolonged or repetitive seizures (status epilepticus) usually require urgent parenteral drug treatment. Intravenous lorazepam is the drug of choice; diazepam can be used but it has a shorter duration of action owing to more rapid tissue redistribution. If intravenous access is not available, then midazolam can be given by the buccal or intranasal route. Diazepam is available as a rectal solution, which may be particularly useful for children or initial treatment out of hospital. Close observation for signs of drug-induced respiratory depression should be maintained after giving a benzodiazepine.

If there is no response after 15 min, or seizures recur, then a slow intravenous injection of phenytoin, or a more rapid injection of fosphenytoin or phenobarbital, should be given. If seizures are still not controlled with these measures, then full anaesthesia using thiopental or propofol (Ch. 17) with assisted respiration in an intensive care unit will be necessary.

PROPHYLAXIS FOR SEIZURES

A diagnosis of epilepsy requires two or more spontaneous seizures. After a single event, up to 80% of people will have a second fit within 3 years. If a predisposing cause cannot be identified and avoided (e.g. alcohol withdrawal, photosensitive epilepsy precipitated by viewing a television from too close a distance), drug treatment will usually be recommended after a second seizure, unless the seizures were separated by very long intervals or were mild.

Treatment should begin with a single drug, the choice depending on the type of epilepsy and relative toxicity of the drugs (Table 23.2). For generalised seizures or unclassifiable seizures, in the absence of factors that would lead to an alternative choice, then sodium valproate is often recommended since it has the broadest spectrum of activity. Lamotrigine is now considered the drug of first choice for partial seizures. The initial drug dose should be low, with gradual titration to minimise unwanted effects. If seizures continue, then the maximum tolerated dose should be taken. If seizures are not controlled with the first-choice drug, it becomes more important to accurately identify the type of seizure. A second single drug should then be introduced while the first is gradually withdrawn (Table 23.2). A single drug will usually control seizures in up to 90% of people with epilepsy, although this may not be achieved with the first drug chosen. However, if the first drug does not control the seizures, then the chance of a second single drug being successful is 13%, and with a third, only 4%.

Refractory epilepsy can indicate poor adherence to treatment, inappropriate drug choice or dosage, or that the seizures are 'pseudoseizures' rather than true epilepsy. Multiple drug treatment (initially with two first-line drugs, or a first- and a second-line drug) should be reserved for seizures that have not been resolved by treatment with two or three drugs given alone. Drugs like tiagabine, vigabatrin and zonisamide are usually used in combination with other agents.

Combination therapy at maximally tolerated doses does not control the seizures in some people with epilepsy, even when there is good adherence to treatment recommendations. Lack of seizure control is more frequent if the onset was at an early age, if there are generalised, atonic or absence seizures, or if there is underlying structural brain damage. Some data suggest that resistance can arise from overexpression of proteins that transport drugs out of the CNS, such as P-glycoprotein. However, the evidence for this is conflicting. Alternatively, resistance may arise from genetic variation affecting targets for drug action. For temporal lobe epilepsy, there is now good evidence that surgical treatment should be considered if more than two consecutive anticonvulsants fail to control the seizures. Surgery for other forms of epilepsy may provide some amelioration of seizure frequency.

It is not usually necessary to monitor plasma drug concentrations to determine whether they are within the 'therapeutic range' unless seizure control is poor, or if poor adherence or drug toxicity is suspected. Good seizure control will often be achieved at plasma drug concentrations that are below the accepted therapeutic range, and under such circumstances an increase in dosage would not be necessary. Conversely, people who continue to have seizures may need plasma drug concentrations above the standard therapeutic range to achieve seizure control,

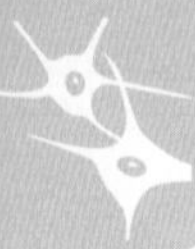

Table 23.2 Drug choice in the treatment of epilepsy

Type of seizure	First-line drugs	Main action of first-line drug[a]	Second-line or adjunctive drugs
Partial seizures	Phenytoin Carbamazepine Valproate Lamotrigine[b] Topiramate	Block Na^+ channel GABA receptor	Phenobarbital[c]/primidone[c] Clonazepam[c]/clobazam[c] Gabapentin[c] (as adjunct) Vigabatrin[c] (as adjunct) Zonisamide[bcd]
Generalised seizures			
Tonic–clonic (grand mal)	Carbamazepine Valproate Lamotrigine[b] Phenytoin	Block Na^+ channel	Phenobarbital[c]/primidone[c] Vigabatrin[c] (as adjunct) Phenytoin
Myoclonic	Valproate Ethosuximide Clonazepam Levetiracetam	Block Na^+ channel Block T-type Ca^{2+} channel	
Absence	Ethosuximide Valproate	Block T-type Ca^{2+} channel Block Na^+ channel	Clonazepam[c] Lamotrigine
Atonic	Valproate Lamotrigine Levetiracetam	Block Na^+ channel	Phenytoin Ethosuximide Clonazepam[c] Phenobarbital[c]

[a]Drugs may also share other sites of action, contributing to the antiepileptic effects.
[b]Also affects glutamate neurotransmission.
[c]Enhances gamma-aminobutyric acid activity.
[d]Blocks Na^+ channels.

provided the drug is well tolerated. The only drug for which monitoring is of proven benefit for dosage adjustment is phenytoin, primarily because metabolism may be saturated at therapeutic doses and the kinetics become non-linear (Fig. 23.1). Adjustment of the dosages of carbamazepine or ethosuximide may be easier if the plasma concentration is known; however, for other drugs, monitoring is only of value to confirm that the drug is being taken.

In the UK, a driving licence is revoked until the individual has been seizure-free for 1 year, or has suffered only nocturnal seizures for 3 years. Driving is not advisable during withdrawal of antiepileptic drugs, or for 6 months afterwards.

Once started, treatment should usually be continued for at least 2–3 years after the last seizure. Treatment should probably be life-long if there is a continuing predisposing condition or the person wishes to continue to drive. If a decision is made to withdraw treatment, then it should be gradual, in order to minimise the risk of rebound seizures. When several drugs are used, one should be withdrawn at a time.

Prophylaxis for seizures is often given for up to 3 months following neurosurgical procedures or head injury, particularly if there was a depressed skull fracture or an associated intracranial haematoma. Evidence that such routine use is beneficial is not secure.

Febrile convulsions occur commonly in infancy and usually do not lead to epilepsy or produce CNS damage. About 4% of children have them and they recur in about one-third. It is important to reduce pyrexia during subsequent febrile episodes, such as by removal of clothes and use of paracetamol (Ch. 29). Routine prophylaxis with antiepileptic drugs is not recommended, but rectal diazepam is sometimes given when a child who has previously had a febrile convulsion becomes pyrexial.

ANTICONVULSANTS IN PREGNANCY

No anticonvulsant has a proven safety record in pregnancy and may carry a high risk of teratogenesis if the fetus is exposed in the first trimester (see Table 56.1). Fetal abnormalities are most frequent if more than one drug is used. Neural tube defects and other problems are particularly common with sodium valproate (malformations in about 10% of pregnancies), and to a lesser extent with carbamazepine and oxcarbazepine (malformations in 2–4% of pregnancies). Developmental abnormalities also occur with phenobarbital, phenytoin and lamotrigine, but there is too little information about many of the other drugs. There is also increasing evidence of language and neurocognitive defects in children born to mothers who are taking antiepileptic drugs. Women taking antiepileptic drugs who wish to become pregnant should be counselled about the risk and offered antenatal screening during pregnancy, with α-fetoprotein measurement (to detect neural tube defects) and second-trimester ultrasound scanning. Folic acid supplements may reduce the risk of neural tube defects and should be advised before and during pregnancy. It is important to advise a potential mother with epilepsy that the risks of uncontrolled seizures during pregnancy, both to her and to the fetus, may be greater than the risk associated with drug therapy.

When the mother is taking carbamazepine, phenobarbital or phenytoin, there is an increased risk of neonatal bleeding. Prophylactic vitamin K_1 should be given to the mother from 36 weeks of pregnancy, and to the newborn immediately after birth.

FURTHER READING

Chen JW, Wasterlain SG (2006) Status epilepticus: pathophysiology and management in adults. *Lancet Neurol* 5, 246–256

Czapiaski P, Blaszczyk B, Czuczwar SJ (2005) Mechanisms of action of antiepileptic drugs. *Curr Top Med Chem* 5, 3–14

Duncan JS, Sander JW, Sisodiya SM et al (2006) Adult epilepsy. *Lancet* 367, 1087–1100

French JA, Pedley TA (2008) Initial management of epilepsy. *N Engl J Med* 359, 166–176

Guerrini R (2006) Epilepsy in children. *Lancet* 367, 499–524

Kalviainen R, Tomson T (2006) Optimising treatment of epilepsy during pregnancy. *Neurology* 67, S59–S63

Marson AG, Al-Kharusi AM, Alwaidh M et al (2007) The SANAD study of effectiveness of carbamazepine, gabapentin, lamotrigine, oxcarbazepine, or topiramate for treatment of partial epilepsy: an unblinded randomised controlled trial. *Lancet* 369, 1000–1015

Marson AG, Al-Kharusi AM, Alwaidh M et al (2007) The SANAD study of effectiveness of valproate, lamotrigine, or topiramate for generalised and unclassified epilepsy: an unblinded randomised controlled trial. *Lancet* 369, 1016–1026

Perruca E (2005) Birth defects after prenatal exposure to antiepileptic drugs. *Lancet Neurol* 4, 781–786

Pohlmann-Eden B, Beghi E, Camfield C et al (2006) The first seizure and its management in adults and children. *BMJ* 332, 339–342

Tatum WO IV, Liporace J, Benbadia SR et al (2004) Updates on the treatment of epilepsy in women. *Arch Intern Med* 164, 137–146

Torbjorn T, Hiilesmaa V (2007) Epilepsy in pregnancy. *BMJ* 335, 769–773

SELF-ASSESSMENT

In questions 1–6, the first statement, in italics, is true. Are the accompanying statements also true?

1. *Generalised seizures involving the whole brain include tonic–clonic seizures (previously called grand mal) and absence seizures (previously called petit mal).* Absence seizures occur mainly in adults.
2. *Partial (or focal) seizures are localised and can involve motor, sensory or psychic symptoms without loss of consciousness.* Generalised muscle contractions do not occur in partial seizures.
3. *The excitatory amino acid glutamate acting on NMDA receptors is increased in some seizures and can lead to excitotoxic damage to cells.*
   a. Inhibition of glutamate release is the primary mechanism of action of several drugs in current use for the treatment of epilepsy.
   b. Drugs that stimulate GABA receptors or enhance GABA stability are useful for treating epilepsy because of their ability to inhibit Na^+ influx.
4. *Two major mechanisms by which drugs act as anticonvulsants is to inhibit Na^+ channels and enhance the activity of GABA.* The metabolism of phenytoin diminishes with regular use.
5. *Phenytoin is highly protein bound.*
   a. Salicylates and sodium valproate reduce the effectiveness of phenytoin.
   b. The plasma concentrations of phenytoin vary in a linear manner with the dose administered over the whole therapeutic dose range.
6. *The abrupt withdrawal of antiepileptics should be avoided.* Vigabatrin is a first-line drug for the treatment of all types of epilepsy.
7. A 10-year-old boy was diagnosed with absence seizures, and the drugs that might be used and their unwanted effects were assessed. Which one of the following statements is **most likely** to apply in this boy?
   A. Phenytoin would be a suitable first-line drug.
   B. Ethosuximide would be a suitable first-line drug.
   C. Valproate, which can be used for the treatment of absence seizures, can be safely given together with ethosuximide.
   D. Ethosuximide acts principally to block Na^+ channels.
   E. The full benefit of sodium valproate is seen within 2 h of administration.
8. Regarding the effects of drugs used in the treatment of epilepsy, choose the one **most appropriate** statement.
   A. Combinations of antiepileptic drugs are preferred in pregnancy because they reduce the incidence of seizures without increasing the risk of teratogenicity.
   B. The effectiveness of phenobarbital diminishes with time.
   C. Plasma concentrations of phenytoin relate linearly to the dose given over a wide dose range.
   D. The anticonvulsant effect of phenytoin is reduced by aspirin.
   E. The main role of diazepam in epilepsy is confined to long-term prophylaxis in tonic–clonic seizures.
9. Case history 1 questions

A 7-year-old boy was described as dreamy by his mother. He was making slow progress at school and his mother and teachers commented that he could not concentrate and had frequent episodes of staring vacantly for a few seconds and then carrying on as normal. Following an electroencephalogram (EEG), a synchronised electrical discharge characteristic of an absence form of epilepsy was demonstrated.

   a. Which of the following drugs would be suitable as a drug of first choice to prescribe: phenytoin, phenobarbital, sodium valproate, ethosuximide?
   b. What are the major relevant unwanted effects of those drugs you could have prescribed in this child?
   c. If control of absence seizures is inadequate with your chosen antiepileptic, can combination therapy be given?

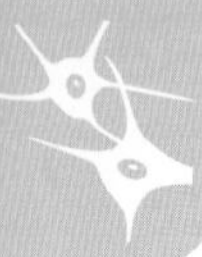

10. Case history 2 questions

A 19-year-old woman had a long-term history of epilepsy of the complex partial seizure type, which often gravitated to generalised seizures. For several years her epilepsy had been well controlled with a stable drug regimen. She now sought advice on contraception.

a. What antiepileptic drugs might be effective in the type of epilepsy this woman has?
b. What suitable options are available for contraception?
c. What potential problems can arise if the woman takes the oral combined contraceptive?
d. Would an injected progestogen contraceptive be worth considering?
e. If the oral combined contraceptive were the chosen method, what strategies should be adopted to ensure its efficacy?
f. Would the progestogen-only contraceptive be a suitable method of contraception?

ANSWERS

1. **False**. Absences, manifested by transient unawareness of surroundings and generally without motor disturbance, occur in children.
2. **False**. In 'jacksonian epilepsy', jerking localised to a particular group of muscles may occur, which can then gradually involve many other muscles.
3. a. **False**. There are currently no drugs whose primary action is to inhibit glutamate transmission, although this may form part of the action of some drugs such as lamotrigine.
   b. **False**. GABA causes hyperpolarisation by increasing Cl^- influx into cells.
4. **False**. Phenytoin induces its own metabolism.
5. a. **False**. Salicylates and valproate displace phenytoin from plasma proteins, to which 80–90% of the drug is bound. This increases the free plasma concentration and the effect of phenytoin.
   b. **False**. Phenytoin exhibits first-order kinetics in the lower region of the therapeutic dose range, but at higher doses the relationship switches to zero-order kinetics after the liver metabolising enzymes have become saturated.
6. **False**. Although vigabatrin is effective in all types of epilepsy, acting by specifically reducing the breakdown of GABA, it is reserved for people who are resistant to other drugs.
7. Answer **B**.
   A. Phenytoin is not used in treating absence seizures, and in a young person should be avoided if possible because it causes hirsutism, gingival hyperplasia, acne and facial coarsening.
   B. Ethosuximide is a first-line drug in absence seizures.
   C. Valproate inhibits liver drug-metabolising enzymes, thus increasing the chance of ethosuximide toxicity.
   D. T-type Ca^{2+} channels are blocked by ethosuximide.
   E. The full benefit of sodium valproate may take several weeks to develop.
8. Answer **B**.
   A. The risk of teratogenesis is increased if more than one drug is given.
   B. Tolerance to the therapeutic effects and unwanted effects of phenobarbital develops with time.
   C. The pharmacokinetics of phenytoin can change from linear to zero order as the dose is increased.
   D. Phenytoin is highly protein bound and can be displaced by salicylates, increasing the concentration of free phenytoin and thus the clinical effect and also the risks of unwanted effects.
   E. Diazepam is sometimes used as an adjunct to other treatments for prophylaxis and alone in status epilepticus.
9. Case history 1 answers
   a. Absence seizures usually respond well to sodium valproate or ethosuximide. Ethosuximide is effective only in absence seizures. Phenytoin and phenobarbital are ineffective in absences.
   b. Sodium valproate causes nausea, reversible transient hair loss and weight gain. Uncommonly, liver damage can occur. Ethosuximide causes nausea, anorexia and headache.
   c. Monotherapy with ethosuximide or sodium valproate should be tried before combining therapies. Compliance should also be checked before combining therapies. Sodium valproate reduces the clearance of ethosuximide and may cause toxicity.
10. Case history 2 answers
   a. A variety of drugs could be used in this person. First-line drugs usually include carbamazepine, lamotrigine or sodium valproate.
   b. Non-hormonal contraceptives such as barrier or intrauterine devices are effective and do not carry the risk of drug interactions. However, many women will want to use a hormonal method.
   c. Carbamazepine, phenytoin, phenobarbital and topiramate all induce liver enzymes that increase the metabolism of sex steroids and reduce efficacy of oral contraceptives.
   d. Injected medroxyprogesterone acetate is affected less than sex steroids administered orally. The interval between injection of medroxyprogesterone acetate should, however, be reduced to 10 weeks. Medroxyprogesterone acetate may also reduce the incidence of epileptic attacks.
   e. Because oestrogen metabolism is enhanced by several antiepileptic drugs (see c above) it is recommended that, if one of these drugs need to be prescribed, at a minimum, fomulations containing a high concentration of oestrogen (50 μg) should be given. Sometimes more than 100 mg oestrogen daily in split doses may be required to prevent breakthrough bleeding. The pill-free period can also be reduced. If any change in medication for her epilepsy is made, additional barrier methods of contraception should be used until medication is stabilised.
   f. No. The progestogen-only oral contraceptive would be unsafe, as its metabolism is increased.

Drugs used to treat epilepsy and status epilepticus

Drug	Half-life (h) and kinetics	Comments
Drugs used for epilepsy		
Drugs given orally, usually once or twice daily, to encourage better compliance		
Acetazolamide	6–15 [R] Negligible metabolism	Low efficacy and used as a second-line drug for partial and tonic–clonic seizures; has a specific role in epilepsy associated with menstruation
Carbamazepine	25–65 (initial) 12–17 (chronic) [M] Good oral bioavailability; epoxide metabolite has anticonvulsant actions; induction of CYP3A4 leads to drug interactions; wide inter-subject variation in the extent of enzyme induction; autoinduction of its metabolism results in a shorter half-life after repeated dosage	Used for partial and secondary generalised tonic–clonic seizures, some primary generalised seizures; also used for trigeminal neuralgia and for bipolar disorder unresponsive to lithium (Ch. 21); given orally or rectally; used for pain control (Ch. 19).
Clobazam	10–50 [M] High oral bioavailability; oxidised in the liver to numerous metabolites; the N-desmethyl metabolite is active and plasma concentrations are 5–10 times those of the parent drug	Used as adjunctive therapy in epilepsy; also used short term for anxiety
Clonazepam	18–45 [M] Oral bioavailability about 80%; metabolites formed by nitro-reduction in the liver have negligible activity	Used in all forms of epilepsy; also used in myoclonus
Ethosuximide	50–60 [M + R] About 80% is metabolised by CYP3A4-mediated hydroxylation and then conjugation; half-life is shorter in children (30 h)	Used for absence seizures, myoclonic seizures and some atypical seizures
Gabapentin	5–7 [R] Absorption from gut is rapid but dose-dependent (possibly because of saturation of active amino acid transporter); oral bioavailability (60%) decreases at high doses; clearance approximates to glomerular filtration rate	Used as adjunctive treatment in partial epilepsy with or without secondary generalised tonic–clonic seizures; also used for neuropathic pain
Lamotrigine	15–60 [M + R] Rapid and complete absorption; metabolised to various products, including a N-glucuronide (unusual reaction)	Used for partial and primary and secondary generalised tonic–clonic seizures
Levetiracetam	7 [R + M] Rapid absorption and 100% bioavailability; eliminated largely by glomerular filtration and some hydrolysis to an inactive carboxylic acid (25%)	Used for partial seizure and generalised myoclonic or atonic seizures
Oxcarbazepine	2 [R] Rapid and complete absorption; reduced in the liver to the active metabolite (10-hydroxy oxcarbazepine), which has a longer half-life (9 h) and is responsible for most of the anti-seizure activity	Used for partial seizures with or without secondary generalised tonic–clonic seizures; oxcarbazepine is the keto analogue of carbamazepine
Phenobarbital	50–150 [M + R] Oral bioavailability >90%; mostly eliminated by hepatic CYP2C9-mediated oxidation; potent inducer of cytochrome P450 isoenzymes, which leads to numerous drug interactions; about 25% is excreted unchanged in urine and renal clearance is increased by alkalinisation of the urine	Used for all forms of epilepsy except absence seizures
Phenytoin	7–60 [M + R] Complete oral bioavailability; dose-dependent elimination because of saturation of metabolism; there is wide inter-subject variation in the concentration at which metabolism is saturated; renal elimination is 7% of dose at low doses; potent inducer of cytochrome P450 isoenzymes, which leads to numerous drug interactions	Can be used for all forms of epilepsy except absence seizures but now little used

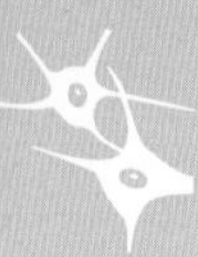

Drugs used to treat epilepsy and status epilepticus

Drug	Half-life (h) and kinetics	Comments
Pregabalin	6 [R] High oral bioavailability (90%); renal clearance is about 50% of glomerular filtration rate	Structural analogue of gabapentin; used as an adjuvant for partial seizures; also used for neuropathic pain
Primidone	4–22 [M] Active metabolites (phenobarbital and phenylethyl malonamide) have longer half-lives than primidone and accumulate; the metabolites account for most activity during chronic treatment; potent inducer of cytochrome P450 isoenzymes, leading to numerous drug interactions	Used for all forms of epilepsy except absence seizures; also used for essential tremor
Tiagabine	5–8 [M] Rapidly and completely absorbed; oxidised by hepatic CYP3A4; does not induce cytochrome P450; elimination is increased by drugs which induce cytochrome P450	Used as adjunctive treatment in partial epilepsy with or without secondary generalised tonic–clonic seizures
Topiramate	20–30 [R + M] Absorbed rapidly with a high bioavailability; about 70% is eliminated unchanged, but there is extensive reabsorption in the renal tubule; there is some metabolism, and elimination is enhanced by cytochrome P450 inducers	Used as monotherapy or adjunctive treatment in generalised tonic–clonic seizures and in partial epilepsy with or without secondary generalisation
Valproate sodium	9–21 [M] Oral bioavailability is >95%; metabolised by oxidation (CYP2C19 and CYP2C9) and by glucuronidation; some metabolites have activity but their importance is not known; interactions with other substrates of CYP2C19 and CYP2C9 have been reported	Used in all forms of epilepsy
Vigabatrin	7–8 [R] Clearance is similar to, and correlates with, glomerular filtration rate; the duration of the effect greatly exceeds the drug half-life	Used under specialist supervision as adjunctive treatment in partial epilepsy with or without secondary generalised tonic–clonic seizures
Zonisamide	60 [M] Good oral absorption; metabolised by acetylation, reduction and conjugation with glucuronic acid	Used as an adjunct for refractory partial seizures
Drugs used primarily for status epilepticus		
These drugs may also be used for other forms of epilepsy		
Clonazepam	See above	Given by intravenous injection or infusion; see above for other information
Diazepam	See Ch. 20 for details	Given rectally or by intravenous injection; see Ch. 20 for other details
Fosphenytoin sodium	0.15–0.25 [M] Metabolised by hydrolysis to phenytoin	Given by intravenous injection or infusion; ester prodrug for phenytoin
Lorazepam	See Ch. 20 for details	Given by intravenous injection; see Ch. 20
Midazolam	See Ch. 20 for details	Given orally; see Ch. 20
Paraldehyde	10 (neonates) [M]	Given rectally using a glass syringe (it dissolves plastic!)
Phenobarbital sodium	See above	Given by intravenous injection
Phenytoin sodium	See above	Given by intravenous injection or infusion; the solution for injection is highly alkaline and venous irritation is reduced by injecting physiological saline before and after drug administration

[M], metabolism; [R], renal excretion.

24 Extrapyramidal movement disorders and spasticity

The group of nuclei in the area of the brain known as the basal ganglia (Fig. 24.1) are part of an integrative loop motor circuit (the cortico-basal ganglia-thalamo-cortical loop). This loop is intimately involved in the coordination of motor function. Nuclei in the basal ganglia feed neuronal output to the cortex and receive input from the cortex. Degeneration of vital neurons in the basal ganglia produces disordered regulation of neuronal activity and dysfunctional motor activity. Treatment for these disorders is directed at restoring the balance among the neurotransmitters in the basal ganglia.

PARKINSON'S DISEASE AND PARKINSONISM

Parkinson's disease and parkinsonism arise from dysfunction in the part of the brain called the basal ganglia, which is involved in the control of movement. The basal ganglia system includes nuclei such as the substantia nigra, the striatum, the globus pallidus and the subthalamic nucleus (Fig. 24.1). Between these nuclei there are many complex *internal neuronal loop circuits* that can use glutamate, dopamine, acetylcholine or gamma-aminobutyric acid (GABA) as neurotransmitters; in addition there are *external loop circuits* that integrate neurons outside of the basal ganglia with the internal circuits of the basal ganglia. For example, basal ganglia nuclei feed into and receive information from the cortex via an external loop (the cortico-basal ganglia-thalamo-cortical loop) that is involved in the control of movement. The precise details of the complex interplay between the neuronal circuits are beyond the scope of this book and only general details are given.

Parkinson's disease is a disorder characterised by a triad of:

- resting tremor
- skeletal muscle rigidity
- bradykinesia (poverty of movement).

There are two clinical subtypes of Parkinson's disease: the akinetic-rigid form and the tremor-dominant type. The trigger for the condition is unknown, but genetic susceptibility and environmental toxins have been implicated.

The underlying pathology involves loss of neurons in the substantia nigra pars compacta and deposition of intracytoplasmic Lewy bodies. Lewy bodies are complex structures that produce functional changes in dopaminergic neurons of the nigrostriatal pathway, possibly involving impaired handling of free radicals generated during dopamine metabolism. This ultimately leads to progressive neuronal death and degeneration of the nigrostriatal pathway (Fig. 24.1). More than 50% of substantia nigra pars compacta neurons must undergo degeneration before symptoms are apparent.

In Parkinson's disease, as a result of degeneration of the nigrostriatal dopaminergic pathways, there is destabilisation of the motor control networks. Denervation of the substantia nigra results in reduced stimulation of D_1 and D_2 receptors in the striatum. The consequence of this is abnormal transmission in other 'internal circuits' in the basal ganglia, leading to the distinctive parkinsonian state with overactive GABAergic stimulation of the thalamus and consequent reduced glutamatergic activation of cortical systems (Fig. 24.1B shows changes in Parkinson's disease *relative* to Fig. 24.1A). At the same time there is hyperactivity in the glutamatergic pathways that connect the cortex to the basal ganglia. Cholinergic transmission in the basal ganglia is also enhanced in Parkinson's disease, contributing to movement disorder and particularly tremor.

In some conditions that have clinical similarities to Parkinson's disease, for example the Steele–Richardson–Olszewski (progressive supranuclear palsy) and Shy–Drager syndromes, the GABA neurons also degenerate, which explains the poor response of these conditions to treatment with dopamine replacement therapy. Drugs that block striatal dopamine receptors, such as antipsychotic drugs (Ch. 21), can produce a parkinsonian syndrome which also responds poorly to dopamine replacement therapy.

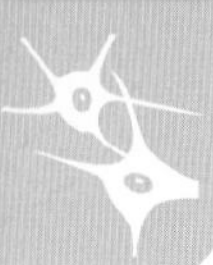

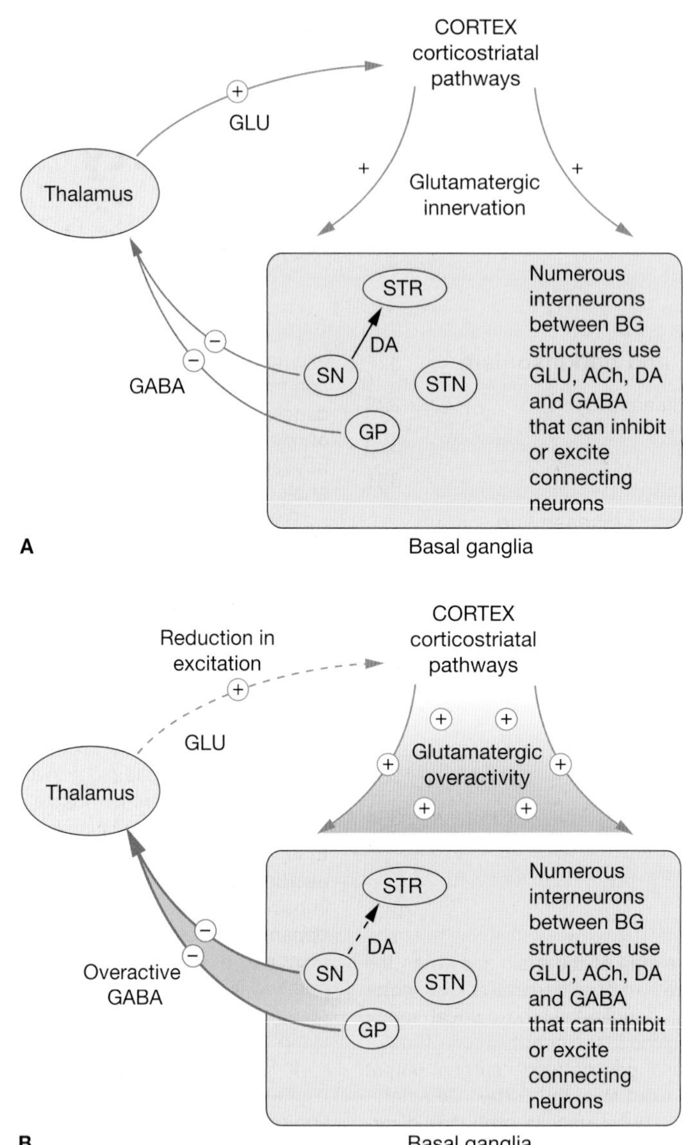

Fig. 24.1 **The cortico-basal ganglia-thalamo-cortical loop.** Panel **A** shows some of the pathways connecting the basal ganglia, the thalamus and the cortex which are involved in movement, and panel **B** indicates how they are disordered in Parkinson's disease *relative to panel **A***. The complex details of interneuronal pathways between the structures of the basal ganglia are omitted for clarity. The nuclei operate together in complex interconnecting loops. The cortico-basal ganglia-thalamo-cortical loop is an important motor network. Internal loops also occur between nuclei within the basal ganglia. Overall in Parkinson's disease the pathological changes in the basal ganglia result in increased inhibitory GABA transmission in pathways from the substantia nigra and the globus pallidus to the thalamus; there is excessive inhibition of thalamic-cortical brainstem motor networks. There is hyperactivity in the glutamatergic cortico-basal ganglia pathways and also in cholinergic pathways in the basal ganglia. BG, basal ganglia; DA, dopamine; GLU, glutamate; GP, globus pallidus; SN, substantia nigra; STN, subthalamic nucleus; STR, striatum; –, inhibition; +, stimulation; ----, reduced activity compared to normal function in control panel A.

DRUGS FOR PARKINSON'S DISEASE

Targets for drug therapy in Parkinson's disease are:

- enhancement of dopaminergic activity
- inhibition of cholinergic activity.

Overactivity in glutamatergic pathways has not yet provided suitable targets for drug therapy.

DOPAMINERGIC DRUGS

Levodopa

Mechanism of action

Dopamine cannot be given to replace the underlying deficiency in the basal ganglia because it does not cross the blood–brain barrier. However, levodopa can be carried into the brain by the large neutral amino acid transporter, where it is taken up into dopaminergic neurons and converted to dopamine by L-aromatic amino acid decarboxylase (Ch. 2).

Pharmacokinetics

Levodopa is absorbed from the small intestine by an active transport mechanism for large neutral amino acids. A similar transport system is used to transfer levodopa across the blood–brain barrier. When it is given alone, levodopa is extensively decarboxylated to dopamine in peripheral tissues such as the gut wall, liver and kidney. This reduces the amount of levodopa that reaches the brain (to about 1% of an oral dose) and the peripheral dopamine produces unwanted effects. Therefore, levodopa is given in combination with a peripheral dopa decarboxylase inhibitor (with carbidopa as co-careldopa or with benserazide as co-beneldopa). The dopa decarboxylase inhibitor does *not* cross the blood–brain barrier and therefore does not inhibit the conversion of levodopa to dopamine within the central nervous system (CNS). Inhibition of the peripheral metabolism of levodopa also increases the amount that crosses the blood–brain barrier to 5–10% of the oral dose.

The half-life of levodopa is short (about 1 h). In the early stages of Parkinson's disease, formation of dopamine in striatal neurons is sufficient to ensure a stable response despite infrequent doses of levodopa. Modified-release formulations of levodopa provide a more continuous supply of drug to the neurons. These formulations are often preferred by people with mild to moderate symptoms who do not experience levodopa-related dyskinesias (see below). Transition from conventional levodopa to a modified-release formulation requires care, because the latter has a lower bioavailability which makes it difficult to estimate the equivalent dose.

Unwanted effects

- Those arising mainly from peripheral dopamine generation, and which are reduced by use of a peripheral decarboxylase inhibitor. These include nausea and vomiting caused by stimulation of the chemoreceptor trigger zone (CTZ) of the medullary vomiting centre which lies outside the blood–brain barrier (Ch. 32), arrhythmias, and postural hypotension and flushing caused by vasodilation.
- Those arising from excessive CNS dopamine generation. These include dyskinetic involuntary movements, especially of the face and neck, or akathisia (restlessness). Psychological disturbance can also occur, including hallucinations, confusion, pathological gambling, increased libido and psychosis.
- Reddish discoloration of urine and other body fluids.
- Sedation, sudden onset of sleep.

Dopamine receptor agonists

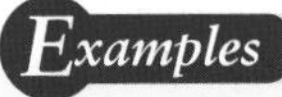

apomorphine, bromocriptine, pergolide, ropinirole, rotigotine

Mechanism of action

In contrast to levodopa, these drugs are direct agonists at central dopaminergic receptors. They have a longer duration of action than levodopa. The orally active drugs act on dopamine D_1, D_2 and D_3 receptors with varying patterns of selectivity (Fig. 24.2). Bromocriptine and pergolide are structurally related to ergot alkaloids (Ch. 26).

Pharmacokinetics

Bromocriptine is incompletely absorbed from the gut and undergoes considerable first-pass metabolism in the liver. Pergolide and ropinirole have higher bioavailability, but are also eliminated by hepatic metabolism. The half-lives vary from short to very long (see compendium).

Apomorphine is given parenterally by subcutaneous injection or continuous infusion, giving a very rapid onset of action. It has a short duration of action because of rapid hepatic metabolism. Rotigotine is only formulated for delivery via a skin patch to provide a more continuous supply of the drug.

Unwanted effects

Gradual dosage titration over several months may limit unwanted effects, which may include:

- Nausea, vomiting, dyspepsia, abdominal pain
- Dyskinesias
- Dizziness, nervousness, fatigue
- Neuropsychiatric effects with hallucinations and confusion are more frequent than with levodopa
- Sedation, sudden onset of sleep
- Skin reactions with transdermal patches
- Peripheral vasospasm with ergot derivatives such as bromocriptine and pergolide, especially in people with Raynaud's phenomenon
- Postural hypotension, peripheral oedema
- Pulmonary, pericardial and retroperitoneal fibrosis with ergot-derived drugs such as bromocriptine and pergolide; cardiac valve lesions also occur
- Respiratory depression with high dosages of apomorphine (an opioid derivative), which is antagonised by naloxone (Ch. 19).

Amantadine

Mechanism of action

Amantadine was introduced originally as an antiviral drug. It is believed to act in Parkinson's disease by stimulating release of dopamine stored in nerve terminals and by reducing reuptake of released dopamine by the presynaptic neuron (Fig. 24.2). Its usefulness tends to be short-lived, because of the development of tolerance. It can be beneficial in treatment of levodopa-induced dyskinesias.

Pharmacokinetics

Amantadine is well absorbed from the gut and has a long half-life (10–15 h). It is excreted unchanged by the kidney.

Unwanted effects

Most are mild and dose-related. They include:

- Anorexia, nausea
- Peripheral oedema

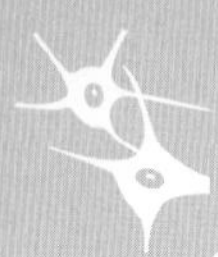

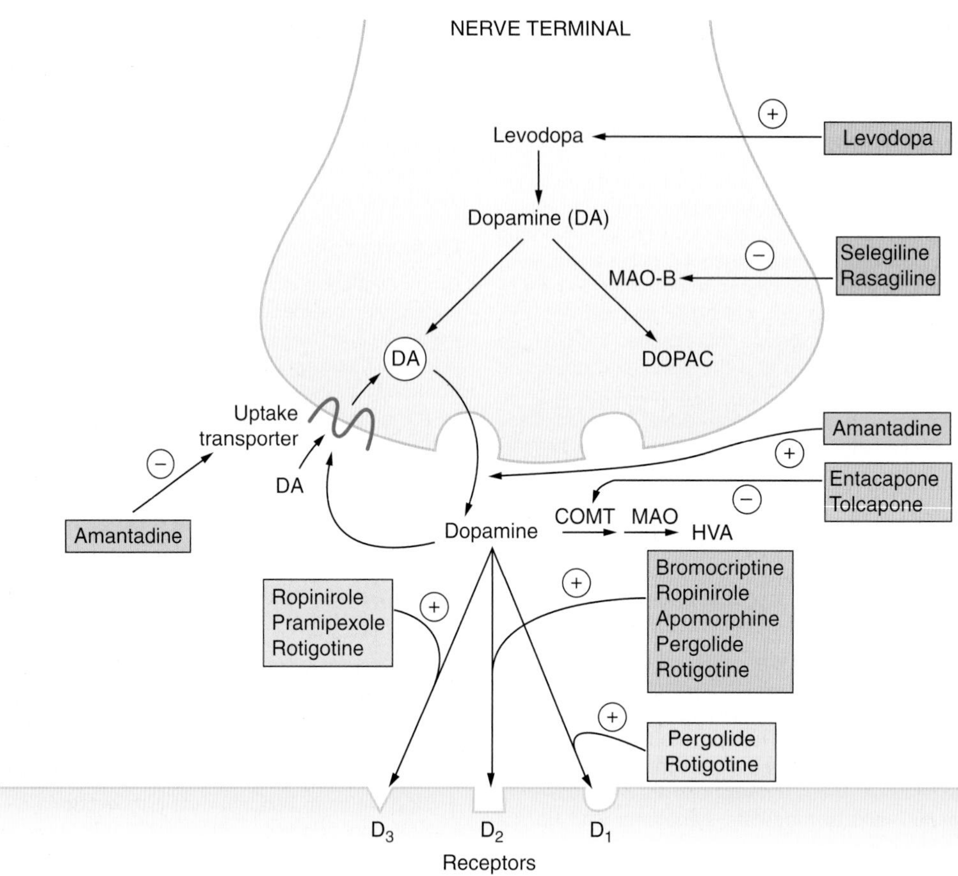

Fig. 24.2 **The major effects of drugs on the dopaminergic nerve terminal.** Drugs act a number of different sites to amplify dopaminergic signalling. COMT, catechol-O-methyltransferase; DA, dopamine; DOPAC, 3,4-dihydroxyphenylacetic acid; HVA, homovanillic acid; MAO-B, monoamine oxidase B; +, stimulation; –, inhibition.

- Nervousness, insomnia, hallucinations, seizures with high doses
- Livedo reticularis (skin vasoconstriction caused by local catecholamine release).

Selective monoamine oxidase type B inhibitors

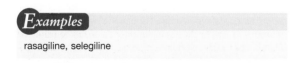

rasagiline, selegiline

Mechanism of action and effects

These drugs are irreversible inhibitors of the enzyme monoamine oxidase (MAO), which is responsible for the intraneuronal degradation of monoamine neurotransmitters (Ch. 4, and Fig. 22.3). They are relatively selective at low doses for the isoenzyme (MAO-B) found in the striatum. This isoenzyme is distinct from MAO-A, which is also present in the gut wall and other peripheral tissues. Interactions with drugs and foods containing tyramine, which is a problem with conventional non-selective MAO inhibitor (MAOI) antidepressants (Ch. 22), do not occur with these MAO-B-selective drugs. They prolong the duration of action of dopamine and reduce the levodopa dosage requirement by about one-third. Selective MAO-B inhibitors produce a small degree of clinical benefit when used alone.

Pharmacokinetics

Selegiline and rasagiline are well absorbed from the gut and both drugs have short half-lives (1–3 h) due to rapid hepatic metabolism. Selegiline undergoes metabolism, in part to the L isomers of amfetamine and methamphetamine, which have long half-lives.

Unwanted effects

- Nausea, dry mouth, constipation, diarrhoea
- Transient dizziness or lightheadedness is common, vertigo
- Insomnia, agitation, confusion, hallucinations caused by production of active amfetamine metabolites (Ch. 54)
- Arthralgia, myalgia.

Catechol-O-methyltransferase inhibitors

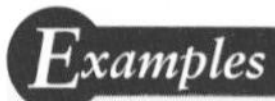

entacapone, tolcapone

Mechanism of action and effects

Catechol-O-methyltransferase (COMT) is responsible for breakdown of between 10% and 30% of levodopa both peripherally and in the CNS (Ch. 4), but, in the presence of a peripheral dopa decarboxylase inhibitor, COMT is responsible for most of the peripheral metabolism of levodopa. Inhibition of COMT doubles the half-life of levodopa (when it is used with a dopa decarboxylase inhibitor) and produces a 50% increase in the motor response. The dose of levodopa may therefore need to be reduced when entacapone or tolcapone is started. Entacapone does not cross the blood–brain barrier, but tolcapone does penetrate the brain and inhibits CNS COMT. The significance of this central action in the management of Parkinson's disease is not known.

Pharmacokinetics

Entacapone is variably absorbed from the gut. It undergoes extensive first-pass metabolism in the liver. Tolcapone is well absorbed from the gut and is metabolised in the liver. Both drugs have short half-lives (2–3 h).

Unwanted effects

- Dry mouth, nausea, vomiting, anorexia, abdominal pain, diarrhoea, constipation
- Dyskinesias, hallucinations, confusion, insomnia
- Discoloration of urine
- Fulminant hepatitis is a rare complication with tolcapone, which is only used if other drugs are inappropriate.

ANTIMUSCARINIC DRUGS

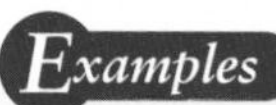

benzatropine, orphenadrine, procyclidine, trihexyphenidyl hydrochloride

Mechanism of action and effects

Drugs that block central muscarinic receptors (Ch. 4) help to restore the balance between cholinergic and dopaminergic activities. They have little effect on bradykinesia, and are less effective than levodopa for treating tremor and rigidity.

Pharmacokinetics

Most antimuscarinic drugs are fairly well absorbed from the gut, and undergo extensive hepatic metabolism. They have half-lives in the range 5–15 h. High lipid solubility ensures that the drug crosses the blood–brain barrier.

Unwanted effects

These are predictable and result from blockade of peripheral muscarinic receptors (Ch. 4). Reduced saliva production can be helpful in some people with Parkinson's disease, in whom sialorrhoea is a problem. Blockade of CNS muscarinic receptors can produce confusion in the elderly.

MANAGEMENT OF PARKINSON'S DISEASE AND PARKINSONIAN SYNDROMES

Treatment is usually avoided in Parkinson's disease until symptoms affect quality of life. Levodopa (with a peripheral decarboxylase inhibitor) is still widely used for the treatment of idiopathic Parkinson's disease, and a useful clinical response is achieved in about 70% of those treated. It is particularly useful for reducing bradykinesia. There is increasing reluctance to use levodopa in the early stages of Parkinson's disease, since it is possible that pulsatile dopaminergic stimulation produced by oral doses of levodopa, with its short half-life, may increase the risk of dyskinesias and response fluctuations developing later in treatment. Various strategies to reduce this problem are under investigation.

There is significantly less risk of response fluctuation or dyskinesias with levodopa in advanced disease if an alternative drug to levodopa is used early in the disease. Therefore a dopamine receptor agonist is often preferred for initial treatment, particularly for younger people. Levodopa is still preferred to a dopamine receptor agonist for older people with Parkinson's disease (over 65 years) or those with cognitive impairment, because of its lower propensity to cause confusion.

Motor complications with levodopa can occur immediately on starting treatment, but become progressively more likely with prolonged use. They can be extremely disabling, and are due to a change from a long-duration response to levodopa to a short-duration response. The duration of symptomatic benefit after each dose may be reduced ('wearing off'), the dose may take longer to work ('delayed on') or it may sometimes fail to produce any improvement ('no on'). The 'on–off' phenomenon with rapid swings between severe bradykinesia and toxic dyskinesias should be treated by a reduction in total levodopa dosage and adding another drug with the aim of maintaining more stable plasma concentrations of levodopa. Successful combinations include levodopa (with a peripheral decarboxylase inhibitor) and an MAO-B inhibitor such as selegiline, or with a COMT inhibitor such as entacapone. Alternatively, a dopaminergic receptor agonist could be added. Poor responses to individual doses of levodopa may be due to interference with absorption by a high protein meal or by delayed gastric emptying, and can be improved by taking the drug before meals. The rapid action of subcutaneous apomorphine can be invaluable to abort the 'off' state, but it is highly emetogenic; this can be prevented by using domperidone, a dopamine receptor blocker that does not cross the blood–brain barrier (Ch. 32). Domperidone should be taken 30 min before apomorphine, but it is often

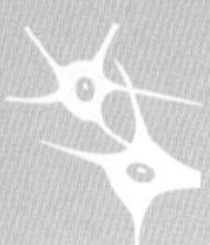

necessary to 'load' with domperidone for 24 h before starting apomorphine. More recently, infusion of levodopa gel into the jejunum via a gastrostomy has been shown to improve motor function in late-stage disease. Amantadine can be helpful to reduce levodopa-associated dyskinesias.

High-frequency bilateral electrical stimulation via implanted electrodes to switch off the subthalamic nuclei is effective for people who respond to levodopa but continue to have marked motor complications despite optimising therapy. It is used as an alternative to ablation of the nuclei since it allows the clinician to vary the site and area of the stimulation with time. Depression may be a problem with this treatment.

Antimuscarinic agents are rarely used, but may be given for tremor that responds inadequately to levodopa. They can also be helpful in reducing excessive salivation.

Symptomatic treatment for a variety of associated symptoms may be necessary in Parkinson's disease. These include treatment of autonomic symptoms such as postural hypotension, vomiting, constipation, urinary frequency and impotence. Parkinsonian psychosis should be treated with an atypical antipsychotic drug (Ch. 21).

Drugs improve symptoms and quality of life in idiopathic Parkinson's disease, but there is little evidence that they alter the underlying rate of neuronal degeneration. Levodopa therapy increases life expectancy, probably by reducing complications. Several studies are underway to look at a potential neuroprotective effect of dopamine receptor agonists. Other neuroprotective strategies, such as with antioxidants or glutamate receptor blocking agents, have so far proved disappointing.

Surgical treatment is sometimes advocated in advanced Parkinson's disease. Severe tremor may respond to stereotactic thalamotomy or pallidotomy. Pallidotomy can also be helpful for severe dyskinesias.

Drug-induced parkinsonism (e.g. with antipsychotics; Ch. 21) responds poorly to levodopa if the causative drug is continued, because blockade of D_2 receptors makes levodopa relatively ineffective. Parkinsonism resulting from antipsychotic drug therapy responds best to drug withdrawal. If this is not possible, then an atypical antipsychotic drug should be used and an antimuscarinic drug given for residual symptoms.

OTHER INVOLUNTARY MOVEMENT DISORDERS (DYSKINESIAS)

Dyskinesias are abnormal involuntary movement disorders that can present in several ways.

- *Tremor* is a rhythmic sinusoidal movement caused by repetitive muscle contractions. It may be an exaggeration of the normal physiological tremor, or an abnormal movement such as seen in Parkinson's disease.
- *Akathisia* is a compulsive need to move, often in stereotyped patterns.
- *Chorea* is irregular, unpredictable, jerky and non-stereotyped movement that involves several different parts of the body.
- *Myoclonus* is rapid shock-like movements that are often repetitive.
- *Tics* are rapid repetitive movements that can sometimes be controlled voluntarily, but with difficulty, for short periods.
- *Dystonias* are sustained spasms of muscle contraction that distort a part of the body into a dystonic posture. The dystonia is often exaggerated by voluntary movement. Examples include spasmodic torticollis (twisted neck) and oculogyric crisis.

Movement disorders have numerous causes, and can be precipitated by drug therapy. For example, a tremor can be caused by lithium, sodium valproate, tricyclic antidepressants and sympathomimetics. Antipsychotic drugs (Ch. 21) are associated with a wide variety of movement disorders, ranging from acute dystonia to akathisia, and tardive dyskinesias (involving choreodystonic movements often of the face and mouth).

Some movement disorders have a genetic origin. One such is Huntington's chorea, an autosomal dominant hereditary disease, which presents in adult life with progressive impairment of motor coordination, bizarre limb movements and dementia. The pathology is a loss of GABA inhibitory neurons within the neostriatum, which connect with the substantia nigra. There is a consequent reduction of inhibitory activity on dopaminergic cells in the substantia nigra and cells in the globus pallidus. Therefore, these cells generate uncoordinated discharges that produce bursts of excess motor activity.

DRUG TREATMENT

Tetrabenazine

Mechanism of action

Tetrabenazine produces selective monoamine depletion from neurons in the CNS. Storage vesicles become leaky and the released contents are degraded by MAO.

Pharmacokinetics

Tetrabenazine has a low oral bioavailability. It is extensively metabolised by first-pass metabolism in the liver to an active derivative. The half-lives of parent drug and metabolite are 7 h and 12 h, respectively.

Unwanted effects

- Gastrointestinal disturbances
- Drowsiness
- Postural hypotension
- Depression
- Dysphagia, which may be caused by extrapyramidal dysfunction.

MANAGEMENT OF DYSKINESIAS

Treatment options depend on the cause. Some common strategies are listed below.

- Cessation of the provoking drug. Symptoms may initially be exacerbated but usually settle. Withdrawal dyskinesias usually respond to gradual drug discontinuation. Tardive dyskinesias associated with antipsychotic treatment may become worse on drug withdrawal, but then slowly improve over many months.
- Exaggerated physiological tremor (e.g. anxiety tremor or tremor of thyrotoxicosis) may respond to a non-selective β-adrenoceptor antagonist such as propranolol (Ch. 5). Benign essential tremor is an action tremor that may benefit from a β-adrenoceptor antagonist or from primidone (Ch. 23). Gabapentin is an alternative second-line treatment (Ch. 23).
- Tetrabenazine is sometimes effective for treatment of choreiform movements.
- Many acute dystonias will respond to an antimuscarinic drug such as trihexyphenidyl given orally, or benzatropine given by intramuscular or intravenous injection for more severe symptoms.
- Enhanced inhibitory GABA neurotransmitter activity with baclofen (see below), sodium valproate or clonazepam (Ch. 23) may help some dystonias.
- Botulinum toxin (Ch. 27), which impairs acetylcholine release from nerve endings in the neuromuscular junction, can be injected into dystonic muscles to provide temporary relief. Spread of the paralytic effect to adjacent muscles can cause problems; for example, dysphagia after injection of neck muscles for torticollis. There are two serologically distinct types of botulinum toxin used therapeutically; some people who are refractory to botulinum toxin A may respond to botulinum toxin B.

SPASTICITY

Spasticity is a state of sustained muscle tone or tension which is often associated with an increase in stretch reflexes. The increase in muscle tone can arise from continued spinal reflex activity in the absence of inhibitory input from the motor cortex, such as can result from a stroke or in multiple sclerosis. Spasticity in skeletal muscles is often associated with partial or complete loss of voluntary movement and can produce painful and deforming contractures. Skeletal muscle relaxants are sometimes used for treatment of spasticity. The primary sites of action of these agents are the spinal reflexes or the release of Ca^{2+} in the muscle fibre, rather than the neuromuscular junction. Drugs that block the neuromuscular junction (Ch. 27) are not used to treat spasticity, because their main effect would be a further loss of voluntary movement.

DRUGS FOR SPASTICITY

Diazepam

Diazepam (and other benzodiazepines) enhances spinal inhibitory pathways by facilitating GABA-mediated opening of Cl^- channels (Ch. 20). The main disadvantage is sedation, as a result of inhibitory activity in higher centres at the doses necessary for a spasmolytic action.

Baclofen

Mechanism of action

Baclofen is an analogue of GABA that inhibits excitatory activity at mono- and polysynaptic reflexes at the spinal level. Its precise mechanism of action is uncertain. However, it binds stereoselectively to, and is an agonist at, $GABA_B$ receptors. This is believed to hyperpolarise neurons by increasing K^+ conductance and increase presynaptic inhibition of reflex pathways by blocking presynaptic Ca^{2+} influx and thus reducing excitatory neurotransmitter release. Baclofen also has an analgesic action, probably by inhibition of the release of substance P (Ch. 19).

Pharmacokinetics

Baclofen is absorbed rapidly from the gastrointestinal tract. It has a short half-life (3–4 h) and is eliminated largely unchanged in the urine. It can be given by intrathecal infusion using an implantable pump if severe spasticity is resistant to oral therapy.

Unwanted effects

- Sedation and drowsiness are common
- Muscle hypotonia
- Nausea
- Urinary disturbances
- Various CNS effects (e.g. lightheadedness, confusion, dizziness, ataxia and headache)
- Hallucinations or other psychiatric disturbance
- Hyperactivity, autonomic dysfunction and seizures can be precipitated by sudden withdrawal.

Tizanidine

Mechanisms of action

Tizanidine is an α_2-adrenoceptor agonist that increases presynaptic inhibition of motor neurons in the spinal cord via descending noradrenergic pathways. Inhibition is greatest in polysynaptic rather than monosynaptic pathways. Tizanidine has only 10% of the antihypertensive activity of the α_2-adrenoceptor agonist clonidine.

Pharmacokinetics

Tizanidine is well absorbed from the gut but undergoes extensive first-pass metabolism in the liver. Its elimination half-life is 2–4 h.

Unwanted effects

These are mainly dose-related, and can be minimised by slow dose titration. They include:

- Drowsiness and fatigue
- Dizziness
- Dry mouth, gastrointestinal disturbances.

Dantrolene

Mechanism of action and uses

Dantrolene is an antagonist at the ryanodine receptor (RYR1) that regulates release of Ca^{2+} from the sarcoplasmic reticulum in muscle cells (Ch. 5). Dantrolene inhibits the release of Ca^{2+} from the sarcoplasmic reticulum of skeletal

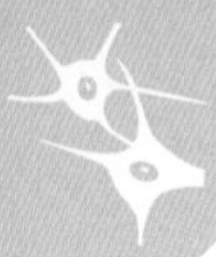

muscles, and uncouples muscle excitation from activation of the contractile apparatus. It is also used for the treatment of malignant hyperthermia (Ch. 17) and as an adjunctive treatment in neuroleptic malignant syndrome (Ch. 21).

Pharmacokinetics

Dantrolene is absorbed slowly from the gut and can also be given by intramuscular or slow intravenous injection. It is metabolised in the liver and has a variable and unpredictable half-life (2–24 h).

Unwanted effects

- Drowsiness, dizziness, weakness and malaise (usually transient)
- Anorexia, nausea, diarrhoea
- Headache
- Rash
- Dose-related risk of hepatitis.

MANAGEMENT OF SPASTICITY

Muscle hypotonia is a common problem in the drug therapy of spasticity. Mild spasticity may be useful, since the increased tone provides support for a weak limb, and should not be treated with drugs. Excessive spasticity following a stroke is most effectively prevented by adequate physiotherapy. Drug therapy, usually with baclofen as a first choice, is most often required for spasticity associated with multiple sclerosis or spinal cord injury. Drugs are most useful for deforming or painful spasticity, particularly if the person is not ambulant. In severe spasticity, intrathecal baclofen infusion may be successful, or intramuscular injection of botulinum toxin (see above, and Ch. 27) can be helpful for up to 3 months.

FURTHER READING

Parkinson's disease

Bhidayasiri R, Truong DD (2008) Motor complications in Parkinson's disease: clinical manifestations and management. *J Neurol Sci* 266, 204–215

Biglan KM, Ravina B (2007) Neuroprotection in Parkinson's disease: an elusive goal. *Semin Neurol* 27, 106–112

Blanchet PJ (2003) Antipsychotic drug-induced movement disorders. *Can J Neurol Sci* 30(suppl 1), S101–S107

Bonsi P, Cuomo D, Picconi B et al (2007) Striatal metabotropic glutamate receptors as a target for pharmacotherapy in Parkinson's disease. *Amino Acids* 32, 189–195

Clarke CE (2007) Parkinson's disease. *BMJ* 335, 441–445

Gerfen CR (2000) Molecular effects of dopamine on striatal-projection pathways. *Trends Neurosci* 23(suppl), S64–S70

Hauser RA, Zesiewicz TA (2007) Advances in the pharmacological management of early Parkinson disease. *Neurologist* 13, 126–132

Hermanowicz N (2007) Drug therapy for Parkinson's disease. *Semin Neurol* 27, 97–105

Hirose G (2006) Drug induced parkinsonism: a review. *J Neurol* 253(suppl 3), iii22–iii24

Lewitt PA (2008) Levodopa for the treatment of Parzinson's disease. *N Engl J Med* 359, 2468–2476

Obeso JA, Rodriguez-Oroz MC, Rodriguez M et al (2002) The basal ganglia and disorders of movement: pathophysiological mechanisms. *News Physiol Sci* 17, 51–55

Ossowska K, Konieczny J, Wardas J et al (2007) The influence of ligands of metabotropic glutamate receptor subtypes on parkinsonism-like symptoms and the striatopallidal pathway in rats. *Amino Acids* 32, 179–188

Schapira AH (2007) Treatment options in the modern management of Parkinson's disease. *Arch Neurol* 64, 1083–1088

Dyskinesias, dystonias and spasticity

Jancovic J (2006) Treatment of dystonia. *Lancet Neurol* 5, 864–872

Kartha N (2006) Dystonia. *Clin Geriatr Med* 22, 899–914

Lorincz MT (2006) Geriatric chorea. *Clin Geriatr Med* 22, 879–897

Louis ED (2001) Essential tremor. *N Engl J Med* 345, 887–891

Meleger AL (2006) Muscle relaxants and antispasticity agents. *Phys Med Rehab Clin North Am* 17, 401–413

Papapetropoulos S, Singer C (2007) Botulinum toxin in movement disorders. *Semin Neurol* 27, 183–194

Tarsey D, Simon DK (2006) Dystonia. *N Engl J Med* 355, 818–829

SELF-ASSESSMENT

In questions 1–4, the first statement, in italics, is true. Are the accompanying statements also true?

1. *In Parkinson's disease, there is abnormally reduced dopaminergic transmission which results in overexpression of GABAergic, and cholinergic transmission.*
   a. Symptoms of Parkinson's disease only become apparent when approximately 25% of dopaminergic neurons have been lost.
   b. Glutamate receptor antagonists are being investigated for use in Parkinson's disease.
   c. Levodopa has a half-life of 24 h.
2. *Treatment with levodopa will usually lead to complications such as dyskinesias and on–off fluctuations after about 5 years in people with young-onset disease (below 40 years of age).*
   a. In very early Parkinson's disease, the dopamine receptor agonist ropinirole is as effective as levodopa.
   b. Antimuscarinic drugs such as trihexyphenidyl have a low incidence of unwanted effects.
3. *The motor complications associated with long-term use of levodopa may be helped by reducing the individual doses and increasing the frequency of administration.*
   a. Bromocriptine is a potent agonist at dopamine (D_2) receptors.

b. Some of the movement disorder in Parkinson's disease arises from abnormalities in non-dopaminergic innervated areas of the brain.
c. The chemoreceptor trigger zone (CTZ) is stimulated by peripheral dopamine, as the CTZ lies outside the blood–brain barrier.
d. The monoamine oxidase inhibitor (MAOI) selegiline causes the 'cheese' reaction with ingestion of tyramine-containing foods.
e. Entacapone acts directly to stimulate dopamine receptors.

4. *Dantrolene is useful in spasticity as it reduces the Ca^{2+} release that contributes to contraction of skeletal muscle.*
   a. Baclofen enhances muscle spasticity.
   b. Botulinum toxin has a duration of action of up to 3 months.
5. A number of drugs are used for the treatment of Parkinson's disease. Which one of the following is a **true** statement about the properties of these drugs?
   A. Levodopa does not slow the progress of Parkinson's disease.
   B. Selegiline is a selective MAO-A inhibitor used for Parkinson's disease.
   C. More than 50% of orally administered levodopa enters the brain unaltered.
   D. Currently used drugs for Parkinson's disease only stimulate D_1-type dopamine receptors.
   E. Carbidopa is an effective dopamine decarboxylase inhibitor in the CNS.
6. Which one of the following adjunctive therapies will **not** increase the levels of dopamine in the brain when given together with levodopa?
   A. Tolcapone
   B. Selegiline
   C. Carbidopa
   D. Benzatropine
   E. Rasagiline
7. Which one of the following unwanted effects is **least likely** to occur following levodopa administration?
   A. Nausea and vomiting
   B. Arrhythmias
   C. Orthostatic hypotension in the elderly
   D. Slowing of heart rate
   E. Dyskinesia
8. Case history 1 questions

> A 75-year-old woman had been suffering from progressive symptoms of Parkinson's disease for 5 years. From the outset she had been treated continuously with levodopa, but problems had developed in controlling the symptoms with this drug.

   a. What is the cause of Parkinson's disease?
   b. What symptoms is this woman likely to have?
   c. Levodopa was given as co-beneldopa. What are the benefits of this formulation compared with levodopa alone?
   d. What difficulties can arise in controlling symptoms with levodopa in the early stages and later stages of treatment, and what changes in therapy could then be considered?
   e. What precautions need to be followed if this woman started to take vitamin supplements?
   f. Could a β-adrenoceptor antagonist be of use as part of this woman's treatment?
   g. Can any treatment protect against progressive deterioration in Parkinson's disease?
9. Case history 2 questions

> A married man aged 40 years was newly diagnosed as suffering from Parkinson's disease. His symptoms were tremor, bradykinesia, hypokinesia and rigidity, which were sufficiently mild that he was still able to carry out his work and pursue his hobbies. He was a security guard and had previously fought as a relatively unsuccessful professional boxer for 10 years, before retiring from the ring at the age of 35.
> Suggest possible treatment regimens for this man, with reasons for your suggestions.

ANSWERS

1. a. **False**. Symptoms develop when more than 50% of neurons have been lost.
   b. **True**. There is overactivity of some glutamatergic neurons in parkinsonism.
   c. **False**. Levodopa has a half-life of 1–2 h and this may contribute to end-of-dose movement disorders; modified-release formulations are available to provide a more continuous supply of the drug.
2. a. **True**. In clinical trials of up to 6 months' duration in early Parkinson's disease, ropinirole has been shown to be as effective as levodopa.
   b. **False**. Trihexyphenidyl can cause minor unwanted effects but also can cause severe confusion, particularly in the elderly.
3. a. **True**. Bromocriptine stimulates dopamine receptors and its half life of 6–8 h is longer than that of levodopa.
   b. **True**. Particularly tremor and rigidity may be partially because of other transmitter substances.
   c. **True**.
   d. **False**. Selegiline only inhibits MAO-B, leaving MAO-A intact to metabolise tyramine in cheese and some other foods.
   e. **False**. Entacapone inhibits the enzyme catechol-O-methyltransferase, which breaks down about 10% of levodopa. It therefore helps to maintain concentrations of levodopa, which has a short half-life.
4. a. **False**. Baclofen is used in the treatment of spasticity by inhibiting excitatory synapses and stimulating responses of the inhibitory transmitter GABA.
   b. **True**. Botulinum toxin is used in spasticity by local injection and inhibits acetylcholine release for up to 3 months.
5. Answer **A**.
   A. **True**.
   B. **False**. Selegiline and rasagiline are selective inhibitors for MAO-B.
   C. **False**. Only 1–2% of an oral dose of levodopa enters the brain in the absence of a decarboxylase inhibitor.

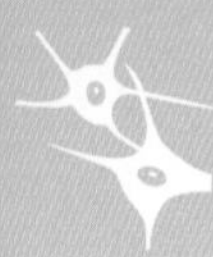

D. **False**. Drugs can stimulate D_1, D_2 or D_3 receptors with different degrees of selectivity (Fig. 24.2).
E. **False**. Carbidopa is a peripheral dopa decarboxylase inhibitor; it does not cross the blood–brain barrier.

6. Answer **D**.
   A. Tolcapone inhibits catechol-O-methyltransferase (COMT), which is one of the enzymes that metabolises dopamine
   B. Selegiline is a selective inhibitor of MAO-B, which, together with MAO-A, participates in the metabolism of dopamine.
   C. Carbidopa is an inhibitor of dopa decarboxylase that does not cross the blood–brain barrier. It therefore increases the amount of levodopa crossing into the brain and the subsequent conversion to dopamine.
   D. Benzatropine is a muscarinic receptor antagonist and will not affect dopamine levels.
   E. Rasagiline is a new irreversible selective MAO-B inhibitor that will increase the concentrations of dopamine in the brain by inhibiting its metabolism.
7. Answer **D**.
   A. Dopamine is a neurotransmitter in the chemoreceptor trigger zone and stimulates the processes of nausea and vomiting.
   B. Dopamine can stimulate β-adrenoceptors in the heart, increasing the likelihood of arrhythmias.
   C. Orthostatic hypotension is common, particularly in the elderly.
   D. Dopamine will not slow the heat rate.
   E. Increased CNS dopamine concentrations are associated with involuntary movements.
8. Case history 1 answers
   a. The cause of Parkinson's disease is uncertain but there is a selective degeneration of dopaminergic neurons in the substantia nigra. The cause of this degeneration is unknown but hypotheses include actions of reactive oxygen species, neurotoxins or immune disturbances. The basal ganglia of patients with Parkinson's disease generally have less than 10% of the normal amount of dopamine. This results in complex neurochemical disturbances. There is inadequate dopaminergic transmission. Cholinergic overactivity results from the removal of the inhibitory effect of dopamine on cholinergic neurons. There is also overactivity of glutamatergic neurons, and control of this may be a target for useful future drugs for the treatment of parkinsonism.
   b. Patients have akinesia, rigidity and tremor possibly from inhibition of the motor cortical system, whereas the descending inhibition of the brainstem locomotor areas may contribute to abnormalities of gait and posture. It leads to difficulty getting going and problems with fine movement, particularly in writing.
   c. Levodopa is the immediate precursor of dopamine and is transported into the CNS by an active transport mechanism. Dopamine does not gain access. Levodopa causes nausea and vomiting because it is metabolised in the periphery to dopamine, which has an effect on the chemoreceptor trigger zone (the blood–brain barrier is deficient in the area postrema). Co-beneldopa is a combination of levodopa and benserazide. Benserazide or another compound, carbidopa, are used because they inhibit peripheral dopa decarboxylase activity and, therefore, prevent the breakdown of levodopa to dopamine. They do not cross the blood–brain barrier, so levodopa is still converted to dopamine in the brain. Protection against peripheral unwanted effects can also be achieved with the peripheral-acting dopamine antagonist domperidone. Unwanted effects of levodopa are nausea and vomiting, postural hypotension, hallucinations and confusion, and unpredictable motor disturbances.
   d. Levodopa remains the most effective treatment for Parkinson's disease. However, there has been extensive debate about when to start therapy with levodopa. There is no convincing evidence that levodopa accelerates neurodegeneration, and survival is reduced if treatment is delayed until greater disability is present. In time, and despite long-term treatment with levodopa, there is an increasing incidence of dyskinesias and on–off fluctuations of effect, although most people continue to derive benefit throughout the duration of their illness. At the end of 5 years of treatment, approximately 50% of those treated will be experiencing reduced effectiveness with levodopa. In people with young-onset disease at or before the age of 40, almost all have developed dyskinesias and on–off problems after 5 years. These motor fluctuations can be as a result of unpredictable pharmacokinetic changes, such as unpredictable absorption across the blood–brain barrier or delayed gastric emptying, or because of progression of the disease process following further loss of dopaminergic neurons. Resolving these problems is highly individual, with dosage adjustments (either up or down) and shortening the interval between doses sometimes being helpful. The dyskinesia and on–off effects may be helped by smaller, more frequent doses of levodopa or perhaps by modified-release formulations. An antimuscarinic drug can be given with levodopa and is particularly useful in the treatment of tremor. However, they have the propensity to cause confusion and hallucinations, particularly in the elderly, so they are often reserved for people suffering from severe tremor. Other drugs which inhibit dopamine metabolism can also be introduced. Selegiline or rasagiline are inhibitors of MAO-B. The use of selegiline was questioned after a study which showed an increase in mortality; however, a second large study has not confirmed this. The catechol-O-methyltransferase inhibitors such as entacapone have also been developed as another way of reducing the metabolsim of levodopa and dopamine. These agents seem to be able to prolong the benefits of levodopa therapy. A direct dopamine agonist could also be added to levodopa treatment for the woman. The ergot derivatives, such as pergolide, are used. A new non-ergot drug, ropinirole, has recently been licensed for the treatment of early Parkinson's disease. Its ability to stimulate D_3 receptors may contribute to its action. Apomorphine given subcutaneously can also be used to counteract the off periods in advanced disease.

e. Vitamin B_6 reduces the central effectiveness of levodopa as it is a cofactor for conversion to dopamine, and, therefore, dopamine formation in the periphery would be enhanced.
f. Beta-adrenoceptor antagonists have been found to be helpful to reduce tremor in some people with parkinsonism.
g. No currently available drug has been proven to reduce disease progression. Studies suggesting that selegiline may be neuroprotective have not been confirmed. It does not delay the onset of dyskinesias during levodopa treatment. An early study that requires confirmation is that ropinirole may delay disease progression.

9. Case history 2 answer
There is extensive debate about when to commence levodopa therapy. The goal should be to improve quality of life and limit long-term unwanted effects. If the degree of disability is not severe and the affected person, carers and clinicians are in agreement, there may be no immediate need for therapy; however, this is controversial, as survival is reduced if treatment with levodopa is delayed until disability develops. If treatment is required, dopamine agonists could be started. These are less likely to produce dyskinesias and could delay the need for levodopa until progressive disabilities start to occur. The possibility of brain damage caused by boxing injury should also be considered. This responds poorly to standard treatments for Parkinson's disease.

Drugs used to treat extrapyramidal movement disorders

Drug	Half-life (h) and kinetics	Comments
Drugs used for Parkinson's disease		
Given orally unless otherwise stated		
Dopamine receptor agonists		
Apomorphine	0.5–1 [M] Undergoes hepatic N-demethylation and also sulphate conjugation to inactive metabolites	D_2 agonist; given by subcutaneous injection; not effective orally, probably as a result of presystemic metabolism
Bromocriptine	3 [M] Low oral bioavailability (about 10%) as a result of poor absorption and first-pass metabolism; extensively metabolised by hydrolysis to inactive products	D_2 receptor agonist; ergot derivative
Cabergoline	60–90 [M + R] Hydrolysed to metabolites that are excreted in bile and urine	D_2 receptor agonist; used as an adjunct to levodopa; ergot derivative
Levodopa	1.3 [M] Complete absorption; metabolised by dopa decarboxylase to dopamine and by *O*-methylation	Precursor of dopamine; normally given with carbidopa or benserazide (see below) to reduce first-pass metabolism and increase duration of action
Pergolide	27 [M] Rapid absorption but high first-pass metabolism; converted to numerous metabolites, some of which retain activity	Agonist at both D_2 and D_1 receptors; ergot derivative
Pramipexole	8–12 [R] High oral bioavailability; eliminated by renal tubular secretion and filtration	Selective agonist at D_3 receptors
Ropinirole	6 [M + R] Bioavailability is about 50%; main metabolic pathway is oxidation by CYP1A2 in the liver	Agonist at D_3 and D_2 receptors
Rotigotine	5–7 [M] Steady-state plasma levels are achieved after 2–3 days; extensively metabolised by N-dealkylation (by multiple isomers of P450) and by conjugation with sulphate and glucuronic acid	Administered via a transdermal patch

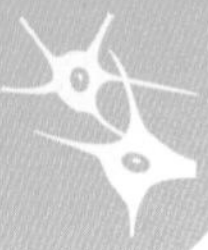

Drugs used to treat extrapyramidal movement disorders

Drug	Half-life (h) and kinetics	Comments
Drugs used in combination with oral levodopa therapy		
Benserazide	? [M] Incomplete absorption; metabolised by hydrolysis	Peripheral decarboxylase inhibitor used in combination with levodopa (co-beneldopa)
Carbidopa	1–3 [M + R] Variable oral bioavailability (40–90%); limited metabolism	Peripheral decarboxylase inhibitor used in combination with levodopa (co-careldopa)
Monoamine oxidase type B inhibitors		
Rasagiline	3 [M] Bioavailability is about 40%; eliminated by hepatic hydroxylation and N-dealkylation; no correlation between half-life and duration of action	Used alone or in combination with levodopa
Selegiline	1–2 [M] High bioavailability; metabolised in the liver to an active desmethyl metabolite and amfetamine analogues	Used alone or in combination with levodopa
Catechol-O-methyltransferase inhibitors		
Entacapone	2–3 [M] Oral bioavailability is about 30–50%; metabolised by glucuronidation	
Tolcapone	2–3 [M] Rapidly absorbed with a bioavailability of 65%; eliminated by CYP3A4-mediated hepatic oxidation	
Other drugs not acting via inhibition of muscarinic receptors		
Amantadine	10–15 [R] Complete oral bioavailability: renal clearance (400 mL min^{-1}) indicates extensive tubular secretion; half-life increases in elderly in relation to changes in renal function	Also used as an antiviral agent
Antimuscarinic drugs		
Benzatropine	? [M] Numerous metabolites found in rat studies	Given orally, or by intramuscular or intravenous injection; few data available
Orphenadrine	14–16 [M + R] Bioavailability is about 70%; eliminated by P450-mediated oxidation	Given orally
Procyclidine	13 [M] About 75% oral bioavailability; eliminated by oxidation and conjugation	Given orally, or by intramuscular or intravenous injection
Trihexyphenidyl hydrochloride	3–7 [M + R] High bioavailability; 56% recovered as hydroxy metabolites within 3 days	
Drugs used for essential tremor, chorea, tics and related disorders		
Given orally		
Chlorpromazine	–	See Ch. 21
Clonidine	–	See Ch. 6
Haloperidol	–	See Ch. 21
Pimozide	–	See Ch. 21
Piracetam	4 [R] Mostly eliminated by glomerular filtration; non-renal elimination (route undefined) accounts for about 30% of elimination	Used as adjunctive treatment for cortical myoclonus

Drugs used to treat extrapyramidal movement disorders

Drug	Half-life (h) and kinetics	Comments
Primidone	–	See Ch. 23
Propranolol	–	See Ch. 8
Sulpiride	–	See Ch. 21
Tetrabenazine	7 [M] Low oral bioavailability (5%); response is probably caused by a metabolite, dihydrotetrabenazine, which is as active as the parent drug and has a longer half-life (12 h)	
Trihexyphenidyl	–	See above
Drugs used to treat spasticity		
Given orally		
Baclofen	3–4 [R + M] Good oral bioavailability (95%); good oral absorption; about 15% undergoes deamination in the liver and the remainder is eliminated by the kidneys	
Dantrolene	4–24 [M] Good oral bioavailability (40–80%); metabolites are largely inactive and eliminated in urine and bile	Also used for malignant hyperthermia and neuroleptic malignant syndrome
Diazepam	–	See Ch. 20
Tizanidine	2–4 [M] Oral bioavailability is about 20–40% because of first-pass metabolism; metabolites are inactive	α_2-Adrenoceptor agonist
Other drugs affecting movement		
Botulinum A toxin	–	Used for torsional dystonias and other involuntary movements; specialist use; given by local intramuscular injection; onset and duration of action depend on the clinical use of the drug
Botulinum B toxin	–	Used for torsional dystonias and other involuntary movements; specialist use; given by local intramuscular injection; onset and duration of action depend on the clinical use of the drug
Carisoprodol	6–8 [M] Rapid absorption; numerous metabolites, including meprobamate, formed by polymorphic CYP2C19	Used for short-term symptomatic relief of muscle spasm; given orally; efficacy uncertain
Methocarbamol	1–2 [M] Complete absorption; extensively metabolised in the liver (more published data for racehorses than for humans!)	Used for short-term symptomatic relief of muscle spasm; given orally; efficacy uncertain
Quinine	8–21 [M] Almost completely absorbed; extensively oxidised in the liver	Used for nocturnal leg cramps; given orally

[M], metabolism; [R], renal excretion.

25 Other neurological disorders: multiple sclerosis, motor neuron disease and Guillain–Barré syndrome

MULTIPLE SCLEROSIS

Multiple sclerosis is characterised by an immunologically mediated inflammatory demyelination of the central nervous system (CNS). The cause is unknown, but it may be initiated by exposure of genetically susceptible individuals to an infective agent with an antigenic structure similar to myelin basic protein (molecular mimicry). This trigger initiates a peripheral immune response, and the blood–brain barrier is then breached by primed T- and B-lymphocytes and macrophages. The initiating agent may also upregulate adhesion molecules (integrins) on T-lymphocytes, promoting their adhesion to cerebrovascular endothelium and transport across the blood–brain barrier. The inflammation in the brain has the characteristics of a Th1-cell autoimmune response (Ch. 38), with the T-cells secreting inflammatory cytokines such as interferon-γ, interleukin (IL)-17 and lymphotoxin (TNFβ). The destruction of myelin is probably initiated by B-cell-derived autoantibodies. Deficient numbers of regulatory T-cells may also contribute to the lack of tolerance to self-antigens.

The T-cell cytokines activate macrophages that phagocytose myelin coated with antimyelin antibody, and destroy the myelin sheath around nerves, particularly in white matter. The immunological damage also affects oligodendrocytes, the cells that produce the myelin. The end result of these processes is the generation of demyelinated plaques that disturb normal conduction of electrical impulses in the CNS. However, the long-term disability in multiple sclerosis is mainly due to axonal damage, which occurs most extensively in the acute stages of the disease. Demyelination may predispose axons to damage from upregulation of Na^+ channels, with subsequent reversal of the Na^+–Ca^{2+} exchanger and Ca^{2+}-induced cytotoxicity. Axon degeneration may also be enhanced by oligodendrocyte dysfunction and failure to remyelinate the nerves.

Multiple sclerosis usually begins in the second or third decades of life and in 85% of cases presents with relapsing and remitting symptoms and signs of multifocal CNS dysfunction. The usual clinical course is initially one of stepwise deterioration, but eventually there is progressive deterioration (secondary progressive multiple sclerosis). In the remainder, the course is slowly progressive from the outset (primary progressive multiple sclerosis). To secure the diagnosis, episodes of neurological dysfunction must be separated in both time and place (more than one episode in more than one area of the brain). A single clinical episode of demyelination with several areas of demyelination on magnetic resonance scanning of the brain that have not caused symptoms is known as clinically isolated syndrome. The areas of the CNS most often involved in multiple sclerosis are the optic nerves, spinal cord, brainstem and cerebellum. Common clinical presentations are optic neuritis, weakness with spasticity, ataxia, and bladder and bowel dysfunction.

DRUG TREATMENT

There is no proven cure for multiple sclerosis, but drugs can be used to reduce the symptoms. There is increasing evidence that modulating the immune response as early as possible in the disease process may reduce disability.

- **Corticosteroids** (Ch. 44) are often used to treat an acute relapse (e.g. intravenous methylprednisolone for 3 days or oral prednisolone for 3 weeks). They probably shorten the duration of an attack but have no effect on long-term outcome.
- **Interferon-β-1a or -1b** reduces the inflammatory response in an acute attack and can reduce the frequency of relapses. They are translocated to cell nuclei and act as transcription factors by binding to enhancer elements, where they stimulate gene expression. Proposed mechanisms for the clinical effect include decreased expression of major histocompatibility complex molecules on antigen-presenting cells (Ch. 38), inhibition of T-cell activation, decreased release of inflammatory cytokines, and enhanced activity of suppressor T-cells. After a single episode of demyelination, about 50% of people will subsequently develop the clinical syndrome of multiple sclerosis. The use of interferon-β at the time of this clinically isolated syndrome significantly reduces the risk of developing multiple sclerosis at 2 years after treatment. Otherwise, the use of interferon-β is reserved for ambulant individuals who have had at least two attacks of relapsing and remitting disease over the previous 2 or 3 years. However, although the drug may reduce relapses by about one-third, it does not prevent ultimate disability. Interferon-β is given by intramuscular or subcutaneous injection. The most frequent unwanted effects are influenza-like symptoms, which occur commonly and may persist for several months, and pain or ulceration at the injection site. Neutralising

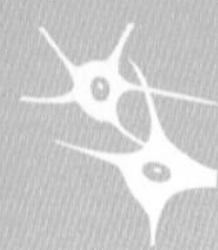

antibodies are produced during repeated administration in 5% of people, which leads to treatment failure within 2 years of starting treatment.

- **Glatiramer acetate** is a synthetic polypeptide immunomodulator that has some structural similarities to myelin basic protein. It may produce immunological tolerance by increasing the number of regulatory T-cells. Its use may reduce the frequency of relapses but, like interferon-β, it does not influence long-term disability. Glatiramer acetate is mainly used when antibodies reduce the effectiveness of interferon-β. It is given by subcutaneous injection. Unwanted effects include flushing, chest pain, palpitation and dyspnoea immediately after injection, and reactions at the injection site.
- **Mitoxantrone,** a cytotoxic antibiotic (Ch. 52), has shown encouraging results in reducing disability when given at 3-monthly intervals. The long-term benefit is uncertain.
- **Natalizumab** is a monoclonal antibody that selectively inhibits the cell surface adhesion molecules α_4-integrins on the surface of T-lymphocytes. This prevents T-cells from interacting with receptors on the vascular endothelium and crossing the blood–brain barrier. Natalizumab reduces relapse rate in relapsing–remitting multiple sclerosis. It increases the risk of infection, and there is a small risk of developing the brain disease *progressive multifocal leucoencephalopathy* when it is used in combination with interferon-β. Natalizumab is currently used when interferon-β or glatiramer acetate has failed, and it is given under close follow-up in specialist units.
- Symptomatic treatment of spasticity may be necessary, for example with baclofen (Ch. 24). A multidisciplinary team approach to the management of the numerous disabling symptoms that may occur is essential.

MOTOR NEURON DISEASE

Motor neuron disease is an uncommon, rapidly progressive disorder of motor neurons that occurs most often in middle-aged males. It leads to both upper motor neuron signs and symptoms (hypertonia, impaired fine movement and hyperreflexia) and lower motor neuron signs and symptoms (fasciculations, muscle cramps, weakness and muscle atrophy). Death from respiratory failure usually occurs 3–5 years from the onset of symptoms. The pathophysiology involves neuronal loss but the cause is unknown; an autoimmune origin is unlikely, since treatment with immunosuppressive drugs is ineffective. There is evidence of excessive activation of excitatory glutamate receptors in the CNS which may lead to prolonged depolarisation of motor neurons, intracellular Ca^{2+} overload, mitochondrial damage and cell death (excitotoxicity). Oxidative stress from excessive free radical generation may be important. Mutations in the genes coding for superoxide dismutase, the cytosolic enzyme that protects against oxidative damage, have been described in motor neuron disease. A third mechanism of neuronal death, accelerated apoptosis, may also be involved.

DRUG TREATMENT

Riluzole is the only available agent that alters the course of motor neuron disease. This crosses the blood–brain barrier and may block the release of glutamate, and is also an indirect antagonist at glutamate NMDA (N-methyl-D-aspartate) receptors. These actions may inhibit glutamate-induced excitotoxicity. Treatment with riluzole does not arrest the disease but may slow its progression to a modest extent, improving survival by an average of 3 months after 18 months of treatment. Unwanted effects of riluzole include nausea, vomiting, diarrhoea, lethargy and dizziness.

Physiotherapists can help with advice on posture and exercise early in the disease, and later with passive movement to reduce musculoskeletal pain. Symptomatic treatment is often necessary for pain, breathlessness or dysphagia.

GUILLAIN–BARRÉ SYNDROME

Guillain–Barré syndrome is usually an autoimmune acute inflammatory demyelinating polyradiculopathy, probably triggered by a bacterial or viral infection. It only affects the peripheral nervous system and it produces rapid onset of limb weakness with loss of tendon reflexes, few sensory signs, and autonomic dysfunction. In about 5% of cases, the problem arises from acute motor or motor and sensory axonal neuropathy. About 10% of affected people die in the acute illness phase and a further 10% have incomplete recovery and are left with severe long-term disability.

The pathological process involves acute lymphocytic infiltration into peripheral nerves and spinal roots. T-lymphocytes and autoantibodies to myelin contribute to the immunological response. T-cells probably activate macrophages, which then invade the myelin sheaths possibly in response to antibody fixation. Axonal degeneration may result from matrix metalloproteinases and toxic nitric oxide radicals released from the macrophages, and frequently results in long-term disability.

MANAGEMENT

There are several aspects to the management of Guillain–Barré syndrome.

- Supportive treatment may be life-saving, and is the cornerstone of management. For example, ventilatory support is necessary for respiratory muscle weakness or paralysis. Haemodynamic disturbance, including significant bradycardia and asystole, can result from autonomic involvement and may require cardiovascular support. Prophylaxis for deep venous thrombosis with subcutaneous heparin (Ch. 11) should be used. Pain may require analgesia and can be reduced by passive limb movement.
- Plasma exchange, when used within 2 weeks of the onset of symptoms, improves the long-term outcome. The benefit is probably due to removal of autoantibodies.
- High-dose intravenous immunoglobulin (IgG) is equally effective as plasma exchange, and is now the preferred treatment. Unwanted effects include malaise, chills and fever.
- Corticosteroids are of no benefit, either alone or in combination with immunoglobulin.

FURTHER READING

Compston A, Coles A (2008) Multiple Sclerosis. *Lancet* 372, 1502–1517

Howard RS, Orrell RW (2002) Management of motor neurone disease. *Postgrad Med J* 78, 736–741

Hughes RAC, Comblath DR (2005) Guillain–Barré syndrome. *Lancet* 366, 1653–1666

Javed A, Reder AT (2006) Therapeutic role of beta-interferons in multiple sclerosis. *Pharmacol Ther* 110, 35–56

Kieseier BC, Wiendl H, Hemmer B, Hartung H-P (2007) Treatment and treatment trials in multiple sclerosis. *Curr Opin Neurol* 20, 286–293

Mitchell JD, Borasio GD (2007) Amyotrophic lateral sclerosis. *Lancet* 369, 2031–2041

Murray TJ (2006) Diagnosis and treatment of multiple sclerosis. *BMJ* 332, 525–527

Ransohoff RM (2007) Natalizumab for multiple sclerosis. *N Engl J Med* 356, 2622–2629

Winer JB (2008) Guillain-Barré syndrome. *BMJ* 337, 227–231

SELF-ASSESSMENT

1. Are the following statements true or false?
   a. Treatment with interferon-γ is of benefit in reducing relapses in multiple sclerosis.
   b. Multiple sclerosis is characterised in the early years by a steady progressive worsening of symptoms in the majority of people.
   c. Glutamate can cause neuronal damage.
   d. Riluzole is of benefit in motor neuron disease by blocking the release of gamma-aminobutyric acid (GABA).
   e. Natalizumab is used in multiple sclerosis as it enhances the action of adhesion molecules, increasing the passage of leucocytes into the central nervous system.
2. The following statements relate to the treatment of multiple sclerosis. Choose the one **most appropriate** statement.
   A. Beta-interferon causes influenza-like symptoms in 1% of those who receive it.
   B. Expert opinion does not recommend glatiramer acetate as a first-line drug for use in multiple sclerosis.
   C. Glatiramer acetate causes few unwanted effects following injection.
   D. Corticosteroid treatment is of benefit in reducing the progression of multiple sclerosis.
   E. Neuronal conduction is unimpaired in multiple sclerosis.

ANSWERS

1. a. **False**. Interferon-β is used in multiple sclerosis and may diminish the production of inflammatory interferon-γ.
   b. **False**. Multiple sclerosis is usually characterised by relapses and remissions over a number of years, although after about 10 years a steady decline sets in.
   c. **True**. Glutamate is an excitatory amino acid neurotransmitter but can cause cell damage and death (excitotoxicity) by a number of mechanisms, including an uncontrolled increase in intracellular Ca^{2+}.
   d. **False**. Riluzole is the only drug that will alter the course of motor neuron disease; it inhibits glutamate release and action, thereby reducing its toxicity.
   e. **False**. Natalizumab is an adhesion molecule inhibitor and reduces the migration of leucocytes into the CNS.
2. Answer **B**.
   A. Influenza-like symptoms can occur in about 50% of people.
   B. The use of glatiramer acetate is usually restricted to people who cannot tolerate interferon-β, or who have developed antibodies to interferon-β.
   C. **False**. Glatiramer acetate can cause flushing, chest tightness, palpitations, anxiety and breathlessness.
   D. **False**.
   E. Long-term disability is due to demyelination of nerves and consequent further axonal damage. Demyelination of nerves results in disordered neuronal conduction.

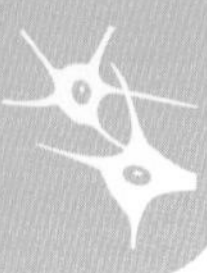

Drugs used to treat multiple sclerosis, motor neuron disease and Guillain–Barré syndrome

Drug	Half-life (h) and kinetics	Comments
Corticosteroids	See Ch. 44	Corticosteroids such as methylprednisolone or prednisolone may be of benefit for acute relapse in people with multiple sclerosis – see Ch. 44
Glatiramer acetate	? [M] Hydrolysed locally at the site of injection and absorbed parent compound and fragments enter the blood and lymphatic system; metabolised by proteolysis	Given by subcutaneous injection to treat multiple sclerosis
Interferon-β	2–4 [M] Rapid elimination due to tissue uptake and catabolism (especially in the liver); metabolised by proteolysis	Given by subcutaneous or intramuscular injection for relapsing, remitting multiple sclerosis
Mitoxantrone	4–220 [R + M]	A cytotoxic antibiotic given by intravenous infusion for the treatment of cancer (Ch. 52); not currently licensed for multiple sclerosis
Natalizumab	11 days [M] Protein clearance; clearance increased by the presence of natalizumab antibodies	A monoclonal antibody; given as an intravenous infusion
Riluzole	12 [M] High oral bioavailability (90%); eliminated by hepatic CYP1A2-mediated oxidation	A glutamate receptor antagonist used for motor neuron disease; given orally

[M], metabolism; [R], renal excretion.

26 Migraine

Headache has many causes, most of which are not produced by any structural abnormality or metabolic disturbance (primary headache) (Box 26.1). Tension is by far the most common primary cause, accounting for about two-thirds of cases, while migraine is the second most frequent cause. When headache is present for a prolonged time, or is recurrent, secondary causes may need to be excluded by a full history and examination for associated neurological symptoms and signs.

Migraine is an episodic headache, typically lasting 4–72 h. The diagnostic features of migraine are listed in Box 26.2. These are the only symptoms in the majority of migraineurs. However, in up to one-third, the headache is preceded or accompanied by focal neurological symptoms (migraine with aura), usually visual disturbances but occasionally more severe focal neurological episodes such as hemiparesis.

PATHOGENESIS OF MIGRAINE

The pathogenesis of migraine is imperfectly understood but involves both neuronal and vascular dysfunction (Fig. 26.1). It is likely that many different factors trigger the migraine process; an important factor is thought to be changes in cortical functioning. The aura that precedes a migraine attack in some people is caused by an initial intense but brief neuronal excitation producing cortical hyperaemia, which may be responsible for the visual aura of flashing or jagged lights. This is followed by a slowly propagated wave of cortical depolarisation that transiently depresses spontaneous and evoked neuronal activity (cortical spreading depression). The depressant wave is associated with vasoconstriction, which is responsible for focal neurological symptoms and signs. Recent evidence indicates that people who do not experience an aura also have a silent cortical spreading depression that precedes the headache. This suppression of electrical activity may therefore be the trigger for the migraine headache. The hallmark of the migraine process is activation of the trigeminal nerve pathway (Fig. 26.1). Under-activity of the sympathetic nervous system, hyperactivity of the parasympathetic nervous system and increased serotonergic neurotransmission are also all thought to contribute to the process. Associated with these dysfunctions, there is altered activity of a wide range of vasoactive and nociceptive mediators (Fig. 26.1).

The migraine process involves dilation and inflammation of the dural blood vessels and dura mater. This results from stimulation of afferents in the trigeminal pathway from the trigeminocervical complex in the brainstem to the dural blood vessels. The inflammation can then stimulate sensory nociceptors on the trigeminal nerves in the dura. The nociceptive impulses are relayed from the dura through the trigeminocervical complex in the brainstem, from where they are transmitted to the thalamus. Thalamic stimulation produces pain, nausea and vomiting. Monoaminergic pathways in the trigeminocervical complex contribute to nociceptive pain modulation (Ch. 19) in afferent nerves to intra- and extracranial blood vessels; there are also reflex parasympathetic connections back to the dural vessels that potentiate vasodilation (Fig. 26.1). Dysfunction of ion channels in the brain stem nuclei of the trigeminocervical complex may be the underlying cause of activation of the pathway. The trigeminocervical complex is rich in serotonin $5HT_{1B/1D}$ receptors, and their stimulation (particularly $5HT_{1B}$ receptors) inhibits neurotransmission to the thalamus.

DRUGS FOR MIGRAINE

SPECIFIC DRUGS FOR THE ACUTE MIGRAINE ATTACK

Triptans

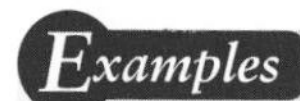

frovatriptan, naratriptan, sumatriptan, zolmitriptan

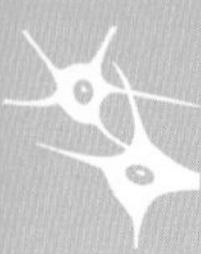

Box 26.1 Causes of headache

Primary headache
Tension-type headache
Migraine
Idiopathic stabbing headache
Exertional headache
Cluster headache

Secondary headache
Systemic infection
Head injury
Drug-induced headache
Vascular disorders
Brain tumour

Box 26.2 Diagnostic features of migraine

Two or more of the following features:

- Unilateral pain
- Throbbing
- Aggravation on movement
- Pain of moderate or severe intensity

and one of the following:

- Nausea or vomiting
- Light or noise sensitivity (photophobia or phonophobia)

Mechanisms of action and effects

The triptans are serotonin $5HT_{1B/1D}$ receptor agonists, with additional activity at $5HT_{1F}$ receptors that may contribute to their actions. Possible mechanisms of action are illustrated in Figure 26.2 and include:

- intracranial vasoconstriction ($5HT_{1B}$)
- inhibition of neurotransmission in the trigeminocervical complex and inhibition of antidromic (i.e. from impulses travelling the 'wrong way' along a nerve fibre) release of pro-inflammatory and vasoactive mediators.

Sumatriptan does not easily cross the blood–brain barrier since it is water-soluble, but this barrier may be impaired during a migraine attack. Naratriptan, zolmitriptan and other 'second-generation' triptans penetrate the blood–brain barrier more readily. These drugs directly inhibit excitability of the trigeminocervical complex in the brainstem, and relieve both the pain and the nausea associated with migraine.

Pharmacokinetics

Absorption of sumatriptan from the gut is rapid but erratic, whereas second-generation triptans such as naratriptan and zolmitriptan have better absorption. Effective plasma concentrations of these drugs are usually reached within 30 min of oral administration. Sumatriptan and zolmitriptan undergo first-pass metabolism by monoamine oxidase A (MAO-A) and have a low oral bioavailability. Sumatriptan is also available for subcutaneous injection and sumatriptan and zolmitriptan for administration by nasal spray, routes which avoid first-pass metabolism and relieve symptoms within 15 min. These routes can be more effective if the headache is accompanied by nausea, because gastric stasis often delays oral drug absorption during a migraine attack. Naratriptan (which is not a substrate for MAO-A) has a high oral bioavailability. Elimination of sumatriptan is by hepatic metabolism via MAO-A and cytochrome P450, while naratriptan and zolmitriptan are partially metabolised and partially excreted unchanged by the kidney. Most triptans have half-lives between 2 and 6 h, but the half-life of frovatriptan is long, at 26 h.

Unwanted effects

The frequency and intensity of unwanted effects is highest after subcutaneous use of sumatriptan:

- Tingling, paraesthesias or sensation of warmth in the head, neck, chest and limbs
- Dizziness or vertigo
- Nausea or vomiting
- Angina caused by coronary artery vasoconstriction (via $5HT_{1B}$ receptor stimulation) in people with pre-existing coronary artery disease
- Chest discomfort or pressure in up to 40% of people who use a triptan; this is probably not caused by myocardial ischaemia
- Pain or irritation at the injection site, or in the nose after local use.

Ergotamine

Mechanism of action

Ergotamine probably has an antimigraine action similar to the triptans by stimulating $5HT_1$ receptors. Unwanted effects arise from agonist activity at several other receptors, including α_1-adrenoceptors and dopamine D_2 receptors.

Pharmacokinetics

Oral administration is often accompanied by nausea, and ergotamine is better tolerated as a rectal suppository. Absorption is poor, erratic and delayed whichever route is chosen. Ergotamine undergoes extensive metabolism in the liver and has a short half-life (2 h). However, tight receptor binding produces a longer duration of action.

Unwanted effects

- Nausea and vomiting are caused by dopamine receptor stimulation at the chemoreceptor trigger zone (Ch. 32).
- Abdominal cramps and diarrhoea.
- Muscle cramps.
- Severe vasoconstriction as a result of α_1-adrenoceptor stimulation can lead to peripheral gangrene (acute ergotism). Ergotamine should be avoided in people with known atheromatous vascular disease (including ischaemic heart disease).
- Chronic intoxication with dependence can occur after prolonged use. Withdrawal then produces nausea and headache similar to an acute migraine attack. For this reason, ergotamine treatment should not be repeated at intervals of less than 4 days and should not be used more than twice a month.

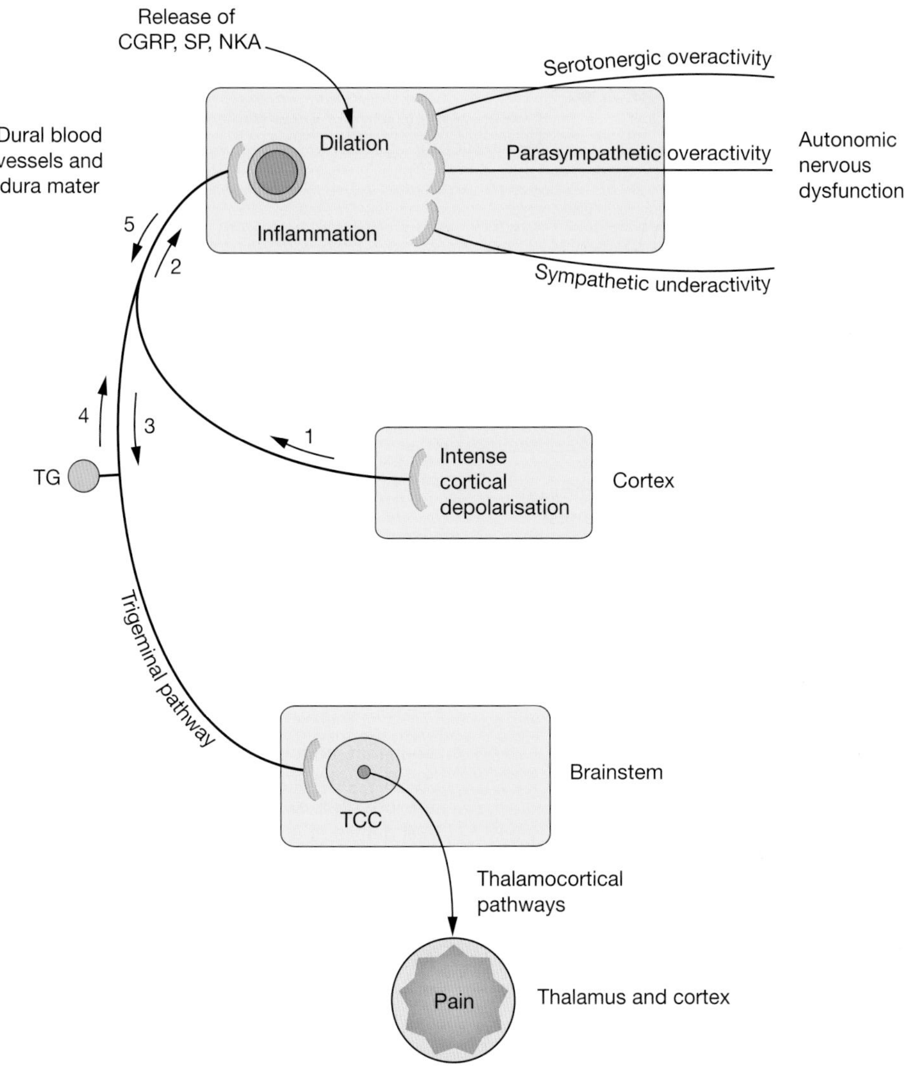

Fig. 26.1 **Proposed mechanisms associated with the processes of migraine.** The sequence and nature of neurogenic and vascular involvement in migraine are vigorously debated and may vary in different kinds of migraine-type headache. One scenario is that the trigger is a wave of cortical depression (1) which sensitizes and stimulates the trigeminal pathway in either direction (2, 3). This results in stimulation of the trigeminocervical complex (TCC) (3) in the brainstem, and onward stimulation of the thalamus and other areas can cause pain and nausea. Other reflex pathways from the brainstem via the superior salivatory nucleus to the dural blood vessels, which result in vasodilation, can also be activated at this stage. The stimulation of trigeminal nerves innervating the dural blood vessels (2, 4) results in the release of mediators such as calcitonin gene-related peptide (CGRP), substance P (SP) and neurokinin A (NKA) which cause vasodilation and participate in inflammation. CGRP and possibly other mediators are able to stimulate nociceptors in the trigeminal nerve endings, resulting in further activation of the pathways to the TCC and thalamus (5) and consequently further pain. Other pathways that may contribute to the migraine process include the sympathetic, parasympathetic and serotonergic systems. *The control of vascular tone in the dural blood vessels is complex. Vasoconstrictor innervation of these vessels is by sympathetic nerves, with co-release of peptides (e.g. neuropeptide Y) and purines (adenosine triphosphate [ATP]). Vasodilation is achieved by parasympathetic innervation, with co-release of vasoactive intestinal peptide, other neuropeptides and possibly nitric oxide. There are also serotonergic pathways that produce vasoconstriction by stimulation of $5HT_{1B}$ receptors and vasodilation via $5HT_2$ receptors. CGRP also has a vasodilator functions and is increased in migraine. TG, trigeminal ganglion.*

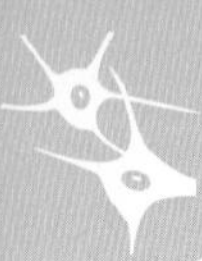

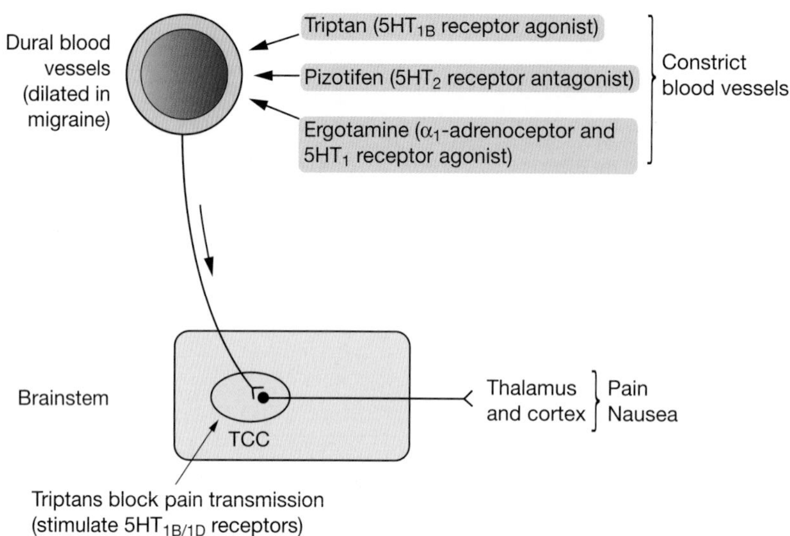

Fig. 26.2 Possible mechanisms of action of triptans in migraine. The trigeminocervical complex (TCC) is rich in $5HT_{1B/1D}$ receptors and their stimulation by some triptans inhibits neurotransmission to the thalamus and cortex. Serotonergic fibres to blood vessels can also cause vasoconstriction as released serotonin stimulates $5HT_{1B}$ receptors and also vasodilation by blocking $5HT_2$ subtype receptors.

PROPHYLACTIC DRUGS

Beta-adrenoceptor antagonists

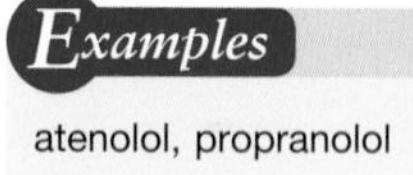

atenolol, propranolol

Mechanism of action in migraine

Full details of the β-adrenoceptor antagonists can be found in Chapter 5. In migraine, drugs with partial agonist activity that cause vasodilation (e.g. pindolol) are ineffective, suggesting that it is the reflex vasoconstriction produced by β-adrenoceptor antagonists that is responsible for their antimigraine action.

Antiepileptic drugs

The mechanism of action of sodium valproate, gabapentin and topiramate in the prophylaxis of migraine is not well understood, and some other antiepileptics that have been studied are ineffective. It is possible that there are multiple mechanisms, one of which may be GABA-mediated suppression of neurotransmission through the trigeminocervical complex in the brainstem. Full details of these drugs can be found in Chapter 23.

Amitriptyline

The mechanism of action in migraine is unknown, but probably relates to multiple neurotransmitter–receptor interactions that modulate the processing of nociceptive impulses. Several other antidepressants have been studied but, with the possible exception of fluoxetine, they are ineffective. Full details of amitriptyline can be found in Chapter 22.

Pizotifen

Mechanism of action

Pizotifen is an antagonist at $5HT_2$ receptors, promoting vasoconstriction of intracranial arteries.

Pharmacokinetics

Oral absorption is almost complete and extensive metabolism occurs in the liver. The half-life of pizotifen is very long, at about 26 h.

Unwanted effects

- Appetite stimulation with weight gain (may be caused by enhanced insulin release)
- Drowsiness.

Methysergide

Mechanism of action

Methysergide has $5HT_2$ receptor antagonist activity and some additional partial agonist activity at $5HT_{1B/1D}$ receptors.

Pharmacokinetics

Oral absorption is complete, and methysergide undergoes extensive first-pass metabolism in the liver. It has a half-life of 10 h.

Unwanted effects

- Restless or painful legs.
- Retroperitoneal fibrosis with long-term use, producing ureteric compression, hydronephrosis and renal failure. This is reversible but methysergide should be given for a maximum of 6 months, followed by a 1-month drug-free interval, to avoid this complication.

MANAGEMENT OF MIGRAINE

THE ACUTE ATTACK

Withdrawal of possible triggers such as cheese, chocolate, citrus fruits or alcoholic drinks may reduce the frequency of attacks by up to 50%. The combined oral hormonal contraceptive is a potential exacerbating factor, although it can be helpful for prevention of menstrual-related migraine.

Simple analgesia with a non-steroidal anti-inflammatory drug (NSAID) such as aspirin or ibuprofen (Ch. 29) may be sufficient for the relief of a mild acute attack of migraine. Nausea frequently accompanies a migraine attack and delays gastric emptying. If this occurs, absorption of the analgesic will be more rapid if an antiemetic such as metoclopramide or domperidone (Ch. 32) is given concurrently. If the person is vomiting, rectal or intramuscular analgesia, for example with an NSAID such as diclofenac or naproxen, can be used combined with rectal domperidone. Analgesics are usually more effective when given early after the onset of pain. Opioid analgesics are not recommended as they are short-acting, produce dependence, and frequent use can also promote 'analgesic headaches' (pain which appears as the effect of the drug wears off). Analgesic headaches are also more common with the use of compound analgesics, especially those that contain caffeine.

If attacks are poorly controlled by simple analgesics or are moderate to severe in intensity, a triptan is usually highly effective. It can relieve pain even if taken more than 4 h after the onset of an attack, but is less effective in those migraineurs who have developed cutaneous allodynia (a form of neuropathic pain; Ch. 19) in the trigeminal nerve distribution in association with the headache. Subcutaneous sumatriptan or intranasal sumatriptan or naratriptan are useful if a rapid response is required or if nausea precludes oral therapy. The response of individuals varies to the different triptans and it may be necessary to try several of them. Headache recurs within 48 h in more than 20–50% of those who gain relief from a triptan, although the risk of recurrence may be less with frovatriptan, which has a long half-life.

Ergotamine can be used to treat acute attacks, but is not recommended concurrently with a triptan. The risk of vasospasm and habituation means that ergotamine should be avoided in older people (who may have cardiovascular disease) and in those with frequent attacks. For these reasons, and because of the frequency of other unwanted effects, ergotamine is now infrequently used.

PROPHYLAXIS

Prophylaxis is usually recommended for people experiencing at least two attacks of migraine each month. Beta-adrenoceptor antagonists are widely held to be the best choice, providing there are no contraindications. The antiepileptic drugs sodium valproate and topiramate are effective second-line alternatives. There is less consistent evidence for the use of gabapentin, which is used as a third-line option. The major disadvantage of these agents is the risk of teratogenicity in women of childbearing age. The acceptability of pizotifen is limited by weight gain, especially in young women. Amitriptyline can be helpful for migraine, and is also effective for tension headache that may coexist with migraine. Methysergide can be given, providing there are brief drug-free periods, and there is some evidence to support the use of the angiotensin receptor antagonist candesartan (Ch. 6). Feverfew (*Tanacetum parthenium*), a herbal remedy, is helpful for some people. Botulinum toxin type A (Ch. 24), by injection into glabellar, frontalis and temporalis muscles, may reduce symptoms for up to 4 months.

The efficacy of all current prophylactic treatments is limited. Although the response to an individual drug class is unpredictable, only about half of all migraineurs can expect to have a 50% reduction in the frequency of attacks.

FURTHER READING

Agostoni E, Frigerio R, Santoro P (2003) Antiepileptic drugs in the treatment of chronic headaches. *Neurol Sci* 249(suppl 2), S128–S131

Ashkenazi A, Silberstein SD (2003) The evolving management of migraine. *Curr Opin Neurol* 16, 341–345

Bolay H, Reuter U, Dunn AK et al (2002) Intrinsic brain activity triggers trigeminal meningeal afferents in a migraine model. *Nat Med* 8, 136–142

Cady RK, Biondi DM (2006) An update on migraine pathophysiology and mechanism-based pharmacotherapeutics for migraine. *Postgrad Med* Apr (Spec No), 5–13

Cutrer FM (2001) Antiepileptic drugs: how they work in headache. *Headache* 41(suppl 1), S3–S10

Dahlöf C (2002) Integrating the triptans into clinical practice. *Curr Opin Neurol* 15, 317–322

Goadsby PJ (2006) Recent advances in the diagnosis and management of migraine. *BMJ* 332, 25–29

Montagna P (2004) The physiopathology of migraine: the contribution of genetics. *Neurol Sci* 25(suppl 3), S93–S96

Rapoport AM, Bigal ME (2004) Preventive migraine therapy: what is new? *Neurol Sci* 25(suppl 3), S177–S185

Silberstein SD (2004) Migraine. *Lancet* 363, 381–391

Snow V, Weiss K, Wall EM et al (2002) Pharmacologic management of acute attacks of migraine and prevention of migraine headache. *Ann Intern Med* 137, 840–849

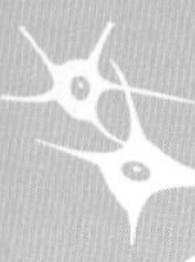

SELF-ASSESSMENT

In the following questions, the first statement, in italics, is true. Are the accompanying statements also true?

1. *Both antagonists at $5HT_2$ receptors and agonists at $5HT_{1B/1D/1F}$ receptors are used for the treatment of migraine.*
   a. Ergotamine is used prophylactically for migraine.
   b. Sumatriptan is useful for acute attacks of migraine as it is slow-acting.
2. *The combined oral hormonal contraceptive can enhance the frequency of migraine attacks in some women.* There is a large release of serotonin (possibly from platelets) in a migraine attack.
3. *Headache in migraine is thought to be caused by stimulation of sensory nerve endings in arteries.*
   a. Pizotifen is used prophylactically and inhibits $5HT_2$ receptors.
   b. Ergotamine is safe to use in ischaemic heart disease.
   c. Sumatriptan causes chest discomfort in 40% of people as a result of coronary vasoconstriction.
   d. Prophylactic treatment for migraine is highly effective.
4. *A variety of drugs such as tricyclic antidepressants, β-adrenoceptor antagonists and pizotifen may be useful in prophylaxis of migraine.* Where migraine is associated with vomiting, metoclopramide and paracetamol given together is a useful combination.
5. *Beta-adrenoceptor antagonists are widely used in the prophylaxis of migraine.* Dietary factors and stress play little part in the precipitation of migraine attacks.

ANSWERS

1. a. **False**. Because of habituation problems and unwanted effects, ergotamine should not be used more than twice a month for acute attacks.
   b. **False**. Sumatriptan is more rapidly absorbed when given by subcutaneous or nasal routes of administration. It gives slower relief when given orally.
2. **True**. Platelet levels of serotonin fall but urinary levels of the serotonin metabolite increase dramatically.
3. a. **True**. By inhibiting $5HT_2$ receptors, there is reduced perivascular inflammation, vasodilation and pain.
   b. **False**. Ergotamine causes vasoconstriction and should be avoided in patients with vascular diseases.
   c. **False**. Although sumatriptan causes chest discomfort and is contraindicated in patients with ischaemic heart disease or angina, the chest discomfort and tightness in people without ischaemic heart disease is probably caused by oesophageal spasm, not myocardial ischaemia.
   d. **False**. The prophylaxis of migraine is effective in only about 40% of individuals.
4. **True**. Metoclopramide is an antiemetic, increases gastric emptying and improves paracetamol absorption.
5. **False**. In some people, stress, chocolate, cheese, alcohol, etc, can provoke migraine attacks.

Drugs used to treat migraine

Drug	Half-life (h) and kinetics	Comments
Analgesics		
Most migraine headaches respond to non-steroidal anti-inflammatory drugs, but reduced gastric emptying and peristalsis may slow the rate of oral absorption; tolfenamic acid is licensed specifically for oral treatment of acute attacks; see Ch. 29		
Antiemetics		
Antiemetics (see Ch. 32) such as metoclopramide or domperidone are often given to relieve the nausea associated with migraine attacks		
$5HT_1$ receptor agonists (triptans)		
Act on $5HT_{1B}$ and $5HT_{1D}$ receptors; may be used during the acute headache phase; preferred treatment for those who fail to respond to analgesics; given orally unless otherwise indicated		
Almotriptan	3–4 [M + R] High oral bioavailability (70%); eliminated by oxidation via monoamine oxidase and P450 and also by renal tubular secretion	
Eletriptan	4–5 [M] Good oral bioavailability (50%); metabolised by CYP3A4; a demethylated metabolite retains the activity and has a longer half-life (13 h) but contributes little to the overall response	
Frovatriptan	26 [M] Oral bioavailability is 20–30%; metabolised by CYP1A2	

Drugs used to treat migraine

Drug	Half-life (h) and kinetics	Comments
Naratriptan	6 [M + R] High oral bioavailability (70%); inactive metabolites; 50% excreted unchanged	
Rizatriptan	2–3 [M + R] More rapid absorption than sumatriptan; good oral bioavailability (45%); oxidised by monoamine oxidase to inactive metabolites	Administration by subcutaneous injection is the treatment of choice for cluster headaches
Sumatriptan	2 [M + R] Low oral bioavailability (15%) but essentially complete availability after subcutaneous injection; eliminated equally by metabolism to inactive products and by renal excretion of the parent drug	Given orally, intranasally or by subcutaneous injection
Zolmitriptan	3 [M + R] Oral bioavailability about 40%; one of the three main metabolites (the N-desmethyl metabolite) is a $5HT_{1D}$ agonist and probably contributes significantly to the activity in vivo; also eliminated by renal excretion of the parent drug	Given orally or intranasally
Ergot alkaloids and related compounds		
Ergotamine	2 [M] Very low oral bioavailability (2%); pathways of metabolism not defined	Given orally or as suppositories
Methysergide	10 [M + R] Rapid and complete absorption but bioavailability is about 15% due to first-pass metabolism; hepatic oxidation and conjugation	Synthetic ergot alkaloid; used orally for prophylaxis but should only be administered under hospital supervision
Other drugs for migraine		
Amitriptyline	See Ch. 22	Used for prophylaxis; see Ch. 22
Antiepileptic drugs	See Ch. 23	Some antiepileptic drugs are used for prophylaxis; see Ch. 23
Beta-adrenoceptor antagonists	See Ch. 8	Some β-adrenoceptor antagonists are used for prophylaxis; see Ch. 8
Clonidine	See Ch. 6	Used orally for prophylaxis but is not recommended; preferred treatment for recurrent migraine; see Ch. 6
Isometheptene	? [M] Metabolised in animals but kinetic data are not available for humans	An indirectly acting sympathomimetic that constricts dilated cranial and cerebral arterioles; used orally for acute attacks
Pizotifen	26 [M] Good oral bioavailability (80%); metabolised to a polar quaternary N-glucuronide (very unusual reaction – see Ch. 2)	Used for prophylaxis; given orally

[M], metabolism; [R], renal excretion.

6

The musculoskeletal system

27 The neuromuscular junction and neuromuscular blockade

NEUROMUSCULAR TRANSMISSION

The neuromuscular junction represents a specialised part of the sarcolemma of skeletal muscle termed the motor endplate (Fig. 27.1a). In mammals, depolarisation of the postsynaptic membrane at the motor endplate causes contraction of the muscle fibre in an all-or-nothing response. Greater contractility is achieved by the stimulation of more motor units.

The neurotransmitter at the neuromuscular junction is acetylcholine (ACh), acting at nicotinic N_2 receptors. The processes of synthesis and release of ACh are described in Chapter 4, in relation to the general properties of neurotransmitters in the nervous system. The presynaptic nerve terminal at the neuromuscular junction contains 300 000 or more vesicles, each of which may contain up to 5000 molecules of ACh (known as a quantum). In response to an action potential, up to 500 vesicles discharge their contents into the synapse over a very short period (0.5 ms). Each N_2 receptor has two binding sites for ACh , and the Na^+ channel in the centre of the receptor opens when both sites are occupied (Ch. 1). This allows an influx of Na^+ into the muscle cell and depolarisation of the motor endplate. If depolarisation is sufficient to reach the firing threshold potential for the cell, then voltage-gated Na^+ channels open, full depolarisation of the muscle cell is triggered and an action potential is generated. Initiation of an action potential requires the release of 50–200 quanta of ACh, which will activate 10–15% of motor endplate N_2 receptors (Fig. 27.1b).

The action potential generated in the skeletal muscle cell passes along the sarcolemma into the T tubules, where Ca^{2+} is released from the sarcoplasmic reticulum. The increased availability of intracellular Ca^{2+} brings about the processes that result in muscle contraction.

The action of ACh on N_2 receptors is very short-lived (about 0.5 ms) because both the junctional cleft and the motor endplate contain large amounts of the extremely potent enzyme acetylcholinesterase (AChE), which degrades ACh extremely rapidly (Ch 4). An esterase called pseudocholinesterase (butyrylcholinesterase, plasma cholinesterase) also exists in plasma and hydrolyses ACh that escapes from the synaptic cleft; it acts more slowly than AChE. Pseudocholinesterase is important pharmacologically because of its ability to metabolise several drugs with ester bonds. Tissue esterases that break down ACh are also present in many cells, notably in the liver.

Although ACh is the neurotransmitter that causes contraction of both skeletal muscle and most smooth muscles, the basic organisation and functioning of these neuroeffector systems are very different, as shown in Table 27.1.

DRUGS ACTING AT THE NEUROMUSCULAR JUNCTION

Acetylcholinesterase inhibitors

Full details of this class of drug are given in Chapter 28.

AChE inhibitors block the breakdown of ACh following its release in neuronal synapses and at neuroeffector junctions. The mechanisms of action of different types of AChE inhibitor are described in Chapter 4, but it is important to remember that they are non-selective and prolong the availability and actions of ACh at all its receptors (nicotinic N_1 and N_2 and muscarinic). An important clinical use for these drugs is in the treatment of myasthenia gravis (Ch. 28).

Inhibitors of release of acetylcholine

Botulinum toxin A from the anaerobic bacillus *Clostridium botulinum* decreases the release of ACh from vesicles. It binds selectively to cholinergic nerve terminals, and, after internalisation via a cell membrane vesicle, it is released into the cell cytoplasm. The toxin cleaves a cytoplasmic protein on the cell membrane that is required for neurotransmitter release. This chemical denervation stimulates collateral axon growth which eventually results in the formation of a new neuromuscular junction. Botulinum toxin is extremely dangerous, as evidenced by the consequences of botulinum poisoning, but it also has clinical roles when injected locally. Two toxin serotypes, A and B, are used in clinical practice as botulinum toxin–haemagglutinin complex. Injection into skeletal muscles produces local muscle paralysis for many weeks, until new nerve terminals develop. It is used to treat involuntary movements such as blepharospasm (spasm of the eyelids) or torticollis (wry-neck) and to relieve spasticity (Ch. 24). It is also used by local injection to reduce excessive sweating, because it acts to inhibit ACh release at sweat glands, and occasionally for the prophylaxis of migraine (Ch. 26). Botulinum toxin is being used increasingly for cosmetic reasons to temporarily remove frown lines and wrinkles.

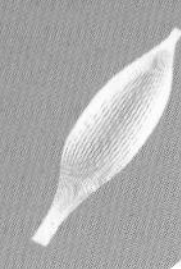

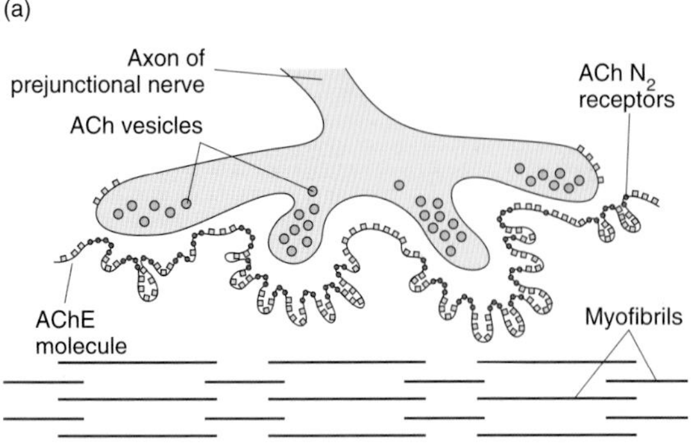

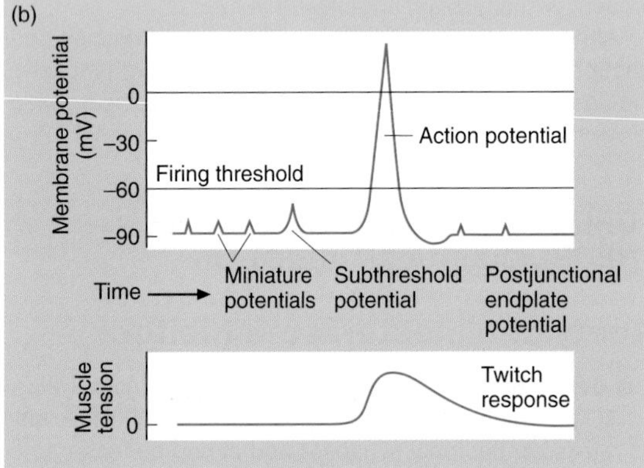

Fig. 27.1 **Acetylcholine (ACh) at the neuromuscular junction.** (a) Released ACh acts upon a postsynaptic nicotinic (N_2) receptor on the motor endplate, opening a cation channel, and an influx of Na^+ occurs, resulting in depolarisation. (b) At rest, insignificant amounts of ACh are released, and miniature endplate potentials generated are insufficient to reach the threshold potential to cause a propagated action potential. If sufficient ACh is released, an action potential is propagated, causing muscle contraction. Non-depolarising muscle relaxants prevent the generation of the action potential by blocking N_2 receptors. AChE, acetylcholinesterase.

Antagonists/blockers at the neuromuscular junction

Skeletal muscle relaxation is achieved by drugs that specifically and reversibly block the actions of ACh on nicotinic N_2 receptors at the neuromuscular junction; they do not affect autonomic nervous system function (i.e. the actions of ACh on muscarinic receptors at postganglionic nerve endings and nicotinic N_1 receptors in ganglia). Drugs that block the neuromuscular junction almost all resemble ACh in that they have a quaternary amino group that binds strongly to the anionic site of the nicotinic N_2 receptor (Fig. 27.2).

A neuromuscular blocker must occupy more than 75% of postsynaptic N_2 receptors before it can start to produce neuromuscular blockade. The potency of a neuromuscular blocker is measured by the ED_{95}, which is the dose required to produce 95% depression of muscular twitch (Table 27.2). About twice this dose is required for muscle relaxation adequate to permit tracheal intubation. The laryngeal

Table 27.1 Comparison of skeletal and smooth muscle innervation

Property	Skeletal muscle fibre	Smooth muscle fibre
Nerves supplying fibre	Single	Multiple
Junction	Highly organised motor endplate	Simple
Neurotransmitter	ACh	ACh
Receptor subtype	Nicotinic N_2	Muscarinic (mainly M_3)
Receptor distribution	Only at motor endplate, only one motor endplate per muscle fibre	Widely on the muscle surface
Effects of stimulation	Single nerve contracts the whole muscle fibre (all-or-none response)	Each nerve contracts part of muscle fibre (graded response)
Overdose by inhibition of AChE	Flaccid paralysis	Spasticity

ACh, acetylcholine; AChE, acetylcholinesterase.

muscles are more rapidly paralysed than other skeletal muscle groups, but the effect is often of shorter duration. This may reflect either the higher blood flow to this muscle, or the greater density of N_2 receptors.

Recovery of muscle action depends on the rate of clearance of the drug from the plasma. After a bolus injection of many neuromuscular blockers, this is largely a result of redistribution to tissues rather than metabolism. Redistribution lowers the plasma concentration (see Ch. 2) and consequently the concentration at the motor endplate. For those drugs which undergo rapid redistribution, the duration of neuromuscular blockade will be more prolonged after repeated boluses or infusions; this is because when equilibrium between plasma and tissue concentrations has been reached, the duration of effect then becomes mainly dependent on metabolism.

Competitive N_2 receptor antagonists (non-depolarising blockers)

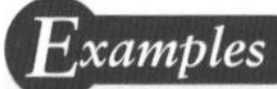

atracurium, cisatracurium, mivacurium, pancuronium, rocuronium, vecuronium

Mechanism of action and effects

Competitive N_2 receptor antagonists bind to the nicotinic N_2 receptor at the neuromuscular junction without causing depolarisation of the postsynaptic membrane. This blocks the depolarising effect of released ACh and leads to muscle relaxation. Inhibition of ACh hydrolysis by an AChE inhibitor (usually neostigmine, see Ch. 28) will prolong the action of ACh and reverse competitive neuromuscular junction

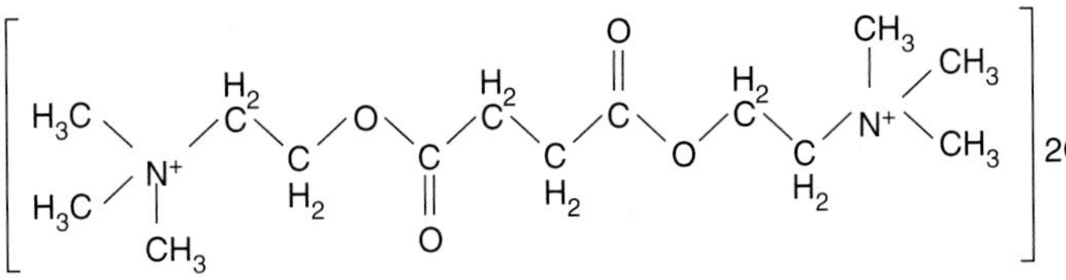

Fig. 27.2 **The structures of pancuronium, a non-depolarising blocking drug, and suxamethonium (succinylcholine), a depolarising blocker.**

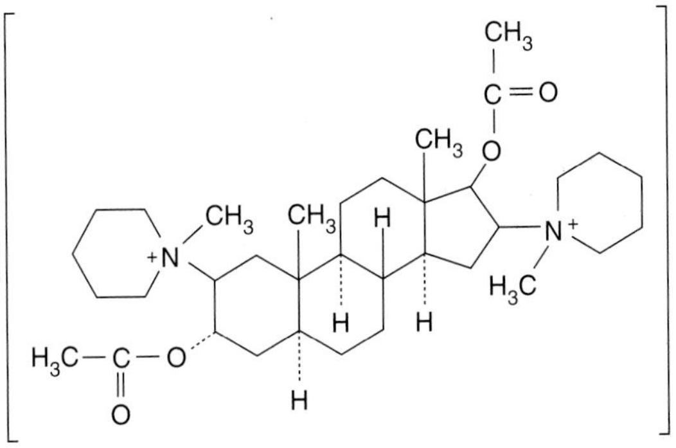

Table 27.2 Properties of some neuromuscular junction blocking drugs

Muscle relaxant	ED_{95} (mg/kg)[a]	Time to max block (min)[b]	Duration (min)[c]	Unwanted effects
Pancuronium	0.06	4–5	90	Tachycardia, hypertension due to sympathetic stimulation; increase in cardiac output
Vecuronium	0.05	3–4	45	Allergy
Atracurium	0.25	3–4	40	Histamine release; increase in heart rate and decrease in SVR, tachycardia, bronchospasm
Cisatracurium	0.05	4.5–5.5	30–40	Low incidence of unwanted effects
Rocuronium	0.4	2–3	30	Increase in heart rate; allergy
Mivacurium	0.08	2–3	15–20	Histamine release; increase in heart rate and decrease in SVR, tachycardia, bronchospasm; prolonged block in people lacking pseudocholinesterase (butyrylcholinesterase, plasma cholinesterase)
Suxamethonium (succinylcholine)		Fast	3–12	Postoperative muscle pain; bradycardia, hyperkalaemia, malignant hyperthermia; after approximately 20 min, some elements of block are those of non-depolarising type; prolonged block in people lacking pseudocholinesterase

[a] ED_{95} is the dose required to suppress muscle twitch by 95%.
[b] Time to maximum block following administration of the dose used for intubation (2 × the ED_{95}).
[c] Time taken to recover to 25% of the original twitch height after an intubation dose (2 × the ED_{95}).
SVR, systemic vascular resistance.

blockade. This principle is used at the end of an operation to aid recovery of the paralysed person.

Pharmacokinetics

Because of their high polarity, conferred by the quaternary N atom (Fig. 27.2), these drugs are not absorbed from the gastrointestinal tract and are given by intravenous injection. They have a low apparent volume of distribution and do not cross the blood–brain barrier. Vecuronium is partially metabolised in the liver but largely excreted unchanged in the bile. Pancuronium and rocuronium are eliminated by a combination of metabolism and renal excretion of unchanged drug. Atracurium (a mixture of 10 isomers) and cisatracurium (a single isomer of atracurium) undergo non-enzymatic spontaneous degradation as well as hydrolysis by non-specific esterases in the plasma, which is an advantage in hepatic or renal impairment. Mivacurium, like suxamethonium (see below), is metabolised by pseudocholinesterase.

The speed of onset of action and duration of action of competitive blockers differ (Table 27.2). Rocuronium has the fastest onset of action, within 2 min, which may make it useful during intubation. With the exception of atracurium and cisatracurium, the duration of action of competitive antagonists at the neuromuscular junction (from about 30 min for vecuronium up to 75 min for pancuronium) is mainly determined by redistribution of the drug into the body tissues. This leads to prolonged action with repeated doses (see above). The duration of effect of atracurium and cisatracurium is about 40 min. This is slightly longer than predicted from their plasma half-lives and may be a consequence of high-affinity binding sites close to the ACh receptor acting as a reservoir for the drug.

Unwanted effects

See Table 27.2.

Depolarising neuromuscular-blocking drugs

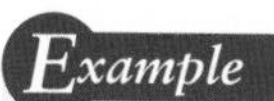

suxamethonium (succinylcholine)

Mechanism of action and effects

Suxamethonium is succinic acid with a choline molecule attached at each carboxylic acid group; it therefore resembles two ACh molecules joined back to back. When two molecules of suxamethonium bind to the nicotinic N_2 receptor, it acts as an agonist and depolarises the motor endplate. However, suxamethonium is not hydrolysed by AChE and therefore produces more prolonged depolarisation than ACh. This leads to a conformational change in the receptor that allows the Na^+ channel to close despite the continued presence of an agonist. As a result, the muscle repolarises and, although it can respond to direct electrical stimulation, it can no longer be stimulated via the neuronal release of ACh. Indeed, if the amount of available synaptic ACh is enhanced (such as occurs with the use of an AChE inhibitor), it will intensify a partial depolarising blockade and not reverse it. After about 20 min of depolarising blockade, suxamethonium exhibits the properties of a 'dual block'. The onset of a non-depolarising competitive type of blockade. At this stage, a partial blockade can be partially reversed by an AChE inhibitor.

Pharmacokinetics

Suxamethonium is a highly polar molecule, is not absorbed orally and must be given intravenously. It has a low volume of distribution and does not cross the blood–brain barrier. Suxamethonium has an onset of action within 1 min, but is rapidly hydrolysed by pseudocholinesterase, which results in a very short duration of action (about 3–12 min). Therefore, an infusion is necessary to produce a prolonged effect. A very prolonged paralysis occurs in about 1 in 2000–3000 individuals, who have a genetically determined deficiency of pseudocholinesterase (see Ch. 2). In this population, the action of suxamethonium is terminated after some 2–3 h by renal excretion.

Unwanted effects

- There is an initial depolarisation of the motor endplates prior to blockade, which results in muscle fasciculation.
- Prolonged apnoea occurs if there is a low circulating concentration of pseudocholinesterase, through either a genetic deficiency or a decreased synthesis of the enzyme in severe liver disease.
- Postoperative muscle pain is common, possibly due to inflammatory prostaglandins synthesised in response to repetitive stimulation of the cell and increased Ca^{2+} availability.
- The use of suxamethonium during anaesthesia has been linked with the development of a rare but potentially fatal disorder of muscles known as malignant hyperthermia, with a rapid rise in temperature, muscle rigidity, tachycardia and acidosis. Predisposition to this condition has an autosomal dominant inheritance. Treatment is with dantrolene (Ch. 24).
- Stimulation of ACh receptors at autonomic ganglia (nicotinic N_1) and muscarinic receptors produces bradycardia, especially with repeated doses.
- Hyperkalaemia, probably due to prolonged muscle depolarization. This is especially marked in the presence of major tissue trauma and severe burns.

INDICATIONS FOR NEUROMUSCULAR-BLOCKING DRUGS

The neuromuscular-blocking drugs are used in both surgical procedures and intensive care. Their administration forms part of the achievement of balanced anaesthesia described in Chapter 17.

Endotracheal intubation

Relaxation of the vocal cords allows easy passage of an endotracheal tube. A rapid onset of action is essential to minimise the risk of aspiration of gastric contents. This is the only current major use for suxamethonium. Because of frequent unwanted effects, suxamethonium is being superseded by rapidly acting non-depolarising blockers such as rocuronium.

During surgical procedures

Neuromuscular blockade produces muscle relaxation for procedures such as abdominal incisions. Selective skeletal muscle relaxation reduces the concentrations of general anaesthetic needed for deep anaesthesia. It can be achieved either by a single injection of a drug or by intravenous infusion for more prolonged surgery. At the end of the operation, the effect of a non-depolarising blocker can be reversed within 1 min by intravenous injection of neostigmine. Glycopyrrolate or atropine (Ch. 4) is given before neostigmine to prevent bradycardia or excessive salivation produced by stimulation of muscarinic receptors.

In intensive care

Neuromuscular blockade is used in addition to analgesia and sedation during mechanical ventilation, particularly if respiratory drive is suppressed (e.g. in adult respiratory distress syndrome), in status asthmaticus, for status epilepticus or tetanus, and for people with elevated intracranial pressure.

FURTHER READING

Bowman WC (2006) Neuromuscular block. *Br J Pharmacol* 147, S277–S286

Denborough M (1998) Malignant hyperthermia. *Lancet* 352, 1131–1136

Moore EW, Hunter JM (2001) The new neuromuscular blocking agents: do they offer any advantages? *Br J Anaesth* 87, 912–925

Münchau A, Bhatia KP (2000) Uses of botulinum toxin injection in medicine today. *BMJ* 320, 161–165

Wiklund RA, Rosenbaum SH (1997) Anesthesiology Part 1. *N Engl J Med* 337, 7132–7141

SELF-ASSESSMENT

In questions 1–4, the initial statement, in italics, is true. Are the accompanying statements also true?

1. *Vecuronium, unlike atracurium, has no haemodynamic effects as it does not cause histamine release.*
   a. Suxamethonium blockade is antagonised by lowered body temperature.
   b. All non-depolarising muscle relaxants cause similar amounts of histamine release.
2. *Malignant hyperthermia is a rare genetically determined disorder that causes hyperthermia and muscle spasms in response to suxamethonium, halothane and some other drugs.*
   a. Dantrolene is used to treat malignant hyperthermia.
   b. A skeletal muscle fibre is innervated by one motor endplate.
   c. The nicotinic receptor on skeletal muscle is identical to the nicotinic receptor in autonomic ganglia.
3. *Except for mivacurium and atracurium, the action of competitive neuromuscular junction blocking drugs is mainly limited by redistribution of the drug.*
   a. Suxamethonium is the only muscle relaxant used for tracheal intubation.
   b. Some competitive neuromuscular-blocking drugs, such as vecuronium, are relatively well absorbed orally.
4. *Botulinum toxin poisoning results from long-lasting blockade of parasympathetic and motor function.*
   a. Botulinum toxin acts postsynaptically to block ACh-induced depolarisation.
   b. Botulinum toxin is administered only by discrete local injection.
   c. Botulinum toxin inhibits pathological excessive sweating as sweat glands are innervated by sympathetic cholinergic nerve fibres.
5. You are evaluating the properties of different neuromuscular-blocking drugs. Choose the **most appropriate** statement from the following options.
   A. Rocuronium will have direct central nervous system effects as it crosses the blood–brain barrier.
   B. Pancuronium is the neuromuscular-blocking drug of choice for a surgical procedure that will take less than 30 min.
   C. Suxamethonium is the only muscle relaxant that can be used for electroconvulsive therapy.
   D. To produce complete block of an evoked twitch, about 50% of nicotinic receptors need to be occupied by a non-depolarising neuromuscular-blocking drug.
   E. Atracurium causes the release of histamine.
6. Case history questions – see the case history questions for Chapter 17.

ANSWERS

1. a. **False**. The depolarising block is enhanced when body temperature is artificially lowered.
   b. **False**. Mivacurium and atracurium are the muscle relaxants with the greatest propensity to cause histamine release and haemodynamic effects.
2. a. **True**. Dantrolene relaxes skeletal muscle by preventing Ca^{2+} release from the sarcoplasmic reticulum.
   b. **True**. Contraction is an all-or-none response of the fibre in response to nerve stimulation.
   c. **False**. The N_2 receptor at skeletal muscle is selectively blocked by non-depolarising and depolarising muscle relaxants. The N_1 receptor at ganglia is selectively blocked by ganglion-blocking drugs. Selectivity is lost if inappropriately large doses of these agents are administered.
3. a. **False**. Short-acting non-depolarising neuromuscular blockers such as rocuronium can be used for intubation. The use of suxamethonium is declining because of the occurrence of malignant hyperthermia.
   b. **False**. Because of the quaternary nature of their structure, they are not absorbed orally. They do not cross the blood–brain barrier or placenta.
4. a. **False**. Botulinum toxin contains two subunits that promote presynaptic binding and long-lasting block of ACh release.
   b. **True**. Botulinum toxin is extremely toxic on systemic absorption.

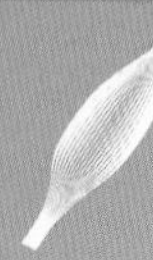

c. **True**. Botulinum toxin only inhibits ACh release. Although sweat glands are sympathetically innervated, the postganglionic neurons are cholinergic and release ACh.

5. Answer **E**.
   A. False. All non-depolarising neuromuscular-blocking drugs have a quaternary ammonium in their structure and will not cross the blood–brain barrier.
   B. False. Pancuronium is a long-acting blocking drug and is used for procedures taking longer than 90 min.
   C. False. Short-acting non-depolarising blocking drugs such as rocuronium or mivacurium are viable alternatives.
   D. False. More than 90% of receptors need to be occupied to produce a complete block of skeletal muscle contractility.
   E. True. Atracurium is one of the most potent neuromuscular-blocking drugs causing the release of histamine.
6. Case history answers – see the case history for Chapter 17.

Drugs acting at the neuromuscular junction

Drug	Half-life (h) and kinetics	Comments
Acetylcholinesterase inhibitors		
Distigmine, Edrophonium, Pyridostigmine		see Ch. 28
Neostigmine	0.4–1.7 (i.v.) [R + M] See Ch. 28 for details	Given i.v. to reverse the effects of a non-depolarising blocker (with atropine to minimise effects of acetylcholine on the parasympathetic system); given orally or by subcutaneous or intramuscular injection for treatment of myasthenia gravis; see Ch. 28
Non-depolarising blockers		
All are used for muscle relaxation for surgery; all have negligible oral absorption and are given by i.v. injection or infusion		
Atracurium	0.3 [M] Spontaneous hydrolysis; very rapidly breaks down within blood; unaffected by hepatic or renal failure	Also used for muscle relaxation during intensive care; a complex mixture of 10 isomers; cardiovascular effects due to histamine release
Cisatracurium	0.5 [unstable] Spontaneous degradation	Also used for muscle relaxation during intensive care; a single isomer of atracurium; does not cause histamine release
Mivacurium	2 min *(trans–trans)*; 50–60 min *(cis–cis)* [M] Hydrolysed by pseudocholinesterase and shows prolonged effect in the rare individuals with a genetic deficiency of this enzyme	Consists of three isomers; the *cis–trans* and *trans–trans* have similar half-lives, are 10 times more potent than the *cis–cis* isomer, and are responsible for the clinical response
Pancuronium	0.5 [R + B + M] Hydrolysed to a product (3-hydroxy metabolite) that retains activity	Often used for long-term muscle relaxation during mechanical ventilation in intensive care; sympathomimetic effects on heart rate and blood pressure can cause tachycardia and hypertension
Rocuronium	1.2 [R + M]	Also used for muscle relaxation during intensive care; most rapid onset of action of drugs in this class; minimal cardiovascular effects
Vecuronium	1.0 [B + M] Bile is major route of elimination (note molecular weight – 638 Da – exceeds the threshold for biliary excretion); lacks cardiovascular effects	
Depolarising blockers		
Suxamethonium (succinylcholine)	2–5 min [M] Hydrolysed by pseudocholinesterase and shows prolonged effect in the rare individuals with a genetic deficiency of this enzyme; half-life shorter in infants and children	Rapid onset but short duration of action; paralysis is preceded by painful fasciculations; prolonged paralysis can cause a so-called dual block in which a non-depolarising block follows the initial depolarising block (edrophonium – see above – can be used to determine the nature of the block); given i.v.

[B], biliary excretion; [M], metabolism; [R], renal excretion; i.v., intravenous.

28 Myasthenia gravis

Myasthenia gravis is a comparatively rare autoimmune disease in which there is an autoantibody to the acetylcholine nicotinic N_2 receptor system. The autoantibody can impair the responsiveness of the neuromuscular junction to acetylcholine (Ch. 27) by three distinct mechanisms:

- increased receptor destruction by complement binding
- cross-linking of receptors, which causes increased receptor internalisation
- receptor blockade by steric hindrance.

The end result is that fewer functional receptors are available for acetylcholine (ACh) to depolarise the muscle cell sufficiently to reach its threshold firing potential. Consequently, in myasthenia gravis there is skeletal muscle weakness. In healthy skeletal muscle, repetitive nerve stimulation leads to a reduction in the numbers of sensitive receptors, but this causes no physiological reduction in muscle activity due to the large number of available receptors. However, in myasthenia gravis, with repetitive stimulation the smaller receptor pool leads to a more rapid reduction than normal in receptor availability, and increasing numbers of muscle fibres fail to fire. This produces the characteristic rapid muscle fatigue on exertion. The earliest symptoms of myasthenia gravis are often diplopia arising from weakness of the extraocular muscles, or ptosis. In 85% of cases, the symptoms progress to involve many other muscle groups, particularly producing bulbar, facial and proximal limb weakness.

The thymus gland plays a part in the genesis of the immune response in myasthenia gravis, although the precise role is as yet uncertain. About 80% of people with myasthenia gravis have an abnormality in the thymus, which is usually lymphoreticular hyperplasia if the onset of the condition is at an early age or thymoma if the onset is over the age of 40 years.

Symptomatic treatment of the weakness in myasthenia gravis is based on prolongation of the action of ACh by inhibiting acetylcholinesterase, the enzyme responsible for its hydrolysis. However, immunosuppression is also important for disease control.

ACETYLCHOLINESTERASE INHIBITORS

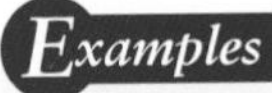

edrophonium, neostigmine, pyridostigmine

Mechanism of action and effects

Acetylcholinesterase (AChE) inhibitors block the breakdown of ACh released from presynaptic neurons, and details of their mechanisms of action are found in Chapter 4. They enhance the effect of ACh at all synaptic connections at which it is the neurotransmitter, but their therapeutic actions in myasthenia gravis are by increasing the longevity of ACh at nicotinic N_2 receptors (Ch. 4). Unwanted effects arise from the excessive actions of ACh at nicotinic N_1 receptors in ganglia and muscarinic receptors at postganglionic nerve endings in the parasympathetic nervous system and at sweat glands in the sympathetic nervous system.

Pharmacokinetics and clinical uses

Neostigmine and pyridostigmine are quaternary amines that are slowly and incompletely absorbed from the gut. As a result, oral doses need to be approximately 10 times greater than parenteral doses to be effective. They have short elimination half-lives (1–2 h), due to a combination of renal tubular secretion and some hepatic metabolism. The effective plasma half-life after oral dosage is longer, due to absorption rate-limited kinetics (Ch. 2). They do not readily cross the blood–brain barrier (see Ch. 9 for AChE inhibitors that cross the blood–brain barrier and are used in Alzheimer's disease). Both neostigmine and pyridostigmine can be used to treat myasthenia gravis, but pyridostigmine is the preferred choice because of its longer duration of action. Neostigmine has a faster onset of action, and is also used by intravenous injection to reverse the effect of competitive neuromuscular blockers (Ch. 27).

Edrophonium is given as an intravenous bolus to test the therapeutic response to AChE inhibitors in myasthenia gravis (see below); it has a very short duration of action (2–5 min), largely owing to tissue redistribution, and is of no value in treatment.

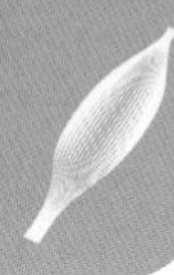

Unwanted effects

Unwanted effects arise because the AChE inhibitors are effective at all sites where ACh is released. Unwanted effects are experienced by up to one-third of people treated, and are more troublesome with neostigmine than with pyridostigmine. Peripheral muscarinic receptor agonist effects, which can be blocked by co-administration of a muscarinic receptor antagonist, include:

- Diarrhoea, abdominal cramps, excessive salivation
- Bradycardia, hypotension (uncommon)
- Miosis and lacrimation
- Bronchoconstriction (see Ch. 12)
- Nausea.

Excessive dosage of AChE inhibitors will lead to a depolarising neuromuscular blockade by ACh. Initially, there may be muscle twitching and cramps, followed by weakness through the build-up of excess ACh (see below).

MANAGEMENT OF MYASTHENIA GRAVIS

Diagnosis

When the diagnosis of myasthenia is suspected, useful information can be obtained rapidly by pharmacological testing. In untreated subjects with myasthenia, an intravenous injection of the short-acting AChE inhibitor edrophonium will produce clinical improvement within 1 min that lasts for about 5 min. Detection of circulating N_2 receptor antibodies, and electromyographic tests that demonstrate abnormal fatigability in multiple muscle fibres, are used to confirm the diagnosis.

Treatment

Symptomatic treatment of myasthenia gravis is with an AChE inhibitor, which reduces the normal rapid breakdown of ACh and thereby enhances the activity of ACh released by nerve stimulation. The type of interaction between the antibody and the receptor probably determines the effectiveness of treatment in an individual. Pyridostigmine is commonly used since its action is more consistent than that of neostigmine, the dosing frequency is less, and there are fewer muscarinic unwanted effects. The onset of action is after about 30–45 min and the duration of action is 3–6 h. An antimuscarinic agent (such as propantheline; may be necessary to block any parasympathomimetic actions of pyridostigmine, especially if large doses are given. Some individuals do not respond well to AChE inhibitors, while unwanted effects may preclude the use of adequate doses in others.

Excessive dosage of an AChE inhibitor can lead to prolonged stimulation of the N_2 receptors by ACh, resulting in a depolarising blockade of the neuromuscular junction similar to that produced by suxamethonium (succinylcholine; Ch. 27). Therefore, muscle weakness in myasthenia gravis can be the result of either inadequate dosage ('myasthenic crisis') or excessive dosage ('cholinergic crisis') with an AChE inhibitor. The safest way to distinguish these problems is to use assisted ventilation and temporarily withdraw the AChE inhibitor. Muscle groups do not all respond equally well to AChE inhibitors; ptosis and diplopia appear to be the most resistant to treatment.

Generalised myasthenia is now usually treated by immunosuppression with a corticosteroid, such as prednisolone (Ch. 44). Corticosteroids are also used for those who are severely ill. They probably act by suppressing T-cell proliferation and reducing antibody synthesis. Initial high-dose corticosteroid therapy can make the weakness worse, particularly in the first few hours, possibly due to a direct effect on neuromuscular transmission. A clinical response is usually apparent after 1 month, but maximum benefit is delayed for up to 9 months. Ciclosporin (alone or with a corticosteroid) or cyclophosphamide with a corticosteroid (Ch. 38) are used if there is a poor response to a corticosteroid alone, but the dosage of ciclosporin is usually limited by significant nephrotoxicity. Long-term immunosuppression is usually necessary, since relapse frequently occurs on withdrawal of therapy.

Plasma exchange to remove circulating acetylcholine receptor antibodies can produce a short-term response in severe disease. With repeated exchanges, improvement is seen after 1 day, with a maximum response after 1–2 weeks that is sustained for 2–8 weeks. An alternative is the use of intravenous immunoglobulin, of which IgG is the active component. It produces improvement after about 4 days, and an optimal response after 1–2 weeks that is sustained for 6–15 weeks. Immunoglobulin treatment is usually better tolerated than plasma exchange.

Thymectomy can induce remission, although this can be delayed for up to 5 years. It is usually used for early-onset disease with positive receptor antibodies, when it produces complete remission within 5 years in about 40% and significant improvement in a further 35%. Thymectomy is also used to remove a thymoma, although the clinical benefit is often less clear-cut.

Some drugs can interfere with neuromuscular transmission and worsen the symptoms of myasthenia gravis. Those most often implicated include aminoglycoside antibiotics (Ch. 51), β-adrenoceptor antagonists (Ch. 5), phenytoin (Ch. 23), chloroquine and penicillamine (Ch. 30). There is also altered sensitivity to neuromuscular junction blockers, with increased response to competitive (non-depolarising) neuromuscular junction blockers but resistance to depolarising neuromuscular junction blockers (Ch. 27).

FURTHER READING

Conti-Fine BM, Milani M, Kaminski HJ (2006) Myasthenia gravis: past, present, and future. *J Clin Invest* 116, 2843–2854

Hart IK, Sathasivam S, Sharshar T (2007) Immunosuppressive agents for myasthenia gravis. *Cochrane Database Syst Rev* (4), CD005224

Newsom-Davis J (2003) Therapy in myasthenia gravis and Lambert–Eaton myasthenic syndrome. *Semin Neurol* 23, 191–197

Nicolle MW (2002) Myasthenia gravis. *The Neurologist* 8, 2–21

Schwendimann RN, Burton E, Minagar A (2005) Management of myasthenia gravis. *Am J Ther* 12, 262–268

SELF-ASSESSMENT

In questions 1 and 2, the first statement, in italics, is true. Are the accompanying statements also true?

1. *Caution is required when administering pyridostigmine to people with asthma.* Overdosage causing respiratory depression can be treated with atropine.
2. *Pyridostigmine produces less muscarinic receptor activity than neostigmine.*
   a. An AChE inhibitor should not be given with depolarising muscle relaxants such as suxamethonium.
   b. A cholinergic crisis should be confirmed by administering pyridostigmine.
3. Regarding a person who has been diagnosed with myasthenia gravis, choose the **most appropriate** statement from the following options.
   A. All people diagnosed with myasthenia gravis have a thymoma.
   B. In order to be effective, anticholinesterases used in treating myasthenia gravis should be able to cross the blood–brain barrier.
   C. Glucocorticoids which can be of benefit in some people with myasthenia gravis are effective because of their anti-inflammatory actions.
   D. Many of the unwanted effects that physostigmine has on the autonomic nervous system can be reduced with a muscarinic receptor blocking drug.
   E. The aim of plasmapheresis is to reduce pseudocholinesterase (butyrylcholinesterase, plasma cholinesterase) which breaks down acetylcholine.
4. Case history questions

A 35-year-old woman with no previous illness noticed that she had ptosis and occasional diplopia. Over a period of time she became aware that she suffered from leg weakness on exertion, although her coordination was normal. Following a sustained upward gaze for a minute, ptosis and diplopia could be elicited. Myasthenia gravis was suspected.

   a. What tests should be performed to verify the diagnosis?
   b. What is the pathogenesis of myasthenia gravis?
   c. Why is edrophonium injection used as a test for myasthenia gravis?

Treatment was commenced following diagnosis.

   d. What principles should treatment follow?

ANSWERS

1. **True**. Atropine-like drugs reduce muscarinic receptor-mediated bronchoconstriction.
2. a. **True**. The neuromuscular blockade with suxamethonium may be prolonged and an extended period of apnoea may result.
   b. **False**. The cholinergic crisis results from the excessive effects of an AChE inhibitor and would be exacerbated by the long-acting pyridostigmine. Assisted ventilation and withdrawal of the treatment should be performed.
3. Answer **D**.
   A. False. About 15% have a thymoma and 60–80% have hyperplasia of the thymus.
   B. False. Neostigmine and pyridostigmine are the main anticholinesterases used in treating myasthenia gravis; they are quaternary amines and do not cross the blood–brain barrier.
   C. False. Glucocorticoids work by suppressing nicotinic receptor antibody production.
   D. True. Muscarinic receptor blockers will prevent the parasympathomimetic effects of pyridostigmine (diarrhoea, urination, miosis, bradycardia, nausea, lacrimation, salivation).
   E. False. Plasmapheresis is carried out to reduce the levels of circulating nicotinic receptor antibodies.
4. Case history answers
   a. Electromyography (Jolly test), single muscle fibre electromyography, anti-acetylcholine receptor (AChR) antibody titres, injection of a short-acting inhibitor of AChE (the Tensilon test, the proprietary name for edrophonium).
   b. AChR antibody blocks nicotinic N_2 receptors; receptors are destroyed and receptors are cross-linked, which causes them to be destroyed more rapidly. The decrease in functional receptors reduces motor endplate potentials and reduces the likelihood of the muscle contracting.
   c. It is short-acting, giving an effect in 30–60 s and effects subsiding in 4–5 min.
   d. Symptomatic treatment with an AChE inhibitor. Immunosuppression with a corticosteroid, or with immunosuppressants such as ciclosporin or azathioprine.

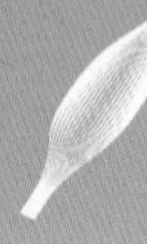

Acetylcholinesterase inhibitors used in myasthenia gravis

Drug	Half-life (h) and kinetics	Comments
Distigmine	? (long) [R + M] Very poor oral bioavailability (1–2%), especially if taken with food; hydrolysed by plasma esterases	Rarely used; also used for urinary retention (Ch. 15); given orally
Edrophonium	1.8 [R?] Pathways of elimination not defined but severe renal impairment reduces total clearance by more than 50%	Very short duration of action and mainly used for diagnosis; given i.v. over 30 s; not given orally
Neostigmine	0.4–1.7 (i.v.) [R + M] Very low oral bioavailability (1–2%); food delays absorption but does not affect AUC (of absorbed drug); elimination after oral dosage is probably longer than after i.v. dosage (absorption rate-limited); metabolised by plasma and hepatic esterases	Given orally or by subcutaneous or i.v. injection
Pyridostigmine	0.4–1.9 (i.v.) [R + M] Low oral bioavailability (10–20%); food delays absorption but does not alter bioavailability; most of the absorbed fraction is excreted in the urine unchanged; terminal half-life after oral dosage is probably longer than after i.v. dosage (absorption rate-limited); longer-acting than neostigmine	Given orally

[M,] metabolism; [R], renal excretion; AUC, area under the plasma concentration versus time curve; i.v., intravenous.

29 Non-steroidal anti-inflammatory drugs

THE ROLE OF CYCLO-OXYGENASE ENZYMES IN THE ACTIONS OF NON-STEROIDAL ANTI-INFLAMMATORY DRUGS

The major therapeutic and unwanted actions of non-steroidal anti-inflammatory drugs (NSAIDs) are achieved because they inhibit the cyclo-oxygenase (COX) enzymes. However, it must not be overlooked that the effects of NSAIDs on other, less well-explored, biochemical mechanisms contribute to both their therapeutic and unwanted effects.

COX enzymes are essential in the production of the prostanoids (prostaglandins and thromboxanes), which are ubiquitous local hormones generated predominantly from the precursor fatty acid arachidonic acid mainly derived from a mixed 'Western' diet (Fig. 29.1). Arachidonic acid can also be converted via the lipoxygenase pathway to leukotrienes. The prostanoids and leukotrienes derived from arachidonic acid are part of the family of eicosanoids, which are polyunsaturated fatty acid derivatives containing 20 carbon atoms. Eicosanoids are local hormones that are generally synthesised and catabolised close to their site of action, and have numerous physiological and pathological actions. Arachidonic acid is mostly formed from dietary linoleic acid, which is found in vegetable oils such as sunflower oil. Linoleic acid is converted in the liver in several steps to arachidonic acid, which is then incorporated into glycerophospholipids in cell membranes. Arachidonic acid is released from glycerophospholipids by lipases such as phospholipase A_2 and can then be converted to eicosanoids (Fig. 29.1).

Prostanoids derived from arachidonic acid all contain two double bonds (e.g. prostaglandin E_2 [PGE_2] or thromboxane A_2 [TXA_2]; Ch. 11); they are synthesised by oxygenation and ring closure of arachidonic acid (which has four double bonds); this is the rate-limiting step and is catalysed by COX enzymes. However, when diets with a high fish intake or supplemented with omega-3 fats (fish oils) are taken, this result in the replacement of some of the arachidonic acid (four double bonds, C20:4) in lipid membranes by eicosapentaenoic acid (EPA; 5 double bonds, C20:5). EPA is a good substrate for COX and gives rise to prostanoids having three instead of two double bonds (e.g. TXA_3 rather than TXA_2, and PGI_3 rather than PGI_2 [prostacyclin]). This manipulation may be of benefit in reducing platelet aggregation (see Ch. 11). It may also be helpful in reducing inflammation, but generally the effects have not been rigorously tested.

The initial products of the action of COX enzymes on arachidonic acid are unstable intermediates known as cyclic endoperoxides. Specific synthases, the presence and abundance of which differ from cell to cell, then convert the endoperoxide PGH_2 to various prostanoids (Fig. 29.1). The products of the COX pathways therefore differ among various tissues depending upon the synthases present, reflecting the diverse nature of their actions and the individual requirements of each cell type. Most cell types can form different prostanoids simultaneously and in different quantities, with the pattern of production determined by various regulatory influences.

COX enzymes occur as at least three isoenzymes, COX-1, COX-2 and COX-3, and other variant enzymes also exist. Until relatively recently it was considered that the different forms of COX had clearly distinct functions. COX-1 was thought to be mainly a constitutive 'housekeeping' enzyme localised to the endoplasmic reticulum. Prostanoids formed via the COX-1 enzyme were thought to be produced in small amounts by many cells in the resting state and to contribute to the regulation of several homeostatic processes such as renal and gastric blood flow, gastric cytoprotection and platelet aggregation (Table 29.1). COX-2 is present in greater concentrations in the nuclear envelope than in the endoplasmic reticulum. It is expressed in significant amounts in many cells such as endothelial cells, macrophages, synovial fibroblasts, mast cells, chondrocytes and osteoblasts, *but only after stimulation, for example by elevated inflammatory cytokine concentrations*. It was originally thought that COX-2-derived prostanoids were formed in large amounts only in pathological situations, giving rise to excessively high levels of prostanoids involved, for example, in inflammation, pain and fever. However, the concept that there is only a pathological role for inducible COX-2-derived prostanoids and a housekeeping physiological role for the constitutive COX-1 enzyme is now recognised as too simplistic. Recent studies have shown that in many biological systems there is no clear separation between the functions of COX-1 and COX-2. This applies particularly to the kidney, central nervous system (CNS), cardiovascular system and reproductive system. Either isoform may be involved in the production of 'physiological' or 'pathological' prostanoids. Table 29.1 shows that there are roles for constitutive COX-2 in

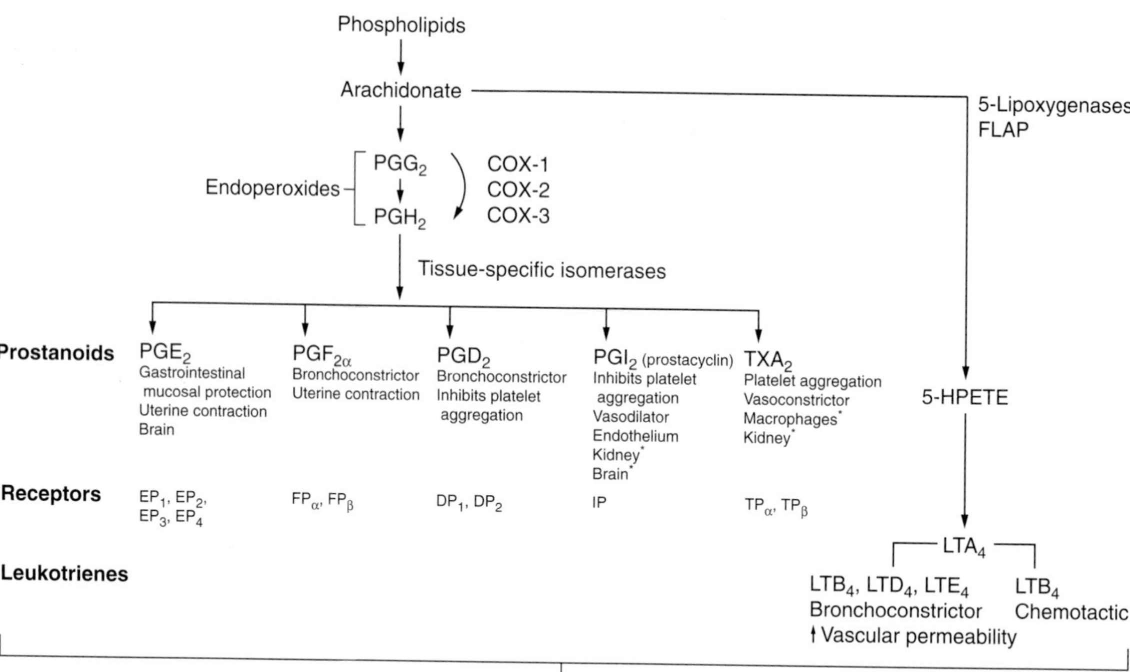

Fig. 29.1 **The arachidonic acid cascade.** Arachidonic acid can be utilised by cyclo-oxygenases (COX) 1, 2 or 3 to form prostanoids (prostaglandins and thromboxanes) having two double bonds in their side-chains or by the lipoxygenase enzyme pathway to form leukotrienes. They have a multitude of actions and stabilities depending upon the product, the site of formation and the amount formed. The receptors they act on are G-protein-coupled. Other properties are shown in Table 29.2 and in the text. FLAP, five (5)-lipoxygenase-activating protein; HPETE, hydroperoxyeicosatetraenoic acid; LT, leukotriene; PG, prostaglandin; TX, thromboxane; *, many different biological actions.

homeostasis in many cell types, and that COX-1 isoenzymes may be involved in some pathological events.

COX-3 is an enzyme variant of COX-1 that retains the entire COX-1 transcript and has an additional conserved intron sequence. It is mainly expressed in the brain and spinal cord and to a lesser extent in the heart, endothelial cells and monocytes. COX-3 may have a role in CNS pain perception, but its precise functions are as yet uncertain.

The actions of prostaglandins and thromboxanes depend upon the circumstances and site of their formation, and whether they are formed in excessive amounts. For example, PGE_2 is generated in low physiological amounts by COX-1 in gastric mucosa and is important for maintaining mucosal integrity by a variety of mechanisms, including bicarbonate production and maintaining mucosal blood flow. During tissue damage, there is increased prostaglandin synthesis via elevated COX-2 expression, and this contributes to inflammation and pain. In particular, production of PGE_2 produces vasodilation, increases vascular permeability and sensitises pain fibre nerve endings to the nociceptive action of bradykinin, serotonin (5-hydroxytryptamine, 5-HT) and other mediators (Ch. 19). However, in the later stages of repair following tissue damage, COX-2-derived prostanoids may contribute to the processes of wound healing.

Prostanoids act via five main classes of G-protein-coupled receptors on cell surfaces (Fig. 29.1; see receptor table at the end of Ch. 1). Some of the actions of prostaglandins are shown in Table 29.2.

The second route for arachidonic acid metabolism is via the lipoxygenase pathway, to produce leukotrienes (Fig. 29.1). These are also involved in the inflammatory process by enhancing vascular permeability (leukotrienes [LT] C_4, D_4 and E_4) and through chemotactic attraction of leucocytes (particularly LTB_4; see also Ch. 12).

NON-STEROIDAL ANTI-INFLAMMATORY DRUGS

Non-steroidal anti-inflammatory drugs (NSAIDs) have three major desirable therapeutic actions: anti-inflammatory, analgesic and antipyretic.

Mechanisms of action

All NSAIDs share a common mode of action by inhibition of the COX isoenzymes (Table 29.3). Different NSAIDs do not inhibit the two main isoenzymes (COX-1 and COX-2) to the same extent, and this partly explains the variations in their therapeutic and unwanted effect profiles. Inhibition of COX reduces the generation of prostanoids but does not

Table 29.1 Some biological roles of cyclo-oxygenase enzymes COX-1 and COX-2[a]

COX-1 'Homeostasis–physiological–housekeeping' roles – constitutive	COX-2 'Homeostasis–physiological–housekeeping' roles – constitutive
Gastrointestinal protection Platelet aggregation Blood flow regulation CNS function	Renal function CNS function Tissue repair and healing (including gastrointestinal) Reproduction Uterine contraction Blood vessel dilation Pancreas Inhibition of platelet aggregation Airways
COX-1 'Pathological roles'	**COX-2 'Pathological roles'**
(Possible involvement in inflammation) Raised blood pressure Pain	Inflammation Pain Fever Blood vessel permeability Reproduction Alzheimer's disease Promote angiogenesis, inhibit apoptosis

[a]The separation of the roles of COX-1- and COX-2-derived prostanoids into 'physiological' and 'pathological' is increasingly indistinct. The actions of the prostanoids may be permissive in allowing and enhancing the actions of other agents while not having marked direct effects themselves.

Table 29.2 Some of the myriad effects of the prostanoids[a]

Tissue	Effect	Eicosanoid
Platelets	Increased aggregation Decreased aggregation	TXA_2 PGI_2, PGD_2
Vascular smooth muscle	Vasodilation Vasoconstriction	PGI_2, PGE_2, PGD_2 TXA_2
Other smooth muscle	Bronchodilation Bronchoconstriction GI tract (contraction/relaxation, depends on muscle type) Uterine contraction	PGE_2 PGD_2, PGF_2, TXA_2, LTC_4, LTD_4, LTE_4 PGF_2, PGE_2, PGI_2, PGD_2 PGE_2, $PGF_{2\alpha}$
Vascular endothelium	Increased permeability Potentiates histamine/bradykinin	LTC_4, LTB_4 PGE_2, PGI_2
Neutrophils/macrophages	Chemotaxis	LTB_4
Gastrointestinal mucosa	Reduced acid secretion Increased mucus secretion Increased blood flow	PGE_2, PGI_2 PGE_2 PGE_2, PGI_2
Nervous system	Inhibition of noradrenaline release Endogenous pyrogen in hypothalamus Sedation, sleep	PGD_2, PGE_2, PGI_2 PGE_2 PGD_2
Endocrine/metabolic	Secretion of ACTH, GH, prolactin, gonadotrophins Inhibition of lipolysis	PGE_2 PGE_2
Kidney	Increased renal blood flow Antagonism of ADH Renin release	PGE_2, PGI_2 PGE_2 PGI_2, PGE_2, PGD_2
Pain	Potentiates pain through bradykinin, serotonin	PGE_2, PGD_2

[a]Only the main prostanoids involved are shown. The prostanoids involved can also vary depending upon the influence of other hormones and mediators.
ACTH, adrenocorticotrophic hormone; ADH, antidiuretic hormone (vasopressin); GH, growth hormone; LT, leukotriene; PG, prostaglandin; TX, thromboxane.

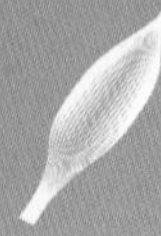

Table 29.3 Drug classes of selected NSAIDs and their approximate rank orders in ratio of inhibition of COX-1 compared with COX-2

Drug class	Example	Ratio of inhibition
PAD	Flurbiprofen	↑ Increasing ratio of selectivity for inhibition of COX-1 compared with COX-2
PAD	Ketoprofen	
HAD	Ketorolac	
Salicylate	Aspirin	
Indole	Indometacin	
PAD	Ibuprofen	
PAD	Naproxen	
PAD	Fenoprofen	Approximately equal ratio of inhibition COX-1 : COX-2
Salicylate	Salicylate	
Enolic acid	Meloxicam	
Enolic acid	Piroxicam	
Indole	Sulindac	
Phenyl acetic acid	Diclofenac	
Sulphonamide (coxib)	Celecoxib	↓ Increasing ratio of selectivity for inhibition of COX-2 compared with COX-1
Bipyridine (coxib)	Etoricoxib	

HAD, heterocyclic acetic acid derivative; PAD, propionic acid derivative.

directly affect the production of leukotrienes, which may as a consequence exert unopposed actions. Leukotriene production may even increase as a result of diversion (shunting) of arachidonic acid into the lipoxygenase pathway. One reason may be reduced synthesis by COX-1 of PGE_2, which normally inhibits leukotriene synthesis; this effect is particularly important in people with aspirin-sensitive asthma (Ch. 12).

The clinical responses observed with individual NSAIDs reflect the ability of the drug to inhibit the different COX isoenzymes involved in the biological actions shown in Tables 29.1 and 29.2. The degree of COX selectivity of each NSAID will depend not only on the type of NSAID but also on the dosage used.

NSAIDs have more complex anti-inflammatory effects than can be explained simply by inhibition of COX. They also have agonist activity at peroxisome proliferator-activated receptor gamma (PPAR-γ). PPARs have a key role in modulation of immune responses by suppressing pro-inflammatory gene expression (for production of tumour necrosis factor alpha [TNFα], interleukin-1 [IL-1] and inducible nitric oxide synthase) in macrophages. This action occurs at higher drug concentrations than are required to produce analgesia. NSAIDs also have complex effects on lymphocytes, including inhibition of T-cell activation and increased T-cell apoptosis, which may reflect PPAR-mediated actions.

Classification of NSAIDs

Table 29.3 shows the principal chemical types of NSAIDs and an indication of the ratios of activity for inhibition of COX-1 or COX-2.

Most NSAIDs bind reversibly to the site in COX that accepts arachidonic acid, but the irreversible inactivation produced by aspirin involves acetylation of a serine residue in the enzyme. Many conventional NSAIDs produce greater inhibition of COX-1 relative to the inhibition of COX-2. Other drugs show greater relative selectivity for COX-2 (Table 29.3). In many clinical conditions the relevance of this selectivity is the subject of active debate.

Actions and effects of non-selective NSAIDs

Some of the properties and actions of a selection of non-opioid analgesic drugs are compared in Table 29.4.

Analgesia

This is in part a peripheral action at the site of pain and is most effective when the pain has an inflammatory origin (see also Ch. 19). It appears to be achieved predominantly through inhibition of COX-2-derived prostaglandins in inflamed or injured tissues. There is also a central compo-

Table 29.4 Properties of some commonly used analgesic drugs

	Aspirin (moderate doses)	Paracetamol	Indometacin	Ibuprofen	Celecoxib
Analgesic	++	++	++	+	+
Anti-inflammatory	+	–	+++	+	+
Antipyretic	+	+	+	+	+
Gastrointestinal bleeding	+	–	+	Low	Low

nent to the analgesic action of NSAIDs which is due to inhibition of COX isoenzymes and reduction of prostaglandin production in the pain pathways of the CNS. The main analgesic effect of prostanoids is thought to be at sensory nerve endings on first-order neurons (Ch. 19). PGE_2 enhances the ability of several mediators (serotonin, substance P, bradykinin) to stimulate Aδ and C nociceptive fibres. COX inhibition may also decrease PGE_2 production in the dorsal horn of the spinal cord, which inhibits neurotransmitter release and reduces the excitability of second-order neurons in the pain relay pathway. The analgesic action of NSAIDs is apparent after the first dose, but does not reach its maximal effect until about 1 week with repeated dosing.

Anti-inflammatory effect

Inhibition of vasodilation and oedema is partly related to a reduction in peripheral COX-2-generated prostaglandin synthesis. However, NSAIDs also affect several other inflammatory processes unrelated to their effects on prostaglandins. For example, they probably reduce harmful superoxide free radical generation by neutrophils. They may also uncouple G-protein-regulated processes in the cell membrane of inflammatory cells. This would reduce cell responsiveness to a variety of agonists released by damaged tissues. The anti-inflammatory effects of NSAIDs develop gradually over about 3 weeks.

Antipyretic effect

Fever is reduced through inhibition of hypothalamic COX-2. Circulating pyrogens such as IL-1 enhance PGE_2 production in the hypothalamus, which depresses the response of temperature-sensitive neurons. NSAIDs do not affect normal body temperature.

Reduction of platelet aggregation

This action is mediated by inhibition of the synthesis of TXA_2 by platelet COX-1; TXA_2 is a potent platelet aggregating agent. This effect is most marked for aspirin, because it has an irreversible action on COX, and platelets are unable to synthesise more enzyme during their life span. The reversible action of most other NSAIDs (with the exception of naproxen) produces weaker platelet inhibition, and highly COX-2-selective NSAIDs do not inhibit platelet aggregation (Table 29.3).

Other actions

Considerable work is being carried out in other areas of medicine to examine the place of NSAIDs. Amongst these are the prevention of various types of cancer and Alzheimer's disease.

Pharmacokinetics

Most NSAIDs are weak acids that undergo some absorption from the stomach due to pH partitioning (Ch. 2). This explains the relatively high drug concentration in cells of the gastric mucosa. However, the majority of the drug is absorbed via the larger surface area of the small bowel. Enteric-coated formulations can be used to reduce release of drug in the stomach and limit direct exposure of the gastric mucosa. Some compounds, such as nabumetone, are inactive prodrugs that are converted to an active metabolite in the liver after absorption (Ch. 2). This avoids direct exposure of the gastric mucosa to the active form of the drug.

Absorption of NSAIDs from the gut is usually fairly rapid from conventional formulations. Some NSAIDs with short half-lives, such as diclofenac, are available as modified-release formulations to prolong their duration of action and reduce dosing frequency. Absorption is slower from these formulations. Certain NSAIDs can be given by intramuscular or intravenous injection for rapid onset of analgesia (such as ketorolac), or rectally to achieve a prolonged action and to reduce direct gastric irritation (such as diclofenac and ketoprofen). Transcutaneous delivery of several NSAIDs, usually as a gel formulation, was introduced with the intention of providing high local drug concentrations while attempting to minimise systemic unwanted effects. However, once the drug has penetrated the skin, it is widely distributed, and this route has little advantage for reducing systemic toxicity.

Most NSAIDs undergo hepatic metabolism to inactive compounds. The compounds differ widely in their elimination half-lives (see drug compendium). Short-acting drugs require frequent dosing to maintain continuous therapeutic effect, although synovial fluid concentrations in joint disease fluctuate less than the plasma concentrations. Piroxicam undergoes enterohepatic cycling, which contributes to its long half-life.

Aspirin (acetylsalicylic acid) is initially converted to an active metabolite, salicylic acid, and finally inactivated by conjugation with glycine and, to some extent, glucuronic acid (Ch. 2). Conjugation with glycine is saturable at higher doses and the metabolism of salicylate then changes from first-order to zero-order elimination kinetics (Ch. 2). This has important implications for aspirin overdose (Ch. 53).

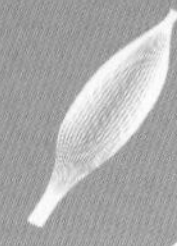

Unwanted effects

Most unwanted effects arise in part from the inhibition of prostaglandin synthesis throughout the body. They are usually dose-related.

Gastrointestinal effects

- *Nausea, dyspepsia, gastric irritation and gastric ulceration* are the most frequent unwanted effects. They occur principally as a result of inhibition of mucosal production of COX-1-generated PGE_2 and PGI_2, although inhibition of COX-2 may interfere with some aspects of tissue healing. PGE_2 has several actions that confer cytoprotection in the stomach (Ch. 33). However, there are many mechanisms by which NSAIDs cause gastric irritation:
  - The hydrophobicity of the mucus gel layer is reduced due to the acidic nature of NSAIDs and their local concentration in gastric mucosal cells; this reduces the barrier effect of the surface layer.
  - Uncoupling of cellular oxidative phosphorylation by the drugs increases mucosal permeability, with consequent back-diffusion of H^+, which is trapped in the mucosal epithelium and leads to cytotoxicity.
  - Reduced mucosal blood flow from inhibition of prostaglandin synthesis, which probably enhances cytotoxicity by producing tissue hypoxia and local free radical generation.
  - Mucus secretion and bicarbonate secretion are reduced and acid secretion increased, also as a result of inhibition of prostaglandin synthesis.
  - Increased local production of leukotrienes may also be involved in the development of gastric toxicity.

NSAIDs accumulate within gastric mucosal cells by direct absorption of the drug from the gastric lumen and also by systemic delivery of the drug to the mucosa. Consequently, rectal or transdermal administration or the use of a prodrug may reduce, but will not eliminate, the risk of gastric damage. Occult blood loss from the bowel is increased during regular treatment with NSAIDs and the risk of overt gastrointestinal bleeding is greater. Management of NSAID-induced gastric damage is considered in Chapter 33.

- Exacerbation of inflammatory bowel disease (Ch. 34).
- Lower gastrointestinal bleeding or perforation.
- Local irritation and bleeding from rectal administration.

Renal effects

- NSAIDs can produce a reversible decline in renal function, with a rise in serum creatinine; prostaglandins (PGE_2, PGI_2) generated by both COX-1 and COX-2 are involved in the maintenance of renal blood flow and have direct effects on the renal tubule, promoting natriuresis (Ch. 14). The adverse consequences of NSAIDs on the kidney are more common if renal function is already impaired (as is often the case in the elderly). There is also an increased risk in the presence of heart failure or cirrhosis, conditions that are associated with reduced effective circulating blood volume, when prostaglandins play a greater role in the maintenance of renal blood flow.
- NSAIDs are associated with salt and water retention even without renal insufficiency. Reduced prostaglandin synthesis in the ascending limb of the loop of Henle decreases expression of the $Na^+/K^+/2Cl^-$ cotransporter complex, and prostaglandins antagonise the action of vasopressin (antidiuretic hormone, ADH; see Ch. 14). Water retention due to the unopposed action of ADH may exceed retention of Na^+, resulting in dilutional hyponatraemia. Suppression of prostaglandin-mediated renin secretion can lead to hypoaldosteronism and hyperkalaemia. Salt and water retention produced by NSAIDs can exacerbate heart failure and raise blood pressure by an average of 3–5 mmHg. In addition, the efficacy of drug treatments for these conditions (e.g. diuretics, angiotensin-converting enzyme inhibitors, β-adrenoceptor antagonists) is blunted by NSAIDs.

Hypersensitivity

Hypersensitivity reactions occasionally produce asthma, urticaria, angioedema and rhinitis. People with nasal polyps and known allergic disorders appear to be most susceptible. Aspirin can precipitate 'pseudo-allergic' asthma in a subgroup of people with asthma, through inhibition of COX-1-generated PGE_2 production in the lung. It is suggested that as many as one in five asthmatics may be affected. Reduction of PGE_2 lowers its partial inhibitory effect on leukotriene synthesis and mast cell degranulation, and is accompanied by increased synthesis of cysteinyl leukotrienes (particularly LTE_4) (Ch. 12).

Other unwanted effects

Other unwanted effects are unrelated to prostaglandin inhibition and are sometimes specific for individual compounds.

- CNS unwanted effects such as headache, dizziness, drowsiness, insomnia and confusion, particularly in the elderly.
- Skin reactions can occasionally be severe, especially with fenbufen.
- Tinnitus in toxic doses; overdose of aspirin can be particularly hazardous (Ch. 53).
- Reye's syndrome in children, a rare condition producing acute encephalopathy and fatty degeneration of the liver with aspirin. Aspirin should be avoided in children under the age of 12 years.
- The risk of myocardial infarction and stroke is increased by diclofenac and high-dose ibuprofen, especially in people with known ischaemic heart disease or at high risk of a cardiovascular event. By contrast, naproxen may be associated with a lower risk.

COX-2-selective inhibitors

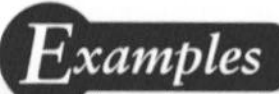

celecoxib, etoricoxib, parecoxib

Mechanism of action

Selective COX-2 inhibitors have less inhibitory action on COX-1, but the degree of selectivity for COX-2 varies among the drugs in this class. Selective COX-2 inhibitors have anti-inflammatory actions similar to conventional non-selective NSAIDs, but there is some evidence that they may be less effective analgesics. This may possibly be due to less inhibition of COX-3 in the brain and spinal cord. Selective COX-2 inhibitors have little direct effect on platelet TXA_2 production and do not impair platelet aggregation; however, they suppress the production of the anti-aggregatory and vasodilator PGI_2 by blood vessels, which may allow thromboxanes to exert unopposed effects on platelets. Selective COX-2-inhibitors also interact with PPARs and impair macrophage activity and T-cell-mediated immune responses (see above).

Pharmacokinetics

Celecoxib and etoricoxib are well absorbed from the gut. They are eliminated by hepatic metabolism. The half-life of celecoxib is 11 h, while that of etoricoxib is longer (25 h). Parecoxib can be given by intramuscular or intravenous injection for control of postoperative pain and has a half-life of 5–9 h.

Unwanted effects

- COX-2-selective inhibitors produce fewer upper gastrointestinal unwanted effects, and reduce the risk of ulcers and ulcer complications by up to 50% compared with conventional NSAIDs. However, there is increasing evidence that the risk of ulceration increases with duration of therapy. Furthermore, if low-dose aspirin is taken concurrently for its antiplatelet benefit, this negates the gastrointestinal-sparing benefits of selective COX-2 inhibitors. Therefore, the strategy of reducing the upper gastrointestinal toxicity of COX inhibition by greater isoenzyme selectivity has limited effectiveness. New molecules that are under investigation may achieve better gastroduodenal tolerability by combining COX inhibition with the protective effects of either lipoxygenase inhibition (COX-LOX inhibitors) or nitric oxide generation (nitric oxide-donating NSAIDs).
- Exacerbation of inflammatory bowel disease (Ch. 34).
- Stomatitis or mouth ulcers.
- Palpitation.
- Selective COX-2 inhibitors are much less likely to induce asthma attacks in NSAID-sensitive individuals.
- Selective COX-2 inhibitors increase the risk of myocardial infarction in people with known ischaemic heart disease or those who are at high risk of a cardiovascular event. They also cause salt and water retention by the kidney. They are contraindicated in people with heart failure, and caution should be exercised if there is a history of left ventricular dysfunction, hypertension, or oedema for any other reason.

Paracetamol

Mechanism of action

Paracetamol (acetaminophen in the USA) is an analgesic without anti-inflammatory activity but is almost always (incorrectly) referred to as an NSAID. It has very little direct inhibitory effect on COX-1 or COX-2 in peripheral tissues, but inhibits COX-3 in the CNS. However, this inhibition is weak and cannot explain all of the effects of paracetamol. Hydroperoxides are generated during the metabolism of arachidonic acid by COX and exert a positive feedback to stimulate COX-2 activity. This feedback is probably blocked by paracetamol, thus inhibiting COX-2.

Other effects may contribute to the analgesic action, such as stimulation of spinal serotonergic neurotransmission via $5HT_{1A}$ receptors. Recent studies have found that paracetamol may affect both cannabinoid (CB_1) and $TRPV_1$ receptors (see also Ch. 19). Paracetamol is metabolised in the brain to N-arachidonyl phenolamine, which is structurally similar to the natural cannabinoid anandamide (arachidonyl ethanolamide). The analgesic action of paracetamol can be attenuated by CB_1 antagonists, suggesting a role for CB_1 receptors. Therefore, the analgesic action of paracetamol may in part depend upon CB_1 stimulation by its arachidonyl metabolite, which also inhibits the neuronal reuptake of anandamide. Lastly, the metabolite stimulates the $TRPV_1$ receptor. At first sight this would be expected to enhance transmission of nociceptive stimuli (Ch. 19); however, prolonged stimulation of the receptor results in desensitisation to many noxious pain stimuli in a similar way to capsaicin (Ch. 19).

Pharmacokinetics

Paracetamol is rapidly absorbed from the gut. It is metabolised mainly by conjugation, but a minor toxic metabolite (N-acetyl-*p*-benzoquinone) is produced by cytochrome P450 in the liver and kidneys. This is detoxified by the limited supply of glutathione in these organs. In overdose, failure to conjugate this reactive metabolite can lead to liver and renal damage (Ch. 53).

Unwanted effects

- Paracetamol is usually well tolerated, and because it does not inhibit peripheral prostaglandin synthesis, it does not cause problems with homeostatic functions of prostanoids, for example gastrointestinal disturbances.
- Hepatic damage and renal failure in overdose (Ch. 53).

Indications for using NSAIDs

NSAIDs are useful for pain relief, particularly for:

- inflammatory conditions affecting joints, soft tissues, etc.
- postoperative pain
- renal colic
- headache
- primary dysmenorrhoea; stimulation of the uterus by prostaglandins can be responsible for the pain in this condition.

About 60% of people will respond to any one NSAID, but those who fail to respond to one may derive benefit from another. Adequate time must be allowed for the full analgesic or anti-inflammatory effect to develop (see above). The choice of NSAID is mainly determined by unwanted effects, particularly on the stomach.

NSAIDs are also used for other conditions not associated with pain:

- as an antipyretic in febrile conditions
- to achieve closure of a patent ductus arteriosus in a neonate where patency may be inappropriately maintained by prostaglandin production; NSAIDs should

not be given to a pregnant mother in the third trimester, to avoid premature closure of the ductus
- for modest reduction of menstrual blood loss in menorrhagia (excessive blood loss at menstruation)
- for prevention of vascular occlusion by inhibition of platelet aggregation (especially low-dose aspirin; Ch. 11)
- for reduction in colonic polyps and prevention of colonic cancer, possibly through suppression of intracellular signalling to reduce the amount of β-catenin (which enhances cell proliferation)
- to possibly reduce the risk of developing Alzheimer's disease (Ch. 9).

Selective COX-2 inhibitors should be used in preference to standard NSAIDs only in people who may be at high risk of developing serious gastrointestinal adverse effects when an NSAID is clearly indicated as part of the management of rheumatoid arthritis or osteoarthritis. They should be taken for the shortest period of time necessary to control symptoms.

FURTHER READING

Bleumink GS, Feenstra J, Sturkenboom CJM et al (2003) Nonsteroidal anti-inflammatory drugs and heart failure. *Drugs* 63, 525–534

Burian M, Geisslinger G (2005) COX-dependent mechanisms involved in the antinociceptive action of NSAIDs at central and peripheral sites. *Pharmacol Ther* 107, 139–154

Camu F, Shi L, Vanlersberghe C (2003) The role of COX-2 inhibitors in pain modulation. *Drugs* 63, 1–7

Epstein M (2002) Non-steroidal anti-inflammatory drugs and the continuum of renal dysfunction. *J Hypertens* 20(suppl 6), S17–S23

Högestätt ED, Jönsson BA, Ermund A et al (2005) Conversion of acetaminophen to the bioactive N-acylphenolamine AM404 via fatty acid amide hydrolase-dependent arachidonic acid conjugation in the nervous system *J Biol Chem* 280, 31405–31412

James MW, Hawkey CJ (2003) Assessment of non-steroidal anti-inflammatory drug (NSAID) damage in the human gastrointestinal tract. *Br J Clin Pharmacol* 56, 146–155

McGettigan P, Henry D (2006) Cardiovascular risk and inhibition of cyclooxygenase. *JAMA* 296, 1633–1644

Micklewright R, Linley SLW, McQuade C et al (2003) NSAIDs, gastroprotection and cyclo-oxygenase-II-selective inhibitors. *Aliment Pharmacol Ther* 17, 321–332

Paccani SR, Boncristiano M, Baldari CT (2003) Molecular mechanisms underlying suppression of lymphocyte responses by nonsteroidal antiinflammatory drugs. *Cell Mol Life Sci* 60, 1071–1083

Parente L, Perretti M (2003) Advances in the pathophysiology of constitutive and inducible cyclooxygenases: two enzymes in the spotlight. *Biochem Pharmacol* 65, 153–159

Strand V (2007) Are COX-2 inhibitors preferable to non-selective non-steroidal anti-inflammatory drugs in patients with risk of cardiovascular events taking low-dose aspirin? *Lancet* 370, 2138–2151

Szallasi A, Cruz F, Geppetti P (2006) TRPV1: a therapeutic target for novel analgesic drugs? *Trends Mol Med* 12, 545–554

Szczeklik A, Stevenson DD (2003) Aspirin-induced asthma: advances in pathogenesis, diagnosis, and management. *J Allergy Clin Immunol* 111, 913–921

Vonkeman HE, Brouwers JRBJ, van de Laar MAFJ (2006) Understanding the NSAID related risk of vascular events. *BMJ* 332, 895–898

Warner TD, Mitchell JA (2008) COX-2 selectivity alone does not define the cardiovascular risk associated with non-steroidal anti-inflammatory drugs. *Lancet* 371, 270–273

SELF-ASSESSMENT

In questions 1–4, the first statement, in italics, is true. Are the accompanying statements also true?

1. *At least three isoenzymes, COX-1, COX-2 and COX-3, are involved in the synthesis of prostaglandins and thromboxanes.*
   a. COX-2 is not found constitutively in cells.
   b. PGE_2 does not cause pain itself but enhances the activity of nociceptive stimuli such as bradykinin.
   c. All NSAIDs inhibit COX-1 and COX-2 isoenzymes with equal potency.
   d. Paracetamol is a potent analgesic and anti-inflammatory agent.
2. *Gastrointestinal complications are the most common unwanted effects of NSAIDs.*
   a. NSAIDs reduce gastric blood flow.
   b. Aspirin and warfarin can be safely administered concurrently.
   c. Celecoxib causes a greater incidence of gastrointestinal symptoms than naproxen.
3. *The PGE_1 analogue misoprostol, if administered with NSAIDs, reduces their potential to cause gastric damage.*
   a. Small daily doses of aspirin (75 mg) can compromise renal function.
   b. The elderly have a greater risk of gastrointestinal adverse events when given NSAIDs.
   c. Ibuprofen is preferred to indometacin or diclofenac as an effective first-choice NSAID in severe rheumatoid arthritis.
   d. Aspirin is a good choice of analgesic therapy for people with asthma.
4. *Celecoxib causes fewer gastrointestinal symptoms on short-term administration.*
   a. Celecoxib is useful for the inhibition of platelet aggregation in patients with myocardial infarction.
   b. Celecoxib is an antipyretic.

5. Extended-matching questions
Choose the one **most appropriate** NSAID A–E that you would initially give in each case scenario 5.1–5.3.
   A. Aspirin
   B. Celecoxib
   C. Diclofenac plus misoprostol
   D. Paracetamol
   E. Indometacin
   5.1. An elderly man with a long history of hypertension, congestive heart failure with oedema, and chronic gastritis has chronic mild knee pain due to osteoarthritic changes which is interrupting his sleep.
   5.2. A 32-year-old severely asthmatic woman with a diagnosis of rheumatoid arthritis and recurrent dyspepsia and no history of heart disease.
   5.3. A 45-year-old man who recently had a myocardial infarction. He was prescribed an angiotensin-converting enzyme inhibitor and simvastatin.

ANSWERS

1. a. **False**. Although COX-2 can be induced by cytokines, endotoxins and other inflammatory mediators in many cells, it is present constitutively in other cells such as in blood vessels and can be induced with appropriate stimuli.
   b. **True**. PGE_2 generated by COX-2 sensitises the sensory pain neurons to bradykinin and other mediators but does not directly stimulate sensory pain fibres.
   c. **False**. There is a wide range in the ratios with which NSAIDs inhibit COX-1/COX-2. This relates approximately, but somewhat loosely, to the extent of their anti-inflammatory effects and gastrointestinal unwanted effects.
   d. **False**. Paracetamol is analgesic and antipyretic but has only a weak anti-inflammatory effect. The reasons for this are imperfectly understood but it may have an inhibitory effect on COX-3 enzymes and other processes in the brain.
2. a. **True**. Reduced blood flow contributes to the gastric damage caused by NSAIDs. They also inhibit bicarbonate and mucus secretion.
   b. **False**. An increase in the risk of haemorrhage can occur.
   c. **False**. The COX-2-selective inhibitor celecoxib is associated with fewer gastrointestinal unwanted effects than is the non-selective naproxen although this difference declines with continued use.
3. a. **False**. Low doses are safe, but long-term use of high doses of aspirin (or paracetamol) can result in renal ischaemia, sodium and water retention, papillary necrosis and chronic renal failure.
   b. **True**. Particularly in those over 75 years of age and in whom there is a history of peptic ulcer.
   c. **False**. Ibuprofen is good in mild to moderate arthritis but other NSAIDs such as indometacin or diclofenac have greater anti-inflammatory potential, although a greater propensity to cause unwanted effects.
   d. **False**. In a subgroup of people with asthma, aspirin induces an asthmatic response through formation of the bronchoconstrictor LTC_4. COX-1-generated prostaglandins are involved and COX-2-selective inhibitors have less potential to cause asthma attacks.
4. a. **False**. Inhibition of platelet aggregation is partly through generation of TXA_2 by COX-1 enzymes. Celecoxib is a selective COX-2 inhibitor. Some studies have suggested that in susceptible individuals the use of selective COX-2 inhibitors is associated with an excess of cardiovascular complications (especially with high doses).
   b. **True**. Pyrexia is caused by elevation of PGE_2 levels under the influence of COX-2.
5. Extended-matching answers
   5.1. Answer **D**. This man's hypertension and heart failure mean that you would not want to give him an NSAID that may result in salt and water retention. Both the COX-2-selective and non-selective NSAIDs contribute to salt and water retention.
   5.2. Answer **B**. The COX-2-selective celecoxib could be prescribed. COX-1 inhibitors such as aspirin or diclofenac may precipitate a hypersensitive asthmatic attack. Paracetamol would not be useful as it has little anti-inflammatory action.
   5.3. Answer **A**. This man should be given low-dose aspirin (75 mg daily). It prevents platelet aggregation by inhibiting TXA_2 synthesis while having a minimal effect on the production of the vasodilator PGI_2 (prostacyclin), which is generated in the vascular endothelium by COX-2. This low dose has been shown to have a beneficial long-term effect on the risk of another infarction.

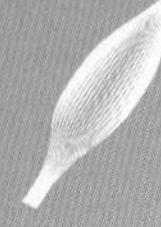

Non-steroidal anti-inflammatory drugs (NSAIDs) and related drugs

Drug	Half-life (h) and kinetics	Comments
NSAIDs		
All drugs have broad indications for pain relief (unless the use is indicated below); all are given orally (unless otherwise stated); many of the drugs are carboxylic acid derivatives which are eliminated as acyl glucuronides		
Aceclofenac	– [M] Slow and incomplete absorption; oxidation in liver by CYP2C9 is the major pathway; a minor hydrolytic pathway results in bioactivation by forming diclofenac	
Acemetacin	1 [M] High oral bioavailability and quantitative conversion to indometacin	Prodrug of indometacin
Aspirin	0.25 [M] Completely absorbed; hydrolysed rapidly to salicylic acid, its active metabolite (half-life 3–20 h)	
Azapropazone	13–17 [R] High oral bioavailability; clearance correlates with creatinine clearance	Use restricted to rheumatoid arthritis, ankylosing spondylitis and acute gout when other NSAIDs have been tried and failed
Celecoxib	11 [M] Good oral absorption; metabolised by polymorphic CYP2C9 to inactive products	A selective COX-2 inhibitor; used for pain and inflammation in osteoarthritis and rheumatoid arthritis
Dexibuprofen	2–4 [M + R] Good oral bioavailability (80%); about 10% is eliminated unchanged by the kidneys and the remainder via metabolism by polymorphic CYP2C9	The active enantiomer of ibuprofen – see below
Dexketoprofen	1–3 [M] High oral bioavailability (90%); glucuronidation is the major route of elimination but the conjugate can be hydrolysed back to the parent drug if elimination is impaired, for example in renal failure	Used for short-term treatment of mild to moderate pain; optical isomer of ketoprofen (see below)
Diclofenac	1–2 [M] Oral bioavailability is about 60%; eliminated by a combination of CYP2C9- and CYP3A4-mediated oxidation and by conjugation	Given orally, rectally, by deep intramuscular injection or intravenous infusion; transdermally or topical to eye; available orally in combined formulation with misoprostol for gastric protection (Ch. 33)
Diflunisal	8–12 [M] Good oral absorption; major route of elimination is conjugation with glucuronic acid	
Etodolac	6–7 [M] Good oral bioavailability (80%); eliminated by both oxidation and conjugation with glucuronic acid	Used for pain and inflammation in osteoarthritis and rheumatoid arthritis
Etoricoxib	25 [M] Good oral bioavailability (90%); eliminated largely by CYP3A4-mediated oxidation	A selective COX-2 inhibitor; used for pain and inflammation in osteoarthritis, rheumatoid arthritis and in acute gout; has not been approved for use in the USA
Felbinac	?	Available for topical application
Fenbufen	10 [M] Rapidly and almost completely absorbed; oxidised to active metabolites, including felbinac, which have a similar half-life	Prodrug
Fenoprofen	2–3 [M] Rapidly and completely absorbed; eliminated by both oxidation and conjugation with glucuronic acid	

Non-steroidal anti-inflammatory drugs (NSAIDs) and related drugs

Drug	Half-life (h) and kinetics	Comments
Flurbiprofen	3–9 [M + R] Rapidly and completely absorbed, metabolised by polymorphic CYP2C9 and also by direct conjugation; about 25% is eliminated unchanged by the kidneys	Given orally, rectally, as lozenge for local treatment of sore throat or topically to eye
Ibuprofen	2–4 [M + R] Good oral bioavailability (80%); about 10% is eliminated unchanged by the kidneys and the remainder via metabolism by polymorphic CYP2C9	Given orally or transdermally
Indometacin	3–5 [M + R] Rapidly and completely absorbed; eliminated by oxidation and conjugation while the remainder is excreted unchanged by the kidneys	Given orally or rectally
Ketoprofen	1–3 [M] High oral bioavailability (90%); glucuronidation is the major route of elimination but the conjugate can be hydrolysed back to the parent drug if elimination is impaired, for example in renal failure	Given orally, rectally, by deep intramuscular injection or transdermally
Ketorolac	3–9 [R + M] Rapid and complete absorption; renal excretion is major route (60% of dose) of elimination; metabolism is by both oxidation and conjugation	Used in short-term management of postoperative pain; given orally, by intramuscular or slow intravenous injection or topically to eye
Lumiracoxib	5–8 [M] High oral bioavailability; extensively metabolised by hepatic CYP2C9	A selective COX-2 inhibitor
Mefenamic acid	3–4 [M] Rapidly and completely absorbed; absorption reduced if taken with food; metabolised by polymorphic CYP2C9 and also by direct conjugation; metabolites are known to be inactive	
Meloxicam	12–20 [M] Absorption is slow but essentially complete; metabolised by polymorphic CYP2C9 to inactive metabolites	Used for pain and inflammation in rheumatoid arthritis, osteoarthritis (short-term) and in ankylosing spondylitis; given orally or rectally
Nabumetone	24 (metabolite) [M] Undergoes complete first-pass metabolism by hydrolysis of methyl ester group to yield an active naphthylacetic acid derivative that is eliminated by hepatic metabolism	Used for pain and inflammation in osteoarthritis and rheumatoid arthritis
Naproxen	12–15 [M] Rapidly and completely absorbed; metabolised by oxidation and conjugation to inactive products	Given orally or rectally
Parecoxib	5–9 [M] Metabolised to a range of products, including valdecoxib	Used in short-term management of postoperative pain; give by deep intramuscular or intravenous injection
Piroxicam	30–60 [M + R] Rapid absorption; metabolised in the liver to inactive products and undergoes enterohepatic circulation; renal excretion accounts for about 10% of dose (99% protein binding minimises glomerular filtration of the drug)	Given orally, rectally or by deep intramuscular injection; restricted use because of incidence of gastrointestinal unwanted effects and serious skin reactions; also unrestricted transdermal use
Sulindac	7–8 [M + R] Good oral absorption; contains a sulphoxide (SO) group that is oxidised to an inactive sulphone (SO_2) and reduced in the liver and lower bowel to active thioether (S) metabolite	Prodrug for active thioether metabolite

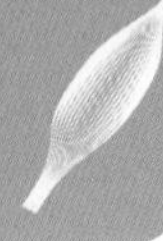

Non-steroidal anti-inflammatory drugs (NSAIDs) and related drugs

Drug	Half-life (h) and kinetics	Comments
Tenoxicam	44–100 [M] Slow absorption after oral dosage; metabolites are known to be inactive	Given orally or by intramuscular or intravenous injection
Tiaprofenic acid	2–4 [M] Good oral bioavailability; oxidised by P450 and metabolites excreted in urine as conjugates	
Tolfenamic acid	2 [M] Complete oral bioavailability; metabolites are eliminated in bile and have a longer half-life (enterohepatic circulation?)	Licensed for the treatment of migraine – see Ch. 26; a potent CYP1A2 inhibitor
Related drugs		
All given orally		
Benorylate	<0.1 [M] Absorbed intact and hydrolysed rapidly in blood and liver to paracetamol and acetylsalicylic acid	Ester of paracetamol and acetylsalicylic acid
Paracetamol (acetaminophen)	3–4 [M] Rapidly and completely absorbed; most is metabolised by conjugation with glucuronic acid and sulphate; a minor oxidation pathway leads to hepatotoxicity – see Ch. 53	The most widely used non-opioid analgesic

[M], metabolism; [R], renal excretion.

30 Rheumatoid arthritis, other inflammatory arthritides and osteoarthritis

RHEUMATOID ARTHRITIS AND OTHER INFLAMMATORY ARTHRITIDES

Rheumatoid arthritis is a chronic inflammatory condition of unknown cause, to which some people are genetically predisposed. The symptoms of rheumatoid arthritis usually appear gradually and most often involve the proximal interphalangeal joints of the fingers, metacarpophalangeal joints and wrists. Other joints such as the ankles and hips may be involved later. The affected joints are warm, swollen and painful. Stiffness is troublesome, particularly in the morning, as a result of an increase in extracellular fluid in and around the joint. Systemic disturbance is common, including general fatigue and malaise, while extra-articular manifestations such as vasculitis and neuropathy can occur.

Autoimmune processes contribute to the maintenance of the rheumatoid arthritis, but it is uncertain whether it is initiated by an autoimmune reaction or by an exogenous antigen. The initiator is believed to bind to Toll-like receptors (TLRs) – pattern recognition molecules that bind to both foreign and self structures – on dendritic cells and macrophages, which initiates a response by the innate immune system. The primary response is lymphoid cell infiltration of the synovium around the joint, formation of new blood vessels and a proliferation of the synovial membrane. The synovium becomes locally invasive (pannus) and osteoclasts destroy joint cartilage and bone. Apart from psoriatic arthritis, other forms of inflammatory arthritis do not produce erosive changes in periarticular bone or marked joint destruction to the same degree.

The chronic inflammatory process is initiated by T-helper 1 (Th1) lymphocytes that migrate into the joint. Failure of suppression of Th1 cells by regulatory T-cells may be important in the pathogenesis of the disease. Activated T-cells produce a gamut of pro-inflammatory cytokines, including tumour necrosis factor alpha (TNFα) and interleukin-1 (IL-1). These cytokines stimulate B-lymphocytes, macrophages, fibroblasts, chondrocytes and osteoclasts (Fig. 30.1). B cells play an important role in the pathology of rheumatoid arthritis. They act as antigen-presenting cells that co-stimulate T-cells, produce inflammatory cytokines such as TNFα and produce rheumatoid factor antibody. Antigen-presenting cells express CD20, CD80 and CD86 surface markers and are involved in the activation of T-cells (Fig. 30.1). TNFα has a prominent role in orchestrating the production of other inflammatory mediators and the recruitment of further immune and inflammatory cells into the joint. This pattern of inflammation differs from most other immune-mediated diseases. The ubiquitous gene transcription factor nuclear factor kappa B (NFκB) is also thought to be involved in many steps in cell activation and cytokine production in the destructive cycle of events.

TNFα and IL-1 aid the recruitment of inflammatory cells such as leucocytes by increasing the expression of adhesion molecules (integrins) on vascular endothelial cells. These cytokines also stimulate synovial fibroblasts, osteoclasts and chondrocytes to release tissue-destroying matrix metalloproteinases (MMPs) and to express chemokine receptors. Activated macrophages, lymphocytes and fibroblasts stimulate angiogenesis in the synovium.

Antibodies are produced to the collagen exposed in the damaged cartilage. Rheumatoid factor (IgM autoantibodies reactive with IgG) is present in the plasma of many people with rheumatoid arthritis. It forms complexes with collagen in damaged cartilage, which then activate the complement pathway. The relevance of this to joint damage is not known. The activated osteoclasts increase bone resorption. The end result of this complex inflammatory process is irreversible destruction of cartilage and erosion of periarticular bone.

The plethora of cells that enter the synovium, and the bewildering array of cytokines that are involved, provide a large number of potential targets for disease-modifying antirheumatic drugs affecting the immune system (Fig 30.1).

DISEASE-MODIFYING ANTIRHEUMATIC DRUGS (DMARDS) FOR RHEUMATOID ARTHRITIS

Non-steroidal anti-inflammatory drugs (NSAIDs – Ch. 29) provide symptomatic relief but do not alter the long-term progression of joint destruction in rheumatoid arthritis. A diverse group of compounds can reduce the rate of progression of joint erosion and destruction, leading to improvement both in symptoms and in the clinical

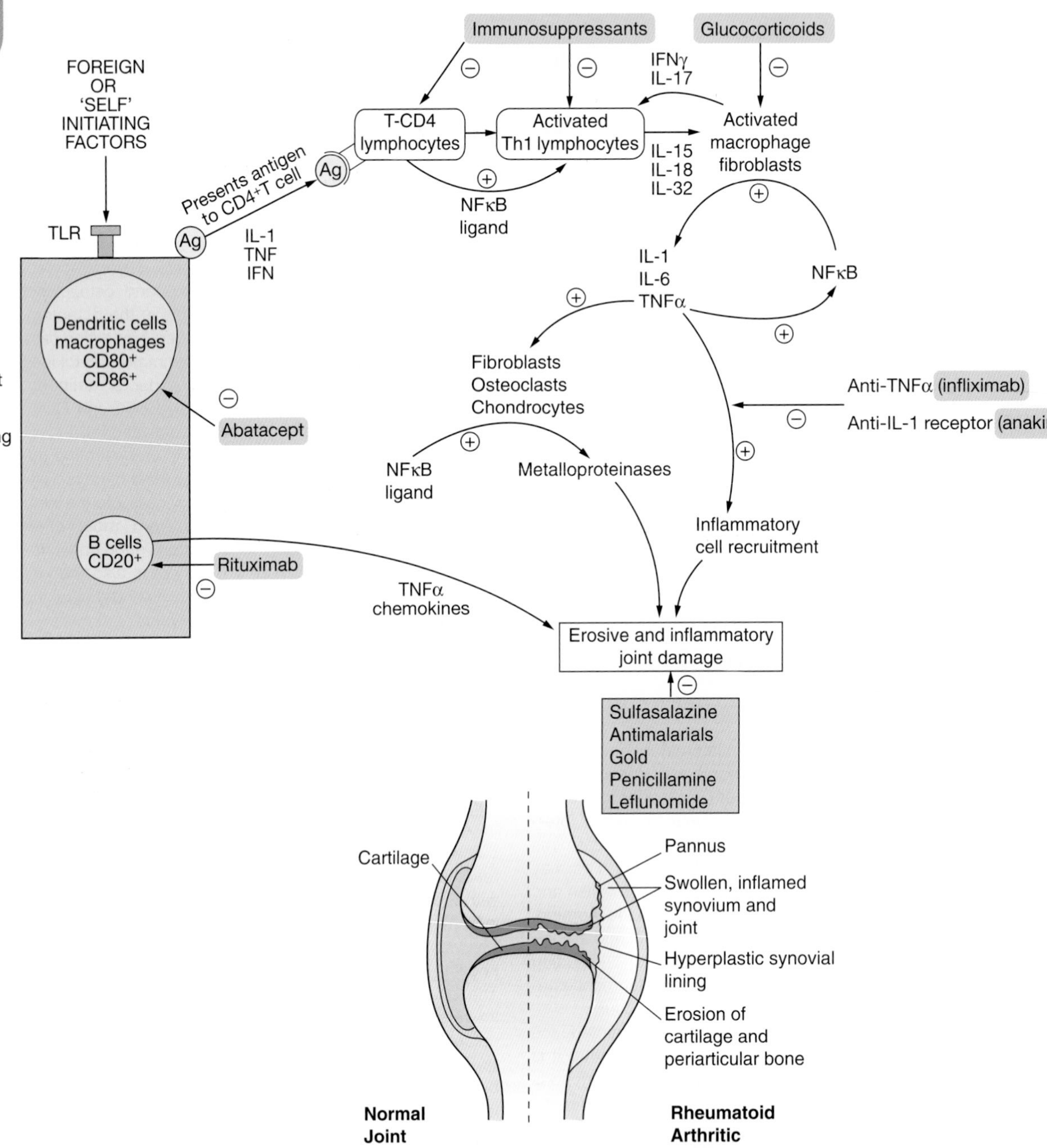

Fig. 30.1 **The biology of rheumatoid arthritis and sites of drug action**. The affected synovial joint is characterised by inflamed and swollen synovium with increased presence of fibroblasts, osteoclasts, plasma cells, mast cells, B-lymphocytes and angiogenesis. The synovial fluid contains increased numbers of polymorphonuclear neutrophil leucocytes. There is erosion of cartilage and adjacent bone. The cascade of self-perpetuating inflammatory events involves many factors, including upregulation of the ubiquitous gene transcription superfamily nuclear factor kappa B (NFκB) which not only can induce gene transcription for many inflammatory, proliferative and remodelling factors but also can be a target for their actions. Many of the drugs shown act at multiple sites. APCs, antigen-presenting cells; IFN, interferon; IL, interleukin; TLR, Toll-like receptor; TNFα, tumour necrosis factor alpha.

and serological markers of rheumatoid arthritis activity. These drugs produce long-term depression of the inflammatory response even though they have little direct anti-inflammatory effect. They all have a slow onset of action, with many producing little improvement until about 3 months after starting treatment. Such drugs are grouped together and known as disease-modifying antirheumatic drugs (DMARDs).

Sulfasalazine

The action of sulfasalazine in arthritis is poorly understood. It is reduced in the colon and split into 5-aminosalicylic acid (which is not believed to contribute to the antirheumatic action) and sulfapyridine. Sulfapyridine in the colon may reduce the absorption of antigens that promote joint inflammation. However, sulfasalazine and sulfapyridine are both absorbed and are found at similar concentrations in synovial fluid. Sulfasalazine can suppress several signal transduction pathways involved in the synthesis of pro-inflammatory cytokines, such as gene transcription mediated by NFκB, which may contribute to its efficacy.

High doses of sulfasalazine are required for the treatment of rheumatoid arthritis and these often produce gastrointestinal upset. This can be minimised by increasing the dose slowly and by using an enteric-coated formulation. Other problems include reversible oligospermia (therefore sulfasalazine should be avoided in males who wish to have a family) and blood dyscrasias. Sulfasalazine is discussed more fully in Chapter 34.

Antimalarials

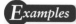

chloroquine, hydroxychloroquine

These antimalarial drugs are believed to reduce T-lymphocyte transformation and chemotaxis. Their weakly basic nature permits their uptake and concentration in cells in a non-ionised form. Having entered the lysosomes inside the cell, the acidic environment traps and concentrates the drug in its ionised state. Macrophages depend on acid proteases in their lysosomes for digestion of phagocytosed protein. Antimalarial drugs slightly increase the pH inside the macrophage lysosomes, which alters the processing of peptide antigens and reduces their subsequent presentation on the cell surface. Thus, the interaction between T-helper cells and antigen-presenting macrophages responsible for joint inflammation is reduced, with a reduction in the inflammatory response. Recent evidence also suggests that these antimalarial drugs reduce the production of several inflammatory cytokines.

The major toxic effect of these drugs is on the retina, although they are relatively safe at the low doses currently recommended. Hydroxychloroquine is better tolerated than chloroquine and is now the preferred agent. Retinal toxicity is a potential problem, and specialist assessment of the eyes is recommended during treatment with hydroxychloroquine if there is a change in visual acuity or blurring of vision or if treatment continues for more than 5 years. The pharmacokinetics and other unwanted effects of these drugs can be found in Chapter 51.

Leflunomide

Mechanism of action and uses

Leflunomide is an isoxazole derivative that inhibits the enzyme dihydroorotate dehydrogenase, a key mitochondrial enzyme in the de novo synthesis of the pyrimidine ribonucleotide uridine monophosphate (UMP). Activated lymphocytes require an eightfold increase in their pyrimidine pool to proliferate. Inadequate provision of UMP increases the expression of the tumour-suppressor molecule p53 which translocates to the cell nucleus and arrests the cell cycle in the G_1 phase. This reduces the expansion of the activated autoimmune T- and B-lymphocyte pool, thereby suppressing immunoglobulin production and cellular immune processes. Other dividing cells can obtain adequate pyrimidines from a separate salvage pathway that reuses existing ribonucleotides and is not affected by leflunomide. There are other potential mechanisms of immunomodulation by leflunomide, such as inhibition of tyrosine kinases and reduced production of transcription factors that regulate inflammatory cytokines, but they are probably of lesser importance.

Pharmacokinetics

Leflunomide is a prodrug. It is well absorbed from the gut and is converted non-enzymatically, mainly in the intestinal mucosa and plasma, to its active metabolite, which has a very long half-life of 15 days. The metabolite is excreted via the bile and kidney, and enterohepatic circulation contributes to the long plasma half-life.

Unwanted effects

- Gastrointestinal upset, especially diarrhoea
- Increase in blood pressure
- Headache, dizziness, lethargy
- Leucopenia
- Skin rash
- Alopecia
- Reversible abnormalities of liver function
- Teratogenicity: it is advised that conception should be avoided for 2 years after stopping treatment in women and for 3 months in men.

Prevention and management of unwanted effects

Monitoring of full blood count (especially white cell count) and liver function should be carried out regularly during treatment. If serious unwanted effects occur, elimination of the drug can be increased by the use of colestyramine (Ch. 48) to bind the active metabolite present in the gut after biliary excretion, thereby interrupting its enterohepatic circulation (Ch. 2).

Immunosuppressant drugs

Several drugs with immunosuppressant actions have been shown to be effective in rheumatoid arthritis. These include:

- antimetabolites: methotrexate, azathioprine (Ch. 38)
- calcineurin inhibitors: ciclosporin, tacrolimus (Ch. 38)
- antiproliferative agents: mycophenolate mofetil (Ch. 38) may be useful in rheumatoid arthritis but is not licensed for this indication in the UK.

Methotrexate is one of the most effective antirheumatic drugs. Although its primary mechanism of action is by folate antagonism, co-administration of folic acid supplements prevents much of the mucosal and gastrointestinal toxicity of the drug but does not reduce its immunomodulatory effect. A possible additional mechanism of action to explain the effect in arthritis is accumulation of adenosine, an intermediate in purine biosynthesis. Methotrexate inhibits the deamination of adenosine, which is a potent anti-inflammatory mediator. Adenosine suppresses neutrophil adhesion and cytokine production, reduces macrophage function and reduces the expression of endothelial adhesion molecules. Methotrexate is usually given orally once a week for the treatment of inflammatory arthritis. It can be given intramuscularly if oral use produces intractable gastrointestinal symptoms or absorption by the oral route is inadequate.

Gold

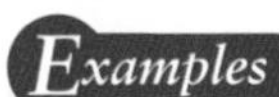

auranofin, sodium aurothiomalate

Mechanism of action

The precise mechanism by which gold compounds act is unknown. A popular concept is that the compound is taken up by mononuclear cells and inhibits their phagocytic function. This will reduce the release of inflammatory mediators and inhibit inflammatory cell proliferation. Production of inflammatory cytokines such as IL-1, IL-6 and TNFα is inhibited, and superoxide generation by neutrophils is reduced. There is also evidence for inhibition of other cell-signalling pathways involved in inflammation, including NFκB.

Oral gold (auranofin) has a rather slower onset of action than intramuscular gold and is less efficacious, but is much better tolerated. The advent of more effective and less toxic drugs has reduced the use of gold salts in current clinical practice.

Pharmacokinetics

The parenteral form of gold (sodium aurothiomalate) is given by deep intramuscular injection. An initial test dose is given to screen for acute toxicity (see below), followed by injections at weekly intervals to gradually achieve a therapeutic concentration in the tissues. Subsequently, a smaller dose is used to maintain remission. Oral gold is taken daily. Gold binds readily to albumin and several tissue proteins and accumulates in many tissues such as the liver, kidney, bone marrow, lymph nodes and spleen. Accumulation also occurs in the synovium of inflamed joints. Elimination is largely by the kidney, and to a lesser extent by biliary excretion. Gold has a half-life of several weeks, probably as a result of its extensive tissue binding.

Unwanted effects

The unwanted effects can be serious and all but the most minor effects should lead to immediate cessation of treatment:

- Oral ulceration
- Proteinuria from membranous glomerulonephritis: this can develop after several weeks of treatment, sometimes progressing to nephrotic syndrome; recovery can take up to 2 years following drug withdrawal
- Blood disorders, especially thrombocytopenia but also agranulocytosis and aplastic anaemia
- Rashes
- Pulmonary fibrosis
- Diarrhoea is common with oral gold.

Prevention and management of unwanted effects

Urine should be checked for protein and a full blood count obtained before each injection of gold, and regularly during oral therapy. Major complications may require treatment with dimercaprol or penicillamine to chelate the gold (Ch. 53) and increase its elimination. Corticosteroids can be helpful to treat blood dyscrasias. Gold should not be used if there is a history of renal or hepatic disease, blood dyscrasias or severe rashes. Gold should be stopped if stomatitis, a pruritic rash, neutropenia, thrombocytopenia or significant proteinuria (>1 g in 24 h) develops.

Penicillamine

Mechanism of action and uses

The mechanisms of action of penicillamine are uncertain. Modulation of the immune system is believed to be important, including a reduction in the number of activated lymphocytes, reduced synthesis of immunoglobulins and stabilisation of lysosomal membranes in inflammatory cells. Penicillamine has not been shown to slow the progression of joint erosions and is no longer widely used for rheumatoid arthritis.

Penicillamine is a thiol compound that can chelate many metals. This is probably of little relevance to its use in arthritis but has given the drug a role in the management of poisoning (Ch. 53) and in Wilson's disease, a genetically determined illness that is associated with copper overload.

Pharmacokinetics

Penicillamine is well absorbed from the gut, although oral iron supplements substantially reduce its absorption. Its half-life is short (1–6 h), but penicillamine binds tightly via disulphide bonds to plasma and tissue proteins. Penicillamine is partially metabolised in the liver, but is also excreted unchanged in the urine.

Unwanted effects

Unwanted effects occur frequently and are responsible for cessation of treatment in about 30% of people. They can be reduced by slow increases in dose. Many unwanted effects resemble those of gold:

- Nausea, vomiting, abdominal discomfort and rashes (often with fever), especially early in treatment

- Loss of taste is common, but may resolve despite continued treatment
- Oral ulceration
- Proteinuria, which is caused by immune-complex glomerulonephritis and is dose-related; nephrotic syndrome can occur
- Blood disorders, especially thrombocytopenia but also neutropenia and, rarely, aplastic anaemia.

Regular monitoring of urine protein and blood counts should be carried out during treatment.

Antibodies against tumour necrosis factor alpha (TNFα)

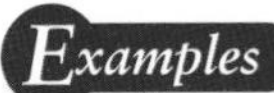

adalimumab, etanercept, infliximab

Mechanism of action

TNFα stimulates several inflammatory processes (see above and Fig. 30.1). It acts by binding to one of two cell surface receptors, p55 and p75, that are found in several tissues. There are several antibody derivatives available that block the action of TNFα.

- Adalimumab is a fully humanised monoclonal antibody specific for TNFα.
- Etanercept is a fusion protein consisting of two recombinant soluble extracellular portions of the human p75 TNF receptor, fused to the constant (Fc) domain of human immunoglobulin (IgG_1). It binds to TNFα and the cytokine lymphotoxin α (also known as TNFβ). Etanercept reduces the pro-inflammatory activity of TNFα, but it is not known whether the effect on lymphotoxin α is of clinical importance.
- Infliximab is a chimeric monoclonal antibody comprising the variable region of a murine antibody, which neutralises TNFα, spliced to the constant region of a human antibody. It does not neutralise lymphotoxin α (TNFβ).

Pharmacokinetics

Adalimumab is given by subcutaneous injection. The very long half-life of about 12 days allows the drug to be given once every 2 weeks. The mechanism of elimination has not been defined, but it is likely to be by proteolysis.

Etanercept is given by twice-weekly subcutaneous injection. It is slowly absorbed from the injection site, and has a very long half-life of about 5 days. It is believed to be metabolised by proteolytic enzymes.

Infliximab is given by intravenous infusion, initially at 2- and 4-week intervals, then every 2 months. It has a very long half-life of 9 days, and its mechanism of elimination is not well understood.

Unwanted effects

- All these drugs can produce gastrointestinal upset, decompensation of heart failure, hypersensitivity reactions, injection site reactions, fever, headache and depression.
- Increased risk of pulmonary tuberculosis: screening for evidence of tuberculosis is recommended before initiation of therapy. Septicaemia and reactivation of hepatitis B virus occur more frequently.

Interleukin-1 receptor antagonists

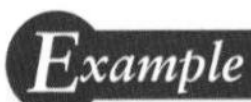

anakinra

Mechanism of action

Anakinra is a recombinant human IL-1 receptor antagonist (Fig. 30.1). IL-1 is actually a family of three cytokines, comprising two agonists (IL-1α and IL-1β) and an IL-1 receptor antagonist. The theoretical basis for the use of anakinra is that joint destruction arises from an imbalance between the agonists and the antagonist. IL-1 agonists are pro-inflammatory cytokines released by macrophages and fibroblasts in inflamed synovium, and by neutrophils in synovial fluid. The IL-1 peptides compete for occupancy of the IL-1 receptor on the membrane of synovial cells, and as little as 2–3% occupancy by the agonists produces maximal pro-inflammatory cell activation. Anakinra blocks the receptors and suppresses the inflammatory response.

Pharmacokinetics

Anakinra is given by daily subcutaneous injection. Elimination is via the kidneys, and it has a short half-life (4–6 h).

Unwanted effects

- Injection site reactions
- Increased risk of serious infections, particularly in people with asthma
- Neutropenia.

T-cell co-stimulation modulator

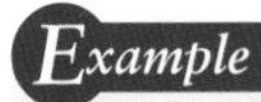

abatacept

Mechanism of action and uses

T-lymphocyte activation requires recognition of a specific antigen carried by an antigen-presenting cell, and a second co-stimulatory signal. A major co-stimulatory signal involves binding of two molecules on the surface of antigen-presenting cells (known as CD80 and CD86) to the CD28 receptor on T-cells. Abatacept is a monoclonal antibody that selectively binds to CD80 and CD86 and blocks the co-stimulatory signal. It therefore reduces the subsequent production of inflammatory mediators and pro-inflammatory cytokines. Abatacept is used for individuals who have failed to respond to, or are intolerant of, a TNFα inhibitor.

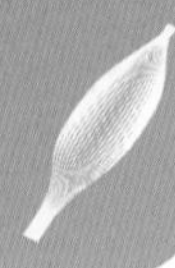

Pharmacokinetics

Abatacept is given by intravenous infusion. Its metabolism is unknown, and it has a very long half-life of about 14 days.

Unwanted effects

- Headache
- Nausea
- Upper respiratory tract infection and, less commonly, other infections.

Anti-CD20 B-cell depleter

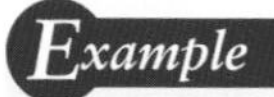

rituximab

Mechanism of action and uses

Rituximab specifically depletes $CD20^+$ B-lymphocytes by binding to the CD20 antigen expressed on the cell surface (Fig. 30.1). The mechanism of action of rituximab in rheumatoid disease is uncertain. Responses usually last for up to 6 months, and relapse corresponds with B-cell repopulation.

Pharmacokinetics

Rituximab is given by intravenous infusion. Its metabolism is unknown, and it has a very long half-life of about 3–8 days.

Unwanted effects

- Cytokine release syndrome with fever, chills, nausea, vomiting and allergic reactions occurs in about one-third of people with the first infusion. Premedication with an antihistamine and sometimes a corticosteroid will reduce these reactions.
- Exacerbation of angina, arrhythmia or heart failure can occur in people with cardiovascular disease.

MANAGEMENT OF RHEUMATOID ARTHRITIS AND OTHER INFLAMMATORY ARTHRITIDES

NSAIDs (Ch. 29) are the mainstay of symptomatic drug treatment for all types of inflammatory arthritis. Physical aids such as splinting and bed rest are important for acute episodes. The choice of NSAID is arbitrary, with considerable variation in individual responses to different drugs. Propionic acid derivatives are often used first; they have a weaker anti-inflammatory activity than other classes of NSAID, but generally have fewer unwanted effects. More powerful drugs such as diclofenac can be used when others fail to control symptoms, although the increased risk of gastrointestinal irritation may limit their use, especially in the elderly. About 60% of people can be expected to respond to the first-choice agent, and most derive some benefit from taking one of the NSAIDs. Predicting which drug will be most effective in an individual is not currently possible. Morning stiffness is often disabling in inflammatory arthritis. This is helped by giving either a late evening dose of an NSAID with a long half-life, a modified-release formulation of a compound with a short half-life, or an NSAID suppository. Topical NSAIDs applied over the affected joint(s) are not usually recommended. Selective COX-2 inhibitors are usually reserved for people who are intolerant of NSAIDs, or who have a higher risk of serious gastrointestinal complications with an NSAID (Ch. 29).

Progressive joint damage is common in rheumatoid arthritis and to a lesser extent in psoriatic arthritis (in contrast to the other seronegative spondylarthritides). There is now a substantial body of evidence that early use of DMARDs leads to a better long-term outcome in these conditions. Indications for DMARDs include:

- the prevention of erosive damage
- the suppression of persistent inflammation that fails to respond to 3 months of treatment with NSAIDs
- intolerance to NSAIDs
- high titre of rheumatoid factor or extra-articular manifestations of rheumatoid disease.

DMARDs are almost always used in combination with NSAIDs in the first few weeks of treatment, since they do not have significant anti-inflammatory action and require 2–3 months before an effect is established. Sulfasalazine is often given initially, because of its perceived low toxicity. Methotrexate is probably the most effective agent and is now the first-choice DMARD of most rheumatologists, since it is well tolerated when used correctly. Hydroxychloroquine can be an effective alternative but is seldom used as monotherapy, while leflunomide is often reserved for those who are intolerant of methotrexate. Gold and penicillamine are now less widely used, due to toxicity and limited efficacy, while immunosuppressant drugs other than methotrexate are generally reserved as third-line agents. Cytotoxic drugs, especially cyclophosphamide, are particularly useful for the management of extra-articular manifestations of rheumatoid disease, such as vasculitis, pericarditis or pleurisy.

Combinations of DMARDs are being used increasingly as standard therapy. Drug combinations are more effective than single agents, and triple therapy may have advantages over two drugs. If a single DMARD is insufficient to suppress disease activity and methotrexate has not been used, then methotrexate should be tried. Combination therapy is used if there is failure to respond to methotrexate within 3 months. If methotrexate has been well tolerated, then another second-line drug such as hydroxychloroquine, sulfasalazine or ciclosporin is usually added. Leflunomide is of comparable efficacy to methotrexate, and is used for people who are intolerant of methotrexate.

The role of corticosteroids in rheumatoid arthritis has been controversial. Intra-articular injections are used for individual inflamed joints (especially knee and shoulder). In active disease, short courses of oral prednisolone or pulsed therapy (repeated high doses over a short period) with intravenous methylprednisolone (Ch. 44) can produce a rapid relief of symptoms before DMARDs work. In early rheumatoid disease, a small dose of oral prednisolone given for 6 months in combination with sulfasalazine or methotrexate retards bone damage and slows disease progression. Pulsed intramuscular corticosteroid therapy is also given for disease flares, or to ameliorate symptoms in the first few weeks after initiating DMARD therapy (because of the slow response).

Anti-TNFα drugs (the most frequently used of the 'biological' agents) for rheumatoid arthritis are usually reserved for those who fail to respond to oral therapies or who are intolerant of several DMARDs. Anti-TNFα drugs are often used in combination with methotrexate, which produces a better response than the biological agent given alone. The combination produces remission and halts disease progression in up to 50% of people who are treated. Increasing evidence suggests that early treatment with a combination of two DMARDs with prednisolone or a biological agent may produce remission of disease which can persist for many months even after drug withdrawal. Anakinra is less effective than anti-TNFα drugs. Abatacept and rituximab have been shown to be effective for people with rheumatoid arthritis who fail to respond to, or who cannot tolerate, a TNFα blocker.

Although most evidence for the use of DMARDs has been obtained in the treatment of rheumatoid arthritis, there is increasing evidence for their efficacy in the seronegative spondylarthritides. Sulfasalazine and methotrexate may be effective for peripheral joint disease in these forms of inflammatory arthritis. Anti-TNFα agents can produce remission of disease in ankylosing spondylitis and psoriatic arthritis in about one-third of those treated, with considerable symptomatic benefit in others.

OSTEOARTHRITIS

Osteoarthritis is the clinical manifestation of joint degeneration that results from loss of articular cartilage and becomes more common with increasing age. Most osteoarthritis is idiopathic (when it can be localised or generalised) but a small proportion is secondary to other conditions such as joint injury or chondrocalcinosis. The cardinal symptom of osteoarthritis is pain during physical activity, which is most pronounced with use of the affected joint and which is relieved by rest. Pain also occurs at rest with advanced disease. Stiffness may be troublesome for short periods after rest. Various joints can be involved, particularly the distal interphalangeal joints of the fingers and the carpometacarpal joint of the thumb. Large joints such as the knee, hip, elbow and shoulder are often asymmetrically affected.

The integrity of articular cartilage depends on the balance of synthetic and catabolic activity of the chondrocytes embedded in the cartilage matrix. Mechanical compression of cartilage produces many physical and biochemical stimuli that influence chondrocyte metabolism. Mechanical overload, the principal cause of secondary osteoarthritis, produces changes that promote matrix destruction and apoptotic chondrocyte death. It remains uncertain whether most osteoarthritis is caused primarily by increased degradation or decreased synthesis of cartilage.

Synthesis of cartilage is promoted by the expression of growth factors by chondrocytes, particularly insulin-like growth factor 1 and transforming growth factor beta. Degradation of cartilage proteins is carried out by matrix metalloproteinases (MMPs), particularly stromelysin 1 (MMP-3) in early osteoarthritis and gelatinase A (MMP-2) and MMP-13 in late disease. MMPs are synthesised by chondrocytes in response to stimulation by the pro-inflammatory cytokines IL-1β and TNFα that are released by inflammatory cells. Synovial inflammation often occurs adjacent to the damaged cartilage. Chondrocytes produce a chemokine, RANTES (regulated upon activation normal T cell expressed and secreted), and synovial cells produce chemokine receptors CXCR4 (chemokine receptor type 4) which interact with molecules on the surface of white blood cells and have a role in recruiting inflammatory cells to the joint.

Loss of matrix leads to disruption of the cartilage, with swelling and fissuring of the surface. Subchondral bone becomes increasingly vascular and new bone is laid down. It is uncertain whether the initiating factors for osteoarthritis originate in the articular cartilage or subchondral bone. However, recent evidence suggests that stiffening of subchondral bone, with less effective shock absorption, may be the trigger for cartilage loss.

MANAGEMENT OF OSTEOARTHRITIS

Treatment of osteoarthritis currently remains symptomatic. Non-pharmacological therapy such as weight loss, exercise, physical therapy and orthotics is often useful. Glucosamine or chondroitin supplements (over-the-counter preparations in the UK) are often used by people with osteoarthritis, but there is little evidence of benefit. If pain is troublesome, simple analgesics should usually be considered as first-line treatment. NSAIDs may be helpful for inflammatory episodes or if paracetamol is ineffective. In vitro studies suggest that some NSAIDs may accelerate the loss of articular cartilage in osteoarthritis; clinical studies are inconclusive, but avoidance of powerful NSAIDs is probably desirable. Intra-articular or periarticular injection of a corticosteroid (Ch. 44) can provide short-term symptomatic relief in osteoarthritis, even if there is little clinical evidence of joint inflammation. Corticosteroids inhibit proinflammatory mediators in synovial tissue, such as IL-1 and TNFα. Joint injection with hyaluronic acid remains a controversial treatment, with conflicting evidence of efficacy from clinical trials.

Compounds under development, particularly matrix metalloproteinase inhibitors and IL-1 receptor antagonists, may offer the possibility of prevention of cartilage degeneration or even promote regeneration.

Long-term management of osteoarthritis may eventually require surgical joint replacement.

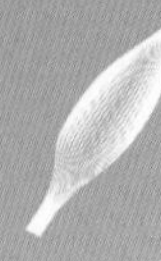

FURTHER READING

Rheumatoid arthritis and other inflammatory arthritides

Braun J, Sieper J (2007) Ankylosing spondylitis. *N Engl J Med* 369, 1379–1390

Brockbank J, Gladman D (2002) Diagnosis and management of psoriatic arthritis. *Drugs* 62, 2447–2457

Conn DL, Lim SS (2003) New role for an old friend: prednisone is a disease-modifying agent in early rheumatoid arthritis. *Curr Opin Rheumatol* 15, 193–196

Donahue KE, Gartlehner G, Jonas DE et al (2008) Systematic review: comparative effectiveness and harms of disease-modifying medications for rheumatoid arthritis. *Ann Intern Med* 148, 162–163

Emery P (2006) Treatment of rheumatoid arthritis. *BMJ* 332, 152–155

Goldblatt F, Isenberg DA (2008) Anti-CD20 monoclonal antibody in rheumatoid arthritis and systemic lupus erythematosus. *Handb Exp Pharmacol* 2008, 163–181

Haringman JJ, Ludikhuize J, Tak PP (2004) Chemokines in joint disease: the key to inflammation? *Ann Rheum Dis* 63, 1186–1194

Katz WA (2002) Use of nonopioid analgesics and adjunctive agents in the management of pain in rheumatic diseases. *Curr Opin Rheumatol* 14, 63–71

Klareskog L, Catrina AI, Paget S (2009) Rheumatoid arthritis. *Lancet* 373, 659–672

O'Dell JR (2004) Therapeutic strategies for rheumatoid arthritis. *N Engl J Med* 350, 2591–2602

Olsen NJ, Stein CM (2004) New drugs for rheumatoid arthritis. *N Engl J Med* 350, 2167–2179

Reveille JD, Arnett FC (2005) Spondyloarthritis: update on pathogenesis and management. *Am J Med* 118, 592–603

Scott DL, Kingsley GH (2006) Tumour necrosis factor inhibitors for rheumatoid arthritis. *N Engl J Med* 355, 704–712

Smolen JS, Aletaha D, Weisman MH et al (2007) New therapies for the treatment of rheumatoid arthritis. *Lancet* 370, 1861–1874

Osteoarthritis

Dieppe P, Brandt KD (2003) What is important in treating osteoarthritis? Whom should we treat and how should we treat them? *Rheum Dis Clin North Am* 29, 687–716

Felson DT (2006) Osteoarthritis of the knee. *N Engl J Med* 354, 841–848

Hunter DJ, Felson DT (2006) Osteoarthritis. *BMJ* 332, 639–642

Sharma S (2002) Nonpharmacological management of osteoarthritis. *Curr Opin Rheumatol* 14, 603–607

SELF-ASSESSMENT

In questions 1–7, the first statement, in italics, is true. Are the following statements also true?

1. *Most disease-modifying antirheumatic drugs (DMARDs) take several weeks for their full effect to take place.*
   a. NSAIDs reduce the symptoms of rheumatoid disease and retard the progress of the disease.
   b. If penicillamine does not lead to clinical benefit within 6 months, it should be stopped.
2. *When tolerated, intramuscular gold is an effective drug for achieving remission in rheumatoid arthritis, but unwanted effects limit tolerability.*
   a. Gold can be given by intramuscular or oral routes.
   b. Intramuscular gold can cause proteinuria.
3. *Methotrexate is often chosen as initial disease-modifying therapy for rheumatoid arthritis partly because of its rapid onset of action (4–6 weeks).*
   a. During methotrexate therapy, folic acid is contraindicated.
   b. The combination of sulfapyridine and 5-aminosalicylic acid formed by the reductive metabolism of sulfasalazine is more effective than either component alone.
   c. Methotrexate has relatively fewer unwanted effects compared with most other DMARDs for rheumatoid arthritis.
4. *Sulfasalazine can scavenge toxic oxygen metabolites (reactive oxygen species) produced by neutrophils, and this may contribute to its effect in rheumatoid arthritis.* Combination therapy with DMARDs should not be used in rheumatoid arthritis.
5. *A major role of corticosteroids is to bridge the gap between starting treatment and the onset of action of the disease-modifying treatments for rheumatoid arthritis.*
   a. Intra-articular injections of corticosteroids slow progression of erosions.
   b. Prolonged treatment with high doses of corticosteroids can cause adrenal atrophy.
6. *Ciclosporin is valuable when used in combination with methotrexate in very active early rheumatoid disease.* The antimalarials chloroquine and hydroxychloroquine are of little benefit in the treatment of rheumatoid arthritis.
7. *In rheumatoid arthritis, B-cells can contribute to the disease by providing co-stimulation of T-cells and secretion of pro-inflammatory cytokines.* Rituximab is an antibody directed at $CD20^+$ B-cells.
8. Case history questions

A 30-year-old woman had gradually developed painful wrists over 4 weeks; she had not experienced similar episodes of pain before. On examination, both wrists and the metacarpophalangeal joints of both hands were tender but not deformed.

a. What course of treatment would you suggest?

There was some initial symptomatic improvement, but subsequently the pain, stiffness and swelling of the hands persisted and 8 weeks later both knees became similarly affected. She saw a rheumatologist, who confirmed that she was suffering from rheumatoid arthritis and altered her treatment.

b. What treatment option would now be appropriate?

She was commenced on treatment that required the supplement folic acid to counteract folate depletion.

c. What drug treatment had been started?

ANSWERS

1. a. **False**. NSAIDs do not slow disease progression; indeed, some evidence suggests they may hasten progress of the disease.
   b. **True**. The second-line drugs take a long time to act (4–6 months) but they should be discontinued if there is no sign of improvement by that time.
2. a. **True**. Sodium aurothiomalate can be given intramuscularly and auranofin by mouth.
   b. **True**. Proteinuria occurs associated with immune-complex nephritis. Only 15% of people continue with treatment after 5–6 years because of unwanted effects.
3. a. **False**. Methotrexate prevents reduction of folic acid to dihydrofolate and tetrahydrofolate (essential for DNA production). Folic acid can be given daily to prevent gastrointestinal and haematological complications.
   b. **True**. Although 5-aminosalicylic acid is the active moiety in the treatment of inflammatory bowel disease, it is less effective than sulfasalazine in treating rheumatoid arthritis.
   c. **True**. More than 50% of people who take methotrexate for rheumatoid arthritis continue taking the drug for 5 years or more, whereas with most other disease-modifying drugs 50% of people have to cease treatment within 2 years.
4. **False**. The combination of methotrexate with ciclosporin, sulfasalazine or hydroxychloroquine has shown significant benefit; it is reserved for people with severe rheumatoid disease.
5. a. **False**. Although corticosteroids can give dramatic relief of symptoms in rheumatoid arthritis, there is no evidence that they slow progression of the disease.
   b. True. Adrenal atrophy can last for many months following treatment.
6. **False**. Chloroquine and hydroxychloroquine can cause remission of rheumatoid arthritis but do not slow the progression of joint damage.
7. **True**. Rituximab is an antibody to $CD20^+$ B-cells. It depletes the numbers of $CD20^+$ B-cells.
8. Case history answers
   a. The brief duration of the symptoms and their mild nature warrant the initial administration of an NSAID such as ibuprofen and follow-up.
   b. The persistence of the symptoms and their spread to the knees suggest that a DMARD should be started. Guidelines now advise that DMARDs should be considered for persistent inflammatory joint disease of more than 8 weeks' duration.
   c. Methotrexate is a DMARD that requires folate supplements (see answer to 3a above). Methotrexate takes 4–6 weeks for its onset of action. Methotrexate and an NSAID should be given to cover this interim period.

Disease-modifying antirheumatic drugs (DMARDs)[a]

Drug	Half-life and kinetics	Comments
Auranofin	17–25 days [M] The available kinetic data are for gold (not the drug form); 13–33% absorbed; the molecule is metabolised rapidly; metabolites eliminated in urine and faeces	Used for active progressive rheumatoid arthritis; given orally
Aurothiomalate (sodium salt)	250 days [M] The available kinetic data are for gold (not the drug form); the drug is probably metabolised and eliminated in urine and faeces	Used for active progressive rheumatoid arthritis and juvenile arthritis; given by deep intramuscular injection
Chloroquine	30–60 days [M] See Ch. 51 for details	Used for moderate active rheumatoid arthritis and juvenile arthritis; given orally; see Ch. 51 for other details
Hydroxychloroquine	18 days [R + M] Extensive oral absorption; metabolised by dealkylation and side-chain oxidation	Used for moderate active rheumatoid arthritis and juvenile arthritis; given orally
Penicillamine	1–6 h [M + F + R] Incomplete oral absorption; the thiol group forms mixed disulphides with cysteine and other thio-compounds	Used for active progressive rheumatoid arthritis; given orally
Sulfasalazine	Parent drug (3–11 h) Sulfapyridine (6–17 h) 5-Aminosalicylate (4–10 h) [M] Parent drug undergoes reductive metabolism – see Ch. 34	Used to suppress the inflammatory activity of rheumatoid arthritis; also used for ulcerative colitis; see Ch. 34 for details

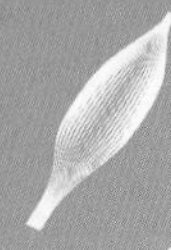

Disease-modifying antirheumatic drugs (DMARDs)

Drug	Half-life and kinetics	Comments
Drugs affecting the immune response		
Abatacept	14 days [M] Pathways of metabolism have not been defined; protein clearance	Monoclonal antibody that selectively binds to $CD80^+$ and $CD86^+$ and blocks the T-cell co-stimulation; given by intravenous infusion; not currently approved in the UK
Azathioprine	3–5 h [M] See Ch. 38 for details	Used for moderate to severe rheumatoid arthritis in people who have not responded to other DMARDs; more toxic than methotrexate and used for patients who have not responded to methotrexate; given orally; see Ch. 38 for other details
Ciclosporin	27 h [M] See Ch. 38 for details	Used for severe active rheumatoid arthritis when conventional second-line therapy is inappropriate or ineffective; given orally or intravenously; see Ch. 38 for other details
Cyclophosphamide	4–10 h [M + R] See Ch. 52 for details	Used for rheumatoid arthritis with severe systemic manifestations when response to other DMARDs has been inadequate; given orally; see Ch. 52 for other details
Leflunomide	2 weeks (the active metabolite) [B + M] Parent drug not detected in plasma; 90% is converted to an active metabolite which is eliminated by biliary excretion and further metabolism; the metabolite has a very long but highly variable half-life	Used for moderate to severe rheumatoid arthritis; more toxic than methotrexate and used for people who have not responded to methotrexate; given orally
Methotrexate	8–10 h [M] See Ch. 52 for details	Used for moderate to severe rheumatoid arthritis; given orally, subcutaneously or intramuscularly; see Ch. 52 for other details
Rituximab	3–8 days Protein clearance	Monoclonal antibody that binds to the antigen $CD20^+$ on the surface of B-lymphocyte precursors and mature B-cells; given by intravenous infusion
Cytokine inhibitors		
Should be used under specialised supervision – recombinant human proteins		
Adalimumab	12 days [M] Protein clearance	Monoclonal antibody against TNFα; used in combination with methotrexate for moderate to severe active rheumatoid arthritis when response to other DMARDs has been inadequate; given by subcutaneous injection
Anakinra	4–6 h [R]	Interleukin-1 receptor antagonist; licensed for use in the UK in combination with methotrexate for rheumatoid arthritis in people who have not responded to methotrexate alone; given by subcutaneous injection
Etanercept	5 days [M] Protein clearance	Monoclonal antibody against TNFα; used for severe, active and progressive rheumatoid arthritis in people who have failed to respond to at least two standard DMARDs; given by subcutaneous injection
Infliximab	8–10 days [M] Protein clearance	Monoclonal antibody against TNFα; used for severe, active and progressive rheumatoid arthritis in people who have failed to respond to at least two standard DMARDs; given by intravenous infusion

[a]Unlike non-steroidal anti-inflammatory drugs, they do not produce a rapid response and may require 4–6 months for a full response.
[F], faecal excretion; [M], metabolism; [R], renal excretion; TNFα, tumour necrosis factor alpha.

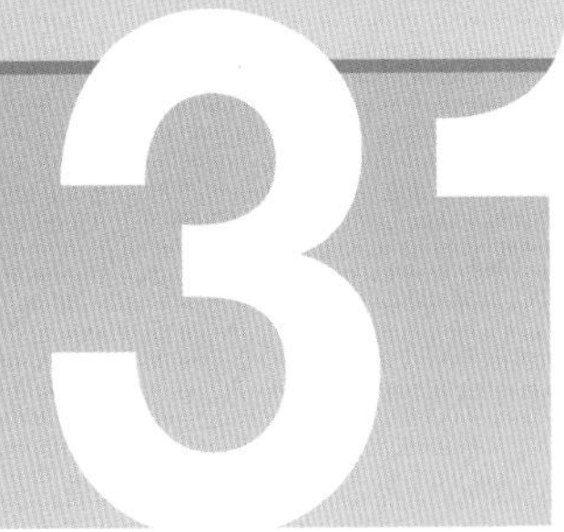

Hyperuricaemia and gout

THE PATHOPHYSIOLOGY OF GOUT

Uric acid is a relatively insoluble product of catabolism of the nucleic acid purine bases guanine and adenine (Fig. 31.1). The immediate precursors of uric acid are xanthine and hypoxanthine, which are more water-soluble. Uric acid is normally eliminated by the kidney. It is filtered at the glomerulus and then reabsorbed from the proximal tubule, and subsequently there is net secretion into the late proximal tubule.

Hyperuricaemia results from:

- *Overproduction of uric acid*: this can arise from
  - excessive cell destruction (e.g. lymphoproliferative or myeloproliferative disorders, especially during treatment for cancer, Ch. 52)
  - inherited defects that increase purine synthesis
  - high purine intake (such as meat, fish and beer)
  - obesity.
- *Reduced renal excretion of uric acid*: the majority of uric acid (>90%) is reabsorbed in the early proximal tubule, but 6–10% is secreted by an active organic acid transporter in the second part of the proximal tubule and this is the main source of urinary uric acid (Ch. 14). Renal failure and certain drugs (e.g. most diuretics, low-dose aspirin, and lactate formed from excess alcohol) can reduce the tubular secretion of uric acid. Reduced excretion accounts for at least 80% of cases of gout.

A high plasma concentration of uric acid is often asymptomatic, but when the plasma concentration exceeds 0.42 mmol L^{-1} (normal about 0.25 mmol L^{-1}) monosodium urate crystals can be deposited in tissues, forming a tophus (a deposit of urate crystals). When monosodium urate crystals are shed from a tophus in the synovial membrane or cartilage of a joint, they produce an extremely painful acute arthritis that presents with the clinical syndrome of gout. In brief, the crystals stimulate phagocytic cells within the synovium by Toll-like receptor signalling. Uric acid crystals also provide a surface on which complement C5 is cleaved, with formation of complement membrane attack complex. In response, phagocytic cells then release mediators such as cytokines, prostaglandins and leukotrienes. The phagocytes also trigger mast cells and activate endothelial cells, leading to the release of other inflammatory mediators such as histamine, tumour necrosis factor alpha (TNFα) and various chemokines (Ch. 30). The activated endothelial cells attract further phagocytic cells, principally neutrophil leucocytes and monocytes. These cells internalise the uric acid crystals, and release proteolytic and lysosomal enzymes that enhance tissue inflammation and destroy cartilage and damage the joint. Attacks of gout are self-limiting, probably in part due to coating of the uric acid crystals with protein, which reduces their irritant properties.

Gout in younger people usually affects a single joint, with repeated acute attacks if the underlying cause is not treated. In the elderly, a chronic arthritis affecting multiple joints can occur. The diagnosis of gout is confirmed by the finding of monosodium urate crystals in the affected joint. With persistent hyperuricaemia, chronic urate deposits are sometimes found in tendon sheaths and soft tissues. Excess uric acid can also be deposited in the interstitium of the kidney or form stones in the renal calyces, both of which can produce progressive renal damage.

There are two components of drug treatment:

- treatment of an acute attack of gout
- reduction of plasma uric acid concentration for prophylaxis against recurrent attacks of gout or to prevent kidney damage.

DRUGS FOR THE TREATMENT OF GOUT AND PREVENTION OF HYPERURICAEMIA

Colchicine

Mechanism of action

Colchicine interferes with several steps in the inflammatory cascade, particularly inhibiting recruitment and actions of neutrophil leucocytes in the gouty joint. It reduces the production of TNFα by macrophages and downregulates TNFα receptors on macrophages and endothelial cells. This may inhibit priming of neutrophil leucocytes before they are activated by monosodium urate crystals. Colchicine inhibits the production of chemotaxins, such as leukotriene B_4 and interleukin-8, which attract leucocytes into inflamed tissue. Colchicine also disrupts the assembly of microtubules in neutrophil leucocytes, by forming a complex with tubulin in the cell. This impairs the adhesion of neutrophils to endothelial cells, which reduces their recruitment into the inflamed joint, and also impairs phagocytosis of crystals if the neutrophil does enter the joint. In addition, if crystals

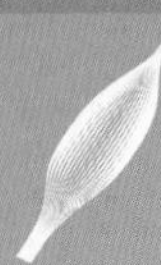

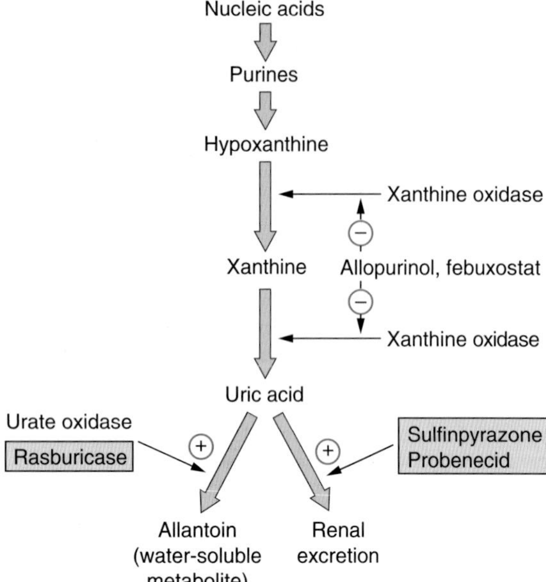

Fig. 31.1 **The pathway for production of uric acid and the sites of action of some of the drugs used in treatment.**

are phagocytosed into the neutrophil, colchicine inhibits the subsequent release of enzymes and free radicals that damage the joint. All of these actions give colchicine a specific anti-inflammatory effect in the gouty joint; it is ineffective in other forms of inflammatory arthritis.

Pharmacokinetics

Colchicine is absorbed from the gut. It is partially eliminated by hepatic metabolism and partially excreted unchanged in the urine and bile. The initial half-life of colchicine is very short, at less than 1 h, but enterohepatic circulation prolongs its action. It is usually given every 8–12 h until symptomatic relief is achieved or unwanted effects occur. Pain relief usually begins after about 18 h and is maximal by 48 h.

Unwanted effects

Colchicine has a low therapeutic index. Unwanted effects include:

- Gut toxicity caused by inhibition of mucosal cell division, which produces abdominal pain, nausea, vomiting and diarrhoea; these effects are common and are often dose-limiting
- Rashes
- Renal and hepatic damage.

Xanthine oxidase inhibitors

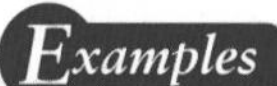

allopurinol, febuxostat

Mechanism of action

Allopurinol is an analogue of hypoxanthine, which is an intermediate in the pathway that generates uric acid. Both allopurinol and its major metabolite competitively inhibit the enzyme xanthine oxidase for which hypoxanthine is the natural substrate, thereby reducing uric acid formation (Fig. 31.1). Febuxostat is a non-purine selective xanthine oxidase inhibitor that inhibits the oxidised and reduced forms of xanthine oxidase. Although plasma xanthine and hypoxanthine concentrations increase, these substances do not crystallise, because of their greater water solubility. Their concentrations remain well below saturation levels even if the concentration of uric acid is reduced to 0.1 mmol L^{-1}. Xanthine and hypoxanthine are reincorporated into the purine synthetic cycle, and this decreases the need for de novo purine formation.

Pharmacokinetics

Allopurinol is well absorbed from the gut and converted in the liver to an active metabolite, oxipurinol (alloxanthine). Both compounds are excreted by the kidney. The half-life of oxipurinol is long (10–40 h), due to tubular reabsorption in the kidney. Febuxostat is well absorbed from the gut and partially metabolised and partially excreted by the kidney. It has a very variable half-life (1–15 h).

Unwanted effects

- Gastrointestinal upset
- There is an increased risk of acute gout during the first few weeks of treatment; this may be caused by fluctuations in plasma uric acid, possibly through uric acid release from tissue deposits
- Allergic reactions with allopurinol, especially rashes, which can be particularly serious in people with renal impairment
- Drug interactions: allopurinol and febuxostat inhibit the metabolism of the cytotoxic drugs mercaptopurine and azathioprine (Ch. 52) because these are also metabolised by xanthine oxidase.

Rasburicase

Mechanism of action

Rasburicase is a recombinant version of the enzyme urate oxidase which catalyses the oxidation of uric acid to a soluble metabolite, allantoin. This enzyme is present in mammals other than humans; the recombinant version is produced by a genetically modified fungal strain. Rasburicase is used for prophylaxis of hyperuricaemia during treatment of malignancies with chemotherapy.

Pharmacokinetics

Rasburicase is given intravenously. It is metabolised by peptide hydrolysis in plasma, and has a long half-life (22 h).

Unwanted effects

- Fever
- Nausea, vomiting, diarrhoea
- Anaphylaxis; rasburicase induces antibody responses in about 10% of those treated, although allergic reactions are rare

- Rashes
- Haemolysis from the production of hydrogen peroxide as a by-product of the formation of allantoin.

Uricosuric agents

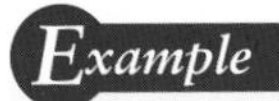

sulfinpyrazone

Mechanism of action

Sulfinpyrazone competitively inhibits the reabsorption of uric acid in the proximal tubule, therefore increasing urine urate concentrations and reducing plasma levels. There is a risk of precipitation of uric acid crystals in the kidney, particularly during the early stages of treatment, which can be prevented by maintaining a high fluid intake and alkaline urine (using potassium citrate or sodium bicarbonate) and carefully titrating the dose. Aspirin and other salicylates should not be given with uricosuric drugs, because low doses of salicylates inhibit tubular uric acid secretion. Probenecid used to be used as a uricosuric agent, but is now only available on a 'named patient' basis in the UK for specific situations.

Pharmacokinetics

Sulfinpyrazone is well absorbed from the gut. It is eliminated partly by metabolism and partly by renal excretion, and has a short half-life of 4–5 h.

Unwanted effects

- Gastrointestinal upset
- Renal uric acid deposition; deterioration of renal function can occur, especially if there is pre-existing impairment
- Allergic rashes.

TREATMENT OF GOUT

Acute gout

Efforts should always be made to identify and remove precipitating causes, particularly enquiring about alcohol intake and reviewing concurrent drug therapy. For acute attacks, non-steroidal anti-inflammatory drugs (NSAIDs; Ch. 29) are the treatment of choice, especially indometacin. Aspirin should be avoided because at low doses it can inhibit renal excretion of uric acid and increase plasma urate concentration. Cyclo-oxygenase 2 (COX-2)-selective anti-inflammatory drugs are as effective as classic NSAIDs (Ch. 29). Colchicine is usually reserved for people who are intolerant of NSAIDs, or who have a contraindication to their use. Intra-articular injection of corticosteroid can be very effective if other treatments are contraindicated. Oral corticosteroids, for example prednisolone (Ch. 44), are reserved for resistant episodes of gout. The dose should be reduced gradually over 8 days to minimise the risk of a rebound flare of symptoms.

Prevention of gout attacks

Allopurinol is given for prophylaxis against recurrent attacks of acute gout, for chronic tophus formation in the tissues, or for the prevention of uric acid-induced renal damage. It is also given prophylactically before cytotoxic chemotherapy, when tissue breakdown releases purines, which generate large amounts of uric acid. To prevent gout, the serum uric acid concentration should be reduced to less than 0.36 mmol L^{-1}, although it may be necessary to go below 0.30 mmol L^{-1} to reabsorb gouty tophi. Allopurinol should not be used during an acute attack of gout since it can prolong the attack. To reduce the risk of provoking an attack when allopurinol is started in someone with hyperuricaemia, a low dosage of an NSAID or colchicine should be given during the first 3 months of treatment. Febuxostat or sulfinpyrazone are reserved for people who do not tolerate allopurinol. Sulphinpyrazone is also used in combination with allopurinol for resistant hyperuricaemia. Sulfinpyrazone should be avoided if there is renal impairment, because of the risk of further renal damage. Low-dose NSAIDs or colchicine are sometimes used long term to prevent gout, although good data on their efficacy are lacking.

Prophylactic treatment should usually be life-long, since recurrence of gout or tophi frequently occurs if treatment is stopped. Short-term prophylaxis is possible when allopurinol is used during cytotoxic chemotherapy. Rasburicase is used when intravenous prophylaxis is required for chemotherapy.

FURTHER READING

Keith MP, Gilliland WR (2007) Update in the management of gout. *Am J Med* 120, 221–224

Stamp LK, O'Donnell JL, Chapman PT (2007) Emerging therapies in the long-term management of hyperuricaemia and gout. *Int Med J* 37, 258–266

Sundy JS, Hershfield MS (2007) Uricase and other novel agents for the management of patients with treatment-failure gout. *Curr Rheumatol Rep* 9, 258–264

Underwood M (2006) Diagnosis and management of gout. *BMJ* 332, 1315–1319

SELF-ASSESSMENT

1. You are investigating the pathophysiology of gout and drugs used in its treatment. Choose the one **most appropriate** statement from the choices A–E.

   A. Sodium urate is more water-soluble than its precursor hypoxanthine.
   B. The cause of joint pain in gout is the high plasma level of urate.
   C. Allopurinol enhances the renal secretion of uric acid.

D. Colchicine is an anti-inflammatory agent that inhibits the release of proteinases that cause joint damage from neutrophils.
E. Aspirin is safe to use in acute attacks of gout to reduce the pain and inflammation.

2. Case history questions

A 56-year-old man awoke in the night with sudden severe pain in his first metatarsophalangeal joint which lasted for a week. Over the next few months, he had similar acute episodes of pain in his ankles and knees, as well as his big toe. He had hypertension but no other vascular disease. The GP suspected gout and referred him to a specialist.

a. What treatment should the GP institute for the acute attacks, prior to the specialist diagnosis?
b. What test could the rheumatologist do to confirm the suspected diagnosis?

The diagnosis of gout was confirmed.

c. What was the cause of his gout?
d. Which drugs would you prescribe and what are the mechanisms by which the drugs act for acute attacks?
e. What would you prescribe for prophylaxis to reduce recurrent attacks and how does this agent act?
f. The chosen treatment was only partially effective; what additional treatment could you prescribe?
g. What might be the consequences of inadequate treatment of this man?

ANSWERS

1. Answer **D**.
   A. Hypoxanthine is more water-soluble than urate; this is the rationale for the use of allopurinol.
   B. It is the sodium urate in the joint that causes the symptoms; plasma uric acid is simply a reflection of the body load.
   C. Drugs like probenecid, not allopurinol, enhance the renal secretion of urate. Allopurinol prevents uric acid formation.
   D. This is one of the anti-inflammatory mechanisms of colchicine.
   E. Aspirin can inhibit the renal secretion of urate, exacerbating the gout.
2. Case history answers
   a. The treatment of choice for an acute attack is an NSAID but not aspirin. Indometacin is often used and is effective within 2 days. If an individual cannot take an NSAID, colchicine or glucocorticoids can be used, but both have significant unwanted effects. Salicylates should be avoided as at low doses they reduce uric acid excretion, although at high doses they are uricosuric.
   b. Plasma uric acid will be raised. An arthrocentesis sample will show sodium urate crystals. Infection should be excluded in an acutely inflamed joint.
   c. Sodium urate crystals in the joint space. People who develop gout have had hyperuricaemia for years. The sodium salt of uric acid is a relatively insoluble metabolic product of purine metabolism. Sardines, liver and kidney are rich in purines, and dietary purines can contribute to gout in some people. In most people, hyperuricaemia is caused by impaired renal clearance of uric acid. Overproduction of uric acid as a result of excessive alcohol consumption can also contribute. Joint trauma, lead toxicity and cool temperatures can decrease uric acid solubility.
   d. NSAIDs are drugs of choice in acute attacks (see a).
   e. Hyperuricaemia is treated after resolution of the acute attack. Allopurinol reduces plasma uric acid by inhibiting xanthine oxidase. This increases concentrations of hypoxanthine and xanthine, which are more water-soluble. People who overproduce uric acid are best treated with allopurinol.
   f. Those that have low renal excretion of uric acid may be treated with a uricosuric drug (probenecid, sulfinpyrazone). Both inhibit the reabsorption of uric acid in the proximal convoluted tubule.
   g. Untreated gout can lead to formation of kidney stones. A significant number of people with gout will have hypertension.

Drugs used for gout and hyperuricaemia

Drug	Half-life (h) and kinetics	Comments
Allopurinol	0.5–2 [M + R] High oral bioavailability; eliminated by metabolism to oxipurinol and unchanged in urine (about 10%); oxipurinol is biologically active and, although less potent than allopurinol, it has a longer half-life (10–40 h) and accumulates on repeated dosage	Used for prophylaxis of gout and of hyperuricaemia associated with cancer chemotherapy; given orally
Colchicine	0.2–1(?) [M + R] Good oral absorption; rapidly eliminated from plasma but the reported half-life may reflect the distribution phase, because the half-life in leucocytes is about 60 h	Used for acute gout and short-term prophylaxis during initial therapy with other drugs; given orally
Febuxostat	1–15 [M + R] Eliminated by glucuronide conjugation and renal excretion (45–50%)	Non-purine xanthine oxidase inhibitor; given orally
Probenecid	4–17 [M + R] Complete oral bioavailability; eliminated by hepatic oxidation, glucuronic acid conjugation and by renal excretion (5–10%); the oxidised metabolites are uricosuric	Used to prevent nephrotoxicity associated with the use of the antiretroviral drug cidofovir; given orally
Rasburicase	22 (data for children) [M] Recombinant peptide and therefore eliminated by metabolism, but pathways have not been defined	Used for the hyperuricaemia arising during the initial chemotherapy of haematological malignancy; a recombinant form of fungal urate oxidase which converts urate to allantoin, which is inactive and soluble; given intravenously
Sulfinpyrazone	4–5 [M] Good oral absorption; metabolised at the SO group to an inactive sulphone (SO_2) and a sulphide (S) analogue (which inhibits platelet aggregation); also metabolised by oxidation and formation of a C-glucuronide (a rare reaction)	Used for gout prophylaxis and hyperuricaemia; given orally

[M], metabolism; [R], renal excretion.

7

The gastrointestinal system

32 Nausea and vomiting

NAUSEA AND VOMITING

Nausea, retching and vomiting (emesis) are part of the body's defence against ingested toxins. Vomiting is a reflex that is integrated by a loose neuronal network known as the 'emetic centre' or 'vomiting centre' in the medulla oblongata of the brainstem. The exact location of the vomiting centre is unclear. It is composed of a series of nuclei in the nucleus tractus solitarius and the dorsal motor nucleus of the vagus. Efferent connections from the vomiting centre include the vagus and phrenic nerves. When stimulated, these nerves relax the fundus and body of the stomach and the lower oesophageal sphincter, and retrograde giant contractions occur in the small intestine. Diaphragmatic and abdominal muscle contractions compress the stomach, and together these factors produce vomiting.

The afferent input to the vomiting centre comes from several sources (Fig. 32.1):

- Abdominal and cardiac vagal afferents, activated by mechano- or chemosensory receptors; some drugs induce vomiting by an effect on gastric chemosensory receptors, such as receptors for acetylcholine, dopamine, serotonin and neurokinins.
- The area postrema in the floor of the 4th ventricle is the location of the chemoreceptor trigger zone (CTZ). This lies outside the blood–brain barrier and responds to stimuli from the cerebrospinal fluid and the systemic circulation. The CTZ has many receptors for neurotransmitters and hormones and has numerous afferent and efferent connections with the underlying nucleus tractus solitarius.
- The vestibular nuclei, which is involved in the emetic response to motion.
- Other brainstem structures, such as the amygdala.
- Higher centres of the cortex and intracranial pressure receptors.

Several neurotransmitter receptors are involved in activation of the vomiting centre and CTZ, including those for dopamine (D_2), serotonin ($5HT_3$ and $5HT_4$), acetylcholine (muscarinic), histamine (H_1) and substance P (neurokinin 1 [NK_1]). There is some evidence that receptors for glutamate (N-methyl-D-aspartate [NMDA]) may also be involved (Fig. 32.1). The roles of these multiple receptors in the triggering of nausea and vomiting are complex. For example, $5HT_3$ receptor antagonists will provide protection against nausea and vomiting induced by cytotoxic drugs and radiation but not by motion or apomorphine. Vomiting can result from the summation of several sub-emetic stimuli, for example in the genesis of postoperative nausea and vomiting.

Many drugs produce vomiting by stimulating the CTZ and they do not have to cross the blood–brain barrier for this action (Box 32.1).

ANTIEMETIC AGENTS

Antihistamines

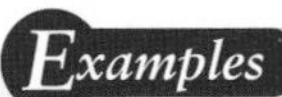

cyclizine, promethazine

Mechanism of action and clinical use

Antihistamines used for the prevention and treatment of vomiting block histamine H_1 receptors (Ch. 39), and many also have antimuscarinic effects. Promethazine also blocks some 5HT receptor subtypes. They are effective against most causes of vomiting, but, apart from the use of cyclizine for drug-induced vomiting, they are rarely treatments of choice. Promethazine is used to treat vomiting in pregnancy since it appears to be free from teratogenic effects.

Pharmacokinetics

These drugs are well absorbed orally; both promethazine and cyclizine can also be given by intramuscular or intravenous injection. After oral dosing, promethazine undergoes extensive first-pass metabolism. They are eliminated by hepatic metabolism; the half-life of promethazine is 7–14 h, while that of cyclizine is longer, at 20 h.

Unwanted effects

- Sedation, particularly with promethazine, and headache
- Antimuscarinic effects (Ch. 4), especially dry mouth, urinary retention and blurred vision.

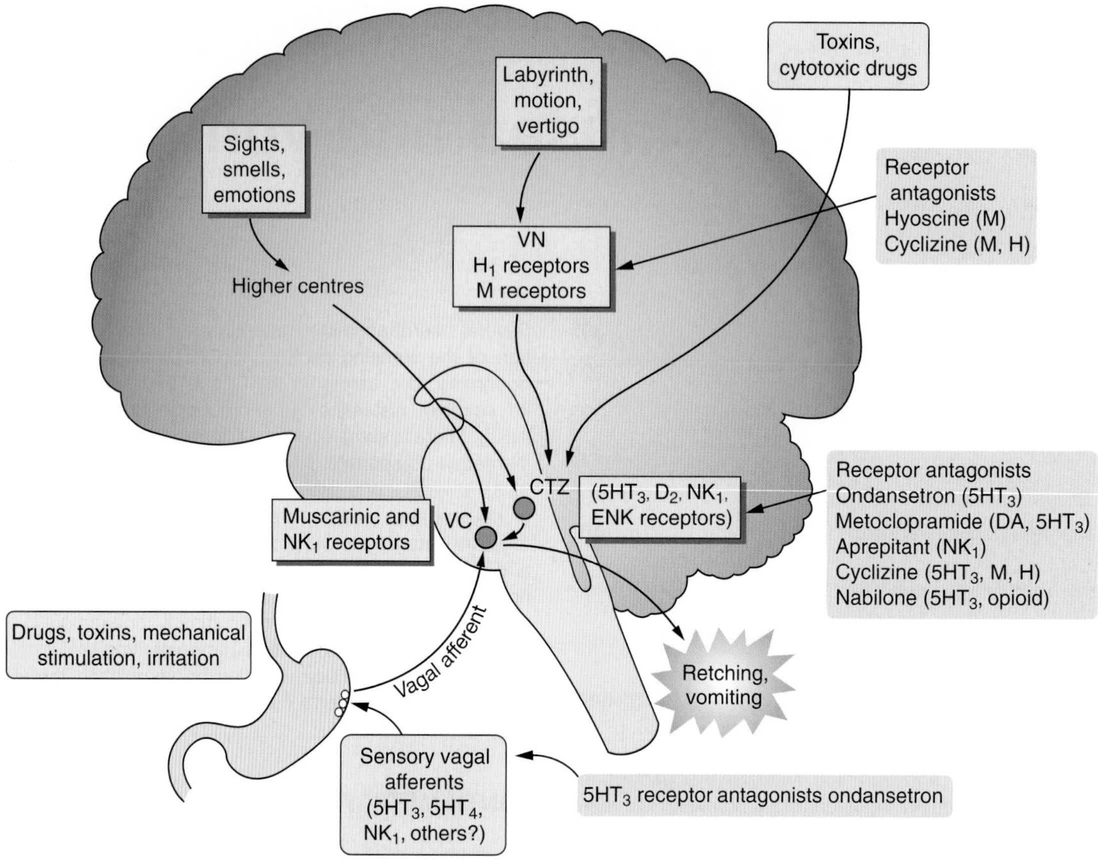

Fig. 32.1 **Some of the neuronal pathways and receptors involved in the control of nausea and vomiting.** The pathways and neurotransmitter receptors involved in nausea and vomiting are complex and only those underpinning the mechanisms of action of the antiemetic drugs are shown. The chemoreceptor trigger zone (CTZ) has neuronal connections to the vomiting centre (VC), which is a collection of nuclei, including the dorsal motor nucleus of the vagus and the nucleus tractus solitarius. $5HT_3$, 5-hydroxytryptamine type 3 receptor; DA, dopamine receptor; ENK, enkephalin (opioid) receptor; H_1, histamine type 1 receptor; M, muscarinic receptor (possibly M_2); NK_1, neurokinin 1 receptor; VN, vestibular nuclei. Other mediators such as glutamate may also be involved.

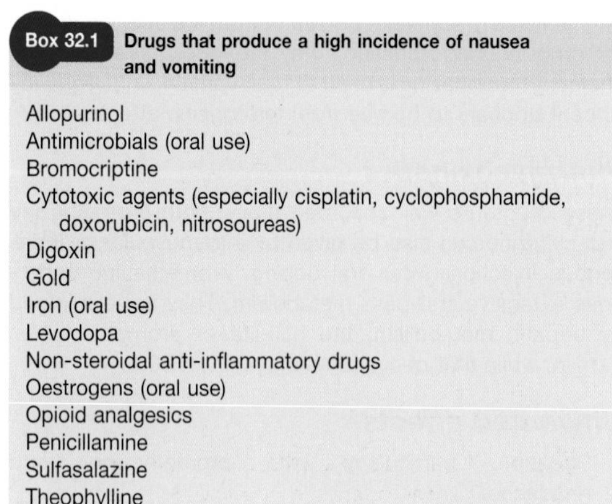

Box 32.1 Drugs that produce a high incidence of nausea and vomiting

Allopurinol
Antimicrobials (oral use)
Bromocriptine
Cytotoxic agents (especially cisplatin, cyclophosphamide, doxorubicin, nitrosoureas)
Digoxin
Gold
Iron (oral use)
Levodopa
Non-steroidal anti-inflammatory drugs
Oestrogens (oral use)
Opioid analgesics
Penicillamine
Sulfasalazine
Theophylline

Antimuscarinic agents

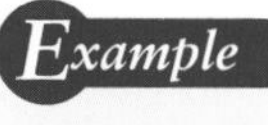

hyoscine

Mechanism of action and clinical use

Muscarinic receptors are involved in the visceral afferent input from the gut to the vomiting centre and in the tract that the VIII cranial nerve takes from the labyrinth to the CTZ via the vestibular nucleus. Hyoscine (known as scopolamine in the USA) is used for the treatment of motion sickness and postoperative vomiting. Some antihistamines such as promethazine and cyclizine (see above), and dopamine receptor antagonists such as prochlorperazine (see below), also have antimuscarinic activity.

Pharmacokinetics

Hyoscine is available for oral, parenteral or transdermal use. Oral absorption is good. The adhesive patch for transdermal delivery can be placed behind the ear and delivers a therapeutic dose for 72 h. Hyoscine is metabolised in the liver and has a half-life of 8 h.

Unwanted effects

- Typical antimuscarinic actions such as dry mouth, urinary retention and blurred vision (Ch. 4)
- Sedation.

Dopamine receptor antagonists

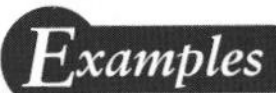

domperidone, metoclopramide, prochlorperazine

Mechanism of action and clinical use

Domperidone, metoclopramide and the antipsychotic drugs block dopamine D_2 receptors and inhibit dopaminergic stimulation of the CTZ (Fig. 32.1).

Their ability to block both dopamine muscarinic receptors also contributes to their antiemetic effects. Antiemetic doses of antipsychotic drugs are generally less than one-third of those used to treat psychoses. The pharmacology of the antipsychotic drugs is discussed in Chapter 21.

Domperidone acts solely by dopamine receptor blockade. Metoclopramide is a dopamine antagonist at usual oral doses, but it also acts as a $5HT_3$ receptor antagonist at higher doses. This enhanced efficacy is utilised by intravenous administration of high doses of metoclopramide to treat the vomiting induced by cytotoxic agents such as cisplatin.

Metoclopramide also has prokinetic actions on the gut that reduce the risk of nausea and vomiting. These include increased tone of the gastro-oesophageal sphincter and enhanced gastric emptying and small intestinal motility. The origin of these effects may be agonist activity at the $5HT_4$ receptor subtype in the enteric nervous system, which indirectly leads to cholinergic stimulation.

Dopamine receptor antagonists are mainly used to reduce vomiting induced by drugs and surgery. Pure dopamine receptor antagonists are ineffective in motion sickness. Antipsychotic drugs, such as prochlorperazine, can also be used to treat vestibular disorders and motion sickness, probably as a result of their antimuscarinic activity.

Pharmacokinetics

Metoclopramide and domperidone are well absorbed orally, but have limited bioavailability due to extensive first-pass metabolism in the liver. Metoclopramide is also available for intravenous or intramuscular use, while domperidone can also be given rectally by suppository. They are eliminated mainly by metabolism in the liver; metoclopramide has a short half-life (3–5 h) and domperidone has a longer half-life (12–16 h). Unlike metoclopramide, domperidone only crosses the blood–brain barrier to a limited extent.

Unwanted effects

Central nervous system (CNS) unwanted effects are produced by metoclopramide and the antipsychotics, but to a lesser extent by domperidone (as a result of lower CNS penetration).

- Acute and chronic extrapyramidal effects from dopamine receptor blockade in the basal ganglia can lead to acute dystonias (especially in children and young adults), akathisia and a parkinsonian-like syndrome. Tardive dyskinesias can be a problem with prolonged use (see also Ch. 24).
- Galactorrhoea and amenorrhoea caused by hyperprolactinaemia from pituitary dopamine receptor blockade.

$5HT_3$ receptor antagonists

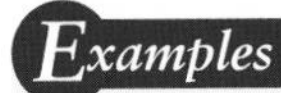

granisetron, ondansetron

Mechanism of action and clinical use

The $5HT_3$ receptor antagonists block the $5HT_3$ receptors in the CTZ and in the gut (Fig. 32.1). They are particularly effective against the acute vomiting induced by highly emetogenic chemotherapeutic agents used for treating cancer (e.g. cisplatin; Ch. 52) and for postoperative vomiting that is resistant to other agents. They are also used when the consequences of vomiting could be particularly deleterious, for example after eye surgery.

Pharmacokinetics

Oral absorption of ondansetron is rapid, and it can also be given by intravenous or intramuscular injection or by rectal suppository. It undergoes partial first-pass metabolism, and is eliminated by metabolism in the liver with a short half-life of 3 h. Granisetron has a similar profile, and is available for oral or intravenous use.

Unwanted effects

- Headache is common
- Constipation, probably caused by $5HT_3$ receptor blockade in the gut
- Flushing.

Neurokinin receptor antagonists

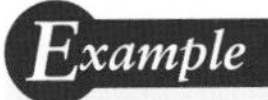

aprepitant

Mechanism of action

Aprepitant blocks CNS NK_1 receptors. It augments the effects of $5HT_3$ receptor antagonists and corticosteroids in preventing the acute and delayed emetic response to the cancer chemotherapeutic agent cisplatin.

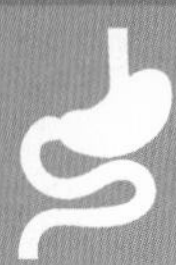

Pharmacokinetics

Aprepitant is well absorbed from the gut. It is extensively metabolised in the liver by the CYP3A4 isoenzyme and has a long half-life (9–13 h).

Unwanted effects

- Fatigue, dizziness, headache, hiccups.
- Anorexia, abdominal pain, diarrhoea.
- Drug interactions: aprepitant is an inhibitor of the liver enzyme CYP3A4, and an inducer of CYP2C9. It may decrease the clinical effect of warfarin.

Cannabinoids

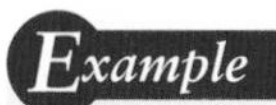

nabilone

Mechanism of action and clinical use

Nabilone, a synthetic derivative of tetrahydrocannabinol (an active substance in cannabis; Ch. 54), is effective in combating vomiting induced by cytotoxic drugs, providing it is given before chemotherapy is started. The mechanism is uncertain, but it may involve inhibition of cortical activity and anxiolysis; cannabinoid receptors are found in several areas of the CNS. Nabilone also inhibits $5HT_3$ receptors; paradoxically, its antiemetic effects can also be inhibited by the opioid receptor antagonist naloxone, which suggests a role for opioid-related mechanisms.

Pharmacokinetics

Nabilone is absorbed from the gut. It is extensively metabolised in the liver and has a short half-life (2 h); some of its metabolites have long half-lives and may contribute to the activity.

Unwanted effects

- Sedation, vertigo, ataxia, sleep disturbance.
- Dry mouth.
- Dysphoric reactions with hallucinations and disorientation are most disturbing to older people. These may be reduced by concurrent use of prochlorperazine (see above).

Corticosteroids

Dexamethasone and methylprednisolone are weak antiemetics. However, they produce additive effects when given with high-dose metoclopramide or with a $5HT_3$ receptor antagonist such as ondansetron. High doses of dexamethasone can be given intravenously before cancer chemotherapy, with subsequent oral doses to prevent delayed emesis. The mechanism of action is unknown but may involve reduction of prostaglandin synthesis or release of endorphins. The pharmacology of corticosteroids is discussed in Chapter 44.

Benzodiazepines

Benzodiazepines, such as lorazepam, have no intrinsic antiemetic activity. They are given orally or intravenously to sedate and produce amnesia before cancer chemotherapy. They are especially useful if there has previously been vomiting with a cytotoxic treatment, since anticipatory nausea and vomiting are then common with subsequent courses. Benzodiazepines are discussed in Chapter 20.

MANAGEMENT OF NAUSEA AND VOMITING

Antiemetics are used in a number of situations where nausea and vomiting can be problematic. Some specific clinical uses are considered in more detail (Table 32.1).

Drug-induced vomiting

It is sometimes necessary to use drugs that carry a high risk of inducing nausea and vomiting (Box 32.1). Cyclizine, prochlorperazine and metoclopramide are often effective for prevention of opioid-induced vomiting.

More problematic are the highly emetogenic agents used for cancer treatment. Cancer chemotherapy is accompanied by an increase in serotonin release in the gut and the brainstem. Serotonin in the gut probably stimulates vomiting via vagal afferent nerve fibres. For treatments that carry a low risk of vomiting, routine prophylaxis is not needed. For moderately emetogenic treatments, a corticosteroid (such as dexamethasone) or domperidone is usually recommended. For highly emetogenic chemotherapy, a $5HT_3$ receptor antagonist such as ondansetron combined with dexamethasone and aprepitant can achieve control in up to 80% of cases. Prochlorperazine, domperidone and

Table 32.1 Common indications for various antiemetic agents

Cause of vomiting	Treatment
Motion sickness	Hyoscine, cyclizine, promethazine
Postoperative vomiting	Hyoscine, metoclopramide, domperidone, prochlorperazine, ondansetron (reserved for resistant vomiting)
Drug-induced vomiting	Prochlorperazine, metoclopramide, cyclizine (particularly for opioid-induced vomiting)
Cytotoxic drug-induced vomiting	Prochlorperazine, metoclopramide, nabilone, ondansetron, aprepitant. Adjunctive treatment, e.g. dexamethasone, benzodiazepines
Pregnancy-induced vomiting	Promethazine, metoclopramide, pyridoxine

nabilone have been used when there is intolerance of $5HT_3$ receptor antagonists or corticosteroids.

Delayed emesis, occurring at least 16 h after the chemotherapy, may be mediated by CNS $5HT_3$ and NK_1 receptors. Dexamethasone combined with aprepitant is recommended for control of delayed emesis, with a $5HT_3$ receptor antagonist being an alternative to aprepitant. Aprepitant is effective for resistant vomiting with cisplatin, given in combination with a $5HT_3$ receptor antagonist and dexamethasone for 3 days and starting immediately before the chemotherapy.

Anticipatory vomiting prior to cycles of chemotherapy usually occurs if previous cycles have been accompanied by nausea and vomiting. It is most effectively prevented by including a benzodiazepine such as lorazepam with the chemotherapy regimen from the start of treatment, to produce amnesia.

Postoperative vomiting

Postoperative nausea and vomiting frequently occur in the first 24 h after anaesthesia and surgery. They are more common in women, in non-smokers and after a previous episode of postoperative nausea and vomiting. They are provoked by inhalational rather than intravenous anaesthesia, more often by abdominal, ophthalmic or ear, nose and throat procedures, by the use of opioid analgesics, and by postoperative pain, hypotension and gastric stasis.

Dexamethasone, prochlorperazine, hyoscine (using a transdermal patch), promethazine and haloperidol are all effective for preventing postoperative vomiting. Antihistamines may be effective in emesis associated with surgery to the middle ear; in contrast, metoclopramide is less effective, and nabilone is ineffective. If vomiting is severe, or if it carries high risk for the individual (e.g. after eye surgery), then a $5HT_3$ receptor antagonist such as ondansetron is particularly effective.

Motion sickness

Hyoscine and cyclizine are often used to treat motion sickness, with promethazine as an alternative. Antimuscarinic unwanted effects or drowsiness may be troublesome with each of these agents.

Vomiting in pregnancy

There is a natural desire to avoid drugs whenever possible if vomiting arises in pregnancy. Psychotherapeutic counselling or hypnotism may be considered, since psychological abnormalities are a frequent trigger. If drugs are necessary, promethazine is the treatment of choice, with metoclopramide as an alternative. Some clinicians advocate a trial of high doses of pyridoxine (vitamin B_6) or of ground ginger in this situation. A Cochrane review in 2006 of the data for vitamin B_6 concluded that there had been few trials and that there was not enough evidence to detect clinical benefits of vitamin B_6 supplementation in pregnancy. Published reviews of clinical trials on the use of ginger have reported evidence of efficacy. There are limited reproductive toxicology data on these substances.

Box 32.2 Causes of vertigo

Ménière's disease
Benign positional vertigo
Migraine
Vestibular neuronitis
Multiple sclerosis
Brainstem ischaemia
Temporal lobe epilepsy
Cerebellopontine angle tumours

VERTIGO

Vertigo is a hallucination of motion, usually perceived as spinning, which is generated in the vestibular system of the inner ear. It is frequently accompanied by nausea and vomiting. There are several causes of vertigo (Box 32.2). The mechanisms of vertigo are poorly understood. Treatment is empirical and involves modulation of neurotransmitters and receptors involved in the vestibular sensory pathway to the oculomotor nucleus. The neurochemistry of vertigo overlaps with that of vomiting, and involves:

- glutamate: excitatory, acting through NMDA receptors on both peripheral and central neurons
- acetylcholine: excitatory, acting through muscarinic M_2 receptors on peripheral and central neurons
- gamma-aminobutyric acid (GABA): inhibitory, acting through $GABA_A$ and $GABA_B$ receptors on central neurons
- histamine: excitatory, acting through H_1 and H_2 receptors on central neurons
- noradrenaline: involved in central modulation of vestibular sensory transmission
- dopamine: excitatory at central neurons.

Ménière's disease is one of the causes of vertigo for which the pathogenesis is better understood. It usually presents with episodic vertigo and associated signs of vagal overactivity such as pallor, sweating, nausea and vomiting. Tinnitus and, later, sensorineural deafness can be troublesome. The basic defect is an excess of endolymph in the membranous labyrinth of the middle ear. There may be a genetic predisposition, while anatomical abnormalities in the middle ear and various immunological, vascular or viral precipitating insults may be involved.

DRUGS FOR TREATMENT OF VERTIGO

- **Antihistamines** (histamine H_1 receptor blockers), e.g. cyclizine, promethazine. These are the most widely used drugs for vertigo.
- **Antimuscarinic agents**. Vestibular suppression can be achieved with hyoscine, and the mechanism of action may be similar to that involved in the treatment of motion sickness.
- **Benzodiazepines**. The use of these agents for short periods may help for severe attacks of vertigo.
- **Cimetidine**. This drug probably produces symptom relief by blockade of histamine H_2 receptors in the CNS (Ch. 33).

- **Histamine receptor agonists.** The use of betahistine to treat Ménière's disease illustrates a paradox that both histaminergic and antihistaminic drugs can be effective in this condition. Betahistine is an analogue of L-histidine, the metabolic precursor of histamine. It is a partial agonist at postsynaptic histamine H_1 receptors and an antagonist at presynaptic H_3 receptors, an action that facilitates central histaminergic neurotransmission. Betahistine also increases blood flow to the inner ear. It is metabolised to an active derivative in the liver, which has a half-life of 5 h. The main unwanted effects are headache and nausea.
- **Dopamine receptor antagonists.** Several antipsychotic drugs such as prochlorperazine are used in vertigo, mainly to treat the associated nausea. Their use for treatment of dizziness in the elderly is not recommended, because of the risk of extrapyramidal effects.

MANAGEMENT OF VERTIGO

Many forms of vertigo are brief and self-limiting. Acute vertigo, such as that caused by vestibular neuronitis, is often treated with antiemetic agents until vestibular compensation occurs, which is usually encouraged by maintaining activity. The antiemetic drug should usually be withdrawn as soon as the acute symptoms subside.

Benign paroxysmal positional vertigo responds poorly to drugs and is most effectively treated by vestibular exercises. Drug therapy should be avoided if possible, since it can blunt the effectiveness of the exercises.

Ménière's disease is often treated initially with sedative antiemetic drugs such as promethazine, cinnarizine or prochlorperazine. Modification of the endolymph production in the inner ear with diuretics such as furosemide or hydrochlorothiazide (Ch. 14) is often attempted for persistent symptoms, although clear evidence of efficacy is lacking. Betahistine is often co-prescribed with a diuretic. For refractory symptoms, the vestibular apparatus can be ablated, for example using local delivery of gentamicin (Ch. 51), which is toxic to the inner ear. Surgical treatment is also used for refractory disease.

Several drugs can cause dizziness or a sensation similar to vertigo. Examples include antihypertensive agents, vasodilators and antiparkinsonian agents. A more serious degree of vestibular damage can be produced by aminoglycosides such as gentamicin (Ch. 51) and high doses of loop diuretics such as furosemide (Ch. 14). This type of vestibular toxicity can be reversible, but is often permanent.

FURTHER READING

Baloh RW (2003) Vestibular neuritis. *N Engl J Med* 348, 1027–1032

Gan TJ, Meyer T, Apfel CC et al (2003) Consensus guidelines for managing postoperative nausea and vomiting. *Anesth Analg* 97, 62–71

Hain TC, Uddin M (2003) Pharmacological treatment of vertigo. *CNS Drugs* 17, 85–100

Hesketh PJ (2008) Drug Therapy-chemotherapy-induced nausea and vomiting. *N Engl J Med* 358, 2482–2494

Jordan K, Sippel C, Schmoll HJ (2007) Guidelines for antiemetic treatment of chemotherapy-induced nausea and vomiting: past, present, and future recommendations. *Oncologist* 12, 1143–1150

Prommer E (2005) Aprepitant (EMEND): the role of substance P in nausea and vomiting *J Pain Palliat Care Pharmacother* 19, 31–39

Saeed SR (1998) Diagnosis and treatment of Ménière's disease. *BMJ* 316, 368–372

Wilhelm SM, Dehoorne-Smith ML, Kale-Pradhan PB (2007) Prevention of postoperative nausea and vomiting. *Ann Pharmacother* 41, 68–78

SELF-ASSESSMENT

In questions 1 and 2, the first statement, in italics, is true. Are the accompanying statements also true?

1. *Nausea and vomiting can be caused by a variety of stimuli that may require different drugs to treat them.*
   a. Toxins need to cross the blood–brain barrier to cause vomiting by stimulating the CTZ (area postrema).
   b. Some antihistamines can be used for motion sickness.
2. *Dopamine antagonists used as antiemetics, such as metoclopramide, can cause extrapyramidal movement abnormalities, particularly in the elderly.* Metoclopramide decreases intestinal motility.
3. Choose the one **correct** statement from the following concerning nausea and vomiting.
   A. Afferents from the stomach to the vomiting centre inhibit vomiting when stimulated.
   B. Selective $5HT_3$ receptor antagonists are particularly effective antiemetics against motion sickness.
   C. Metoclopramide inhibits the nausea and vomiting caused by opioids.
   D. Stimulation of NK_1 receptors on the CTZ inhibits nausea.
   E. Digoxin inhibits nausea.
4. Case history questions

A 35-year-old man was diagnosed with non-Hodgkin's lymphoma requiring many sessions of treatment with combined cytotoxic therapy, including cyclophosphamide, vincristine and prednisolone.

a. Why was this man likely to experience nausea and vomiting?

Nausea and vomiting started several hours after each course of treatment and continued for 4 to 5 days.

b. What planned antiemetic treatment prior to the first course of chemotherapy could be beneficial?
c. How do the treatments you have chosen work?

This man became very distressed by the severity of the nausea and vomiting and developed intense nausea and vomiting prior to the administration of the chemotherapeutic agents.

d. What treatment could be given to reduce the anticipatory nausea and vomiting?

ANSWERS

1. a. **False**. The CTZ is outside the blood–brain barrier. Moreover, toxins can also cause vomiting by stimulating vagal afferents in the stomach.
   b. **True**. Common antihistamines like promethazine have antimuscarinic activity and inhibit activity in the vomiting centre and in the vestibular nuclei. It is not certain whether the antihistamine component plays a role.
2. **False**. Metoclopramide increases stomach and intestinal motility (prokinetic activity), which can add to its antiemetic effects.
3. Answer **C**.
   A. Incorrect. The vagal afferents from the stomach are emetogenic and respond to toxins, etc.
   B. Incorrect. Selective $5HT_3$ receptor antagonists are not effective against motion sickness, where a drug with antimuscarinic actions, e.g. hyoscine or promethazine, should be used.
   C. Correct.
   D. Incorrect. The effect of stimulating NK_1 receptors in the CTZ is to cause vomiting.
   E. Incorrect. Digoxin causes nausea and vomiting.
4. Case history answers
   a. Cyclophosphamide induces nausea and vomiting in almost all people, but vincristine is much less emetogenic. The vomiting arises from stimulation of the CTZ.
   b. A selective $5HT_3$ receptor antagonist such as ondansetron, alone or together with a corticosteroid, would be beneficial.
   c. Ondansetron inhibits $5HT_3$ receptors in the CTZ and also $5HT_3$ receptors in the stomach. In the stomach, some cancer chemotherapeutic agents can cause damage and release of serotonin, which stimulates vagal afferents to the vomiting centre. It is uncertain how corticosteroids work, but they have an antiemetic effect which is additive with ondansetron.
   d. Anticipatory nausea and vomiting is poorly treated with antiemetic drugs. Treatment with benzodiazepines prior to the course of chemotherapy treatment can be helpful.

Antiemetic agents

Drug	Half-life (h) and kinetics	Comments
Antihistamines		
These drugs have sedating properties		
Cinnarizine	3 [M] Very variable absorption; numerous metabolites which are eliminated in the urine and faeces	Used for vestibular disorders and motion sickness; also used for peripheral vascular disease; given orally
Cyclizine	20 [M] Few data are available; demethylated metabolite has no activity	Used for a wide range of indications; given orally or by intramuscular or intravenous injection
Meclozine (meclizine)	6 [M] Undergoes extensive metabolism and eliminated in urine as metabolites and in faeces as parent drug (incomplete absorption?)	Given orally for motion sickness
Promethazine	7–14 [M] Low bioavailability (25%); bile is a major route of elimination of the (inactive) metabolites	Given orally, by deep intramuscular injection or by slow intravenous injection for a wide range of indications
Dopamine receptor antagonists		
Phenothiazine and related drugs		
Chlorpromazine	8–35 [M] Incomplete oral bioavailability (10–33%); numerous pathways of metabolism; see Ch. 21	Used for nausea and vomiting associated with terminal illness; given orally, rectally or by deep intramuscular injection
Perphenazine	9 [M] Low oral bioavailability (30–40%); undergoes extensive hepatic metabolism; see Ch. 21	Given orally for severe nausea and vomiting
Prochlorperazine	6–7 [M] Variable absorption of oral doses; undergoes extensive hepatic metabolism; see Ch. 21	Given orally or by deep intramuscular injection for severe nausea and vomiting

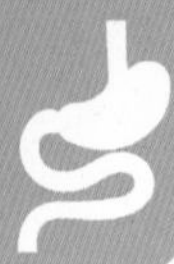

Antiemetic agents

Drug	Half-life (h) and kinetics	Comments
Trifluoperazine	14 (7–18) [M] Variable absorption but oral bioavailability has not been defined; numerous inactive metabolites formed; see Ch. 21	Given orally for severe nausea and vomiting
Domperidone and metoclopramide		
Domperidone	12–16 [M] Low bioavailability (about 15%); oxidised in liver to metabolites, which are excreted in urine and faeces	Used for a wide range of indications; given orally or rectally
Metoclopramide	3–5 [M + R] Oral bioavailability is variable (40–100%); eliminated by N-sulphation (a rare reaction) and renal excretion	Used for a wide range of indications; given orally or by intramuscular injection or intravenous injection over 1–2 min
$5HT_3$ receptor antagonists		
Dolasetron	0.1–0.3 [M] Undergoes extensive first-pass metabolism after oral dosage; the alcohol analogue, formed by reduction of the carbonyl group, is the major circulating metabolite; this metabolite has greater affinity for $5HT_3$ receptors, has a longer half-life (7 h), and is probably responsible for most of the in vivo activity	Used to prevent nausea and vomiting induced by cytotoxic chemotherapy or surgery; given orally or by intravenous injection or infusion
Granisetron	4 (3–9) [M + R] Oral bioavailability is 40–70%; metabolised by CYP3A4 with wide inter-individual variability in kinetics	Used to prevent nausea and vomiting induced by cytotoxic chemotherapy or radiotherapy; given orally or by intravenous injection or infusion
Ondansetron	3 [M] Oral bioavailability is 60%; oxidised in liver by CYP3A4 plus CYP2D6 (but no in vivo difference in kinetics between extensive and poor metabolisers of debrisoquine)	Used to prevent nausea and vomiting induced by cytotoxic chemotherapy or radiotherapy; given orally, rectally, by intramuscular injection or by slow intravenous infusion
Palonosetron	40 [M + R] Eliminated slowly by a combination of renal excretion and metabolism (by CYP2D6 and, to a lesser extent, CYP3A4 and CYP1A2)	Given by intravenous injection for nausea and vomiting associated with severely emetogenic chemotherapy
Tropisetron	6–7 [M] Metabolised by CYP2D6, and poor metabolisers show an increased incidence of unwanted effects	Used to prevent nausea and vomiting induced by cytotoxic chemotherapy; given by slow intravenous injection or infusion followed by oral dosage
Neurokinin (NK_1) receptor antagonists		
Aprepitant	9–13 [M] Oral bioavailability is good (65%); eliminated by hepatic metabolism (mostly CYP3A4)	Given orally as an adjunct for preventing nausea and vomiting associated with severely emetogenic chemotherapy
Cannabinoids		
Nabilone	2 [M] Completely absorbed; metabolised in the liver by multiple P450 isoenzymes to metabolites that may contribute to the long duration of action	Given orally to prevent nausea and vomiting induced by cytotoxic chemotherapy which is unresponsive to conventional antiemetics
Antimuscarinics		
Hyoscine (scopolamine)	8 [M] Radiolabelled studies indicate incomplete oral absorption (but good activity orally); hydrolysed to inactive products	Given as a transdermal patch for motion sickness and as premedication; also given by subcutaneous or intramuscular injection
Other drugs used for treatment and prevention of nausea and vomiting		
Benzodiazepines	–	See Ch. 20
Betahistine	5 (metabolite) [M] Undergoes almost complete first-pass metabolism to 2-pyridylacetic acid, which has a half-life of 5 h	Given orally for vertigo and tinnitus associated with Ménière's disease
Corticosteroids	–	See Ch. 44

[M], metabolism; [R], renal excretion.

33 Dyspepsia and peptic ulcer disease

THE SPECTRUM OF DISEASE

DYSPEPSIA AND PEPTIC ULCER DISEASE

Dyspepsia is the term used for a group of symptoms that arise from the upper gastrointestinal tract. They include heartburn, abdominal pain or discomfort, belching and nausea. Dyspepsia can occur alone or in association with a number of upper gastrointestinal disorders.

Peptic ulceration can occur in the stomach or duodenum. Characteristic symptoms include epigastric pain, which is relieved by antacids or by food and often is worse at night, and vomiting. Peptic ulcer disease is more common in males and in smokers, and there is often a family history of the disorder. It is also more common in people who use non-steroidal anti-inflammatory drugs (NSAIDs; Ch. 29) or who have a high alcohol intake. Women more often develop gastric rather than duodenal ulceration. Symptoms are a poor guide to the location of an ulcer, although with gastric ulcer the pain may be made worse by food and it is more likely than duodenal ulcer to be associated with weight loss, anorexia and nausea.

A proportion of those who present with peptic ulcer symptoms, especially over the age of 45 years, will have a gastric cancer. Investigation by upper gastrointestinal endoscopy above this age is important, since drug treatment for peptic ulcer can produce symptomatic improvement in early gastric cancer.

Aetiology of peptic ulceration

The precise aetiology of peptic ulceration is not known but there are many contributory factors. A major risk factor associated with peptic ulceration is gastric and duodenal infection with *Helicobacter pylori*.

The incidence of *H. pylori* in the gastric mucosa varies widely in the adult population in different countries, with about 10–15% of the UK population infected. Infection is usually acquired in childhood and persists unless treated. Infection with *H. pylori* is an acknowledged risk factor for gastritis, peptic ulcer, gastric cancer and mucosa-associated lymphoid tissue (MALT) lymphoma. Only a small percentage of infected individuals develop *H. pylori*-associated disease; the reasons for this are not resolved but depend upon a number of factors, including the host response to the infection and whether the infecting strain carries particular factors for high virulence. Infection with *H. pylori* is found in about 80% of people with duodenal ulcer and somewhat fewer with gastric ulcer. *H. pylori* secrete the enzyme urease, which contributes to its survival during brief exposure to gastric acid by producing ammonia from urea.

Gastric ulceration

The healthy stomach mucosa is able to resist acid digestion. There is an adherent layer of viscoelastic mucus that acts as a physical barrier, and HCO_3^- is secreted into the mucus to neutralise acid locally. In addition, there is a high electrical resistance of, and tight junctions between, gastric mucosal cells, which make the mucosa relatively impermeable to luminal contents. Gastric mucosal blood flow provides an extra layer of defence, by delivering HCO_3^- to buffer any H^+ ions that penetrate the mucosa. Many of these protective functions are dependent on the synthesis by gastric mucosal cells of prostaglandins PGE_2 and PGI_2 (Ch. 29) (Table 33.1).

If a gastric ulcer is present, this is often associated with *H. pylori* infection of the corpus of the stomach or both the corpus and antrum (pangastritis). Moreover, unlike the situation in duodenal ulceration, there is a decrease or at least no increase in acid secretion. The reason for this is that infection of the corpus is associated with atrophy of acid-secreting cells and metaplasia of the gastric mucosa, which lead to gastric ulceration and increases the risk of gastric cancer.

NSAID-induced gastric ulceration often occurs in the absence of *H. pylori*. The mechanisms are distinct, and

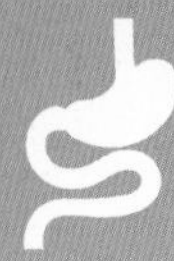

Table 33.1 Some of the many factors associated with protection and damage of the intestinal mucosa[a]

Factors associated with peptic ulcer disease	Factors associated with peptic ulcer protection and healing
Thin or breached mucus layer	Intact mucus layer
Helicobacter pylori and host immune response	Adequate blood flow
Reduced bicarbonate secretion	Bicarbonate in mucus layer
Reduced mucosal blood flow	Prostaglandins (generated by COX-1 and COX-2 isoenzymes)
Stress	Hydrophobicity of phospholipid layer of epithelial cells
Smoking	Regrowth of epithelial cell layer following damage (restitution)
Alcohol	Growth factors
Acid	Nitric oxide
Pepsin	
Iatrogenic, e.g. NSAIDs	

[a]The factors shown are associated with ulcer disease but it is uncertain which are causative. Many factors are interlinked; for example, prostaglandins can increase mucus secretion, blood flow and epithelial healing and can decrease acid secretion.

relate to inhibition of prostaglandin formation and intracellular trapping of NSAID in the gastric mucosa (Ch. 29).

The prevalence of non-*H. pylori*, non-NSAID-associated gastric ulcers appears to be increasing in Western societies. The pathogenesis of these ulcers is poorly understood.

Duodenal ulceration

The duodenal mucosa is protected by a layer of viscoelastic mucus, but the mucosal cells are highly permeable, permitting absorption of luminal nutrients. The mucosal cells secrete HCO_3^-, which accumulates in the mucus layer (the mucosal barrier) and buffers the pulses of gastric acid released from the stomach.

With duodenal ulceration, *H. pylori* infection is predominantly in the stomach and confined to the antral mucosa and there is more often excess acid secretion; exposure of duodenal cells to excess acid alters the structure of some of them, making them gastric-like and allowing them to be colonized by *H. pylori*; in addition, the likelihood of antral gastritis eventually leading to duodenal ulceration may depend upon the virulence of the strain of *H. pylori*, which is widely variable. Unless the *H. pylori* are eradicated, about 80% of duodenal ulcers will reoccur within a year after healing with proton pump inhibitors alone. The recurrence rate is low if *H. pylori* are eradicated.

Duodenal bicarbonate secretion is often deficient in duodenal ulceration.

GASTRO-OESOPHAGEAL REFLUX DISEASE

Gastro-oesophageal reflux disease (GORD) can produce heartburn, pain or difficulty in swallowing, and regurgitation of gastric contents into the oesophagus and even the mouth (reflux). If associated with oesophagitis, there may be more prolonged chest pain and chronic bleeding. Reflux is produced by transient lower oesophageal sphincter relaxations (TLOSRs) in the absence of swallowing. TLOSRs occur in response to stimulation of gastric vagal mechanoreceptors and allow gastric acid, pepsin and bile to come into contact with the vulnerable epithelium of the oesophagus. Oesophageal hypomotility and abnormal patterns of oesophageal contractility often coexist with GORD, and reduce clearance of refluxed material. The disturbance of normal motility may reflect a sensory abnormality in the oesophageal mucosa.

Oesophageal spasm is a distinct disorder, in which oesophageal pain is often not accompanied by any change in luminal pH. The pain often occurs without obvious dysmotility, and this syndrome is probably due to a combination of local sensory disturbances and psychological factors.

Up to 50% of people with symptoms of GORD have no apparent oesophagitis at endoscopy, whereas severe oesophagitis may produce few symptoms unless complications such as stricture or anaemia arise. GORD has an association with asthma, through microaspiration of gastric contents into the lungs and triggering of vagal oesophagobronchial reflexes. GORD is also associated with chronic cough.

The relationship of *H. pylori* infection to GORD is not straightforward: antral infection appears to predispose to GORD by promoting greater amounts of gastric acid secretion, while corporal gastritis is protective partly because the acid content of the stomach may be reduced. Symptoms in GORD are usually chronic and relapsing, with at least two-thirds of those diagnosed still taking continuous or intermittent treatment after 10 years. Relapse rates on stopping treatment are directly related to the initial severity of the disease. It is now believed that there are three distinct clinical groups of GORD rather than a steady progression of severity. These are possibly determined by genetic factors and the immunological response to reflux. The groups are:

- non-erosive reflux disease
- erosive oesophagitis, an acute inflammatory T-helper cell 1 (Th1) response (Ch. 38)
- Barrett's oesophagus (intestinal metaplasia of oesophageal mucosal cells) with increased risk of cancer; this is a Th2-type response (Ch. 38).

CONTROL OF GASTRIC ACID SECRETION

Acid secretion into the canaliculi of gastric parietal cells is caused by the activity of a membrane-bound proton pump which exchanges K^+ and H^+ across the cell membrane (H^+/K^+-ATPase). Hydrogen ions are obtained from carbonic acid (H_2CO_3) by the enzyme carbonic anhydrase, and HCO_3^- enters the plasma in exchange for Cl^-. Chloride ions are then secreted into the stomach lumen with H^+ via a symport carrier. The activity of the proton pump is influenced by several mediators, including histamine, gastrin and acetylcholine (Fig. 33.1).

DRUGS FOR TREATING DYSPEPSIA, PEPTIC ULCER AND GASTRO-OESOPHAGEAL REFLUX DISEASE

ANTISECRETORY DRUGS

It is only necessary to raise intragastric pH above 3 for a few hours each day to promote healing of most peptic ulcers. However, rapid healing requires acid suppression for a minimum of 18–20 h per day. The duration of acid suppression determines the rate of healing but not the eventual proportion of ulcers healed. Several classes of drug have antisecretory actions on the gastric mucosa.

Proton pump inhibitors

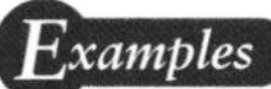

esomeprazole, lansoprazole, omeprazole, pantoprazole

Mechanism of action

Since the proton pump (H^+/K^+-ATPase) is the final common pathway for acid secretion in gastric parietal cells, inhibition of the pump almost completely blocks acid secretion (Fig. 33.1). Proton pump inhibitors are irreversible inhibitors of H^+/K^+-ATPase, and the return of acid secretion is dependent on the synthesis of new proton pumps. The drugs are weak bases that are concentrated from the general circulation into the acid environment of the secretory canaliculi of the gastric parietal cell. The drug is then protonated and structurally transforms into the active derivative that covalently binds to and irreversibly inhibits the proton pump. Because the active derivative is only formed at acid pH, these drugs have a selective action on gastric cells, and proton pumps elsewhere in the body are not inhibited. Acid production is inhibited by about 90% for approximately 24 h with a single dose.

Pharmacokinetics

Omeprazole is a prodrug that is unstable in acid, and is given orally as an enteric-coated formulation. Absorption is variable and incomplete, although it improves with repeated dosing. It is also available in an intravenous formulation. Elimination is by hepatic metabolism, largely by CYP2C19-mediated oxidation. Omeprazole has a short plasma half-life (1 h), but, because of the irreversible mechanism of action, this bears no relationship to the long biological duration of action. This is also a feature of other proton pump inhibitors that all have similar short half-lives. Esomeprazole is the S-isomer of omeprazole and has lower clearance and therefore slightly higher plasma levels and a longer half-life than omeprazole (1–2 h).

Lansoprazole is well absorbed from the gut. It is metabolised in the liver and has a short half-life (1–2 h). Pantoprazole is available in both oral and intravenous formulations. It is well absorbed from the gut and undergoes extensive hepatic metabolism. Once again, it has a short half-life (1–2 h).

Unwanted effects

- Gastrointestinal upset, such as nausea, vomiting, abdominal pain, diarrhea, constipation
- Headache, dizziness
- Omeprazole and some other proton pump inhibitors are inhibitors of CYP2C9 and CYP2C19 in the liver; this can give rise to drug interactions with other substrates of these isoenzymes, e.g. decreasing the metabolism and increasing the clinical effects of warfarin or phenytoin (see Table 2.9).

Concerns that substantial reductions of gastric acid, and the associated rise in gastrin secretion, might predispose to an increased incidence of gastric cancer (cf. the risk in pernicious anaemia) appear to be unfounded. These drugs do not completely abolish acid secretion and intragastric pH can still fall below 4 during part of the day, the critical pH below which bacterial populations that predispose to cancer are thought not to become established.

Histamine H_2 receptor antagonists

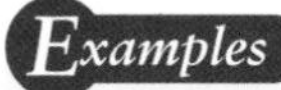

cimetidine, ranitidine

Mechanism of action

Histamine H_2 receptor antagonists act competitively at receptors on gastric parietal cells. They reduce basal acid secretion and pepsin production, and prevent the increase in secretion that occurs in response to several secretory stimuli. Overall, acid secretion is reduced by about 60% (Fig. 33.1).

Pharmacokinetics

Absorption of cimetidine and ranitidine from the gut is almost complete but both undergo limited first-pass metabolism. The drugs are mainly eliminated unchanged by the kidney, in part through active tubular transport. Their half-lives are between 1 and 4 h.

Unwanted effects

- Diarrhoea and other gastrointestinal disturbances
- Headache, dizziness, tiredness
- Rash
- Drug interactions: cimetidine is an inhibitor of hepatic P450 isoenzymes (see Table 2.9) and can increase the plasma concentrations and actions of drugs such as warfarin, phenytoin and theophylline.

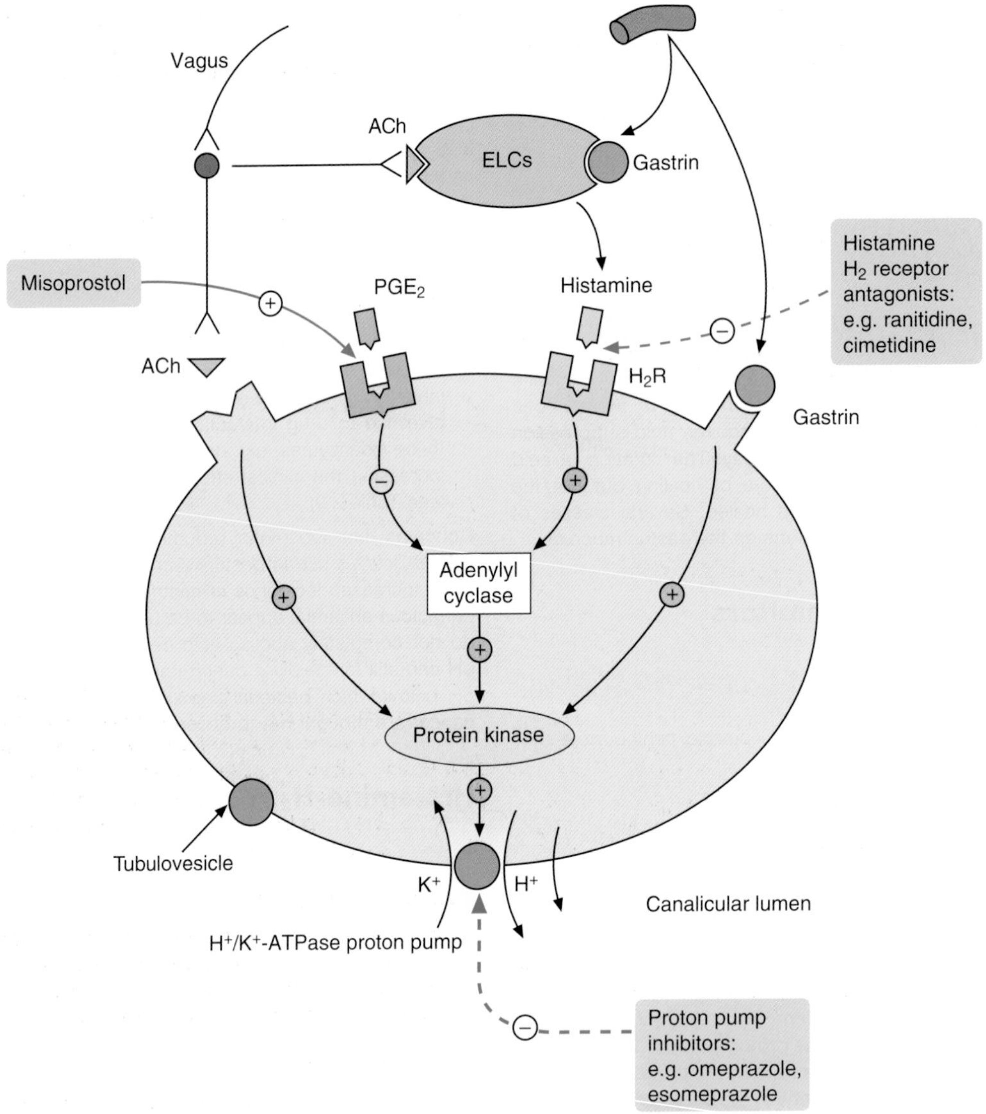

Fig. 33.1 **Control of gastric acid secretion from the parietal cell.** Acid secretion from the parietal cell is stimulated by acetylcholine (ACh), histamine and gastrin. Gastrin and ACh also reinforce acid secretion by causing the release of histamine from the enterochromaffin-like cells (ECLs) which lie close to the parietal cells in the gastric pits. Prostaglandin E_2 (PGE_2) reduces acid secretion. The sites of action of the main drugs used to inhibit acid secretion from the parietal cell are shown. There are no useful inhibitors of gastrin action, and the muscarinic receptor inhibitor pirenzepine is no longer available in the UK. H_2R, histamine type 2 receptor.

ANTACIDS

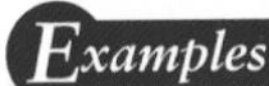

aluminium hydroxide, magnesium trisilicate

Mechanism of action

Antacids neutralise gastric acid; magnesium salts do so much more rapidly than aluminium salts. They have a more prolonged effect if taken after food; if used without food, the effect lasts no more than an hour because of rapid gastric emptying. Antacids quickly produce symptom relief in peptic ulcer disease, but large doses are required to heal ulcers. Liquid preparations work more rapidly, but tablets are more convenient to use. Most antacids are relatively poorly absorbed from the gut.

Unwanted effects

- Constipation can occur with aluminium salts, and diarrhoea with magnesium salts; mixtures may have less effect on stool consistency

- Systemic alkalosis can occur with very large doses
- Retention of absorbed aluminium may contribute to metabolic bone disease and encephalopathy in advanced renal failure, requiring dialysis
- Drug interactions: aluminium salts can bind to NSAIDs and tetracyclines in the gut and reduce their absorption.

Antacids with alginic acid

Alginic acid is an inert substance. It is claimed that it forms a raft of high-pH foam which floats on the gastric contents and will protect the oesophageal mucosa during reflux. All proprietary preparations combine alginic acid with an antacid, which is probably responsible for much of the clinical effect. Some formulations contain a high Na^+ concentration and these should be used with caution in people with heart failure.

CYTOPROTECTIVE DRUGS

Sucralfate

Mechanism of action

Sucralfate is a complex of aluminium hydroxide and sucrose octasulphate. It dissociates in the acid environment of the stomach to its anionic form, which binds to the ulcer base. This creates a protective barrier to pepsin and bile and inhibits the diffusion of gastric acid. Sucralfate also stimulates the gastric secretion of bicarbonate and prostaglandins.

Pharmacokinetics

Sucralfate is only slightly absorbed from the gut. The absorbed fraction is excreted unchanged by the kidney.

Unwanted effects

- Constipation.

Bismuth salts

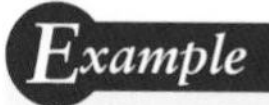

tripotassium dicitratobismuthate

Mechanism of action

Bismuth salts precipitate in the acid environment of the stomach and then bind to glycoprotein on the base of an ulcer. The resulting complex adheres to the ulcer and has similar local effects to sucralfate. Bismuth salts, in combination with antibiotics, were the first effective anti-*Helicobacter* agents and this effect may have accounted for their ulcer-healing properties. They have now largely been superseded by proton pump inhibitor combinations for this purpose; however, when triple therapy with two antibacterials and a proton pump inhibitor fails, bismuth is included as part of the treatment regimen (see below). A combination product with ranitidine (as ranitidine bismuth citrate) is still available.

Pharmacokinetics

Bismuth compounds are poorly soluble and only slightly absorbed from the gut. The absorbed fraction is excreted by the kidney, and has a very long half-life of 5 days.

Unwanted effects

- Blackened stools and darkened tongue.

Prostaglandin analogues

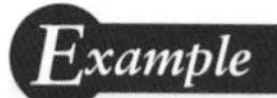

misoprostol

Mechanism of action

Misoprostol is an analogue of PGE_1 and has several actions that protect the gastric and duodenal mucosae (see Ch. 29). Misoprostol limits the damage to superficial mucosal cells caused by agents such as acid and alcohol. It is most widely used to reduce NSAID-induced gastric damage, and is available in combination products with diclofenac or naproxen (Ch. 29).

Pharmacokinetics

Misoprostol is an ester that is well absorbed from the gut and undergoes essentially complete first-pass metabolism to an acid. Elimination of the acid is mainly by hepatic metabolism, and it has a very short half-life (<1 h).

Unwanted effects

- Diarrhoea and abdominal cramps are common
- Uterine contractions, therefore avoid in pregnancy
- Menorrhagia and postmenopausal bleeding.

PROKINETIC DRUGS

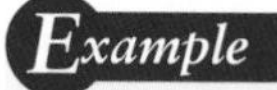

metoclopramide

Mechanism of action

Metoclopramide is a dopamine receptor antagonist and is discussed in Chapter 32. It enhances gastric motility, increases the rate of gastric emptying and increases lower gastro-oesophageal sphincter tone.

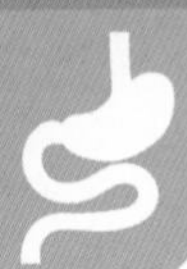

MANAGEMENT OF DYSPEPSIA, PEPTIC ULCER AND GASTRO-OESOPHAGEAL REFLUX DISEASE

Non-ulcer dyspepsia

Most people with dyspepsia do not have significant underlying disease (non-ulcer or functional dyspepsia). In all cases, efforts should be made to remove causative agents, for example smoking, excess alcohol, or NSAIDs. Several functional abnormalities in gastrointestinal motility, increased gastroduodenal sensitivity to mechanical distention, and increased acid sensitivity in the duodenum have been described in people with non-ulcer dyspepsia. For persistent symptoms, antacids provide symptomatic relief. Younger people (especially under 55 years of age) who do not have 'ALARM' symptoms (**A**naemia, **L**oss of weight, **A**norexia, **R**ecent onset of progressive symptoms, **M**elaena, haematemesis or dysphagia) are often treated symptomatically without investigation by upper gastrointestinal endoscopy. A proton pump inhibitor is more effective than a histamine H_2 receptor antagonist for symptom relief. Treatment should be given for 4–6 weeks, followed by clinical review with the intention of reducing the dose of drug or moving to intermittent or on-demand therapy for symptom relief.

Confirmed peptic ulceration

Proton pump inhibitors produce the fastest rate of healing (over 90% of ulcers heal within 4 weeks). Histamine H_2 receptor antagonists usually give symptomatic relief for both gastric and duodenal ulcers within a week, but healing of the ulcer is much slower, requiring up to 8 weeks for duodenal ulcer or 12 weeks for gastric ulcer. Other agents such as colloidal bismuth and sucralfate will heal ulcers in a similar proportion of people, but are used less often, since they do not improve symptoms as quickly.

Identification and eradication of *H. pylori* infection enhances ulcer healing and reduces relapse, so that maintenance therapy with acid-suppressing drugs is often unnecessary for uncomplicated ulcers. If *H. pylori* is not eradicated, 80% of ulcers will reoccur within a year, whereas following successful eradication the recurrence is less than 20%.

Eradication of *Helicobacter pylori*

Several indications for eradication have been proposed (Box 33.1). Many eradication regimens are available: the highest eradication rates are achieved by treatment with high dosage of a proton pump inhibitor combined with two antibacterials (to maximise efficacy and minimise resistance) given for 1 week. Treatment for 2 weeks has a higher eradication rate, but unwanted effects often reduce adherence to the regimen, which reduces the success rate. The incidence of resistance to metronidazole (up to 50% in some places) and to clarithromycin is increasing. If in vitro clarithromycin resistance is detected, then this is always reflected in a reduced ability to eliminate the bacterium clinically; in contrast, eradication may be successful even when laboratory resistance to metronidazole is demonstrated. Resistance to amoxicillin is less common, and resistance to tinidazole is currently lower than to metronidazole.

Resistance to triple therapy is now widespread in some localities, with a failure to eradicate *H. pylori* in up to 20% of people treated. Quadruple therapy can be used for resistant bacteria. One recommended regimen is a proton pump inhibitor plus bismuth plus metronidazole plus tetracycline for 7 days (Fig. 33.2). Other regimens are also used following the results of microbiological tests on biopsy specimens. These quadruple-therapy regimens achieve an eradication rate of 93–98%. More complicated and longer treatment regimens may become the norm in the future.

Box 33.1 Indications for eradication of *Helicobacter pylori*

Eradication recommended
Proven peptic ulcer
Low-grade mucosa-associated lymphoid tissue (MALT) gastric lymphoma
Severe gastritis
After resection of early gastric cancer

Eradication suggested (less certain indications)
Functional dyspepsia
Family history of gastric cancer
Non-steroidal anti-inflammatory drug (NSAID) therapy
Intended long-term proton pump inhibitor therapy

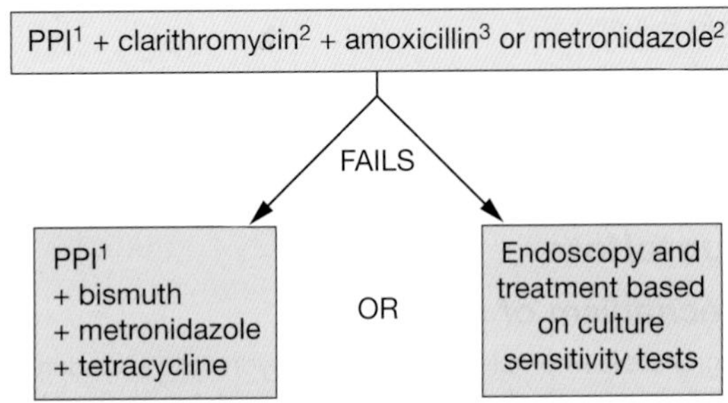

[1] If PPI not tolerated, ranitidine bismuth citrate or an H_2 receptor antagonist could be substituted
[2] Resistance is common
[3] Resistance is not common
Triple regimens are increasingly unsuccessful due to resistant strains.

Fig. 33.2 **Recommended regimens for the eradication of *Helicobacter pylori*.** Many regimens exist, dictated by local patterns of sensitivity and resistance. Increasing resistance is reducing the success rate of the triple regimen. PPI, proton pump inhibitor.

Maintenance therapy with acid-suppressant treatment is only required if symptoms continue despite eradication of *H. pylori* and after exclusion of more serious conditions.

PEPTIC ULCERATION ASSOCIATED WITH NON-STEROIDAL ANTI-INFLAMMATORY DRUGS

If the NSAID cannot be withdrawn, then ulcers will often heal if an ulcer-healing agent is co-prescribed. Continued use of NSAIDs can slow ulcer healing by histamine H_2 receptor antagonists, but probably not by proton pump inhibitors. Eradication of *H. pylori* infection is recommended if an NSAID must be continued in someone who has had previous peptic ulceration, although this may be more effective in preventing ulcers early in treatment with NSAIDs, and less effective during long-term use.

Misoprostol provides effective prophylaxis against gastric or duodenal ulceration, but a high dosage is necessary for prevention of ulcer recurrence and ulcer complications. At such doses, unwanted effects often reduce adherence to treatment. Proton pump inhibitors are effective for prophylaxis against recurrent gastric and duodenal ulcers. Standard doses of a histamine H_2 receptor antagonist protect against NSAID-induced duodenal ulcers, but not against gastric ulceration. Double doses of a histamine H_2 receptor antagonist or standard doses of a proton pump inhibitor protect against both gastric and duodenal ulceration, and are better tolerated than misoprostol.

When an NSAID is first used, careful assessment is recommended before prophylaxis against ulceration is given in the absence of upper gastrointestinal symptoms. Those at higher risk of NSAID-induced ulceration are the elderly (>65 years), smokers, heavy alcohol users and people with a history of previous ulceration. The use of cyclo-oxygenase 2 (COX-2)-selective inhibitors has been advocated for people at higher risk of ulceration. The use of a conventional NSAID with a proton pump inhibitor may be as effective as a COX-2-selective drug alone for reducing risk. There is limited evidence to support the use of a COX-2-selective inhibitor with a proton pump inhibitor as a strategy to further reduce the risk of peptic ulceration in people at high risk of ulceration. The combination of a COX-2 inhibitor with low-dose aspirin carries the same risk of ulceration as a conventional NSAID and should be avoided.

GASTRO-OESOPHAGEAL REFLUX DISEASE

Initial measures against GORD include avoidance of tight clothing, smoking, alcohol and caffeine, and encouraging weight loss. Raising the head of the bed by 15 cm on wooden blocks can promote symptom relief and mucosal healing. For mild persistent symptoms, reduction of gastric acid with antacids, with or without the addition of an alginate to provide a mechanical barrier, is often helpful. Alginates should be taken after meals to reduce their clearance by rapid gastric emptying. Histamine H_2 receptor antagonists often relieve troublesome symptoms but may not produce mucosal healing; heartburn is relieved in up to 50% of cases after 4 weeks, but oesophagitis only heals in about 20%. Better response rates can often be achieved by using these drugs at high dosages, which will produce healing in 70–80% of people by 8–12 weeks. Proton pump inhibitors are the most effective treatment for severe resistant or relapsing GORD. They will rapidly ease symptoms and heal oesophagitis in up to 85% of those treated by 8 weeks. Acid secretion may break through at night during treatment with a proton pump inhibitor. This may be important in severe erosive oesophagitis or Barrett's oesophagus, and esomeprazole may be more effective than other proton pump inhibitors for severe oesophagitis. Failure to heal oesophagitis with a proton pump inhibitor often indicates bile rather than acid reflux.

An alternative approach to the relief of symptoms is to enhance oesophageal motility with a prokinetic drug such as metoclopramide. Metoclopramide encourages normal peristalsis in the upper gastrointestinal tract and produces similar symptomatic relief to histamine H_2 receptor antagonists. However, it does not heal oesophagitis, and should only be used alone for non-erosive disease.

Intermittent therapy with healing agents, or use of an alginate after healing, often controls recurrent symptoms. More severe disease requires continuous drug treatment. Long-term use of a proton pump inhibitor is the only effective treatment for severe or resistant reflux disease. About 60% of people will need only a low maintenance dose after healing has occurred. Eradication of *H. pylori* in GORD does not improve symptoms.

Laparoscopic antireflux surgery is increasingly used for GORD, particularly if there is high-volume reflux.

Pain due to oesophageal spasm sometimes responds to smooth muscle relaxants such as calcium channel blockers (Ch. 5), nitrates (Ch. 5) or sildenafil (Ch. 16). Local injection of botulinum toxin (Ch. 24) has also been successful in limited studies.

FURTHER READING

Atherton JC (2006) The pathogenesis of *Helicobacter pylori*-induced gastro-duodenal diseases. *Ann Rev Pathol* 1, 63–96

Chan FKL, Leung WK (2002) Peptic-ulcer disease. *Lancet* 360, 933–941

Collins J, Ali-Ibrahim A, Smoot DT (2006) Antibiotic therapy for *Helicobacter pylori*. *Med Clin North Am* 90, 1125–1140

Coron E, Hatlebakk JG, Galmiche JP (2007) Medical therapy of gastroesophageal reflux disease. *Curr Opin Gastroenterol* 23, 434–439

Delaney B, McColl K (2005) Review article: *Helicobacter pylori* and gastro-oesophageal reflux disease. *Aliment Pharmacol Ther* 22(suppl 1), 32–40

Fass R (2007) Erosive and nonerosive reflux disease (NERD): comparison of epidemiologic, physiologic, and therapeutic characteristics. *J Clin Gastroenterol* 41, 131–137

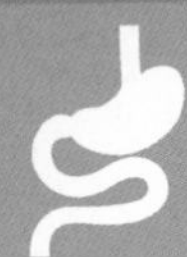

Fuccio LL, Zagari RM, Cennamo V et al (2008) Treatment of Helicobacter pylori infection. *BMJ* 337, 746–750

Hawkey CJ, Langman MJS (2003) Non-steroidal anti-inflammatory drugs: overall risks and management. Complementary roles for COX-2 inhibitors and proton pump inhibitors. *Gut* 52, 600–608

Kahrilas PJ (2008) Gastroesophageal reflux disease. *N Engl J Med* 359, 1700–1707

Kaunitz JD, Akiba Y. (2006) Review article: duodenal bicarbonate – mucosal protection, luminal chemosensing and acid–base balance. *Aliment Pharmacol Ther* 24(suppl 4), 169–176

Louw JSA (2006) Peptic ulcer disease. *Curr Opin Gastroenterol* 22, 607–611

Parfitt JR, Driman DK (2007) Pathological effects of drugs on the gastrointestinal tract: a review. *Hum Pathol* 38, 527–536

Seager JM, Hawkey CJ (2001) Indigestion and non-steroidal anti-inflammatory drugs. *BMJ* 323, 1236–1239

Stanghellini V, De Ponti F, De Giorgio R et al (2003) New developments in the treatment of functional dyspepsia. *Drugs* 63, 869–892

Storr M, Allescher H-D, Classen M (2001) Current concepts on pathophysiology, diagnosis and treatment of diffuse oesophageal spasm. *Drugs* 61, 579–591

Suerbaum S, Michetti P (2002) *Helicobacter pylori* infection. *N Engl J Med* 347, 1175–1186

Wallace JL (2005) Recent advances in gastric ulcer therapeutics. *Curr Opin Pharmacol* 5, 573–577

SELF-ASSESSMENT

In questions 1–6, the first statements, in italics, are true. Are the accompanying statements also true?

1. H. pylori *infection induces a spectrum of consequences. Some individuals with infection predominantly in the gastric corpus have persistently reduced or no change in acid secretion, whereas if infection is in the gastric antrum people have enhanced acid secretion.*
   a. *H. pylori* infection can be found in the duodenum in people with duodenal ulcers.
   b. Recurrence of duodenal ulcers following healing with proton pump inhibitors is approximately 20% over a year if *H. pylori* is not eliminated.
   c. *H. pylori* is a risk factor for the development of certain types of gastric cancer.
   d. Gastric acid inhibits bacterial growth.
   e. There is little risk of *H. pylori* developing resistance to antibacterial treatment.
   f. Omeprazole is a prodrug.
   g. Histamine acts on H_1 receptors on the parietal cell to stimulate acid secretion.
   h. Vagal stimulation of the parietal cell increases acid secretion.
2. *An unwanted effect of antacids containing magnesium salts is diarrhoea.* Antacids are not effective in healing peptic ulcers.
3. *Therapeutic doses of cimetidine, but not ranitidine, can potentiate the effects of other drugs by inhibiting hepatic cytochrome P450 enzymes.*
   a. Ranitidine is associated with a lower incidence of gynaecomastia than cimetidine.
   b. Cimetidine reduces acid secretion by more than 90%.
   c. The active metabolite of omeprazole is a reversible inhibitor of the H^+/K^+-ATPase proton pump.
4. *Omeprazole is converted to its active form at acid pH.* Omeprazole inhibits the cytochrome P450 system in the liver.
5. *Misoprostol helps prevent mucosal damage by NSAIDs.*
   a. PGI_2 reduces gastric mucosal blood flow.
   b. Misoprostol causes constipation.
   c. Histamine H_2 receptor antagonists and proton pump inhibitors are not useful for treatment of ulcers induced by NSAIDs.
6. *Proton pump inhibitors are first-line drugs in the treatment of GORD.* Metoclopramide increases the rate of gastric emptying and raises lower oesophageal sphincter tone.
7. Choose the one **most appropriate** option from the following statements relating to peptic ulcer disease.
   A. *H. pylori* organisms are not found in the duodenum.
   B. Resistance to clarithromycin is not a problem in the treatment of *H. pylori* infection.
   C. Cimetidine increases the plasma levels of warfarin.
   D. One test for *H. pylori* is to incubate a gastric biopsy with a solution containing a pH indicator and urease.
   E. The duration of action of omeprazole is about 2 h.
8. Case history questions

A 47-year-old man, Mr TK, was newly appointed as headmaster of a large comprehensive school and he was experiencing some difficulties with the increasing demands of the job. He increased his smoking from 5 to 20 cigarettes a day and he drank 10 units of alcohol a week. He had a good, varied diet. He had suffered intermittently from dyspepsia for some years, taking proprietary antacids when required. His symptoms then increased and the pain caused him to wake most nights. He bought a supply of ranitidine from the local chemist without consultation with the pharmacist. Following 2 weeks of treatment, his symptoms were successfully relieved and he was symptom-free for 3 months. His symptoms then returned and he took further treatment with ranitidine for 2 weeks. He was symptom-free for a further month, but when symptoms returned again he consulted his GP.

   a. Why did his symptoms return?
   b. Would his symptoms have been less likely to return following a short course of a proton pump inhibitor?
   c. What should be the GP's course of action?

An endoscopic examination revealed a duodenal ulcer.

d. Why do some people infected with *H. pylori* develop gastric ulcer and some duodenal ulcer?
e. What eradication therapy for *H. pylori* should be given, and is a proton pump inhibitor beneficial when given with antibacterial therapy?

The eradication therapy given was 7 days with omeprazole, amoxicillin and clarithromycin. Mr TK was symptom-free for 6 weeks but then his symptoms returned.

f. What were the possible reasons for the return of the symptoms?
g. What treatment could be given?

ANSWERS

1. a. **True**. Although the organism appears to live only on gastric mucosa, it is known that changes in duodenal mucosa occur in response to low pH, enabling duodenal colonisation.
   b. **False**. Approximately 80% of duodenal ulcers recur if *H. pylori* is not eliminated.
   c. **True**. Although the relationship between *H. pylori* and gastric cancer is somewhat difficult to prove, it has been estimated from epidemiological studies that this infection may increase the risk of developing gastric adenocarcinoma by five- to sixfold. It is possible that acquiring the infection at a young age may be important in the development of gastric cancer.
   d. **True**. The relevance of this to *H. pylori* is that when infection is associated with pangastritis, glandular atrophy and reduced gastric acid secretion occurs. This can then result in bacterial overgrowth and the formation of N-nitroso compounds that are mutagenic. Although *H. pylori* can resist acid transiently because of its ability to produce ammonia, it is destroyed by longer exposure.
   e. **False**. In some countries the resistance to metronidazole is as high as 90% and in some locations resistance to erythromycin is as high as 17%.
   f. **True**. Omeprazole has to be converted to its active form by protonation in acid. This is why it is active on the proton pump in the parietal cell but not other proton pumps in the body that operate at higher pH. This contributes to its selectivity.
   g. **False**. Histamine acts on H_2 receptors on parietal cells to stimulate acid secretion. This is the basis for the selective action of histamine H_2 receptor antagonists such as ranitidine and cimetidine.
   h. **True**. Acetylcholine stimulates muscarinic receptors, which, by increasing Ca^{2+}, causes increased acid secretion. Selective vagotomy has been used to treat ulcer disease.
2. **False**. Antacids do heal peptic ulcers but their effects are slower than with proton pump inhibitors or histamine H_2 receptor antagonists.
3. a. **True**. Cimetidine causes gynaecomastia. This is because of its greater anti-androgenic effect.
   b. **False**. Histamine H_2 antagonists reduce acid secretion by about 60%. The actions of other agents that promote acid secretion, for example gastrin and acetylcholine, are unaffected by histamine H_2 receptor antagonists.
   c. **False**. The active metabolite irreversibly inhibits the proton pump and fresh protein must be synthesised to replace the inhibited pump. This is the explanation for the very long duration of action of omeprazole.
4. **True**. Omeprazole is a substrate for CYP2C19 and can inhibit the metabolism of drugs such as warfarin or phenytoin by both CYP2C9 and CYP2C19. Lansoprazole is a weaker enzyme inhibitor.
5. a. **False**. Part of the way that prostaglandins protect the mucosa is by increasing gastric mucosal blood flow, removing back-secreted H^+ and providing HCO_3^-. Prostaglandins additionally increase mucus secretion, decrease acid secretion and increase HCO_3^- secretion.
   b. **False**. Prostaglandin (particularly PGI_2) in large doses can increase gastrointestinal motility and increase gastrointestinal secretions.
   c. **False**. Healing can be brought about by both of these anti-ulcer drugs. Omeprazole may produce more rapid healing since the rate of healing is probably related to the degree of acid suppression.
6. **True**. This is the mechanism for its usefulness in the treatment of oesophageal reflux disease. Metoclopramide and similar drugs are most effectively used as adjuncts to proton pump inhibitors and H_2 receptor antagonists.
7. Answer **C**.
   A. False. *H. pylori* is found in the duodenum associated with colonisation by gastric metaplasia of the duodenal mucosa.
   B. False. Increasingly, resistance of *H. pylori* to clarithromycin is developing.
   C. True. Cimetidine inhibits the cytochrome P450 metabolising enzymes that break down warfarin, hence increasing the plasma levels of warfarin.
   D. False. The solution contains urea not urease. The urease associated with *H. pylori* then converts the urea to ammonia, which causes a colour change in the pH indicator.
   E. False. Although the plasma half-life of omeprazole is about 2 h, its biological half-life is much longer, as it is converted to an active metabolite which irreversibly inhibits the parietal cell proton pump.
8. Case history answers
   a. This man could be experiencing non-ulcer dyspepsia or have peptic ulceration. Whichever he has, if his symptoms are associated with *H. pylori* infection, they will return, as *H. pylori* has not been eradicated. Ranitidine for only 2 weeks of treatment is available without prescription. If ranitidine had been continued, the symptoms would probably have been suppressed for longer. Failure to eradicate *H. pylori* results in a recurrence of peptic ulcer disease in 80% of people within a year. At this stage, of course, it is not known if peptic ulcer disease is present. However, even if he has non-ulcer dyspepsia and is *H. pylori*-positive, it is likely that he will develop peptic ulcer disease in the future.
   b. No. If *H. pylori* is present, the symptoms will still recur in a high percentage of individuals.

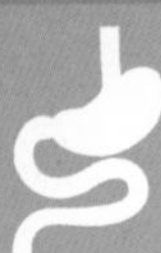

c. It is recommended that any person over 45 years of age should be endoscopically examined, and he should be referred for this procedure. The GP could assess for *H. pylori* infection serologically using a blood test; alternatively, this could be done in hospital with urea breath test or bacteriological culture on a gastric antral biopsy. Intake of any NSAIDs, smoking and alcohol intake should be assessed, as these are strongly contributory to ulcer disease. (An endoscopic examination revealed a duodenal ulcer.)
d. The answer to this is complex and imperfectly understood. If there is only antral inflammation and *H. pylori* is present, more gastrin and therefore excess acid is produced, resulting in duodenal ulcers. If a pangastritis exists, it is associated with corporal atrophy, lower levels of acid secretion, and gastric ulcers.
e. Numerous treatment regimens have being evaluated. Seven days therapy with a proton pump inhibitor or ranitidine (if intolerant) plus two antimicrobials (either metronidazole or amoxicillin plus clarithromycin in a combination dictated by local sensitivities) results in 70–90% eradication rate.
f. It is possible that the strain of *H. pylori* was resistant to the antibiotics used. In some places, clarithromycin resistance is 17%. Tests should be carried out to see if *H. pylori* is still present after treatment. If necessary, quadruple therapy or longer treatment periods should be used.
g. Culture sensitivities of the *H. pylori* in a biopsy specimen could be sought. Quadruple therapy, which has 93–98% success, could be used – for example, a proton pump inhibitor or ranitidine plus bismuth plus metronidazole plus tetracycline (Fig. 33.2). With resistance developing rapidly, this type of regimen may become the norm.

Drugs used for dyspepsia and peptic ulcer disease

Drug	Half-life (h) and kinetics	Comments
Antisecretory agents		
H_2 receptor antagonists		
Cimetidine	1–3 [R] Incomplete oral absorption; cleared by renal tubular secretion; weak relationship between blood levels and therapeutic response; inhibits cytochrome P450 enzymes	May be given orally, by intramuscular injection, or by slow intravenous injection or infusion
Famotidine	3–4 [R + B + M] Incomplete absorption; weak relationship between blood levels and response; does not affect cytochrome P450 enzymes	Given orally
Nizatidine	1.5–1.6 [R + M] Almost complete oral bioavailability; mostly eliminated by glomerular filtration and secretion; does not affect cytochrome P450 enzymes	Given orally or by intravenous infusion
Ranitidine	2–3 [R + M] Oral bioavailability is about 50% due to first-pass metabolism; cleared by renal tubular secretion and oxidation; no effect on cytochrome P450 enzymes	May be given orally, by intramuscular injection, or by slow intravenous injection or infusion
Ranitidine bismuth citrate	Dissociates in stomach contents to ranitidine (see above) and soluble and insoluble forms of bismuth. Bismuth shows variable and incomplete absorption; the absorbed fraction is largely eliminated in the bile with a terminal half-life of 11–28 days	Given orally only
Proton pump inhibitors		
These drugs have longer durations of action than indicated by the half-life of the parent compound; they are inhibitors of CYP2C19 but may cause weak induction of CYP1A2		
Esomeprazole	1–2 [M] Kinetic properties are similar to omeprazole (see below) but it gives higher plasma levels and has a slightly longer half-life than the racemate because the S-isomer has a lower clearance	The S-isomer of omeprazole (both isomers are active); given orally, or by intravenous injection or infusion
Lansoprazole	1.3–1.7 [M] High oral bioavailability (80%); eliminated by hepatic metabolism via CYP2C19 and CYP3A4	Given orally

Drugs used for dyspepsia and peptic ulcer disease

Drug	Half-life (h) and kinetics	Comments
Omeprazole	1 [M] Almost complete oral bioavailability; metabolised by CYP2C19; poor metabolisers have plasma AUC values 20-fold higher than fast metabolisers; no data available on plasma concentration–response relationship; potent inhibitor of CYP2C19 but induces cytochrome CYP1A2	Given orally or by slow intravenous injection (over 5 min) or infusion
Pantoprazole	1 [M] Well absorbed with about 20% hepatic first-pass metabolism; eliminated by CYP2C19-mediated metabolism; longer half-life (4–10 h) in poor metabolisers; lower affinity for CYP2C19 and possibly fewer drug interactions than omeprazole	Given orally or by slow intravenous injection (over 2 min) or infusion
Rabeprazole	1–2 [M] Bioavailability is about 50%; extensively metabolised in the liver (mostly by CYP3A4 rather than CYP2C19) to inactive products; fewer drug interactions than omeprazole	Given orally; shows limited activity against *H. pylori*
Cytoprotective agents		
Given orally		
Misoprostol	0.3 (acid) [M] Misoprostol per se is not detectable in blood after oral dosage because of essentially complete first-pass metabolism to misoprostol acid	A prostaglandin analogue; misoprostol is a methyl ester of misoprostol acid
Sucralfate	Minimal absorption (2% or less); no data on the fate of absorbed material (the high polarity would probably result in rapid renal excretion)	
Tripotassium dicitratobismuthate	Minimal absorption; absorbed bismuth is eliminated very slowly in the urine	
Prokinetic drugs		
Metoclopramide	3–5 [M + R] Oral bioavailability is variable (40–100%); eliminated by N-sulphation (a rare reaction) and renal excretion	Used for a wide range of indications; given orally or by intramuscular injection or intravenous injection over 1–2 min
Other drugs		
Alginic acid	–	Produces local effects within the stomach
Antacids	Their absorption and systemic fates are not of therapeutic importance	Antacids include aluminium hydroxide, magnesium trisilicate, hydrocalcite (mixed aluminium/magnesium preparation) and sodium carbonate; produce local effects within the stomach
Antimicrobials	See Ch. 51	Used to eliminate *H. pylori*

AUC, area under the curve for plasma concentration versus time; [B], biliary excretion; [M], metabolism; [R], renal excretion.

34 Inflammatory bowel disease

Crohn's disease and **ulcerative colitis** are chronic inflammatory disorders of the gastrointestinal tract which together are termed 'inflammatory bowel disease' (IBD); however, this common terminology conceals many differences in predisposition and in pathogenesis between the two conditions. It is also likely that within each category there are different individual disease phenotypes.

Ulcerative colitis is a disorder that is confined to the mucosa and submucosa, with inflammation usually confined to the large bowel. The extent of colonic involvement varies, but the rectum is always involved and mucosal inflammation is continuous, not patchy. Symptoms include bloody diarrhoea, fever and weight loss. Ulcerative colitis can be associated with extracolonic manifestations such as uveitis, sacroiliitis and various skin disorders.

Crohn's disease is a transmural granulomatous condition that can involve any part of the gut. The bowel involvement is discontinuous and segmental, often sparing the rectum. Fistula formation, small-bowel strictures and perianal disease such as abscesses and fissures are common. Clinical features of colonic involvement include diarrhoea, abdominal pain and fatigue. Involvement of more proximal parts of the gut produces various symptoms depending on the site of the disease, and diarrhoea need not be present.

The aetiologies of IBD are unclear, although several susceptibility genes have been identified (Fig. 34.1). The genetic predisposition is stronger in Crohn's disease, but both conditions can occur in the same families. The trigger for disease in susceptible individuals is unknown but a failure of development of immune tolerance in the gut may be important, and IBD may arise from impaired handling of microbial antigens by the intestinal immune system. The abnormal immune response involves an excess number of T-helper type 1 (Th1) lymphocytes in Crohn's disease, and T-helper type 2 (Th2) lymphocytes in ulcerative colitis (Ch. 38). Recently, T-helper type 17 (Th17) lymphocytes have been identified that are involved in immunity, inflammation and tissue damage and may be involved in the pathogeneses of both Crohn's disease and ulcerative colitis. Regulatory T-cells are probably deficient, and excess production of inflammatory cytokines results in the secretion of large amounts of tumour necrosis factor alpha (TNFα) and interleukin (IL)-1 and IL-6 by macrophages. Natural killer T-cells and neutrophil leucocytes also contribute to the inflammatory response. There is a close interaction between the immune system and the enteric nervous system that contributes to initiation and maintenance of inflammation, motility disturbance in the bowel and pain. Cigarette smoking increases the risk of Crohn's disease and the frequency of exacerbations, but slightly decreases the risk of ulcerative colitis. Inflammatory bowel disease can undergo periods of relapse and remission over many years. The symptoms associated with Crohn's disease and ulcerative colitis are shown in Box 34.1. Which clearly points out the fact that IBD causes pathological events in organs other than the bowel.

Treatment of both types of IBD is intended to induce and maintain remission. The drugs used for these two conditions are broadly similar, but Crohn's disease is less responsive to some of the widely used drugs, especially when it involves the small intestine. Better understanding of the pathogenic mechanisms in IBD has resulted in advances in treatment, although much still needs to be learned.

DRUGS FOR INFLAMMATORY BOWEL DISEASE

Aminosalicylates

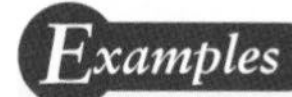

balsalazide, mesalazine, olsalazine, sulfasalazine

Mechanism of action and effects

The active anti-inflammatory constituent of all the aminosalicylates is 5-aminosalicylic acid (5-ASA). The different aminosalicylate drugs are formulated in a variety of ways; they are all designed to deliver 5-ASA to the lower bowel (see below). Sulfasalazine was the first aminosalicylate shown to be effective in treating IBD. Colonic bacteria cleave sulfasalazine into its constituent parts, 5-ASA and sulfapyridine. Sulfapyridine is responsible for many of the unwanted effects of this drug; in contrast to its role in inflammatory arthritis (Ch. 30), sulfapyridine has no therapeutic value in IBD. The mechanisms of action of aminosalicylates are not clear, but they may involve inhibition of leucocyte chemotaxis by reducing cytokine formation, reduced free radical generation and inhibition of the production of inflammatory mediators (such as prostaglandins, thromboxanes, leukotrienes and platelet activating factor). Aminosalicylates are increasingly used as first-line treatment of mild to moderate ulcerative colitis, and are highly effective for reducing relapse rate. Their efficacy in Crohn's disease is less well established, particularly for non-colonic disease. They are

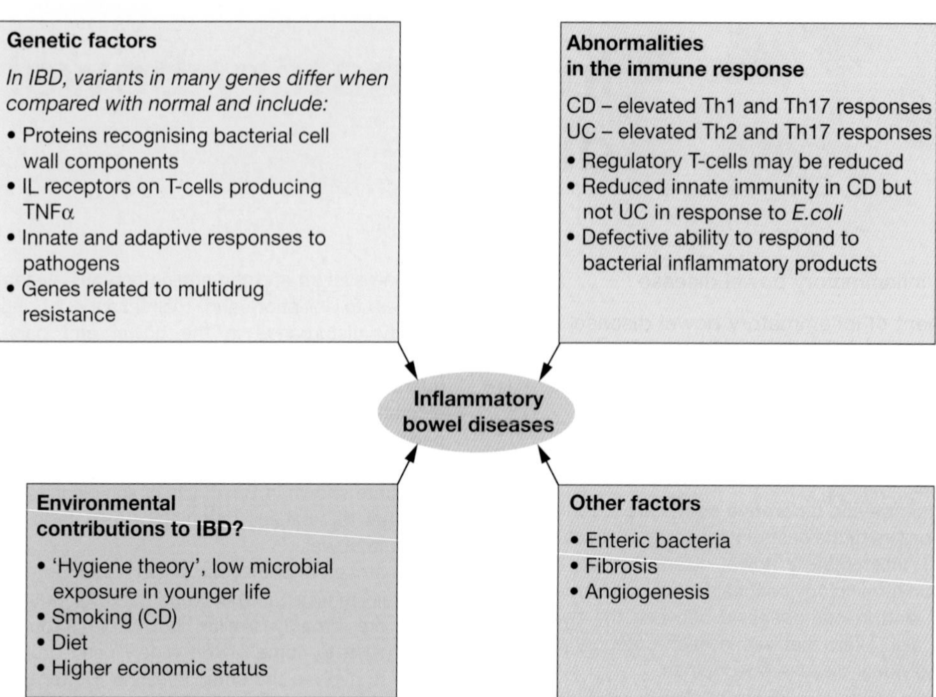

Fig. 34.1 **Some factors associated with inflammatory bowel disease**. Investigations into the aetiology of inflammatory bowel disease have confirmed the multiplicity of factors that might be involved. The association of some events is strong while others are weak. Some changes may occur as a consequence of the disease rather than being involved in the cause. CD, Crohn's disease; IBD, inflammatory bowel disease; IL, interleukin; TNFα, tumour necrosis factor alpha; UC, ulcerative colitis.

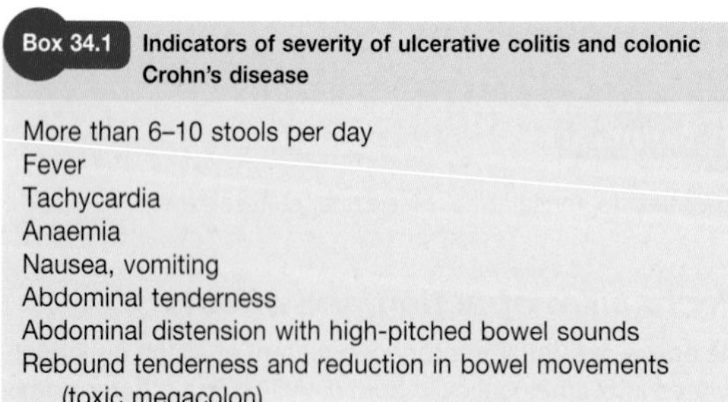

Box 34.1 Indicators of severity of ulcerative colitis and colonic Crohn's disease

More than 6–10 stools per day
Fever
Tachycardia
Anaemia
Nausea, vomiting
Abdominal tenderness
Abdominal distension with high-pitched bowel sounds
Rebound tenderness and reduction in bowel movements (toxic megacolon)

less effective in ameliorating sudden exacerbations of active IBD.

Pharmacokinetics

Sulfasalazine is partially absorbed from the gut intact, but most reaches the colon, where it undergoes reduction by gut bacteria to sulfapyridine and 5-ASA. Sulfapyridine and about 20% of the 5-ASA are absorbed from the colon, and then metabolised in the liver. Both have plasma half-lives of about 5–10 h. There are several ways of delivering 5-ASA to the mucosa of the lower gut without also giving sulfapyridine. Mesalazine (5-ASA itself) is given as an enteric-coated or modified-release formulation to limit absorption from the small bowel and deliver adequate drug to the colon. Olsalazine is a drug comprising two 5-ASA molecules joined by an azo bond. It is not absorbed from the upper gut and 5-ASA is released after reductive splitting of the azo bond by the colonic flora. Balsalazide is a prodrug in which 5-ASA is linked to a carrier molecule (4-aminobenzoyl-β-alanine) by an azo bond, which is cleaved by bacterial reduction in the large bowel.

Mesalazine and sulfasalazine can be given rectally (by suppository or enema) to treat distal disease in the colon.

Unwanted effects

These occur in up to 45% of people treated with sulfasalazine, but only 15% of those who take mesalazine. They include:

- Nausea, vomiting, diarrhoea, abdominal pain
- Headache
- Rashes
- Blood dyscrasias, especially agranulocytosis and thrombocytopenia
- Anorexia, fever, oligospermia with sulfasalazine.

Corticosteroids

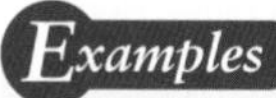

budesonide, hydrocortisone, prednisolone

Corticosteroids (Ch. 44) are very effective for inducing remission in active IBD; however, there is little evidence that they prevent relapse when used at doses that do not produce major unwanted effects. Newer corticosteroids formulated for topical use, such as budesonide (see also Ch. 44), have limited systemic unwanted effects and are useful alternatives to the older drugs. Topical treatment with liquid or foam enemas or suppositories is used for localised rectal disease, but oral or parenteral administration is needed for more severe or extensive disease.

Cytokine inhibitors (TNFα antibodies)

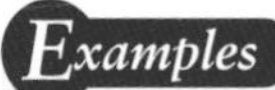

adalimumab, infliximab

Mechanisms and uses

Infliximab was the first monoclonal antibody to be approved for the treatment of Crohn's disease. Adalimumab is effective when infliximab is poorly tolerated or for those who have become refractory to treatment. Other TNFα antibodies used for inflammatory arthritis (Ch. 30) are not yet licensed for the treatment of IBD. Inhibition of the binding of TNFα to its receptors reduces pro-inflammatory cytokine (e.g. IL-1 and IL-6) production, leucocyte migration and infiltration, and neutrophil and eosinophil activation. Infliximab may also be useful for treatment of severe attacks of ulcerative colitis. Unwanted effects of TNFα antibodies are discussed in Chapter 30.

Immunosuppressants

Azathioprine and, less often, mercaptopurine are useful in some people with active IBD and may enable corticosteroid doses to be reduced. Azathioprine should be considered if control of IBD requires more than two 6-week courses of oral corticosteroid therapy per year, or if the disease relapses as the dose of corticosteroid is reduced. Mercaptopurine is more frequently used in North America; it may be a little less effective but perhaps with a lower rate of nausea than found with azathioprine. Maximum efficacy is not achieved with either drug for about 6–12 weeks. Nausea, vomiting, rashes and a hypersensitivity syndrome affect about 10% of people during the first 6 weeks of therapy. Pancreatitis and liver toxicity are rare but serious complications.

Methotrexate is useful in both ulcerative colitis (an unlicensed indication in the UK) and Crohn's disease. It is given intramuscularly and is only used when azathioprine has failed. Ciclosporin may induce remission in corticosteroid-resistant ulcerative colitis but has no long-term efficacy. More details of these drugs are found in Chapter 38.

Antibacterials

Metronidazole (Ch. 51) is moderately effective for treatment of some aspects of Crohn's disease, particularly perianal disease, although the mechanism of action is uncertain. Data on the use of other antibacterials such as clarithromycin and ciprofloxacin are conflicting.

MANAGEMENT OF INFLAMMATORY BOWEL DISEASE

ULCERATIVE COLITIS

Treatment is determined by the extent and severity of disease. Non-steroidal anti-inflammatory drugs (NSAIDs) and also selective cyclo-oxygenase 2 (COX-2) inhibitors (Ch. 29), can exacerbate symptoms in severe colitis and should not be used. Opioids (Ch. 35) should be avoided in the treatment of diarrhoea in extensive colitis since they can precipitate the life-threatening complication toxic megacolon.

Rectal drug delivery is often successful if the disease is limited to the rectum or left side of the colon (distal colitis). For mild symptoms, topical mesalazine is more effective than topical corticosteroid. Foam enemas or suppositories will treat inflammation up to 12–20 cm from the anus, while liquid enemas are effective up to 30–60 cm (i.e. to the splenic flexure). An oral aminosalicylate is an alternative approach for more severe disease. An oral corticosteroids may be necessary to induce remission, with gradual dosage reduction when control is achieved to minimise unwanted effects. Once symptoms are quiescent, maintenance treatment with topical mesalazine or an oral aminosalicylate should be life-long and reduces the relapse rate by two-thirds.

More extensive colitis will settle with an oral aminosalicylate if symptoms are mild to moderate, but the response can take 6–8 weeks. Oral corticosteroids induce remission more quickly. Severe colitis requires intensive fluid and electrolyte replacement; anaemia should be corrected by transfusion, and large doses of parenteral corticosteroid should be given. Infliximab can be used for severe refractory disease, and for subsequent maintenance therapy. Surgery is required in about 20% of people with ulcerative colitis.

The indications for immunosuppressants in the treatment of ulcerative colitis are the same as for Crohn's disease (see below). Azathioprine is the only agent with a good evidence base for long-term therapy of ulcerative colitis. Intravenous ciclosporin may induce remission in refractory cases.

CROHN'S DISEASE

Corticosteroid therapy is the mainstay of medical treatment for active Crohn's disease, usually with oral prednisolone. Maintenance corticosteroid therapy does not reduce the risk of relapse, and every effort should be made to withdraw the drug once the disease activity has been controlled. Immunosuppressive drugs such as azathioprine may be useful to aid this process, especially in chronically active Crohn's disease, where corticosteroid dependence occurs in 40–50% of people who take the drug to induce remission. Disease confined to the distal colon can respond to topical

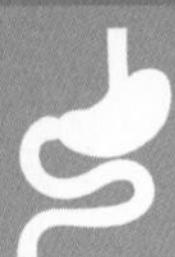

therapy with a corticosteroid, and an oral aminosalicylate such as sulfasalazine can also be useful (see management of ulcerative colitis).

Metronidazole is also effective in some aspects of Crohn's disease, and is particularly useful for perianal disease, where it probably has both an antibacterial and anti-inflammatory effect. Infliximab has been successfully used to induce and maintain remission in Crohn's disease that is resistant to conventional therapy. An infusion of infliximab can induce remission in Crohn's disease for up to 3 months. Intermittent 2-monthly maintenance infusions can reduce the severity of the disease. Antibody formation, which may cause allergic reactions and/or loss of efficacy, is less likely to occur with this regimen, and can be further reduced by corticosteroid pretreatment and maintenance immunosuppressant therapy.

Surgery may be necessary for disease refractory to medical therapy. Intestinal obstruction can require bowel resection, or abscesses may need drainage. A defunctioning ileostomy to 'rest' the bowel may allow active inflammation to settle with medical therapy in refractory disease, but colonic disease usually recurs after closure of the stoma. Surgery should be an integral part of the management plan, and is required in up to 80% of people with Crohn's disease. It should not be considered as failure or a last resort.

FURTHER READING

Baumgart DC, Sandborn WJ (2007) Inflammatory bowel disease: clinical aspects and established and evolving therapies. *Lancet* 369, 1641–1657

Behm BW, Bickston SJ (2008) Tumor necrosis factor-alpha antibody for maintenance of remission in Crohn's disease. *Cochrane Database Syst Rev* (1), CD006893

Collins P, Rhodes J (2006) Ulcerative colitis: diagnosis and management. *BMJ* 333, 340–343

Cummings JFR, Keshav S, Travis SPL (2008) Medical management of Crohn's disease. *BMJ* 336, 1062–1066

Katz JA (2007) Management of inflammatory bowel disease in adults. *J Dig Dis* 8, 65–71

Panés J, Gomollón F, Taxonera C et al (2007) Crohn's disease: a review of current treatment with a focus on biologics. *Drugs* 67, 2511–2537

Peyrin-Biroulet L, Desreumaux P, Sandborn WJ et al Crohn's disease: beyond antagonists of tumour necrosis factor. *Lancet* 372, 67–81

Scaldaferri F, Fiocchi C (2007) Inflammatory bowel disease: progress and current concepts of etiopathogenesis. *J Dig Dis* 8, 171–178

Tamboli CP (2007) Current medical therapy for chronic inflammatory bowel disease. *Surg Clin North Am* 87, 697–725

SELF-ASSESSMENT

In questions 1 and 2, the first statement, in italics, is true. Are the accompanying statements also true?

1. *Inflammatory bowel disease can be treated with pro-drugs of 5-aminosalicylic acid (5-ASA).*
   a. The active constituent of sulfasalazine is 5-ASA.
   b. Mesalazine (5-ASA) can be given rectally.
2. *The cause of inflammatory bowel disease is uncertain.*
   a. Cigarette smoking increases the risk of Crohn's disease.
   b. Mesalazine is equally useful in the treatment of Crohn's disease involving the colon or the small bowel.
   c. Corticosteroids are effective for maintaining remission in ulcerative colitis.
   d. Immunosuppressants such as azathioprine are ineffective for the treatment of Crohn's disease.
3. Choose the one **most appropriate** option from the following statements concerning treatment of inflammatory bowel disease.
   A. Crohn's lesions are transmural and confined only to the small bowel.
   B. Sulfapyridine is the active constituent in sulfasalazine that is used to treat inflammatory bowel disease.
   C. Azathioprine is the first-line drug of choice in treating mild Crohn's disease.
   D. Infliximab is antibody directed against interleukin-10.
   E. Metronidazole can be used in the treatment of inflammatory bowel disease.
4. Case history questions

A 35-year-old man presented with a 3-week period of frequent diarrhoea with mucus but no blood in the stool. Stool analysis for infective agents was negative. Sigmoidoscopy indicated gross thickening of the mucosa, with inflammation and linear ulcers. Changes were present in restricted areas (skip lesions) with intervening normal mucosa. Histology was diagnostic of Crohn's disease and investigation suggested that the condition was confined to the sigmoid colon and rectum.

a. What is the cause of Crohn's disease?
b. How should this man be treated initially?
c. How do corticosteroids act in Crohn's disease?
d. How should the corticosteroid be given, and why?
e. Why should the corticosteroid dosage be reduced slowly at the end of treatment?
f. How can remission be maintained in this man?
g. What alternative therapies can be given to try to reduce the risk of corticosteroid dependence?

ANSWERS

1. a. **True**. Sulfasalazine consists of sulfapyridine and 5-ASA linked by an azo bond. The azo bond is cleaved by bacterial reduction to release the active 5-ASA. Sulfapyridine probably produces many of the unwanted effects of sulfasalazine.

b. **True**. Modified-release formulations are available for rectal administration to deliver the drug to the distal colonic mucosa. About 20% of the mesalazine administered in this way is absorbed into the circulation.

2. a. **True**. There is increased risk of Crohn's disease in smokers but a slightly decreased risk of ulcerative colitis.
   b. **False**. Although mesalazine may be of some benefit in colonic Crohn's disease, it is not very effective for small-bowel Crohn's disease.
   c. **False**. Although they are effective for inducing remission, there is little evidence that corticosteroids prevent relapse.
   d. **False**. People with chronic Crohn's disease can become corticosteroid-dependent, and immunosuppressants such as azathioprine can be useful in reducing this dependence. Many months of treatment are required before they are fully effective.
3. Answer **E**.
   A. Crohn's disease is transmural but can affect any part of the gastrointestinal tract.
   B. Sulfasalazine is composed of 5-ASA, which is the active constituent, linked by an azo bond to sulfapyridine, which is responsible for many of the unwanted effects.
   C. Azathioprine is usually given in corticosteroid-refractory disease or when people are having frequent courses of corticosteroids for treatment (more than two 6-week courses per year).
   D. Infliximab is a TNFα antibody given systemically for the treatment of refractory disease.
   E. Antibacterials such as metronidazole can be useful in treating Crohn's disease, particularly if there is perianal disease.
4. Case history answers
   a. The cause of Crohn's disease is unknown. Several hypotheses have implicated a number of risk factors, including infection, altered immune response to infection and environmental factors (see Fig. 34.1)
   b. Initial treatment is with corticosteroids. Because the Crohn's disease is confined to the distal colon, topical treatment with corticosteroids, such as budesonide, could be used to limit systemic unwanted effects. If, however, there was involvement of the proximal large bowel or small bowel, it would be necessary to give an oral corticosteroid, such as prednisolone.
   c. Corticosteroids have a variety of actions. They can alter the release of inflammatory mediators such as arachidonic acid metabolites, kinins and cytokines. They can alter cell-mediated cytotoxicity, antibody production, adhesion molecule expression, phagocytic function, leucocyte chemotaxis and leucocyte adherence.
   d. Corticosteroids should be given until remission occurs. If possible, the corticosteroid should be administered locally to keep the plasma concentration low, but for individuals who experience systemic symptoms of IBD (such as fatigue, anorexia or weight loss) oral therapy is indicated.
   e. Systemic corticosteroids suppress the hypothalamic–pituitary–adrenal axis and can reduce the circulating levels of endogenous adrenal glucocorticoids (see Ch. 44). Gradual reduction of the dose of therapeutically administered glucocorticoid allows recovery of the production of endogenous corticosteroids.
   f. If the colitis is restricted to the distal colon, topical administration of mesalazine or an oral formulation that delivers 5-ASA to the colon could be used. 5-ASA is, however, less effective in Crohn's disease, particularly if it involves the small bowel.
   g. Continuous corticosteroid therapy for periods of 6 months or longer is eventually required in 40–50% of people with Crohn's disease. If more than two 6-week courses of corticosteroid per year are required to maintain control of symptoms, immunosuppressive therapy should be considered. Immunosuppressive therapy is usually with azathioprine or 6-mercaptopurine: prolonged treatment with these drugs is usually required (up to 6 months) before a clinical response occurs. TNFα antibody treatment is also of benefit in severe disease that is not responsive to other therapies.

Drugs used in inflammatory bowel disease (all drugs given orally, unless otherwise indicated)

Drug	Half-life (h) and kinetics	Comments
Aminosalicylates[a]		
Balsalazide	– [M] Bacterial azoreductases in the colon cleave the compound to release 5-aminosalicylic acid (5-ASA), the therapeutically active metabolite, and 4-aminobenzoyl-β-alanine; half-life not reported due to wide inter-individual variations	Used for mild to moderate ulcerative colitis and maintenance of remission; a prodrug which is converted to an active metabolite locally in the colon
Mesalazine (mesalamine; 5-aminosalicylic acid; 5-ASA)	0.5–1.0 [M + R + F] Uncoated tablets are well absorbed in the upper intestine after oral dosage; poor absorption after rectal administration; the absorbed fraction is eliminated largely as acetyl metabolite and partly as parent compound	Used for mild to moderate ulcerative colitis and maintenance of remission; given orally, or rectally as a foam enema or a suppository; poorly absorbed from the gut; may be more effective than sulfasalazine in the presence of diarrhoea, because there is no requirement for reduction by the gut flora

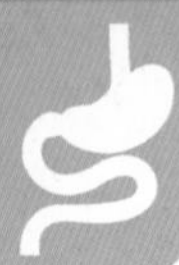

Drugs used in inflammatory bowel disease (all drugs given orally, unless otherwise indicated)

Drug	Half-life (h) and kinetics	Comments
Olsalazine	1 [M + R + F] Only 3% is absorbed in the upper intestine; bacterial azoreduction generates 5-aminosalicylate, which is partly absorbed and excreted in urine as parent drug and acetyl metabolite	Used for mild ulcerative colitis and maintenance of remission
Sulfasalazine	3–11 (parent drug) [M] About 20–30% absorbed in the small intestine; remainder passes down to anaerobic intestinal bacteria which convert it to active metabolites 6–17 (sulfapyridine) [M] Absorbed and undergoes acetylation and oxidation in the liver 4–10 (5-aminosalicylate) [M + R +F] Poor absorption from the colon; acetylated in the colonic wall and liver	Used for mild to moderate and severe ulcerative colitis and for Crohn's disease; given orally, or rectally as a retention enema or a suppository; reduced by gut bacteria to two active metabolites, sulfapyridine and 5-aminosalicylic acid, which have local actions; sulfapyridine is probably the cause of many of the unwanted effects
Cytokine inhibitors (TNFα antibodies)		
TNFα antibodies other than infliximab and adalimumab (e.g. etanercept) which are used for rheumatoid arthritis (see Ch. 30) are not currently approved for IBD		
Adalimumab	12 days [M] Protein clearance	Monoclonal antibody against TNFα; given by subcutaneous injection to those in whom infliximab is not tolerated or is ineffective
Infliximab	9.5 days [M] Metabolised by cellular uptake and proteolysis; no evidence of accumulation on repeated infusion	Monoclonal antibody against TNFα; given by intravenous infusion
Immunosuppressants		
Azathioprine	3–5 [M] Metabolised to 6-mercaptopurine which represents a bioactivation process (see Ch. 38)	Used in resistant and frequently relapsing cases of ulcerative colitis or Crohn's disease
Ciclosporin	27 [M] A lipid-soluble peptide oxidised by CYP3A4 (see Ch. 38)	Used for short-term treatment of ulcerative colitis (an unlicensed indication in the UK)
Corticosteroids	(see Ch. 44)	Budesonide, hydrocortisone and prednisolone; not suitable for maintenance treatment because of unwanted effects
Mercaptopurine	1–1.5 [M] Low oral bioavailability owing to first-pass metabolism (about 20%); bioactivated by intracellular phosphorylation; inactivated by xanthine oxidase (interaction with allopurinol – see Ch. 31)	Used in resistant and frequently relapsing cases of ulcerative colitis or Crohn's disease; main use is as an anticancer drug (see Ch. 52);
Methotrexate	8–10 [M] (see Ch. 52 for details)	May be given weekly in unresponsive or chronically active Crohn's disease; see Ch. 52 for other details
Antibiotics		
Metronidazole	6–9 [M] Complete oral bioavailability; metabolites are eliminated slowly, primarily in the urine	May be beneficial for the treatment of active Crohn's disease; used in people who fail to respond to sulfasalazine; see Ch. 51

[a]The elimination half-life of the absorbed drug is not related to the amount at the site of action.
[F], faecal excretion; [M], metabolism; [R], renal excretion.

35 Constipation, diarrhoea and irritable bowel syndrome

CONSTIPATION

Humans normally defecate with a frequency ranging from three times a day to once every 3 days (or sometimes less often). Maintenance of 'regular' bowel habits is a preoccupation of Western societies, and is best achieved by increasing dietary fibre. Nevertheless, laxative drugs are widely prescribed or taken without prescription, and are frequently abused.

Constipation affects 10% of the population, and is the passage of hard, small stools less frequently than the patient's own normal function. It is often associated with straining. There are many causes (Box 35.1).

Irritable bowel syndrome (IBS) can be constipation-predominant or diarrhoea-predominant and associated with frequent bowel movement but the sensation of incomplete evacuation (see below).

Underlying organic disease should be excluded when there is persistent constipation or if there has been a recent change in bowel habit.

LAXATIVES

The mechanisms of action of common laxatives are shown in Figure 35.1. There is overlap between the mechanisms of action of these drugs, and they are classified by their principal action.

Bulking agents

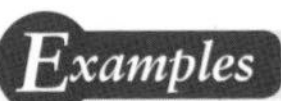

bran, ispaghula husk, methylcellulose, sterculia

Bulking agents include various natural polysaccharides, usually of plant origin, such as unprocessed wheat bran, ispaghula husk and sterculia, and methylcellulose, all of which are poorly broken down by digestive processes. They have several mechanisms of action:

- a hydrophilic action causing retention of water in the gut lumen, which expands and softens the faeces
- stimulation of colonic mucosal receptors by the increased bulk, promoting peristalsis
- proliferation of colonic bacteria, which further increases faecal bulk
- sterculia also contains polysaccharides which are degraded to substances that have an osmotic effect.

Bulking agents take at least 24 h after ingestion to work. A liberal fluid intake is important to lubricate the colon and minimise the risk of obstruction. Bulking agents are useful for establishing a regular bowel habit in chronic constipation, diverticular disease and IBS, but they should be avoided if the colon is atonic or there is faecal impaction. Regular fibre intake may also be of benefit for treatment of diarrhoea.

Unwanted effects include a sensation of bloating, flatulence or griping abdominal pain.

Osmotic laxatives

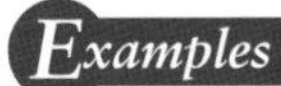

lactulose, macrogols, magnesium salts, sodium acid phosphate

Magnesium compounds, such as the sulphate (Epsom salts) and hydroxide, and lactulose are most frequently used. Magnesium salts are poorly absorbed from the gut, and act as osmotically active solutes that retain water in the colonic lumen. They may also stimulate cholecystokinin release from the small-intestinal mucosa, which increases intestinal secretions and enhances colonic motility (Fig. 35.1). These actions result in more rapid transit of gut contents into the large bowel, where distension promotes evacuation within 3 h. About 20% of ingested magnesium is absorbed and has central nervous system (CNS), cardiovascular and neuromuscular-blocking activity if it is retained in the circulation in large enough amounts, as can occur in renal failure. Magnesium hydroxide is a mild laxative, while the action of magnesium sulphate can be quite fierce, associated with considerable abdominal discomfort.

Lactulose is a disaccharide of fructose and galactose. In the colon, bacterial action releases fructose and galactose, which are fermented to lactic and acetic acids with release of gas. The fermentation products are osmotically

Box 35.1 Causes of constipation

Diet low in fibre or fluid
Disease, e.g. colonic cancer, myxoedema, hypercalcaemia
Drug-induced – frequent causes include:

- opioid analgesics (this chapter and Ch. 19)
- antimuscarinic agents, e.g. oxybutynin (Ch. 15), orphenadrine (Ch. 24), cyclizine (Ch. 32)
- antacids containing calcium or aluminium salts (Ch. 33)
- calcium channel blockers (Ch. 5)
- iron salts (Ch. 47)
- tricyclic antidepressants (Ch. 22)
- phenothiazines (Ch. 21)

Slow gut transit, especially in young women
Immobility
Hypotonic colon in the elderly or following chronic laxative abuse

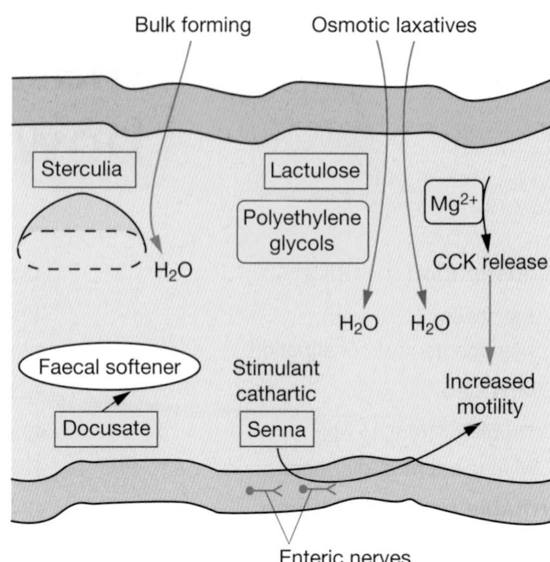

Fig. 35.1 **Sites of action of the major types of laxative drug.** CCK, cholecystokinin.

active. They also lower intestinal pH, which favours overgrowth of some selected colonic flora but inhibits the proliferation of ammonia-producing bacteria. This is useful in the treatment of hepatic encephalopathy (Ch. 36). Unwanted effects include flatulence and abdominal cramps. Lactulose can take more than 24 h to act.

Macrogols (polyethylene glycols) are large, inert molecules that are not absorbed from the gut and exert an osmotic effect in the colon; the available preparations also contain sodium salts. They are as effective as other osmotic agents, but the Na^+ content may be hazardous for people with impaired cardiac function.

Sodium acid phosphate and sodium citrate are osmotic preparations that are given as an enema or suppository, usually for bowel preparation before local procedures or surgery.

Irritant and stimulant laxatives

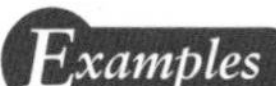

bisacodyl, dantron, senna, sodium picosulfate

These include the anthraquinones senna and dantron, and the polyphenolic compounds bisacodyl and sodium picosulfate. They act by a variety of mechanisms, including stimulation of local reflexes through myenteric nerve plexuses in the gut, which enhances gut motility and increases water and electrolyte transfer into the lower gut. Stimulant laxatives are useful for more severe forms of constipation, but tolerance is common with regular use and they can produce abdominal cramps. Given orally, they stimulate defecation after about 6–12 h.

- Senna has the most gentle purgative action of this group. Given orally, it is hydrolysed by colonic bacteria to release the irritant anthracene glycoside derivatives sennosides A and B.
- Dantron is available as co-danthramer, a combination with the surface wetting agent poloxamer '188', and as co-danthrusate, a combination with the mildly stimulant and faecal softening agent docusate (see below). Dantron is carcinogenic at high doses in animals, and it is recommended that its use in humans should be limited to the elderly or terminally ill.
- Bisacodyl can be given orally or, for a more rapid action (15–30 min), rectally; it undergoes enterohepatic circulation.
- Sodium picosulfate is a powerful irritant and is used to prepare the bowel for surgery or colonoscopy and generally acts in less than 6 h.

The chronic use of stimulant laxatives has been suspected to cause progressive deterioration of normal colonic function, with eventual atony ('cathartic colon'). It is now recognised that the condition probably arises from severe, refractory constipation, not from the treatment.

Faecal softeners

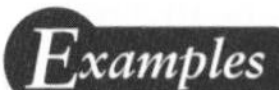

arachis oil, docusate sodium

Docusate sodium has detergent properties which may soften stools by increasing fluid and fat penetration into hard stool; it has some stimulant activity but overall it is a relatively ineffective laxative. It is given rectally or orally, alone or in combination with dantron (co-danthrusate). Arachis oil can be given rectally, or liquid paraffin orally. Liquid paraffin is not recommended since it impairs the absorption of fat-soluble vitamins, can cause anal seepage with anal pruritus, and accidental inhalation produces lipoid pneumonia.

MANAGEMENT OF CONSTIPATION

For simple constipation, adopting a high-fibre diet, supplemented by bulking agents when necessary, is recommended. Exercise and an adequate fluid intake are also important. For short-term use, a stimulant laxative such as senna or bisacodyl can be taken orally at night to give a morning bowel action. Suppositories will give a more rapid effect. For longer-term therapy, regular magnesium salts or macrogols are usually well tolerated and effective.

Senna, magnesium salts and docusate appear to be safe in pregnancy. Bisacodyl, co-danthramer and co-danthrusate are suitable for the elderly or for the terminally ill with opioid-induced constipation. The peripheral opioid receptor antagonist, methylnaltrexone, can be added if laxatives are ineffective (Ch. 19). Lactulose is useful as a second-line agent and specifically to treat constipation associated with hepatic encephalopathy (Chs 36 and 56). For people in whom neurological disease is the cause of constipation, a faecal softener should be used, with regular enemas or rectal washouts.

Refractory idiopathic constipation is a condition almost exclusively found in women, starting at a young age. Long-term use of stimulant laxatives, often at high dosage, may be necessary. Bulk laxatives are ineffective, and a high-fibre diet usually increases abdominal distension and discomfort. Biofeedback can help in up to 80% of people with the condition. For those who fail with these approaches, surgical intervention with colectomy may be the only option.

DIARRHOEA

Diarrhoea is frequent watery bowel movements, with or without gas and cramping. Severe acute diarrhoea is usually a result of gastrointestinal infection, and it can be the consequence of both reduced absorption of fluid and an increase in intestinal secretions. Viral gastroenteritis is much more common than bacterial causes of diarrhoea in children, but viral and bacterial causes are both important in adults. Traveller's diarrhoea is a particularly common problem because of exposure of the traveller to organisms which have not been encountered before. Common causes include enterotoxin-producing *Escherichia coli*, *Clostridium jejuni* and *Salmonella* and *Shigella* species. Parasites such as *Giardia lamblia*, *Cryptosporidium* species and *Cyclospora cayetanensis* are less commonly involved. Diarrhoea may result from local release of bacterial enterotoxins, which have a variety of actions on gut mucosal cells, including stimulation of intracellular cAMP synthesis, which causes excess Cl^- secretion into the bowel.

Drugs that can produce diarrhoea include magnesium salts (see above), cytotoxic agents (Ch. 52), α- and β-adrenoceptor antagonists (Chs 5 and 6), and broad-spectrum antibacterial drugs, which produce diarrhoea by altering colonic flora (Ch. 51). Antibacterial treatment can be associated with *Clostridium difficile* colitis.

Chronic diarrhoea requires full investigation for non-infectious causes such as carcinoma of the colon, inflammatory bowel disease and coeliac disease. Irritable bowel syndrome is often accompanied by faecal frequency, loose stool and a sensation of incomplete evacuation (see below).

DRUGS FOR TREATING DIARRHOEA

Opioids

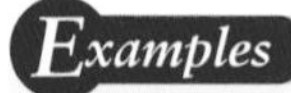

codeine phosphate, diphenoxylate, loperamide

The anti-motility action of opioids is a result of binding to μ-receptors on neurons in the submucosal neural plexus of the intestinal wall (Ch. 19). This enhances segmental contractions in the colon, inhibits propulsive movements of the small intestine and colon, and prolongs the transit time of intestinal contents. These actions provide the opportunity for enhanced absorption of fluids. The opioids most often used to treat diarrhoea are codeine, loperamide and diphenoxylate (used in combination with atropine as co-phenotrope). Most have short half-lives (<5 h). Loperamide has a more rapid onset of action, and a longer half-life (11 h), giving it a longer duration of action. It is more selective for the gut because high first-pass metabolism limits systemic absorption and, in contrast to other opioids, dependence is not a problem. Loperamide has additional antimuscarinic activity that also inhibits peristalsis (also achieved by atropine in co-phenotrope) and it increases anal tone. Morphine is sometimes used to treat diarrhoea in combination with kaolin (see below). Unwanted effects of opioid drugs are discussed in Chapter 19.

Adsorbent and bulking agents

Kaolin is an adsorbent that is relatively ineffective, and is not recommended for the treatment of acute diarrhoea. Ispaghula and methylcellulose are bulking agents that can help to control faecal consistency in diarrhoea-predominant irritable bowel syndrome, or for people with an ileostomy or colostomy. They are not recommended for treatment of acute diarrhoea.

MANAGEMENT OF DIARRHOEA

In developed countries, most people with acute infective diarrhoea who are otherwise fit generally require only high oral fluid intake. Fluid and electrolyte balance are particularly important in young children and the elderly, as they can dehydrate more quickly. Specially formulated powders containing electrolytes (particularly Na^+ and K^+) and glucose are available, which, when correctly reconstituted with clean water, provide a balanced rehydration solution. Replacement of electrolytes is as important as fluid replacement. Intravenous fluids may be required in severe dehydration.

If drug treatment is required, an opioid is useful for mild to moderate diarrhoea. They should be avoided in dysentery, when prolonging contact of the organism with the gut mucosa can be detrimental. In young children, ileus with severe abdominal distention can occur with opioids, and it is recommended that they are not used in this age group.

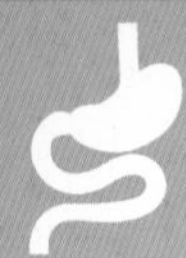

Antibacterial prophylaxis can be used to prevent traveller's diarrhoea in people visiting high-risk areas. Co-trimoxazole or ciprofloxacin are most often recommended (Ch. 51), depending on the area to which the person is travelling. Alternatively, the antibacterial can be taken at the first sign of illness, and it will usually shorten the duration of the attack to less than 24 h.

Antibacterial-induced diarrhoea usually resolves rapidly on stopping the provoking drug. In prolonged, severe cases, or when *Clostridium difficile* colitis is suspected or *Clostridium difficile* toxin has been detected in the stool, treatment with oral metronidazole or vancomycin should be given (Ch. 51).

Diarrhoea in inflammatory bowel disease should be treated by management of the underlying condition. Antidiarrhoeals should not be used in active inflammatory bowel disease, because of the risk of precipitating toxic megacolon (see Ch. 34).

IRRITABLE BOWEL SYNDROME

Irritable bowel syndrome (IBS) is said to occur in 15% of the population. IBS is characterised by abdominal distension, bloating and alteration in bowel habit. There are two overlapping clinical presentations, constipation-predominant and diarrhoea-predominant. Abdominal discomfort may be relieved by defecation, but there is a sensation of incomplete evacuation and mucus is often passed per rectum. The cause is unknown, but a generalised motor and/or sensory disorder of the gastrointestinal tract is likely. A strong psychological component is also evident and the brain–gut axis is thought to play an important role. However, studies examining the role of the autonomic nervous system, the hypothalamic–pituitary–adrenal axis and disordered gut motility have shown variable results.

DRUGS FOR TREATING IRRITABLE BOWEL SYNDROME

Antimuscarinic drugs

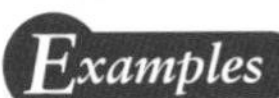

dicycloverine, propantheline

Mechanism of action

Antimuscarinic drugs reduce colonic motility by inhibiting parasympathetic stimulation of the myenteric and submucosal neural plexuses. They also inhibit gastric emptying.

Pharmacokinetics

Oral absorption of dicycloverine is good and it is metabolised in the liver. The half-life is 9–10 h. Propantheline is a poorly absorbed quaternary amine; most is hydrolysed in the bowel. Further details of these drugs can be found in Chapter 4.

Other antispasmodic agents

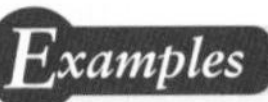

alverine citrate, mebeverine, peppermint oil

Mechanism of action

These antispasmodic agents have direct smooth muscle relaxant properties (possibly by phosphodiesterase inhibition). They can relieve gut spasm and the associated pain.

Pharmacokinetics

Oral absorption of mebeverine is rapid and it undergoes extensive first-pass metabolism. The half-life of the main metabolite is short. Little is known about the pharmacokinetics of alverine citrate and peppermint oil.

Unwanted effects

These are rare but include:

- Gastrointestinal disturbances
- Headache
- Insomnia with mebeverine.

MANAGEMENT OF IRRITABLE BOWEL SYNDROME

Drug therapy should form only part of the treatment, supplemented by counselling, relaxation and hypnotherapy where appropriate. Hypnosis is effective in up to 60% of people, but should be given by a properly trained therapist. Reductions in tea and coffee consumption and smoking, and modification of diet may be helpful, and studies with probiotics containing lactobacilli or bifidobacteria look promising.

Constipation can be treated with bulking agents such as ispaghula husk, or, if colonic transit time is very prolonged, an osmotic laxative may be effective. Diarrhoea can be ameliorated with an opioid. Loperamide is useful in true diarrhoea-predominant IBS because it has a rapid onset of action and enables people to control their bowels, particularly when out of their normal environment or in other circumstances where diarrhoea would be socially disruptive. Care has to be taken with other opioids because of the risks of dependency and opioid-induced abdominal pain. Regular use of small doses of a laxative or antidiarrhoeal drug may be preferable to intermittent use.

Treatments for diarrhoea in IBS do not usually reduce the abdominal pain. There may be benefit from antispasmodic agents or low-dose tricyclic antidepressants or, possibly, selective serotonin reuptake inhibitors (Ch. 22). Proton pump inhibitors (Ch. 33) may relieve diarrhoea by reducing the gastro-colic reflex.

Overall, current treatment of IBS is unsatisfactory. Serotonin $5HT_3$ receptor antagonists (for diarrhoea-predominant IBS) and $5HT_4$ receptor agonists (for constipation-predominant IBS) are available in some countries, but currently not in the UK. Ischaemic colitis has been a problem with some $5HT_3$ receptor antagonists. Agents acting at 5HT receptors give only modest improvement. Novel therapeutic approaches to the management of IBS may be developed as our understanding of the physiology of the gut, and the neurotransmitters that regulate it, improves.

FURTHER READING

Andresen V, Camilleri M (2006) Irritable bowel syndrome. Recent and novel therapeutic approaches. *Drugs* 66, 1073–1088

Barbara G, De Giorgio R, Stanghellini V et al (2004) New pathophysiological mechanisms in irritable bowel syndrome. *Aliment Pharmacol Ther* 20(suppl 2), 1–9

Lembo A, Camilleri M (2003) Chronic constipation. *N Engl J Med* 349, 1360–1368

Mayer EA (2008) Irritable bowel syndrome. *N Engl J Med* 358, 1692–1699

Spiller R (2007) Clinical update: irritable bowel syndrome. *Lancet* 369, 1586–1588

Spiller R, Aziz Q, Creed F et al (2007) Guidelines on the irritable bowel syndrome: mechanisms and practical management. *Gut* 56, 1770–1798

Thielman NM (2004) Acute infectious diarrhea. *N Engl J Med* 350, 38–47

Thomas J, Karver S, Cooney GA (2008) Methylnaltrexone for opioid-induced constipation in advanced illness. *New Engl J Med* 358, 2332–2343

Wald A (2007) Appropriate use of laxatives in the management of constipation. *Curr Gastroenterol Rep* 9, 410–414

SELF-ASSESSMENT

In questions 1–4, the first statement, in italics, is true. Are the accompanying statements also true?

1. *Regulation of gastrocolonic motility involves the CNS, the enteric nervous system and gastrointestinal hormones.*
   a. Defecation of stools of normal form and consistency once every 3 days in the absence of any organic disease requires investigation.
   b. The majority of cases of 'simple' constipation can be treated by lifestyle changes.
   c. Chronic intake of senna causes progressive hyperactivity of colonic motility.
2. *A drug history is important in investigation of people with chronic constipation or diarrhoea.*
   a. Antacids containing aluminium salts can cause constipation.
   b. All laxatives act to stimulate bowel movements within 3–6 h.
3. *The causes of diarrhoea are many but can be largely of psychological origin in some people.*
   a. In infants (<2 years), infectious diarrhoea is mainly caused by bacteria.
   b. Pseudomembranous colitis may result from the use of broad-spectrum antibacterial drugs.
   c. The use of antidiarrhoeal agents may increase the residence of entero-invasive bacteria in the gut.
4. *In industrialised countries, the use of antibacterials to treat acute episodes of diarrhoea is rarely necessary.*
   a. There is little resistance among *Vibrio cholera* strains to tetracycline.
   b. Oral rehydration powders must be reconstituted with water to give a hypertonic solution.
5. Choose the one **correct** option from the following statements concerning laxatives.
   A. The use of bulk laxatives should be accompanied by drinking plenty of water.
   B. Magnesium sulphate acts as a laxative by inhibiting cholecystokinin release.
   C. Lactulose works by stimulating the enteric nerves.
   D. Aluminium hydroxide can cause diarrhoea.
   E. Sterculia acts as a laxative within 12 h.
6. Choose the one **incorrect** option from the following statements about diarrhoea.
   A. Rotavirus is an uncommon cause of diarrhoea in adults.
   B. *Campylobacter jejuni* is a Gram-negative microaerophilic bacterium.
   C. In developed countries, *Campylobacter jejuni* is the commonest cause of bacterial gastroenteritis.
   D. Loperamide decreases the gut residence time of the infective organism.
   E. In the UK, oral fluid replacement is all that is generally required for treating acute diarrhoea in otherwise healthy adults.

ANSWERS

1. a. **False**. Defecation once every 3 days or three times a day is not abnormal.
   b. **True**. Increased fibre intake and exercise will help in the majority of cases of 'simple' constipation.
   c. **False**. Chronic use has been associated with loss of colonic function, with damage to the myenteric plexus (cathartic colon). It was long considered that this condition was caused by the inappropriate prolonged use of stimulant laxatives; however, it is now thought that it is probably due to the refractory constipation rather than to drug use.
2. a. **True**. Aluminium salts cause constipation, as do many other drugs, including some antidepressants, opioid analgesics and calcium channel blockers.
   b. **False**. Some laxatives (magnesium salts) can act within 6 h, whereas lactulose and docusate take considerably longer to exert their activity.
3. a. **False**. Viral gastroenteritis is a major cause of infant diarrhoea and rotavirus predominates.
   b. **True**. Overgrowth of the anaerobe *Clostridium difficile* following usage of broad-spectrum antibacterials can occur and is increasingly resistant to metronidazole treatment.

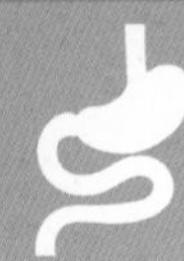

   c. **True**. However, the clinical importance of this is debated.
4. a. **False**. There are now frequent epidemics of cholera that are resistant to tetracycline.
   b. **False**. A hypertonic solution will have an osmotic action drawing water into the bowel; the formulated solution should be isotonic or slightly hypotonic.
5. Answer **A**.
   A. Correct. Adequate water intake is necessary when constipation is treated with bulk laxatives.
   B. Incorrect. Magnesium sulphate is an osmotic laxative but also stimulates cholecystokinin release, which stimulates enteric nerves.
   C. Incorrect. Lactulose is an osmotic laxative.
   D. Incorrect. Aluminium hydroxide causes constipation.
   E. Incorrect. Sterculia is a bulking laxative and takes more than 24 h to act.
6. Answer **D**.
   A. Correct. Rotavirus causes diarrhoea in young children but is a very uncommon cause in adults.
   B. Correct. *Campylobacter jejuni* is a Gram-negative microaerophilic bacterium.
   C. Correct. *Campylobacter jejuni* is the commonest cause of gastroenteritis in adults in developed countries.
   D. Incorrect. Loperamide inhibits gut contractility and may increase the residence of invasive organisms.
   E. Correct. In otherwise healthy individuals, oral rehydration is all that is required; in the very young or elderly, intravenous rehydration may be required.

Drugs used in constipation, diarrhoea and irritable bowel syndrome (all given orally unless otherwise indicated)

Drug	Half-life (h) and kinetics	Comments
Constipation		
Bulk and osmotic laxatives	–	Act because of their lack of absorption; uptake and systemic disposition is not relevant to their therapeutic effects (*brans, ispaghula husk, sterculia, lactitol, lactulose, macrogols [polyethylene glycol], magnesium salts and rectal phosphates or sodium citrate*); bulking agents may affect the absorption of nutrients and minerals
Gut stimulants	–	Some gut stimulants may undergo significant absorption and produce unwanted systemic effects, for example *dantron* produce liver damage; *senna compounds* such as sennoside are degraded by the gut microflora and produce local effects; *bisacodyl* is a stimulant laxative that can be given orally or rectally; *sodium picosulfate* acts as a poorly absorbed stimulant often used before bowel surgery and colonoscopy
Faecal-softening agents	–	*Docusate sodium* probably acts as both a softening agent and a stimulant; *glycerol* or *arachis oil* may be given as a suppository or enema, respectively, to produce a local softening effect; oral liquid paraffin can be used to produce softening, but long-term treatment is not recommended and can result in anal leakage and irritation
Diarrhoea		
Anti-motility drugs such as opioids should be used for treatment of acute uncomplicated diarrhoea in adults but not in young children		
Adsorbents	–	Kaolin is given orally and acts because of its lack of absorption
Codeine	3–4 [M] Oxidised to morphine (about 5%) by CYP2D6; see Ch. 19	Opioid
Diphenoxylate	2–3 [M] Oral bioavailability limited; metabolised in liver to an active metabolite, diphenoxylic acid, which has a half-life of 3–14 h; see Ch. 19	Opioid; given as co-phenotrope (co-formulation with atropine)
Loperamide	11 [M] Oral bioavailability is 40%; undergoes hepatic metabolism mainly by CYP2C8 and CYP3A4; 30% excreted unchanged in faeces; see Ch. 19	Opioid; main effect is due to parent drug prior to absorption

Drugs used in constipation, diarrhoea and irritable bowel syndrome (all given orally unless otherwise indicated)

Drug	Half-life (h) and kinetics	Comments
Morphine	1–5 [M] Oral bioavailability is low (10–50%); eliminated by conjugation with glucuronic acid; see Ch. 19	Opioid; used in combination with kaolin for short-term treatment of diarrhoea
Irritable bowel syndrome		
Treatment comprises antispasmodic drugs, including antimuscarinic drugs (all are shown for completeness)		
Alverine citrate	? Few data available	Smooth muscle relaxant used for irritable bowel disease, as an adjunct in disorders characterised by spasm, and also for dysmenorrhoea
Atropine	12 [M + R] Rapidly absorbed and crosses the blood–brain barrier and the placenta; metabolised in the liver to tropic acid and other metabolites	Antimuscarinic used for symptom relief in disorders characterised by spasm of the gastrointestinal tract, also used for mydriasis and cycloplegia and as a premedication; good oral absorption; significant antimuscarinic unwanted effects limit use
Dicycloverine	9–10 [R] Rapidly absorbed; oral bioavailability about 50%; eliminated in urine	Antimuscarinic used for symptom relief in disorders characterised by spasm of the gastrointestinal tract, including irritable bowel disease; less severe antimuscarinic unwanted effects than atropine
Hyoscine	8 [M] Radiolabelled studies indicate incomplete oral absorption (but good activity orally); hydrolysed to inactive products	Antimuscarinic used for symptom relief in disorders characterised by spasm of the gastrointestinal tract and smooth muscle spasm in genitourinary disorders; can be given orally or by intramuscular or intravenous injection; poor oral absorption; antimuscarinic unwanted effects limit use
Mebeverine	? [M] Negligible absorption intact due to first-pass metabolism; metabolised rapidly by oxidation to mebeverine alcohol, and then to the acid (half-life of 1 h)	Smooth muscle relaxant used for irritable bowel disease and in disorders characterised by spasm of the gastrointestinal tract
Propantheline	1.5–2 [M] Incomplete oral absorption (10–25%); metabolites excreted as glucuronic acid conjugates	Antimuscarinic used for symptom relief in disorders characterised by spasm of the gastrointestinal tract, including irritable bowel disease

[M], metabolism; [R], renal excretion.

36 Liver disease

ACUTE AND SUBACUTE LIVER FAILURE

Liver failure arises from a number of insults to liver cells, principally viral infection (such as hepatitis B) or the toxic effects of drugs and chemicals. In the UK, paracetamol poisoning (Ch. 53) is the most common cause of acute liver failure.

Presenting symptoms of liver failure are often non-specific, with malaise, nausea and abdominal pain. As the syndrome progresses, signs of impairment of brain function occur (hepatic encephalopathy) with initial confusion followed by drowsiness and coma. These clinical features reflect alterations in neurotransmitter synthesis and increased central nervous system (CNS) neuroinhibition, caused by endogenous toxins that the liver fails to remove.

The syndrome of liver failure can be categorised by the speed of onset of encephalopathy after the onset of jaundice:

- hyperacute – onset within 7 days
- acute – onset between 7 and 28 days
- subacute – onset between 29 days and 12 weeks; in this form, ascites and renal failure may also be prominent.

MANAGEMENT

Acetylcysteine should be given if paracetamol was the precipitant (Ch. 53) and it may be useful in other forms of acute liver failure through beneficial effects on microcirculatory haemodynamics. Other management is supportive and includes:

- prevention of bacterial and fungal infection with broad-spectrum antibacterial and antifungal agents
- prevention of cerebral oedema by appropriate fluid management; if cerebral oedema arises, then mechanical ventilation and infusion of mannitol (Ch. 14) can reduce the resulting oedema
- prevention of hypoglycaemia with intravenous dextrose
- control of coagulopathy with intravenous vitamin K (Ch. 11), or fresh frozen plasma or cryoprecipitate if there is active bleeding
- treatment of shock, often with vasoconstrictors such as terlipressin (see below)
- artificial support for renal failure by maintaining circulating blood volume, and, if necessary, with haemofiltration or haemodialysis.

Liver transplantation is necessary for many people.

CHRONIC LIVER DISEASE

There are many causes of chronic liver disease, most of which ultimately lead to fibrotic changes in the liver that eventually alter the liver architecture and lead to distortion of the vasculature within the liver. This advanced change is called cirrhosis, and in the UK is most often caused by alcohol or hepatitis C. Hepatitis B is the most common cause in many developing countries. Other causes include autoimmune hepatitis, haemochromatosis, Wilson's disease and α_1-antitrypsin deficiency. The diagnosis of liver cirrhosis is often made when complications arise (often referred to as decompensated cirrhosis), which include variceal haemorrhage, spontaneous bacterial peritonitis and hepatic encephalopathy (see below).

AUTOIMMUNE LIVER DISEASE

There are three principal forms of autoimmune liver disease: autoimmune hepatitis, primary biliary cirrhosis (PBC), and primary sclerosing cholangitis, which is less common. The pathogenesis of these diseases is poorly understood, but the occurrence of autoimmune phenomena (such as circulating autoantibodies) and histological evidence of immunologically competent cells in the inflammatory infiltrate in the

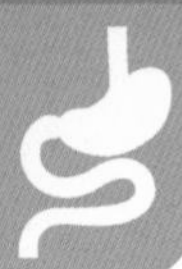

liver has encouraged the use of immunosuppressant treatments. Without treatment, autoimmune hepatitis usually progresses to cirrhosis.

MANAGEMENT

There are several therapeutic options for autoimmune hepatitis.

- Corticosteroids, usually prednisolone (Ch. 44), induce remission in 85% of people with autoimmune hepatitis, but, when used alone, up to 50% of those treated will still have developed cirrhosis after 10 years.
- Azathioprine (Ch. 38) has a corticosteroid-sparing action in autoimmune hepatitis and is widely used in combination with corticosteroids, both to induce remission and for maintenance therapy.
- Ciclosporin, tacrolimus or mycophenolate (Ch. 38) are used for autoimmune hepatitis that has not responded to corticosteroids. Evidence for their effectiveness is limited.
- Treatment of PBC is less satisfactory because immunosuppression is ineffective. Ursodeoxycholic acid is the only drug licensed for use in PBC in the UK. This is a bile acid that is produced by bacterial oxidation of chenodeoxycholic acid. It retards progression of the disease by a cytoprotective effect (by reducing nitric oxide synthesis), immune modulation and suppression of the cytotoxic effects of other bile acids. The main unwanted effect is diarrhoea. About one-third of people treated will have a response, with reduction in elevated liver enzymes, and a reduced risk of either death or the need for liver transplantation.
- Supportive therapy is necessary to reduce the complications that can arise from malabsorption of fat-soluble vitamins. Vitamin D (Ch. 42) and vitamin A supplements are most often needed.
- Primary sclerosing cholangitis is also responsive to ursodeoxycholic acid, but, unlike PBC, it may also respond to immunosuppression with prednisolone or azathioprine.
- Liver transplantation is necessary for end-stage disease in all autoimmune liver disease, and it has good long-term results.

CHRONIC VIRAL HEPATITIS

There are two important hepatic viral infections that can cause chronic hepatitis: hepatitis B virus (HBV; a DNA virus) and hepatitis C virus (HCV; an RNA virus). The end result of the chronic inflammation produced by these viruses is cirrhosis.

DRUGS FOR TREATMENT OF VIRAL HEPATITIS

Interferon alfa

Mechanism of action and effects

Interferons are glycoprotein cytokines that are produced by virus-infected cells, and protect uninfected cells of the same type. Interferon alfa binds to cell surface receptors and stimulates production of enzymes in the host cell that inhibit viral mRNA translation by host ribosomes. This inhibits viral replication, and augments viral clearance from infected hepatocytes (Ch. 51). There are two forms of Interferon alfa: Interferon alfa-2a has lysine in position 23, while alfa-2b has methionine in this position. Interferons are obtained either by recombinant DNA technology or from virus-stimulated leucocytes.

Pharmacokinetics

Interferon alfa is given by subcutaneous injection three times a week for 4–6 months. It is metabolised in the kidney, and has a short half-life (3–4 h). Pegylated (polyethylene glycol-conjugated) derivatives of interferon alfa are available that prolong the presence of the interferon in the blood, and these are given once weekly.

Unwanted effects

- Immediate effects are almost universal and include headache, myalgia, fever and rigors, usually occurring 4–6 h after injection. Tolerance occurs with repeated use.
- Delayed effects include fatigue and anorexia.
- Bone marrow suppression.

Nucleoside analogues

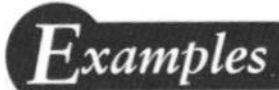

adefovir dipivoxil, entecavir, lamivudine, ribavirin

Mechanism of action and uses

Nucleoside analogues inhibit viral polymerase, reduce RNA and protein synthesis, and suppress viral replication (Ch. 51). Lamivudine is a cytidine nucleoside analogue and has similar efficacy to interferon alfa in chronic hepatitis B. Resistance of HBV to lamivudine is found in 10–25% of people who are treated for 1 year. Adefovir is an adenosine nucleoside analogue used for treatment of hepatitis B. It is effective against viruses that have become resistant to lamivudine. Adefovir additionally enhances immune responsiveness through stimulation of the production of endogenous tumour necrosis factor alpha. Entecavir is a guanosine nucleotide analogue that is also used in hepatitis B for viruses that have become resistant to lamivudine. Ribavirin is a synthetic nucleoside analogue with activity against some RNA and DNA viruses. It inhibits viral RNA synthesis by blocking incorporation of uridine and cytidine. It also increases the production of antiviral cytokines. Ribavirin has little effect on viral replication when used alone, but it enhances the efficacy of interferon alfa against HCV. Ribavirin is also used by inhalation to treat respiratory syncytial virus infection.

Pharmacokinetics

Nucleoside analogues are well absorbed from the gut. They are inactive prodrugs that are metabolised intracellularly to the active phosphorylated derivatives, and then eliminated by the kidney. The half-lives of lamivudine and adefovir are 5–7 h and 8 h, respectively, whereas entcavir and ribavarin have very long half-lives, varying from 5 to 14 days.

Unwanted effects

- Anorexia, abdominal pain, nausea, vomiting, diarrhoea
- Cough, dyspnoea
- Headache, dizziness, insomnia, fatigue
- Rashes
- Muscle disorders with lamivudine
- Accumulation of ribavirin in red cells produces haemolysis
- Interstitial pneumonitis, palpitation, chest pain, syncope with ribavirin
- Renal failure with adefovir.

MANAGEMENT OF CHRONIC VIRAL HEPATITIS

Chronic hepatitis B

There is no role for drug treatment in acute hepatitis B, which usually resolves spontaneously. Chronic infection is characterised by persistence of hepatitis B surface antigen (HBsAg) and other immunological markers at least 6 months after the acute infection. Antiviral treatment should be used if there is evidence of active chronic infection with ongoing liver damage and high viral replication (high titre of HBV-DNA). This is usually, but not always, associated with hepatitis Be antigen (HBeAg) in plasma as a marker of active viral replication. The criteria for successful treatment are a matter of debate. Seroconversion to HBe antibody only occurs in a minority of those who are treated, and even fewer seroconvert to HBsAg, which is the ideal outcome. Measurement of HBV-DNA is a sensitive way to monitor treatment and detect drug resistance. Interferon alfa achieves seroconversion in about one-third of cases, with no difference between the pegylated and non-pegylated forms of the drug. About 40% of those treated will show a conversion to low viral replication, and about 10% will have complete eradication. Treatment should be stopped after 3–4 months if there is no response, or continued for up to a year if suppression of viral replication is achieved. A further course of treatment with interferon alfa can be given for relapse after initial successful therapy.

If cirrhosis is more advanced, or if interferon alfa therapy has been unsuccessful or poorly tolerated, then lamivudine is usually used. Complete eradication of the virus by lamivudine is unusual, but about two-thirds of people who take lamivudine will show viral suppression after 3 years of treatment. Long-term treatment is given to people with cirrhosis. The relapse rate on withdrawal of lamivudine is high, with only about 10% of people showing long-term responses once treatment is discontinued. Emergence of viral strains with drug resistance to lamivudine is common and occurs progressively, with a 15–30% prevalence of resistant strains after 1 year of treatment. Adefovir or entecavir is used to treat viruses that develop resistance to lamivudine, or for those who cannot tolerate lamivudine. Viral resistance to adefovir or entecavir is unusual.

Chronic hepatitis C

The aim of treatment is eradication of the virus. If left untreated, about 85% of people who are infected develop chronic infection, and of these up to 30% will develop cirrhosis. Treatment with pegylated interferon alfa alone can eradicate the virus, with a 15% sustained response rate. It can also prevent liver damage even if eradication is not successful [treatment duration and success depend on the viral strain, or genotype of which three are found in Europe]. The addition of ribavirin increases the overall response rate to 45% for genotype 1 and 80% for genotype 2 or 3, and the combination is standard therapy for all people who can tolerate both drugs. For genotypes 2 or 3, 24 weeks' treatment is sufficient for a maximal response, while treatment for genotype 1 (the most common type in developed countries) should be continued for 48 weeks in those who have a response in the first 24 weeks. Pegylated interferons produce up to a 10% higher response rate than the conventional interferons. There is no treatment currently available for those who fail to respond to a combination of interferon alfa and ribavirin, although other antiviral drugs are being evaluated in clinical trials.

CHRONIC HEPATIC ENCEPHALOPATHY

Many chronic liver diseases predispose to the neuropsychiatric disturbance known as chronic hepatic encephalopathy. The clinical features are similar to those occurring in acute liver failure. Spontaneous bacterial peritonitis is a common cause of deterioration in previously compensated liver failure. In people with chronic encephalopathy nutritional support may be necessary, and malabsorption of fat-soluble vitamins can be a particular problem if there is cholestasis. Osteoporosis can result, made worse by the use of corticosteroids.

MANAGEMENT

- Lactulose (Ch. 35) can be given orally to reduce colonic production of neurotoxins (particularly ammonia) by decreasing intestinal transit time and increasing nitrogen fixation by colonic bacteria. The evidence that lactulose is effective has recently been challenged.
- Oral antibacterials such as neomycin or metronidazole (Ch. 51) reduce bacterial ammonia production in the colon. Neomycin is less favoured because of its potential to cause nephrotoxicity and ototoxicity, even though little is absorbed from the gut.
- Careful attention to nutrition is required, especially an appropriate carbohydrate and protein intake.
- Fat malabsorption can be treated with medium-chain triglyceride supplements, and sufficient calorie intake should be ensured. Fat-soluble vitamin supplements (A, D, E, K) may be needed. Metabolic bone disease may require treatment with bisphosphonates (Ch. 42).
- Sepsis, including spontaneous bacterial peritonitis, is often due to bowel flora and should be treated with intravenous broad-spectrum antibacterial drugs, such as cefuroxime with metronidazole (Ch. 51).

VARICEAL HAEMORRHAGE

Gastro-oesophageal varices are large collateral venous communications that develop in portal hypertension, often

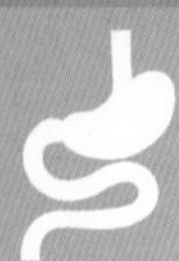

at the gastro-oesophageal junction but also at other places such as the rectum. They arise from a combination of increases in splanchnic blood flow and in the resistance to portal blood flow within the liver. Varices are found in 70% of people with cirrhosis and they carry a high risk of haemorrhage, from which mortality is 30–50%. Varices form after the hepatic venous pressure gradient rises above 10 mmHg, and the probability of rupture is high when the pressure gradient reaches 12 mmHg.

MANAGEMENT

Management of bleeding gastro-oesophageal varices

- Repletion of blood volume can be carried out with colloid solution, or preferably with whole blood. Impaired coagulation and thrombocytopenia are common findings in advanced liver disease, and transfusion of platelet concentrates and fresh frozen plasma may be necessary. The risk of bacterial infections is high in acute variceal bleeding, and short-term antibacterial prophylaxis with an agent such as ciprofloxacin (Ch. 51) should be given.
- Endoscopic variceal injection with a sclerosant is successful in up to 95% of cases. The main complications are oesophageal ulceration, increased risk of infections, and pleural effusions. Variceal band ligation is as effective as sclerosant therapy, and is now preferred in many centres.
- Endoscopic variceal injection of a cyanoacrylate tissue adhesive is effective for bleeding gastric varices, and is successful in 80% of cases. It is also an option for oesophageal varices. These compounds are tissue glues that polymerise on contact with water or blood.
- Balloon tamponade to compress the bleeding point achieves control in 80–90% of bleeding varices. It is often used to treat re-bleeding after endoscopic sclerosant therapy or as a holding measure, and is rarely used as a first-line treatment.
- A transjugular intrahepatic portosystemic shunt (TIPS) is used as rescue therapy when sclerosant therapy has failed.
- Terlipressin (N-triglycyl-8-lysine-vasopressin) is a synthetic vasopressin analogue (Ch. 43). Given intravenously, it produces splanchnic vasoconstriction, reduces portal pressure and reduces bleeding from varices. Terlipressin is a prodrug that is slowly converted to lypressin, and can be given by bolus injection. Unwanted effects are uncommon. It is mainly used when endoscopic sclerosant therapy is not immediately available. Vasopressin also has been used to treat bleeding varices, but has a shorter duration of action than terlipressin and must be given by intravenous infusion. Systemic vasoconstriction causes ischaemic complications in up to 50% of those treated with vasopressin. It is therefore little used, although co-administration of the vasodilator glyceryl trinitrate (Ch. 5) reduces the systemic complication rate.
- Octreotide (Ch. 43) and somatostatin (Ch. 43) are probably as effective as vasopressin for stopping haemorrhage, but there is less convincing evidence compared with terlipressin. They also work by reducing portal venous pressure.

Prevention of variceal re-bleeding

- Splanchnic vasoconstrictors that lower portal flow and reduce portal pressure by at least 20% will reduce the risk of re-bleeding to about 10% at 2 years. This is most often achieved by the use of a non-selective β-adrenoceptor antagonist such as propranolol (Ch. 5). Sometimes, isosorbide mononitrate (Ch. 5) is added to vasodilate the portal circulation and further reduce portal flow. However, this can produce systemic hypotension and worsen salt and water retention.
- Local treatment of the varices, for example by banding, will reduce the risk of re-bleeding, but does not reduce portal pressure. In about 50% of cases, the varices will recur within 2 years. Banding is usually reserved for those who do not respond to drug therapy.
- TIPS is most commonly used for elective prevention of further bleeding. It can lead to chronic encephalopathy and other significant adverse effects, so is only undertaken in specialist centres. Surgical creation of a portosystemic shunt is an alternative to TIPS. This is used when the previous treatments have failed.

ASCITES

Ascites in chronic liver disease arises largely as a result of splanchnic vasodilation. Portal hypertension results in local production of vasodilators, which reduce effective circulating blood volume. This promotes salt and water retention in the kidney due to activation of the renin–angiotensin system. The increased portal pressure combined with vasodilation leads to transudation of fluid into the peritoneal cavity. Spontaneous bacterial peritonitis can complicate ascites associated with liver disease and make the ascites resistant to treatment.

MANAGEMENT

The presence of ascites in chronic liver disease is associated with a poor prognosis, with a 5-year survival of 30–40%, unless there is liver transplantation. Management of ascites includes:

- reduction of salt intake
- diuretic therapy, starting with a potassium-sparing diuretic such as spironolactone or amiloride (Ch. 14); a low dose of furosemide can be added after a few days, with care taken to avoid hypovolaemia and consequent prerenal failure
- large-volume ascites usually requires drainage by paracentesis in addition to diuretics as maintenance therapy; paracentesis should be accompanied by plasma expansion with albumin to maintain circulating blood volume
- refractory ascites that fails to respond to high doses of diuretics or recurs rapidly after paracentesis may need repeated large-volume paracentesis with intravenous albumin replacement.

FURTHER READING

Bass NM (2007) The current pharmacological therapies for hepatic encephalopathy. *Aliment Pharmacol Ther* 25(suppl 1), 23–31

Bosch J, Garcia-Pagan JC (2003) Prevention of variceal rebleeding. *Lancet* 361, 952–954

Chapman R (2003) The management of primary sclerosing cholangitis. *Curr Gastroenterol Rep* 5, 9–17

Dienstag JL (2008) Drug Therapy: hepatitis B virus infection. *N Engl J Med* 359, 1486–1500

Ferguson JW, Tripathi D, Hayes PC (2006) Review article: the management of acute variceal bleeding. *Aliment Pharmacol Ther* 18, 253–262

Ginès P, Cárdenas A, Arroyo V et al (2004) Management of cirrhosis and ascites. *N Engl J Med* 350, 1646–1654

Khan SA, Shah N, Williams R et al (2006) Acute liver failure: a review. *Clin Liver Dis* 10, 239–258

Lata J, Hulek P, Vanasek T (2003) Management of acute variceal bleeding. *Dig Dis* 21, 6–15

Liaw Y-F, Chu GM (2009) Hepatitis B virus infection. *Lancet* 373, 582–592

Medina J, Garcia-Buey L, Moreno-Otero R (2003) Review article: immunopathogenetic and therapeutic aspects of autoimmune hepatitis. *Aliment Pharmacol Ther* 17, 1–16

Patel K, Muir AJ, McHutchison JC (2006) Diagnosis and treatment of chronic hepatitis C infection. *BMJ* 332, 1013–1017

Schiødt FV, Lee WM (2003) Fulminant liver disease. *Clin Liver Dis* 7, 331–349

Schuppan D, Afdhal NH (2008) Liver cirrhosis. *Lancet* 371, 838–851

Shah VH, Kamath P (2006) Management of portal hypertension. *Postgrad Med* 119, 14–18

Talwalkar JA, Lindor KD (2003) Primary biliary cirrhosis. *Lancet* 362, 53–61

Tripathi D, Ferguson JW, Therapondos G et al (2007) Recent advances in the management of bleeding gastric varices. *Aliment Pharmacol Ther* 24, 1–17

SELF-ASSESSMENT

1. A 45-year-old woman was admitted to the accident and emergency department in a London hospital with acute liver failure. Choose the one **incorrect** statement concerning her condition.
   A. Paracetamol overdose should be excluded.
   B. Paracetamol-induced hepatocellular liver damage is not reversible.
   C. Mannitol could be used to reduce the cerebral oedema associated with acute liver failure.
   D. Warfarin could be used to manage the coagulopathy which can occur.
   E. Terlipressin could be given as a vasoconstrictor to treat shock.
2. Choose the one **incorrect** statement concerning the following antiviral treatments.
   A. Interferon alfa protects against viral hepatitis.
   B. Pegylated interferon alfa (polyethylene glycol conjugate with interferon alfa) is cleared from the plasma at the same rate as the non-pegylated interferon alfa.
   C. Pegylated interferon alfa is inactive if given orally.
   D. Lamivudine is a prodrug.
   E. Combination therapy with ribavirin and interferon alfa is recommended for the treatment of hepatitis C.
3. Case history questions

Mr S was a 61-year-old publican who presented ‘feeling as though I am 9 months’ pregnant’. His abdominal swelling was caused by ascites, which was drained. A liver biopsy was performed, which showed micronodular cirrhosis. He commenced treatment with oral spironolactone.

a. Was this a good choice of diuretic?

He remained well on this regimen for 5 years but continued to imbibe large quantities of alcohol. He re-presented as an emergency, having had a haematemesis and melaena. At the time he was slightly jaundiced and demonstrated signs of hepatic encephalopathy. In addition, there was gynaecomastia and testicular atrophy. The liver edge was palpable 8 cm below the right costal margin. Investigations showed a bilirubin of 27 mmol L^{-1} (normal <17) and an albumin of 30 g L^{-1} (normal 32–50). A gastroscopy was performed under sedation with intravenous diazepam, and revealed oesophageal varices.

b. What evidence was there to indicate diminished hepatic reserve in this man?
c. In what way(s) would the pharmacodynamics and pharmacokinetics of diazepam be altered in this man? Was diazepam a good choice?
d. What alterations to the dosage of diazepam might be necessary when compared with its use in someone without liver disease?

It has been shown that the incidence of re-bleeding from oesophageal varices can be reduced by the oral administration of propranolol (by reducing portal venous pressure).

e. What effect is this man’s liver disease likely to have on the pharmacodynamics and pharmacokinetics of propranolol? Specifically, in what way will the free fraction of the drug in plasma be affected; how will its bioavailability be influenced; and what, if any, would be the effects on the drug’s half-life?
f. People with hepatic cirrhosis are often treated with colestyramine and/or lactulose. How do these drugs work and what benefits are produced?
g. What would you use for pain relief in someone with established liver cirrhosis?

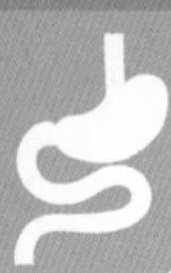

ANSWERS

1. Answer **D**.
   A. In the UK, paracetamol poisoning is the most common cause of acute liver failure.
   B. True.
   C. Mannitol is an osmotic diuretic (Ch. 14). It has few uses, but one is for the reduction of cerebral oedema.
   D. The coagulopathy which occurs is inadequate clotting due to a reduction in vitamin K-dependent clotting factors. Vitamin K should be given, not warfarin, which will make the problem worse.
   E. Terlipressin is an analogue of vasopressin; it causes vasoconstriction and can be given to treat shock.
2. Answer **B**.
   A. Interferon alfa prevents virus replication (Ch. 52) and can augment the immune system.
   B. The polyethylene glycol conjugated with interferon alfa (pegylated interferon alfa) has a plasma half-life of about 80 h, compared with 3–4 h for the non-conjugated form.
   C. It is ineffective orally and is given by subcutaneous injection.
   D. Lamivudine is converted to its active triphosphate form by phosphorylation with viral enzymes.
   E. Combined ribavirin and interferon alfa is recommended by NICE for the treatment of hepatitis C, giving better results than either treatment alone.
3. Case history answers
   a. Spironolactone would be a reasonable choice as any changes in serum K^+ should be avoided because such people are easily tipped into encephalopathy/coma by electrolyte imbalances; therefore avoid furosemide/thiazides initially, although after a few days they could be cautiously given. There is an increase in circulating aldosterone, probably because of decreased metabolism and renin stimulation secondary to low plasma volume. This probably contributes to fluid retention; therefore, spironolactone or amiloride is usually chosen.
   b. Diminished hepatic reserve is indicated by four factors: (i) increased plasma bilirubin, which will be a combination of unconjugated bilirubin (because of impaired glucuronidation) plus conjugated bilirubin (because of impaired biliary excretion); (ii) decreased plasma albumin, caused by decreased synthesis, which will lower the osmotic pressure of blood and, therefore, draw less water back out of tissues, leading to oedema/ascites; (iii) decreased clotting factors, caused by decreased synthesis, which may contribute to oesophageal bleeding (note, a proton pump inhibitor, such as omeprazole, is often used to reduce risk of a gastrointestinal bleed); (iv) increased oestrogenic activity, as evidenced by gynaecomastia and testicular atrophy, possibly caused by decreased inactivation of oestrogenic steroids in the liver.
   c. The long-acting diazepam is probably not a good choice. People with cirrhosis are more susceptible to the effects of CNS depressant drugs and diazepam is likely to give an increased response. The general mechanism is not known (may be change in blood–brain barrier). The metabolism of diazepam by cytochrome P450 will be reduced and, therefore, there will be an increased plasma concentration. (Note: there will be decreased formation of the desmethyl metabolite, which has similar activity to diazepam.) A short-acting benzodiazepine without active metabolites would be better, e.g. midazolam.
   d. If diazepam was administered, a much lower dose than usual should be given and slower recovery would be expected. In some cases it may be necessary to reverse the effect by giving flumazenil, a benzodiazepine antagonist.
   e. There will be decreased albumin and α_1-acid glycoprotein in the plasma; therefore, less protein binding of propranolol can occur and there will be more free drug in blood, leading to an increased response. Decreased first-pass metabolism means that the bioavailability will increase (from about 30% up to 70–80%). This is because of decreased cytochrome P450 activity and increased portocaval shunting of blood. The elimination half-life is independent of bioavailability but it will be longer because the reduced cytochrome P450 results in a decrease in plasma clearance.
   f. Colestyramine is a non-absorbed anion exchange resin that adsorbs bile acids in the gastrointestinal lumen. In liver cirrhosis, fibrosis reduces outflow from bile canaliculi and there is decreased bile flow. This leads to a build-up of bile salts in blood and deposition in the skin, which causes itching. Adsorption of bile salts in the gut onto colestyramine lowers blood bile salts by reducing enterohepatic circulation. Lactulose is used to modify the gut flora. A possible cause of encephalopathy is the failure of the liver to detoxify bacterial products formed in the large bowel. (Encephalopathy is more common during constipation). Possible bacterial metabolites of importance are ammonia and tyramine. Lactulose is not absorbed in the upper gastrointestinal tract but is fermented in the lower bowel; the metabolic product (Ch. 35) lowers lumen pH and may act by altering the microbial metabolism, with decreased formation of ammonia and tyramine. It also prevents constipation.
   g. Analgesia in cirrhosis is a problem, and there is no ideal answer. Opioids should usually be avoided because of the risk of encephalopathy, but reduced doses could be given. NSAIDs are best avoided, to reduce the risk of haemorrhage from oesophageal varices. Paracetamol is a possible risk because it is hepatotoxic: however, it is well tolerated in people with cirrhosis, probably because the decreases in effective perfusion of hepatocytes and reduced activity of cytochrome P450 outweigh the decrease in conjugation with glucuronic acid, sulphate and glutathione.

Drugs used in liver disease

Drug	Half-life (h) and kinetics	Comments
Autoimmune liver disease		
Azathioprine	3–5 [M] Converted to active metabolite, 6-mercaptopurine, which is metabolised to nucleoside and uric acid analogues (therefore interaction with allopurinol) (Ch. 38)	Has a corticosteroid-sparing action and is used in combination with corticosteroids; oral or intravenous dosage
Corticosteroids	(see Ch. 44)	Usually prednisolone is used
Ursodeoxycholic acid	? days [M] Most is absorbed in the small intestine; metabolised and eliminated in bile as glycine and taurine conjugates (like a bile acid); slow elimination due to enterohepatic circulation	The only drug licensed for use in primary biliary cirrhosis; produced by bacterial oxidation of chenodeoxycholic acid; given orally
Other drugs		Ciclosporin, tacrolimus or mycophenolate (see Ch. 38) are used for autoimmune hepatitis that has not responded to corticosteroids
Viral hepatitis		
Interferons		
Interferon alfa	3–4 [M]	Used in the treatment of chronic hepatitis B, but response rate is less than 50%; given by subcutaneous, intramuscular or intravenous injection; peak levels appear 4–8 h after subcutaneous or intramuscular injection; taken up by kidney and catabolised
Peginterferon alfa	80 [M]	Used in combination with ribavirin for chronic hepatitis C; polyethylene glycol-conjugated form of interferon alfa which gives more prolonged blood levels after dosage; given by subcutaneous injection; prolonged duration of action compared with interferon alfa
Nucleoside analogues		
Adefovir dipivoxil	8 [M] (adefovir) A diester prodrug that undergoes hydrolysis to adefovir; adefovir is an acyclic nucleotide analogue which undergoes intracellular phosphorylation to the active diphosphate; adefovir is eliminated by the kidneys	Used in chronic hepatitis B infection with *either* compensated liver disease with evidence of viral replication and histologically documented active liver inflammation and fibrosis, *or* decompensated liver disease; given orally
Entecavir	≈130 [R] Complete oral bioavailability; eliminated by glomerular filtration and tubular secretion	Used in chronic hepatitis B infection with compensated liver disease, evidence of viral replication and histologically documented active liver inflammation or fibrosis
Lamivudine	5–7 [R + M] Rapid absorption with about 70% bioavailability; undergoes intracellular phosphorylation to an active triphosphate; eliminated by the kidneys and limited sulphoxidation	Antiviral reverse transcriptase inhibitor used in the initial treatment of hepatitis B, and for decompensated liver disease; given orally
Ribavirin	7–21 days [M + R] Oral bioavailability is 50%; metabolised by hydrolysis of ribosyl group from triazole moiety, which is then excreted in urine; very slowly cleared from erythrocytes and tissue compartments (short half-lives are reported after single doses)	Given orally
Tenofovir	17 [R] Low oral bioavailability (about 25%); undergoes intracellular phosphorylation to its active metabolite, tenofovir diphosphate; eliminated by a combination of glomerular filtration and active renal tubular secretion	Used for people requiring treatment for both HIV and chronic hepatitis B; given orally as tenofovir disoproxil fumarate

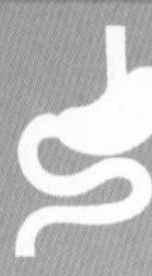

Drugs used in liver disease

Drug	Half-life (h) and kinetics	Comments
Drugs used for oesophageal varices		
Octreotide	1.7 [R + M] Eliminated by renal excretion (about 40%) and probably by tissue uptake and metabolism	Given by subcutaneous injection, or by intravenous injection if a more rapid response is required
Terlipressin	0.5 [M] Triglycyl prodrug of lysine-vasopressin; metabolised by hydrolysis to the active form (which then has a formation rate-limited half-life of 0.5 h)	Given by intravenous injection

[M], metabolism; [R], renal excretion.

37 Obesity

Obesity is defined as a body mass index (BMI) above 30 kg m^{-2}, compared with the ideal range of 18.5–24.9 kg m^{-2}. A BMI of 25–29.9 kg m^{-2} is considered overweight. The prevalence of obesity is increasing in the Western world; it varies from less than 10% in the Netherlands to about 50% in some parts of Eastern Europe. In the UK, it is currently about 15%, but over half the British population is now overweight.

The health consequences of obesity are considerable (Box 37.1). Obesity decreases life expectancy by 7 years at the age of 40 years. Recent data suggest that waist circumference above 102 cm in males or 88 cm in females is more closely correlated than BMI with the cluster of atherogenic risk factors known as the metabolic syndrome. Metabolic syndrome is the presence of at least two of the following characteristic features in association with large waist circumference:

- abnormally raised triglyceride
- decreased high-density lipoprotein (HDL) cholesterol
- raised fasting blood glucose (as a result of insulin resistance)
- hypertension.

Excess calories are stored as fat in adipose tissue. Intra-abdominal (visceral) fat is most closely associated with the metabolic and atherogenic consequences of obesity. The association between central obesity and atherothrombosis is related to enlarged visceral adipocytes. These adipocytes secrete numerous inflammatory, pro-atherogenic and pro-coagulant cytokines such as interleukin-6, tumour necrosis factor alpha and plasminogen activator inhibitor-1, but secrete reduced amounts of the anti-inflammatory and anti-atherogenic hormone adiponectin. Cytokines produced by omental adipocytes enter the portal circulation and alter many aspects of hepatic metabolism.

PATHOGENESIS OF OBESITY

Food intake is controlled by numerous hormonal, societal, genetic and psychological factors. Obesity usually develops gradually, and results when energy input exceeds output. This is determined by the balance between energy intake and exercise, or muscular work, and a small imbalance is all that is required for progressive weight gain. The recent epidemic of obesity in the Western world suggests that major environmental factors (reduced activity and dietary changes) are responsible, rather than biological causes, although there are polygenic influences that determine who is more susceptible to weight gain. For a few individuals, obesity arises from hormonal disturbances, or from neurological conditions that lead to behavioural change. There are several drugs that are associated with weight gain, such as antipsychotics, tricyclic antidepressants, corticosteroids, anticonvulsants, antihistamines and antidiabetic drugs.

Energy balance is regulated in the hypothalamus, which integrates neural, hormonal and circulating nutrient stimuli, and sends signals to higher centres to trigger feelings of satiety or hunger. The hypothalamus also regulates sympathetic nervous system function (which controls lipolysis and thermogenesis) and pituitary hormones that help to regulate energy expenditure. The body has two types of adipose tissue: brown adipose tissue is responsible for thermogenesis, and white adipose tissue for lipolysis. White adipose tissue is a target for insulin, and there is resistance to the action of insulin in obese people leading to accumulation of fat.

The biochemical factors that underlie the regulation of weight are increasingly well characterised (Fig. 37.1). The control of food intake is regulated by the brain (particularly the hypothalamus). Signals that reduce food intake (satiety signals) are provided by a number of hormones produced by the endocrine cells of the gut, adipose tissue and the pancreas. Leptin, which is released from adipocytes, and insulin both signal via specific hypothalamic receptors to indicate the degree of filling of adipocytes and induce the sensation of satiety. Leptin, insulin and a number of gut-derived peptides (see below) all act on the hypothalamus to *inhibit* several hypothalamic appetite-stimulating (orexigenic) neurotransmitters, including neuropeptide Y (NPY) and agouti-related protein (AGRP), and they also *stimulate* the hypothalamic appetite-suppressing substances alpha melanocyte-stimulating hormone (α-MSH) and cocaine- and amphetamine-regulated transcript (CART). Perversely, circulating concentrations of leptin are usually high in obesity; this is interpreted by some as representing hypothalamic resistance to the hormone that may arise from saturation of the transport system for leptin across the blood–brain barrier; alternatively, the high plasma leptin could simply reflect the excess fat accumulation. Hypothalamic resistance to satiety cues when faced with palatable food may be the principal cause of obesity.

Several gut-derived peptides act as short-term appetite regulators. Ghrelin is released by the stomach

Box 37.1 Adverse health consequences of obesity

Metabolic consequences
Hypertension
Hyperlipidaemia (raised VLDL cholesterol, reduced HDL cholesterol)
Hyperuricaemia
Insulin resistance

Clinical consequences
Coronary artery disease (BMI >29 kg m^{-2} increases risk fourfold)
Non-insulin-dependent diabetes mellitus (BMI >35 kg m^{-2} increase risk 40-fold)
Stroke
Osteoarthritis
Sleep apnoea
Large bowel and endometrial cancer (BMI >30 kg m^{-2} increases risk two- to fivefold)
Low self-esteem

BMI, body mass index: HDL, high-density lipoprotein; VLDL, very-low-density lipoprotein.

pre-prandially, and *stimulates* orexigenic peptides. Oxyntomodulin, glucagon-like peptide-1 (GLP-1), cholecystokinin and peptide YY_{3-36} (PYY) are released from the small intestine and colon in response to carbohydrates and lipids, and *inhibit* release of orexigenic peptides in the hypothalamus. Other neurotransmitters and hormones that influence appetite include the appetite inhibitors serotonin and dopamine, while cannabinoids, cortisol and growth hormone-releasing hormone stimulate appetite.

The role of the endocannabinoid system in regulating appetite has received increased attention in recent years. Acting via CB_1 receptors, the natural agonists such as anandamide and 2-arachidonylglycerol have both central nervous system (CNS) and peripheral actions. Endocannabinoids in the CNS are released from postsynaptic neurons, and act on presynaptic receptors to inhibit neurotransmitter release. They stimulate appetite by actions at the hypothalamus and nucleus accumbens. Peripherally, endocannabinoids have effects on gastrointestinal motility that reduce satiety signals.

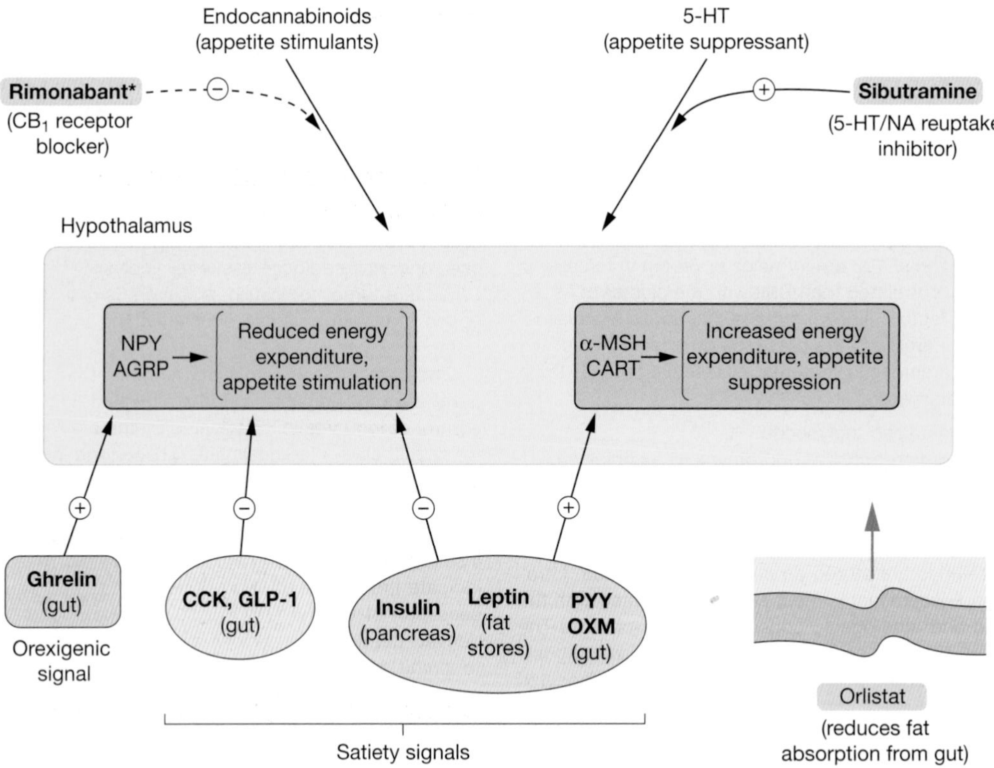

Fig. 37.1 **Some factors involved in the regulation of food intake.** Feedback loops between the periphery and the brain control food intake. The hypothalamus sends signals to higher centres, indicating satiety or hunger. The sources of the peripheral orexigenic and satiety signals are shown in italics. Peripheral signals stimulate or inhibit transmitters in the arcuate nucleus of the hypothalamus (in yellow) that control appetite and energy expenditure. These neurons send further messages to the paraventricular nucleus. For clarity, other interlinking signalling mechanisms are not shown. Cannabinoid receptors are involved in stimulating appetite, and the CB_1 receptor is blocked by rimonabant. Serotonin (5-hydroxytryptamine, 5HT) acts on the hypothalamus to suppress appetite and this action is reinforced by sibutramine. Orlistat reduces fat absorption from the gut. AGRP, agouti-related protein; CART, cocaine- and amphetamine-regulated transcript; CCK, cholecystokinin; GLP-1, glucagon-like peptide-1; α-MSH, melanocyte-stimulating hormone; NA, noradrenaline; NPY, neuropeptide Y; OXM, oxyntomodulin; PYY, polypeptide YY. *Rimonabant has been withdrawn due to unwanted effects but other drugs of this class are under development.

Improved understanding of the biochemical signals that regulate appetite has led to the development of several new pharmacological approaches to the management of obesity that are currently undergoing clinical trials.

DRUGS FOR TREATMENT OF OBESITY

DRUGS ACTING ON THE GASTROINTESTINAL TRACT

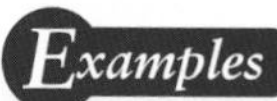

methylcellulose, orlistat

Mechanisms of action

Methylcellulose is taken before meals and swells when hydrated and produces a sense of satiety. There is little evidence to support its ability to reduce appetite, and has little use in the treatment of obesity. It is also used in constipation as a bulk-forming faecal softener.

Orlistat acts by binding to pancreatic lipase in the gut and inhibiting its action. It reduces triglyceride digestion and, therefore, energy intake from dietary fat. An effect on energy intake is seen after 24–48 h, and orlistat achieves sustained weight loss when used as an adjunct to dietary restriction and exercise. However, only about 20% of people will lose more than 5% of body weight. Continuous use of orlistat for more than 2 years is not recommended.

Pharmacokinetics

Methylcellulose and orlistat undergo minimal absorption after oral administration, and are largely excreted unchanged in the faeces.

Unwanted effects

- Orlistat produces gastrointestinal upset, including flatulence, faecal urgency and faecal soiling. These are most common with poor adherence to a low-fat diet while taking the drug, and result in discontinuation of treatment by one-third of people. There is also impaired absorption of fat-soluble vitamins, especially vitamin D.
- Methylcellulose swells rapidly when hydrated and should be taken carefully with water to avoid oesophageal obstruction. As a bulk-forming faecal softener, it may have a laxative effect.

CENTRALLY ACTING APPETITE SUPPRESSANTS

Serotonin and noradrenaline reuptake inhibitors

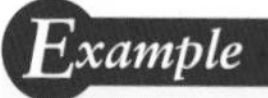

sibutramine

Mechanism of action

Sibutramine inhibits the reuptake of noradrenaline and serotonin in the CNS. The increase in synaptic serotonin acts on the hypothalamus to produce appetite suppression. About one-third of people will lose more than 5% of body weight when use of the drug is combined with behavioural changes. It is only licensed for use for up to 1 year, and rapid rebound weight gain often follows withdrawal. Several other centrally acting appetite suppressants such as dexfenfluramine, fenfluramine and phentermine, which also act to increase amine levels in the areas of the brain controlling appetite, have been withdrawn because of the increased risks of valvular heart disease and pulmonary hypertension.

Pharmacokinetics

Sibutramine is well absorbed from the gut and undergoes extensive first-pass metabolism in the liver, generating active derivatives. Elimination of the metabolites is by further hepatic metabolism, and the active metabolites have long half-lives (15 h).

Unwanted effects

- Constipation, anorexia, nausea, dry mouth
- Insomnia, anxiety, headache
- Tachycardia, palpitation, hypertension.

Endocannabinoid receptor antagonists

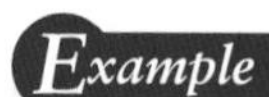

rimonabant

Mechanism of action

Rimonabant is a selective CB_1 receptor antagonist that suppresses appetite by an effect on the hypothalamus. Peripherally, it enhances thermogenesis by increasing oxygen consumption in skeletal muscle, decreases hepatic and adipocyte lipogenesis, and potentiates cholecystokinin and vagal satiety signals. Rimonabant has been withdrawn due to psychological disturbances.

MANAGEMENT OF OBESITY

Weight loss reduces the morbidity associated with obesity, but it is not known whether it prolongs life. Weight loss can be difficult to achieve and to maintain. Obesity is not caused by psychological disturbances, but these commonly arise in obese people. The social prejudice against obesity, concern about body image, and the depression and irritability that arise from dieting are all contributory factors.

The cornerstone of management of obesity is to reduce energy intake by 500–600 kcal below daily requirements. Fat is ‘energy dense’ and should be particularly restricted. However, dietary restriction alone is usually inadequate to achieve weight loss, and increased exercise combined

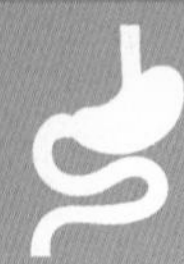

with diet is more effective than either alone. Exercise need not be vigorous, provided it is maintained long-term; walking or cycling is usually enough if performed daily. Behaviour modification is essential for long-term adherence to treatment.

Drug treatment should be restricted to individuals with a BMI >27 kg m^{-2} who have not achieved target weight through behavioural change but who have lost at least 2.5 kg body weight by diet and exercise in the preceding month. There is no clear guidance on the choice of drug – tolerability and comorbidities may reduce the suitability of one or more of the available agents. A major disadvantage is that weight gain often follows cessation of drug therapy. The use of thyroxine to encourage weight loss by increasing metabolic rate is not recommended due to long-term risks such as osteoporosis. Bulking agents such as methylcellulose are usually ineffective for reducing food intake. Bariatric surgery to restrict the size of the stomach (gastroplasty) or gastric bypass (such as Roux-en-Y) are used in the morbidly obese (BMI >40 kg m^{-2}), or those with a BMI >35 kg m^{-2} and an obesity-related medical condition.

Current drug and lifestyle treatments for obesity can be expected to produce weight loss of about 10–15%, which is often enough to ameliorate obesity-related metabolic disorders and their accompanying clinical manifestations. Bariatric surgery produces average weight loss of 25–30%. The management of obesity should be carried out by a multidisciplinary team, who can advise on lifestyle and other treatment options. Treatments under investigation that interfere with the many neurotransmitter systems that regulate weight promise to offer more effective pharmacotherapy than the current limited range of options.

FURTHER READING

Berthoud HR, Sutton GM, Townsend RL et al (2006) Brainstem mechanisms integrating gut-derived satiety signals and descending forebrain information in the control of meal size. *Physiol Behav* 89, 517–524

Eckel RH (2008) Non surgical management of obesity. *N Engl J Med* 358, 1941–1950.

Haslam DW, James WPT (2005) Obesity. *Lancet* 366, 1197–1209

Kamiji MM, Inui A (2007) Neuropeptide Y receptor selective ligands in the treatment of obesity. *Endocrine Rev* 28, 664–684

Padwal RS, Majumdar SR (2007) Drug treatments for obesity: orlistat, sibutramine, and rimonabant. *Lancet* 369, 71–77

Woods SC (2007) Role of the endocannabinoid system in regulating cardiovascular and metabolic risk factors. *Am J Med* 120 (3 suppl 1), S19–S25

SELF-ASSESSMENT

1. Are the following statements true or false?
   a. Drug treatment for obesity should be restricted to those who fail to lose a realistic amount of weight by other means, for example diet and exercise.
   b. Courses of appetite suppressant drugs are virtually all followed by a rebound weight gain.
   c. The appetite suppressant sibutramine inhibits the actions of released noradrenaline.
   d. One of the brain centres that controls appetite is in the posterior pituitary.
   e. Leptin is a peptide that is produced by fat cells and stimulates appetite.
2. Concerning drugs used in obesity, choose the one correct answer from the following options.
   A. There is no association between obesity and symptoms of depression.
   B. An anti-obesity drug should only be considered for people with a BMI in excess of 27 kg m^{-2} who are losing weight but who are failing to reach target weight following a regimen managed by health professionals.
   C. Combination therapy with anti-obesity drugs should be tried if weight loss with one drug fails.
   D. Sibutramine causes virtually no unwanted effects.
   E. Orlistat acts centrally to inhibit naturally occurring appetite-stimulating neurotransmitters.

ANSWERS

1. a. **True**.
   b. **True**.
   c. **False**. Sibutramine inhibits the neuronal reuptake of released noradrenaline and serotonin.
   d. **False**. The hypothalamus controls appetite, and naturally occurring appetite suppressants and stimulants have been identified.
   e. **False**. Leptin is produced in adipose tissue and reduces the production of the appetite-stimulant neurotransmitter neuropeptide Y.
2. Answer **B**.
   A. Depression and other psychosocial problems have been shown to be associated with obesity in some people.
   B. This is the expert advice given to prescribers in the *British National Formulary*.
   C. Combination therapy with more than one anti-obesity drug is contraindicated.
   D. Sibutramine can cause headaches, hypertension and other unwanted effects, and blood pressure should be monitored.
   E. Orlistat inhibits pancreatic lipase in the gut, reducing triglyceride absorption.

Drugs used in obesity

Drug	Half-life (h) and kinetics	Comments
Drugs acting on the gastrointestinal tract		
Methylcellulose	– Not absorbed	Taken before meals to produce a sense of satiety; preparations that swell should be taken carefully with water to avoid oesophageal obstruction; little evidence to support efficacy
Orlistat	1–2 [M] Negligible absorption (about 1%) and low systemic exposure in clinical use; systemic disposition is unimportant	Pancreatic lipase inhibitor acting within the intestine; taken orally before, during or immediately after a meal; no significant effects on the absorption of other drugs
Centrally acting appetite suppressants		
Recommended if BMI is ≥30 kg m^{-2} and no comorbidity, or ≥27 kg m^{-2} in the presence of risk factors, such as diabetes or dyslipidaemia		
Sibutramine	1 [M] Undergoes extensive first-pass metabolism by CYP3A4 to a number of metabolites, two of which are active; the active metabolites have longer half-lives (about 15 h) than the parent drug	Serotonin/noradrenaline reuptake inhibitor; used in the adjunctive treatment of obesity for a maximum of 12 months; taken orally

[M], metabolism.

8

The immune system

38 The immune response and immunosuppressant drugs

BIOLOGICAL BASIS OF THE IMMUNE RESPONSE

The immune system is composed of innate (natural) and adaptive components, which protect the host against a wide variety of pathogens and tumour cells. The adaptive system is further divided into *humoral* and *cell-mediated* immunity. Overall the immune system has the ability to distinguish between 'self' and 'non-self' proteins and to protect the host ('self') against 'non-self' infectious and other pathogenic agents.

INNATE IMMUNITY

The term *innate immunity (*sometimes called *natural immunity)* was used because it is an inherited system and is part of our genetic make-up. It is made up of several generally *non-specific* protective mechanisms, some of which do not involve the immune system; all foreign pathogens are recognised approximately equally by pattern recognition receptors on cells involved in the system. Pattern recognition receptors are proteins expressed by cells in the immune system to identify pathogenic 'groups' such as bacterial lipopolysaccharides and bacterial DNA rather than responding to individual antigens. The innate immune system has an important role in processing foreign pathogens and triggering the highly selective adaptive system described below.

The innate immune system incorporates the following processes:

- physicochemical barriers, e.g. intact skin and mucous membrane, low stomach pH, antibacterial agents (lysozyme) in skin and tear secretions
- macrophages and dendritic cells, particularly in lungs, liver, lymph nodes and spleen, phagocytose pathogenic material and produce antigens (short peptides of approximately 8–25 amino acids) from the pathogenic material which they then display on their surfaces; the cells are then described as antigen-presenting cells (APCs) and are necessary for the presentation of the antigen to T-lymphocytes and the triggering of the adaptive immune system (see below)
- attraction of immune cells to sites of inflammation by substances such as cytokines
- phagocytosis of bacteria and parasites by granulocytes, including neutrophils, monocytes and macrophages
- actions of natural killer cells
- binding of antigens to IgE antibody on mast cells and basophils and subsequent response by the cell
- fever
- complement activation.

The innate immune system may be an adequate defence to deal with the many pathogens, but, unlike adaptive immunity, long-term immune protection following initial exposure to a pathogen does not occur.

ADAPTIVE IMMUNITY

Adaptive immunity is superimposed upon the innate mechanisms. It is evolutionarily more recent and differs from innate immunity in that it is slower to respond, offers long-term protection and has exquisite specificity in recognising individual 'non-self' molecules. Adaptive immunity has two basic complementary and interacting mechanisms, *cell-mediated immunity* and *humoral immunity* (Figs 38.1 and 38.2).

Essential components of the adaptive system are the two populations of lymphocytes:

- *T-lymphocytes* are produced in the bone marrow and migrate to the thymus, where they express receptors for antigens and interact with immunogenic 'self' peptides. T-cells are selected in the thymus for low or high avidity for 'self' peptides, and those showing high avidity are destroyed. The surviving T-cells retain the potential to cross-react with multiple foreign 'non-self' antigens but not 'self' molecules.
- *B-lymphocytes* make up about 10% of the lymphocyte population and mature in the bone marrow.

T-cells and B-cells are coated with vast numbers of clusters of antigen receptors against foreign molecules on their surfaces. An individual cluster can recognise and bind antigens of a foreign protein. Clusters can be defined by antibody

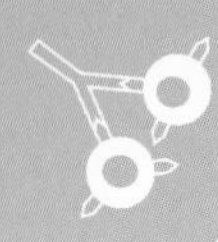

Cytotoxic (CD8+) T-cells are activated
TCR
Clonal proliferation
Destroys pathogenic cell infected with virus (or other pathogen) which is expressing MHC class I antigen
Antigen fragments on class I MHC
Ag
Ciclosporin
Tacrolimus
Co-stimulatory signals
Co-stimulatory signals
Th1 (CD4+) cells are activated
TCR recognises specific antigen
Cell proliferation
Ag
Ca2+ → Calcineurin
TCR
DNA replication
IL-2
Macrophages are activated
B-cells are stimulated (Fig. 38.2)
Cytokines are produced
Memory cells are produced
Chemotactic agents are released
Antigen-presenting cell
Purine
Corticosteroid
Corticosteroids
IL–2R
Sirolimus
Mycophenolate mofetil
Azathioprine
Basiliximab
Daclizumab

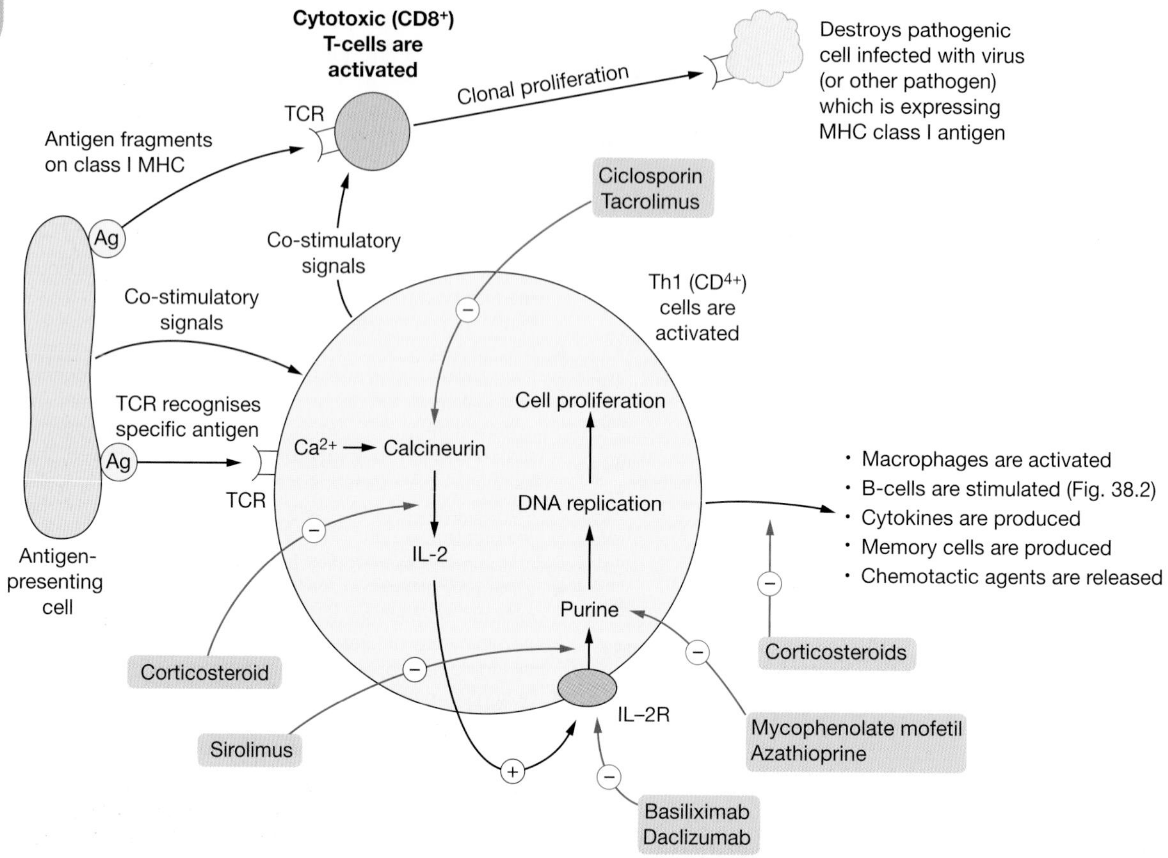

Fig. 38.1 **Aspects of cell-mediated immunity.** This shows in simplified form some steps in T-cell activation following antigen presentation to the T-cell receptor (TCR) and subsequent events that may contribute to cell-mediated immunity. Pathogenic antigens are presented by antigen-presenting cells to the uncommitted CD4⁺ lymphocyte which carries the specific receptor to the antigen; under the influence of interleukin-2 (IL-2), Th1 cells are formed which have a variety of roles in cell-mediated immunity. They activate macrophages, which are then responsible for some of the cell-mediated immune response. Antigens can also be presented to CD8⁺ lymphocytes that have the correct antigen receptors, which mature into cytotoxic T-cells. Drugs used as immunosuppressants (red arrows) act at the sites shown. Corticosteroids act at many sites (see also Fig. 38.2 and Ch. 44). Ag, antigen; IL-2R, interleukin-2 receptor; MHC, major histocompatibility complex; Th, T-helper cell.

typing and are called $CD2^+$, $CD4^+$, $CD8^+$, etc. This means that the surface of the particular cells expresses **C**luster of **D**ifferentiation (CD) antigens of the type 2, 4, 8, etc. When T-cells leave the thymus they are considered naïve or uncommitted since they have not yet been exposed to the 'non-self' antigens. At this stage, naïve T-cells consist of two major populations, known as helper (Th [$CD4^+$]) and cytotoxic or killer (Tc [$CD8^+$]) T-cells (Fig. 38.1). Immunogenic peptides are presented to T-cells within the cleft of major histocompatibility complex (MHC) type II molecules on the surface of APCs. The $CD4^+$ (Th) cells have high affinity for class II MHC which binds antigen peptides, while $CD8^+$ (Tc) cells have an affinity for class I MHC.

The $CD4^+$ Th-cell is activated if its receptors recognise and bind avidly to an antigen; this leads to a series of complex processes resulting in general preparation of the cell for its immune role and commitment of the cell to become a type 1 Th-cell (Th1) or a type 2 Th cell (Th2); the details of these events are rapidly evolving. When appropriately activated, Th-cells orchestrate the immune response and secrete cytokines that stimulate cytotoxic Tc-cells and B cells to grow and divide, attract neutrophils and enhance (activate) the phagocytic activity of macrophages.

Co-stimulatory signals are deemed increasingly important processes in T-cell function, particularly in the activation of cytotoxic Tc-cells. CD40 and CD45 antigenic protein molecule clusters on T-cells have co-stimulatory roles in T-cell activation. Interactions between CD28 antigenic molecules on Th-cells and CD80, CD86 and CD20 antigenic molecule clusters on APCs are also important, CD20 being restricted to the surface of B-cells. The importance of co-stimulatory molecules has been recognised and targeted in the development of drugs for the treatment of arthritis: abatacept is an antibody that binds to CD80 and CD86 antigenic clusters on APCs and rituximab is an antibody that binds to CD20 on B-cells, thus modulating the destructive immune responsiveness against 'self' molecules in this disease (Ch. 30, Fig. 30.1).

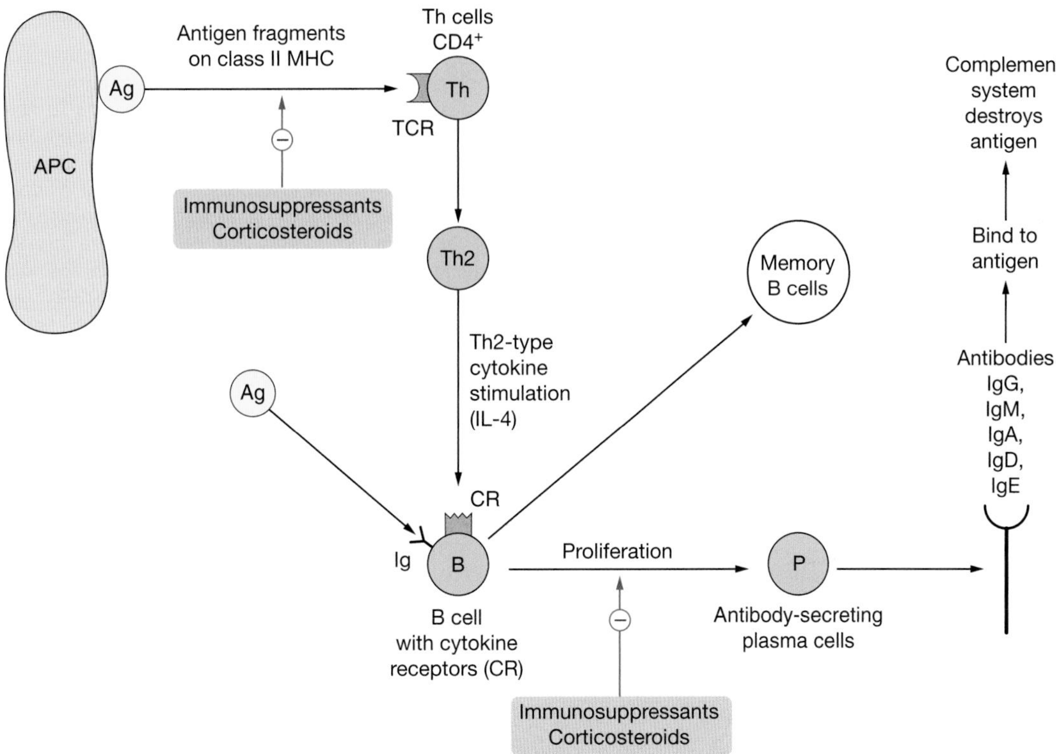

Fig. 38.2 **Aspects of humoral immunity.** Adaptive immunity can result in production of antibodies (humoral response) or a cell-mediated response (Fig. 38.1). Antigens on bacteria or bacterial toxins bind to immunoglobulins on B cells. Before proliferation and antibody production can occur, the B cell also has to be stimulated by activated T-cell cytokine production, usually of the Th2 type. Antigen fragments can be presented on the major histocompatibility complex (MHC) to T-cells via a T-cell receptor (TCR) that recognises the antigen. T-cells undergo clonal proliferation and produce cytokines and stimulate B cells to produce antibodies (IgG, IgM, IgA, IgD and IgE) – humoral immunity. In atopic individuals, the T-cells are tipped towards the Th2 type and produce IL-4, IL-5, IL-10 and TGF-β, which induce the B cells to produce IgE. Ag, antigen; APC, antigen-presenting cell; CR, cytokine receptor; P, plasma cell; Th, T-helper cell.

Th1- and Th2-cell subsets are programmed to produce different arrays of cytokines which have varied effects on the immune system (Figs 38.1 and 38.2). It is a complex issue to decide whether predominantly Th1- or Th2-mediated immune responses are involved in a particular disease; in part this is due to the fact that Th2 cytokines can inhibit Th1-cell functions. Th1-mediated immune responses are significantly involved in rheumatoid arthritis (Ch. 30) and in the formation of atheroma (Ch. 48), and Th2-mediated responses are important in mild to moderate asthma but with increasing participation of Th1-mediated responses in severe asthma (Ch. 12).

Immature B cells can bind antigen with the cooperation of T-cells, but on subsequent exposure antigen binds directly to immunoglobulins on the B cell (Fig. 38.2)

Cell-mediated immunity

Cell-mediated immunity is largely T-cell-driven, utilising Th1 and cytotoxic T-cell (Tc) subtypes, and is involved in responses to viral infection, graft rejection, chronic inflammation and tumour immunity. Figure 38.1 shows schematically the basic processes occurring in cell-mediated immunity. T-cells that possess the receptor to the antigen of the invasive pathogen that is presented on APCs are stimulated to express interleukin-2 (IL-2) and the IL-2 receptor. For clarity, the many co-stimulatory processes that are described in the text above are not shown in the figure.

Stimulation of the IL-2 receptor induces the Th cell to:

- activate macrophages to phagocytose the pathogen
- stimulate cytotoxic Tc cells to grow and divide
- stimulate B cells to grow and divide
- attract macrophages and neutrophils to the site
- produce memory B cells that respond rapidly to the pathogen on future exposure.

Cytotoxic T-cells ($CD8^+$) that recognise the foreign antigen presented on MHC type 1 on APCs are activated to proliferate and attack pathogens expressing the antigen. Co-stimulation from Th1 cells also occurs. When cytotoxic cells bind to an antigen on a pathogenic cell they release a variety of proteases or lysins to destroy the cell.

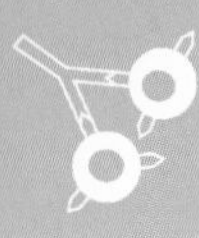

Humoral immunity

Figure 38.2 illustrates the basic processes in humoral immunity. The foreign antigen is recognised by immunoglobulin (Ig) molecules or specific receptors to that antigen on the surface of a specific clone of B-cells. The presence of nearby Th2-cells that have been activated to secrete IL-4 is required. The secreted IL-4 causes B-cell clonal proliferation, and converts B-cells into active plasma cells that can secrete antibodies of the IgG, IgM, IgA, IgD and IgE classes which bind to and destroy pathogenic antigens.

On encountering an antigen, the primary immune response consists of IgM, replaced later by IgG. B-cells that are primed to produce specific antibodies survive as memory B-cells. On a further encounter with the antigen, the secondary immune response occurs more rapidly and consists of large amounts of IgG produced by plasma cells derived from reactivation of memory B-cells.

UNWANTED IMMUNE REACTIONS

The processes of inflammation and immunity described above are essential to protect the host against pathogens and other damage, but excessive, inappropriately prolonged or misdirected immune responses can cause disease, including hypersensitivity reactions, graft rejection and autoimmune diseases.

Hypersensitivity reactions

Hypersensitivity reactions were classified by Gell and Coombs in the late 1950s.

Type 1 (acute, immediate)

This includes hayfever and acute asthma. IgE molecules on the surface of mast cells and basophils are cross-linked by harmless antigens (allergens such as pollens or house-dust mites), leading to the synthesis and/or release of inflammatory mediators. These include cysteinyl leukotrienes, prostaglandins, histamine, platelet-activating factor, proteases and cytokines.

Type 2 (cytotoxic)

Cell surface antigens, including microbial proteins and drug molecules haptenised onto cell surfaces, are recognised and bound by IgG and IgM antibodies (opsonisation), leading to activation of complement (classic pathway) and cytolysis of the target cell. Examples include destruction of red cells after incompatible blood transfusion, and haemolytic anaemia caused by binding of some drugs to host cells (see Ch. 53).

Type 3 (complex-mediated)

Soluble antigens react with excess circulating antibodies to form complexes that precipitate in small blood vessels, causing vasculitis and organ damage. Pigeon fancier's lung and farmer's lung are systemic type 3 reactions, while the Arthus reaction is a local response to an injected antigen (e.g. non-human insulins).

Type 4 (cell-mediated, delayed-type hypersensitivity)

Inappropriate regulation of cell-mediated immunity may cause damaging chronic inflammation, leading to fibrosis and granuloma formation. Cell-mediated immunity misdirected against harmless foreign proteins (allergens) can lead to chronic allergic inflammation (such as occurs in eczema), or cause contact sensitivity in the skin to haptenising metals and chemicals. In allergy, Th2-cells secrete cytokines, including IL-4, IL-5 and IL-13, which promote eosinophilic inflammation and overproduction of IgE by B-cells.

Transplant rejection

In blood transfusion, rejection usually occurs because non-self antigens on the transfused red blood cells (ABO system) trigger a type 2 hypersensitivity reaction in the recipient. In immunodeficient people, transfused T-cells react against recipient antigens (graft-versus-host reactions). For organ transplants, hyperacute rejection can occur if there is ABO incompatibility, or host-versus-graft reactions can arise later with foreign MHC molecules (human leucocyte antigens, HLA). The latter can be reduced by HLA tissue-typing to increase the chance of selecting a graft that is compatible with the host tissues. This will reduce the rate of tissue destruction but not prevent chronic rejection. The immune response and its place in the rejection of a transplanted organ is complex. The antigens on the graft are recognised as foreign, and the cascaded responses outlined in Figures 38.1 and 38.2 occur, with increased production of B-cells, cytotoxic T-cells, and monocyte/macrophages. Graft destruction occurs from antibody production against the graft, lysis of graft cells and delayed hypersensitivity responses. Rejection can be immediate (days), acute (weeks) or chronic (years).

Autoimmunity

Normally the immune system is tolerant of 'self' antigens. T-cells in the thymus that express receptors with high avidity for self peptides are normally destroyed in a process known as negative selection (see above). If this self-tolerance breaks down, then autoimmune disorders result. Numerous mechanisms can trigger autoimmune diseases, including viral infection of host cells, binding of drug molecules to host cells (e.g. penicillin), antigens shared between host cells and microbes, and sequestered antigens liberated by cell damage. Examples of autoimmune disease include haemolytic anaemia, type 1 diabetes mellitus, Addison's disease, rheumatoid arthritis, myasthenia gravis, systemic lupus erythematosus and Graves' disease.

IMMUNOSUPPRESSANT DRUGS

The immune system presents a large number of potential molecular targets for therapeutic intervention. Present drugs tend to be non-specific immunosuppressants with a range of unwanted effects. Immunosuppressant drugs are widely used in many diseases; examples include rheumatoid arthritis, psoriasis and inflammatory bowel disease.

Their benefit is achieved both through modulation of the immune system and, in some cases, through their anti-inflammatory properties. In addition to the drugs discussed in this chapter, others, such as methotrexate and cyclophosphamide, which are used for their cytotoxic actions in cancer chemotherapy (Ch. 52), are also used for their immunosuppressant properties in various disease states. Methotrexate and cyclophosphamide have immunosuppressant properties at doses much lower than those required to treat malignancy (Ch. 52). Corticosteroids (e.g. dexamethasone and prednisone; Ch. 44) are highly effective anti-inflammatory drugs that can be used systemically to suppress type 4 hypersensitivity reactions, autoimmune diseases and graft rejection. They are also used topically for inflammatory skin disease (Ch. 49) and inflammatory bowel disease (Ch. 34) and by inhalation for asthma (e.g. beclometasone, fluticasone; Ch. 12).

Inflammatory mediators released during immune reactions can be blocked by antagonists at their receptors on target cells, or by inhibiting their synthesis. Anti-mediator drugs include histamine H_1 receptor antagonists (antihistamines), cysteinyl-leukotriene receptor antagonists (LTRA) and cyclo-oxygenase inhibitors (non-steroidal anti-inflammatory drugs [NSAIDs]). Topical and systemic antihistamines (e.g. loratadine and cetirizine) are used in the control of hayfever and eczema (Ch. 39), while oral leukotriene receptor antagonists (e.g. montelukast and zafirlukast) are used in asthma (Ch. 12). Oral NSAIDs block the synthesis of prostaglandins and are extensively used in inflammatory arthritis (Chs 29 and 30).

CALCINEURIN INHIBITORS

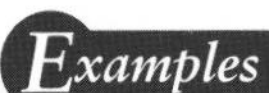

ciclosporin, tacrolimus

Ciclosporin

Mechanism of action

Ciclosporin is a fungal cyclic peptide which inhibits T-cell division. It binds in the cell cytoplasm to the protein cyclophilin, and the complex inhibits calcineurin, a calmodulin-Ca^{2+}-dependent phosphatase which is a key component in T-cell activation (Fig. 38.1). Activated calcineurin is produced in response to an antigenic signal at T-cell receptors and dephosphorylates nuclear factor of activation in T-cells (NFAT). NFAT then enters the cell nucleus and binds to a promoter region of the IL-2 gene. IL-2 stimulates T-cell division. By inhibiting calcineurin, ciclosporin prevents dephosphorylation of NFAT, which remains in the cytoplasm. This inhibits IL-2 production, and the T-cell division cycle is arrested between G_0 and G_1.

Ciclosporin also inhibits other cellular mitogen-activated protein kinases (such as c-Jun N-terminal kinase and p38 kinases) triggered by the inflammatory cytokines tumour necrosis factor alpha (TNFα), IL-1, and various other cellular factors. These kinases phosphorylate transcription factors involved in upregulation of *c-Fos*-mediated gene transcription, a process that is involved in many cell responses to inflammation.

Ciclosporin also stimulates the production of transforming growth factor beta (TGF-β), possibly by releasing an inhibitory effect of calcineurin on gene transcription. This may be responsible for some of the unwanted effects of the drug.

Pharmacokinetics

Oral absorption of a standard formulation of ciclosporin is variable and incomplete, requiring initial dispersion by bile salts. For this reason, a microemulsion formulation has replaced it for oral use. This emulsifies when it comes into contact with water in the gut, increasing the surface area for absorption, which then becomes independent of bile production. After absorption, ciclosporin selectively concentrates in some tissues, including liver, kidney, several endocrine glands, lymph nodes, spleen and bone marrow. Ciclosporin is extensively metabolised in the liver by the CYP3A4 isoenzyme and has a long half-life (27 h). Ciclosporin can also be given by intravenous infusion. Trough plasma drug concentration monitoring has traditionally been used to guide dosage for optimal effectiveness and to minimise toxicity. However, recent evidence suggests that a blood concentration 2 h post-dose may be a better guide to graft survival and reduced toxicity.

Unwanted effects

- Nephrotoxicity almost always occurs, with a dose-dependent increase in serum creatinine in the first few weeks. The acute effect is due to intrarenal vasoconstriction that may persist and contribute to the less common long-term sequelae, which include interstitial fibrosis and tubular atrophy. Induction of TGF-β may be a contributory factor. The decline in renal glomerular function is usually reversible, but permanent renal impairment can result.
- Hypertension, often associated with fluid retention, occurs in up to 50% of people, and especially after heart transplantation. It usually responds to standard antihypertensive drug treatment.
- Hepatic dysfunction.
- Tremor, headache, fatigue.
- Hypertrichosis (excessive hair growth) and gum hypertrophy are common.
- Gastrointestinal disturbance, including anorexia, nausea and vomiting.
- Hyperlipidaemia.
- Drug interactions can be dangerous and caution should be taken when ciclosporin is used with other nephrotoxic drugs, such as aminoglycoside antimicrobials and amphotericin (Ch. 51) and NSAIDs (Ch. 29). Drugs that induce hepatic CYP3A4, such as phenytoin and carbamazepine, can reduce the plasma concentrations of ciclosporin to sub-therapeutic levels. Drugs that inhibit cytochrome P450, such as erythromycin and ketoconazole (Ch. 51), can increase ciclosporin concentrations and provoke toxicity.

Tacrolimus

Mechanism of action and effects

Tacrolimus inhibits calcineurin, and therefore T-cell proliferation, by arresting the cell cycle between G_0 and G_1 in a similar manner to ciclosporin. After binding to a receptor

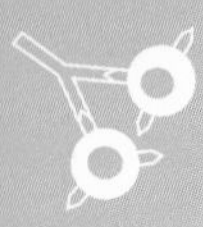

protein called FK-binding protein-12, the complex binds to calcineurin and inhibits Ca^{2+}-dependent calcineurin activation. Tacrolimus also inhibits c-Jun N-terminal kinase and p38 kinases. Unlike ciclosporin, tacrolimus does not stimulate production of TGF-β.

Pharmacokinetics

Tacrolimus is more water-soluble than ciclosporin and undergoes more predictable, though poor, absorption from the gut. It is metabolised by the liver and has a highly variable half-life (4–41 h). Monitoring of the trough blood concentration of tacrolimus is essential for appropriate dose adjustment, especially early in treatment.

Unwanted effects

These are similar to those of ciclosporin except that tacrolimus causes less hypertension, hirsutism and gum hyperplasia. Effects that are more common with tacrolimus include:

- Pleural and pericardial effusions
- Cardiomyopathy in children, who should be monitored by echocardiography.

mTOR (TARGET OF RAPAMYCIN) INHIBITORS

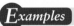

sirolimus

Mechanism of action and effects

Sirolimus (previously known as rapamycin) is a natural fungal fermentation product that inhibits T-cell proliferation by arresting the cell between the G_1 and S phases. It binds to intracellular FK-binding protein-12, and the complex inhibits the action of mTOR, a cytoplasmic kinase. mTOR is a key step in a series of intracellular Ca^{2+}-independent events that transduce signals from the cell surface IL-2 receptor and other growth factor receptors to cell cycle regulators that promote DNA and protein synthesis and mitogenesis. The action of sirolimus therefore differs from that of tacrolimus, despite binding to the same intracellular receptor.

Pharmacokinetics

Sirolimus is rapidly absorbed from the gut, and the absorption is modulated by P-glycoproteins. It is metabolised by intestinal and hepatic cytochrome P450 (CYP3A4), and has a very long half-life (60 h).

Unwanted effects

- Lymphocele
- Oedema, tachycardia
- Abdominal pain, diarrhoea, stomatitis
- Anaemia, thrombocytopenia, neutropenia
- Hyperlipidaemia
- Hypokalaemia
- Arthralgia
- Rash
- Drug interactions: rifampicin reduces plasma sirolimus concentrations by induction of CYP3A4; the antifungal agents itraconazole and ketoconazole increase plasma concentrations of sirolimus by enzyme inhibition.

ANTIPROLIFERATIVE AGENTS

azathioprine, mycophenolate mofetil

Azathioprine

Mechanism of action

Azathioprine is widely used for immunosuppression. Most of the effects result from cleavage to the active derivative 6-mercaptopurine (Ch. 52). Both cell- and antibody-mediated immune reactions are suppressed (Figs 38.1 and 38.2). Effects on the immune response include impaired synthesis of immunoglobulins by B-lymphocytes, and inhibition of the infiltration of mononuclear cells into inflamed tissue. These arise from the antimetabolite action of 6-mercaptopurine, which interferes with purine biosynthesis, thus impairing DNA synthesis in the S-phase of the cell cycle (Figs 52.1 and 52.2).

Pharmacokinetics

Oral absorption is almost complete. Azathioprine is a prodrug that is metabolised in the liver to produce the active compound 6-mercaptopurine, which is further metabolised to inactive compounds. The half-lives of azathioprine and 6-mercaptopurine are short (3–5 h). Azathioprine can be given by intravenous injection, but the solution is alkaline and very irritant.

Unwanted effects

- Dose-dependent bone marrow suppression, especially leucopenia and thrombocytopenia. Regular monitoring of the full blood count (at least every 3 months) is essential.
- Hypersensitivity reactions, with malaise, dizziness, vomiting, diarrhoea, fever, myalgia, arthralgia, rash and hypotension. The drug should be stopped immediately if these arise.
- Increased susceptibility to infection, often with 'opportunistic' organisms.
- Alopecia.
- There is a small risk of carcinogenicity, especially lymphomas.
- Drug interactions: the most important interaction is with allopurinol (Ch. 31). Allopurinol inhibits the enzyme xanthine oxidase, which is involved in the catabolism of 6-mercaptopurine, the active metabolite of azathioprine, and the dose of azathioprine should be reduced by 75% if the drugs are used together. Rifampicin may reduce the efficacy of azathioprine by inducing cytochrome P450.

Mycophenolate mofetil

Mechanism of action and effects

Mycophenolic acid reduces purine synthesis by reversible non-competitive inhibition of the enzymes inosine monophosphate (IMP) dehydrogenase and guanylyl synthase. These enzymes are involved in the conversion of IMP to xanthylate, and then to guanylyl. Guanylyl is the precursor of guanosine triphosphate that is involved in RNA, DNA and protein synthesis. Inhibition of these enzymes depletes the cell of guanine nucleotides and inhibits cellular DNA synthesis. T-cells, B-cells and monocytes rely on de novo purine nucleotide synthesis, unlike neutrophils, which can use pre-formed guanine released from the breakdown of pre-formed nucleic acids (the salvage pathway). Mycophenolate mofetil therefore is a selective inhibitor of lymphocyte function.

A further action of mycophenolate mofetil is inhibition of smooth muscle proliferation in arterial walls, which may also help to reduce graft rejection that arises from obliterative arteriopathy.

Pharmacokinetics

Mycophenolate mofetil is a prodrug ester of mycophenolic acid. It is almost completely absorbed from the gut, and hydrolysed rapidly to the acid derivative after absorption. Elimination of the active metabolite is via hepatic metabolism, and it has a long half-life (18 h) due to enterohepatic circulation. Mycophenolate mofetil can be given by intravenous infusion.

Unwanted effects

- Gastrointestinal upset is very common, including nausea, vomiting, diarrhoea, abdominal cramps and, occasionally, hepatitis or pancreatitis. Tolerance to the gastrointestinal symptoms often occurs.
- Hypertension, oedema, tachycardia, chest pain.
- Dyspnoea, cough.
- Dizziness, insomnia, headache, tremor.
- Bone marrow suppression resulting in leucopenia, thrombocytopenia and anaemia
- Opportunistic infections may be increased, especially with cytomegalovirus, herpes simplex, aspergillus and candida, as well as bacterial urinary tract infection and pneumonia.
- Lymphoproliferative disease and skin cancer.

INTERLEUKIN-2 RECEPTOR ANTIBODIES

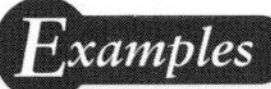

basiliximab, daclizumab

Basiliximab is a chimeric monoclonal antibody with murine sequences in the hypervariable region that bind to the α-subunit of the IL-2 receptor on activated T-cells and prevent T-cell proliferation. Daclizumab is a humanised antibody to IL-2 receptors with fewer than 10% murine sequences, making it less immunogenic. Both drugs are used to treat acute transplant rejection.

Pharmacokinetics

Basiliximab is given by intravenous infusion immediately before and again 4 days after surgery. Daclizumab is given immediately before surgery and then every 2 weeks for a total of five doses. Both drugs have very long half-lives (1–3 weeks).

Unwanted effects

Hypersensitivity reactions occur rarely.

IMMUNOSUPPRESSION IN ORGAN TRANSPLANTATION

Immunosuppressant drugs block rejection at the steps of T-cell activation, T-cell proliferation and cytokine production (Fig. 38.1). A major direction of current research is to find a regimen that will induce immune tolerance and allow eventual withdrawal of immunosuppressant drugs.

Effective immunosuppression has improved the early survival of kidney, liver, heart, heart–lung and haematopoietic stem-cell transplants. However, suppression of acute rejection is more effective than prevention of chronic rejection, which responds poorly to immunosuppressant therapy. Regimens for immunosuppression vary among transplant units and according to the immunogenicity of the transplanted tissue. Combination therapy with a corticosteroid, calcineurin inhibitor and an antiproliferative agent is commonly used.

For kidney transplantation, the corticosteroid prednisolone (Ch. 44) with ciclosporin (or sometimes tacrolimus) is widely employed; some units add azathioprine to this regimen. Initial acute rejection is reduced by treatment with the IL-2 receptor antibodies basiliximab or daclizumab. With such regimens, more than 85% of cadaveric kidney grafts will survive beyond 1 year. Only half of those that fail are lost due to rejection, and the rest from thrombosis of the graft blood supply. Progressive graft loss continues after the first year, with only 60% of grafts surviving at 10 years. Grafts from living donors have better survival rates of 95% at 1 year and 70% at 10 years. Most of the late graft losses are as a result of chronic vascular rejection. If this occurs, increasing the dosages of the primary immunosuppressant drugs may help; however, there is continuing uncertainty about whether chronic rejection reflects nephrotoxicity from long-term use of calcineurin inhibitors or inadequate immunosuppression. It is possible that drugs such as sirolimus or mycophenolate mofetil may reduce the incidence of chronic rejection, but there are few long-term data on outcome. Late acute rejection is a less common problem. It can sometimes be overcome by high-dose corticosteroid or the use of polyclonal antilymphocytic globulin or monoclonal antilymphocytic antibody (although the use of these is associated with an increased risk of opportunistic infection and long-term malignancy). Tacrolimus or mycophenolate mofetil can also be used successfully as a rescue treatment during late episodes of acute rejection.

In contrast to renal transplants, pancreatic transplants are more immunogenic and quadruple immunosuppressant regimens are widely used. Induction treatment with antilymphocytic globulin is then followed by ciclosporin, azathioprine and a corticosteroid. Mycophenolate mofetil is sometimes substituted for azathioprine, or tacrolimus for ciclosporin. Despite these treatments, 5-year graft survival is only about 60% and the risk of post-transplant infection is high.

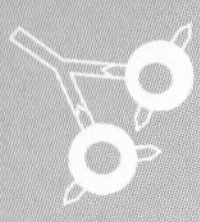

Triple immunosuppressant therapy is used for heart (50% 10-year survival), heart–lung (30% 10-year survival), liver (70% 10-year survival) and intestinal (40–50% 3-year survival) transplants, often with initial use of an IL-2 receptor antibody. In addition to prednisolone, tacrolimus is often included in these regimens in place of ciclosporin. The use of azathioprine is diminishing due to recent evidence that it may add little benefit but increase toxicity, and mycophenolate mofetil as an alternative may reduce acute rejection rates but there is less evidence for an impact on chronic rejection.

With haematopoietic stem-cell transplantation, graft-versus-host disease (GVHD) is the major barrier. This usually begins at least 3 months after the transplant, and has three phases. The first phase involves damage to intestinal mucosa and the liver, with activation of host cells and release of inflammatory cytokines. These cytokines upregulate major histocompatibility (MHC) antigens on the host cells, which are recognised by the donor T-cells. The second phase involves activation and proliferation of donor T-cells, and the third phase includes tissue destruction by monocytes primed by inflammatory cytokines and lipopolysaccharide from T-cells and damaged intestinal mucosa. GVHD can be prevented by inhibition of phase one, using a calcineurin inhibitor such as ciclosporin or tacrolimus, or possibly mycophenolate mofetil. Acute GVHD can be treated by a corticosteroid with ciclosporin, and possibly daclizumab.

IMMUNOSUPPRESSION IN OTHER DISORDERS

Immunosuppressant therapy is used for several diseases in which autoimmunity may contribute to the pathogenesis. These include many connective tissue diseases such as vasculitis and systemic lupus erythematosus, certain types of glomerulonephritis, chronic active hepatitis, psoriasis, inflammatory bowel disease and some haematological disorders. Immunosuppressant drugs may be given alone or in combination. Those most widely used include corticosteroids, azathioprine, methotrexate and cyclophosphamide (Ch. 52). Ciclosporin and mycophenolate mofetil have also been used in disorders such as asthma, inflammatory bowel disease and psoriasis, with some success.

FURTHER READING

Fernandez EJ, Lolis E (2002) Structure, function and inhibition of chemokines. *Annu Rev Pharmacol Toxicol* 42, 469–499

Fishbein TM (2009) Current concepts: intestinal transplantation. *N Engl J Med* 361, 998–1008

Hirose R, Vincenti F (2006) Immunosuppression: today, tomorrow and withdrawal. *Semin Liver Dis* 26, 201–210

Jacobsohn DA, Vogelsang GB (2002) Novel pharmacotherapeutic approaches to prevention and treatment of GVHD. *Drugs* 62, 879–889

Jørgensen KA, Koefoed-Nielsen PB, Karamperis N (2002) Calcineurin phosphatase activity and immunosuppression. A review on the role of calcineurin phosphatase activity and the immunosuppressant effect of cyclosporin A and tacrolimus. *Scand J Immunol* 57, 93–98

Kobashigawa JA, Patel JK (2006) Immunosuppression for heart transplantation: where are we now? *Nat Clin Pract Cardiovasc Med* 3, 203–212

Mascarell L, Truffa-Bachi P (2003) New aspects of cyclosporin A mode of action: from gene silencing to gene up-regulation. *Min Rev Med Chem* 3, 205–214

Neuhaus P, Klupp J, Langrehr JM (2001) mTOR inhibitors: an overview. *Liver Transpl* 7, 473–484

Snell GI, Westall GP (2007) Immunosuppression for lung transplantation: evidence to date. *Drugs* 67, 1531–1539

Tang IY, Meier-Kriesche HU, Kaplan B (2007) Immunosuppressive strategies to improve outcomes of kidney transplantation. *Semin Nephrol* 27, 377–392

Webber SA, McCurry K, Keevi A (2006) Heart and lung transplantation in children. *Lancet* 368, 53–69

SELF-ASSESSMENT

In questions 1–3, the first statement, in italics, is true. Are the accompanying statements also true?

1. *Ciclosporin, tacrolimus and corticosteroids decrease maturation of cytotoxic T-cells by suppressing IL-2 transcription.*
   a. Ciclosporin does not cause bone marrow suppression.
   b. Careful assessment of renal function is required with ciclosporin administration.
2. *Immunosuppression induced by corticosteroids involves their effects on T-cells and inflammation.* Tacrolimus enhances the actions of calcineurin.
3. *Using smaller doses than for cancer chemotherapy, drugs such as cyclophosphamide, methotrexate and azathioprine are immunosuppressant.* Azathioprine suppresses antibody-mediated immune responses.
4. Concerning the pharmacology of corticosteroids, choose the one **most appropriate** answer from the following.
   A. Act within the nucleus to inhibit the expression of genes responsible for the generation of some inflammatory mediators.
   B. Promote leukotriene synthesis in mast cells.
   C. Reduce blood sugar by increasing glucose uptake into cells.
   D. Promote growth in children.
   E. Promote cytokine-mediated macrophage activation.

5. Case history questions

> A 35-year-old woman was about to receive her second kidney transplant. The previous transplant had lasted 5 years but, despite immunosuppression with prednisolone and ciclosporin, it was eventually rejected.

a. How might the chances of acute rejection of the second transplant be reduced?
b. What could be the long-term risks of combination chemotherapy with corticosteroids, tacrolimus and azathioprine?

ANSWERS

1. a. **True**.
   b. **True**. Ciclosporin is nephrotoxic and renal monitoring is necessary.
2. **False**. Tacrolimus is a calcineurin inhibitor.
3. **True**. Azathioprine has a toxic action on cells and proliferation of antibody-producing cells is inhibited. Proliferation of cells involved in cell-mediated immunity is also inhibited.
4. Answer **A**.
   A. True. Corticosteroids decrease the expression of genes involved in the production of some inflammatory mediators.
   B. False. Corticosteroids inhibit the production of leukotrienes by inhibiting phospholipase A_2-mediated release of the precursor arachidonic acid from membrane glycerophospholipids.
   C. False. Corticosteroids can cause increased blood sugar levels due to increased gluconeogenesis and insulin resistance.
   D. False. Corticosteroids will inhibit growth in children. Growth is inhibited at multiple levels, including inhibition of growth hormone release.
   E. False. Corticosteroids inhibit macrophage activation in delayed hypersensitivity.
5. Case history answers
   a. Basiliximab given before and 4 days after surgery has been shown to reduce acute rejection by 35%. Reduction of acute rejection is also achieved with combination therapy (a calcineurin inhibitor such as ciclosporin and an antiproliferative immunosuppressant such as azathioprine) and corticosteroids. When used in combination, lower doses of the drugs can be administered than when giving the drugs alone. Intensive monitoring of liver and renal functions is important.
   b. Oversuppression of the immune response brings with it problems of opportunistic infections associated with reduced immunity. Additional 'steroid effects' as described for iatrogenic Cushing-like syndrome may be apparent.

Immunosuppressant drugs[a]

Drug	Half-life (h) and kinetics	Comment
Calcineurin inhibitors		
Ciclosporin	27 (10–40) [M] Oral bioavailability is 40%; lipid-soluble cyclic peptide metabolised by CYP3A4 in liver and gut wall to at least 25 metabolites, some of which retain biological activity	Used in organ and tissue transplantation; oral or intravenous dosage
Tacrolimus	9 (4–41) [M] Low oral bioavailability (about 20%); substrate for P-glycoprotein in the intestine; metabolised by CYP3A4 in liver and gut wall; low bioavailability combined with low systemic clearance indicate that it undergoes extensive first-pass metabolism in the gut wall but not the liver; metabolites are mostly inactive (see Ch. 2)	Used for prophylaxis to prevent kidney and liver transplant rejection; oral or intravenous dosage
mTOR (target of rapamycin) inhibitors		
Sirolimus	60 [M] Low oral bioavailability (<30%) which is increased by giving with fatty food; substrate for and inhibitor of intestinal P-glycoprotein and metabolised by CYP3A4, which contributes to low oral bioavailability	Potent non-calcineurin-inhibiting immunosuppressant; used for prophylaxis to prevent kidney transplant rejection; inhibits T-cell activation and proliferation; given orally as an oil solution
Antiproliferative agents		
Azathioprine	3–5 [M] Good oral absorption; converted to active metabolite, 6-mercaptopurine, which is converted to nucleoside and uric acid analogues (therefore interaction with allopurinol)	Antiproliferative immunosuppressant used for transplant recipients, for autoimmune conditions and for rheumatoid arthritis; oral or intravenous dosage

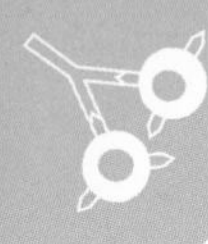

Immunosuppressant drugs

Drug	Half-life (h) and kinetics	Comment
Mycophenolate mofetil	18 (as MPA) [M] Rapidly absorbed after oral dosage; very rapidly hydrolysed (within minutes) to the active form, mycophenolic acid (MPA); oral and intravenous doses undergo essentially quantitative conversion to MPA; MPA is eliminated as a glucuronide conjugate	Used for prophylaxis to prevent acute transplant rejection; oral or intravenous dosage
Interleukin-2 receptor antibodies		
Basiliximab	7–11 days [M] Binding to interleukin-2 receptor α-chain is maintained for 1 to 2 weeks after dosage	Monoclonal antibody that prevents T-lymphocyte proliferation; used for prophylaxis to prevent kidney transplant rejection; given by intravenous infusion with ciclosporin and corticosteroid regimens
Daclizumab	20 days [M] Low clearance from the circulation	Monoclonal antibody that prevents T-lymphocyte proliferation; used for prophylaxis to prevent kidney transplant rejection; given by intravenous infusion with ciclosporin and corticosteroid regimens; normally given every 2 weeks for a total of five doses

[a]Corticosteroids, such as prednisolone, have important immunosuppressant properties. Immunostimulants are covered in Ch. 52 (Chemotherapy of malignancy). See also the inflammatory arthritides (Ch. 30).
[M], metabolism.

39 Antihistamines and allergic disease

ATOPY, ALLERGIC DISORDERS AND ANAPHYLAXIS

Allergic responses occur in atopic individuals who are predisposed to produce antigen-specific immunoglobulin E (IgE) when exposed to common, normally harmless environmental allergens such as house-dust mite, grass pollen or animal dander. Re-exposure to the allergen then results in the antigen cross-linking IgE on mast cells and basophils and triggering an allergic response as explained below. The control of antibody production in the immune response is shown in Figure 38.2. The key to the allergic reaction is that there is a preponderance of IgE production, rather than other antibodies. This is because when atopic individuals are exposed to allergens it provokes a T-helper type 2 (Th2) lymphocyte response, rather than the usually dominant Th1-cell response (Ch. 38). The production of the Th2 profile of interleukins, including IL-4, IL-10 and IL-13, by the Th2-cell type then causes the B-cells to produce IgE rather than IgG; this phenomenon is known as class switching. Dominance of Th1 or Th2 response is partially programmed in early life, with exposure to microbial antigens promoting the normal Th1 dominance.

Most allergic reactions are predominantly of the type 1 (immediate) hypersensitivity category (see Ch. 38 for definitions). Immediate hypersensitivity to an allergen in a person with atopy produces a weal and flare reaction in the skin, or sneezing and a runny nose, or wheezing, within minutes. Pre-formed and newly synthesised mediators of the allergic response are released from mast cells and basophils after allergen cross-links IgE bound to cell surface receptors. The mediators include histamine, tryptase, platelet-activating factor, prostaglandin D_2, and the cysteinyl leukotrienes LTC_4, LTD_4 and LTE_4 (Ch. 29). Tryptase activates receptors on endothelial and epithelial cells to upregulate adhesion molecules that attract inflammatory cells. Some allergic reactions, such as those that produce contact allergy and eczema, and a component of other allergic responses are driven by T-cell-mediated inflammatory processes. Many atopic individuals have coexisting allergic diseases such as asthma, hayfever and eczema, although these are not invariably associated with atopy.

A prolonged inflammatory reaction (delayed-type hypersensitivity) may follow the initial allergic response, reaching a peak 6–9 h later. Depending on the site of the reaction, this produces an oedematous, red, indurated swelling in the skin, or sustained blockage in the nose, or further wheezing. This delayed reaction is associated with initial tissue accumulation of eosinophils and neutrophils, followed by T-cells and basophils. Some delayed reactions can arise without an immediate phase, and may be triggered by activation of T-cells rather than mast cells. Chronic allergic inflammation is maintained by production of several Th2-type cytokines, such as IL-4, IL-5, IL-9, IL-10 and IL-13, which promote the development of mast cells and eosinophils, stimulate adhesion molecules and enhance the production of IgE. Eosinophils release toxic basic proteins, cysteinyl leukotrienes and platelet-activating factor. T-cells, mast cells and eosinophils also produce neurotrophins that release neuropeptides such as substance P, calcitonin gene-related peptide and neurokinin A from sensory neurons. These contribute to the inflammatory response by producing vasodilation with increased vascular permeability, and smooth muscle contraction and mucus secretion in the lung.

Allergic reactions to antigens vary in severity. At the most severe end of the spectrum is anaphylaxis, a systemic allergic reaction which is life-threatening because of respiratory obstruction and/or hypotension. Severe anaphylactic reactions can occur within minutes of exposure to the allergen. There are several causes of anaphylaxis (Box 39.1). Drugs can also act directly on mast cells to release mediators without the involvement of IgE. Such reactions are called anaphylactoid, and they present in the same way as true anaphylaxis. If the allergen exposure is via systemic injection, then hypotension and shock will predominate. Foods are more likely to cause facial and laryngeal oedema with prominent respiratory problems.

HISTAMINE AS AN AUTACOID

Histamine is a heterocyclic amine that functions as a local hormone (autacoid). It is found in mast cells, particularly in tissues that come into contact with the outside world, for example skin, lungs and gut, where it forms part of the tissue defence mechanisms. It is also present in circulating basophils, where it may have a similar role. Histamine is found also in enterochromaffin-like cells in the stomach, where it participates in acid secretion (Ch. 33), and in the brain, where it acts as a neurotransmitter (Ch. 4).

Histamine is synthesised in mast cells and basophils from dietary histidine by decarboxylation. After release from the cells it is rapidly metabolised (see Ch. 4). Its effects are mediated by four distinct types of G-protein-coupled receptors known as H_1, H_2, H_3 and H_4 (see receptor table at end

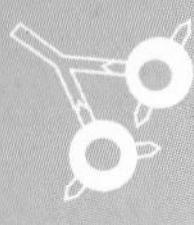

Box 39.1 Causes of anaphylaxis

Foods: especially peanuts, tree nuts, fish, shellfish, eggs, milk
Drugs: especially penicillin, intravenous anaesthetic agents, aspirin and other non-steroidal anti-inflammatory drugs, intravenous contrast media, morphine
Bee and wasp stings
Latex rubber

of Ch. 1). In general, H_1 receptors are involved in the 'defensive' actions of histamine and act through intracellular Ca^{2+} as a second messenger. Gastric acid secretion is mediated by H_2 receptors that generate cyclic adenosine monophosphate (cAMP) as a second messenger (Ch. 33). These receptors are also involved in cardiac function (stimulation of rate and force of contraction) and are inhibitory post-synaptic receptors in the brain. There also H_3 and H_4 receptors in various locations (see Ch. 1, Ch. 4).

Allergic reactions involve the action of histamine at H_1 receptors. Histamine H_1 receptors are coupled to inositol phospholipid intracellular signalling pathways. They also activate the ubiquitous gene transcription factor nuclear factor kappa B (NF-κB) (Ch. 30). NF-κB stimulates production of pro-inflammatory cytokines (particularly tumour necrosis factor alpha [TNFα] and IL-6 and IL-8) and expression of epithelial and endothelial adhesion molecules (such as intercellular adhesion molecule [ICAM]-1) that attract inflammatory cells. The following are the major consequences of H_1 receptor stimulation.

- Capillary and venous dilation can produce marked hypotension. In the skin, histamine contributes to the weal and flare response; an axon reflex via H_1 receptors is responsible for the spread of vasodilation or flare from the oedematous weal.
- Increased capillary permeability can produce oedema. This can lead to urticaria, angioedema and laryngeal oedema. The consequent loss of circulating blood volume contributes to hypotension.
- Smooth muscle contraction can occur, especially in bronchioles and the intestine.
- Skin itching (in combination with kinins and prostaglandins).
- Pain from stimulation of nociceptors.

HISTAMINE H_1 RECEPTOR ANTAGONISTS (ANTIHISTAMINES)

Examples

First-generation (sedating) antihistamines: chlorphenamine, ketotifen, promethazine
Second-generation (non-sedating) antihistamines: cetirizine, fexofenadine, loratadine, mizolastine

Mechanisms of action and effects

The antihistamines are selective for histamine H_1 receptors; antagonists at other histamine receptors are traditionally not called antihistamines. They are competitive inverse agonists (see Ch. 1) that reduce the basal level of spontaneous activity at histamine H_1 receptors as well as blocking the effects of histamine. Useful actions of antihistamines include:

- suppression of many of the vascular effects of histamine
- inhibition of inflammatory cell accumulation in tissues by second-generation antihistamines; this may result from downregulation of the activation of NF-κB in tissues at the site of an allergic response.

First-generation antihistamines have other actions that can be used therapeutically. They are lipophilic and cross the blood–brain barrier, producing sedation. They also have central antimuscarinic effects that may be clinically useful in suppressing nausea in motion sickness (e.g. cyclizine [no longer used as an antihistamine], promethazine; Ch. 32).

Second-generation (non-sedating) antihistamines such as cetirizine, fexofenadine, loratadine and mizolastine are more hydrophilic or more ionised at physiological pH; they do not penetrate the blood–brain barrier well, and have little sedative effect. They also have little antimuscarinic action.

So-called 'third-generation' antihistamines, such as desloratadine, are active metabolites of second-generation drugs. They have similar efficacy to second-generation drugs but may have a different profile of unwanted effects.

Pharmacokinetics

Chlorphenamine is slowly absorbed from the gut, while promethazine is more rapidly absorbed. Both undergo considerable first-pass metabolism in the liver to inactive compounds and have half-lives of 10–20 h. Formulations of chlorphenamine and promethazine are available for administration by intravenous or intramuscular injection in medical emergencies.

Most second-generation antihistamines are rapidly absorbed from the gut and metabolised in the liver to active compounds with half-lives ranging from 2 to 20 h. Cetirizine and fexofenadine undergo little metabolism and are mainly eliminated unchanged by the kidneys.

Several topical formulations of antihistamines exist, including nasal sprays for allergic rhinitis, topical skin preparations for insect stings (but see unwanted effects) and eye drops for allergic conjunctivitis.

Unwanted effects

- Drowsiness or psychomotor impairment, especially with first-generation compounds, although paradoxical stimulation can occur in children and the elderly
- Headache
- Dry mouth, blurred vision, urinary retention and gastrointestinal upset from the antimuscarinic effects of first-generation compounds
- Topical antihistamines for use on the skin commonly cause hypersensitivity reactions.

MANAGEMENT OF ALLERGIC DISORDERS

Most allergic reactions involve a complex series of chemical processes. However, the mainstay of treatment for many conditions is based on the use of antihistamines. Their efficacy indicates the importance of histamine as a mediator of allergic responses.

Anaphylaxis

This is a medical emergency and requires rapidly acting treatments. The person should be laid flat with their feet raised if there is hypotension. Adrenaline (epinephrine; Ch. 4) should be given intramuscularly and doses repeated every 10 min until the clinical state is stable. People known to have allergies that cause anaphylaxis can carry a pre-loaded adrenaline (epinephrine) syringe for emergencies, accompanied by detailed instructions on its appropriate use. Intravenous adrenaline (epinephrine) should only be given if there is profound shock, and then in a very dilute solution with close cardiac monitoring. Intravenous use carries a risk of arrhythmias and intense vasoconstriction with myocardial ischaemic damage.

Once adrenaline (epinephrine) has been given, late relapse can be prevented by intramuscular injection or slow intravenous injection of chlorphenamine and hydrocortisone (Ch. 44). Oxygen should be given in high concentration, and an inhaled β_2-adrenoceptor agonist such as salbutamol (Ch. 12) administered if there is marked bronchospasm. This can be particularly useful if a β-adrenoceptor antagonist has previously been taken, when adrenaline (epinephrine) may be less effective on the airways. If there is persistent hypotension, intravenous fluid should be given rapidly, preferably a colloid such as gelatin or dextran (or saline if a colloid is unavailable).

Seasonal and perennial rhinitis

The symptoms of rhinitis include nasal obstruction, sneezing, itching and inflammation of the lining of the nose. These result from increased glandular secretions producing nasal obstruction and mucous rhinorrhoea, as well as afferent nerve stimulation which is responsible for itching and sneezing. Allergies can cause both perennial (usually house-dust mite) and seasonal (pollens and moulds) rhinitis. The allergic response makes individuals more susceptible to the nasal irritant effects of non-specific stimuli, such as tobacco smoke and changes in temperature. Rhinitis also has several non-allergic causes, including acute infection and chronic sinus infection. Aspirin can produce rhinitis (as well as asthma [Ch. 12]) in sensitive subjects, probably by enhancing leukotriene generation. Prolonged use of nasal decongestants such as the α_1-adrenoceptor agonist oxymetazoline (see below) can also cause rhinitis. Less frequent causes include β-adrenoceptor antagonists (Ch. 5) and angiotensin-converting enzyme (ACE) inhibitors (Ch. 6).

Oral antihistamines are useful for reducing itching, sneezing and rhinorrhoea, but they are less effective for nasal obstruction. They can also suppress associated allergic conjunctivitis. Topical antihistamines such as azelastine (Ch. 50) are also available as a nasal spray. For more severe allergic rhinitis, a topical intranasal corticosteroid spray (Ch. 44) is the treatment of choice, providing relief from most symptoms. Topical sodium cromoglicate or nedocromil (Ch. 12) can be useful in atopic subjects, but they are less effective than antihistamines or topical corticosteroids and are no longer preferred treatments. The antimuscarinic drug ipratropium bromide (Ch. 12) can also be used topically for relief of rhinorrhoea. Nasal decongestants have a short-term role in treatment. These are solutions for topical application that contain α-adrenoceptor agonists such as ephedrine or xylometazoline. They work by producing local vasoconstriction, but prolonged use impairs ciliary activity in the nasal mucosa. They should not be taken long-term because of the risk of rebound nasal congestion. Oral corticosteroids are reserved for the most severe symptoms. If drugs fail, then the possibility of structural abnormalities such as nasal polyps, hypertrophied inferior turbinates or a deviated nasal septum should be considered, since surgery may be helpful.

Urticaria

Acute urticarial reactions often occur to the same allergens that cause anaphylaxis. Antihistamines are the treatment of choice, with an oral corticosteroid (Ch. 44) for more severe episodes.

Chronic urticaria can be provoked by physical factors such as cold, sun, scratching the skin or exercise, or it can be caused by urticarial vasculitis in association with connective tissue diseases such as systemic lupus erythematosus. In some cases, the cause may be autoimmune, caused by IgG autoantibodies to the IgE receptors on mast cells and basophils. Antihistamines can be useful to suppress the itch from urticaria, but often they have little effect on the weal. About 15% of the histamine receptors in the skin are H_2, and a histamine H_2 receptor blocker (Ch. 33) may be useful in addition to an antihistamine. Leukotriene antagonists such as montelukast (Ch. 12) may be helpful for some people. Corticosteroids (Ch. 44) can be used in high dosage for severe symptoms, but long-term use should be avoided because of the unwanted effects. Immunosuppression with ciclosporin (Ch. 38) has been used successfully for some severe autoimmune urticarias.

Allergic conjunctivitis

Topical treatment with antihistamines, such as azelastine or levocabastine, or with sodium cromoglicate or nedocromil is usually successful (see Ch. 50).

Contact and atopic eczema

Contact and atopic eczemas are considered in Chapter 49.

Asthma

Although asthma often has an allergic component, antihistamines have little or no role. The management of asthma is considered in Chapter 12.

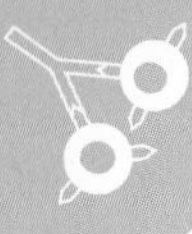

FURTHER READING

Al Suleimani YM, Walker MJA (2007) Allergic rhinitis and its pharmacology. *Pharmacol Ther* 114, 233–260

Charlesworth EN, Beltrani VS (2002) Pruritic dermatoses: overview of etiology and therapy. *Am J Med* 113(suppl 9A), 25S–33S

de Groot H, Brand PLP, Fokkens WF et al (2007) Allergic rhinoconjunctivitis in children. *BMJ* 335, 985–988

del Cuvillo A, Mullol J, Bartra J et al (2006) Comparative pharmacology of the H_1 antihistamines. *J Invest Allergol Clin Immunol* 16(suppl 1), 3–12

Ellis AK, Day JH (2003) Diagnosis and management of anaphylaxis. *CMAJ* 169, 307–311

Holgate ST, Canonica GW, Simons FE et al (2003) Consensus group on new-generation antihistamines (CONGA): present status and recommendations. *Clin Exp Allergy* 33, 1305–1324

Kaplan AP (2002) Chronic urticaria and angioedema. *N Engl J Med* 346, 175–179

Kemp SF (2007) Office approach to anaphylaxis: sooner better than later. *Am J Med* 120, 664–668

Leurs R, Church MK, Taglialatela M (2002) H_1-antihistamines: inverse agonism, anti-inflammatory actions and cardiac effects. *Clin Exp Allergy* 32, 489–498

Plaut M, Valentine MD (2005) Allergic rhinitis. *N Engl J Med* 353, 1934–1944

Saleh HA, Durham SR (2007) Perennial rhinitis. *BMJ* 335, 502–507

Simons FER (2002) Comparative pharmacology of H_1 antihistamines: clinical relevance. *Am J Med* 113(suppl 9A), 38S–46S

SELF-ASSESSMENT

In questions 1 and 2, the first statement, in italics, is true. Are the accompanying statements also true?

1. *Antihistamines such as fexofenadine and loratadine are non-sedating.*
   a. Fexofenadine is associated with electrocardiographic (ECG) changes.
   b. Antihistamines reduce acid secretion from the gastric parietal cell.
   c. Fexofenadine reduces the release of histamine from mast cells.
2. *The allergic response in mast cells from atopic individuals can cause the release of leukotrienes, histamine and prostaglandins from sensitised mast cells.*
   a. Corticosteroids are ineffective for treating allergic rhinitis.
   b. Histamine is the only mediator that causes symptoms in rhinitis.
3. In an atopic individual, which **one** of the following would contribute to an allergic response to an allergen?
   A. Increased production of cytokines from Th1-cell response.
   B. Increased production of IgM.
   C. Stabilisation of mast cells.
   D. Histamine release acting on both H_1- and H_2-type receptors.
   E. Reduction in leukotriene production from mast cells.
4. Regarding the properties of antihistamines, choose the one **correct** answer from the following.
   A. First- and second-generation antihistamines are equally sedating.
   B. Second-generation antihistamines have less antimuscarinic activity than first-generation antihistamines.
   C. First-generation antihistamines are the preferred first-line treatment for cytotoxic drug-related vomiting.
   D. Second-generation antihistamines readily cross the blood–brain barrier.
   E. Antihistamines cause vasodilation.
5. Case history questions

A 10-year-old boy visited his doctor with his mother in the spring. His current symptoms of rhinorrhoea, nasal congestion, sneezing and itching eyes were interfering with his schoolwork. He gave a history of repeated episodes of recurrent otitis media, rhinorrhoea, nasal congestion, sneezing and itching eyes occurring over a 3-year period, but predominantly in the spring and autumn. He had had three episodes of otitis media over the previous 2 years, the last being 6 months before, which were treated with antibiotics because of prolonged residence of fluid in the middle ear. The boy had suffered from atopic dermatitis as an infant. He had no history of asthma; his mother had allergic rhinitis; they had two cats. Other than antibacterial drug treatment for his otitis media, he had taken no medication. Examination of the ears revealed healthy tympanic membranes with no current otitis media. He had no hearing loss. He was otherwise fit.

   a. What was the likely diagnosis?
   b. Were the boy's symptoms related to the history of otitis media?

Allergen skin testing showed him to be responsive to cat dander and house-dust mite.

   c. What treatment would you give?

ANSWERS

1. a. **False**. The original parent drug, terfenadine, was associated with ventricular arrhythmias in high doses and has now been withdrawn. Fexofenadine, a metabolite of terfenidine retains the parent drug's antihistamine activity without having unwanted effects on the heart.
   b. **False**. The histamine receptors on the parietal cell are H_2 subtype and are not affected by these anti-

histamines, which act on H_1 receptors. H_2 receptor antagonists such as cimetidine are used.

c. **False**. Fexofenadine acts only on the H_1 receptors.

2. a. **False**. Nasal corticosteroids are very effective.
   b. **False**. Prostaglandins and leukotrienes can also be released from mast cells and contribute to symptoms.
3. Answer **D**.
   A. False. In atopy there is a predominance of a Th2 response profile which is partially genetically determined.
   B. False. The Th2 response leads to increased production of IgE.
   C. False. Mast cells degranulate following allergen cross-linking of IgE on mast cells.
   D. True. Although the main effect of histamine in allergy is on the H_1 receptor, actions on H_2 receptors also contribute to the allergic symptoms.
   E. False. Leukotriene synthesis in mast cells increases, contributing to the allergic response.
4. Answer **B**.
   A. False. First-generation drugs such as promethazine are more sedating than second-generation drugs such as fexofenadine.
   B. True.
   C. False. Antihistamines can be effective in motion sickness but not vomiting caused by cancer chemotherapeutic agents.
   D. False. Second-generation antihistamines cross the blood–brain barrier less readily than the first-generation antihistamines.
   E. False. Antihistamines reduce vasodilation induced by the action of histamine at the H_1 receptor which contributes to the wheal and flare response.
5. Case history answers
   a. The family history of atopy and the child's atopic dermatitis as an infant increase the likelihood that he would have had allergies. He is likely to have had seasonal allergic rhinitis but he may also have had sensitisation to cat and/or dust mite or other allergens. His fitness and lack of current drug intake suggest that it is not non-allergic rhinitis, which may arise because of infections, drugs, etc.
   b. Yes. As many as 50% of children older than 3 years with recurrent otitis media have confirmed allergic rhinitis.
   c. It was important to carry out sensitivity testing, and sensitivity to cat dander and house-dust mite was identified in this boy. Avoidance of exposure to allergens is advisable and should be actively pursued in the home and school environment. If pharmacological treatment is required, a non-sedating oral antihistamine should reduce rhinorrhoea, sneezing and itching but will have little effect on nasal congestion. A short course of nasal inhaled corticosteroids can be effective in controlling symptoms of allergic rhinitis, including congestion. Nasal cromoglicate may also offer symptom relief but is not the preferred treatment.

Antihistamines[a]

Drug	Half-life (h) and kinetics	Comments
Non-sedating antihistamines		
All drugs are given orally and used for symptomatic relief of allergic conditions such as hayfever and urticaria		
Acrivastine	2 [R + M] Rapidly absorbed; renal excretion of unchanged drug accounts for 60% of an oral dose, indicating high bioavailability; about 15% is converted to an active metabolite which has a half-life of 4 h	
Cetirizine	6–10 [R] Complete oral bioavailability; clearance is by both glomerular filtration and active renal tubular secretion; undergoes limited metabolism	
Desloratadine	20–30 [M] Undergoes hydroxylation in the liver and the product is conjugated with glucuronic acid and excreted in urine; slow metabolisers have been identified who show longer half-life and elimination via the urine rather than metabolism	The active metabolite of loratadine
Fexofenadine	14 [R] Oral bioavailability has not been defined; about 1% only is metabolised (by CYP3A4); mostly eliminated in faeces, possibly due to incomplete absorption	The active metabolite of terfenadine (no longer used)
Levocetirizine	8–9 [R + M] Rapidly absorbed; about 14% is metabolised by CYP3A4 and the remainder excreted in urine unchanged	The levo-isomer of cetirizine

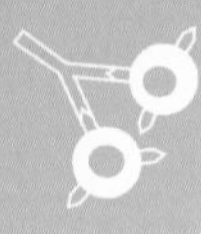

Antihistamines[a]

Drug	Half-life (h) and kinetics	Comments
Loratadine	8 [M] Oral bioavailability (about 10%) increased by food; it is a prodrug which undergoes extensive first-pass metabolism by CYP3A4 and CYP2D6 to the active desloratadine, which has a half-life of 20–30 h	
Mizolastine	15 [M] Oral bioavailability is about 70%; active metabolites have not been detected	
Sedating antihistamines		
All drugs are given orally unless otherwise indicated		
Alimemazine	4–7 [R + M] Undergoes hepatic metabolism via S-oxidation and N-dealkylation (which produces an active metabolite)	Used for urticaria and pruritus and as a premedication
Chlorphenamine	22 [R + M] Oral bioavailability is about 50%; some metabolism via CYP2D6; renal excretion is more important than metabolism	Used orally for symptomatic relief of hayfever and urticaria and by slow intravenous injection as an adjunct to adrenaline (epinephrine) for the emergency treatment of anaphylaxis and angioedema
Clemastine	21 [M] Oral bioavailability is 40%; earlier data indicated a half-life of 4–6 h	Used for symptomatic relief of hayfever and urticaria; metabolised by oxidation
Cyproheptadine	1–4 [M] Eliminated by oxidative metabolism; few kinetic data are available; duration of action is about 12 h	Used for symptomatic relief of hayfever and urticaria and in the treatment of migraine
Hydroxyzine	About 20 [M] Rapidly absorbed; metabolised to an active metabolite, cetirizine, which has a formation rate limited half-life, i.e. it is determined by the half-life of hydroxyzine	Used for pruritus and for the short-term treatment of anxiety
Ketotifen	22 [M] Rapidly absorbed but bioavailability is 50% due to first-pass metabolism; eliminated by oxidation and conjugation (as an N-glucuronide)	Used for allergic conjunctivitis and allergic rhinitis
Promethazine	10–14 [M] Low oral bioavailability (25%); converted to inactive metabolites in the liver; bile is the major route of elimination of metabolites	Used orally for symptomatic relief of hayfever and urticaria and by slow intravenous injection as an adjunct to adrenaline (epinephrine) for the emergency treatment of anaphylaxis and angioedema; also used for motion sickness and as a premedication before anaesthesia; can also be given by deep intramuscular injection

[a]Antihistamines may also be given topically in the eye, nose and on the skin. Drugs with antihistamine actions which are not used to treat allergic conditions, such as cinnarizine and cyclizine and meclozine (see Ch. 32), are used for the treatment of vestibular disorders and nausea and vomiting, especially motion sickness.
[M], metabolism; [R], renal excretion.

9

The endocrine system and metabolism

40 Diabetes mellitus

CONTROL OF BLOOD GLUCOSE

Glucose occupies a central position in metabolism as the predominant substrate for energy production. Cells receive their supply of glucose from blood, and control mechanisms ensure that blood glucose concentrations remain within narrow limits. Glucose enters the blood by absorption from the gut and from breakdown of stored glycogen or gluconeogenesis in the liver. At physiological concentrations, glucose is transferred from the blood into cells almost entirely by active transport: in most tissues, this transfer is dependent on the action of the polypeptide hormone insulin.

Insulin is a protein that is rapidly secreted from the beta cells of the islets of Langerhans in the pancreas in response to a small rise in blood glucose; its secretion is inhibited by a fall in blood glucose (Table 40.1). Insulin consists of two peptide chains, A and B, connected by two disulphide bridges. In the beta cell, insulin aggregates into hexamers with zinc, and after release it dissociates into dimers and eventually the active monomeric form.

The presence of nutrients in the small intestine stimulates the release from gut endocrine cells of peptide hormones called incretins, which stimulate insulin secretion. The principal incretins are glucose-dependent insulinotropic peptide (GIP) secreted by the upper gut, and glucagon-like peptide-1 (GLP-1) that is released from the lower intestine. Incretins are probably responsible for about 60% of the insulin that is secreted in response to a meal. GLP-1 has several actions that regulate glucose homeostasis:

- enhanced glucose-dependent insulin secretion
- suppression of glucagon secretion
- reduced gastric emptying
- promotion of satiety by an action on the hypothalamus (Ch. 37).

The actions of GLP-1 and GIP are brief as they have very short plasma half-lives owing to rapid degradation by the enzyme dipeptidyl peptidase-IV (DPP-IV).

Insulin is secreted into the blood under fasting conditions, with pulses every 10–14 min, and a slower cycle of release every 105–120 min. In response to a rise in plasma glucose (both the actual concentration and the rate of change), there is a superimposed biphasic pattern of insulin release.

- The **first phase** of release occurs within seconds, peaks at 3–5 min, and lasts for about 10 min. This is achieved by the release of a small pool of insulin in secretory vesicles.
- The **second phase** is more gradual, rising to a lower peak than in phase 1, and is partly due to release of a stored insulin pool, and partly to synthesis of new insulin.

In the pancreatic beta cells there are K^+ channels in the cell membrane that are sensitive to ATP (K_{ATP} channels) which can indirectly affect insulin secretion. The K_{ATP} channel is associated with a regulatory protein (SUR1) which is the site of action for the sulphonylurea drugs (see below) and is stimulated by ATP. A rise in the plasma glucose concentration increases the intracellular adenosine triphosphate (ATP) concentration in the beta cell. Activation of the receptor by ATP closes the K_{ATP} channel; this reduces membrane K^+ efflux, which depolarises the beta cell. Depolarisation opens voltage-dependent L-type Ca^{2+} channels in the cell membrane, and an influx of Ca^{2+} ions into the cell triggers exocytosis of insulin granules. (See Fig. 5.4 for description of the K_{ATP} channel in vascular smooth muscle.) In addition to glucose, many other factors influence insulin secretion (Table 40.1).

Peripheral tissues express specific cell surface receptors for insulin that are linked to a tyrosine kinase (insulin receptor kinase) (Ch. 1). Stimulation of these receptors leads to translocation of the glucose transporter (Glut 4) to the cell surface, allowing glucose uptake, and activates numerous other intracellular lipid and protein kinase enzymes. Metabolic effects of insulin include:

- Inhibition of the conversion of amino acids to glucose (gluconeogenesis) in the liver, enhanced glucose storage as glycogen, and inhibition of the breakdown of

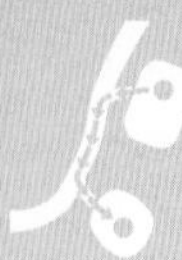

Table 40.1 Control of insulin release from pancreatic islets of Langerhans beta cells

Stimulants of insulin release	Inhibitors of insulin release
Parasympathetic stimulation (muscarinic receptors)	Sympathetic stimulation of α_2-adrenoceptors
Glucose	Somatostatin
Amino acids	Decreased glucose
Fatty acids	
Cortisol	
Gastrin	
Secretin	
Glucagon	
Incretins: glucagon-like peptide-1 (GLP-1) glucose-dependent insulinotropic peptide (GIP)	

glycogen (glycogenolysis). The overall effect is to increase glycogen stores.

- Promotion of active transport of glucose into the cell, particularly in skeletal muscle, accompanied by K^+.
- Reduced plasma free fatty acids and increased adipocyte triglyceride storage. Insulin inhibits lipases and prevents triglyceride breakdown in adipose tissue. It also increases hydrolysis of circulating triglycerides from lipoproteins by enhancing the activity of lipoprotein lipase. Glucose entry into adipocytes provides glycerol phosphate for esterification of fatty acids.
- Effects on protein metabolism, with inhibition of the catabolism of amino acids in the liver and, to a lesser extent, increased amino acid transport into muscle and enhanced protein synthesis.

The effects of insulin on different tissues are summarised in Table 40.2.

Several hormones inhibit the anabolic actions of insulin, particularly on carbohydrate metabolism, although effects on protein metabolism vary. These include glucagon, growth hormone, cortisol and catecholamines. Most of these hormones are released in stressful situations that require the breakdown of glycogen reserves for energy.

DIABETES MELLITUS

Failure to secrete sufficient insulin to control the normal level of blood glucose results in diabetes mellitus. The condition is diagnosed when the fasting plasma glucose concentration exceeds 7 mmol L^{-1}. The long-term consequences include increased risk of the development of vascular and neuropathic disease (Table 40.3). Two patterns of diabetes mellitus are recognised: type 1 and type 2. There is still dispute over whether they represent distinct entities, or different manifestations of the same disease process. There is a strong genetic predisposition for both conditions.

Table 40.2 Metabolic effects of insulin

Liver	Increased glucose storage as glycogen Decreased protein catabolism Increased protein synthesis Decreased gluconeogenesis
Muscle	Increased protein synthesis Increased glycogen synthesis Increased glucose uptake Increased amino acid uptake
Adipose tissue	Increased triglyceride storage Increased triglyceride synthesis Decreased lipolysis

Table 40.3 Complications of diabetes

Complication	Consequences
Microvascular	
Nephropathy	Microalbuminuria, macroalbuminuria, renal failure
Retinopathy	Background retinopathy, proliferative retinopathy leading to visual impairment
Peripheral neuropathy	Loss of peripheral sensation Pain, ulceration
Autonomic neuropathy	Impotence Gastrointestinal disturbance Orthostatic hypotension
Macrovascular	
Cardiovascular disease	Hypertension Ischaemic heart disease
Cerebrovascular disease	Stroke

TYPE 1 (OR INSULIN-DEPENDENT) DIABETES MELLITUS; IDDM

Type 1 diabetes represents a severe deficiency of insulin production and usually presents in younger people. There is destruction of pancreatic beta cells, usually as part of an autoimmune process, although the cause in some cases is unknown. Individuals with type 1 diabetes typically present with a history of feeling tired and unwell, together with weight loss; they develop polyuria and polydipsia, and are prone to ketoacidosis because of breakdown of fatty acids and amino acids in the liver.

TYPE 2 (OR NON-INSULIN-DEPENDENT) DIABETES MELLITUS; NIDDM

Type 2 diabetes, which usually presents later in life, is the consequence of a relative deficiency of insulin. It accounts for 90% of cases of diabetes in the Western world. In established type 2 diabetes, the first phase of insulin secretion is absent or attenuated, and the second phase is slowed. Evidence of beta-cell dysfunction, such as an abnormal glucose tolerance test, precedes overt diabetes by up to 10 years. Maximum insulin release is reduced by up to 50% in type 2 diabetes, particularly in non-obese people, in whom reduced insulin secretion is more important than the reduced ability of insulin to promote glucose uptake into tissues (tissue insulin resistance; see below).

There are many reasons for impaired insulin secretion in type 2 diabetes, including high circulating free fatty acids, and the production of reactive oxygen species in response to a sustained high plasma glucose concentration. Enhanced free fatty acid oxidation in diabetes also contributes to the development of insulin resistance by inhibition of enzymes in the glycolytic pathway and attenuation of transmembrane glucose transport. In type 2 diabetes, there is reduced or absent GLP-1 secretion in response to oral glucose, and a reduced sensitivity to the peptide at pancreatic beta cells.

People with type 2 diabetes are often overweight (the average body mass index at diagnosis is 30 kg m^{-2}), and this increases cellular resistance to insulin in the liver and peripheral tissues. Insulin resistance characteristically precedes overt diabetes by several years, but for some time insulin secretion by the pancreas is sufficient to overcome cellular resistance. Beta-cell dysfunction with loss of the early-phase insulin response to a glucose load results in loss of compensation for insulin resistance. As a result, there is both reduced tissue uptake of glucose and an inability to adequately suppress hepatic glucose output. In type 2 diabetes, postprandial hyperglycaemia is the major defect in blood glucose control.

People with type 2 diabetes do not usually develop ketoacidosis, because sufficient glucose enters cells to permit adequate energy production for most situations. The main problem is excess glucose outside the cells rather than a shortage inside. The ideal approach to treatment would be an intervention that restores the early phase of insulin secretion in response to a glucose load.

INSULINS AND INSULIN ANALOGUES

Normal insulin secretion from the pancreas is into the portal circulation and is strictly related to metabolic needs. Sixty per cent of the insulin that is released from the pancreas is extracted by the liver before it reaches the systemic circulation. In contrast, therapeutic delivery of insulin is to the systemic circulation, and the relationship to metabolic needs can only be approximated by the dosages used and their timing in relation to meals.

Natural insulin formulations

Insulins for therapeutic administration were formerly extracted from either bovine or pig pancreas. Bovine insulin differs chemically from human insulin in three amino acid residues, and porcine in one, but their actions are very similar to human insulin. Human-sequence insulin is produced either by enzymatic modification of porcine insulin, or by recombinant DNA technology using bacteria or yeast. Human-sequence insulin preparations have largely superseded those of animal origin. All current insulin preparations have a low content of impurities, which have caused problems in the past, and have low immunogenic potential.

Pharmacokinetics

Currently available insulins must be given parenterally, because insulin is a protein and would otherwise be digested in the gut. At present, subcutaneous injection is used for routine treatment, and intravenous infusion for emergency situations. An inhaled formulation of insulin was marketed and then withdrawn, but several others are in development. The half-life of insulin in plasma is very short (about 8–16 min), and to avoid the need for frequent injections during maintenance treatment, the absorption of insulin from injection sites must be prolonged. Insulin is formulated either in a soluble preparation or is complexed with a substance to delay absorption from the injection site (Table 40.4). After subcutaneous injection, the maximum plasma concentration of soluble insulin (also called neutral insulin) is achieved about 2 h later, compared with minutes after intravenous injection. To limit the increase in plasma glucose concentration generated by a meal, subcutaneous insulin must be given at least 30 min before eating. The action of intravenous soluble insulin lasts less than an hour and is mainly terminated by degradation in the kidney. Continued absorption from a subcutaneous injection site prolongs the duration of action after injection to about 5 h.

Recommended subcutaneous injection sites include upper arms, thigh, buttocks and abdomen. Absorption is faster from the abdomen than from the limbs, although strenuous exercise can increase absorption from the limbs.

To generate intermediate- or long-acting formulations, insulin is complexed with:

- **Protamine**: to create the intermediate-acting complex. This can be given as a ready-mixed preparation that consists of a complex of protamine with bovine, porcine or human insulin (*isophane insulin*). It can also be formulated as a mixture of isophane insulin together with a non-complexed solution of insulin from the same species (*biphasic isophane insulin*). The ratio of soluble to isophane insulin in biphasic insulin varies from 10:90, through 20:80; 30:70, 40:60, to 50:50.
- **Zinc**: to create the intermediate-acting *insulin zinc* suspension or the long-acting *crystalline insulin zinc* suspension. Insulin molecules form hexamers, and the size of these molecular aggregates determines the rate of diffusion from the site of injection. Such complexes act as modified-release formulations for subcutaneous administration (Table 40.4).
- **Protamine and zinc**: to create the long-acting *protamine–zinc* insulin. This is now rarely used because it binds soluble insulin if given in the same syringe.

Unwanted effects

- The main problem is an excessive action producing hypoglycaemia. Neuroglycopenia with confusion and coma can occur. Treatment is by intravenous injection of 20% glucose if the person is unconscious, or sugary foods or drinks, oral glucose or glucose gel (Hypostop®; 10–20 g) if conscious. Glucagon (see below) can be given intramuscularly if the person is unconscious and venous access is not available, followed by a sugary

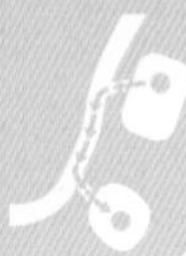

Table 40.4 Comparisons among insulins following subcutaneous administration

Type	Onset of action	Peak activity (h)	Duration (h)	
Insulin formulations				
Neutral (regular or soluble)	0.5 h	1–3	7	Short-acting
Isophane[a]	1 h	2–6	20	Intermediate-/long-acting
Zinc	2 h	6–14	22	Long-acting
Protamine–zinc	4 h	12–24	30	Long-acting
Insulin analogues				
Insulin lispro	10–20 min	0.5–0.75	2–5	Short-acting
Insulin aspart	10–20 min	0.6–0.7	2–4	Short-acting
Insulin glulisine	10–20 min	1	5	Short-acting
Insulin glargine	Plateau (4–24 h)		15–30	Long-acting
Insulin detemir	Plateau (7–24 h)		>20	Long-acting

[a]Sometimes called NPH insulin (neutral protamine Hagedorn).

drink on waking. All people with diabetes who take insulin should carry a card with details of their treatment. Although most get warning symptoms of hypoglycaemia, some do not and are prone to sudden and severe hypoglycaemic coma. More frequent hypoglycaemic attacks reduce the awareness of their onset.

- Rebound hyperglycaemia can occur after an episode of hypoglycaemia, especially at night (Somogyi effect). This results from the compensatory release of hormones such as adrenaline. It can produce ketonuria, leading to a mistaken belief that too little insulin has been given.
- Animal insulins produce circulating antibodies, although this is less common with current highly purified preparations. These could diminish the activity of the insulin (insulin resistance) or produce local reactions (lipoatrophy) at injection sites.
- Insulins can cause local fat hypertrophy at the injection site; rotating the site of injection reduces this.

Insulin analogues

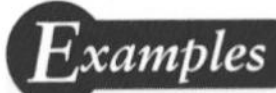

Short-acting: insulin aspart, insulin glulisine, insulin lispro
Long-acting: insulin detemir, insulin glargine

Mechanism of action and effects

The insulin analogues are recombinant chemical modifications of naturally occurring insulin. These changes have no effect on the binding of the molecule to cellular insulin receptors.

Short-acting insulin analogues

These do not readily form dimers and hexamers, and therefore they are rapidly absorbed from an injection site.

- Insulin aspart has one amino acid substitution of aspartic acid for proline at position B28.
- Insulin glulisine has two amino acid changes involving substitution with glutamic acid for lysine at B29 and lysine for asparagine at B3.
- Insulin lispro has the amino acids lysine and proline reversed at positions B28 and B29.

Long-acting insulin analogues

- Insulin detemir has threonine at B30 omitted and a fatty acid chain added to the amino acid B29.This increases the formation of insulin complexes and enhances binding to albumin, both actions which slow absorption from the injection site.
- Insulin glargine has two amino acid changes involving substitution of glycine for asparagine at A21 and addition of two arginines to the C-terminus of the B chain. This makes the molecule more soluble at acid pH, and less soluble at physiological pH. Insulin glargine precipitates after subcutaneous injection, slowly redissolves and is then absorbed.

Pharmacokinetics

Compared with standard soluble insulin, absorption of short-acting insulin analogues from a subcutaneous injection site occurs faster and leads to an early and high peak plasma concentration (Table 40.4). The duration of action is also shorter, at almost 3 h. They are usually given just before a meal, but can be used immediately after eating. They can be mixed with long-acting standard insulins, and are also available as biphasic formulations (insulin aspart with insulin aspart protamine in a 30:70 ratio; insulin lispro with insulin lispro protamine in a 25:75 ratio). Insulin aspart can be given by subcutaneous injection or infusion, and insulin lispro by subcutaneous injection or infusion, intravenous injection or intravenous infusion.

Long-acting insulin analogues are slowly and uniformly absorbed after subcutaneous injection, which avoids plasma insulin peaks.

Unwanted effects

- These are similar to those of other insulins. Despite the structural modifications, there is no reported excess of immunogenic reactions compared with standard insulin.
- There is a slightly reduced frequency of hypoglycaemia with insulin aspart or lispro compared with soluble insulin, because of the shorter duration of action.

THERAPEUTIC REGIMENS FOR INSULIN

The choice of regimen for insulin administration depends on the age, lifestyle, circumstances and preference of the individual. The general principle is to maintain a background (basal) level of insulin with boluses prior to meals to deal with the glucose load (basal-bolus regimens). Options include the following:

- **Single daily injections before breakfast or at bedtime**: used mainly for elderly people with type 2 diabetes who require insulin, and in whom the long-term complications of diabetes are less relevant. An intermediate- or long-acting insulin is used which can be combined with a short-acting one to optimise control.
- **Twice-daily injections before breakfast and evening meal**: suitable for people who have a reasonably stable pattern of activity and eating habits. Short- and intermediate-acting insulins are combined, either in fixed ratios provided by the manufacturers (see above), or in varying ratios according to individual requirements.
- **Multiple injections before breakfast and evening meal and at bedtime** are increasingly used in younger, active people who require more flexibility in their lifestyle. A number of tailored regimens can be employed using short- and intermediate-acting insulins. One regimen is short-acting insulin before breakfast, midday and evening meal, with an intermediate-acting insulin at bedtime to ensure a 'background' level during the night. A second regimen is short-acting insulin given before breakfast and evening meal and the amount adjusted for the size of the meal. To ensure a 'background' effect of insulin throughout the 24 h, intermediate-acting insulin may be added at breakfast and at bedtime, depending upon individual insulin requirements.

  There are also situations in which a basal-bolus regimen is not appropriate:
- **Continuous subcutaneous infusion** of a short-acting insulin via a portable infusion pump is sometimes used if there is a problem with recurrent or unpredictable hypoglycaemia despite optimisation of a multiple-injection insulin regimen
- **Intravenous infusion**: used for treatment of ketoacidotic crises, in labour, during and after surgery, or at other times when the person's usual routine cannot be adhered to. Short-acting insulin is infused in 5% dextrose solution with added potassium chloride (unless there is hyperkalaemia).
- **Intraperitoneal infusion**: people with diabetes who are being treated for chronic renal failure by continuous ambulatory peritoneal dialysis can add their insulin to the dialysis fluid. Some implantable insulin pumps also use this route. This is the only therapeutic regimen in which insulin has direct access to the portal circulation.

OTHER PARENTERAL HYPOGLYCAEMIC DRUGS

Synthetic incretin mimetic

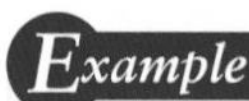

exenatide

Mechanism of action

Exenatide is a peptide that shares part of its amino acid sequence with the naturally occurring incretin, glucagon-like peptide-1 (GLP-1), but was developed from a peptide called exendin-4 found in the saliva of a North American lizard called the Gila monster. Exenatide binds to and activates the GLP-1 receptor, leading to an increase in glucose-dependent synthesis of insulin and secretion of insulin from beta cells. Exenatide restores the first-phase insulin response to an oral glucose load and, unlike insulin, promotes weight loss.

Pharmacokinetics

Exenatide is given by subcutaneous injection. It is eliminated by the kidney and has a short half-life of about 2 h.

Unwanted effects

- Nausea, vomiting, diarrhoea, abdominal pain
- Dizziness, headache, fatigue
- Injection site reactions.

ORAL HYPOGLYCAEMIC DRUGS

The main sites of action of oral hypoglycaemic drugs are shown in Figure 40.1.

Sulphonylureas

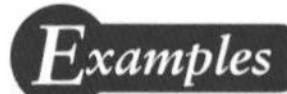

glibenclamide, gliclazide, glimepiride, glipizide, tolbutamide

Mechanism of action

Sulphonylureas act mainly by increasing the release of insulin from the pancreatic beta cells in response to stimulation by glucose (Fig. 40.1). They bind to the SUR1 receptor and inhibit the K_{ATP} (K_{ir}) channel in the cell membrane. The resultant membrane depolarisation increases both first- and second-phase insulin secretion in response to glucose and amino acids. Compounds with a short duration of action are usually preferred, to minimise the risk of hypoglycaemia.

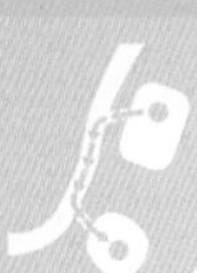

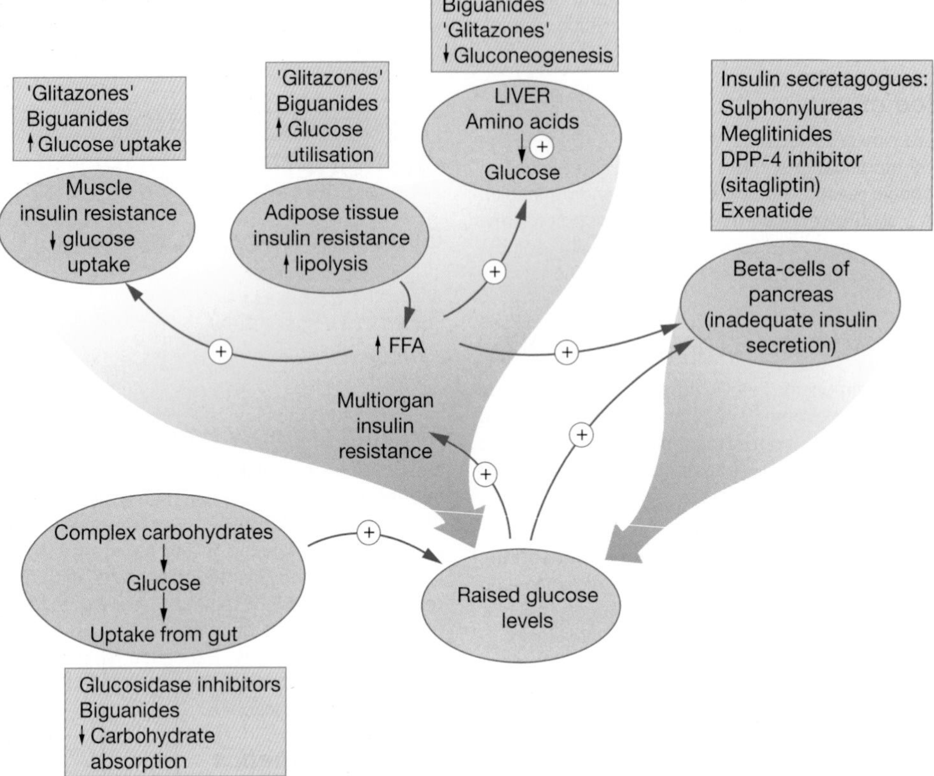

Fig. 40.1 **Metabolic dysfunctions in type 2 diabetes and sites of drug action**. The metabolic dysfunctions seen in type 2 diabetes are illustrated in blue areas; these result from inadequate insulin secretion and tissue resistance to the effects of insulin. Orally active drug classes that are used to overcome the metabolic dysfunctions are 'insulin sensitisers' or increase insulin secretion and are shown in the orange boxes together with their actions. DPP-4, dipeptidyl peptidase-4; FFA, free fatty acids.

Pharmacokinetics

Sulphonylureas are structurally related to sulphonamides. They are absorbed rapidly (although the rate of absorption is reduced when taken with food), are highly protein bound, and are metabolised by the liver. Tolbutamide, glipizide, glimepiride and gliclazide have half-lives of <10 h and short durations of action.

Glibenclamide has a longer duration of action than would be predicted from its short plasma half-life, because of slow dissociation from the SUR1 receptor. It is not recommended for treatment of the elderly.

Unwanted effects

- Gastrointestinal disturbance, with nausea, vomiting, diarrhoea, constipation.
- Hypoglycaemia (particularly nocturnal) is most frequent with the longer-acting drugs or with excessive dosage since the drugs continue to work at low plasma glucose concentrations. Long-acting drugs should be avoided in the elderly.
- Weight gain is almost inevitable unless dietary restrictions are observed.
- Hypersensitivity reactions (usually in the first 6–8 weeks of therapy) include skin rashes and, rarely, blood disorders.
- Glipizide occasionally increases renal sensitivity to antidiuretic hormone and can produce water retention with dilutional hyponatraemia.
- Sulphonylureas (apart from glipizide) should be avoided in individuals with acute porphyria.
- Concerns have been raised that sulphonylureas might increase cardiovascular mortality in type 2 diabetes, possibly as a result of binding to the SUR2 receptor and inhibiting K_{ATP} channels in the heart. These channels have a cardioprotective role in ischaemic tissue, preventing cell depolarisation to conserve intracellular energy stores. Inhibition of the channels could lead to arrhythmias in diabetics with ischaemic heart disease (see Ch. 5). However, recent clinical studies have failed to confirm the original concerns about cardiovascular mortality. Glimepiride and gliclazide bind less avidly than other sulphonylureas to cardiac SUR2 receptors.
- There is some evidence that sulphonylureas may accelerate the rate of pancreatic beta-cell loss.

Meglitinides (also called 'meglinides' or 'glinides')

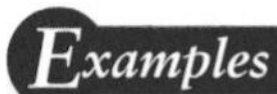

nateglinide, repaglinide

Mechanism of action

Nateglinide and repaglinide chemically resemble the sulphonylurea moiety of glibenclamide; this moiety is called meglitinide and the currently available glinides are derived from this. Nateglinide binds to the sulphonylurea receptor on the beta cell, while repaglinide binds to a different nearby site. They stimulate insulin release in the same way as sulphonylureas. Nateglinide, unlike repaglinide, has a greater effect on insulin secretion when plasma glucose levels are rising and therefore produces little stimulation of insulin secretion in the fasting state. They have a rapid onset of action and a short duration of activity, and thus are taken shortly before main meals.

Pharmacokinetics

Both nateglinide and repaglinide are rapidly and well absorbed from the gut, and are given immediately before a meal. They are metabolised in the liver to inactive metabolites and have short half-lives (1–2 h).

Unwanted effects

- Gastrointestinal upset, including nausea, vomiting, abdominal pain, diarrhoea or constipation, with repaglinide.
- Hypoglycaemia, but much less than with sulphonylureas owing to the short duration of action. This also reduces the need to snack between meals, so weight gain is not usual.
- Hypersensitivity reactions with rashes and urticaria.

Biguanides

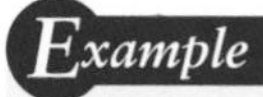

metformin

Mechanism of action and effects

Metformin does not affect insulin secretion. The molecular target of metformin is unknown, but it requires the hepatic enzyme AMP-activated protein kinase which is a key regulator of the metabolism of fat and glucose. The major actions are as follows:

- Partial suppression of hepatic gluconeogenesis is the most important effect. Since some gluconeogenic activity remains, the risk of hypoglycaemia is minimal.
- Facilitation of glucose uptake in skeletal muscle and adipocytes. The full effect requires the presence of insulin. Metformin inhibits mitochondrial respiratory chain oxidation, which increases cell surface expression and activity of the membrane glucose transporters GLU1 and 4, but this effect is relatively weak.
- Improvement in the adverse plasma lipid profile found in diabetes. Metformin reduces free fatty acid oxidation, which raises plasma high-density lipoprotein (HDL) cholesterol and reduces plasma triglycerides (Ch. 48).
- A variety of effects unrelated to glucose control, including potential anti-atherosclerotic and anti-thrombotic actions. Improved endothelial function and an anti-apoptotic effect may underlie some of these actions.

Metformin can suppress appetite and causes less weight gain than with sulphonylureas, which is useful in overweight people with diabetes.

Pharmacokinetics

Metformin is slowly and incompletely absorbed from the gut and is excreted unchanged by the kidney. It has a short half-life (2–4 h).

Unwanted effects

- Gastrointestinal upset, including anorexia, nausea, abdominal discomfort and diarrhoea (usually transient).
- Metallic taste.
- Decreased vitamin B_{12} absorption.
- Inhibition of pyruvate metabolism encourages lactate accumulation. Lactic acidosis can result in situations that lead to an increase in anaerobic metabolism (e.g. shock with hypoxaemia), and metformin should be avoided in these situations. Lactic acidosis is more common in the presence of renal impairment, although the degree of renal impairment at which this becomes a significant risk is unclear.

Thiazolidinediones (also called 'glitazones')

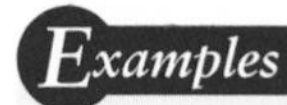

pioglitazone, rosiglitazone

Mechanisms of action and effects

Thiazolidinediones have no effect on insulin secretion but are insulin sensitisers. The effects are mediated through binding to peroxisome proliferator-activated receptor gamma (PPAR-γ) in the cell nucleus. PPAR-γ associates as a heterodimer with the retinoid X receptor (RXR) (Ch. 1) in the cell nucleus and binds to PPAR-γ response elements in the promoter domains of target genes. In the absence of a ligand, this heterodimer is further associated with a multi-protein co-repressor complex that contains histone deacetylase activity and inhibits gene transcription. When a PPAR ligand binds to the PPAR/RXR heterodimer, the co-repressor complex dissociates and a co-activator complex with histone acetylase activity is recruited. In the case of PPAR-γ, this results in the expression of genes that control adipocyte differentiation, and may increase the number of small adipocytes which are more insulin-sensitive.

The actions of thiazolidinediones include:

- Enhanced insulin sensitivity and glucose utilisation in peripheral tissues, especially in adipocytes but also skeletal muscle and hepatocytes. Adipose tissue more

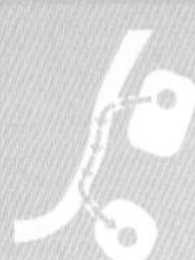

readily takes up triglycerides from the blood, and as a secondary effect reduced availability of non-esterified fatty acids to muscle improves insulin sensitivity in muscle cells. Other effects on adipocyte cell signalling may also influence tissue insulin sensitivity. These include reduced synthesis of pro-inflammatory cytokines that interfere with the insulin signalling cascade, such as tumour necrosis factor alpha and interleukin-6, and an increase in the insulin-sensitising and anti-inflammatory cytokine adiponectin.

- Suppression of gluconeogenesis in the liver by inhibition of the enzyme fructose-1,6-bisphosphatase.
- In addition to reducing the plasma glucose concentration, the effect on triglycerides also improves diabetic dyslipidaemia. Pioglitazone, in particular, increases plasma HDL cholesterol concentrations, due to increased lipolysis of triglycerides in very-low-density lipoprotein (VLDL). The plasma low-density lipoprotein (LDL) fraction may also become larger and less dense, which may further reduce atherogenesis (Ch. 48). Overall, fat is redistributed from visceral to subcutaneous stores.
- A small reduction in blood pressure, possibly by improving endothelial function and reducing sympathetic nervous system activity. They also reduce diabetic microalbuminuria.

Pharmacokinetics

Pioglitazone and rosiglitazone are well absorbed from the gut and are metabolised in the liver. They have half-lives of 3–7 h, but this is not related to the duration of action. Since the mechanism of action involves gene transcription, the onset of the hypoglycaemic effect is gradual over 6–8 weeks.

Unwanted effects

- Gastrointestinal disturbances
- Headache
- Anaemia
- Hypoglycaemia
- Fluid retention leading to oedema; this can cause decompensation in controlled heart failure
- Weight gain because of fat-cell differentiation
- Rosiglitazone has been associated with an increased risk of myocardial infarction, and should be avoided in people with ischaemic heart disease or peripheral vascular disease
- Liver dysfunction has been reported rarely, and liver function tests should be monitored during treatment.

Dipeptidyl peptidase-4 (DPP-4) inhibitors

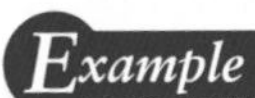

sitagliptin

Mechanism of action

Sitagliptin is a reversible competitive inhibitor of DPP-4, and reduces the ability of the enzyme to inactivate the incretin hormones GLP-1 and GIP. As a consequence, insulin synthesis and secretion is increased and therefore glucose levels are decreased and beta-cell function improved.

Pharmacokinetics

Sitagliptin is well absorbed from the gut. It is excreted by the kidney, and has a half-life of about 12 h.

Unwanted effects

- Nausea
- Oedema
- Nasopharyngitis.

Glucosidase inhibitors

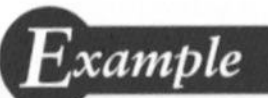

acarbose

Mechanism of action and effects

Carbohydrate digestion in the intestine involves several enzymes that sequentially degrade complex polysaccharides such as starch into monosaccharides like glucose. Initial digestion of carbohydrates in the gut lumen is carried out by amylases from the saliva and pancreas. The final digestion of oligosaccharides is carried out by β-galactosidases (including lactase) and various α-glucosidase enzymes (such as maltase, isomaltase, glucoamylase and sucrase, which hydrolyse oligosaccharides) in the small-intestinal brush border. Acarbose competes with dietary oligosaccharides for α-glucosidase enzymes, and has a higher affinity for these enzymes. Binding to the enzymes is reversible, so that digestion and absorption of glucose after a meal is slower than usual but not prevented. As a result, the postprandial peak of blood glucose is reduced and blood glucose concentrations are more stable through the day. Acarbose has no effect on insulin secretion or its tissue action and is less effective for achieving glycaemic control than are other oral hypoglycaemic agents. Its use is limited by the high incidence of unwanted effects.

Pharmacokinetics

Oral absorption of acarbose is very poor. Only about 2% of the active parent drug reaches the circulation. Inactive metabolites are formed in the gut lumen by enzymic degradation. About one-third of the oral dose is absorbed as inactive metabolite and most of this is excreted in the faeces. The absorbed parent compound is eliminated in the urine.

Unwanted effects

Gastrointestinal effects include flatulence, abdominal distension and diarrhoea, owing to fermentation of unabsorbed carbohydrate in the bowel. These effects are dose-related and often transient.

DRUGS TO INCREASE PLASMA GLUCOSE LEVELS

Glucagon

Mechanism of action and use

Glucagon is a polypeptide that is synthesised by the alpha cells of the pancreatic islets of Langerhans. It binds to

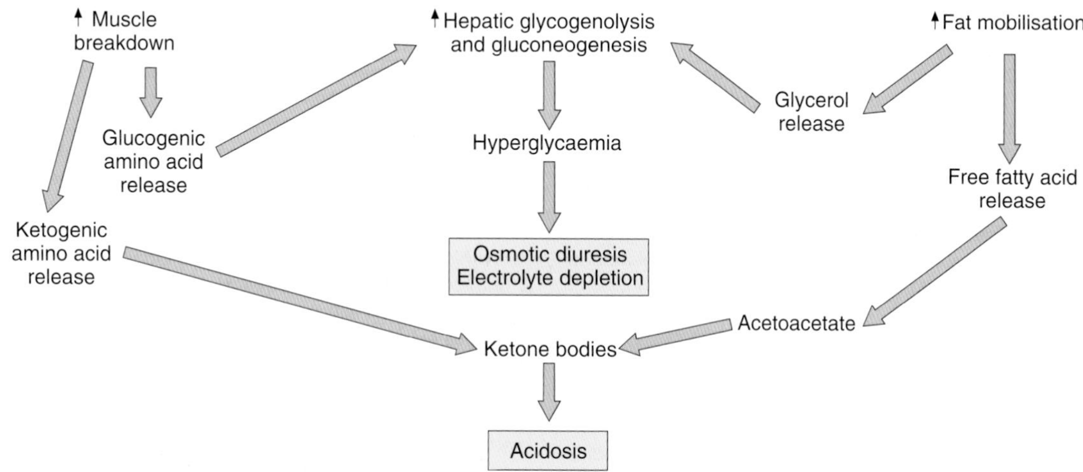

Fig. 40.2 **Pathophysiology of diabetic ketoacidosis.**

specific hepatocyte receptors and activates membrane-bound adenylyl cyclase. The consequent increase in intracellular cyclic adenosine monophosphate (cAMP) leads to inhibition of glycogen synthase. This blocks the effect of insulin on hepatocytes and mobilises stored liver glycogen. Glucagon is used to raise blood glucose in severe acute insulin-induced hypoglycaemia.

Pharmacokinetics

Glucagon must be given by intramuscular, subcutaneous or intravenous injection, and acts within 10–20 min. It is degraded rapidly by enzymes in the plasma, liver and kidney.

Unwanted effects

These are not usually troublesome with a single injection but include nausea, vomiting and diarrhoea.

MANAGEMENT OF TYPE 1 DIABETES

The aim of treatment is to maintain a plasma glucose concentration as close to normal as possible. Maintenance treatment of type 1 diabetes should include an appropriate diet with a regulated carbohydrate intake distributed throughout the day. Excess dietary saturated fat should be avoided. The complications of type 1 diabetes can be reduced by close control of the blood sugar concentration using insulin in an appropriate regimen (see above).

The success of the chosen approach can be monitored by measurement of the blood sugar concentrations, often carried out on a finger-prick blood specimen using a blood glucose reagent strip. If peak or trough blood glucose estimations are outside an acceptable range, the insulin regimen should be adjusted, although this should not be done more than once or twice a week. Long-term control of diabetes is usually assessed by the plasma concentration of glycosylated haemoglobin (HbA_{1c}). An HbA_{1c} level greater than 7% or greater than 53 mmol/mol (upper limit of normal is 6.0%) is associated with a higher risk of developing microvascular and neuropathic complications. Hyperglycaemia leads to the glycosylation of proteins which inhibits their function and may promote vascular and neurological damage. Several other mechanisms of vascular and neurological damage may also contribute to the complications of hyperglycaemia. In older people with type 1 diabetes, management of cardiovasular risk factors (see type 2 diabetes below) becomes increasingly important.

The most dramatic complication of untreated or poorly controlled type 1 diabetes is diabetic ketoacidosis (Fig. 40.2), which can lead to coma if it is severe. Systemic infection, dietary indiscretion, or inappropriate insulin dose reduction or omission can precipitate ketoacidosis in a person with treated type 1 diabetes. Apart from the treatment of any precipitating cause, the management of ketoacidosis includes the following.

- Restoration of extracellular volume: hyperglycaemia leads to an osmotic diuresis with excessive urinary salt and water loss. Replacement by physiological (0.9%) saline is essential.
- Potassium replacement: the osmotic diuresis results in excessive urinary potassium loss. Potassium is also shifted from within cells into extracellular fluid in exchange for hydrogen ions in the ketoacidotic state. Correction of the extracellular acidosis reverses this shift and can produce profound hypokalaemia. Once a good urine flow has been established, intravenous potassium supplements are usually required.
- Intravenous insulin until the ketosis is abolished and the plasma glucose is below 15 mmol L^{-1}. The metabolic acidosis will usually correct with treatment of the hyperglycaemia and fluid replacement. Intravenous sodium bicarbonate is occasionally required if the arterial pH is less than 7.0, but should be used with caution.

MANAGEMENT OF TYPE 1 DIABETES IN SPECIAL SITUATIONS

- Close attention to diabetic control is important before conception and during pregnancy because poor control

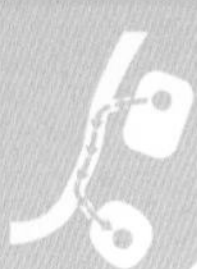

will affect the fetus, leading to increased intrauterine and perinatal mortality.

- At times of intercurrent illness, the dose of insulin will need to be increased, guided by blood sugar monitoring, to counteract the hyperglycaemic action of hormones released during stress reactions.
- During and after surgery, soluble insulin should be given in 5% dextrose solution by intravenous infusion, dosage being guided by the blood glucose concentrations. Subcutaneous insulin can be restarted when the person is able to eat and drink.

MANAGEMENT OF TYPE 2 DIABETES

The mainstays of treatment are lifestyle and dietary modifications. As for type 1 diabetes, close control of the blood sugar concentration in type 2 diabetes reduces the risk of microvascular complications, although the effect on macrovascular complications such as myocardial infarction is less convincing.

More than 75% of people with newly diagnosed type 2 diabetes are obese. Weight reduction not only improves blood glucose levels but also reduces other cardiovascular disease risk factors. Dietary advice should include:

- reducing energy intake if obese (an average weight loss of 18 kg is required to control blood sugar)
- eating small regular meals
- ensuring that more than half the total energy intake is from carbohydrates, total fat contributing less than 35% of total energy intake
- encouraging high-fibre foods and limiting sucrose and alcohol intake.

This should be combined with advice to exercise regularly and to stop smoking (because of the contribution to vascular disease) as appropriate. Underweight people with type 2 diabetes often require early treatment with an oral hypoglycaemic agent, usually a sulphonylurea, whereas lifestyle and dietary advice should initially be encouraged for obese people, with use of metformin if this fails. There is some evidence that metformin may reduce the risk of cardiovascular disease in obese people with type 2 diabetes. Combination therapy with a sulphonylurea and metformin can be useful if a single drug is insufficient to reduce the blood glucose concentration. The thiazolidinediones (glitazones) should be considered if there is intolerance to combination therapy with metformin plus a sulphonylurea (replacing the drug to which there is intolerance with a glitazone). Failure of such combinations usually indicates declining insulin release and the need for exogenous insulin, although for some overweight people the combination of a sulphonylurea, metformin and a glitazone may be helpful. The metiglinides are used alone for non-obese people with diabetes or those in whom metformin is contraindicated. In other individuals metiglinides can be given in combination with metformin. Sitagliptin may be considered when metformin alone is inadequate, but preferably in people without marked obesity.

Within 3 years of diagnosis, 50% of individuals with type 2 diabetes will need combination therapy to achieve glycaemic control. Failure of oral treatment usually implies 'beta-cell exhaustion', and up to 30% of those with type 2 diabetes require insulin with or without an oral hypoglycaemic drug. The most effective combination is a basal dose of intermediate-acting insulin at bedtime combined with metformin during the day. A sulphonylurea can be used if metformin is contraindicated, but with a greater risk of hypoglycaemia and eventual loss of efficacy as beta-cell exhaustion develops. Combination therapy with insulin and a glitazone or a meglinide has not been well studied. There is some evidence that insulin therapy is more likely to be successful if used early in type 2 diabetes to preserve beta-cell function. Exenatide is probably most appropriate for obese people for whom insulin is being considered; it is less likely to be effective if the diabetes has been present for many years, because beta-cell exhaustion is often present.

Acarbose is of limited value when used alone or in combination with metformin. It may be most effective in early diabetes, when there is still sufficient insulin secretion for it to influence glycaemic control.

Intensive management of risk factors for cardiovascular disease is of crucial importance because the major complications of type 2 diabetes are vascular. In particular, control of raised blood pressure reduces both microvascular and macrovascular complications. There is little to choose between antihypertensive drugs for use in diabetes, except that thiazides and β-adrenoceptor antagonists may aggravate diabetes and should probably be avoided in people who are managed with dietary control alone. An angiotensin-converting enzyme (ACE) inhibitor or an angiotensin receptor antagonist (alone and in combination) reduces the risk of renal failure when there is evidence of diabetic nephropathy (either overt or with microalbuminuria) (Ch. 6). Treatment of the abnormal atherogenic plasma lipid profile that is common in type 2 diabetes is recommended for people over the age of 40 years (Ch. 48). Once a person with diabetes has developed coronary artery disease, management of risk factors (Ch. 48) will reduce the risk of subsequent myocardial infarction or death to the same extent as for someone without diabetes.

FURTHER READING

Beckman JA, Creager MA, Libby P (2002) Diabetes and atherosclerosis. Epidemiology, pathophysiology, and management. *JAMA* 287, 2570–2581

Blood Pressure Lowering Treatment Trialists' Collaboration (2005) Effects of different blood pressure-lowering regimens on major cardiovascular events in individuals with and without diabetes mellitus. *Arch Intern Med* 165, 1410–1419

Brunton S (2008) Insulin delivery systems: reducing barriers to insulin therapy and advancing diabetes mellitus treatment. *Am J Med* 121(suppl 1), S35–S41

Daneman D (2006) Type 1 diabetes. *Lancet* 367, 847–858

De Witt DE, Dugdale DC (2003) Using new insulin strategies in the outpatient treatment of diabetes: clinical applications. *JAMA* 289, 2265–2269

De Witt DE, Hirsch IB (2003) Outpatient insulin therapy in type 1 and type 2 diabetes mellitus. *JAMA* 289, 2254–2264

Heine RJ, Diamant M, Mbanya J-C et al (2006) Management of hyperglycaemia in type 2 diabetes. *BMJ* 333, 1200–1204

Holmboe ES (2002) Oral antihyperglycaemic therapy for type 2 diabetes. Clinical applications. *JAMA* 287, 373–376

Inzucchi SE (2002) Oral antihyperglycaemic therapy for type 2 diabetes. Scientific review. *JAMA* 287, 360–372

Kirpichinikov D, McFarlane SI, Sowers JR (2002) Metformin: an update. *Ann Intern Med* 137, 25–33

Klein L, Gheorghiade M (2004) Management of the patient with diabetes mellitus and myocardial infarction: clinical trials update. *Am J Med* 116(suppl 5A), 47S–63S

Lenhard MJ, Reeves GD (2001) Continuous subcutaneous insulin infusion. *Arch Intern Med* 161, 2293–2300

Metchick LN, Petit WA Jr, Inzucchi SE (2002) Inpatient management of diabetes mellitus. *Am J Med* 113, 317–323

Mooradian AD (2003) Cardiovascular disease in type 2 diabetes. Current management guidelines. *Arch Intern Med* 163, 33–40

Mudaliar S, Henry RR (2002) PPAR agonists in health and disease: a pathophysiological and clinical overview. *Curr Opin Endocrinol Diabetes* 9, 285–302

Nathan DM (2002) Initial management of glycaemia in type 2 diabetes mellitus. *N Engl J Med* 347, 1342–1349

Plank J, Siebenhofer A, Berghold A et al (2005) Systematic review and meta-analysis of short-acting insulin analogues in patients with diabetes mellitus. *Arch Intern Med* 165, 1337–1344

Rosenstock J (2004) Basal insulin supplementation in type 2 diabetes: refining the tactics. *Am J Med* 116(suppl 3A), 10S–16S

Selvin E, Bolen S, Yeh H-C et al (2008) Cardiovascular outcomes in trials of oral diabetes medications: a systematic review. *JAMA* 168, 2070–2080

Snow V, Weiss KB, Mottur-Pilson C et al (2003) Evidence for tight blood pressure control in type 2 diabetes mellitus. *Ann Intern Med* 138, 587–592

Stafylas PC, Sarafidis PA, Lasaridis AN (2009) The controversial effects of thiazolidinediones on cardiovascular morbidity and mortality. *Int J Cardiol* 131, 298–304

Stumvoll M, Goldstein BJ, van Haeften TW (2005) Type 2 diabetes: principles of pathogenesis and therapy. *Lancet* 365, 1333–1346

Verspohl EJ (2009) Novel therapeutics for type 2 diabetes: incretin hormone mimetics (glucagon-like peptide-1 receptor agonists) and dipeptidyl peptidase-4 inhibitors. *Pharmacol Ther* 124, 113–138

Wang C-HW, Weisel RD, Fedak PWM et al (2003) Glitazones and heart failure. *Circulation* 107, 1350–1353

SELF-ASSESSMENT

In questions 1–4, the first statement, in italics, is true. Are the accompanying statements also true?

1. *Oral hypoglycaemic drugs (sulphonylureas, biguanides, thiazolidinediones, acarbose) are only used in type 2 diabetes and act by different mechanisms to control glucose levels.*
   a. Glibenclamide is the drug of choice when there is no residual insulin secretion.
   b. Sulphonylureas should be administered in conjunction with a dietary regimen, particularly in obese people.
   c. Glibenclamide can cause hypoglycaemia, particularly in the elderly, and should be used very cautiously in this age group.
2. *Hyperglycaemia results from uncontrolled glucose output from the liver and reduced uptake of glucose into muscle and other tissues.* The oral hypoglycaemic drugs metformin and gliclazide can be taken together.
3. *Untreated diabetes during pregnancy results in increased intrauterine and perinatal mortality.*
   a. Oral hypoglycaemics given to a pregnant mother can cause hypoglycaemia in the fetus and are normally substituted with insulin in pregnancy.
   b. Sulphonylureas should not be given together with the antibacterial trimethoprim.
4. *Different formulations of insulin are available that have varied peak effects and durations of action.* Insulin lispro has a longer duration of action than isophane insulin.
5. Ms JJ is a 55-year-old housewife with a body mass index of 35 kg m^{-2}. She was diagnosed with diabetes. Which **one** of the following statements is **correct**?
   A. The mainstay of treatment is diet and exercise.
   B. Diabetes presenting in this way is a medical emergency.
   C. A sulphonylurea would be the drug of first choice for Ms JJ.
   D. Rosiglitazone would be the drug of first choice.
   E. Treatment with metformin can increase the risk of heart disease.
6. Case history questions

A 25-year-old teacher, Mr JAH, was admitted to hospital as an emergency. He had developed a sore throat a week previously. His GP prescribed penicillin, but the soreness persisted and Mr JAH noticed profuse white spots on the back of his throat. He drank fluids copiously and passed more urine than usual. Two days before admission, he began to vomit. The day before admission, he became drowsy and confused. He had lost approximately 2 stones in weight, despite eating more than usual. His great uncle had diabetes mellitus. Mr JAH was clinically dehydrated and ketones could be smelt on his breath. Results of blood tests indicated that he had diabetic ketoacidosis.

a. Which type of diabetes does Mr JAH have?
b. What was the significance of his sore throat?
c. Was it significant that his great uncle suffered from diabetes mellitus?
d. Explain his polydipsia and polyuria.
e. What treatments should have been rapidly instituted?
f. After he had recovered from the acute illness, what general advice should have been given about diet?
g. Mr JAH was a 'three meals a day' man whose only exercise was walking a mile to work and back each day. Although insulin regimens vary widely, suggest a possible regimen and the types of insulin that could be given.
h. How long before meals should subcutaneous injection of soluble insulin have been given?
i. In addition to glucose levels, what other indicator could have been measured to signify good control in diabetes?

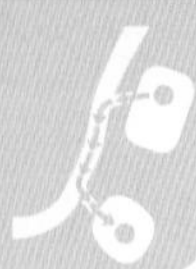

Mr JAH became more active, joined a health club and met a partner who liked to party. His eating became more irregular with hurried meals. His glycaemic control deteriorated.

j. What alterations to his insulin regimen could have been helpful?

ANSWERS

1. a. **False**. Glibenclamide is a sulphonylurea which stimulates insulin secretion from the beta cells of the islets and would be ineffective in the absence of any insulin-secreting ability.
   b. **True**. Sulphonylureas cause weight gain partly by stimulating appetite: metformin might be a better choice.
   c. **True**. Glibenclamide has a long duration of action and active metabolites can increase when renal function declines. Hypoglycaemia is a greater problem in the elderly.
2. **True**. These drugs act in part by different mechanisms. Additionally, metformin does not stimulate appetite; indeed, it may suppress appetite.
3. a. **True**. Neonates born to diabetic mothers who were taking oral hypoglycaemics in pregnancy have problems with hypoglycaemia.
   b. **True**. Sulphonylureas have some structural similarities to the sulphonamides and trimethoprim and can produce severe hypoglycaemia when given together.
4. **False**. Isophane insulin is complexed with protamine and has a duration of action of 20 h, whereas synthetic insulin lispro is modified structurally and has a faster onset of action and shorter duration.
5. Answer **A**.
   A. Correct. A trial of this for 3 months should be tried before suggesting other treatments.
   B. Incorrect. Treatment, support and advice should take place over many months.
   C. Incorrect. Sulphonylureas can stimulate appetite by increasing insulin secretion and causing further weight gain.
   D. Incorrect. The use of a glitazone (pioglitazone or rosiglitazone) as second-line therapy added to either metformin or a sulphonylurea is not recommended, except for people who are unable to tolerate metformin and sulphonylurea combination therapy, or people in whom either metformin or a sulphonylurea is contraindicated; in such cases, the thiazolidinedione should replace whichever drug in the combination is poorly tolerated or contraindicated.
   E. Incorrect. Metformin has a cardioprotective effect which can only in part be explained by its effects on glucose and may be due to improvements in the lipid profile.
6. Case history answers
   a. Type 1.
   b. An upper respiratory infection can be all that is necessary to tip someone into ketoacidosis. Aggravating factors include candidiasis in the throat, and overbreathing causing dryness.
   c. There is a familial tendency, but neither type 1 nor type 2 diabetes mellitus is a single gene disorder, so there is no classic pattern of inheritance.
   d. Once the tubular transport maximum for glucose reabsorption in the kidneys is exceeded, the glucose in the distal tubules causes an osmotic diuresis, leading to polyuria, and then to thirst.
   e. Insulin, fluids and salts to correct dehydration, glucose levels, ketoacidosis and electrolyte imbalances. Ketoacidosis can lead to coma.
   f. A dietary regimen should be agreed to create a stable pattern of eating habits commensurate with his lifestyle. Diets low in animal fat and high in fibre are recommended, ideally with carbohydrate intake distributed throughout the day.
   g. Initiate a stable pattern of eating habit and activity, and twice-daily subcutaneous insulin injections before breakfast and evening meal. The insulin regimen would contain a mixture of short- and long-acting insulins, the ratios of which vary depending upon his glucose levels. Insulins frequently used are soluble insulin and isophane insulin.
   h. The time to onset of activity of neutral soluble insulin is 30 min, with peak activity at 1–3 h.
   i. The amount of glycosylated haemoglobin (HbA_{1C}) can be measured. High concentrations are indicative of increased risk for microvascular and neuropathic complications.
   j. Newer, rapid-acting monomeric insulin lispro may be helpful. This has a time to onset of only 15 min and a time to peak plasma levels of 0.5–0.75 h. It should, therefore, be given immediately before a meal. A possible altered regimen may involve insulin lispro during the day with insulin isophane given in the evening. However, overall education about eating and lifestyle would probably provide greater benefit than a change of insulin regimen.

Drugs used in diabetes mellitus

Drug	Half-life (h) and kinetics	Comments
Treatment of hyperglycaemia		
Insulins		
Normally given by subcutaneous injection or subcutaneous infusion; onset and duration of action depend on the formulation used, many of which are combinations containing bovine, porcine or human insulin, e.g. insulin zinc suspension, isophane insulin, protamine–zinc insulin, or recombinant human insulin analogues such as biphasic insulin aspart, biphasic insulin lispro and biphasic isophane insulin		
Short-acting insulins		
Soluble insulin	See text [M]	A sterile solution of bovine, porcine or human insulin; may also be given by intramuscular or i.v. injection or by i.v. infusion, depending on requirements
Insulin aspart	See text [M]	A recombinant human insulin analogue; may also be given by i.v. injection or infusion, depending on requirements
Insulin glulisine	See text [M]	A recombinant human insulin analogue
Insulin lispro	See text [M]	A recombinant human insulin analogue; may also be given by i.v. injection or infusion, depending on requirements
Intermediate- and long-acting insulins		
Insulin detemir	See text [M]	A long-lasting recombinant human insulin analogue
Insulin glargine	See text [M]	A long-lasting recombinant human insulin analogue that has a longer duration of action than soluble insulin
Insulin complexes – see text		
Sulfonylureas		
All are given orally for the treatment of type 2 diabetes mellitus		
Chlorpropamide	25–60 [M + R] Complete oral bioavailability; eliminated by oxidative metabolism to inactive metabolites and by renal excretion (about 20%)	Because of unwanted effects this is no longer recommended
Glibenclamide	2–4 [M] Complete oral bioavailability; metabolised in liver to active hydroxyl metabolites that have a longer duration of action than the parent drug (one study has reported a terminal half-life for the parent drug of 10 h)	
Gliclazide	6–14 [M + R] Variable absorption between patients, probably linked to differences in first-pass metabolism; eliminated largely by oxidative metabolism in the liver, with 10% excreted unchanged	
Glimepiride	5–9 [M] Complete bioavailability; oxidised by P450 to hydroxy and carboxy metabolites, the former of which retains activity; drug clearance increases at low creatinine clearance (probably because of decreased plasma protein binding)	
Glipizide	2–4 [M] Complete oral bioavailability; oxidised in the liver to inactive hydroxy metabolite	
Tolbutamide	4–37 [M] Complete oral bioavailability; about 1 in 500 people has severely impaired metabolism of tolbutamide; metabolised by the polymorphic CYP2C9	

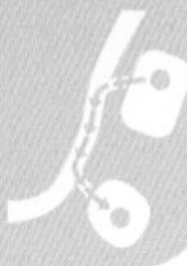

Drugs used in diabetes mellitus

Drug	Half-life (h) and kinetics	Comments
Biguanides		
Given orally for the treatment of type 2 diabetes mellitus		
Metformin	2–4 [R] Oral bioavailability is 50–60% owing to incomplete absorption; eliminated largely unchanged by renal tubular secretion	
Meglitinides (also called 'glinides')		
Given orally for the treatment of type 2 diabetes mellitus		
Nateglinide	1.5 [M + R] Good oral bioavailability (70%); metabolised by CYP2C9 and CYP3A4, and metabolites eliminated as glucuronic acid conjugates	Given in combination with metformin when metformin alone is inadequate
Repaglinide	1 [M] Good oral bioavailability (60%); eliminated by CYP3A4 oxidation to metabolites that are eliminated in the faeces	Given alone, or in combination with metformin when metformin alone is inadequate
Thiazolidinediones (also called 'glitazones')		
All drugs given orally for the treatment of type 2 diabetes mellitus		
Pioglitazone	3–7 [M] Rapidly absorbed; metabolised by CYP2C8 and CYP3A4; metabolites contribute to in vivo activity due to their long half-lives (16–24 h)	Used alone or in combination with metformin or a sulphonylurea only as a second-line drug when there is intolerance to one of these
Rosiglitazone	3–4 [M] Complete oral bioavailability; oxidised by CYP2C8 to hydroxy and demethylated metabolites	Used alone or in combination with metformin or a sulphonylurea only as a second-line drug when there is intolerance to one of these
Other hypoglycaemics		
Acarbose	3 [R] Negligible oral absorption (1–2%); main action is in the intestinal tract; the systemic disposition data given are largely irrelevant to therapeutic use	Given orally for diabetes mellitus inadequately controlled by diet with or without other oral hypoglycaemic drugs; α-glycoside hydrolase inhibitor
Exenatide	2 [M] Filtered in the glomerulus and metabolised in the kidney	Binds to the GLP-1 receptor, increasing glucose-dependent synthesis of insulin; given by subcutaneous injection
Guar gum	Not relevant	Given orally; acts in gut lumen to inhibit glucose absorption
Sitagliptin	12 [R] High oral bioavailability; limited metabolism by CYP3A4; most is excreted unchanged in urine by renal tubular secretion	Reversible competitive inhibitor of DPP-4; given orally in combination with metformin
Treatment of hypoglycaemia		
Glucagon	5–10 min [M] A protein that is rapidly and extensively degraded by liver and kidneys	Used for acute insulin-induced hypoglycaemia and *is not used* for chronic hypoglycaemia; given by subcutaneous, intramuscular or intravenous injection

[M], metabolism; [R], renal excretion; i.v., intravenous.

41 The thyroid and control of metabolic rate

THYROID FUNCTION

The main functions of thyroid hormones – triiodothyronine (T_3) and thyroxine (T_4) – are in the control of metabolism, growth and development. The term 'basal metabolism' refers to the energy-utilising biochemical processes of the body at rest. Basal metabolic rate is controlled by thyroid hormones, which stimulate tissue oxygen consumption and regulate energy and heat production, mainly by stimulating an increase in the metabolism of fats, carbohydrates and proteins. Most of these functions are a result of thyroid hormones acting in combination with other hormones such as insulin. Thyroid hormones have a thermogenic action on brown fat in infants, increasing synthesis of uncoupling proteins that divert the energy released during lipolysis into heat rather than high-energy phosphate synthesis. Thyroid hormones also promote gluconeogenesis, obtaining the substrate for glucose formation from amino acids in tissues such as muscle and bone. Thyroid hormones facilitate the development of the nervous system, somatic growth and puberty. They also regulate the synthesis of proteins involved in hepatic, cardiac, neurological and muscular functions. Thyroid hormones interact with the sympathetic nervous system, in particular enhancing the effects of β-adrenoceptor stimulation (Ch. 4).

T_3 is mainly responsible for effects at a cellular level, while T_4 is now considered to be a prohormone. T_3 and T_4 are synthesised in the thyroid gland (Fig. 41.1), where inorganic iodide is trapped with great avidity by an enzyme-dependent process. The iodide is then oxidised and incorporated into tyrosine (as tyrosyl residues of the glycoprotein thyroglobulin) to form mono-iodotyrosine and di-iodotyrosine residues. Two di-iodinated tyrosine molecules or one di-iodinated molecule with one mono-iodinated tyrosine molecule are joined by a coupling reaction to form T_4 and T_3, respectively. The enzyme thyroxine peroxidase is important both in the initial oxidation and in the final combination steps of the synthetic process (Fig. 41.1). Proteolytic enzymes from thyroid lysosomes then degrade thyroglobulin and release thyroid hormone into the circulation.

The synthesis and release of thyroid hormones are controlled by the anterior pituitary hormone thyrotrophin (thyroid-stimulating hormone, TSH). This in turn is controlled by the hypothalamus, which secretes thyrotrophin-releasing hormone (TRH). Circulating T_3 and T_4 exert a negative feedback on both the hypothalamic and pituitary hormones (Fig. 41.2).

Circulating thyroid hormones are highly protein bound, mostly to thyroxine-binding globulin (TBG) (particularly T_4, of which less than 0.1% is free). Only the free fraction of hormone can bind to specific cell receptors. The thyroid secretes mainly T_4 (thyroxine) and a small amount of T_3. Most T_3 is derived from peripheral deiodination of T_4 by the enzyme thyroxine 5′-deiodinase, which is found in the liver, kidney, brain and brown adipose tissue. About 35% of T_4 is converted to T_3, while about 40% is converted to reverse T_3 (a metabolically inactive isomer of T_3). T_3 has a half-life in the circulation of about 1.5 days compared with about 7 days for T_4. Elimination of T_3 and T_4 is by conjugation, mainly in the liver.

The cellular actions of thyroid hormone are due to interaction with thyroid hormone receptors (TR) (Ch. 1) which belong to the superfamily of nuclear receptors. Thyroid hormone receptors usually repress target genes, but, following T_3 binding, the complex is able to activate transcription and enhance protein synthesis. Thyroid hormone receptors are expressed in most tissues, but there are three isoforms of the receptor, which differ in their tissue distribution. Recent evidence suggests that these isoforms mediate different effects of T_3. T_3 also has non-genomic actions that include stimulation of cellular uptake of amino acids and glucose, and interactions with G-protein-coupled membrane receptors with activation of the mitogen-activated protein kinase (MAPK) pathway.

HYPERTHYROIDISM

The commonest form of hyperthyroidism (often, and interchangeably, called thyrotoxicosis) is Graves' disease, an autoimmune condition in which thyroid-stimulating immunoglobulin binds to thyrotrophin (TSH) receptors on thyroid cells and initiates signal transduction. There is often an immunologically mediated inflammatory reaction in the extrinsic muscles and fat of the orbit, causing swelling and

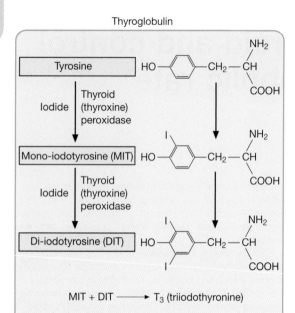

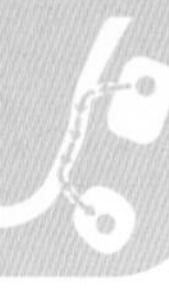

Thyroglobulin

Tyrosine — HO–C$_6$H$_4$–CH$_2$–CH(NH$_2$)COOH

Iodide — Thyroid (thyroxine) peroxidase

Mono-iodotyrosine (MIT) — HO–C$_6$H$_3$I–CH$_2$–CH(NH$_2$)COOH

Iodide — Thyroid (thyroxine) peroxidase

Di-iodotyrosine (DIT) — HO–C$_6$H$_2$I$_2$–CH$_2$–CH(NH$_2$)COOH

MIT + DIT ⟶ T_3 (triiodothyronine)

DIT + DIT ⟶ T_4 (thyroxine)

Release of T_4 and T_3 from thyroglobulin by proteolysis

T_3 HO–C$_6$H$_3$I–O–C$_6$H$_2$I$_2$–CH$_2$CH(NH$_2$)COOH

T_4 HO–C$_6$H$_2$I$_2$–O–C$_6$H$_2$I$_2$–CH$_2$CH(NH$_2$)COOH

Fig. 41.1 **The sequence of the synthesis of thyroid hormones.** Peroxidation of iodide results in its incorporation into tyrosine residues of thyroglobulin, the colloidal substance that fills the lumen of the thyroid follicles. MIT and DIT are formed by a subsequent peroxidation reaction on the iodinated thyroglobulin.

the characteristic exophthalmos. Toxic multinodular goitre, thyroid adenomas (toxic nodule) and various forms of thyroiditis are much less common causes of hyperthyroidism. Rarely, the condition arises from ectopic production of thyrotrophin or thyroxine or it can be induced by treatment with amiodarone (Ch. 8). Symptoms of hyperthyroidism include weight loss, palpitation, sweating, fatigue, nervousness, heat sensitivity and tremor. These are in part mediated by the action of excess thyroid hormone, and partly by excess sensitivity of tissues to β-adrenoceptor stimulation. Signs are often less marked in the elderly, who are more likely to present with atrial fibrillation that is resistant to treatment.

DRUGS FOR TREATMENT OF HYPERTHYROIDISM

Thionamides

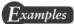

carbimazole, propylthiouracil

Mechanism of action

Thionamides inhibit thyroxine peroxidase, and, therefore, the synthesis of thyroid hormone (Fig. 41.2). The long half-life of T_4 means that changes in the rate of synthesis take 4–6 weeks to lower circulating T_4 and T_3 concentrations to normal. These drugs also appear to have an immunosuppressant effect in individuals with autoimmune thyroid disease. They reduce the levels of thyroid-stimulating immunoglobulin, although the clinical importance of this is uncertain. Large doses of propylthiouracil also decrease peripheral conversion of T_4 to T_3.

Pharmacokinetics

Carbimazole is almost completely absorbed from the gut and rapidly converted by first-pass metabolism to the active derivative methimazole. Methimazole has a short half-life (3–5 h) and is inactivated by hepatic metabolism. Propylthiouracil has only about one-tenth of the activity of methimazole and has a short half-life (1–3 h) due to rapid liver metabolism. It is usually reserved for individuals intolerant to carbimazole. Although the antithyroid drugs have short half-lives, they accumulate in the thyroid, which extends their duration of action.

Unwanted effects

- Gastrointestinal upset (especially nausea and epigastric discomfort), headache, arthralgia and pruritic rashes are common in the first 8 weeks of treatment.
- Allergic reactions, including vasculitis, a lupus-like syndrome, myopathy, cholestatic jaundice and nephritis. Some cross-sensitivity occurs between carbimazole and propylthiouracil.
- Bone marrow suppression, especially agranulocytosis, is an important unwanted effect and is probably immunologically mediated. A severe sore throat with fever is often the presenting complaint, and the occurrence of this, or any other infection, should be immediately reported by patients to their doctor. The onset is sudden, and routine blood counts are unhelpful. The risk is higher with propylthiouracil than with carbimazole. The blood count usually recovers about 3 weeks after drug withdrawal.
- Placental transfer of the active metabolite of carbimazole can produce neonatal hypothyroidism, but propylthiouracil does not transfer in large enough quantities to cause problems. However, in Graves' disease, the thyroid-stimulating antibody crosses the placenta and causes fetal thyrotoxicosis; therefore, carbimazole is the treatment of choice for maternal Graves' disease. Carbimazole is secreted in breast milk but rarely produces hypothyroidism in the infant.

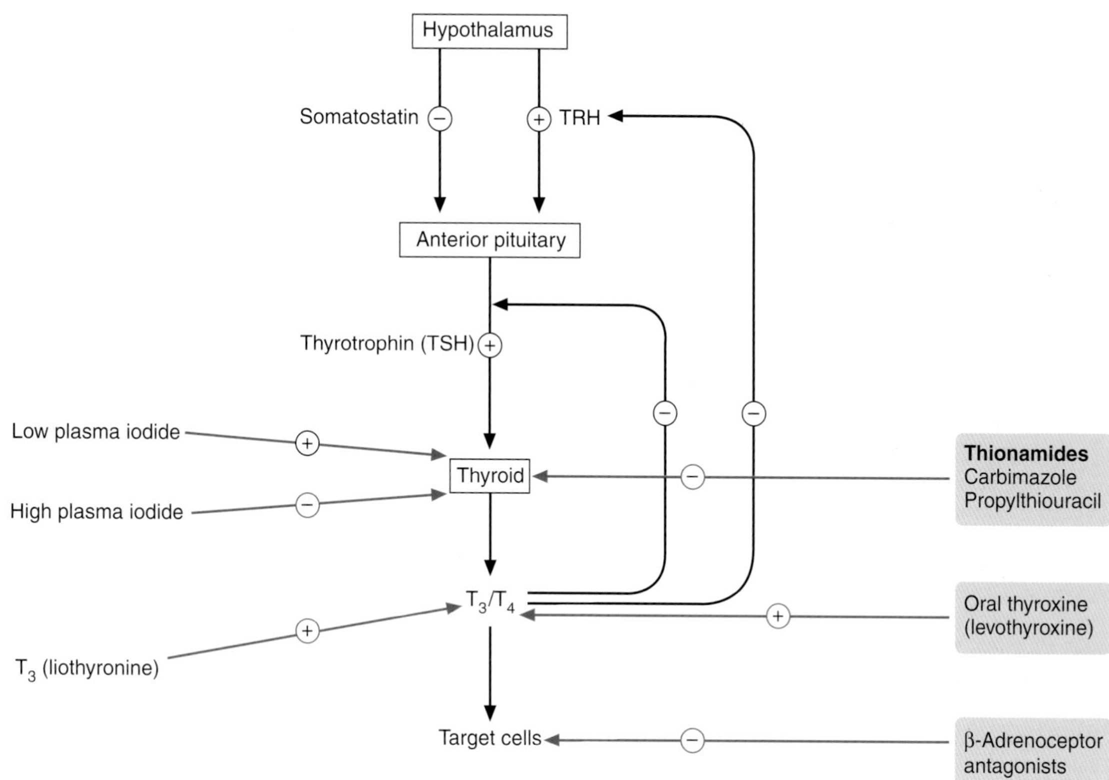

Fig. 41.2 **Control of thyroid hormone synthesis and release, and sites of action of drugs acting on the thyroid.** TSH (thyroid-stimulating hormone, thyrotrophin) and TRH (thyrotrophin-releasing hormone) are inhibited by circulating levels of T_3 and T_4. The actions of drugs used are shown by red arrows.

MANAGEMENT OF HYPERTHYROIDISM

Graves' disease

Carbimazole is the drug of choice for Graves' hyperthyroidism, and will usually decrease the thyroid hormone concentration to normal levels over 4–12 weeks. It is usual to start treatment with a high dosage for 4–6 weeks, unless the thyrotoxicosis is mild, when smaller initial doses may be more appropriate. The dosage is then gradually reduced every 4–6 weeks, provided the serum T_4 concentration remains within the normal range, to reach the lowest possible dose that controls the serum T_4. Initially, treatment should be continued for 12–18 months, then the dose can be tapered or treatment withdrawn. Occasionally, a block–replace regimen is used, giving a high dosage of carbimazole in conjunction with thyroxine replacement for 6–12 months. This maintains normal thyroid function regardless of the dose of carbimazole.

Beta-adrenoceptor antagonists (especially propranolol, Ch. 5) are particularly useful for symptomatic relief from tremor, anxiety or palpitation during the early period of treatment with carbimazole. They have immediate effects on symptoms but do not alter the rate of thyroid hormone synthesis or secretion.

Exophthalmos associated with Graves' disease usually responds poorly to treatment with antithyroid drugs, since it is caused by TSH receptor antibody. Severe thyroid eye disease can be helped by treatment with oral prednisolone if antithyroid treatment is not improving the condition.

Approximately 50% of individuals with Graves' disease have a single episode that is cured by drug treatment. Those who relapse will usually do so within 6 months, and thereafter repeat relapses are common. Most subjects are then offered definitive treatment by either a subtotal thyroidectomy (for a large goitre) or a therapeutic dose of radioactive iodine (^{131}I).

Radioiodine can be used as first-line treatment for Graves' disease or for relapse after antithyroid drug treatment. Radioiodine may make thyroid ophthalmopathy worse, but this can be prevented by treatment with a corticosteroid for 2–3 months. Before radioiodine treatment, it is often recommended that the thyrotoxicosis should be stabilised with carbimazole to reduce the risk of exacerbation of hyperthyroidism from radiation thyroiditis immediately after isotope treatment. However, antithyroid drug treatment must be stopped 3–5 days before radioactive iodine is given or it will prevent uptake of the radioiodine by the thyroid cells. Beta-adrenoceptor antagonists can be useful in this period to prevent symptomatic relapse. Carbimazole can be restarted 2–4 days after radioiodine, to cover the period of up to 8 weeks before radioiodine is fully effective. Between 10% and 20% of individuals will require a second dose of radioiodine to achieve euthyroid status. Following radioiodine treatment, permanent hypothyroidism can occur. Up to 1 year after treatment, the incidence of

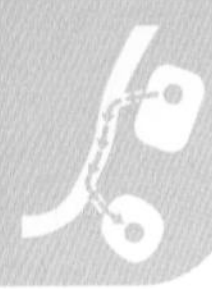

hypothyroidism is related to the initial dose of radioactivity; thereafter, the risk is 2–3% annually. The theoretical increase in risk of cancer or leukaemia following radioiodine treatment has not been substantiated in clinical studies.

Surgery in Graves' disease is used if there is a poor response to antithyroid drugs, a very large goitre, for coexisting thyroid malignancy or if the person expresses a preference for this treatment. Before surgery, carbimazole is usually used to achieve a euthyroid state. If the thyrotoxicosis is drug-resistant, oral potassium iodide can be used for up to 2 weeks prior to surgery to inhibit thyroxine synthesis and release and to reduce the vascularity of the hyperplastic thyroid gland. Hypothyroidism, often delayed by several months or years, is common after surgery.

Toxic nodular goitre

Radioiodine is also used for toxic multinodular goitre. A solitary toxic thyroid nodule can be removed surgically, but radioactive iodine is extremely effective, because the isotope is taken up only by the abnormal tissue (the remainder is suppressed by the absence of thyrotrophin in the circulation). Carbimazole is unsuitable as sole treatment for these conditions, since spontaneous remission does not occur. However, some elderly people may choose to continue treatment with carbimazole for life.

Amiodarone-induced thyrotoxicosis

Treatment of amiodarone-induced thyroiditis (Ch. 8) depends on the clinical subtype. Type 1 is provoked by the iodide contained in the drug in people with an underlying multinodular goitre, and responds to antithyroid drug treatment. Type 2 is an inflammatory thyroiditis that arises from a direct toxic effect of the drug on the gland, and responds well to treatment with a corticosteroid.

HYPOTHYROIDISM

Hypothyroidism is usually caused by primary thyroid failure, and the low circulating T_4 concentration is accompanied by a raised plasma thyrotrophin (TSH) concentration. Autoimmune thyroiditis is the commonest cause, but hypothyroidism is occasionally congenital or can follow treatment for hyperthyroidism by surgery or radioiodine. Rarely, hypothyroidism can be secondary to pituitary or hypothalamic failure, when the circulating TSH concentrations will be low. Drug therapy with lithium (Ch. 22) or amiodarone (Ch. 8) can produce hypothyroidism.

Typical symptoms of hypothyroidism in an adult are non-specific and include lethargy, slowing of mental processes, cold intolerance, dry skin, hoarseness, weight gain, constipation and menorrhagia. Severe hypothyroidism (myxoedema) produces marked coarsening of the facial appearance and may ultimately lead to a hypothermic, comatose state. In children, hypothyroidism stunts mental and physical development, resulting in a condition known as cretinism.

MANAGEMENT OF HYPOTHYROIDISM

Standard treatment is with oral thyroxine (levothyroxine, T_4). Although its absorption is incomplete and variable, sufficient T_3 will be formed by peripheral deiodination of T_4, although the proportion of circulating T_3 is usually lower than normal. Therefore, circulating levels of T_4 will often need to be higher than those in healthy individuals in order to obtain a satisfactory response. In some people, particularly those with ischaemic heart disease, a rapid increase in metabolic activity with thyroxine replacement can cause excessive cardiac stimulation, and therefore thyroxine should be introduced gradually in those at risk of cardiac complications. In others, the anticipated weight-related maintenance dose can be given from the start. Because of its long half-life, steady-state plasma concentrations of thyroxine will not be achieved with constant dosage for 4–5 weeks. The adequacy of thyroxine replacement therapy is best monitored by measurement of the serum TSH concentration 4–6 weeks after a change in dose of thyroxine. When the TSH concentration is within the normal range, the plasma T_4 will usually be slightly high or in the upper part of the normal range. Once the dose is correct, an annual check of serum TSH is sufficient, unless there are symptoms suggesting hypo- or hyperthyroidism. When the hypothyroidism is caused by drug treatment, the precipitating drug can be continued while thyroxine is given. Problems with thyroid replacement preparations are uncommon unless excessive doses are used, but allergic reactions have been reported, and transient scalp hair loss can occur in the first few weeks of treatment.

Some drugs interfere with the absorption of thyroxine from the gut. These include iron, calcium carbonate, mineral supplements, colestyramine (Ch. 48) and sucralfate (Ch. 33). The metabolism of thyroxine is accelerated by the concurrent use of the hepatic enzyme-inducing drugs phenobarbital, phenytoin, carbamazepine (Ch. 23) and rifampicin (Ch. 51). The therapeutic response to thyroxine may be impaired in all of these situations.

Liothyronine (T_3, triiodothyronine) is usually reserved for intravenous use in severe hypothyroidism (myxoedema coma), when its potency, more rapid effect and shorter half-life allow more rapid attainment of a therapeutic blood concentration. However, even in this situation, a large dose of thyroxine has been successfully used, and may be associated with a lower mortality. An oral formulation is also available for rapid response in severe hypothyroid states.

FURTHER READING

Brent GA (2008) Graves disease. *N Engl J Med* 358, 2594–2605

Cooper DS (2003) Hyperthyroidism. *Lancet* 362, 459–468

Pearce EN (2006) Diagnosis and management of thyrotoxicosis. *BMJ* 332, 1369–1373

Roberts CGP, Ladenson PW (2004) Hypothyroidism. *Lancet* 363, 793–803

Toft AD (2001) Subclinical hyperthyroidism. *N Engl J Med* 345, 512–516

SELF-ASSESSMENT

In questions 1 and 2, the first statement, in italics, is true. Are the accompanying statements also true?

1. *Synthesis and secretion of T_3 and T_4 are controlled by hypothalamic hormones, thyrotrophin-releasing hormone and somatostatin, by the anterior pituitary hormone thyrotrophin and by plasma iodide.*
   a. Most circulating T_3 and T_4 is highly bound to albumin.
   b. Thyroxine (T_4) has a long residence time in the body.
   c. At target cells, T_4 is converted to T_3, which then binds to specific nuclear receptors.
   d. Hyperthyroidism will be made worse by iodine administration.
2. *Severe hypothyroidism causes 'myxoedema' in adults and cretinism in children; its origins are immunological.*
   a. Therapy with ^{131}I can cause hypothyroidism.
   b. Hypothyroidism is treated with oral thyroxine.
   c. When thyroxine is taken, it reaches steady-state plasma concentrations after about 5 weeks.
3. Mr RH was diagnosed with thyrotoxicosis and was about to be prescribed carbimazole. Choose the one **incorrect** answer from the following.
   A. It will take 5 weeks to reduce the circulating T_4 and T_3 concentrations to normal.
   B. Carbimazole is a prodrug.
   C. An unwanted effect of carbimazole is bone marrow suppression.
   D. Carbimazole inhibits the stimulant action of thyrotrophin on the thyroid.
   E. Carbimazole has a long duration of action.
4. Mrs JH was diagnosed with hypothyroidism and ischaemic heart disease and treatment for her hypothyroidism was started. Choose the one **correct** answer from the following statements about her condition and her treatment.
   A. Low circulating T_4 levels in hypothyroidism are accompanied by low levels of thyrotrophin.
   B. Treatment should be with oral levothyroxine.
   C. During regular dosing, steady-state plasma levels of levothyroxine are reached within 7 days.
   D. No special precautions are required when prescribing levothyroxine to Mrs JH.
   E. Oxygen consumption in metabolically active tissues is unaffected by levothyroxine.
5. Case history questions

A 45-year-old man suffered from weight loss, palpitations, tremor, anxiety and sweating, plus eyelid retraction, and orbital and ocular inflammation. Blood tests showed increased levels of free and bound T_3 and T_4. A diagnosis of Graves' thyrotoxicosis was made. An electrocardiogram showed atrial fibrillation.

   a. What is Graves' disease?
   b. What other blood tests could be done to confirm this diagnosis?
   c. Why were the free, rather than total, plasma T_3 and T_4 measured?
   d. How could the symptoms be controlled?
   e. What drug could be given to control the hyperthyroidism?

With treatment, he became euthyroid, but relapsed in the following year. A decision was made to treat him with ^{131}I.

   f. What treatment should be given before administering the ^{131}I and what are the reasons for this?
   g. How long after treatment will benefit be seen?

ANSWERS

1. a. **False**. T_3 and T_4 are largely bound to thyroxin-binding globulin (TBG).
   b. **True**. Thyroxine has a half-life of about 7 days.
   c. **True**. The T_3–receptor complex activates transcription and protein synthesis.
   d. **False**. Iodine is converted to iodide and inhibits T_3 and T_4 release.
2. a. **True**.
   b. **True**. Levothyroxine is the standard treatment.
   c. **True**. Thyroxine has a very long half-life.
3. Answer **D**.
   A. Correct. The long half-life of T_4 (about 7 days) means that it takes 5–6 weeks to reduce thyroid hormone levels to normal.
   B. Correct. The metabolite methimazole is the active component.
   C. Correct. The Committee on Safety of Medicines warns that signs of bone marrow suppression should be watched for; these include symptoms and signs suggestive of infection, especially sore throat. A white blood cell count should be performed if there is any clinical evidence of infection. Carbimazole should be stopped promptly if there is clinical or laboratory evidence of neutropenia.
   D. Incorrect. Carbimazole inhibits the action of thyroxine peroxidase.
   E. Correct. Carbimazole accumulates in the thyroid and needs to be given only once a day.
4. Answer **B**.
   A. Incorrect. If T_4 levels were low, then thyrotrophin levels would be raised, as the negative feedback effect of T_4 on thyrotrophin release would be reduced.
   B. Correct. Normal treatment is with T_4 (levothyroxine).
   C. Incorrect. The half-life of levothyroxine is 6–7 days; therefore, steady state would not be reached until 5–7 weeks of administration.
   D. Incorrect. Special care is required, as a rapid increase in metabolic activity can cause excessive heart stimulation.
   E. Incorrect. Levothyroxine stimulates oxygen consumption in metabolically active tissues.
5. Case history answers
   a. An autoimmune disease in which antibodies to TSH are generated and bind to and activate TSH receptors on the thyroid, promoting thyroid hormone release.
   b. TSH (thyrotrophin) levels could be measured. It will be low due to the negative feedback effect of elevated T_3 and T_4.

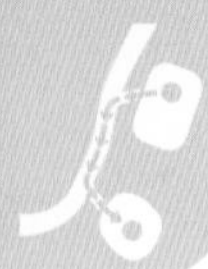

c. Bound T_3 and T_4 levels may be high due to increased binding capacity of binding proteins or increased levels of binding proteins rather than actual elevated levels of free T_3 and T_4.
d. Drugs of choice for controlling symptoms are β-adrenoceptor antagonists, although they do not improve fatigue and muscle weakness. Digoxin should be given for the atrial fibrillation (Ch. 8), and anticoagulation with warfarin to prevent thromboembolism, which has an increased incidence in people with both atrial fibrillation and thyrotoxicosis.
e. Carbimazole is the drug of choice, given in a high dose, then reducing over 4–6 weeks.
f. The clinical state should be stabilised with carbimazole and a β-adrenoceptor antagonist. Carbimazole is stopped 3–4 days before radioiodine is given, as it can prevent the uptake of iodine by thyroid cells.
g. It can take several months for maximum benefit of ^{131}I to occur.

Thyroid and antithyroid drugs

Drug	Half-life (h) and kinetics	Comments
Thyroid hormones		
Levothyroxine/thyroxine (T_4)	6–7 days [M] Oral bioavailability is 50–80% (with some variability between brands); metabolised by deiodination in peripheral tissues to T_3 (which has a half-life of 1–2 days)	Treatment of choice for maintenance therapy; given orally
Liothyronine (L-tri-iodothyronine) (T_3)	1–2 days [M] Almost complete oral bioavailability; metabolised by deiodination and conjugation with glucuronic acid and sulphate	More rapid onset of action than levothyroxine and can be used for severe hypothyroid states; given orally or by slow intravenous injection (for hypothyroid coma)
Antithyroid drugs[a]		
All drugs given orally once-daily, because of their long-term effects on the thyroid		
Carbimazole	3–5 [M] (methimazole) Complete absorption with complete presystemic metabolism to the active form methimazole; methimazole is eliminated by metabolism plus some renal excretion	
Iodine and iodide	– [R] Complete oral absorption; incorporated into thyroid hormones; excreted largely in urine	Used as an adjunct to antithyroid drugs for 10–14 days before partial thyroidectomy, but should not be given for long-term treatment
Propylthiouracil	1–3 [M] Bioavailability is 50–75% due to poor absorption; the main metabolic route is formation of an S-glucuronide	

[a]Beta-adrenoceptor antagonists, such as propranolol, can be used to treat the symptoms of thyrotoxicosis.
[M], metabolism; [R], renal excretion.

42 Calcium metabolism and metabolic bone disease

REGULATION OF CALCIUM METABOLISM

Calcium ions play a part in a large number of cellular activities, including stimulus–response coupling in striated and smooth muscle, and in endocrine and exocrine glands. Calcium modulates the actions of intracellular cyclic adenosine monophosphate (cAMP) and is a cofactor for numerous intracellular enzymes and for blood clotting. However, more than 98% of Ca^{2+} in the body is in the form of hydroxyapatite crystals deposited on the protein matrix of bone, which provides its mechanical strength.

Calcium circulates in plasma partly bound to protein (approximately 50%) and partly in the free ionised (and therefore 'active') form. The free fraction in plasma is precisely maintained within narrow limits principally by the actions of parathyroid hormone (PTH) and 1,25-dihydroxyvitamin D_3 (calcitriol). Calcitonin secretion (see below) also reacts to changing plasma Ca^{2+} concentrations but it is less important in overall control of Ca^{2+} homeostasis. Calcium in plasma is in dynamic exchange with Ca^{2+} in the gut, renal tubules and bone. This is illustrated, with the main controlling factors, in Figure 42.1.

PTH is a polypeptide hormone which is the main physiological regulator of Ca^{2+} in blood. Its secretion from parathyroid chief cells is stimulated by a reduction of ionised Ca^{2+} in plasma. PTH secretion is inhibited when the plasma Ca^{2+} concentration rises.

The main actions of PTH relating to calcium homeostasis are:

- stimulation of the synthesis of the biologically active form of vitamin D (calcitriol) in the kidney.
- facilitation of reabsorption of Ca^{2+} from the kidney tubules and enhancement of urinary phosphate excretion
- mobilisation of calcium and phosphate from bone through stimulation of osteoclasts, which increases bone resorption; PTH also enhances osteoblastic activity, resulting in some bone repair.

The effect of PTH on the kidney occurs within minutes of PTH release, while that on bone begins after 1–2 h.

Vitamin D (calciferol) is a prohormone that is metabolised to several active compounds (Box 42.1) that have steroid nuclei. Ergocalciferol (vitamin D_2), a precursor of active vitamin D, is absorbed from the gut. However, given adequate UVB sunlight, the major source of vitamin D is conversion of 7-dehydrocholesterol in the skin to cholecalciferol (vitamin D_3). Therefore, cholecalciferol is really a skin-derived hormone rather than a vitamin but this source was discovered after the dietary origins. Vitamins D_2 and D_3 are further metabolised in the liver to 25-hydroxy D_3 (calcidiol), and then in the kidney to 1,25-dihydroxy D_3 (calcitriol). 1α-Hydroxylation is an essential step for activation of vitamin D, and PTH stimulates 1α-hydroxylase activity in the kidney, increasing the formation of calcitriol. Calcitriol binds to specific steroid receptors in the cell cytoplasm (Ch. 1). The resulting complex migrates to the nucleus and increases the synthesis of an intracellular Ca^{2+}-binding protein. The main effect of active forms of vitamin D is to increase the plasma concentration of Ca^{2+} by:

- facilitating absorption of Ca^{2+} from the small intestine
- enhancing Ca^{2+} mobilisation out of bone by increasing osteoclastic activity.

Vitamin D also inhibits the transcription of the gene coding for PTH.

In the kidney, vitamin D promotes phosphate retention, in contrast to the action of PTH. These actions of vitamin D affect Ca^{2+} turnover in bone over periods of days to weeks.

Calcitonin is a peptide secreted by the parafollicular cells of the thyroid when the calcium-sensing receptor detects a rise in plasma Ca^{2+}. The main target cell for calcitonin is the osteoclast, which it inhibits by stimulation of adenylyl cyclase, thus reducing bone turnover. Calcitonin also decreases Ca^{2+} and phosphate reabsorption by the kidney, thereby increasing their excretion.

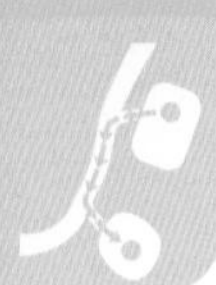

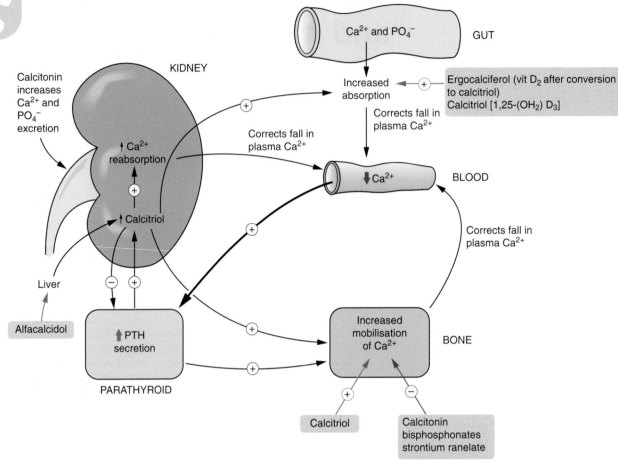

Ca^{2+} and PO_4^-
GUT
KIDNEY
Calcitonin increases Ca^{2+} and PO_4^- excretion
Increased absorption
Ergocalciferol (vit D_2 after conversion to calcitriol)
Calcitriol [1,25-(OH_2) D_3]
Corrects fall in plasma Ca^{2+}
Corrects fall in plasma Ca^{2+}
↑ Ca^{2+} reabsorption
↓ Ca^{2+}
BLOOD
↑ Calcitriol
Corrects fall in plasma Ca^{2+}
Liver
Alfacalcidol
↑ PTH secretion
PARATHYROID
Increased mobilisation of Ca^{2+}
BONE
Calcitriol
Calcitonin
bisphosphonates
strontium ranelate

Fig. 42.1 **Regulation of calcium metabolism.** This illustrates the response to a fall in plasma Ca^{2+}. This leads to an increase in the release of parathyroid hormone (PTH) production from the parathyroid gland. This increases calcitriol [1,25-(OH_2) D_3] formation in the kidney. This in turn increases gut absorption of Ca^{2+}. PTH further increases bone mobilisation of Ca^{2+} to return plasma Ca^{2+} to normal. An increase in plasma Ca^{2+}, conversely, decreases PTH secretion. Calcitonin, secreted by the thyroid, decreases Ca^{2+} reabsorption from the kidney and decreases bone turnover. Drugs used for hypercalcaemia are indicated by arrows in green. Drugs for hypocalcaemia are indicated by arrows in red.

Box 42.1 Vitamin D and its natural metabolites

Vitamin D (calciferol) is a group of prohormones converted in the body to compounds with a range of biological activities. The most active compounds relevant to mineral homeostasis are:

vitamin D_2 (ergocalciferol) and vitamin D_3 (cholecalciferol)
calcitriol (1,25-dihydroxy D_3), which is an active metabolite of vitamin D_3
alfacalcidol (1α-hydroxycholecalciferol), which is converted to the active calcitriol

Confusingly, in the literature, vitamin D is used to refer to D_2 or D_3 and active metabolites!

HYPERCALCAEMIA

The main causes of hypercalcaemia are:

- increased resorption of Ca^{2+} from bone – for example, primary hyperparathyroidism, secretion of parathyroid-related hormone by cancer cells, bony metastases
- increased absorption of Ca^{2+} from the gut through excessive use of vitamin D or sarcoidosis (a disease of the lymph nodes of unknown origin)
- reduced renal excretion of Ca^{2+} – for example, as caused by thiazide diuretics (Ch. 14).

Hypercalcaemia occurs when the mobilisation of Ca^{2+} into the extracellular space exceeds the capacity to remove it. Chronic moderate hypercalcaemia leads to a progressive decline in renal function, formation of renal stones, and ectopic calcification (e.g. cornea, blood vessels). Severe hypercalcaemia causes anorexia, nausea, vomiting, constipation, drowsiness and confusion, eventually leading to coma. Hypercalcaemia impairs the ability of the kidney to reabsorb salt and water; in conjunction with vomiting, this can lead to depletion of plasma volume and renal failure. Urgent treatment is indicated when the plasma Ca^{2+} concentration rises above 3.5 mmol L^{-1} (normal usually <2.6 mmol L^{-1}), since sudden death from cardiac arrest can occur.

ANTIRESORPTIVE DRUGS FOR HYPERCALCAEMIA

Bisphosphonates

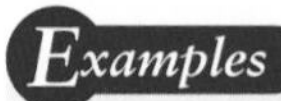

alendronic acid, sodium clondronate, disodium etidronate, disodium pamidronate, ibandronic acid, risedronate sodium, zoledronic acid

Mechanisms of action and effects

Bisphosphonates are pyrophosphate analogues that bind to hydroxyapatite crystals in bone matrix. They are preferentially deposited under osteoclasts, and are taken up by these cells and inhibit their resorptive action on bone. There are two different cellular actions of the drugs on osteoclasts, depending on the structure of the bisphosphonate:

- metabolism within the cell to form a toxic analogue of adenosine triphosphate (ATP) that induces osteoclast apoptosis (non-nitrogen-containing drugs: clodronate, etidronate)
- inhibition of the ATP-dependent enzyme farnesyl pyrophosphate synthase in the synthetic pathway from mevalonic acid to cholesterol; this reduces the production of lipids that are essential for osteoclast function, and leads to impaired differentiation of osteoclast precursors, reduced ability of mature osteoclasts to reabsorb bone by altering the permeability of osteoclast membranes to small ions, and, eventually, osteoclast apoptosis (nitrogen-containing drugs: alendronate, ibandronate, pamidronate, risedronate, zoledronate).

The actions of most bisphosphonates are relatively short-lived, but zoledronic acid can suppress bone resorption for up to a year after a single dose.

Pharmacokinetics

Bisphosphonates are poorly absorbed from the gut (less than 10% of the ingested dose). Oral formulations are best taken with the stomach empty, to avoid binding by Ca^{2+} in food. Alendronic acid, disodium etidronate and risedronate sodium are only available in an oral formulation, disodium pamidronate and zoledronic acid are only formulated for intravenous use, while ibandronic acid and sodium clodronate are available for oral or intravenous dosage. Removal of most bisphosphonates from blood is rapid via the kidney, but their effect is prolonged since they remain bound to Ca^{2+} in bone.

Unwanted effects

- Gastrointestinal disturbance, particularly nausea, abdominal pain, diarrhoea or constipation with the oral treatments.
- Headache, dizziness.
- Alendronic acid and risedronate sodium can cause severe oesophagitis and oesophageal strictures. To reduce the risk, the tablets should be taken whole with a full glass of water at least 30 min before food and the person should then stand or sit (but not lie down) for at least 30 min after ingestion. Once-weekly dosing also reduces the risk of oesophageal damage.
- Transient pyrexia and influenza-like symptoms after intravenous infusion.
- Osteonecrosis of the jaw, especially after intravenous use.

Calcitonin

Mechanism of action and effects

The actions of calcitonin on bone and the kidney to reduce plasma Ca^{2+} concentrations have been discussed above. Calcitonin begins to act within a few hours of administration, with a maximum effect within 12–24 h. However, the hypocalcaemic effect produced by repeated administrations only lasts between 2 and 3 days. This loss of clinical response results from downregulation of calcitonin receptors on osteoclasts, leading to a rebound increase in bone resorption.

Pharmacokinetics

Salmon calcitonin (salcatonin) is now used exclusively, since it is less immunogenic than the earlier preparation of porcine calcitonin. It is usually given by intramuscular or subcutaneous injection, although intravenous infusion can be used. A nasal spray formulation is also available. The half-life is very short (about 20 min), and it is broken down to inactive fragments by enzymic degradation in plasma and in the kidney.

Unwanted effects

- Facial flushing occurs in most people
- Headache, dizziness
- Nausea, vomiting, abdominal pain, diarrhoea
- Taste disturbance
- Nose and throat irritation with nasal spray.

TREATMENT OF HYPERCALCAEMIA

When possible, the primary cause should be corrected, for example removal of a parathyroid adenoma or treatment of myeloma. Oral Ca^{2+} supplements, vitamin D and thiazide diuretics should be discontinued. Additional measures may include correction of dehydration, enhancing renal excretion of Ca^{2+} and inhibiting bone resorption.

Most people with severe hypercalcaemia are fluid-depleted at presentation. Rehydration with intravenous saline is essential; this also promotes a sodium-linked Ca^{2+} diuresis in the proximal and distal renal tubules. Loop diuretics such as furosemide (Ch. 14) increase renal Ca^{2+} elimination but should be given with high volumes of intravenous normal saline and intensive monitoring of fluid balance to avoid dehydration.

A bisphosphonate such as ibandronate, pamidronate or zoledronate, especially given by intravenous infusion, is the drug treatment of first choice for severe hypercalcaemia. Initial intravenous rehydration is essential to avoid precipitation of calcium bisphosphonate in the kidney. Oral bisphosphonate treatment may be sufficient for less severe

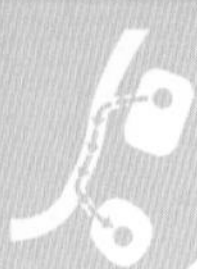

hypercalcaemia. Following a single intravenous infusion of bisphosphonate, the plasma Ca^{2+} concentration falls gradually after 2–4 days, with a maximum effect after 4–7 days and a response that persists for 1–4 weeks after treatment. Because of the delay in onset of action of the bisphosphonates, calcitonin can be given concurrently for an early effect. Corticosteroids such as prednisolone (Ch. 44) are effective for lowering plasma Ca^{2+} when vitamin D excess is an important factor, for example in sarcoidosis and for acute treatment of vitamin D overdose, or for hypercalcaemia associated with haematological malignancy such as myeloma or lymphoma. Corticosteroids probably act by reducing the effect of vitamin D on intestinal Ca^{2+} transport, but can take several days to work.

HYPOCALCAEMIA

There are two major underlying causes of hypocalcaemia:

- deficiency of PTH – for example, idiopathic hypoparathyroidism, after surgical parathyroid removal
- deficiency of vitamin D – for example, dietary deficiency, limited exposure to sunlight, renal failure (failure of 1α-hydroxylation).

Hypocalcaemia produces neuromuscular irritability with paraesthesiae of the extremities or around the mouth, muscle cramps and tetany. When severe, it can produce seizures. Chronic hypocalcaemia, especially in congenital hypoparathyroidism, is associated with mental deficiency, seizures, intracranial calcification (e.g. choroid plexus) and ocular cataracts.

DRUGS FOR HYPOCALCAEMIA

Vitamin D compounds

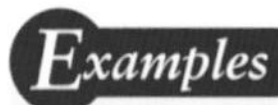

alfacalcidol (1α-hydroxycholecalciferol), calcitriol (1,25-dihydroxy D_3 or 1,25-dihydroxycholecalciferol), ergocalciferol (vitamin D_2), paricalcitol

Mechanism of action

This is discussed above. A dose-related increase in Ca^{2+} and phosphate absorption from the gut occurs at lower concentrations than those which stimulate bone resorption. Ergocalciferol is inactive and can only be used if 1α-hydroxylation by the kidney is intact. In renal impairment, the hydroxylated active forms alfacalcidol or calcitriol should be used. Paricalcitol is a synthetic vitamin D analogue used in chronic renal failure; it binds to the vitamin D receptor and inhibits PTH synthesis and secretion, but has less effect than natural vitamin D on the plasma Ca^{2+} concentration.

Pharmacokinetics

The fat-soluble D vitamins are well absorbed orally in the presence of bile. They can also be given intravenously. Both alfacalcidol and calcitriol are active forms of vitamin D; they have short half-lives (about 3 h) and are metabolised and excreted mainly in the bile. Paricalcitol requires intravenous injection. It is metabolised in the liver, and has a half-life of about 5 h.

Unwanted effects

- Excessive dosing will produce hypercalcaemia.
- Excretion of vitamin D supplements in breast milk can cause hypercalcaemia in a suckling infant.

TREATMENT OF HYPOCALCAEMIA

Mild hypocalcaemia can be treated with oral Ca^{2+} supplements, taken between meals to avoid binding to dietary phosphate and oxalate which forms salts that are poorly absorbed. In the absence of reversible pathology such as malabsorption due to coeliac disease, the mainstay of treatment for more severe hypocalcaemia is vitamin D supplements. The few individuals who have vitamin D deficiency from inadequate diet or lack of exposure to sunlight (such as may be found in Asian women in the UK) will respond to small doses of vitamin D. Most causes of hypocalcaemia, however, require much larger doses (usually given as ergocalciferol) to maintain normocalcaemia. Oral Ca^{2+} supplements (as carbonate or citrate salts) are often used with vitamin D for the treatment of chronic hypocalcaemia.

For treatment of hypoparathyroidism, alfacalcidol is given; PTH is not used for replacement therapy (although PTH and a synthetic PTH fragment, teriparatide, are now licensed for treatment of osteoporosis; see below). Large doses of ergocalciferol could be used, but carry a risk of hypercalcaemia. The action of vitamin D begins after 2–4 weeks of treatment, because there is deficient renal hydroxylation of vitamin D in hypoparathyroidism; the action of calcitriol is much more rapid, beginning after 1–2 days, but it is rarely required unless a very rapid onset of action is necessary.

Acute severe hypocalcaemia (sometimes occurring after parathyroidectomy) must be treated with intravenous Ca^{2+} (as gluconate, gluceptate or chloride salt).

METABOLIC BONE DISEASE

OSTEOMALACIA

Osteomalacia is the bone disease resulting from failure of adequate bone mineralisation due to lack of vitamin D. Bone pain is prominent, and low plasma Ca^{2+} and phosphate concentrations produce muscle weakness. In developing children, the bones become distorted (rickets). Treatment is with vitamin D (ergocalciferol) supplements, but it will take at least a year to achieve a normal bone structure.

RENAL BONE DISEASE

Chronic renal disease is associated with deficient activation of vitamin D, and hypocalcaemia. At the same time, reduced renal phosphate excretion leads to hyperphosphataemia. The low serum Ca^{2+} leads to secondary hyperparathyroidism in an attempt to maintain the plasma Ca^{2+} concentration. The result is demineralisation of bone (renal bone disease) and soft tissue calcification from the increased calcium–

phosphorus product. Vascular calcification is associated with increased cardiovascular disease and mortality.

Treatment of renal bone disease is with a 1α-hydroxylated vitamin D derivative (such as alfacalcidol or calcitriol), but this will increase plasma Ca^{2+} without affecting the plasma phosphate. An oral non-Ca^{2+}-containing phosphate binder such as aluminium hydroxide will be necessary to reduce the plasma phosphate concentration. People who are receiving haemodialysis or ambulatory peritoneal dialysis cannot readily excrete absorbed aluminium, and an alternative phosphate binder such as sevelamer or lanthanum is used. Despite the symptomatic benefit of vitamin D in renal disease, there is little evidence for any improvement in long-term mortality.

OSTEOPOROSIS

Osteoporosis is the loss of bone mass due to reduced organic bone matrix and, consequently, mineral content, which decreases the mechanical strength of bone. It is a natural and inevitable part of the ageing process, and in females a marked increase in bone loss occurs after the menopause. Other predisposing factors include smoking, heavy alcohol intake and lack of exercise. Osteoporosis in younger people is associated with trabecular bone loss and predisposes to spontaneous vertebral fractures. In older people, cortical bone is also lost, increasing the risk of low-impact traumatic fracture, particularly of the neck of the femur. Sometimes osteoporosis is secondary to other conditions such as myeloma or thyrotoxicosis or occurs as a result of corticosteroid therapy (Ch. 44). Once established, osteoporosis is extremely difficult to reverse, and emphasis should be placed on prevention where possible. Management of osteoporosis includes:

- non-pharmacological approaches
- the use of either antiresorptive therapies (with an associated decrease in markers of bone formation and bone resorption: bisphosphonates, raloxifene, oestrogen) or
- anabolic therapies that lay down new bone (with increases in markers of bone formation and bone resorption: calcitonin, teriparatide).
- Treatment with vitamin D which increases the laying down of hydroxyapatite on bone collagen organic matrix.
- Strontium ranelate which does not conform to these patterns of effect on bone metabolism (see below).

Prevention of osteoporosis

- **Oral calcium supplements** increases bone mineral density in the spine, but with an uncertain effect on the risk of vertebral fractures in postmenopausal women. The addition of **vitamin D** (ergocalciferol) confers greater benefit, with a reduction in the risk of non-vertebral fractures. Recently, concern has been raised that high-dose Ca^{2+} supplements may increase the risk of myocardial infarction.
- **Oral bisphosphonates** (see above) are the treatment of choice for prevention of postmenopausal osteoporosis and corticosteroid-induced osteoporosis.
- **Raloxifene** is a selective oestrogen receptor (ER) modulator. It shows tissue specificity since, although it binds to both types of oestrogen receptor (ERα and ERβ; Ch. 45), it is an antagonist of ERβ by recruiting co-repressor molecules, but a partial agonist of ERα. Raloxifene has oestrogen receptor agonist effects on bone and lipids but acts as an anti-oestrogen on the breast and endometrium (Ch. 45). Raloxifene reduces the risk of oestrogen receptor-positive breast cancer, but its effects on pre-existing breast cancer are unknown. It is used in postmenopausal women to reduce the risk of osteoporosis but does not reduce menopausal vasomotor symptoms. Raloxifene reduces the risk of vertebral fractures by 40%, but has no effect on non-vertebral fractures, which may reflect the tissue distribution of oestrogen receptor subtypes. It is recommended for women who cannot take a bisphosphonate, or who have a fragility fracture after at least 1 year of treatment with a bisphosphonate. Raloxifene is well absorbed orally, and is metabolised in the liver. Enterohepatic cycling gives it a very long half-life (28 h). Unwanted effects include hot flushes and leg cramps. In addition, raloxifene increases the risk of venous thromboembolism, particularly during the first 4 months of treatment.
- The use of **hormone replacement therapy (HRT)** with oestrogen (Ch. 45) in peri- and postmenopausal women was once the mainstay of preventative treatment for osteoporosis. However, 5–10 years of oestrogen therapy may be required and long-term use of HRT increases the risk of breast cancer and thromboembolic events. As a consequence, the use of HRT for this indication has declined.

Treatments for established osteoporosis

The choice of treatment depends on the clinical circumstances. Pain relief is important if there are fractures, but drug treatment to prevent bone loss can reduce the risk of further fractures by up to 50%. Options include the following.

- **Oral bisphosphonates** produce an increase in bone density. Most studies have been carried out in postmenopausal women. Alendronic acid and risedronate sodium have been shown to reduce hip, vertebral and wrist fractures. Bisphosphonates are also first-line treatment for the management of corticosteroid-induced osteoporosis. If there has been a good response in bone mineral density after 5 years, then stopping treatment for 3–5 years while monitoring markers of bone turnover may not increase the risk of subsequent fractures.
- **Raloxifene** is useful for the management of vertebral fractures in postmenopausal women.
- **Salmon calcitonin** given subcutaneously or intranasally produces a modest increase in bone mass. Calcitonin can also produce pain relief when used for up to 3 months after a vertebral fracture.
- **Teriparatide** is a synthetic recombinant fraction of PTH (amino acids 1–34) that is effective for the treatment of postmenopausal osteoporosis. It is given daily by subcutaneous injection. The most common unwanted effects are nausea, oesophageal reflux, postural hypotension, dyspnoea, depression and dizziness. It is recommended for postmenopausal women who cannot tolerate a bisphosphonate. There is also evidence that it is effective for osteoporosis treatment in men, and corticosteroid-induced osteoporosis. Recombinant human parathyroid hormone is now also available for subcutaneous administration.

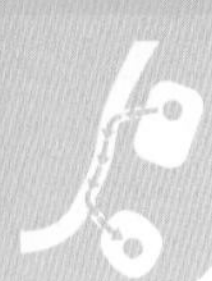

- **Strontium ranelate** is preferentially taken up by trabecular bone and incorporated into bone in the same way as Ca^{2+}. It stimulates osteoblast activity and inhibits osteoclast differentiation and resorptive activity. Strontium ranelate reduces the risk of both hip and vertebral fractures. The pattern of bone remodelling, with increases in markers of bone formation and a decrease in bone resorption, differs from that seen with both antiresorptive and anabolic therapies. It is taken orally and is eliminated by the kidneys with a very long effective half-life of 60 h. Unwanted effects include nausea, diarrhoea, headache and rashes. Strontium ranelate is recommended for use in postmenopausal women who cannot tolerate a bisphosphonate, and may be the first-choice treatment for women older than 80 years.
- **Calcitriol** is effective when bisphosphonates are unsuitable, including for corticosteroid-induced osteoporosis.
- **Testosterone** (Ch. 46) is used for prophylaxis and treatment of corticosteroid-induced osteoporosis in men.
- **Oral fluoride supplements** increase bone formation in osteoporotic bone but also produce a defect in mineralisation of cortical bone. This can be minimised by giving Ca^{2+} supplements, but the ability of fluoride to prevent fractures is unproven.

PAGET'S DISEASE OF BONE

Paget's disease of bone is a disturbance of bone remodelling characterised by both excessive bone reabsorption by osteoclasts and an increase in formation of poor-quality bone. The new bone matrix is non-lamellar woven bone with areas of osteosclerosis, leaving bone that is structurally weakened. Paget's disease mainly affects the skull and long bones. The aetiology is unknown but a slow virus infection may initiate the disease.

About a third of the bone lesions are asymptomatic, but they can produce bone pain and deformity, nerve entrapment and pathological fractures. Active treatment should be given if symptoms are present or a risk of complications is identified. Apart from symptomatic measures such as analgesics, two main treatments are used:

- **Bisphosphonates** are effective for treatment and primarily inhibit bone resorption, but long-term use can also impair bone mineralisation and carries the risk of producing osteomalacia by creating secondary hyperparathyroidism. Oral treatment is usually sufficient, with intravenous treatment reserved for severe disease. Calcium and vitamin D supplements reduce the risk of hypocalcaemia.
- **Calcitonin**, by reducing osteoclastic bone resorption, can reduce pain and then improve the structural abnormalities in Pagetic bone. Pain relief usually begins within 2 weeks, but treatment may be necessary for several months to improve bone modelling. Approximately 50% of people will relapse on stopping treatment. Calcitonin is often reserved for initial treatment while awaiting a response to a bisphosphonate.

FURTHER READING

Andress DL, Coyne DW, Kalantar-Zadeh K et al (2008) Management of secondary hyperparathyroidism in stages 3 and 4 chronic kidney disease. *Endocr Pract* 14, 18–27

Canalis E, Giustina A, Bilezikian JP (2007) Mechanisms of anabolic therapies for osteoporosis. *N Engl J Med* 357, 905–916

Cooper MS, Gittoes NJL (2008) Diagnosis and management of hypocalcaemia. *BMJ* 336, 1298–1302

Ebeling PR (2008) Osteoporosis in men *N Engl J Med* 358, 1474–1482

Holick MF (2007) Vitamin D deficiency. *N Engl J Med* 357, 266–281

Laroche M (2008) Treatment of osteoporosis: all the questions we still cannot answer. *Am J Med* 121, 744–747

MacLean C, Newberry S, Maglione M et al (2008) Systematic review: comparative effectiveness of treatments to prevent fractures in men and women with low bone density or osteoporosis. *Ann Intern Med* 148, 197–213

Mallick S, Kanthety R, Rahman M (2009) Vitamin D: bone and beyond, rationale and recommendations for supplementation. *Am J Med* 122, 793–802

Palmer SC, McGregor DO, Macaskill P et al (2007) Meta-analysis: vitamin D compounds in chronic kidney disease. *Ann Intern Med* 147, 840–853

Poole KES, Compston JE (2006) Osteoporosis and its management. *BMJ* 333, 1251–1256

Potts JT (2005) Parathyroid hormone: past and present. *J Endocrinol* 187, 311–325

Ralston SH, Langston AL, Reid IR (2008) Pathogenesis and management of Paget's disease of bone. *Lancet* 372, 155–163

Rosen CJ (2005) Postmenopausal osteoporosis. *N Engl J Med* 353, 595–603

Russell RG (2006) Bisphosphonates: from bench to bedside. *Ann NY Acad Sci* 1068, 367–401

Shoback D (2008) Hypoparathyroidism. *N Engl J Med* 359, 391–403

Sitges-Serra A, Bergenfelz A (2007) Clinical update: sporadic primary hyperparathyroidism. *Lancet* 370, 468–470

Stewart AF (2005) Hypercalcemia associated with cancer. *N Engl J Med* 352, 373–379

Whyte MP (2006) Paget's disease of bone. *N Engl J Med* 355, 593–600

SELF-ASSESSMENT

In questions 1 and 2, the first statement, in italics, is true. Are the accompanying statements also true?

1. *Hypocalcaemia develops when there is a deficiency in PTH or vitamin D, or when target organs do not respond to these hormones.*
   a. Vitamin D deficiency can lead to hypoparathyroidism.
   b. Calcitonin decreases Ca^{2+} resorption in the kidney.
   c. Bisphosphonates lower blood Ca^{2+} levels rapidly.
2. *Hormone replacement therapy in postmenopausal women is beneficial in preventing bone density loss.*
   a. Oestrogens maintain bone density by directly enhancing Ca^{2+} absorption from the intestine.

b. Raloxifene stimulates oestrogen receptors on bone, breast and uterine tissue.

3. The following statements concern osteoporosis. Choose the one **incorrect** statement.
   A. High doses of oral prednisolone increase the risk of osteoporosis.
   B. Raloxifene has oestrogenic activity at all oestrogen receptors.
   C. Oral bisphosphonates reduce Ca^{2+} mobilisation in bone.
   D. Raloxifene causes hot flushes in some women.
   E. Lack of exercise increases the risk of osteoporosis.
4. The following statements concern osteomalacia and rickets. Choose the one **incorrect** statement.
   A. Lack of sunlight can contribute to osteomalacia.
   B. Renal failure may reduce the effectiveness of ergocalciferol treatment in osteomalacia.
   C. Intestinal absorption of Ca^{2+} will be decreased in osteomalacia.
   D. Osteomalacia results in low levels of PTH
   E. Vitamin D promotes bone mineralisation.

ANSWERS

1. a. **False**. Vitamin D deficiency leads to hyperparathyroidism, which may assist in reducing the worst excesses of vitamin D deficiency. PTH increases calcitriol formation and calcitriol has a negative feedback effect on PTH.
   b. **True**. Calcitonin reduces Ca^{2+} resorption and inhibits bone turnover.
   c. **False**. Bisphosphonates inhibit bone dissolution, and effects occur slowly; plasma Ca^{2+} concentrations fall slowly, with a maximum effect after about a week.
2. a. **False**. Oestrogens inhibit the cytokines that recruit the bone-resorbing osteoclasts. Oestrogens also inhibit the actions of PTH.
   b. **False**. Raloxifene has been licensed to reduce bone density loss in postmenopausal women. It is an oestrogen receptor agonist selective for its actions on oestrogen receptors in bone and without stimulant effects on oestrogen receptors in breast and uterus.
3. Answer **B**.
   A. Correct. Corticosteroids can reduce the number of bone-forming cellular units (osteoclasts/osteoblasts), decrease Ca^{2+} absorption even at low doses, increase renal Ca^{2+} excretion, decrease gonadal hormone levels and increase bone resorption.
   B. Incorrect. Raloxifene is oestrogenic on bone but anti-oestrogenic on receptors in the breast and uterus.
   C. Correct. Bisphosphonates reduce bone Ca^{2+} mobilisation and are particularly useful in corticosteroid-induced osteoporosis.
   D. Correct. The anti-oestrogenic effects of raloxifene can result in hot flushes and thromboembolism in some women.
   E. Correct. Load-bearing exercises increase bone turnover.
4. Answer **D**.
   A. Correct. Sunlight is involved in the formation of cholecalciferol in the skin, which is then converted to active vitamin D compounds in the liver and kidneys.
   B. Correct. Ergocalciferol is hydroxylated in the kidney to calcitriol before it can exert its biological activity. In renal failure, if 1α-hydroxylase activity is defective, alfacalcidol or calcitriol may have to be substituted.
   C. Correct. Because of the lack of vitamin D compounds formed in the kidney, less Ca^{2+} and phosphate will be absorbed from the gut.
   D. Incorrect. Low levels of Ca^{2+} and lack of vitamin D may result in higher levels of parathyroid hormone (secondary hyperparathyroidism).
   E. Correct. Vitamin D promotes bone mineralisation by promoting the laying down of hydroxyapatite on the collagen organic matrix.

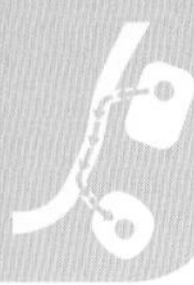

Drugs used to regulate calcium metabolism and in metabolic bone disease

Drug	Half-life (h) and kinetics	Comments
Calcitonin and parathyroid hormone		
Calcitonin (salmon)/ salcatonin	12–21 min [M] Peak plasma concentrations are seen 15–45 min after subcutaneous injection; rapidly metabolised by the kidney (note, biological effects are prolonged for hours or days)	Involved with parathyroid hormone in the regulation of bone turnover; used to lower plasma Ca^{2+} in hypercalcaemia and for the treatment of Paget's disease; given intranasally, by subcutaneous or intramuscular injection or by slow intravenous infusion
Parathyroid hormone	? [M?] New drug; few data available; pharmacokinetics are probably similar to teriparatide (see below)	Human recombinant parathyroid hormone; given by subcutaneous injection for the treatment of postmenopausal osteoporosis
Teriparatide	5 min [M] Clearance exceeds hepatic plasma flow, indicating a role for extrahepatic metabolism; the half-life from a subcutaneous injection is about 1 h owing to absorption rate-limited kinetics (see Ch. 2)	A recombinant fragment of parathyroid hormone used for the treatment of postmenopausal osteoporosis; given by subcutaneous injection
Bisphosphonates		
All these drugs are adsorbed onto hydroxyapatite crystals and reduce bone turnover; there is an extremely long half-life of release from binding to bone and essentially all of the drugs share similar fates in the body; they are all used for osteoporosis; the drugs are highly polar and most of the dose is eliminated in the faeces after oral administration; elimination of absorbed drug is by renal excretion, and care should be taken in subjects with renal impairment		
Alendronic acid (alendronate)	11 years (bone) [R] Very low oral bioavailability (<1%) reduced even further by food; the absorbed fraction is eliminated by glomerular filtration; about 40% of an intravenous dose is eliminated and the remainder retained and eliminated very slowly, due to binding to bone	First-line option for the prevention and treatment of osteoporosis; given orally
Clodronate (sodium)	6 [R] Published half-life probably reflects the rate of bone uptake and renal excretion and does not reflect the release due to bone turnover (which is probably years)	Used for hypercalcaemia of malignancy; given orally or by slow intravenous infusion
Etidronate (disodium)	2–6 (plasma), very long (bone) [R] Low absorption (1–9%); about 50% of intravenous dose is eliminated in the urine within 24 h, but the remainder is retained in bone and elimination is dependent on bone turnover (presumably about 11 years as for alendronate, see above)	Used for prevention and treatment of osteoporosis; given orally
Ibandronic acid	10–60 [R] Published half-life probably reflects the rate of bone uptake and renal excretion and does not reflect the release due to bone turnover (which is probably years)	Potent bisphosphonate used for hypercalcaemia of malignancy and prevention and treatment of osteoporosis (given every 3 months for osteoporosis); given orally or by intravenous infusion
Pamidronate (disodium)	0.5 (plasma), very long (bone) [R] Fate is similar to alendronate (see above) and the half-life given is the distribution from plasma to tissues; the half-life in bone depends on bone turnover (and has been reported to be about 2 years)	Used for hypercalcaemia of malignancy and Paget's disease; given by slow intravenous infusion
Risedronate sodium	10 days [R] High oral bioavailability (about 60%) due to the presence of a lipophilic pyridinyl side-chain; bioavailability is reduced if taken with food; the published half-life probably reflects the rate of bone uptake and renal excretion and does not reflect the release due to bone turnover (which is probably years)	Potent bisphosphonate which is used for the prevention and treatment of osteoporosis and Paget's disease; given orally

Drugs used to regulate calcium metabolism and in metabolic bone disease

Drug	Half-life (h) and kinetics	Comments
Tiludronic acid	Very long (bone) [R] Oral bioavailability is highly variable (between and within individuals) and low (about 6%); fate in the body is probably similar to that of alendronate	Used for Paget's disease; given orally for 12 weeks, then at least 6 months without treatment
Zoledronic acid	7 days [R] Fate in the body is probably similar to that of alendronate	Used for hypercalcaemia of malignancy and prevention and treatment of osteoporosis; given by intravenous infusion only used once a year for osteoporosis
Vitamin D		
Because vitamin D requires metabolic activation in the kidneys, alfacalcidol or calcitriol should be used in cases of severe renal impairment		
Alfacalcidol	3 [M] High oral bioavailability; undergoes side-chain oxidation by a 25-hydroxylase to calcitriol, which is the active form	1α-Hydroxycholecalciferol; given orally or by intravenous injection
Calcitriol	3–6 [M] Rapidly and completely absorbed; oxidised to inactive hydroxy-metabolites	1α,25-Dihydroxycholecalciferol; given orally or by intravenous injection
Cholecalciferol (vitamin D_3)	Not defined [M] High oral bioavailability; oxidised at 25-position to 25-hydroxycholecalciferol, which is oxidised to the active 1,25-dihydroxy compound in the kidney	Given orally or by intravenous injection
Dihydrotachysterol	10 (?) [M] Peak concentrations are at 4 h after dosage; few kinetic data available	Synthetic analogue of vitamin D_2; given orally
Ergocalciferol (calciferol; vitamin D_2)	19–24 [M] High oral bioavailability; metabolic precursor of cholecalciferol; metabolised to 1,25-dihydroxycholecalciferol (calcitriol) in liver and kidney	Given orally or by intravenous injection
Paricalcitol	4–6 [M] Oxidised by CYP3A4 and conjugated with glucuronic acid; metabolites eliminated in bile	19-Nor-1α-25-dihydroxyvitamin D_2; binds to the vitamin D receptor and inhibits PTH synthesis and secretion; given by slow intravenous injection
Other drugs affecting bone metabolism		
Strontium ranelate	60 [R] Bioavailability 25%; steady state achieved after 2 weeks of treatment	Two atoms of stable strontium complexed with one molecule of ranelic acid; given orally
Raloxifene	28 [M] Rapidly absorbed; undergoes extensive first-pass conjugation with glucuronic acid and enterohepatic cycling	Used for the treatment and prevention of postmenopausal osteoporosis; does not affect menopausal vasomotor symptoms; given orally

[M], metabolism; [R], renal excretion.

43 Pituitary and hypothalamic hormones

ANTERIOR PITUITARY AND HYPOTHALAMIC HORMONES

Thyrotrophin and thyrotrophin-releasing hormone (TRH) are considered in Chapter 41.

GROWTH HORMONE

Growth hormone (GH), or somatotrophin, is a 191-amino acid peptide that is synthesised in specific cells in the anterior pituitary. Its secretion is controlled by the hypothalamus via a releasing hormone (GHRH) and dopamine (Fig. 43.1) and also modulated by a growth hormone release inhibiting hormone (GHRIH [somatostatin]) via specific somatostatin receptors (SSTs). GH is released in pulses repeatedly throughout both day and night. Like other peptide hormones, GH binds to cell surface receptors and activates adenylyl cyclase, and has direct metabolic effects on several tissues. In addition it produces other effects via the production of insulin-like growth factor 1 (IGF-1, a somatomedin); IGF-1 is synthesised by the liver in response to GH stimulation, and is highly protein bound in plasma.

The effects of GH are anabolic in relation to protein metabolism, especially in skeletal muscle, and in epiphyseal cartilage, where the proliferating effects stimulate bone growth. These actions are mediated by IGF-1. IGF-1 also has effects on the liver via the insulin receptor, and decreases hepatic glucose production. However, GH has an opposing direct effect on carbohydrate metabolism, reducing glucose uptake by skeletal muscle and adipose tissue, creating an insulin-resistant state (Box 43.1).

The effect of GH on fat is catabolic, with a direct action on adipocytes that promotes lipolysis and reduces lipogenesis. This action may be mediated in part by the β_3-adrenoceptor as well as by GH receptors. IGF-1, by contrast, has an antilipolytic effect in mature adipocytes, but these cells have few IGF-1 receptors.

GROWTH HORMONE FOR THERAPEUTIC USE

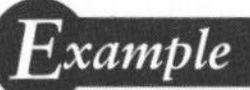

somatropin (synthetic form of GH)

Since 1985, biosynthetic human-sequence GH (somatropin), which was developed using recombinant DNA techniques, has replaced GH derived from human cadaveric pituitary origin, because the latter could transmit the prion-mediated Creutzfeldt–Jakob disease. Therapeutic uses of somatropin in children include:

- children with proven GH deficiency (who usually lack GHRH: pituitary dwarfism) to improve linear growth
- chronic renal insufficiency before puberty
- Turner's syndrome
- Prader–Willi syndrome.

To be effective, the hormone must be given before the closure of the epiphyses in long bones. If growth velocity does not increase by at least 50% from baseline, then treatment should be stopped.

Adult GH deficiency may warrant treatment with somatropin if all the following criteria are fulfilled:

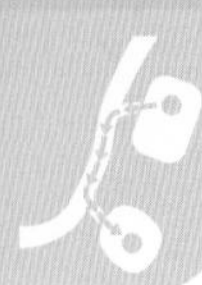

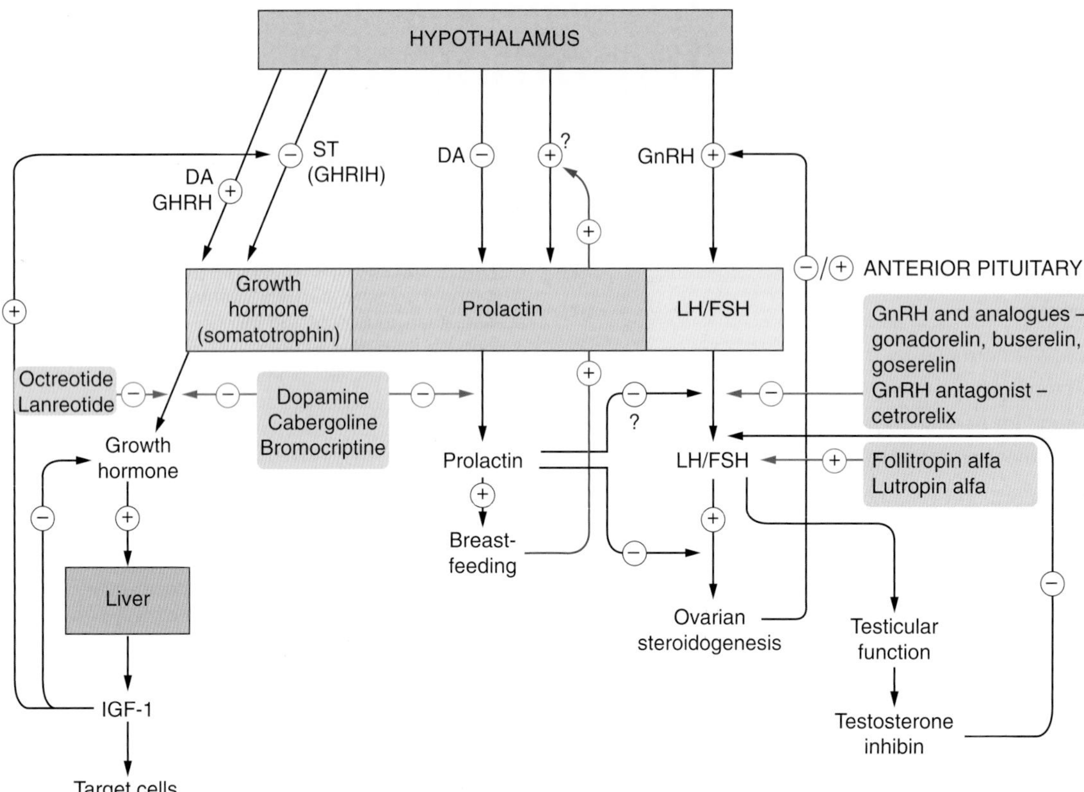

Fig. 43.1 **Control mechanisms for the release of growth hormone, gonadotrophins and prolactin from the anterior pituitary.** For control of other hormones, see Ch. 41 (thyroid), Ch. 44 (adrenocorticotrophic hormones) and Ch. 24 (dopamine agonists). Oestrogen effects on GnRH are shown as both positive and negative because oestrogen suppresses LH secretion in the early follicular phase but enhances secretion around ovulation (Ch. 45). Gonadorelin is synthetic but identical to GnRH. Pulsatile administration of GnRH or analogues enhances LH/FSH. On continuous administration, it rapidly downregulates the GnRH receptors, inhibiting LH/FSH release. The actions of drugs are shown by red arrows. DA, dopamine; FSH, follicle-stimulating hormone; GHRH, growth hormone-releasing hormone; GnRH, gonadotrophin-releasing hormone; IGF-1 insulin-like growth factor 1; LH, luteinising hormone; ST, somatostatin (also called GHRIH, growth hormone release inhibiting hormone); octreotide is synthetic somatostatin; ? = regulating hormone not yet established. Note: dopamine stimulates GH release in healthy individuals, but paradoxically in acromegaly it inhibits release.

Box 43.1 Effects of growth hormone

- Multiple effects through cAMP activation
- Anabolic effects on protein synthesis in muscle
- Increases bone growth, mineralisation and Ca^{2+} retention
- Increases fat catabolism
- Stimulates the growth of most internal organs
- Reduces liver uptake of glucose and promotes gluconeogenesis
- Stimulates the immune system

- severe GH deficiency
- impaired quality of life
- already receiving treatment for another pituitary hormone deficiency.

Pharmacokinetics

Somatropin has a very short half-life (0.5 h). Somatropin is usually given by subcutaneous injection, although the intramuscular route can be used. Plasma concentrations fluctuate widely following both routes, although the latter gives more stable levels because of slower uptake into the circulation. By contrast, concentrations of IGF-1 are much more constant, due to its high protein binding. As a consequence, three doses of somatropin per week give good clinical results, although daily dosing is often used.

Unwanted effects

- Headache, occasionally associated with visual problems, nausea and vomiting, and papilloedema, from benign intracranial hypertension
- Fluid retention with peripheral oedema
- Arthralgia, myalgia, carpal tunnel syndrome
- There is a transient insulin-like action which occasionally produces hypoglycaemia
- If excessive doses are used (as may happen during illicit use by athletes), there is a risk of diabetes mellitus in predisposed individuals
- Pain at the injection site.

ACROMEGALY

Acromegaly results from excessive production of GH, almost always by an adenoma in the anterior pituitary, which also secretes prolactin in one-third of cases (Fig. 43.1). The most common clinical features arise from excessive growth of bone and soft tissue. Complex metabolic consequences include insulin resistance with diabetes and hypertension.

The morbidity and mortality of acromegaly vary according to its severity. Untreated acromegalic individuals have a life expectancy approximately half that of people without acromegaly, due to an excess incidence of cardiovascular and respiratory disease and of carcinoma of the colon. Acromegaly is therefore usually treated actively.

DRUGS FOR ACROMEGALY

Somatostatin analogues

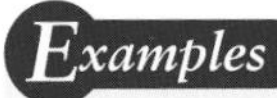

lanreotide, octreotide

Mechanisms of action and uses

The synthetic derivatives of somatostatin (GHRIH) are both more potent and longer-acting inhibitors of GH secretion than is the native compound. They are selective for the SST receptor subtypes that are highly expressed on GH-secreting adenomas. Like somatostatin, they also inhibit the release of gastro-entero-pancreatic peptide hormones, such as insulin, glucagon and gastrin, via intestinal receptors which generate intracellular cyclic adenosine monophosphate (cAMP) and promote Ca^{2+} influx into the cell. These actions make somatostatin analogues useful also for the treatment of a variety of conditions that are associated with excess secretion of gut hormones.

Uses of somatostatin analogues include:

- management of acromegaly
- management of other endocrine tumours, for example carcinoid tumours (to reduce flushing and diarrhoea), VIPoma (to reduce diarrhoea) and glucagonoma (to improve the characteristic necrolytic rash)
- management of thyroid tumours (lanreotide) and prevention of complications following pancreatic surgery (octreotide)
- octreotide is sometimes used to stop bleeding from oesophageal varices (Ch. 36).

Pharmacokinetics

Octreotide is given by subcutaneous injection. It has a short half-life (1–2 h) but suppresses GH secretion for up to 8 h, and it is therefore given three times daily. A depot preparation is available in which octreotide is adsorbed onto microspheres and given by deep intramuscular injection; the duration of action of this preparation is about 4 weeks. The depot preparation is used once control has been achieved by the use of the conventional formulation. Lanreotide also has a short half-life (1–2 h) and is formulated as a sustained-release preparation that is given by subcutaneous or intramuscular injection every 2–4 weeks, depending on the formulation.

Unwanted effects

- Gastrointestinal upset is common, especially anorexia, nausea, vomiting, abdominal pain, bloating and diarrhoea. It usually resolves with continued treatment
- Impaired postprandial glucose tolerance.
- Gallstones, due to suppression of cholecystokinin secretion with decreased gallbladder motility. In addition, an increase in bowel transit time alters colonic flora and makes bile salts more lithogenic.
- Pain at the injection site.

Growth hormone receptor antagonists

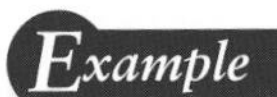

pegvisomant

Mechanism of action

Pegvisomant is a pegylated synthetic analogue of growth hormone that acts as a highly selective GH receptor antagonist.

Pharmacokinetics

Pegvisomant is given by subcutaneous injection. The mechanism of its clearance is unknown; the half-life is very long, at 6 days.

Unwanted effects

- Nausea, vomiting, dyspepsia, abdominal distension, diarrhoea, constipation
- Hypertension
- Headache, dizziness, fatigue, drowsiness, tremor, sleep disturbance
- Influenza-like symptoms, arthralgia, myalgia
- Weight gain, hypo- or hyperglycaemia.

Dopamine receptor agonists

(see Ch. 24)

In healthy people, dopaminergic receptor stimulation increases the secretion of GH, but in acromegaly there is a paradoxical decrease. Bromocriptine was originally used to treat acromegaly, but the clinical response was unpredictable and control of plasma IGF-1 was achieved in only about 20% of cases. It has been superseded by better-tolerated drugs such as cabergoline, which adequately suppress IGF-1 concentrations in about 40% of people with acromegaly. Further details of these drugs and compendium entries can be found in Chapter 24.

TREATMENT OF ACROMEGALY

Surgery by the trans-sphenoidal route is the usual treatment of choice, sometimes followed by external radiotherapy if the tumour was large.

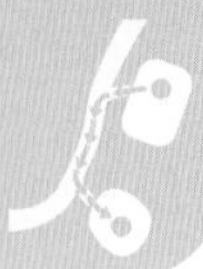

Three groups may be suitable for drug treatment:

- those in whom an excess of GH persists despite surgery and radiotherapy; after radiotherapy, the plasma GH concentration can take 1–2 years to fall
- those with mild acromegaly
- the elderly.

Somatostatin analogues are the first-line treatment, with pegvisomant used when there is intolerance or failure to respond. Cabergoline is sometimes used with a somatostatin analogue when there is resistance to other treatments. The effectiveness of treatment is monitored by the plasma concentration of IGF-1.

ADRENOCORTICOTROPHIC HORMONE (ACTH)

ACTH is a straight-chain polypeptide with 39 amino acids, of which the 24 that form the N-terminal are essential for full biological activity. It promotes steroidogenesis in adrenocortical cells by occupying cell surface receptors and stimulating adenylyl cyclase. Release of ACTH occurs in response to the hypothalamic peptide corticotrophin-releasing factor (CRF). CRF secretion is pulsatile and has a diurnal rhythm, with maximal release in the morning around the time of waking (see further detail in Ch. 44). The release of CRF is affected by other factors, including chemical (e.g. antidiuretic hormone, opioid peptides), physical (e.g. heat, cold, injury) and psychological influences. The main inhibitory influence on ACTH release is negative feedback control by circulating glucocorticoids. This occurs at both hypothalamic and pituitary levels. Adrenal androgens, although stimulated by ACTH, play no part in feedback control.

ACTH FOR THERAPEUTIC USE

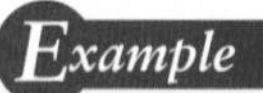

tetracosactide

ACTH preparations of animal origin have been replaced by a less allergenic synthetic peptide analogue, tetracosactide, which consists of the active N1–24 amino acid section of the ACTH molecule.

Pharmacokinetics

There are two formulations of tetracosactide:

- a rapid-acting form that increases steroidogenesis for about an hour and is suitable for tests of adrenocortical function. In adrenal insufficiency, there is a subnormal or no rise of plasma cortisol 30 min after intramuscular or intravenous injection of tetracosactide.
- a depot form that is absorbed slowly into the circulation over several hours and can be used as an alternative to exogenous corticosteroid therapy. However, the unpredictable response means that the therapeutic value of this drug is limited.

Once absorbed into the circulation, tetracosactide is metabolised rapidly with a very short half-life (0.2 h).

Unwanted effects

Prolonged use will produce all the features of corticosteroid excess (Ch. 44).

PROLACTIN

Prolactin is a glycoprotein similar in structure to growth hormone but secreted by distinct cells in the anterior pituitary (Fig. 43.1). The major hypothalamic control mechanism is inhibition by dopamine via D_2 receptors on the prolactin-secretory cells of the anterior pituitary (Ch. 45). The main target tissue for prolactin – a key hormone in lactation – is the breast, which secretes milk in response to prolactin if the mammary glands have been primed by ovarian and other hormones. At delivery, the maternal plasma prolactin concentration is high. Release of further prolactin continues as long as suckling continues. Prolactin-releasing peptide from the hypothalamus and both TRH and TSH are involved in stimulating prolactin release. A high plasma concentration of prolactin leads to a failure of ovarian follicle growth and a low oestrogen state in the female. It may also interfere with gonadotrophin release. Plasma prolactin is raised during lactation, and this may explain the relative subfertility of women who are breastfeeding.

HYPERPROLACTINAEMIA

Persistent hyperprolactinaemia is usually caused by a microadenoma of the anterior pituitary or by the action of dopamine receptor antagonist drugs such as phenothiazines (Ch. 21). In younger women, hyperprolactinaemia can produce amenorrhoea, infertility, and signs and symptoms of oestrogen deficiency (e.g. vaginal dryness and dyspareunia, galactorrhoea and osteoporosis). In men, it may cause hypogonadism. A dopamine D_2 receptor agonist such as cabergoline (Ch. 24) can be used to suppress prolactin secretion. Pituitary surgery may be considered for treatment failure.

GONADOTROPHIN-RELEASING HORMONE (GnRH)

GnRH is a decapeptide that is synthesised in the hypothalamus and is transported by neuronal axons to the pituitary. It is then released in a pulsatile fashion into the capillaries of the pituitary-portal circulation and positively controls the synthesis and release of both luteinising hormone (LH) and follicle-stimulating hormone (FSH) from the anterior pituitary (Fig. 43.1). The cell surface receptors for GnRH are G-protein linked and are found widely in the body as well as on the gonadotrophic cells in the anterior pituitary. The receptors are induced by repeated stimulation with GnRH, but pulsatile exposure is essential to maintain responsiveness. There is rapid tolerance to constant-rate infusions of GnRH because of downregulation of cell surface receptors; both pulsatile stimulation and receptor downregulation can be achieved with different patterns of therapeutic administration, and these have different clinical uses, as described below. There is negative feedback control of GnRH release via neural pathways and sex steroids (Fig. 43.1).

GnRH-RELATED PRODUCTS FOR THERAPEUTIC USE

Synthetic GnRH (gonadorelin)

Synthetic GnRH is available for treatment of female infertility. In women with amenorrhoea due to impaired release of GnRH, repeated pulses of exogenous gonadorelin will often lead to normal pituitary–gonadal function, including a regular menstrual cycle and ovulation. The hormone is usually infused subcutaneously in pulses every 90 min (to avoid receptor downregulation) from a portable syringe-driving pump. Unwanted effects are unusual, but include nausea, headaches and abdominal pain.

Gonadorelin analogues

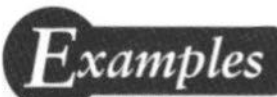

buserelin, goserelin

Mechanism of action

Structurally similar to the natural hormone, gonadorelin analogues (see Ch. 52 for detail) initially stimulate GnRH receptors, but rapidly promote receptor downregulation, which then inhibits further gonadotrophin production. The end result is reduced production of oestrogen or androgen. This latter action underlies their clinical uses.

Clinical uses of gonadorelin analogues

- The main use is to reduce testosterone secretion to castration levels in men with prostatic cancer. An initial rise in testosterone from receptor stimulation can produce tumour 'flare' in the first 1–2 weeks of treatment (Ch. 52). An anti-androgen (Ch. 46) is usually given to counteract this effect.
- Treatment of endometriosis by reducing oestrogen secretion.
- Treatment of advanced breast cancer in women by reducing oestrogen secretion.
- To achieve reduction in endometrial thickness for 3–4 months prior to intrauterine surgery.
- For women undergoing preparation for assisted conception by methods such as in vitro fertilisation (IVF) (see below).

Pharmacokinetics

Buserelin can be given either by subcutaneous injection or by nasal spray. It has a short half-life (1–1.5 h). Goserelin, which has a half-life of 4 h, must be given by subcutaneous injection and is available as an oily depot preparation. Depot formulations inhibit gonadotrophin production for up to 4 weeks after a single injection.

Unwanted effects

- Menopausal effects in women, with hot flushes, sweating, vaginal dryness and loss of libido
- Orchidectomy-like effects in men, with loss of libido, gynaecomastia and vasomotor instability
- Headache
- Hypersensitivity reactions, including skin rashes, asthma and anaphylaxis
- Osteoporosis with repeated courses
- Local reactions at injection sites, or intranasally with spray.

GnRH antagonists

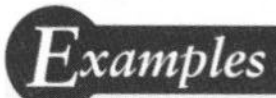

cetrorelix, ganirelix

Mechanism of action and uses

These drugs are competitive receptor antagonists that produce immediate, reversible suppression of gonadotrophin secretion. They are used in assisted reproduction techniques in the management of female infertility (IVF; see below). They have advantages compared with gonadorelin analogues in this role, since there is no initial surge of LH release (which can lead to cancellation of the IVF in about 20% of cycles).

Pharmacokinetics

Both cetrorelix and ganirelix are given by subcutaneous injection, and inactivated by hepatic metabolism. They have long half-lives (>12 h).

Unwanted effects

- Nausea
- Headache
- Injection site reactions.

GONADOTROPHINS

LH and FSH are glycoproteins which are released from the anterior pituitary when it is stimulated by pulsatile exposure to GnRH. Negative feedback by inhibin, a hormone produced by the gonads, selectively inhibits FSH secretion. In addition, both gonadotrophins are subject to negative feedback from gonadal steroids, including progesterone (Ch. 45).

In the male, LH acts on specific receptors on the surface of the Leydig cells in the testes and stimulates adenylyl cyclase, leading to the production of testosterone. FSH acts in a similar way on the Sertoli cells of the seminiferous tubules, stimulating the formation of a specific androgen-binding protein.

In the female, receptors for FSH and LH are found in granulosa cells of ovarian follicles. FSH is responsible for follicular development. The rising oestradiol concentration in the late follicular phase has a positive-feedback effect on

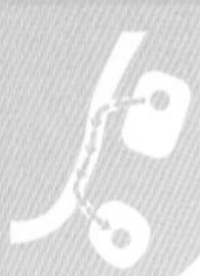

secretion of LH, and produces a short-lived surge of LH release. This triggers rupture of the follicle, release of the ovum and formation of the corpus luteum (Ch. 45). Both FSH and LH, like human chorionic gonadotrophic hormone (HCG), are also produced in large quantities by the placenta during pregnancy.

GONADOTROPHINS FOR THERAPEUTIC USE

- Human menopausal gonadotrophins (HMG) are FSH and LH (in a 1 : 1 ratio, also known as menotrophin) extracted from urine obtained from postmenopausal women.
- Chorionic gonadotrophin (HCG) contains large quantities of LH with little FSH. It is secreted by the placenta and extracted from the urine of pregnant women. An alternative preparation is human choriogonadotropin alfa (recombinant human chorionic gonadotropin).
- Follitropin alfa and beta (recombinant human FSH) (Fig. 43.1).
- Lutropin alfa (recombinant human LH) (Fig. 43.1).

Gonadotrophins are given by intramuscular or subcutaneous injection.

Unwanted effects

- Nausea and vomiting
- Abdominal and pelvic pain
- Headache
- In women, the most serious problem is ovarian hyperstimulation syndrome, in which the ovaries can become grossly enlarged as a result of multiple follicle stimulation, leading to considerable abdominal pain, ascites and even pleural effusions
- In men, the commonest problem is gynaecomastia or oedema with prolonged use.

CLINICAL USES OF GONADOTROPHINS

- Treatment of infertility in women with hypopituitarism.
- Treatment of infertility after failure of clomifene treatment (see below).
- For superovulation treatment for assisted conception (such as IVF).
- In men with hypogonadotrophic hypogonadism and oligospermia. This requires long courses of gonadotrophin injections, initially to achieve external sexual maturation and then to maintain satisfactory sperm production. Spermatozoa take 70–80 days to mature, and a year or more of treatment may be needed to achieve optimal response. A combination of HMG and HCG is usually given.

DRUG TREATMENT OF FEMALE INFERTILITY

Infertility is said to be present after 1 year of unprotected intercourse without conception. It has several causes, which need full evaluation before treatment is given or IVF considered.

If there is hyperprolactinaemia, then bromocriptine or one of the newer longer-acting dopamine agonists should suppress prolactin levels and permit ovulation in 70–80% of women. The management of polycystic ovary syndrome is considered below.

When deficiency of gonadal stimulation by gonadotrophin is the limiting factor, treatment with GnRH (gonadorelin) is given in a pulsatile fashion subcutaneously via a syringe pump. Conception rates are similar to those in the normal population. Alternatively, FSH (follitropin) can be given with LH (HMG), or combined as HCG to encourage the development of a single mature ovarian follicle (see Ch. 45). Ovarian hyperstimulation can be a problem.

If the hypothalamic–pituitary axis is normal, the anti-oestrogen clomifene blocks oestrogen receptors in the pituitary, which decreases the negative feedback on FSH (Fig. 43.1), giving increased FSH concentrations that stimulate follicle growth. There is a small risk of ovarian hyperstimulation, and multiple fetuses develop in about 11% of those who become pregnant.

Clomifene

Mechanism of action and use

Clomifene is an agent with both oestrogenic and anti-oestrogenic properties. The latter are related to its ability to block pituitary oestrogen receptors and increase gonadotrophin secretion. It is used to stimulate ovulation in anovulatory infertility.

Pharmacokinetics

Clomifene is well absorbed from the gut. It is metabolised in the liver, and has a very long half-life (5 days).

Unwanted effects

- Reversible ovarian enlargement and cyst formation
- Hot flushes
- Abdominal or pelvic pain
- Nausea, vomiting
- Breast tenderness, weight gain.

Preparation for assisted conception (IVF)

Ovulation is targeted on a particular date, and initial inhalation of a gonadorelin analogue or use of a GnRH antagonist will 'switch off' natural cyclical menstrual activity. Ovarian stimulation treatment is then begun to achieve maturation of oocytes at the time chosen for egg recovery prior to IVF. This involves giving large doses of human chorionic gonadotrophin or human menopausal gonadotrophin to stimulate the maturation of several follicles (superovulation treatment). These ova are then 'harvested' by aspiration of the follicles.

POLYCYSTIC OVARY SYNDROME

This is a common cause of infertility, affecting 5–10% of women of reproductive age. It is characterised by abnormal ovarian function with hyperandrogenism. Other complaints include menstrual disturbance, hirsutism and acne. It is often associated with obesity and insulin resistance in adipose and muscle tissue, conferring an increased risk of diabetes and cardiovascular disease in later life.

Metformin (Ch. 40) is a first-line treatment, and the resulting improvement in insulin sensitivity reduces androgen concentrations. This leads to weight loss, reduction of the consequences of hyperandrogenisation, and improved fertility. If fertility is not restored, then clomifene can be added. Because of the absence of good safety data, metformin is usually stopped during pregnancy. There is potential for the use of newer insulin sensitisers such as the thiazolidinediones (Ch. 40) in polycystic ovary syndrome, and promising results have been obtained with these agents.

Alternative approaches to treatment include a combined hormonal contraceptive (Ch. 45) or anti-androgen therapy with cyproterone acetate (Ch. 46) or high doses of the steroidal diuretic spironolactone (Ch. 14). Topical therapies are available for managing hirsutism associated with polycystic ovary syndrome. These include minoxidil cream (Ch. 6) to reverse male pattern hair loss, and eflornithine cream (an ornithine decarboxylase inhibitor) to slow facial hair growth.

POSTERIOR PITUITARY HORMONES

VASOPRESSIN (ANTIDIURETIC HORMONE)

Vasopressin is a nonapeptide, sometimes referred to as arginine vasopressin (AVP) because human vasopressin has an arginine residue in position 8. It is also known as antidiuretic hormone (ADH). Vasopressin is released from neurosecretory cells of the hypothalamus and transported down the axons of the nerve cells that form the pituitary stalk. It is stored in the nerve endings in the posterior pituitary and released in response to stimulation of the hypothalamus via osmoreceptors, sodium receptors and volume receptors. Vasopressin has two main target tissues.

- Stimulation of vascular smooth muscle via V1 receptors leads to Ca^{2+} influx and vasoconstriction. Vasoconstriction sufficient to raise blood pressure only occurs at high plasma vasopressin concentrations.
- At the collecting ducts of the kidney nephron, stimulation of V2 receptors leads to intracellular cAMP production which facilitates water reabsorption to produce more concentrated urine.

Vasopressin is metabolised in many tissues, including the liver and kidney, and has a very short half-life of about 10 min. It is given therapeutically by subcutaneous or intramuscular injection or by intravenous infusion.

Vasopressin analogues

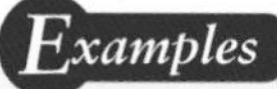

desmopressin, terlipressin

Vasopressin has a short duration of action. Desmopressin (DDAVP, des-amino-D-arginine vasopressin) has an increased diuretic potency and reduced pressor activity compared with vasopressin. It is absorbed through the nasal mucosa and is most conveniently administered by a metered-dose nasal spray. It can also be given by subcutaneous, intramuscular or intravenous injection. An additional action of parenteral desmopressin is to increase clotting factor VIII concentration in blood (Ch. 11).

Terlipressin is also a vasopressin analogue that is used to treat bleeding oesophageal varices. It is discussed in Chapter 36.

Pharmacokinetics

Like vasopressin, desmopressin is metabolised in the liver and kidney, but it has a longer half-life (0.5–2 h). Terlipressin is a prodrug of lysine-vasopressin, and is hydrolysed to the active form, which then has a formation rate-limited half-life of 0.5 h.

Unwanted effects

- Excessive water retention, producing dilutional hyponatraemia
- Headache
- Nausea, vomiting and abdominal pain.

CLINICAL USES OF VASOPRESSIN AND ITS ANALOGUES

- Treatment of cranial diabetes insipidus (see below), although the long-acting derivative desmopressin is usually used for maintenance treatment.
- Vasopressin can be given intranasally for primary nocturnal enuresis.
- To control bleeding from oesophageal varices in portal hypertension (Ch. 36). Terlipressin is now preferred to vasopressin for this indication.
- Desmopressin by injection is used to boost factor VIII concentration and reduce bleeding in mild to moderate haemophilia.
- Desmopressin can be given to test for urine concentrating ability in suspected diabetes insipidus (see below).
- Vasopressin is given for its pressor activity in the treatment of shock associated with hypotension, when it also increases vascular sensitivity to noradrenaline.

DIABETES INSIPIDUS

Diabetes insipidus is usually caused by a failure of secretion of vasopressin in the hypothalamus ('cranial' diabetes insipidus). Tumours, inflammatory conditions, granulomatous conditions such as sarcoidosis, and trauma to the hypothalamus are the main causes. A distinct condition known as nephrogenic diabetes insipidus occurs when the kidney is unresponsive to vasopressin. It can result from a hereditary deficiency of renal vasopressin receptors, or from drug therapy, particularly with lithium (Ch. 22) or the tetracycline demeclocycline. Diabetes insipidus presents clinically with thirst, polyuria, and a tendency to high plasma osmolality together with an inappropriately low urine osmolality.

Vasopressin produces concentrated urine in people with cranial diabetes insipidus, desmopressin is used for long-term treatment. Treatment of nephrogenic diabetes insipidus is more difficult, because the kidney does not respond to vasopressin. Paradoxically, thiazide diuretics

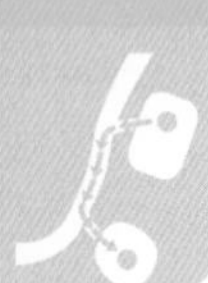

(Ch. 14) can reduce the polyuria. This may be due to initial contraction in extracellular volume, with subsequent increase in proximal tubular salt and water retention. Carbamazepine (Ch. 23) is also effective, by sensitising the renal tubule to the effect of vasopressin.

VASOPRESSIN V2 RECEPTOR ANTAGONIST

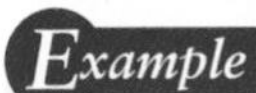

tolvaptan

Mechanism of action and uses

Tolvaptan is a competitive antagonist at Vasopressin V2 receptors. Its major action is in the renal collecting ducts to reduce water reabsorption and produce aquaresis without sodium loss, thus increasing free water clearance, and correcting dilutional hyponatraemia. In the UK, tolvaptan is currently licenced for the treatment of hyponatraemia secondary to inappropriate ADH secretion. However, it is also effective for correction of hyponatraemia in cirrhosis and heart failure arising from diuretic use. In all these situations, tolvaptan is not suitable for urgent treatment of severe hyponatraemia, when there is a risk of significant neurological complications. When initiating treatment, it is important to monitor the rise in serum sodium to avoid rapid correction and precipitation of osmotic demyelination syndrome.

Pharmacokinetics

Tolvaptan is fairly well absorbed from the gut, and eliminated by metabolism via cytochrome P450 (CYP 3A). It has a half-life of about 12 h.

Unwanted effects

- thirst, dry mouth, polyuria
- hypotension
- hypernatraemia
- hypoglycaemia

SYNDROME OF INAPPROPRIATE ANTIDIURESIS

This is a condition caused by inappropriately high secretion of vasopressin, resulting in excess water retention and a dilutional hyponatraemia. There are many causes, including malignant tumours that secrete vasopressin, pulmonary disorders (including infection), and various disorders of the central nervous system. Drugs such as antidepressants (Ch. 22), carbamazepine (Ch. 23) and various cytotoxic agents can also produce the syndrome.

Severe hyponatraemia can cause confusion, seizures and coma. Slow correction of the serum Na^+ concentration with intravenous normal saline is the mainstay of treatment. Rapid correction can disturb the osmotic balance across neurons and cause irreversible damage known as central pontine myelinolysis which produces dysarthria, spastic quadriparesis and pseudobulbar palsy.

Less severe hyponatraemia may respond to fluid restriction. Demeclocycline, a tetracycline antimicrobial agent that reduces the sensitivity of the collecting ducts to vasopressin, can also be used. The vasopressin V2 receptor antagonist tolvaptan is used, but not for urgent treatment when there is a risk of neurological complications.

OXYTOCIN

Oxytocin is discussed in Chapter 45.

HYPOPITUITARISM

Pituitary insufficiency can arise from traumatic brain injury and subarachnoid haemorrhage, when a single hormonal axis is often affected. Pituitary irradiation or surgery, by contrast, often affects multiple axes. Less common causes include both pituitary and non-pituitary intracranial tumours, and ischaemic damage.

Replacement of a deficiency of glucocorticoid (Ch. 44) and thyroid (Ch. 41) hormonal function is essential. Female sex hormone (Ch. 45) or testosterone (Ch. 46) replacement can be important to restore libido and bone mass. In some individuals, deficiency of growth hormone or vasopressin may also require replacement.

FURTHER READING

Balen AH, Rutherford AJ (2007) Management of infertility. *BMJ* 335, 608–611

Balen AH, Rutherford AJ (2007) Managing anovulatory infertility and polycystic ovary syndrome. *BMJ* 335, 663–666

Colao A, Arnaldi D, Beck-Peccoz P et al (2007) Pegvisomant in acromegaly: why, when, how. *J Endocrinol Invest* 30, 693–699

Danzig J (2007) Acromegaly. *BMJ* 335, 824–825

Dattani M, Preece M (2004) Growth hormone deficiency and related disorders: insights into causation, diagnosis, and treatment. *Lancet* 363, 1977–1987

Ehrmann DA (2005) Polycystic ovary syndrome. *N Engl J Med* 352, 1223–1236

Ellison DH, Beri T (2007) The syndrome of inappropriate antidiuresis. *N Engl J Med* 356, 2064–2072

Evers JLH (2002) Female subfertility. *Lancet* 360, 151–159

Huirne JAF, Lambalk CB (2001) Gonadotropin-releasing-hormone-receptor antagonists. *Lancet* 358, 1793–1803

Khanna A (2006) Acquired nephrogenic diabetes insipidus. *Semin Nephrol* 26, 244–248

Melmed S (2006) Acromegaly. *N Engl J Med* 355, 2558–2573

Norman RJ, Dewailly D, Legro RS et al (2007) Polycystic ovary syndrome. *Lancet* 370, 685–697

Olive DL (2008) Gonadotropin–releasing hormone agonists for endometriosis. *N Engl J Med* 359, 1136–1142

Sands JM, Bichet DG (2006) Nephrogenic diabetes insipidus. *Ann Intern Med* 144, 186–194

Schneider HJ, Almaretti G, Kreitschmann-Andermahr I et al (2007) Hypopituitarism. *Lancet* 369, 1461–1470

Setji TJ, Brown AJ (2007) Polycystic ovary syndrome: diagnosis and treatment. *Am J Med* 120, 128–132

Van Voorhis BJ (2007) In vitro fertilization. *N Engl J Med* 356, 379–388

SELF-ASSESSMENT

In questions 1–3, the first statement, in italics, is true. Are the accompanying statements also true?

1. *The release of GH (somatotrophin) is reduced by somatostatin (GHRIH).*
   a. Somatostatin stimulates GH release.
   b. Somatostatin is produced only from the hypothalamus.
   c. The inhibition of GH release by bromocriptine in people with acromegaly is paradoxical.
   d. Octreotide is a useful drug for the treatment of acromegaly.
2. *Prolactin is an anterior pituitary hormone that is an essential hormone for milk secretion by the mammary gland; it also contributes to reduced fertility by suppressing steroidogenesis.*
   a. Bromocriptine reduces prolactin secretion.
   b. Continuous administration of analogues of gonadotrophin stimulates sex steroid synthesis.
   c. The gonadotrophin analogue gonadorelin has no clinical use in males.
   d. Gonadorelin is used for the treatment of endometriosis.
   e. Follitropin alfa is a genetically engineered FSH used in preparation for in vitro fertilisation.
3. *Vasopressin is an antidiuretic hormone and acts on the collecting ducts to facilitate water reabsorption. The response to vasopressin is impaired in nephrogenic diabetes insipidus.*
   a. Vasopressin is a peptide.
   b. Nephrogenic diabetes insipidus is a condition in which there is a failure of secretion of vasopressin (ADH).
   c. In nephrogenic diabetes insipidus, thiazide diuretics increase the polyuria.
4. Choose the one **incorrect** statement from the following options about GH.
   A. The release of GH is constant through a 24-h period.
   B. GH acts by stimulation of IGF-1 release.
   C. In acromegaly, the dopamine receptor agonist cabergoline reduces IGF-1 levels.
   D. IGF-1 has a negative feedback effect on GH release.
   E. Somatropin that is used for GH deficiency in children is obtained by recombinant DNA techniques.
5. Choose the one **incorrect** statement from these options about GnRH.
   A. GnRH used in IVF needs to be given by continuous high-dose infusion to stimulate sufficient gonadotrophin release to induce both follicle growth and ovulation.
   B. GnRH reduces testosterone secretion in men with prostate cancer.
   C. GnRH given in high dose produces a menopausal-like effect.
   D. Clomifene stimulates FSH secretion by having an anti-oestrogenic effect.
   E. Continuous GnRH administration produces a surge in gonadotrophins before blocking FSH and LH release.
6. Case history questions

An assessment of a 10-year-old girl with short stature showed that she had abnormally low levels of GHRH and GH.

   a. Was this girl too old to benefit from treatment?
   b. If it was considered that treatment would be of benefit, what treatment would you recommend and how would you administer it?
   c. What unwanted effects might occur?

ANSWERS

1. a. **False**. Somatostatin is an inhibitor of GH release.
   b. **False**. Somatostatin is also produced from intestinal and pancreatic cells.
   c. **True**. Bromocriptine is a dopamine receptor agonist and is a stimulant of GH release in healthy individuals but paradoxically inhibits GH release in acromegaly.
   d. **True**. Octreotide is a long-acting analogue of somatostatin and inhibits GH release.
2. a. **True**. It is a dopamine receptor agonist and inhibits prolactin release from the anterior pituitary. It can be used to improve fertility in women with high levels of prolactin.
   b. **False**. Although brief administration of gonadotrophins stimulates sex steroid synthesis, on continued administration, gonadotrophin receptors are rapidly downregulated and sex steroid synthesis declines.
   c. **False**. Gonadorelin is used to inhibit testosterone synthesis in prostate cancer and reduce the size of the prostate.
   d. **True**. Gonadorelin, synthetic GnRH, reduces oestrogen synthesis, which inhibits endometriosis.
   e. **True**. Follitropin alfa promotes follicle growth.
3. a. **True**. Vasopressin is a nonapeptide released from the posterior pituitary although it is synthesised in the hypothalamus.
   b. **False**. In nephrogenic diabetes insipidus, the kidney is unresponsive to vasopressin.
   c. **False**. Paradoxically, in diabetes insipidus, the response to thiazide diuretics is a reduction in polyuria.

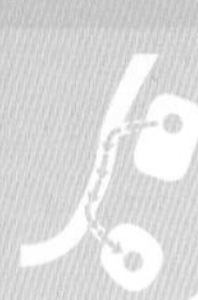

4. Answer **A**.
   A. Incorrect. GH is released in a pulsatile manner and is higher particularly during deep sleep in children.
   B. Correct. GH stimulates IGF-1 release from the liver, which then acts on receptors in many tissues and in concert with other hormones.
   C. Correct. Cabergoline is a dopamine agonist. Although in normal individuals dopamine and its analogues stimulate GH release, in acromegaly they paradoxically inhibit release.
   D. Correct IGF-1 inhibits GH release and also stimulates somatostatin release from the hypothalamus, which further inhibits GH release.
   E. Correct. GH is now obtained by recombinant DNA techniques to avoid transmission of Creutzfeldt–Jakob disease.
5. Answer **A**.
   A. Incorrect. GnRH is given in a pulsatile manner to stimulate FSH and LH release. If given continuously, there is soon a downregulation of gonadotrophin receptors and inhibition of gonadotrophin release.
   B. Correct. Given continuously, testosterone will be inhibited, although an initial stimulation of release may precede this. This effect is used to shrink prostate cancers.
   C. Correct. As mentioned in part A, gonadotrophin secretion is inhibited by high-dose continuous GnRH and ovulatory synthesis of oestrogens and progesterone is inhibited.
   D. Correct. Clomifene is an anti-oestrogen. Early in the menstrual cycle, low levels of oestrogen inhibit gonadotrophin secretion and therefore temporary oestrogen inhibition will promote gonadotrophin secretion and follicle growth.
   E. Correct. Downregulation of receptors is preceded by stimulation of gonadotrophin release.
6. Case history answers
   a. No. Epiphyseal closure occurs much later, so treatment at this age can increase growth.
   b. Biosynthetic GH (somatropin) has a half-life of only 25 min and levels fluctuate widely. However, high protein binding of the IGF-1 that is released under the action of GH means that three injections a week are sufficient to maintain IGF-1 at required levels.
   c. Insulin-like effects can produce hypoglycaemia and there is pain at the site of injection. Headache and oedema can also occur.

Pituitary and hypothalamic hormones

Drug	Half-life (h) and kinetics	Comments
Hypothalamic hormones and antagonists		
Gonadotrophin-releasing hormone (GnRH)		
Gonadorelin	4 min [M + R] Very short half-life probably reflects tissue uptake and intracellular metabolism	Synthetic preparation identical to GnRH; synthetic analogues are used for endometriosis (Ch. 45) and breast and prostate cancer (Ch. 52); given by subcutaneous or intravenous injection
Gonadorelin analogues		
Buserelin	(see Ch. 52)	Used for prostate cancer (see Ch. 52)
Goserelin	(see Ch. 52)	Used for prostate cancer (see Ch. 52)
Leuprorelin acetate	(see Ch. 52)	Used for prostate cancer (see Ch. 52)
Nafarelin	(see Ch. 45)	Used for endometriosis (see Ch. 45)
Triptorelin	(see Ch. 52)	Used for prostate cancer (see Ch. 52)
Gonadotrophin-releasing hormone (GnRH) antagonists		
Inhibit the release of gonadotrophins (LH and FSH); used to inhibit premature LH surges in the treatment of female infertility (under specialist supervision)		
Cetrorelix	20–60 [M] Metabolised by peptidases; some is eliminated unchanged in urine and bile	A synthetic decapeptide given by subcutaneous injection
Ganirelix	16 [M] Metabolised by peptidases to oligopeptide products; some is eliminated unchanged in urine and bile	Given by subcutaneous injection

Pituitary and hypothalamic hormones

Drug	Half-life (h) and kinetics	Comments
Drugs that interfere with gonadotrophin release (anti-oestrogens)		
Used in the treatment of female infertility due to oligomenorrhoea or secondary amenorrhoea; they occupy oestrogen receptors and interfere with feedback mechanisms inducing gonadotrophin release		
Clomifene	5 days [M + B] A racemate with the more active isomer (zuclomifene) accumulating over the first few days of treatment; undergoes enterohepatic circulation	Given orally
Tamoxifen	7 days [M]	Main use is in breast cancer – see Ch. 52
Growth hormone-releasing hormone (GHRH) analogues		
Sermorelin	1 (GHRH) [M]	Analogue of GHRH; used as a diagnostic test of secretion of growth hormone (GH); given by intravenous injection; half-life is for GHRH; the time for the release and removal of GH after GHRH are about 10 min and 20–30 min, respectively
Growth hormone release inhibiting hormone (GHRIH; somatostatin) analogues		
Lanreotide	1.3 [R + M] Eliminated by renal excretion and probably by tissue uptake and metabolism	Used for acromegaly and neuroendocrine tumours and for the treatment of thyroid tumours; given by intramuscular or deep subcutaneous injection
Octreotide	1.7 [R + M] Eliminated by renal excretion (about 40%) and probably by tissue uptake and metabolism	Used for acromegaly and neuroendocrine tumours, and for reducing vomiting in palliative care and stopping oesophageal variceal bleeds; given by subcutaneous injection or by intravenous injection if a more rapid response is required
Thyrotrophin-releasing hormone (TRH)		
Protirelin (TRH)	4 min (TRH) [M] Rapidly metabolised by tissues and serum	Thyrotrophin-releasing hormone; used for assessment of thyroid function; given by intravenous injection
Anterior pituitary hormones and antagonists		
Corticotrophins		
Tetracosactide (cosyntropin)	0.2 [M] Metabolised by endopeptidases in serum	Corticotrophin (ACTH) analogue; used largely as a test of adrenocortical function (formerly given by intramuscular injection for conditions such as Crohn's diseases and rheumatoid arthritis); given by intramuscular or intravenous injection; slower release from intramuscular injection
Gonadotrophins (FSH, LH and HCG) and analogues		
Follitropin alfa and beta (FSH)	24 (alfa), 30–40 (beta) [M + R] Absorption rate-limited half-life; mostly eliminated by metabolism but pathway has not been defined	Recombinant human FSH; given by subcutaneous or intramuscular injection
Lutropin alfa (LH)	14 [M] About 50% is absorbed from the injection site as the active drug; limited data available	Recombinant human LH; given by subcutaneous injection
Human menopausal gonadotrophins (menotrophin) (FSH + LH)	7–10 (FSH) 3 (LH) [M] Peak concentrations seen at 4–6 h after administration; metabolites eliminated in urine	Contains a 1:1 mixture of pituitary-derived FSH and LH; given by deep intramuscular or subcutaneous injection

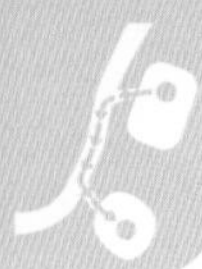

Pituitary and hypothalamic hormones

Drug	Half-life (h) and kinetics	Comments
Chorionic gonadotrophin; human chorionic gonadotrophin (HCG)	30–35 [M + R] The half-life is longer after subcutaneous or intramuscular injection (30–35 h) because of slow release from the site of injection	Glycoprotein extracted from the urine of pregnant women; given by subcutaneous or intramuscular injection
Choriogonadotropin alfa	29 [M + R] Routes of metabolism have not been defined; about 10% is excreted in urine	Recombinant human chorionic gonadotrophin; given by subcutaneous injection
Growth hormone		
Somatropin	0.5 (i.v.) [M] Serum half-life after subcutaneous administration (usual route) is 4 h due to absorption rate-limited elimination	Synthetic form of growth hormone (somatotrophin); given by subcutaneous or intramuscular injection
Growth hormone receptor antagonists		
Pegvisomant	6 days [?] Route of elimination has not been defined (but not unchanged in urine)	Pegylated synthetic analogue of growth hormone; given by subcutaneous injection
Prolactin antagonists		
Used to suppress lactation		
Bromocriptine	3 [M] Extensively metabolised by hydrolysis to inactive products	D_2 receptor agonist; given orally; (see Ch. 24)
Cabergoline	60–90 [M + R] Hydrolysed to metabolites that are excreted in bile and urine (see Ch. 24)	D_2 receptor agonist; better tolerated than bromocriptine; given orally (see Ch. 24)
Quinagolide	? Kinetic data have not been identified	Non-ergot D_2 receptor agonist; better tolerated than bromocriptine; given orally
Thyroid stimulating hormone (TSH)		
Thyrotropin alfa	25 [M + R] Few kinetic data available	Recombinant form of TSH; used to detect thyroid remnants post-thyroidectomy; given by intramuscular injection
Posterior pituitary hormones and antagonists		
Demeclocycline	10–15 [R + B] Oral bioavailability is 66% (due to poor absorption)	Has anti-ADH action possibly due to blockade of renal tubular effects of ADH; used for treatment of hyponatraemia resulting from inappropriate secretion of ADH; given orally
Desmopressin	0.5–2 [M] Poor oral bioavailability due to presystemic metabolism; metabolised by liver, kidney and plasma to inactive products	Vasopressin analogue; used for treatment of pituitary diabetes insipidus; given orally, intranasally, or by subcutaneous, intramuscular or intravenous injection
Terlipressin	0.5 [M] Triglycyl prodrug of lysine-vasopressin which is metabolised by hydrolysis to the active form (which then has a formation rate-limited half-life of 0.5 h)	Used for treatment of oesophageal varices; given by intravenous injection
Tolvaptan	12 [M] metabolised by CYP3A	Has anti-ADH action by blocking vasopressin V2 receptors in the renal collecting ducts. Used for treating hyponatraemia; given orally.
Vasopressin (ADH)	5–15 min [M] Rapidly metabolised in kidney, liver, brain and placenta	Used for treatment of pituitary diabetes insipidus and bleeding oesophageal varices; given by subcutaneous or intramuscular injection or by intravenous infusion

[B], biliary excretion; [M], metabolism; [R], renal excretion.

44 Corticosteroids (glucocorticoids and mineralocorticoids)

STRUCTURE AND SYNTHESIS OF STEROID HORMONES

Steroid hormones comprise several compounds synthesised mainly in the adrenal cortex and the gonads. They are derived from cholesterol and share a common nucleus (Fig. 44.1). The pathways of steroid hormone synthesis are shown in Figure 44.2. The steroid hormones responsible for phenotypic gender differences are known as the sex hormones; these compounds are considered in Chapters 45 and 46.

This chapter considers steroid hormones derived predominantly from the adrenal cortex that are known as adrenal corticosteroids. They have two distinct classes of action (see below and Table 44.1):

- glucocorticoid activity, which affects carbohydrate and protein metabolism
- mineralocorticoid activity, which affects water and electrolyte balance.

The natural glucocorticoid cortisol (also known as hydrocortisone) has a hydroxyl grouping at position 17 and has small structural differences from the natural mineralocorticoid aldosterone, which has an aldehyde grouping at position 18. There is variation in the spectrum of activity among different synthetic corticosteroids; hydrocortisone has approximately equal glucocorticoid and mineralocorticoid activity, whereas synthetic corticosteroids have been modified structurally to enhance either the glucocorticoid or mineralocorticoid activity.

Glucocorticoid (and, to a lesser extent, mineralocorticoid) secretion is controlled by the hypothalamic–pituitary–adrenal axis (Fig. 44.3). An increase in the plasma glucocorticoid concentration feeds back to reduce the release of corticotrophin-releasing factor (CRF).

MODE OF ACTION OF STEROID HORMONES

All steroid hormones have similar receptor mechanisms, but there are distinct receptors for the different structural variants (Ch. 1). The distribution of the various receptors among tissues gives tissue specificity to each type of steroid hormone and defines its activity. In the circulation, steroid hormones are bound to specific globulins. Steroids are highly lipophilic and cross cell membranes by diffusion and bind to a specific cytoplasmic receptor (Ch. 1). In the absence of a steroid molecule, the receptor is retained in the cytoplasm and prevented from migrating to the cell nucleus because it is associated with a heat shock protein (HSP). Binding of the steroid to the receptor dissociates the complex from the HSP, and the steroid–receptor complex then enters the nucleus and binds to a steroid-response element on the target genes (see Fig. 1.8). The binding usually involves the presence of other proteins, called chaperone proteins, and can lead to either increased or decreased transcription of proteins, depending on the target cell. Some genes are activated by simple interaction of the steroid receptor with the steroid-response element, but the rate of gene transcription is modulated by recruitment of various intranuclear co-regulator proteins and complexes.

The corticosteroid receptor only interacts with the response element for a matter of seconds before dissociating, and appears to have a 'hit and run' effect on gene transcription. When corticosteroids are given for a therapeutic effect, the response is delayed by many hours due to the time taken for modulation of protein synthesis.

However, some actions of glucocorticoids are relatively rapid in onset and do not require gene transcription (non-genomic signalling pathways). There is direct activation of various intracellular kinases by the ligand-activated glucocorticoid receptor, leading to effects such as endothelial nitric oxide production.

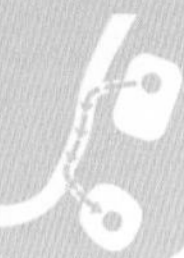

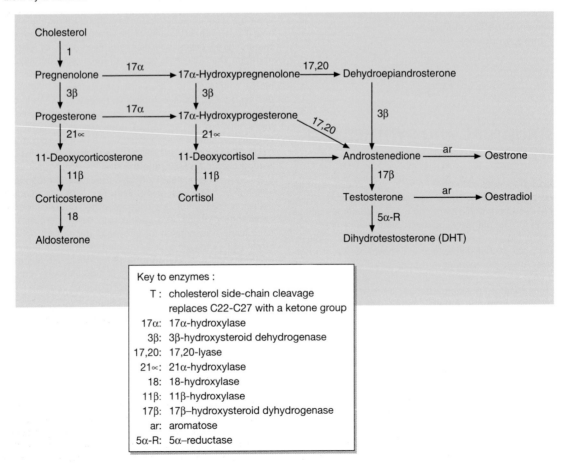

GLUCOCORTICOIDS

Examples

betamethasone, dexamethasone, hydrocortisone, prednisolone

Hydrocortisone (cortisol) is the main natural glucocorticoid in humans. It is synthesised in the adrenal cortex in response to adrenocorticotrophic hormone (ACTH) secreted from the anterior pituitary (Ch. 43). Glucocorticoid receptors are found in most tissues, giving hydrocortisone a wide range of actions. Although hydrocortisone and various synthetic derivatives are used for their glucocorticoid activity, they are frequently referred to as 'corticosteroids' or less accurately as 'steroids'. In this chapter, the distinction between glucocorticoid and mineralocorticoid is emphasised. In the rest of the book drugs with mainly glucocorticoid activity are usually referred to as corticosteroids.

Fig. 44.1 **The 'core' structure of steroid hormones is derived from the cholesterol molecule shown.** Note: the four rings are each identified by a letter, and each carbon atom by a number.

ACTIONS OF GLUCOCORTICOIDS

Immunosuppressant and anti-inflammatory actions

Glucocorticoids have important immunomodulatory actions that underpin many of their therapeutic uses. These arise predominantly from inhibition of the activity of pro-inflammatory transcription factors such as activator protein-1 (AP-1) and nuclear factor kappa B (NF-κB) (gene transrepression). The activated glucocorticoid receptors recruit histone deacetylases to the transcription complex of genes that have been activated by inflammatory stimuli. The deacetylation of core histones at the transcription complex silences these genes. Glucocorticoids also activate anti-inflammatory genes (gene transactivation), which contributes to their immunomodulatory action.

Cholesterol → (1) Pregnenolone
Pregnenolone → (17α) 17α-Hydroxypregnenolone → (17,20) Dehydroepiandrosterone
Pregnenolone → (3β) Progesterone; 17α-Hydroxypregnenolone → (3β) 17α-Hydroxyprogesterone; Dehydroepiandrosterone → (3β) Androstenedione
Progesterone → (17α) 17α-Hydroxyprogesterone → (17,20) Androstenedione
Progesterone → (21∝) 11-Deoxycorticosterone → (11β) Corticosterone → (18) Aldosterone
17α-Hydroxyprogesterone → (21∝) 11-Deoxycortisol → (11β) Cortisol
11-Deoxycortisol → Androstenedione
Androstenedione → (ar) Oestrone
Androstenedione → (17β) Testosterone → (ar) Oestradiol
Testosterone → (5α-R) Dihydrotestosterone (DHT)

Key to enzymes :
T: cholesterol side-chain cleavage replaces C22-C27 with a ketone group
17α: 17α-hydroxylase
3β: 3β-hydroxysteroid dehydrogenase
17,20: 17,20-lyase
21∝: 21α-hydroxylase
18: 18-hydroxylase
11β: 11β-hydroxylase
17β: 17β–hydroxysteroid dyhydrogenase
ar: aromatose
5α-R: 5α–reductase

Fig. 44.2 **Pathways of steroid hormone biosynthesis.**

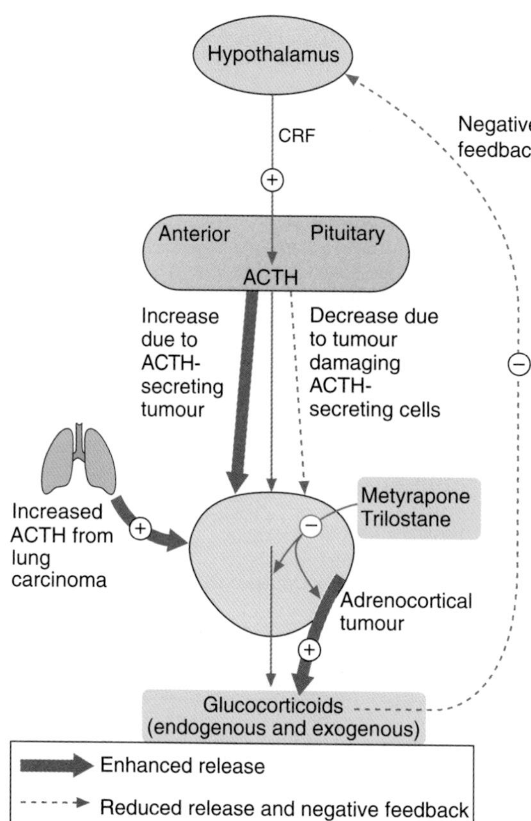

Fig. 44.3 **Control of secretion of glucocorticoids.** Stimulation by corticotrophin-releasing factor (CRF) and adrenocorticotrophic hormone (ACTH) increases the release of glucocorticoids. The level of glucocorticoids in the blood feeds back and negatively controls the release of CRF and ACTH. Synthetic glucocorticoids have the same action, suppressing the hypothalamic–pituitary axis. In conditions in which excess glucocorticoids are released, e.g. in ACTH-secreting tumours or adrenocortical tumours, glucocorticoid synthesis and release can be reduced by drug therapy, shown in red. In patients with tumours that result in hormone-induced reduction in glucocorticoids, synthetic glucocorticoids can be administered.

As a result of the above actions, glucocorticoids:

- inhibit mononuclear cell and neutrophil leucocyte migration and their adhesion to inflamed capillary endothelium; the ability of these inflammatory cells to phagocytose and destroy micro-organisms and to release oxygen free radicals is also reduced (Ch. 38)
- reduce the synthesis of inflammatory prostaglandins and leukotrienes (Ch. 29)
- impair fibroblast activity with reduced collagen synthesis and inhibition of matrix metalloproteinases, which impairs wound repair
- decrease capillary permeability, which has a protective effect on blood volume and raises blood pressure; the sensitivity of vascular walls to the vasoconstrictor actions of catecholamines and angiotensin II is also enhanced.

Glucocorticoids act at several sites to reduce the immune response (Ch. 38). These include:

- inhibition of genes synthesising many cytokines, including interleukin (IL)-1, IL-2 and interferon-gamma (IFN-γ) resulting in reduced T-lymphocyte proliferation involved in cell-mediated immunity (Ch. 38)
- inhibition of humoral immunity by reducing B-lymphocyte proliferation, T-cell activation, and Ig production, particularly IgG (Ch. 38).

Metabolic effects

The metabolic effects of glucocorticoids are on carbohydrate and protein metabolism.

- Gluconeogenesis, particularly in the liver, is increased; storage of glycogen in the liver and, to a lesser extent, in muscle is increased; and tissue uptake and utilisation of glucose is impaired. These actions promote hyperglycaemia.
- Protein is degraded, particularly in muscle, to enable synthesis of glucose and to increase the available pool of amino acids, while protein synthesis is inhibited. As a result, there is an overall negative nitrogen balance.
- Fat is redistributed from the glucocorticoid-sensitive fat stores in the limbs to the glucocorticoid-resistant stores in the face, neck and trunk. This action results from enhancement of the lipolytic response to catecholamines.
- Osteoblast formation is decreased, and apoptosis of mature osteoblasts is increased. The function of mature osteoblasts is inhibited by reducing production of osteocalcin, a key extracellular matrix protein in bone that promotes bone mineralisation. Activity of osteoclasts is increased. These actions lead to bone demineralisation.
- Inhibition of the proliferation and differentiation of chondrocytes at the epiphyseal end of the growth plate of long bones reduces bone growth in children.

Central nervous system effects

Plasma cortisol concentrations rise to a peak at the time of awakening and are lowest during sleep. In general, high circulating concentrations of hydrocortisone are associated with alertness, but severe disturbances of mood may occur with abnormally high levels of glucocorticoid. Low concentrations produce a feeling of lethargy.

Mineralocorticoid effects

Natural glucocorticoids also have mineralocorticoid activity, although this has minimal impact at physiological doses (see below). Synthetic glucocorticoid compounds are altered structurally to minimise the amount of mineralocorticoid activity (Table 44.1).

PHARMACOKINETICS OF GLUCOCORTICOIDS

Both hydrocortisone and synthetic glucocorticoids are used in clinical practice. They are readily absorbed from the gut. Hydrocortisone binds to corticosteroid-binding globulin and to albumin in the blood; it is extensively metabolised in the gut wall and liver. Synthetic glucocorticoids are more potent than hydrocortisone and bind to albumin but not

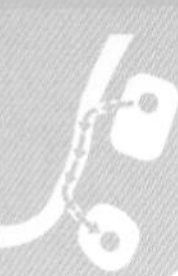

Table 44.1 Relative glucocorticoid and mineralocorticoid activities of some natural and synthetic corticosteroid hormones

	Glucocorticoid	Mineralocorticoid
Cortisol (hydrocortisone)	1	1
Prednisolone	4	0.8
Dexamethasone	30	Negligible
Betamethasone	30	Negligible
Aldosterone	0	80
Fludrocortisone	10	125

All potencies are relative to the glucocorticoid and mineralocorticoid activities of cortisol assigned arbitrary values of 1. Due to intracellular metabolism by 11β-hydroxysteroid dehydrogenase in aldosterone-sensitive cells, cortisol has about one thousandth of the mineralocorticoid activity of aldosterone in vivo.

to corticosteroid-binding globulin. They are more slowly metabolised in the liver, giving them a longer duration of action. Substantial amounts are excreted via the kidneys as metabolites. Of the many synthetic glucocorticoids, dexamethasone is the most potent and has the least mineralocorticoid activity.

Most glucocorticoids are available in formulations for parenteral use. This does not appreciably shorten the time to onset of action, which is delayed by up to 8 h while protein synthesis is modulated intracellularly. Some glucocorticoids are available in preparations for local use (e.g. beclometasone, budesonide and fluticasone by inhaler for asthma) and this reduces their systemic actions, although systemic unwanted effects can occur, particularly with high doses (see Chs 12 and 34).

The plasma half-lives vary, but, because of their mechanism of action – via gene transcription and changes in protein synthesis – their biological (i.e. effective) half-lives are long (varying from 12 h for hydrocortisone to 2 days for dexamethasone).

Box 44.1 Examples of diseases for which systemic glucocorticoid therapy is useful

Replacement therapy in corticosteroid deficiency
Acute inflammatory disease
- Bronchial asthma
- Anaphylaxis and angioedema
- Acute fibrosing alveolitis

Chronic inflammatory disease
- Connective tissue disorders, e.g. systemic lupus erythematosus, polymyositis, vasculitis
- Renal disorders, e.g. glomerulonephritis
- Hepatic disorders, e.g. chronic active hepatitis
- Bowel disorders, e.g. inflammatory bowel disease
- Eye disorders, e.g. posterior uveitis

Neoplastic disease
- Myeloma
- Lymphomas
- Lymphocytic leukaemias

Miscellaneous disorders
- Bell's palsy
- Sarcoidosis
- Organ transplantation
- Antiemetic therapy (for cytotoxic chemotherapy)

Table 44.2 Examples of topical corticosteroid administration

Disease	Mode of administration	Chapter
Asthma	Aerosol	12
Vasomotor rhinitis	Aerosol	39
Eczema	Ointment or cream	49
Superficial ocular inflammation	Aqueous solution	50
Ulcerative colitis	Aqueous solution or foam enema	34
Proctitis	Suppository	34
Arthritis	Aqueous solution by intra-articular injection	30

CLINICAL USES OF SYSTEMICALLY ADMINISTERED GLUCOCORTICOIDS

The anti-inflammatory and immunosuppressive effects of glucocorticoids are used for various inflammatory diseases (especially those which are immunologically mediated) and neoplastic conditions, particularly when they involve lymphoid tissue (Box 44.1). Powerful glucocorticoids with little mineralocorticoid activity, such as prednisolone, are usually chosen. Dexamethasone is often used to reduce oedema around malignant tumours in the brain and those compressing the spinal cord. It is also used in some antiemetic regimens during cancer chemotherapy (Ch. 32).

Physiological replacement therapy for corticosteroid deficiency

Hydrocortisone or an equivalent synthetic glucocorticoid is given orally twice or three times daily in doses as close as possible to the amount normally secreted by the adrenal cortex. The dose must be doubled or tripled in stressful situations, for example intercurrent infection. Acute adrenal insufficiency requires immediate treatment with high-dose intravenous hydrocortisone. Conditions that can give rise to corticosteroid deficiency are shown in Box 44.3.

For uses of ACTH and its analogues, see Chapter 43.

CLINICAL USES OF TOPICALLY ADMINISTERED GLUCOCORTICOIDS

Topical use of glucocorticoids can deliver high concentrations to a target site and reduce systemic unwanted effects. However, significant absorption into the blood can occur at higher doses. Examples of the clinical uses of topical corticosteroids are given in Table 44.2.

UNWANTED EFFECTS OF GLUCOCORTICOIDS

Pharmacological doses of glucocorticoids given over long periods will produce the typical features of adrenocortical

Box 44.2 Unwanted effects of glucocorticoids

- Central obesity with 'buffalo hump', moon face and abdominal striae.
- Loss of supporting tissue in skin with skin atrophy, bruising, and poor wound healing. Local atrophy can be marked at the site of topical corticosteroid application.
- Osteoporosis due to catabolism of protein matrix in the bone and defective mineralisation.
- Proximal (i.e. shoulder and hip girdle) muscle wasting and weakness.
- Hyperglycaemia, which may lead to overt diabetes mellitus (Ch. 40).
- Peptic ulceration due to inhibition of gastrointestinal prostaglandin (Ch. 33).
- Mood changes, including euphoria and occasionally psychosis.
- Posterior capsular cataracts in the eye, and exacerbation of glaucoma.
- Increased susceptibility to infection with bacteria, viruses or fungi. Activation of latent infection such as tuberculosis can also occur.
- Growth retardation in children, with reduced linear bone growth and premature epiphyseal closure.
- After long-term treatment, sudden withdrawal can produce an acute adrenal crisis due to suppression of the hypothalamic–pituitary–adrenal axis and adrenal atrophy. Recovery of adrenal responsiveness can take several months. Basal cortisol secretion is restored before maximal responses, leaving patients at risk during stress and intercurrent infection.
- Mineralocorticoid effects (which vary among the different drugs).

Box 44.3 Causes of glucocorticoid excess (Cushing's syndrome) and corticosteroid deficiency

Causes of Cushing's syndrome

- Excessive secretion of ACTH by the anterior pituitary (pituitary adenoma) (Cushing's disease)
- Excessive secretion of ACTH from an ectopic source (most commonly carcinoma of the bronchus)
- A tumour of the adrenal cortex secreting predominantly cortisol
- Iatrogenic: administration of glucocorticoid or ACTH in pharmacological doses

Causes of corticosteroid deficiency

- Primary adrenal insufficiency (Addison's disease)
  - autoimmune adrenalitis
  - infections, e.g. tuberculosis, various fungi, opportunistic infections in AIDS
  - metastatic carcinoma
- Secondary adrenocortical failure (deficient ACTH from the anterior pituitary)
  - pituitary tumour
  - sarcoidosis
  - suppression of the hypothalamic–pituitary–adrenal axis by prolonged glucocorticoid treatment at pharmacological doses
- Various enzyme defects in cortisol synthesis (congenital adrenal hyperplasia)

overactivity (Cushing's syndrome). Unwanted glucocorticoid actions are shown in Box 44.2.

CUSHING'S SYNDROME

Cushing's syndrome is characterised by excessive glucocorticoid effects (Box 44.2). There are four possible causes (Box 44.3).

Surgery is the definitive treatment for excessive pituitary secretion of ACTH (usually from an adenoma) and for unilateral adrenal tumours, with subsequent radiotherapy for some pituitary tumours.

Drug treatment to reduce corticosteroid secretion is desirable for several weeks before surgery, in order to reverse the excessive tissue catabolism and correct the metabolic disturbances. This is usually achieved with metyrapone, which reduces corticosteroid biosynthesis by competitive inhibition of 11β-hydroxylase (Fig. 44.2). It also inhibits cytochrome P450 in the liver, which can produce important drug interactions (Ch. 2). Oral absorption of metyrapone is variable, and extensive metabolism occurs in the liver. Gastrointestinal upset is the main unwanted effect. Trilostane is a less effective alternative to metyrapone, and is a reversible inhibitor of the earlier enzyme in the synthesis of corticosteroids, 3β-hydroxysteroid dehydrogenase (Fig. 44.2). The antifungal agent ketoconazole (Ch. 51) reduces cortisol synthesis by inhibition of 11β-hydroxylase, but its onset of action is slower than that of metyrapone; it also inhibits sex steroid production and therefore often causes gynaecomastia and decreased libido in males and hirsutism in females. Ketoconazole can be used alone or in combination with metyrapone. All these drugs have relatively short-lived benefit, with loss of control (escape) when increased ACTH secretion is the cause of the syndrome.

Mitotane is a chemotherapeutic drug (Ch. 52) that causes more profound suppression of glucocorticoid synthesis with no escape. It can be used for long-term control of symptoms for people who are unwilling or too unfit to undergo surgery. Glucocorticoid replacement therapy is usually necessary.

Ectopic ACTH secretion is not usually amenable to surgical cure, but palliative drug treatment can be helpful (Fig. 44.3).

MINERALOCORTICOIDS

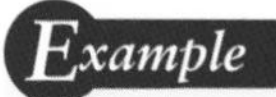

fludrocortisone

Aldosterone is the principal mineralocorticoid and is secreted from the zona glomerulosa of the adrenal cortex. Aldosterone secretion is regulated by several factors, of which angiotensin II (Ch. 6), low plasma Na^+ and high plasma K^+ are the most important. Angiotensin II acts via specific angiotensin II receptors (AT_1 and AT_2) (see Ch. 1 and Ch. 6), of which the AT_1 receptor induces aldosterone release. ACTH has some stimulatory effect on aldosterone secretion. Mineralocorticoid receptors are found in fewer tissues than are glucocorticoid receptors. The main target cells are in the distal renal tubule and collecting duct, where aldosterone increases the permeability of the luminal tubular

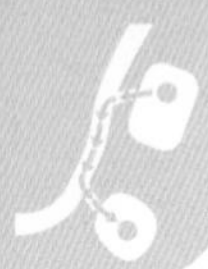

membrane to Na^+ by increasing the number of Na^+ channels. It also stimulates the Na^+/K^+-ATPase pump in the basolateral membrane, which leads to active Na^+ reabsorption and loss of K^+ into tubular urine (Ch. 14). Water is passively reabsorbed with Na^+, so that extracellular fluid volume and blood pressure are both increased. Target cells for aldosterone, especially in the renal tubule, contain the enzyme 11β-hydroxysteroid dehydrogenase which metabolises hydrocortisone to cortisone. Cortisone has very low affinity for the mineralocorticoid receptor and this ensures that aldosterone-responsive tissues are not stimulated by endogenous glucocorticoids.

FLUDROCORTISONE

Pharmacokinetics

Aldosterone is almost completely inactivated on its first passage through the liver and is therefore unsuitable for oral use. 9α-Fluorohydrocortisone (fludrocortisone) is a synthetic alternative which is well absorbed from the gut, but only about 10% escapes first-pass metabolism. The half-life is short (0.5 h) due to rapid hepatic metabolism.

Clinical uses

- Fludrocortisone is given as replacement therapy for defective aldosterone production. This is usually the result of primary adrenal pathology with destruction of all three zones of the cortex (Addison's disease).
- Expansion of blood volume by fludrocortisone can be used to raise blood pressure in postural hypotension resulting from autonomic neuropathy. However, it often produces supine hypertension without fully eliminating the postural fall in blood pressure.

Unwanted effects

Excessive Na^+ retention and K^+ loss can occur with pharmacological doses of fludrocortisone. Hypertension can result, but the expansion of blood volume stimulates cardiac stretch receptors, leading to secretion of natriuretic peptides. This results in an 'escape' natriuresis which establishes a new equilibrium between Na^+ intake and excretion at a higher blood volume. Consequently, oedema does not usually occur.

PRIMARY HYPERALDOSTERONISM (CONN'S SYNDROME)

Autonomous oversecretion of aldosterone causes hypertension and a hypokalaemic alkalosis. Some cases are caused by an adenoma in the zona glomerulosa of the adrenal cortex and are treated surgically. The majority are caused by hyperplasia of both zonae glomerulosa. This usually causes less marked clinical consequences, and a potassium-sparing diuretic (usually spironolactone) is the treatment of choice to preserve the plasma K^+ concentration and reduce blood pressure (Ch. 14).

FURTHER READING

Adcock IA (2003) Glucocorticoids: new mechanisms and future agents. *Curr Allergy Asthma Rep* 3, 249–257

Canalis E (2003) Mechanisms of glucocorticoid-induced osteoporosis. *Curr Opin Rheumatol* 15, 454–457

Lipworth BS (1999) Systemic adverse effects of inhaled corticosteroid therapy. *Arch Intern Med* 159, 941–955

Lovas K, Husebye ES (2003) Replacement therapy in Addison's disease. *Expert Opin Pharmacother* 4, 2145–2149

Newell-Price J, Bertagna X, Grossman AB et al (2006) Cushing's syndrome. *Lancet* 367, 1605–1617

Nieman LK, Ilias I (2005) Evaluation and treatment of Cushing's syndrome. *Am J Med* 118, 1340–1346

Rhen T, Cidlowski JA (2005) Antiinflammatory effects of glucocorticoids – new mechanisms for old drugs. *N Engl J Med* 353, 1711–1723

Young WF Jr (2003) Minireview: primary aldosteronism – changing concepts in diagnosis and treatment. *Endocrinology* 144, 2208–2213

SELF-ASSESSMENT

In questions 1–4, the first statement, in italics, is true. Are the accompanying statements also true?

1. *In maximum recommended doses, inhaled corticosteroids can cause systemic unwanted effects.*
   a. Oral fludrocortisone is a useful anti-inflammatory corticosteroid in severe asthma.
   b. Beclometasone is not used orally.
2. *Corticosteroids take many hours to produce their clinical effects because they act by modulating gene transcription and cellular production of proteins.*
   a. Hypoglycaemia is common during glucocorticoid administration.
   b. If prolonged administration of prednisolone results in unwanted effects, it is appropriate to withdraw the drug slowly.
3. *Mineralocorticoid secretion is decreased in Addison's disease which can be caused by autoimmune disease or drugs such as ketoconazole.*
   a. Aldosterone secretion is inhibited by angiotensin II.
   b. Aldosterone and cortisol secretion are regulated by ACTH.
4. *Glucocorticoids affect all inflammatory responses caused by infection, chemical or altered immune stimuli.*
   a. Dexamethasone causes vomiting.
   b. Glucocorticoids delay wound healing.
   c. Before giving an intra-articular injection of glucocorticoid in gout, infection of the joint should be excluded.

5. Case history 1

A 35-year-old woman showed signs of cortisol excess, including centripetal obesity, muscle weakness, easy bruising and amenorrhoea.

a. What were the possible causes?

She was not taking corticosteroids, eliminating an iatrogenic cause. The cortisol level in a 24-h urine collection was elevated. Plasma ACTH levels were also high.

b. What did these results indicate?

A single high dose of dexamethasone was administered and resulted in only marginal suppression of plasma cortisol.

c. What did this result indicate?

A computed tomography scan and other tests showed an inoperable carcinoma of the bronchus.

d. What treatment could be given?

6. Case history 2 questions

Mr BFG, a 69-year-old man, suffered from late-onset asthma, which was poorly controlled by β_2-adrenoceptor agonists. His GP prescribed an inhaled corticosteroid (low-dose) which helped him initially.

a. Which corticosteroids could have been given by aerosol?
b. What were the possible unwanted effects of inhaled corticosteroid?

Mr BFG then had a particularly severe attack (acute severe asthma or status asthmaticus) which led to his admission to hospital as an emergency.

c. Amongst the drugs he was given was a corticosteroid. Which drug was likely to have been given, by what route, and what was the objective of its use?

Mr BFG's status asthmaticus resolved and he was then prescribed a course of oral corticosteroid while in hospital and subsequently sent home with high-dose inhaled corticosteroid.

d. Which corticosteroid could have been used for oral therapy?
e. Comment on the principles that should be followed for the initiation and duration of the course of treatment with the oral corticosteroid.
f. Compare the unwanted effects resulting from high-dose oral corticosteroid with those of the low-dose aerosol.

Mr BFG's asthma was poorly controlled by high-dose inhaled corticosteroid and it was decided to recommence oral therapy.

g. Why would oral therapy likely to have been better than inhaled therapy in more severe asthma?
h. How would you have determined the dose to be used and monitor its appropriateness?

After many months of this therapy, Mr BFG started to complain of apparently unrelated problems, including: recurrent minor infections; minor epigastric discomfort, especially on an empty stomach; weight gain and increased appetite; a tendency to bruise easily; and severe back pain after a minor fall.

Examination revealed a cushingoid appearance, and investigation showed a raised plasma glucose level and decreased plasma levels of cortisol and ACTH.

i. Discuss the reasons for Mr BFG's symptoms.

ANSWERS

1. a. **False**. Fludrocortisone is a synthetic mineralocorticoid with a salt-retaining:anti-inflammatory ratio of about 12.5:1. The glucocorticoid prednisolone should be used orally.
   b. **True**. Beclometasone is used by inhalation for its local effects on the airways in the treatment of asthma (Ch. 12).
2. a. **False**. Corticosteroids lead to reduced tissue uptake of glucose and increased gluconeogenesis, leading to 'steroid-induced diabetes'.
   b. **True**. After prolonged administration it is possible that the hypothalamic–pituitary–adrenal axis (secretion of both CRF and ACTH) will be suppressed (Fig. 44.3), i.e. endogenous cortisol levels are low. Slow withdrawal allows the adrenals to recover their normal cortisol secretion and avoids corticosteroid deficiency.
3. a. **False**. Reduced plasma sodium results in stimulation of renin secretion, which is converted to angiotensin II. This then stimulates aldosterone release from the adrenal cortex, which acts to increase Na^+ reabsorption in the distal part of the distal tubule.
   b. **True**. ACTH stimulates both cortisol and aldosterone secretion by the adrenal cortex.
4. a. **False**. Dexamethasone can inhibit vomiting and will add to the antiemetic actions of agents such as ondansetron in vomiting caused by cancer chemotherapy (Ch. 32).
   b. **True**. Because of their catabolic effect on proteins, they delay the healing of wounds.
   c. **True**. Immunosuppressant effects of glucocorticoids can exacerbate an underlying infection.
5. Case history 1 answers
   a. Possible causes include:
      (i) a tumour of the adrenal cortex secreting cortisol
      (ii) excess secretion of ACTH by a pituitary tumour

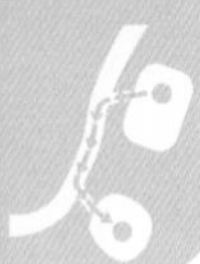

(iii) excess secretion of ACTH by a non-pituitary tumour (commonly small-cell carcinoma of the lung, medullary or thyroid carcinoma)
(iv) iatrogenic, from therapeutic administration of glucocorticoids or ACTH.

b. The cause could not be a primary cortisol-secreting adrenocortical tumour or glucocorticoid administration, as the ACTH levels would be low due to negative feedback of glucocorticoid on the anterior pituitary and hypothalamus. The possibility is an ACTH-secreting pituitary adenoma or ACTH-secreting non-pituitary tumour.
c. The dexamethasone suppression test is not definitive; it has been shown to suppress ACTH of pituitary origin but not from ectopic ACTH-producing tumours or adrenocortical tumours. The result might therefore exclude a tumour of pituitary origin.
d. Control by inhibitors of adrenal corticosteroid synthesis, e.g. trilostane or metyrapone. (Note: she would probably also show signs of excess mineralocorticoid activity, which should also be treated in parallel with spironolactone.)

6. Case history 2 answers
   a. Beclometasone, budesonide and fluticasone are all available for inhalation (see Ch. 12). They are systemically absorbed; however, with low doses, amounts reaching the systemic circulation are insufficient to have significant systemically mediated effects. This does not apply with high doses, where systemic unwanted effects may sometimes be evident.
   b. Although systemic unwanted effects may be few with low doses, local problems such as oral candidiasis or other fungal infections may arise, but this could be managed with a spacer and good oral hygiene. High doses may lead to iatrogenic 'cushingoid' signs and symptoms (see below).
   c. Hydrocortisone intravenously. This is a lipid-soluble corticosteroid; giving it intravenously would minimise the time to onset of action, which can still, however, take hours. The objective is to reduce both the acute and chronic inflammation accompanying this acute exacerbation of asthma.
   d. Oral prednisolone is often used.
   e. Give a short course of high-dose prednisolone and then gradually tail off the dose over the following 1–2 weeks in order to allow the return of normal hypothalamic–pituitary–adrenal axis function, which may have been suppressed by the high-dose prednisolone.
   f. Systemic unwanted effects are less with inhaled corticosteroids than with oral corticosteroids.
   g. A high concentration of drug is needed at target cells, and poor technique, inflammation, mucus, etc., might prevent inhaled drugs reaching their target. Systemic prednisolone following oral administration reaches the target cells more effectively than following inhalation of a corticosteroid.
   h. For long-term oral treatment, use the lowest possible dose of corticosteroid to prevent unwanted effects. The dose may vary with the severity of the asthma. Therefore, monitor peak expiratory flow rate (usually done at home each morning). Relatively frequent dose adjustments may be needed.
   i. Corticosteroids have a wide range of metabolic effects in addition to their anti-inflammatory and immunomodulatory actions. The cushingoid symptoms described can all be attributed to actions on carbohydrate, protein and lipid metabolism and suppression of the hypothalamic–pituitary–adrenal axis.

Corticosteroids[a]

Drug	Half-life (h) and kinetics	Comments
Glucocorticoids		
The durations of action ('biological half-lives') of corticosteroids greatly exceed their chemical half-lives because of their mechanism of action		
Betamethasone	35–55 [M] Ester prodrugs are hydrolysed to betamethasone; betamethasone per se is rapidly absorbed if given orally; inactivated by hepatic metabolism	Used for suppression of inflammatory and allergic disorders, congenital adrenal hyperplasia and cerebral oedema; given orally, topically, by intramuscular or slow intravenous injection, or by intravenous infusion; phosphate ester prodrug used for injections
Cortisone acetate	1–2 (HC) [M] Oral bioavailability is 20–90%; rapidly hydrolysed and converted to cortisol (hydrocortisone) which is inactivated by oxidation to cortisone and reduction to tetrahydrocortisol	Formerly used for replacement therapy; given orally
Deflazacort	1 [M] Bioavailability not affected by food (absolute bioavailability not defined); hydrolysed to the active 21-desacetyl metabolite (21-hydroxy compound)	Used for suppression of inflammatory and allergic disorders; given orally

Corticosteroids[a]

Drug	Half-life (h) and kinetics	Comments
Dexamethasone	2–4 [M] High but variable oral bioavailability possibly due to intestinal CYP3A metabolism; metabolised in the liver by CYP3A4-mediated oxidation to the 6-hydroxy compound	Used for suppression of inflammatory and allergic disorders, congenital adrenal hyperplasia and cerebral oedema, and diagnosis of Cushing's disease; given orally, by intramuscular or slow intravenous injection, or by intravenous infusion; antiemetic; phosphate ester prodrug used for injections
Hydrocortisone (cortisol)	1–2 [M] Variable absorption (30–90%) due to first-pass metabolism; metabolised by oxidation to cortisone and reduction to dihydro- and tetrahydrocortisol	Numerous anti-inflammatory and anti-allergic uses; given orally, by intramuscular or slow intravenous injection, or by intravenous infusion; phosphate ester prodrug used for injections
Methylprednisolone	1–3 [M] High oral bioavailability (80–90%); esters are very rapidly hydrolysed; metabolised in liver and kidney by reduction to 20-hydroxy compound	Used for suppression of inflammatory and allergic disorders, cerebral oedema and connective tissue disease; given orally, by intramuscular or slow intravenous injection, or by intravenous infusion; injectable forms are lipid-soluble esters in solvents
Prednisolone	2–4 [M] High oral bioavailability (70–80%); extensively metabolised but all pathways have not been defined	Used for suppression of numerous inflammatory and allergic disorders; given orally, topically and by intramuscular injection; injectable form is the acetate ester as an aqueous suspension
Triamcinolone	2–5 [M] Oxidised in the liver to inactive metabolites	Used for suppression of inflammatory and allergic disorders; given by deep intramuscular injection as an aqueous suspension
Mineralocorticoids		
The durations of action ('biological half-lives') of corticosteroids greatly exceed their chemical half-lives because of their mechanism of action		
Fludrocortisone acetate	0.5 [M] Low bioavailability (10%) due to first-pass metabolism; hydrolysed to fludrocortisol, which is reduced and eliminated as conjugated metabolites	Mineralocorticoid used in combination with hydrocortisone for adrenocortical insufficiency; given orally
Inhibitors of steroid metabolism		
Metyrapone	2 [M] Rapid oral absorption; metabolised to an active alcohol metabolite – metyrapol; both metyrapone and metyrapol are eliminated as glucuronide conjugates	Competitive inhibitor of 11β-hydroxylation in the adrenal cortex; used to control the symptoms of Cushing's syndrome, especially prior to surgery; given orally
Trilostane	? [M] Eliminated by oxidation to a keto analogue which has slightly more activity than the parent drug	Reversible inhibitor of 3β-hydroxysteroid dehydrogenase, causing inhibition of the synthesis of both glucocorticoids and mineralocorticoids; used in Cushing's syndrome (but is less effective than metyrapone) and primary hyperaldosteronism; given orally

[a]Additional corticosteroids used for specific purposes are covered in other chapters.
[M], metabolism.

45 Female reproduction

PHYSIOLOGY OF THE MENSTRUAL CYCLE AND PREGNANCY

The endocrine function of the hypothalamic–pituitary–ovarian axis acts through a series of feedback loops to control the reproductive processes of the menstrual cycle (Fig. 45.1). The menstrual cycle begins with the uterus shedding its lining (**menstrual phase:** days 1 to 3–5 of the menstrual cycle). Following the shedding of the endometrium, a group of 5–7 follicles in the ovary that have been growing for up to a year start to mature. This occurs under the influence of the gonadotrophic hormones follicle-stimulating hormone (FSH) and luteinising hormone (LH) secreted from the anterior pituitary (**follicular phase**: approximately days 5–13 of the menstrual cycle). Release of the gonadotrophic hormones (FSH and LH) is controlled by pulsatile secretion of gonadotrophin-releasing hormone (GnRH) from the hypothalamus. The increase in FSH during the early follicular phase is a result of the low levels of oestrogen during the first half of the follicular phase. The prolonged release of low levels of FSH and LH results in the selection and ongoing maturation of a single (occasionally two) dominant ovarian follicle. This is prepared for ovulation at the expense of the remaining follicles, which regress, possibly from a lack of gonadotrophin receptors on the unsuccessful follicles. FSH also stimulates the release of the follicle-derived peptide inhibin, which in turn controls FSH release.

The developing ovarian follicle is driven by FSH and LH to convert androgens produced by its thecal cells into oestradiol (Fig. 44.2) within its granulosa cells, possibly following the stimulation of DNA synthesis by FSH. Oestrogen secretion from the follicle slowly rises as the follicle matures. In the window of time between the early to mid follicular phase of the menstrual cycle, the modest amount of oestrogen secreted by the follicle exerts a negative feedback on both the hypothalamus and pituitary to keep gonadotrophin secretion low (Fig. 43.1). The low plasma concentration of progesterone also weakly suppresses gonadotrophin secretion in the early follicular phase. Although the circulating FSH concentration remains low, oestradiol enhances the effectiveness of the action of gonadotrophin on the ovary to stimulate further oestradiol synthesis.

In the late follicular phase, a cohort of granulosa cells in the maturing ovarian follicle differentiates under the influence of FSH and starts to express LH receptors. These granulosa cells can then be stimulated by LH to secrete progesterone and are destined to become the corpus luteum after ovulation. In the mid to late follicular phase, the circulating oestradiol concentration rises dramatically as

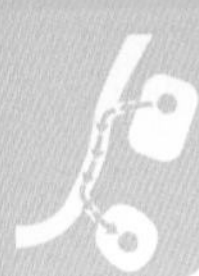

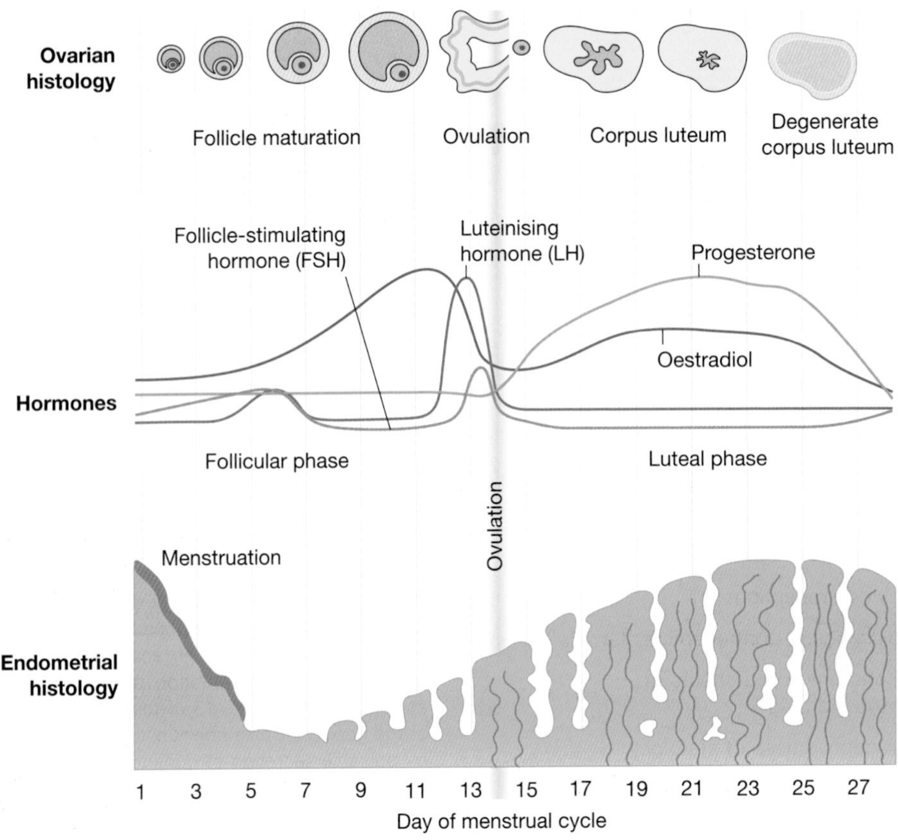

Fig. 45.1 **Endocrine control of the menstrual cycle.**

the follicle secretes more of the hormone under the influence of FSH. Eventually, the plasma oestradiol reaches a critical concentration of about 200 pg mL^{-1} for 48 h. This sustained concentration of oestradiol, and the relatively rapid rate of increase in oestradiol, triggers a switch from a negative feedback to a positive feedback of oestradiol upon the pituitary and hypothalamus. As a result, there is an acute mid-cycle surge of LH and, to a lesser extent, FSH, which is essential for ovulation.

Following **ovulation** (about day 14 of the menstrual cycle), the residual follicle transforms into the corpus luteum under the influence of the pituitary gonadotrophins. The plasma LH concentration falls rapidly and remains low throughout the **secretory** (**luteal**) **phase** (days 15–26 of the menstrual cycle). The reason for this is that granulosa cells containing LH receptors proliferate in the corpus luteum and produce increasing amounts of progesterone. Progesterone suppresses LH and FSH production by negative feedback on the hypothalamus and pituitary. The plasma concentrations of progesterone and oestrogen rise as they are produced by the corpus luteum. Progesterone is produced from the inner granulosa lutein layer and oestrogen from the outer thecal lutein layer. If implantation of a fertilised ovum does not occur, the corpus luteum regresses after about 10 days, possibly under the influence of local synthesis of vasoconstrictor prostaglandin ($PGF_{2\alpha}$), although there is little direct confirmation of this in humans. From day 5 to late in the menstrual cycle, the gradually increasing plasma concentrations of oestrogens and progesterone, which are produced as the menstrual cycle progresses, result in proliferation and vascularisation of endometrial cells that are able to secrete a variety of fluids and nutrients aimed at making the endometrium receptive for implantation. The temporal precision of the change in receptivity is critical if successful implantation of a fertilised oocyte is to occur. Oestrogen and progesterone cause the endometrium to become oedematous, and its glands secrete increasing quantities of amino acids, sugars and glycoproteins in a viscous liquid. At the end of the menstrual cycle, the decreasing circulating levels of progesterone and oestrogen eventually fall to levels that no longer support the endometrium. Deprived of hormonal support, the endometrial spiral arteries go into spasm and the endometrial cells die, producing digestive enzymes (**ischaemic phase**: days 27–28 of the menstrual cycle). As a consequence of this and other changes, the endometrium is shed during menstruation.

The cervical mucus is also influenced by oestrogen and progesterone concentrations. Under the dominant influence of progesterone, cervical mucus is viscid and less penetrable by sperm, whereas at ovulation, the high plasma oestradiol concentration results in thinner and more elastic mucus that is easily penetrable by sperm. Progesterone also inhibits the motility of the fallopian tube, altering the transport of sperm, and the fertilised or unfertilised oocyte. Excess progesterone may alter the chance of fertilisation occurring or the embryo may reach the uterine cavity when the endometrium is not receptive to implantation. Oestrogens have the opposite action, increasing tubal motility, and may accelerate the transport of the ovum into the uterine cavity.

Pregnancy is accompanied by considerable hormonal changes. The corpus luteum is essential for the maintenance of pregnancy during the first 6–8 weeks, after which, placental production of hormones takes over. During the early weeks the continuation of the pregnancy depends implicitly on the sex steroids and gonadotrophins secreted by the corpus luteum. Thereafter, the combined feto-placental unit produces progressively greater quantities of oestrogen and progesterone which reach the maternal circulation. The placenta also produces human chorionic gonadotrophin (HCG) (Ch. 43), which reaches a peak circulating concentration at about 50–60 days of gestation and then falls. HCG stimulates progesterone and oestrogen production from the corpus luteum. The increasing placental production of oestrogens, progesterone and human placental lactogen as pregnancy advances results in the development of duct and milk-secreting cells in the breast. The precise balance of sex steroids also contributes to quiescence of the uterus during pregnancy and the onset of labour at term.

MECHANISM OF ACTION OF OESTROGENS AND PROGESTOGENS

In common with other steroid hormones, both oestrogens and progestogens act by influencing gene transcription. They passively diffuse into the cell and bind to specific receptors in either the cytoplasm or cell nucleus (see Fig. 1.8). The receptors are probably associated with 'chaperone' molecules when in their unbound state, which are displaced by the hormone. Oestrogen binds to two specific cytoplasmic receptors (ERα and ERβ) which have different tissue distributions. The steroid–receptor complex enters the cell nucleus and associates with the oestrogen response elements of oestrogen-responsive genes. This leads to recruitment of co-activator molecules to the complex, and produces gene activation. Progesterone also has two specific receptors (PR-A and PR-B) that regulate progesterone-responsive genes. Oestrogen increases and progesterone decreases the expression of the progesterone receptors.

STEROIDAL CONTRACEPTIVES

Oral hormonal contraceptives ('the pill') are the most widely used form of contraception and contain either a combination of a synthetic oestrogen plus a synthetic progestogen (a C19 synthetic progesterone derivative) or a progestogen alone.

MECHANISMS OF HORMONAL CONTRACEPTION

Elevated circulating concentrations of synthetic oestrogen and progestogen prevent the precise cyclic pattern of hormone-related events seen in the normal menstrual cycle (Fig. 45.2).

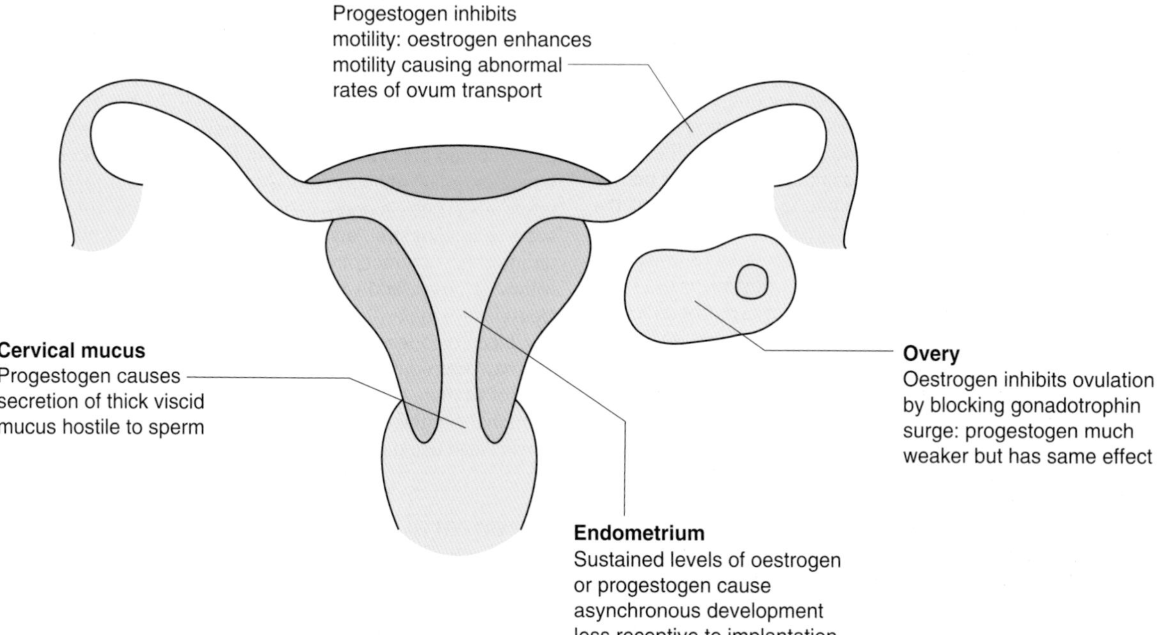
Fallopian tube
Progestogen inhibits motility: oestrogen enhances motility causing abnormal rates of ovum transport
Cervical mucus
Progestogen causes secretion of thick viscid mucus hostile to sperm
Overy
Oestrogen inhibits ovulation by blocking gonadotrophin surge: progestogen much weaker but has same effect
Endometrium
Sustained levels of oestrogen or progestogen cause asynchronous development less receptive to implantation

Fig. 45.2 **The contraceptive actions of the synthetic oestrogen and progestogen in the contraceptive pill.** Gn, gonadotrophin (LH and FSH).

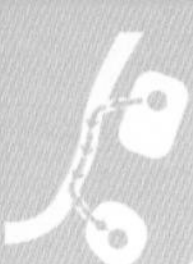

- The combination of oestrogen and progestogen exerts its contraceptive effect mainly through suppression of mid-cycle FSH release and inhibition of the LH surge that causes ovulation.
- The sustained levels of oestrogen and, to a lesser extent, progestogen suppress LH and FSH secretion and inhibit follicular development.
- Progestogen produces asynchronous development of the endometrium with stromal thinning, which makes it less receptive to implantation. Fallopian tube motility is increased by oestrogens and decreased by progestogens; this may affect fertility by altering the rate of transport of the ovum.
- Progestogen alters cervical mucus, making it thicker and less copious, thereby creating an environment more hostile to sperm penetration. Progestogens alone inhibit ovulation in only about 25% of women; contraception must therefore rely upon the other actions of the hormone.

THE 'COMBINED' HORMONAL CONTRACEPTIVE

Combined hormonal contraceptives contain both a synthetic oestrogen and progestogen. The oestrogen component is usually ethinylestradiol (an oestrogen that is alkylated at C17 to slow its metabolism), but in some combinations is mestranol, a compound that is metabolised in the liver to ethinylestradiol. Over the years since the oral combined hormonal contraceptive was introduced, the dose of the oestrogen component has been reduced. 'Second-generation' combined hormonal contraceptives have a lower oestrogen concentration than first-generation combined hormonal contraceptives, which are no longer used.

The progestogen component of the second-generation oral combined hormonal contraceptives is either levonorgestrel (the active isomer of norgestrel) or norethisterone; these compounds are testosterone analogues that also possess androgenic activity. 'Third-generation' oral combined hormonal contraceptives contain modified progestogens that have less androgenic activity; these are desogestrel, gestodene, norgestimate (which are all derivatives of norgestrel) and drospirenone (a derivative of the aldosterone antagonist spironolactone). Modified progestogens are used if there are unacceptable unwanted effects with the second-generation progestogens.

Other differences and similarities between second- and third-generation combined hormonal contraceptives are discussed later.

Monophasic preparations

Monophasic preparations contain fixed amounts of oestrogen and progestogen. They are taken daily for the first 21 days of the menstrual cycle, followed by 7 contraceptive-free days with tablets containing an inactive substance, such as lactose. The oestrogen concentration should be the lowest that maintains good cycle control and produces minimal unwanted effects. There is a choice of:

- low-strength preparations that contain 20 μg ethinylestradiol
- standard-strength preparations that contain 30 or 35 μg ethinylestradiol, or mestranol.

The monophasic oral combined hormonal contraceptive contains one of several progestogens (see above). In some women it may be necessary to change the formulation to reduce minor unwanted effects, such as breakthrough bleeding or weight gain during the menstrual cycle. The degree of androgenic activity possessed by different progestogens (see combined hormonal contraceptive section above) may influence the suitability of an individual preparation for a particular woman.

A transdermal patch formulation of low-strength ethinylestradiol with the progestogen norelgestromin is also available; this is applied weekly for 3 weeks followed by a 7-day patch-free interval.

Biphasic and triphasic preparations

Biphasic and triphasic preparations are designed to mimic more closely the changes in sex hormone concentrations that occur during the natural menstrual cycle. The total sex hormone intake through the cycle is no less than with monophasic preparations. Several preparations are available, all of which contain ethinylestradiol in combination with levonorgestrel, norethisterone or gestodene. The dose of ethinylestradiol is either kept constant throughout, as in the monophasic pills, or increased during days 7–12. Progestogen doses are increased once (biphasic) or twice (triphasic) as the menstrual cycle proceeds.

PROGESTOGEN-ONLY CONTRACEPTIVES

Oral progestogen-only contraceptives

The progestogen-only contraceptive is particularly useful for women in whom the administration of oestrogen is considered to be undesirable, for example if there is a history of thromboembolic disorders (see below). It is as effective as combined hormonal contraceptives containing 30 μg of ethinylestradiol, although some reports say that pregnancy rates are slightly higher. Various progestogens are used, such as desogestrel, etynodiol, levonorgestrel or norethisterone. The contraceptive tablet must be taken regularly, without a break, and within 3 h of the usual time every day (see efficacy below). Because the dose of progestogen is low, bleeding does occur at approximately monthly intervals but may be irregular. Breakthrough bleeding occurs in up to 40% of women; this is much higher than with the combined hormonal contraceptive. Some women become amenorrhoeic while using progestogen-only contraception.

Parenteral progestogen-only contraceptives

Intramuscular injection of a progestogen, either medroxyprogesterone acetate or norethisterone, can provide contraception for up to 8–12 weeks. Ovulation is reliably inhibited, unlike with the oral progestogen-only contraceptives, and therefore there is a low incidence of ectopic pregnancy. The contraceptive effect is fully reversible, but there is a high incidence of amenorrhoea when its effect wears off. Prolonged use of medroxyprogesterone acetate can reduce bone mineral density and cause osteoporosis. The loss of bone mineral density occurs over the first 2–3 years of use, and then stabilises. Prolonged use of medroxyprogesterone acetate beyond 2 years, or its use in adolescents or people with other risk factors for osteoporosis, is discouraged.

A subcutaneous implant of etonogestrel provides contraception for up to 3 years, after which time it should be replaced; the progestogen is released from a flexible rod inserted subdermally on the lower surface of the upper arm. Unwanted effects are the same as those experienced with the oral progestogen-only contraceptive, but lower doses of progestogen are needed because first-pass metabolism in the gut and liver is avoided.

Intrauterine progestogen-only device

A plastic intrauterine contraceptive device (IUCD) with a levonorgestrel-releasing system from a silicone reservoir provides effective contraception with reduced menstrual blood loss compared with copper IUCDs that do not contain a progestogen. The progestogen is released from the device for a period of 5 years.

EFFICACY OF HORMONAL CONTRACEPTION

When taken according to the recommended schedule, the failure rate for the combined hormonal contraceptive is 0.2%. With the oral combined hormonal preparations, contraceptive protection is reduced if there is a delay of more than 12 h in taking the daily dose. In such circumstances, the missed dose should be taken and additional contraceptive measures should be used for 7 days.

Failure of the progestogen-only oral contraceptive is age-related and is up to 5% in young women, falling with decreasing fertility to about 0.3% at the age of 40 years. With the oral progestogen-only contraceptive, other contraceptive precautions should be taken for 2 days if there is a delay of only 3 h or more after the normal time of taking the daily dose.

EMERGENCY CONTRACEPTION

This can be carried out with a single dose of 1.5 mg levonorgestrel taken as soon as possible after unprotected intercourse, and preferably within 12 h. The mechanism of action may be to accelerate transport of the fertilised ovum so that it reaches the uterine cavity before the endometrium is receptive. Implantation is therefore prevented, and the action is considered to be contraceptive rather than as an abortifacient. The treatment is successful in up to 99% of cases, but the efficacy is greatly reduced if used between 72 and 120 h after unprotected intercourse. Nausea is a frequent unwanted effect, occurring in up to 22% of people; vomiting can occur and an antiemetic (e.g. domperidone; Ch. 32) may be needed. Absorption takes 2 h, and vomiting after this time will not affect the efficacy of treatment. A larger dose may be required if drugs that induce drug-metabolising enzymes in the liver are being taken. In the UK, levonorgestrel can be purchased without prescription by women over the age of 16 years. In other countries, preparations containing levonorgestrel and ethinylestradiol are also available with prescription. Mifepristone, a progesterone antagonist (see below), is also used in some parts of the world as emergency contraception.

Insertion of an IUCD is an alternative strategy that is more effective than a progestogen, and retains its efficacy even when inserted up to 120 h after unprotected intercourse.

PHARMACOKINETICS OF CONTRACEPTIVE STEROIDS

The synthetic oestrogens, like the naturally occurring estradiol-17β (estradiol), and progestogens are highly lipid-soluble molecules and are rapidly and completely absorbed from the gut lumen after oral administration. Pharmacologically active synthetic parent drugs (see drug compendium) are metabolised more slowly than the natural hormones estradiol (half-life, 1–2 h) and progesterone (half-life, 5–20 min). Some synthetic compounds are prodrugs that undergo first-pass metabolism to the active entity. Active natural parent compounds with short half-lives due to rapid metabolism, such as estradiol, also have a low oral bioavailability because of extensive first-pass hepatic metabolism; in contrast, synthetic drugs with longer half-lives usually undergo slower metabolism and also limited first-pass metabolism. Oestrogens and progestogens (see drug compendium) are eliminated by hepatic metabolism, often involving CYP3A4-mediated oxidation and/or conjugation with glucuronic acid and/or sulphate. The conjugates may undergo enterohepatic cycling. There is considerable inter-individual variation in plasma levels of oestrogen and progestogen after ingestion of the combined hormonal contraceptive.

The metabolism and kinetics of oestrogens and progestogens can be affected by the administration of other drugs. Contraceptive failure may occur if there is concomitant treatment with anticonvulsants (e.g. barbiturates, carbamazepine or phenytoin), antiretroviral drugs such as nelfinavir, nevirapine or ritonavir, or the antibacterials rifampicin and rifabutin (Ch. 51) which induce liver cytochrome P450 enzymes (Table 2.9). A dose of at least 50 μg of ethinylestradiol (using multiple tablets) should be used if these drugs are given long term. Some antibacterials, for example ampicillin, doxycycline and rifampicin (Ch. 51), alter the gut flora and thereby decrease the enterohepatic circulation of ethinylestradiol. Alternative methods of contraception should be used for the duration of treatment with these broad-spectrum antibacterials and for 7 days thereafter (but 4 weeks in the case of rifampicin because of additional effects on liver enzymes).

The pharmacokinetics of individual synthetic oestrogens and progestogens vary widely and data on ethinylestradiol and norethisterone only are summarised here.

Ethinylestradiol is absorbed rapidly from the gut, and undergoes some first-pass metabolism, but this is low (about 20%) compared with estradiol (90–95%), and it has a half-life of 8–24 h. Enterohepatic cycling of

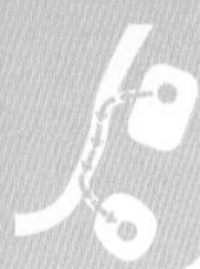

ethinylestradiol is responsible for maintaining effective plasma concentrations with low-dose formulations. Norethisterone is rapidly absorbed from the gut and eliminated by hepatic metabolism, with the metabolites eliminated in urine and bile; it has a half-life of 5–12 h.

BENEFICIAL AND UNWANTED EFFECTS OF CONTRACEPTIVE STEROIDS

Beneficial effects

- *Cancer*: there is a 40% reduction in the risk of ovarian cancer, seen after 5 years of use and persisting for up to 15 years after stopping. Endometrial cancer is reduced by 50%, with a similar duration of protection.
- *Acne* can be treated with oral combined hormonal contraceptives, since they reduce the concentration of free testosterone (Ch. 49). A combination of ethinylestradiol with cyproterone acetate, a weak progestogen with antiandrogenic activity (Ch. 46), is sometimes used for this purpose.
- *Dysfunctional uterine bleeding*, e.g. menorrhagia, is reduced by the combined oral contraceptive.

Unwanted effects

Both oestrogen and progestogen have a number of minor and major unwanted effects, but the incidence of the major effects, although important, is relatively low.

- Thromboembolism: the incidence of venous thromboembolic disease is increased in some subgroups of women taking the combined hormonal contraceptive. The mechanisms are complex but include procoagulant activity from increased production of clotting factors X and II and decreased production of the protective antithrombin (Ch. 11). Fibrinolysis is impaired, while reduced prostacyclin generation enhances platelet aggregation (Ch. 11). The risk of thromboembolism increases with age, and is greater in women who smoke (because smoking increases the risk of thrombogenesis) and in those with a thrombophilic tendency such as deficiency of protein C or protein S or the presence of factor V Leiden. The baseline risk of venous thromboembolism in women of reproductive age not taking the combined oral hormonal contraceptive is ≤5 or per 100 000. The excess risk in women taking second-generation preparations is 6–12 per 100 000 (depending on age) and in those taking preparations containing desogestrel or gestodene (third-generation) is 16–30 per 100 000. It is important that these risks are put into context, because there was considerable public concern when these findings were published in the media, following which some women stopped taking their combined hormonal contraceptive and became pregnant: the risk of venous thromboembolism in pregnancy is 60 per 100 000.
- Ischaemic heart disease and ischaemic stroke: analysis of data in women largely taking the second- and third-generation combined hormonal contraceptive shows that there is no significantly increased risk of myocardial infarction or ischaemic stroke for women who are non-smokers and who have normal blood pressure, irrespective of age. However, there is an increased risk of myocardial infarction and stroke in women taking the combined hormonal contraceptive who smoke or who are hypertensive, particularly in those over the age of 35 years. The added risk in those over 40 years is 20 per 100 000 for smokers and 29 per 100 000 for hypertensives. It has been suggested that enhanced thrombogenesis rather than premature atherogenesis is responsible for the excess cardiovascular risk with the combined hormonal contraceptive. It is uncertain whether the risk is different for the newer progestogens. If older women use the combined hormonal contraceptive, then the lowest possible dose of oestrogen should be given.
- Increase in blood pressure: a small increase in blood pressure is common during use of the combined hormonal contraceptive. A significant rise can occur in about 5% of women with previously normal blood pressure and in up to 15% of women with pre-existing hypertension. The mechanism is probably an increase in plasma renin substrate (Ch. 6) produced by oestrogen and, to a lesser extent, progestogen. Blood pressure may remain elevated for some months after the combined hormonal contraceptive has been stopped. Regular monitoring of blood pressure is advisable during use of the combined hormonal contraceptive.
- Cancer: despite numerous studies, the question of an association between combined hormonal contraceptives and breast cancer remains unresolved, and a small excess risk cannot be ruled out. The effect on the incidence of cervical cancer is uncertain, but it may be slightly increased by combined hormonal contraceptives in the presence of human papillomavirus infection.
- Nausea, mastalgia, depression, headache, weight gain and provocation of migraine may be minimised by prescribing preparations with low oestrogen content, or by changing the progestogen to desogestrel, drospirenone or gestodene.
- Breakthrough bleeding occurs frequently in some women, whereas in others withdrawal bleeding fails to occur. Gestodene-containing pills or triphasic preparations probably give the best cycle control. Amenorrhoea after stopping the combined hormonal contraceptive can last beyond a few months in about 5% of women, and a small number can experience amenorrhoea for more than a year. A history of irregular periods before taking the combined hormonal contraceptive increases the chance of prolonged amenorrhoea.
- Metabolic effects: oestrogens alone increase protective plasma high-density lipoprotein (HDL) cholesterol, decrease low-density lipoprotein (LDL) cholesterol and increase plasma triglycerides (see also Ch. 48). When used in combination with progestogens in the second-generation combined hormonal contraceptive, HDL cholesterol is reduced. Oestrogens increase vascular prostacyclin and nitric oxide synthesis, inhibit platelet adhesion, and suppress smooth muscle cell proliferation. They have been shown to reduce cholesterol accumulation in the arterial walls of cholesterol-fed animals. Some progestogens such as norethisterone and medroxyprogesterone acetate may oppose the beneficial effects of oestrogens on the arterial wall. The third-generation combined hormonal contraceptives

containing gestodene and desogestrel increase plasma triglycerides but, unlike the progestogens in the second-generation pills, they increase HDL cholesterol. Although the latter could be advantageous, the benefit may be illusory, because there is little evidence that the second-generation combined hormonal contraceptive actually promotes atherosclerosis.

- Increased skin pigmentation can occur in some women who take oestrogens. The androgenic progestogens can sometimes cause or aggravate hirsutism and acne or produce weight gain. In women with hyperandrogenaemia (such as occurs with polycystic ovary syndrome), a third-generation combined hormonal contraceptive would be preferred, as gestodene and desogestrel have little androgenic activity.
- Effects on the liver are occasionally seen. Cholestatic jaundice can be produced by progestogens, and oestrogens increase the risk of gallstones.
- Drug interactions: drugs that alter the metabolism of oestrogen may cause a reduction in the efficacy of the combined hormonal contraceptive, which may result in breakthrough bleeding and contraceptive failure (see above).

NON-CONTRACEPTIVE USES OF STEROIDAL CONTRACEPTIVES

The combined hormonal contraceptive can be used:

- to reduce excessive blood loss from menorrhagia
- to reduce the pain of dysmenorrhoea
- to treat premenstrual tension
- to treat endometriosis
- to treat acne in women.

Menorrhagia

Excessive menstrual blood loss is a common gynaecological problem. Menstrual loss can be reduced to a variable extent by non-steroidal anti-inflammatory drugs (NSAIDs; Ch. 29), and numerous different NSAIDs have been used. They are taken only during the time of menstruation. The combined hormonal contraceptives and the progestogen-only contraceptives can also reduce excessive menstrual loss. For the progestogen-only contraceptive to be useful, it has to be taken for 3 weeks at a fairly high dose. A more effective way of giving the progestogen is from an IUCD, which reduces blood loss by up to 90%.

The antifibrinolytic agent tranexamic acid (Ch. 11) can also reduce blood loss by up to 50%. Its effect is rapid in onset and therapy is only required during the time of menstruation.

Dysmenorrhoea

Primary dysmenorrhoea (pain associated with menstruation) has an unknown aetiology; many explanations have been proposed, including uterine hyperactivity, excessive prostaglandin or leukotriene generation, and excessive production of vasopressin. Various NSAIDs (Ch. 29) have been used for the relief of dysmenorrhoea, with approximately 70% of women being relieved of their symptoms. However, there are differences in efficacy among the NSAIDs which are poorly understood and do not seem to be simply related to their analgesic or anti-inflammatory activity. NSAIDs with a licence for this indication in the UK include dexibuprofen, dexketoprofen, flurbiprofen, ibuprofen, indometacin, ketoprofen, mefenamic acid and naproxen.

The combined hormonal contraceptive and the progestogen-only contraceptive are effective in reducing symptoms of dysmenorrhoea. Small studies suggest that calcium channel blockers (Ch. 5) and β_2-adrenoceptor agonists (Ch. 12) have some beneficial effect.

Endometriosis

Endometriosis is the presence and proliferation of endometrial tissue outside the uterine cavity. It may arise from retrograde menstrual flow through the fallopian tubes. The main consequences are pelvic pain, dysmenorrhoea, dyspareunia and infertility. Treatment is either medical or surgical.

Medical treatment can be given to suppress ovarian activity and create a hypo-oestrogenic anovulatory state, and does not restore fertility. Symptoms often improve in pregnancy, and the combined hormonal contraceptive or a progestogen-only contraceptive are often effective. Alternative strategies include induction of a pseudo-postmenopausal state with the use of danazol (Ch. 46) or gonadotrophin-releasing hormone (GnRH) analogues (Ch. 43). Treatment is usually necessary for at least 6 months, but up to 50% of women have recurrence of painful symptoms in the 2 years after it is stopped.

If fertility is the major problem, then treatment involves surgery or in vitro fertilisation techniques (Ch. 43).

HORMONE REPLACEMENT THERAPY (HRT)

The menopausal transition from regular periods to amenorrhoea takes place over about 4 years, during which time the plasma oestrogen concentration falls markedly, with a rise in plasma FSH. After the menopause, the ovaries do not produce oestrogen or progesterone, but continue to produce testosterone. Some oestrogen is still produced by conversion of adrenal corticosteroids to oestradiol in peripheral adipose tissue. The consequences of oestrogen deficiency during and after the menopause include the following:

- symptoms such as vasomotor instability (hot flushes and night sweats), and altered sexual and urinary function. Vasomotor instability results from resetting of the hypothalamic temperature set-point so that it perceives that the body is warmer than it is. Vasodilation and sweating represent an attempt to disperse heat. The mechanism is uncertain but may be due to either reduced oestrogen or increased FSH leading to a reduction in noradrenergic or serotonergic neurotransmission in the hypothalamus. Loss of connective tissue in the vagina and trigone of the bladder, and a less acidic vaginal pH underlie many of the other problems. These include vaginal dryness, discomfort and itching,

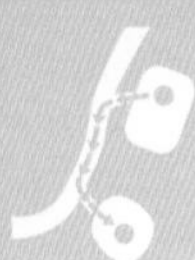

dyspareunia, and urinary urgency, frequency and incontinence. Other postmenopausal symptoms such as irritability and depression are less clearly related to oestrogen deficiency.

- Bone loss leading to osteoporosis (Ch. 42) and an increased susceptibility to fragility fracture occur after the menopause. The ERβ receptor is present in higher concentrations in developing cancellous bone (such as vertebrae), and the ERα receptor in developing cortical bone (such as the hip). Oestrogen deficiency increases bone turnover, with bone resorption increasing more than formation.
- Cardiovascular disease and cerebrovascular disease are more common. The cause is uncertain. Unfavourable changes in lipids may be part of the explanation, due to a reduced HDL_2 cholesterol subfraction and increased LDL cholesterol (Ch. 48). However, an independent effect of oestrogen in reducing plasma fibrinogen (a factor in thrombogenesis) may be more important. Oestrogen receptors are found on the cells of the arterial wall, and stimulation decreases arterial resistance and increases vessel compliance, which may also be relevant.

Treatment with oestrogens during the peri- and postmenopausal period is often advocated to try to reverse the effects of oestrogen deficiency, but recent evidence of both lack of efficacy and potential harm has limited their use (see benefits and risks below).

ORAL HORMONE REPLACEMENT THERAPY (HRT) AND OTHER DRUGS USED FOR POSTMENOPAUSAL CONDITIONS

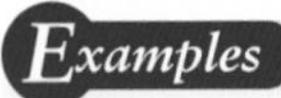

estradiol, raloxifene, tibolone

Oral oestrogens and progestogens

For HRT, oestrogens are given at much lower doses than are used for contraception. If oestrogen is given alone for more than a few weeks to a woman who has a uterus, then cystic hyperplasia of the endometrium can occur. Progestogen is given concurrently to avoid this, and is used for 12 days each calendar month or continuously if withdrawal bleeding is to be avoided. Oestrogen can be used alone if the woman has had a hysterectomy.

The majority of oral HRT preparations contain the natural estradiol as the oestrogen, although preparations with conjugated equine oestrogens are also available. Synthetic progestogens are used: dydrogesterone, medroxyprogesterone, norethisterone, levonorgestrel or drospirenone.

Oral oestrogen replacement will reduce the symptoms of postmenopausal oestrogen deficiency, although relief may take up to 3 months. Treatment for symptom relief probably should be given for at least 6 months to perimenopausal women, after which, withdrawal can be attempted to see if symptoms have spontaneously resolved.

Raloxifene

Raloxifene is a tissue-selective oestrogen receptor modulator which has oestrogenic effects on bone but anti-oestrogenic actions on breast and uterine receptors. It increases bone mineral density in postmenopausal osteoporosis; more details on raloxifene and osteoporosis are given in Chapter 42.

Pharmacokinetics

Raloxifene is rapidly absorbed and is metabolised by conjugation and excreted in bile; it has a long half-life (28 h).

Unwanted effects

- Headache
- Dizziness
- Nausea
- Rash
- Weight gain
- Increased risk of breast cancer, but less than with combined HRT.

Tibolone

Tibolone is a synthetic molecule with combined weak oestrogenic, progestogenic and androgenic properties. The global effects are predominantly oestrogenic, although in breast tissue it inhibits the enzyme responsible for activation of its metabolites, giving a low incidence of breast tenderness. In the endometrium it activates progesterone and androgen receptors, and the effects are mainly progestogenic, without stimulation of the endometrium or producing bleeding. Tibolone reduces postmenopausal symptoms and prevents postmenopausal bone loss. Vaginal bleeding can occur in women who still produce some endogenous oestrogen, and therefore tibolone is not usually given to women who are within 12 months of their last period.

Pharmacokinetics

Tibolone is a prodrug that is well absorbed from the gut and is metabolised in the liver to active metabolites (data on the half-life are not available).

Unwanted effects

- Hot flushes
- Leg cramps
- Venous thromboembolism.

VAGINAL OESTROGEN

Oestrogen cream (usually estradiol) or pessaries can be used to treat vaginal atrophy and dyspareunia and can relieve perimenopausal urinary symptoms such as frequency and dysuria. Considerable systemic absorption occurs with some formulations, and an oral progestogen may be needed to prevent endometrial hyperplasia. Creams or pessaries are used daily for 2–3 weeks initially and then applied twice weekly for as long as required.

SUBCUTANEOUS OESTROGEN IMPLANTS

Estradiol can be surgically implanted as pellets which release drug for up to 6 months. The major use for this option is when tolerance of oral oestrogen is poor, perhaps because of nausea. Oral progestogen must also be taken for 10–12 days each month if the woman has a uterus, and continued for up to 2 years after stopping oestrogen, to prevent vaginal bleeding from persistently high oestrogen levels.

TRANSDERMAL OESTROGEN WITH PROGESTOGEN

A variety of transdermal patches that deliver sex steroids are available. In some preparations, oestrogen alone is delivered by patches twice weekly for 2 weeks, followed by patches delivering oestrogen plus progestogen for 2 weeks. In other regimens, progestogen is taken orally for at least 12 days of the cycle while continuing with the patch-delivered oestrogen. Patches delivering continuous oestrogen plus progestogen (levonorgestrel or norethisterone) are also available. This route avoids first-pass metabolism so that a lower dose of progestogen can be used transdermally, which might reduce unwanted effects. Estradiol gels applied twice daily are also available and require co-administration of progestogen for 12 days per month in women with a uterus. It is recommended that patches are applied below the waistline, and not close to the breasts.

BENEFITS AND RISKS OF HORMONE REPLACEMENT THERAPY

The benefits and risks of oestrogen-based HRT are highly individual for the patient. For most women, it is recommended that HRT is reserved for short-term alleviation of menopausal symptoms. Any treatment should be reviewed at least annually. Tibolone (see above) or alternative approaches to the treatment of menopausal symptoms (see below) should be considered. Atrophic vaginitis may respond to a short course of topical oestrogen.

HRT reduces the risk of vertebral and non-vertebral osteoporotic fractures. However, because of the potential risks of treatment, HRT is not considered to be first-line treatment except for women with early natural or surgical menopause before the age of 45 years. It is not recommended that treatment should continue beyond age 50 years if osteoporosis is the main concern, because alternative approaches are more appropriate (Ch. 42).

UNWANTED EFFECTS OF HORMONE REPLACEMENT THERAPY

- Breakthrough bleeding can be troublesome, and regular withdrawal bleeds during the cycle are common unless continuous progestogen is used. These may be preceded by symptoms of premenstrual tension.
- Breast pain and abdominal or leg cramps.
- Nausea and vomiting.
- Headache, dizziness.
- Depression, irritability, loss of energy, and poor concentration due to progestogen.
- Transdermal delivery can cause contact sensitisation.
- Increased risk of venous thromboembolism, especially in the first year. The risk after 5 years of use is increased by about 40% for combined HRT (added risk is 4 cases per 1000 for combined HRT, and 1 case per 1000 for oestrogen-only HRT over 5 years if aged 50–59 years; the excess risk is more than doubled between 60 and 69 years). Limited evidence suggests that transdermal oestrogen replacement may not increase the risk of venous thromboembolism.
- Increased risk of stroke (excess risk is 1 case per 1000 for combined HRT and 2 cases per 1000 for oestrogen-only HRT over 5 years if aged 50–59 years; this excess risk is tripled between 60 and 69 years).
- HRT does not prevent coronary heart disease, and may increase the risk in the first year of treatment.
- Increased risk of breast cancer within 1–2 years of starting use, increasing further with duration of use. The excess risk is lost 5 years after stopping HRT. Taking combined HRT for 10 years leads to a 40% increase in the risk of developing breast cancer in women aged 50–64 years (excess 6 cases per 1000). Oestrogen-only HRT carries about one-quarter of this excess risk.
- The risk of endometrial cancer is increased by 160% over 10 years with oestrogen-only HRT (excess risk 5 cases per 1000).

ALTERNATIVE TREATMENTS FOR MENOPAUSAL SYMPTOMS

Oestrogens are by far the most effective treatment for menopausal symptoms. Vasomotor symptoms may be alleviated by the use of high doses of progestogens but unwanted effects are common. There is limited evidence for the use of antidepressants that modulate monoaminergic neurotransmission, such as selective serotonin reuptake inhibitors (SSRIs) and serotonin–noradrenaline reuptake inhibitors (SNRIs) (Ch. 22). The anticonvulsant gabapentin (Ch. 23) has also shown modest efficacy in treating hot flushes.

THE ONSET AND INDUCTION OF LABOUR

The aetiology of the induction of labour is still uncertain. (Fig. 45.3). The actual onset may be multifactorial in nature and it is probable that prostaglandins, oxytocin, progesterone, oestrogen and corticosteroids are among the agents involved. Our lack of knowledge about the mechanisms that underpin the onset of labour is directly reflected in our poor ability to prevent preterm labour, where at best we can delay parturition for short periods of time only (see below).

CORTICOTROPHIN-RELEASING HORMONE

The critical factor in the timing of birth in humans is development of the placenta, and particularly expression of the gene for corticotrophin-releasing hormone (CRH) by the placenta. In late pregnancy, placental CRH production increases exponentially and at the end of pregnancy the

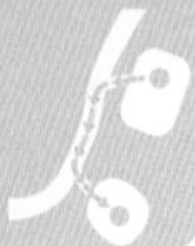

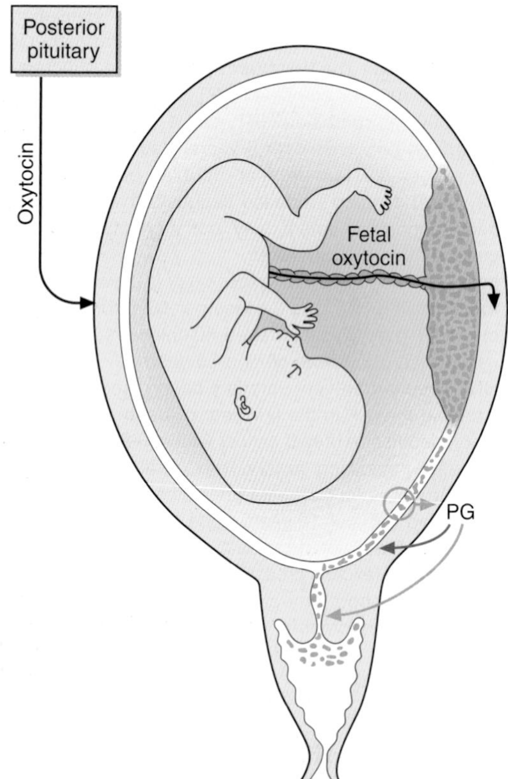

Fig. 45.3 **Induction of labour.** The mechanisms involved in the onset of labour in man are uncertain but it is likely to be multifactorial. Prostaglandin (PG) is synthesised by the amnion and the decidua and can act to stimulate the uterus and soften the cervix. Fetal and maternal oxytocin and prostaglandins may be involved in the processes of labour; their role in the *initiation* of labour is uncertain.

concentration of CRH-binding protein in plasma falls. The resulting increase in active CRH drives the hypothalamic–pituitary–adrenal axis to produce corticosteroids (Ch. 43). In the fetus, CRH and cortisol stimulate the fetal lung to produce surfactant protein A (Ch. 13), which enters amniotic fluid and then the amnion, where it stimulates synthesis of prostaglandin E_2 (PGE_2). In the mother, the formation of myometrial $PGF_{2\alpha}$ is also increased.

PROSTAGLANDINS

$PGF_{2\alpha}$ and PGE_2 have many actions that could contribute to labour. They are synthesised by the cells of the amnion and decidua. Uterine contraction sensitivity to prostaglandins is increased at term, when it is approximately 10-fold higher than in earlier pregnancy. The contractility of the uterus during labour commences at the utero-tubular junction and progresses through the body of the uterus to the cervix, thus promoting efficient labour. This type of synchronous contractile pattern, which does not occur in early pregnancy, is caused by prostaglandins and oestrogens promoting the synthesis of 'contraction-associated proteins' and increasing connectivity between myometrial cells. Gap junctions are specialised connections between the smooth muscle cells allowing excitatory impulses to pass between cells. The 'right type' of uterine contractions that result in efficient progress of labour can only occur in uterine muscle cells that are rich in gap junctions. The progesterone-dominated uterus has few gap junctions. Prostaglandins also increase the release of Ca^{2+} from intracellular stores in myometrial cells, which promotes muscle contraction.

PGE_2 softens the cervix, an essential prerequisite for the smooth passage of labour. Prostaglandins also increase the synthesis of oxytocin from the posterior pituitary.

OXYTOCIN

Oxytocin is a peptide produced by the posterior pituitary (Ch. 43). There is a marked increase in the expression of uterine oxytocin receptors from about 35 weeks of pregnancy onwards, so that oxytocin has a marked uterotonic action at term but is much less effective earlier in pregnancy. Oxytocin acts synergistically with prostaglandins to release Ca^{2+} from intracellular stores in the myometrial cells and promote muscle contraction. The oxytocin concentration in the maternal circulation does not increase until the second stage of labour.

SEX STEROID HORMONES

Oestrogens and progesterone both increase during pregnancy. Overall, the actions of oestradiol promote uterine contractility while progesterone decreases contractility.

- **Progesterone:** decreases gap junctions, diminishes uterine pacemaker activity and decreases the sensitivity of the uterus to oxytocin and prostaglandins. At the onset of labour there is reduced responsiveness of progesterone receptors which blocks the cellular action of the hormone.
- **Estradiol:** increases the number of uterine oxytocin receptors and increases oxytocin release from the posterior pituitary. It increases gap junctions, and fundal dominance of uterine contractility is increased by an effect on the functional pacemaker at the utero-tubular junction. Estradiol increases the synthesis of prostaglandins and increases the sensitivity of the uterus to their effects. Estradiol also has a softening effect on the cervix.

DRUGS USED FOR INDUCING LABOUR

Oxytocin and prostaglandins are the only drugs currently used to induce labour.

Oxytocin

Oxytocin is used for the induction of labour and to augment contractions in inadequate labour. It is given by slow intravenous infusion to induce labour. The concentration given depends upon the response: the aim is to produce regular coordinated contractions at intervals of approximately 1.5–2 min with complete relaxation between contractions. Oxytocin is an effective uterine stimulant in women at term, and labour will usually proceed well if the cervix is partially dilated and softened prior to its use. Inappropriately high concentrations of oxytocin can cause uterine hypertonus, in which the uterus does not relax between contractions, and fetal distress can occur. As labour progresses and the woman's 'endogenous' induction mechanisms come into play, the concentration of oxytocin may need to be reduced. Following delivery, oxytocin can also be useful to reduce postpartum haemorrhage (see below). Oxytocin, unlike prostaglandins, does not soften the cervix and is now often used after intravaginal prostaglandin (usually dinoprostone) has been given for this purpose (see below). Oxytocin in high doses has a weak antidiuretic activity as it is related to vasopressin (Ch. 43).

Dinoprostone

Dinoprostone (the name for exogenous PGE_2) causes contractions of both the non-pregnant and the pregnant uterus. The sensitivity of the uterus to prostaglandins is higher than to oxytocin prior to term. Like oxytocin, correct doses of prostaglandins can produce contractions that are indistinguishable from spontaneous labour, but prostaglandins have the advantage of softening the cervix. Thus, they can be used for induction of labour before term. Dinoprostone is given as vaginal tablets, pessaries or gels for induction of labour or for priming of the uterus prior to rupture of membranes and induction by oxytocin. In some women dinoprostone will result only in ripening of the cervix, whereas others will go into labour. Intravenous dinoprostone is now far less commonly used for the induction of labour.

Unwanted effects

- Gastrointestinal disturbances, particularly nausea, vomiting and diarrhoea
- Uterine hypertonus
- Flushing
- Bronchospasm.

INDUCTION OF ABORTION

Prostaglandin derivatives

Prostaglandins are widely used for the induction of abortion. In the second trimester, their use results in fewer complications than surgical abortion. Gemeprost (PGE_1 analogue), given as an intravaginal pessary, is used for the medical induction of late therapeutic abortion. Misoprostol (Ch. 33), given orally or vaginally, is also used for the induction of second trimester abortion. Mifepristone pretreatment (see below) is increasingly used before vaginal administration of a prostaglandin. Extra-amniotic dinoprostone is now rarely used for this indication. The mechanism of action of these drugs is to produce prolonged uterine contraction. Gemeprost is also given as a pessary to ripen and soften the cervix prior to early surgical abortion and together with mifepristone for early medical abortion (see below).

Mifepristone

Mechanism of action and uses

Mifepristone is a potent progesterone antagonist that binds to the progesterone receptor. It is given orally and sensitises the uterus to prostaglandin-induced contractions and softens the cervix. In early pregnancy and in later pregnancy up to 24 weeks' gestation, mifepristone is given as a single oral dose followed 36 h later by either oral gemeprost, or oral or vaginal misoprostol (Ch. 33). It can also be given alone to soften the cervix 36 h before surgical termination of early pregnancy. Mifepristone is also given orally following spontaneous fetal death in utero.

The softening effect on the uterine cervix can also be used for cervical ripening prior to the induction of labour at term, although there is little information on fetal outcome or maternal unwanted effects and it is not licensed in the UK for this purpose.

Pharmacokinetics

Mifepristone is well absorbed from the gut and is metabolised slowly in the liver by CYP3A4, generating three main metabolites, one of which retains pharmacological activity; the metabolites are largely excreted in bile and eliminated in faeces. Mifepristone has a long half-life (18 h).

Unwanted effects

- Nausea, vomiting
- Vaginal bleeding
- Uterine pain (that can be severe)
- Malaise, faintness, headache.

POSTPARTUM HAEMORRHAGE

Bleeding can arise after incomplete abortion, or after a normal delivery. In the latter situation, preventative treatment is routinely given to avoid excessive blood loss.

Ergometrine maleate

Ergometrine causes hypertonic contractions of the uterus and is therefore not used for induction of labour as it would result in fetal distress and poor progress in labour. The effect of hypertonus is to squeeze the uterine blood vessels after placental separation, thereby reducing blood loss; it also causes vasoconstriction through α-adrenoceptor stimulation (see ergotamine Ch. 26), which further limits haemorrhage.

Pharmacokinetics

Ergometrine is given intramuscularly, and works within 2–7 min. Elimination is by hepatic metabolism.

Unwanted effects

- Nausea, vomiting
- Headache, dizziness, tinnitus
- Abdominal or chest pain
- Peripheral vasoconstriction.

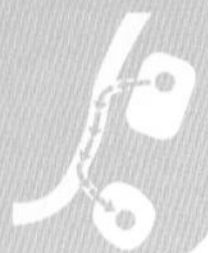

Management of postpartum haemorrhage

To minimise bleeding after delivery, ergometrine should be given together with oxytocin by intramuscular injection on delivery of the anterior shoulder. Following delivery of the baby, postpartum haemorrhage can also be reduced by increasing the concentrations of intravenous oxytocin being administered. This causes hypertonic contraction of the uterus and compresses intrauterine blood vessels. If bleeding continues, the prostaglandin carboprost (15-methyl $PGF_{2\alpha}$, a compound related to dinoprostone) is given by intramuscular injection.

MYOMETRIAL RELAXANTS (TOCOLYTICS) AND PRETERM LABOUR

Preterm birth is a delivery that occurs before 37 weeks of gestation, and affects more than 10% of pregnancies. It is possible that preterm labour is multifactorial. Factors that may contribute to preterm birth are excessive myometrial and fetal membrane overdistension (as may occur with multiple fetuses), early fetal endocrine activation, decidual haemorrhage, and intrauterine infection or inflammation.

Prematurity is the largest cause of neonatal morbidity and mortality, but relatively poor pharmacological tools are available currently to prevent it. Therapeutic strategies have concentrated on inhibition of myometrial contractions (tocolysis). Tocolytics have not been shown statistically to improve fetal morbidity or mortality, but they provide a limited time for treatment with corticosteroids to enhance lung maturation (Ch. 13), or for transfer of the mother to a specialist unit. Prophylactic treatment with antibacterials may improve outcome in particular at-risk groups but has not been widely adopted.

Atosiban

Mechanism of action

Atosiban is a peptide analogue of oxytocin and is an oxytocin receptor antagonist. It binds to the oxytocin receptors in the decidua and myometrium, and reduces the release of intracellular Ca^{2+}. Recent evidence suggests that the use of atosiban may be associated with a lower birth weight.

Pharmacokinetics

Atosiban is given by intravenous injection or infusion. It is metabolised to an active derivative, and has a very short half-life (about 15 min).

Unwanted effects

- Nausea, vomiting
- Headache, dizziness
- Tachycardia, hypotension
- Hyperglycaemia.

Beta$_2$-adrenoceptor agonists

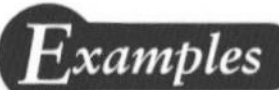

ritodrine, salbutamol, terbutaline

Beta$_2$-adrenoceptor agonists inhibit uterine contractility by increasing the intracellular concentration of cyclic adenosine monophosphate (cAMP). Ritodrine, salbutamol and terbutaline are used in the UK, and are given for up to 48 h following the start of preterm labour, after which the risks to the mother increase with no benefit to the fetus. They are used for uncomplicated premature labour between 24 and 33 weeks of gestation. β_2-adrenoceptor agonists can be administered intravenously or orally. Unwanted effects include nausea, vomiting, flushing, and maternal and fetal tachycardia with hypotension (see also Ch. 12).

Calcium channel blockers

Nifedipine (Ch. 5) is used orally and is as effective as other tocolytics, with fewer unwanted effects than β_2-adrenoceptor agonists. The use of nifedipine may improve fetal outcome.

Other agents for preterm labour

Magnesium sulphate has been widely used in the USA for treating women in preterm labour. Recent evidence indicates that it may be no better than placebo, and may be associated with worse fetal outcomes. Intravenous or transdermal glyceryl trinitrate (Ch. 5) may be effective through nitric oxide generation in smooth muscle, but is not widely used.

The NSAID indometacin (Ch. 29) can be successful for delaying delivery, but there are concerns about transient neonatal renal impairment and premature closure of the ductus arteriosus.

FURTHER READING

Boulvain M, Kelly A, Irion O (2008) Intracervical prostaglandins for induction of labour. *Cochrane Database Syst Rev* (1), CD006971

Davison S, Davis SR (2003) Hormone replacement therapy: current controversies. *Clin Endocrinol* 58, 249–261

Farquhar C (2007) Endometriosis. *BMJ* 334, 249–253

Franco V, Oparil F (2002) Hormone replacement therapy and hypertension. *Curr Opin Nephrol Hypertens* 11, 229–235

Grady D (2006) Management of the menopause. *N Engl J Med* 355, 2338–2347

Gruber CJ, Tschuggel W, Schneeberger C et al (2002) Production and actions of estrogens. *N Engl J Med* 346, 340–352

Hickey M, Davis SR, Sturdee DW (2005) Treatment of menopausal symptoms: what shall we do now? *Lancet* 366, 409–421

Kaunitz AM (2008) Hormonal contraception in women of older reproductive age. *N Engl J Med* 358, 1262–1270

Nelson HD, Humphrey LL, Nygren P et al (2002) Postmenopausal hormone replacement therapy. Scientific review. *JAMA* 288, 872–881

Norwitz ER, Robinson JN, Shallis JRG (1999) The control of labor. *N Engl J Med* 341, 660–666

Peterson HB, Curtis KM (2005) Long-acting methods of contraception. *N Engl J Med* 353, 2169–2175

Petitti DB (2003) Combination estrogen–progestin oral contraceptives. *N Engl J Med* 349, 1443–1450

Prentice A (1999) Medical management of menorrhagia. *BMJ* 319, 1343–1345

Riggs BL, Hartmann LC (2003) Selective estrogen-receptor modulators. Mechanisms of action and application to clinical practice. *N Engl J Med* 348, 618–629

Sanchez-Ramos L (2005) Induction of labor. *Obstet Gynecol Clin North Am* 32, 181–200

Simhan HN, Caritis SN (2007) Prevention of preterm delivery. *N Engl J Med* 357, 477–487

Stearns V, Ullmer L, Lopez JF et al (2002) Hot flushes. *Lancet* 360, 1851–1861

Stubblefield PG, Carr-Ellis S, Borgatta L (2004) Methods for induced abortion. *Obstet Gynecol* 104, 174–185

Westhoff C (2003) Emergency contraception. *N Engl J Med* 349, 1830–1835

SELF-ASSESSMENT

In questions 1–9, the first statements, in italics, are true. Are the accompanying statements also true?

1. *The mid-cycle surge in LH and FSH is essential for ovulation to occur.*
   a. Oestrogen has a negative feedback effect on LH and FSH secretion from the anterior pituitary throughout the follicular phase.
   b. The elevated level of progesterone in the secretory phase is under the control of gonadotrophins.
2. *Progesterone causes cervical mucus to be viscous and hostile to the passage of sperm. This is an important contraceptive action of the oral progestogen-only contraceptive.*
   a. The oral progestogen-only contraceptive inhibits ovulation in 90% of women.
   b. Both oestrogen and progesterone inhibit the motility of the fallopian tube, altering the rate of transport of sperm and the oocyte.
   c. The functioning corpus luteum is essential for the maintenance of pregnancy for about the first 6–8 weeks following implantation.
3. *The term 'second-generation' combined hormonal contraceptives refers to those that have low concentrations of ethinylestradiol and generally either levonorgestrel or norethisterone as the progestogenic component. The 'third-generation' combined hormonal contraceptives contain progestogens such as gestodene or desogestrel.*
   a. There is little to choose between the different progestogens in a combined hormonal contraceptive in terms of their androgenic activity.
   b. The oral combined hormonal contraceptive administered in a biphasic or triphasic pattern results in the overall administration of less oestrogen and progestogen.
   c. Plasma concentrations of administered ethinylestradiol are lower than anticipated because ethinylestradiol undergoes enterohepatic cycling.
   d. With the oral combined hormonal contraceptive or the progestogen-only contraceptive, effective protection may be lost if there is a delay of more than 3 h in taking the daily dose.
4. *The antibacterials rifampicin and ampicillin can lower the effective concentrations of ethinylestradiol in the plasma.* Antiepileptic drugs such as carbamazepine can reduce the plasma concentrations of oestrogens and progestogens.
5. *There is no significant increased risk of myocardial infarction irrespective of age in women who are non-smokers taking the combined hormonal contraceptive pill.*
   a. Mortality from venous thromboembolism in those who use the oral combined hormonal contraceptive is increased in women who smoke, particularly those over the age of 35 years.
   b. The second- and third-generation oral combined hormonal contraceptives can impair glucose tolerance.
6. *In women who have not had a hysterectomy, unopposed oestrogen treatment, such as HRT can result in endometrial hyperplasia and an increased risk of endometrial cancer.*
   a. Postmenopausal women taking continuous therapy containing both oestrogen and progestogens do not experience breakthrough bleeding.
   b. Oestrogens and progestogens can be given by skin patches to reduce the level of first-pass metabolism.
   c. Raloxifene is a selective oestrogen receptor modulating agent.
   d. Tibolone reduces bone loss in postmenopausal women.
7. *Unlike oxytocin, the prostaglandins have a softening effect on the cervix.*
   a. Oxytocin is preferred to prostaglandins for the induction of labour in a woman at 34 weeks' gestation.
   b. Progesterone increases the number of gap junctions in the uterus.
   c. Natural prostaglandins are produced from the posterior pituitary during labour.
8. *For the induction of abortion, mifepristone should be given 24–48 h before the administration of prostaglandins.*
   a. Prostaglandins given for the induction of labour do not produce hypertonic uterine activity.
   b. Ergometrine can be used for the induction of labour.

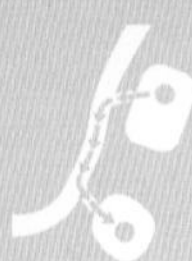

9. *NSAIDs are used in treating dysmenorrhoea.* The oral combined hormonal contraceptive is ineffective for relieving the symptoms of dysmenorrhoea.
10. You are discussing the benefits and drawbacks of oral contraception with a 35-year-old woman who smokes 40 cigarettes a day and, despite treatment, has not been able to stop smoking. Choose the one **most appropriate** option from the following.
    A. The oral combined hormonal contraceptive will be suitable for her contraception.
    B. The oral combined hormonal contraceptive increases the risk of endometrial cancer.
    C. The intrauterine contraceptive device has a higher failure rate than the oral combined hormonal contraceptive.
    D. The progestogen-only contraceptive will provide adequate contraception and does not increase the risk of venous thromboembolic disease.
    E. An injection of medroxyprogesterone acetate will give contraceptive protection for more than 6 months.
11. You are discussing with a medical student the drugs that are used during labour and abortion. Choose the one **incorrect** option from the following.
    A. Mifepristone acts to induce abortion and is an antagonist at progesterone receptors.
    B. PGE_2 is preferred to oxytocin for induction of labour at 35 weeks of gestation in a woman with intact membranes.
    C. Oxytocin has less potential than prostaglandins to cause uterine hypertonus.
    D. β_2-Adrenoceptor agonists are ineffective in reducing morbidity or mortality in children born preterm.
    E. Ergometrine reduces postpartum haemorrhage by acting on uterine blood vessel α_1-adrenoceptors to cause vasoconstriction.

ANSWERS

1. a. **False**. Until the middle to late part of the follicular phase, oestrogens do have a negative feedback effect, but at a level of approximately 200 pg mL^{-1} oestradiol, there is a switch to positive feedback and the mid-cycle LH and FSH surge results.
   b. **True**. Although the LH levels fall precipitously after the mid-cycle surge, they are high enough to support the secretion of progesterone.
2. a. **False**. The inhibition of ovulation is seen in between 25% and 40% of women with the progestogen-only contraceptive; other effects such as thickening of cervical mucus are responsible for its contraceptive action. In women given medroxyprogesterone acetate by injection, however, the percentage in whom inhibition of ovulation occurs is almost 100%.
   b. **False**. Progesterone inhibits the motility of the fallopian tube, whereas oestrogens have the opposite action. An imbalance of either may alter the rate of ovum transport and the chances of fertilisation and implantation.
   c. **True**. Removal of the corpus luteum before 6–8 weeks of pregnancy results in abortion, whereas after that time the placental production of sex steroids under the influence of HCG is sufficient to maintain the pregnancy.
3. a. **False**. Although the progestogens in the second-generation combined hormonal contraceptives have variable androgenic activity, the progestogens gestodene and desogestrel have weak or no androgenic activity.
   b. **False**. Although there are some small variations, overall the biphasic and triphasic patterns of application mimic more closely the steroidal changes in the menstrual cycle. However, they do not reduce the sex steroid load overall.
   c. **False**. The fact that ethinylestradiol undergoes enterohepatic cycling serves to maintain plasma concentrations.
   d. **False**. Although protection is reduced if there is a delay of more than 12 h in taking the combined hormonal contraceptive, with the progesterone-only contraceptive this can occur with a delay of only 3 h.
4. **True**. By inducing liver microsomal enzymes, the effective concentrations may be reduced as metabolism is enhanced.
5. a. **True**. The excess risk of thromboembolic disease in women taking the combined hormonal contraceptive is significantly greater in smokers who are over the age of 35 years.
   b. **True**. Moreover there is little evidence for any difference on carbohydrate metabolism between second-generation combined hormonal contraceptives containing progestogens such as levonorgestrel and the third-generation progestogens such as gestodene.
6. a. **False**. Breakthrough bleeding frequently occurs, particularly in the first 6 months of treatment.
   b. **True**. Both sex steroids undergo first-pass metabolism and this can be avoided by absorption through the skin.
   c. **True**. Raloxifene stimulates oestrogen receptors in bone and liver but not breast and reproductive tissue.
   d. **True**. Tibolone has weak oestrogenic and progestogenic activity and has been shown to reduce bone loss.
7. a. **False**. Oxytocin is less effective in earlier pregnancy compared with term. In this case it is probable that an intravaginal pessary of prostaglandin would be used, as this causes uterine contractility and also softens the cervix. This may be followed by oxytocin.
   b. **False**. Oestrogens increase the gap junctions in the uterus, thus facilitating the transmission of the uterine contractility from the fundal region through the body of the uterus. Progesterone prevents the action of oestrogens.
   c. **False**. The source of the prostaglandins during labour is the uterine amnion membranes and the decidua.
8. a. **False**. Uterine hypertonus can occur in some women with the administration of prostaglandins in doses that are inappropriate.
   b. **False**. Ergometrine is given alone or together with oxytocin at the time of delivery and produces hypertonic uterine activity and reduces postpartum haem-

orrhage. It should not be given for labour induction.

9. **False**. The reason is not known but the combined hormonal contraceptive does relieve dysmenorrhoea in some women.

10. Answer **D**.
   A. False. In a woman of 35 years of age who smokes, it has been shown that the combined oral contraceptive results in a significant increase in cardiovascular complications. It would therefore not be a good choice.
   B. False. The combined hormonal contraceptive reduces the risk of endometrial cancer.
   C. False. The IUCD is as effective as the combined hormonal contraceptive.
   D. True. The increase in risk of thromboembolic complications is related to the oestrogen content of the pill.
   E. False. Medroxyprogesterone acetate given intramuscularly is effective for 8–12 weeks.

11. Answer **C**.
   A. Correct. Mifepristone is a progesterone receptor antagonist; inhibition of the actions of progesterone results in abortion, although the precise mechanisms are uncertain.
   B. Correct. Guidelines advise that all women with intact membranes should be initially given intravaginal prostaglandins to soften the cervix prior to rupture of the membranes, and then given intravenous oxytocin if required.
   C. Incorrect. Both oxytocin and prostaglandins can cause uterine hypertonus and potentially fetal anoxia if given in inappropriate amounts.
   D. Correct. Although β_2-adrenoceptor agonists may delay labour for 48 h, overall they have not been shown to decrease morbidity or mortality in the preterm newborn child.
   E. Correct. It can also cause uterine hypertonus, reducing uterine blood loss postpartum.

Drugs acting on the female reproductive system

Drug	Half-life (h) and kinetics	Comments
Oestrogens		
Components of oral contraceptives and for HRT; all compounds are lipid-soluble and rapidly absorbed after oral dosage; other uses are specified		
Conjugated oestrogen (equine)	– [M] Components are absorbed both intact and after hydrolysis; excreted as sulphate conjugates	Given as sulphate conjugates of >10 equine oestrogens; used as a component of oral HRT
Estradiol	1–2 [M] Rapidly absorbed and metabolised by the liver during absorption to estrone and estriol, the major circulating forms in the serum, by 17β-hydroxysteroid dehydrogenase; estrone undergoes P450 oxidation; estriol is conjugated and excreted	
Estradiol valerate	– [M] Assumed to be a prodrug for estradiol	
Ethinylestradiol	8–24 [M] Oral bioavailability is 83%; undergoes both oxidation and direct conjugation with glucuronic acid and sulphate	Component of oral combined hormonal contraceptive; has been replaced by other oestrogens for the treatment of menopausal symptoms; limited use for the management of hereditary haemorrhagic telangiectasia
Mestranol	8–24 [M] More than 50% is converted to ethinylestradiol, in part during first-pass metabolism	
Progestogens		
Components of oral contraceptives and for HRT; other uses are specified		
Desogestrel	30 [M] Undergoes P450-mediated oxidation in gut wall and liver to 3-keto-desogestrel, the active metabolite responsible for the pharmacological actions	Component of oral hormonal contraceptives; termed a *third-generation progestogen*
Drospirenone	36–42 [M] Oral bioavailability is about 80%; oxidised in the liver to inactive metabolites that are conjugated and eliminated in urine and faeces	Component of oral hormonal contraceptives; termed a *third-generation progestogen*

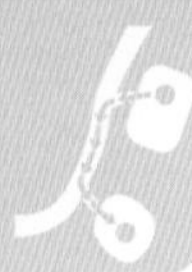

Drugs acting on the female reproductive system

Drug	Half-life (h) and kinetics	Comments
Dydrogesterone	5–7 [M] Metabolised by reduction to 20-dihydrodydrogesterone which retains progestogenic activity and has a half-life of 14 h	Progesterone analogue used for the treatment of endometriosis, infertility, recurrent miscarriage, premenstrual syndrome, amenorrhoea and dysmenorrhoea
Etonogestrel	29 [M] Metabolised by CYP3A4; activity of metabolites is not known	Etonogestrel-releasing implant can be inserted subdermally to give prolonged contraception
Etynodiol (ethynodiol)	5–14 (as norethindrone) [M] Rapidly absorbed and undergoes complete hepatic first-pass metabolism; metabolised to norethindrone, the active metabolite responsible for its actions	Used in progestogen-only oral contraceptives
Gestodene	18 [M] Metabolised by oxidation plus reduction reactions; metabolism by CYP3A4 results in irreversible inhibition of the enzyme	Component of oral hormonal contraceptives; termed a *third-generation progestogen*
Levonorgestrel	8–30 [M] Bioavailability is 100%; undergoes oxidation followed by conjugation plus some reduction	Component of oral combined hormonal contraceptive; effective emergency contraception if used within 72 h of unprotected intercourse; also present in an intrauterine device that is used for contraception and for primary menorrhagia
Medroxyprogesterone acetate	30 days [M] Undergoes oxidation and reduction reactions to give 26 essentially inactive metabolites	A long-acting progestogen; given as an aqueous suspension by deep intramuscular injection
Norelgestromin	? [M] Use of a transdermal patch gives sustained blood levels	Progestogen: used as a once-weekly transdermal patch, that also contains ethinylestradiol; applied for 3 weeks in every 4
Norethisterone	5–12 [M] Major routes of metabolism are reduction of unsaturated A ring and ketone group; the metabolites are eliminated in urine and via the bile into faeces	Testosterone analogue used for the treatment of endometriosis, premenstrual syndrome, dysmenorrhoea and postponement of menstruation; component of oral hormonal contraceptives
Norethisterone acetate	10 (NEth) [M] Hydrolysed to norethisterone (NEth)	Component of oral hormonal contraceptives
Norethisterone enantate	10 (NEth) [M] Prodrug of norethisterone (NEth) which is formed on hydrolysis	A long-acting progestogen; given as an oil solution by very slow deep intramuscular injection
Norgestimate	8–30 (metabolites) [M] A prodrug that is converted to active metabolites including 17-deacetyl norgestimate (norelgestromin) and levonorgestrel	Component of oral hormonal contraceptives; a prodrug
Norgestrel	20 [M] Undergoes hepatic metabolism	Component of oral hormonal contraceptives
Progesterone	5–20 min [M] Metabolised in the liver to pregnanediol and conjugated with glucuronic acid	Given as rectal or vaginal pessaries for the treatment of infertility, premenstrual syndrome and postnatal depression, or by injection for the treatment of dysmenorrhoea

Drugs acting on the female reproductive system

Drug	Half-life (h) and kinetics	Comments
Drugs used primarily for endometriosis		
Other uses are specified		
Danazol	4–5 [M] Metabolised by oxidation in the liver	Anti-gonadotrophic drug with androgenic, anti-oestrogenic and anti-progestogenic effects; anti-gonadotrophic effects are due to parent drug; also used for severe pain in benign fibrocystic breast disease and hereditary angioedema; synthetic steroid; given orally
Gestrinone	27 [M] Oxidised to less active products, which are excreted as conjugates	Actions are similar to danazol; given orally
Gonadorelin	4 min [M + R] The half-life probably reflects tissue distribution and binding at therapeutic doses rather than excretion and metabolism; see Ch. 43	Gonadotrophin-releasing hormone (Ch. 43); complex peptide given by intravenous injection for assessment of pituitary function, but of questionable value
Gonadorelin analogues		
Produce downregulation of gonadotrophin-releasing hormone receptors and thereby reduce the release of gonadotrophins; used for endometriosis, infertility, and before intrauterine surgery; other uses are specified		
Buserelin	1–1.5 [M + R] Metabolism plus some excreted in urine	Used for prostate cancer (see Ch. 52); complex peptide; given nasally for endometriosis and by subcutaneous injection
Goserelin	4 [M] Metabolised by cell peptidases	Used for prostate cancer and early and advanced breast cancer (see Ch. 52); complex peptide; given by subcutaneous implant
Leuprorelin acetate	3 [M] Metabolised by cell peptidases	Used for prostate cancer (see Ch. 52); complex peptide; given by subcutaneous or intramuscular injection
Nafarelin	3–4 [M] Slow hydrolysis; inactive metabolites have long half-lives (85 h)	Used for endometriosis; given as a nasal spray
Triptorelin	3 [M] Metabolism and routes of elimination are not known	Used for prostate cancer (see Ch. 52); given by intramuscular injection
Drugs used for menopausal symptoms and/or osteoporosis		
Given orally		
Raloxifene	28 [M] Rapidly absorbed; undergoes extensive first-pass conjugation with glucuronic acid and enterohepatic cycling	Used in the treatment of postmenopausal osteoporosis (Ch. 42)
Tibolone	? [M] Rapidly and extensively metabolised by reduction of 3-keto group, and isomerisation to three active metabolites, two of which have oestrogenic activity and half-lives of about 7 h	Used for the short-term treatment and prevention of menopausal vasomotor symptoms and postmenopausal osteoporosis; shows oestrogenic, progestogenic and weak androgenic activities

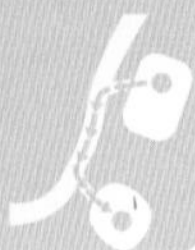

Drugs acting on the female reproductive system

Drug	Half-life (h) and kinetics	Comments
Anti-oestrogens		
Induce gonadotrophin release		
Clomifene	5 days [M] Z-isomer is eliminated more slowly and is detectable in plasma 1 month after treatment; see Ch. 43	Used for the treatment of female infertility associated with oligomenorrhoea or secondary amenorrhoea; exists as two isomers of which the Z (cis) is active and the E (trans) is inactive; given orally
Tamoxifen	7 days [M] High bioavailability; oxidised by CYP2C and CYP3A isoenzymes	Main use is in breast cancer – see Ch. 52
Drugs used to treat mastalgia		
Bromocriptine	–	See Chs 24 and 43
Danazol	–	See above
Tamoxifen	–	See Ch. 52
Prostaglandins, oxytocics and drugs used to reduce postpartum haemorrhage		
Carbetocin	40 min [M] Routes of metabolism have not been defined	Used for uterine atony and postpartum haemorrhage after caesarean section; given by intravenous injection
Carboprost	8 min [M] Metabolised slowly compared with prostaglandin $F_{2\alpha}$	15-Methyl derivative of prostaglandin $F_{2\alpha}$; used for postpartum haemorrhage due to uterine atony; given by deep intramuscular injection
Dinoprostone (PGE_2)	30 s [M] Metabolised by dehydrogenation	Used for the induction of labour; given intravaginally (or rarely by intravenous injection)
Ergometrine (ergonovine)	2 [M] Eliminated by hepatic metabolism	Used to prevent and treat postpartum haemorrhage; given by intramuscular injection
Gemeprost	? [M] Systemic half-life not known; very rapidly hydrolysed (within minutes) and subsequently oxidised	Used to soften the cervix in labour induction and to induce abortion; given intravaginally
Oxytocin	2–10 min [M] Rapid metabolism via reduction of the intramolecular disulphide bond followed by peptidase hydrolysis	Used for the induction of labour; given by slow intravenous injection or infusion
Drugs used for effects on ductus arteriosus		
Alprostadil (PGE_1)	30 s [M] Metabolised by dehydrogenation	Used to maintain patency of the ductus arteriosus in neonates with congenital heart defects; given as an intravenous infusion
Indometacin	3–5 [M] Metabolised by conjugation and oxidation (see Ch. 29)	Used to close the ductus arteriosus in premature babies; given by intravenous injection
Drugs used primarily for therapeutic abortions		
Gemeprost (PGE_1 analogue)	? [M] Peak plasma levels occur at 2–3 h and remain detectable until about 8 h; predicted to be eliminated by metabolism	Used for the medical induction of late therapeutic abortion; given as an intravaginal pessary
Mifepristone	18 [M + B] Metabolised by CYP3A4-mediated demethylation and hydroxylation; long half-life due in part to enterohepatic cycling	Given orally or vaginally prior to therapeutic abortion to sensitise the uterus to the actions of prostaglandins

Drugs acting on the female reproductive system

Drug	Half-life (h) and kinetics	Comments
Misoprostol	? [M] Rapidly and extensively absorbed by either route; eliminated in urine as metabolites	Used for the induction of second trimester abortion; given orally or vaginally
Myometrial relaxant drugs		
Atosiban	0.25 [M] Metabolised to an active derivative	An oxytocin receptor antagonist used for the inhibition of uncomplicated premature labour between 24 and 33 weeks of gestation; given by intravenous injection or infusion
Nifedipine	2–4 [M] Oral bioavailability is about 40% owing to first-pass metabolism by CYP3A4 in gut wall and liver	A calcium channel blocker (see Ch. 5); given orally
Ritodrine	15–20 [M] Conjugated with sulphate and glucuronic acid	β_2-Adrenoceptor agonist used for the inhibition of uncomplicated premature labour between 24 and 33 weeks of gestation; given orally or by intravenous infusion
Salbutamol	3–5 [M + R] Eliminated in urine as the sulphate conjugate	β_2-Adrenoceptor agonist used for the inhibition of uncomplicated premature labour between 24 and 33 weeks of gestation; given by intravenous infusion and then orally
Terbutaline	14–18 [M + R] (see Ch. 12)	β_2-Adrenoceptor agonist used for the inhibition of uncomplicated premature labour between 24 and 33 weeks of gestation; given orally or by subcutaneous or intravenous infusion

[B], biliary excretion; [M], metabolism; [R], renal excretion.
Some oestrogens (diethylstilbestrol and ethinylestradiol), progestogens (gestonorone, medroxyprogesterone, megestrol and norethisterone) and oestrogen receptor antagonists (tamoxifen and toremifene) are used for the treatment of malignant disease – see Chapter 52.

46 Androgens and anabolic steroids

ANDROGENS

Naturally occurring androgens are 19-carbon steroid hormones that are synthesised in the adrenal cortex and gonads (see Fig. 44.2). They have characteristic actions on the reproductive tract and other tissues as well as an anabolic effect on metabolism. A number of synthetic androgenic steroids have been developed. The term 'anabolic steroid' is used when the predominant action of the compound is anabolic rather than reproductive. Although there are a few medical uses for anabolic steroids, they have achieved notoriety because of their abuse by athletes to enhance muscle development.

Testosterone is secreted by the Leydig cells of the testis, and its synthesis and release are stimulated by the gonadotrophin luteinising hormone (Ch. 43). Androgens are also released from the adrenal cortex, in response to stimulation by adrenocorticotrophic hormone (ACTH); these are mainly dehydroepiandrosterone and androstenedione (see Fig. 44.2).

The cellular mechanism of action of steroid hormones is discussed in Chapters 1 and 44. Androgens act mainly through genomic effects on protein synthesis via the cytoplasmic androgen receptor, although rapid-onset non-genomic actions have also been described. The latter may be mediated by cell surface receptors; an example of a non-genomic action of testosterone is vasodilation through direct effects on Ca^{2+} channels.

MALE SEX HORMONES

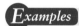

mesterolone (methyltestosterone), testosterone

Actions of testosterone

The actions of testosterone are in part due to its metabolite dihydrotestosterone (DHT). This is produced from testosterone in the prostate, skin and reproductive tissues by the action of the enzyme 5α-reductase (Fig. 44.2). Dihydrotestosterone has a higher affinity than testosterone for the androgen receptor. Actions of androgens include the following:

- sexual differentiation in the fetus.
- sexual development of the male testis, penis, epididymis, seminal vesicles and prostate at puberty, and maintenance of these tissues in adults.
- spermatogenesis in adults.
- stimulation and maintenance of sexual function and behaviour.
- metabolic actions. Testosterone is a powerful anabolic agent producing a positive nitrogen balance with an increase in the bulk of tissues such as muscle and bone. In the skin, sebum production is increased, which can provoke acne. Growth of axillary, pubic, facial and chest hair is stimulated. In the liver, testosterone increases the synthesis of several proteins, including clotting factors, but decreases high-density lipoprotein (HDL) synthesis (Ch. 48). Testosterone also induces several liver enzymes, including steroid hydroxylases.
- haematological actions. Testosterone stimulates the production of erythropoietin by the kidneys, leading to higher haemoglobin concentrations in men than in women.

Pharmacokinetics

- Oral preparations. Testosterone is well absorbed from the gut but is almost completely degraded by first-pass metabolism in the gut wall and liver. Oral absorption can be enhanced by esterification of testosterone to create hydrophobic compounds, such as testosterone undecanoate, which are absorbed via lacteals into the lymphatic system, thus avoiding hepatic metabolism. Mesterolone is a testosterone derivative that has a greater oral bioavailability than testosterone.

- Depot injection. The most popular form of therapy for hypogonadism in men is an intramuscular injection of a testosterone ester, usually in oily solution, given at intervals from 2–3 weeks up to 10–14 weeks depending on the formulation. Testosterone is absorbed gradually after ester hydrolysis at the site of injection. Examples include testosterone enantate, isocaproate, propionate, phenylpropionate and undecanoate.
- Transdermal delivery. A transdermal delivery patch containing testosterone can be used to treat hypogonadism. It is usually applied to the back, abdomen, upper arm or thigh, rotating the site daily to avoid skin irritation. Testosterone gel is an alternative way to deliver the drug transdermally.
- Buccal delivery. A buccal tablet which softens to a gel and adheres to the mucosa has recently been introduced for transmucosal delivery and gives sustained slow release of testosterone, and avoids hepatic first-pass metabolism.
- Subcutaneous implant. A pellet of pure crystalline testosterone provides a reservoir for gradual absorption of testosterone into the systemic circulation for 4–5 months. A minor surgical procedure is necessary, and therefore this method of delivery is rarely used.

Circulating androgens are bound largely to a specific transport protein, sex hormone-binding globulin (SHBG), which has a greater affinity for androgens than for oestrogen. Testosterone is metabolised in the liver to androstenedione, and then to inactive compounds. Some testosterone undergoes conversion in specific organs by 5α-reductase to dihydrotestosterone, and a small amount undergoes aromatisation to oestrogenic derivatives. Mesterolone is not metabolised to oestrogenic compounds. The half-lives of testosterone and methyltestosterone are 2–4 h.

Unwanted effects

- In hypogonadal adolescents, initial nitrogen retention and a spurt in linear growth is followed by premature epiphyseal closure and short stature. A short course can be used for the treatment of delayed puberty without inducing epiphyseal closure.
- Headache.
- Anxiety, depression.
- Nausea, gastrointestinal bleeding.
- Sodium retention with oedema and hypertension.
- Hirsutism, male-pattern baldness, acne; virilisation occurs in women given testosterone.
- Conversion to oestrogens by aromatase can produce gynaecomastia (see Fig. 44.2). This is less likely to occur with mesterolone.
- Suppression of gonadotrophin release with diminished testicular size and reduced spermatogenesis. Hypogonadal men will not regain fertility while taking androgens.
- Cholestatic jaundice. Liver tumours are a rare complication.

Clinical uses of testosterone

- The main clinical use is as hormone replacement therapy for primary hypogonadism in adult males.
- It can be used briefly in constitutionally delayed puberty, even in the absence of hypogonadism.
- Androgens are occasionally beneficial for promoting erythropoiesis in some forms of aplastic anaemia.

DANAZOL

Mechanism of action

Danazol is an androgen derivative described as an 'impeded' androgen. It is weakly androgenic on peripheral tissues; It has no oestrogenic activity as, unlike testosterone, it is not converted into an oestrogen by aromatases. Indeed, its main property is feedback inhibition of gonadotrophin and gonadotrophin-releasing hormone secretion. It therefore has anti-oestrogenic and anti-progestogenic actions.

Pharmacokinetics

Danazol is well absorbed orally, metabolised in the liver and has a short half-life (3 h).

Unwanted effects

- Nausea, epigastric pain
- Acne, hirsutism, oedema, hair loss or deepening of voice, due to androgenic effects
- Depression, anxiety
- Dizziness, headache
- Vaginal dryness, reduction in breast size, changes in libido, amenorrhoea, hot flushes.

Clinical uses of danazol

- Treatment of endometriosis (Ch. 45)
- Treatment of menorrhagia (Ch. 45)
- Management of gynaecomastia (Ch. 45)
- Long-term management of hereditary angioedema.

ANABOLIC STEROIDS

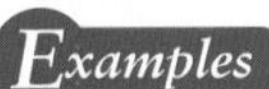

nandrolone, oxymetholone

Anabolic steroids are most frequently encountered as drugs of abuse to improve athletic performance. In medical practice, there are few indications for these compounds, and there is little evidence for efficacy in many conditions where their use has been advocated.

Pharmacokinetics

Nandrolone is given as a decanoate ester depot formulation by intramuscular injection every 3 weeks.

Unwanted effects

Androgenic effects may be troublesome in women.

Clinical uses

- Promotion of erythropoiesis in aplastic anaemias
- Itching associated with chronic biliary obstruction in palliative care.

Abuse of anabolic steroids

The ability of androgens to promote an increase in muscle mass has led to their abuse to improve physical performance by athletes, weightlifters and bodybuilders. Often, several different androgens are used for prolonged periods, perhaps with a brief 'drug-free' period. Abused compounds include testosterone, nandrolone and oxymetholone and many that are licensed only for veterinary use. The consequences of abuse include:

- weight gain from muscle hypertrophy and fluid retention
- acne in adolescent and young men
- decreased testicular size and reduced sperm count
- hepatotoxicity with cholestasis, hepatitis or, occasionally, hepatocellular tumours
- atherogenic changes in the plasma lipids with a rise in plasma LDL cholesterol and a fall in HDL cholesterol (Ch. 48); these changes may predispose to premature vascular disease
- psychological disturbance, including changes in libido, increased aggression, and psychotic symptoms.

ANTI-ANDROGENS

BICALUTAMIDE AND FLUTAMIDE

Mechanism of action

Bicalutamide and flutamide are non-steroidal, relatively pure anti-androgens. They may inhibit the dissociation of androgen receptors from heat shock protein in the cell cytoplasm, and prevent their translocation to the site of action in the nucleus.

Pharmacokinetics

Bicalutamide and flutamide are well absorbed orally, and are metabolised in the liver. Bicalutamide has a very long half-life of 7–10 days, while that of flutamide is 8 h. The major metabolite of flutamide, 2-hydroxyflutamide, is more active than the parent compound and also has a short half-life.

Unwanted effects

- Anti-androgenic effects, for example gynaecomastia
- Gastrointestinal upset
- Insomnia.

CYPROTERONE ACETATE

Mechanism of action

Cyproterone acetate, a 21-carbon steroid, is a progestogen and a weak glucocorticoid (Ch. 44). Its progestational activity produces feedback inhibition of gonadotrophin secretion (Ch. 45). At high doses, cyproterone is an anti-androgen, which inhibits androgen binding to its receptors.

Pharmacokinetics

Cyproterone acetate is well absorbed orally, metabolised in the liver, and has a very long half-life of 2 days.

Unwanted effects

- Anti-androgenic effects, for example gynaecomastia
- Inhibition of spermatogenesis
- Reduction in libido and potency in males
- Hepatotoxicity with long-term use, causing hepatitis and, occasionally, hepatic failure.

CLINICAL USES OF ANTI-ANDROGENS

- The main use of anti-androgens is in the treatment of carcinoma of the prostate (Ch. 52), usually in conjunction with a gonadorelin analogue (Ch. 43).
- Cyproterone acetate is used in male sexual offenders as 'chemical castration'.
- Cyproterone acetate can be given for manifestations of hyper-androgenisation in females, such as acne and hirsutism, in conjunction with ethinylestradiol in an oral combined hormonal contraceptive (Ch. 45).

5α-REDUCTASE INHIBITORS

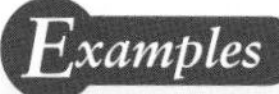

dutasteride, finasteride

Mechanism of action and effects

Dutasteride and finasteride reduce the formation of androgens rather than inhibiting androgen receptors.

5α-Reductase is an enzyme associated with androgen-dependent target cells. It is responsible for the conversion of testosterone to dihydrotestosterone, which is the hormone responsible for prostatic growth (Fig. 44.2). In the adult male, finasteride and dutasteride can produce regression of benign prostatic hypertrophy and improve the symptoms of prostatism (Ch. 15).

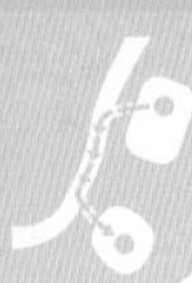

FURTHER READING

Basaria S, Wahlstrom JT, Dobs AS (2001) Anabolic-androgenic steroid therapy in the treatment of chronic diseases. *J Clin Endocrinol Metab* 86, 5108–5117

Conway AJ, Handelsman DJ, Lording DW et al (2000) Use, misuse and abuse of androgens. *Med J Aust* 172, 220–224

Di Luigi L, Romanelli F, Lenzi A (2005) Androgenic-anabolic steroids abuse in males. *J Endocrinol Invest* 28(suppl 3), 81–84

Jones TH (2007) Testosterone replacement therapy. *Br J Hosp Med* 68, 547–553

Kazi M, Geraci SA, Koch CA (2007) Considerations for the diagnosis and treatment of testosterone deficiency in elderly men. *Am J Med* 120, 835–840

Rhoden EL, Morgentaler A (2004) Risks of testosterone-replacement therapy and recommendations for monitoring. *N Engl J Med* 350, 482–492

Schneider HPG (2003) Androgens and antiandrogens. *Ann NY Acad Sci* 997, 292–306

SELF-ASSESSMENT

In questions 1 and 2, the first statement, in italics, is true. Are the accompanying statements also true?

1. *Mature men with androgen deficiency may have decreased libido, impotence, reduced muscle mass and reduced body hair.*
   a. Testosterone cannot be given orally.
   b. Testosterone alone cannot stimulate spermatogenesis.
   c. Nandrolone causes less virilisation in women than testosterone.
2. *The anti-androgen cyproterone acetate is used as an adjunct to the treatment of prostate cancer and hirsutism.* Anti-androgens can cause gynaecomastia.
3. Regarding drugs that affect androgenic and anabolic activities, choose the one **most appropriate** option from the following.
   A. 5α-Reductase inactivates dihydrotestosterone.
   B. Cyproterone acetate promotes spermatogenesis.
   C. Nandrolone reduces muscle mass.
   D. Danazol is used in the treatment of endometriosis.
   E. Testosterone has marked anti-anabolic activity.

ANSWERS

1. a. **True**. Testosterone is well absorbed orally but undergoes very extensive first-pass metabolism to inactive metabolites.
   b. **True**. Other treatments are required, including the administration of HCG and other gonadotrophins.
   c. **True**. Nandrolone has fewer androgenic effects than testosterone, but has many other unwanted effects.
2. **True**.
3. Answer **D**.
   A. False. 5α-Reductase converts testosterone to the active dihydrotestosterone.
   B. False. Cyproterone is an anti-androgen; it inhibits spermatogenesis and is used as a form of chemical castration.
   C. False. Nandrolone is an androgen and promotes an increase in muscle mass.
   D. True. Danazol has anti-androgen, anti-oestrogen and anti-progesterone activity and is used in the treatment of endometriosis.
   E. False. Testosterone is markedly anabolic, increasing turnover and growth in many tissues and cells.

Drugs acting on the male reproductive system and anabolic agents

Drug	Half-life and kinetics	Comment
Androgens		
Danazol	See Ch. 45	Inhibits pituitary gonadotrophins; clinically used for endometriosis (see Ch. 45)
Mesterolone (methyltestosterone)	3 h [M] Oral bioavailability is 50%; eliminated as glucuronide and sulphate conjugates	Used for androgen deficiency and male infertility associated with hypogonadism; given orally
Testosterone and esters	2–4 h [M] Low oral bioavailability due to first-pass metabolism; very rapidly cleared from blood; the different dosage methods act as modified-release' preparations that maintain blood testosterone concentrations despite its rapid elimination	Used for androgen deficiency and breast cancer in women; given orally (as undecanoate), by intramuscular injection (as enantate or propionate), as an implant (as testosterone) or as patches (as testosterone); testosterone per se is inactive orally

Drugs acting on the male reproductive system and anabolic agents

Drug	Half-life and kinetics	Comment
Anabolic steroids		
Nandrolone decanoate	5–17 days [M] (from injection) The in vivo half-life is dependent on release from the depot injection, since the half-life for hydrolysis and the elimination of nandrolone from the circulation is only 4 h	Not used for effects on male reproductive system; used for aplastic anaemia, and has been used for osteoporosis in postmenopausal women (but is not advocated for this purpose); given as deep intramuscular injection (modified release – see testosterone)
Oxymetholone		Given for 3–6 months for aplastic anaemia (see Ch. 47); given orally
Gonadorelin analogues		
Given for advanced prostate cancer (see Ch. 52), and for actions on the female reproductive system (see Ch. 45)		
Buserelin	(see Ch. 45)	Given by subcutaneous injection followed by intranasal dosage
Goserelin	(see Ch. 45)	Given by subcutaneous implant
Leuprorelin acetate	(see Ch. 45)	Given by subcutaneous or intramuscular injection
Triptorelin	(see Ch. 45)	Given by subcutaneous or intramuscular injection
Anti-androgens		
Bicalutamide	7–10 days[M] Metabolised by oxidation and conjugation, with the metabolites excreted in urine and bile	Used for advanced prostate cancer; given orally
Cyproterone acetate	2 days [M] Hydrolysed and conjugated with glucuronic acid and sulphate; metabolites eliminated in urine and bile	Used as an adjunct for prostate cancer, for hirsutism and acne in women, and for severe hypersexuality and sexual deviation in men; given orally
Flutamide	8 h [M] Essentially complete oral bioavailability; rapid oxidation in the liver to an active hydroxy metabolite	Used for advanced prostate cancer; acts by inhibition of the uptake and/or nuclear binding of testosterone and dihydrotestosterone by prostatic tissue; given orally
5α-Reductase inhibitors		
Inhibit 5α-reductase, the enzyme which converts testosterone to 5α-dihydrotestosterone (DHT), the primary androgen that stimulates the development of prostatic tissue		
Dutasteride	5 weeks [M] Oral bioavailability about 60%; metabolised by CYP3A4 to largely inactive products; long half-life results in slow accumulation to steady state (by about 6 months)	Used for benign prostatic hyperplasia; selective inhibitor of type I and type II 5α-reductase; given orally
Finasteride	5–6 h [M] Metabolised by hepatic oxidation	Used for benign prostatic hyperplasia and male-pattern baldness in men; selective inhibitor of type II 5α-reductase; given orally

[M], metabolism.

47 Anaemia and haematopoietic colony-stimulating factors

ANAEMIA

The definition of anaemia is rather arbitrary, and the absolute normal ranges for the haemoglobin concentration in blood vary among laboratories. In adults, anaemia equates to a blood concentration of haemoglobin in males below about 135 g L^{-1} (normal is about 154 g L^{-1}) or in females below about 115 g L^{-1} (normal is about 135 g L^{-1}). Many individuals, however, have concentrations below these arbitrary values without apparent detriment. Lower concentrations can be normal in children. Anaemia can cause many symptoms, including shortness of breath and fatigue. There are many causes of anaemia (Box 47.1).

Anaemias are classified by red cell size and haemoglobin content (Box 47.2). There are three key dietary factors that are required for normal red cell synthesis, referred to as haematinics:

- iron
- folic acid
- vitamin B_{12}.

IRON

Dietary iron is absorbed from the duodenum and upper jejunum. In an omnivorous diet, most iron is absorbed from meat, in which it is present as haem. Haem is the ferrous form of iron (Fe^{2+}) complexed with a porphyrin ring. Haem is readily absorbed from the gut, but non-haem iron in a vegetarian diet, which is mainly in the ferric state (Fe^{3+}), is inefficiently absorbed. Absorption of Fe^{3+} is facilitated by several factors:

- gastric acid, which increases its solubility.
- conversion to ferrous iron, which is aided by reducing agents such as ascorbic acid, fructose and some amino acids.
- intestinal absorption of non-haem iron occurs mainly in the duodenum, and is mediated by the divalent metal transporter (DMT-1). Expression of the transporter is increased in iron deficiency and in hereditary haemochromatosis.

In the circulation, ferric iron is bound to the globulin transferrin and transported to the bone marrow and iron stores. Cellular iron uptake occurs via transferrin receptors, and within most cells iron is stored as a complex with the protein ferritin. In some tissues, iron is also found as an insoluble degraded form of ferritin, known as haemosiderin. Two-thirds of the iron in the body is present in circulating red cells, and about half of the remainder is stored in macrophages, reticuloendothelial cells and hepatocytes. The rest is present in myoglobin in muscle cells or associated with various intracellular enzymes.

When ageing red cells are broken down by the reticuloendothelial system, most of the released iron is recycled for further erythropoiesis. Iron loss from the body is normally low, and occurs through shedding of mucosal cells containing ferritin; there is negligible renal loss of iron.

IRON DEFICIENCY

The main cause of iron deficiency in the UK is abnormal loss of blood, particularly from the gut or from exaggerated menstrual loss. Iron malabsorption can result from disease of the upper small intestine, for example coeliac disease, or following partial gastrectomy. Dietary deficiency is rarely a major cause in Western societies, although worldwide a

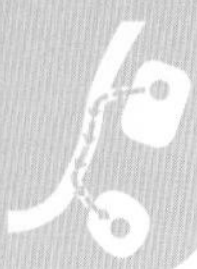

Box 47.1 Causes of anaemia

Reduced red cell production
- Defective precursor proliferation, e.g. iron deficiency, anaemia of chronic disorder, marrow aplasia or infiltration
- Defective precursor maturation, e.g. vitamin B_{12} or folate deficiency, myelodysplastic syndrome, toxins

Increased rate of red cell destruction
- Haemolysis

Loss of circulating red cells
- Bleeding

Box 47.2 Classification of anaemias by red cell characteristics

Hypochromic, microcytic (small-size cells)
- Genetic, e.g. thalassaemia, sideroblastic anaemia
- Acquired, e.g. iron deficiency, sideroblastic anaemia

Normochromic, macrocytic (large-size cells)
- With megaloblastic marrow: vitamin B_{12} or folate deficiency
- With normoblastic marrow: alcohol, myelodysplasia

Polychromatophilic, macrocytic
- Haemolysis

Normochromic, normocytic (normal-size cells)
- Chronic disorders, e.g. infection, malignancy, autoimmune disease
- Renal failure
- Bone marrow failure

vegetarian diet low in absorbable forms of iron is the commonest contributory cause of iron deficiency.

THERAPEUTIC IRON PREPARATIONS

Oral iron

Oral supplements are preferred and are given as ferrous salts – for example, ferrous sulphate, fumarate or gluconate. Tablets are normally used, but some people find that a syrup is more acceptable. In the presence of iron deficiency, a daily oral dose equivalent to 100–200 mg of elemental iron produces the maximum rate of rise of haemoglobin (200 mg ferrous sulphate contains 65 mg iron). About one-third of this dose will be absorbed. Gastrointestinal intolerance to oral iron is common, but unwanted effects can be minimised by taking iron supplements with food or by reducing the dose. Modified-release iron formulations have been developed to improve tolerability, but much of the iron is released beyond the region of the bowel where it is best absorbed. These formulations should only be used when other methods for improving iron tolerance are ineffective. Some oral preparations contain vitamin C, but the therapeutic advantage is minimal compared to the ferrous salt alone.

Unwanted effects

- Gastrointestinal intolerance, especially nausea and dyspepsia. The prevalence of these effects depends both on the dose of elemental iron and on psychological factors, rather than on the iron salt used. Diarrhoea or constipation also occur, but are not dose-related.
- Oral iron turns stools black.

Parenteral iron

Iron can be given parenterally by deep intramuscular injection, or more commonly by slow intravenous injection or infusion. Iron sucrose (a complex of ferric hydroxide with sucrose; only formulated for intravenous use) or iron dextran (a complex of ferric hydroxide with dextrans) is used. The iron in these formulations is not bound to transferrin but accumulates in reticuloendothelial cells. When calculating the amount of iron to give, the approximate total body iron deficit (haemoglobin and body stores) is estimated from the person's size and haemoglobin concentration.

Unwanted effects

- Nausea, vomiting, diarrhoea
- Flushing, fever
- Headache
- Bronchospasm
- Chest pains, arthralgia, myalgia
- Urticaria
- Anaphylactoid/anaphylactic reactions, including cardiovascular collapse; facilities for resuscitation should always be available.

THERAPEUTIC USE OF IRON

The cause of iron deficiency should always be sought before resorting to symptomatic treatment with iron. If this is not done, then serious disorders such as gastrointestinal malignancy can be overlooked. Oral iron supplements are adequate for most mild or moderate iron-deficiency anaemias. After an initial delay of a few days while new red cells are formed, oral iron supplements should raise the blood haemoglobin concentration by about 20 g L^{-1} over the first 3–4 weeks, and about 10 g L^{-1} per week thereafter. Oral iron supplements should be continued for 3 months after the haemoglobin concentration has been restored, in order to replenish tissue iron stores.

Failure to respond to oral iron can be caused by several factors:

- incorrect diagnosis, e.g. anaemia of chronic disorder, thalassaemia
- poor adherence to oral iron therapy
- inadequate iron dosage, e.g. in some modified-release formulations
- continuing excessive blood loss
- malabsorption
- concurrent deficiency of other substances necessary for haemoglobin synthesis.

Parenteral iron preparations are used if there are intractable unwanted effects from oral preparations, if there is severe uncorrectable malabsorption or continuing heavy blood loss, and when adherence to oral treatment is poor. Parenteral iron does not raise the haemoglobin concentration any faster than oral iron, except in severe renal failure during haemodialysis.

Oral iron supplements are occasionally given for prophylaxis against iron deficiency at times of high demand for iron, e.g. pregnancy, menorrhagia, or if there is a poor dietary intake. The reduced iron absorption after subtotal or total gastrectomy can also be overcome by long-term iron supplements.

FOLIC ACID

Folate is required for a number of cellular biochemical processes, including DNA synthesis, and is essential for cell replication, including the formation of red cells. Folic acid (pteroylglutamic acid) is ingested as conjugated folate polyglutamates, found mainly in fresh leaf vegetables (in which it is heat-labile) and in liver (where it is more heat-stable). Before absorption, the polyglutamates are deconjugated to the monoglutamate. Folate monoglutamate is absorbed principally in the duodenum and jejunum, and is methylated and reduced to 5-methyltetrahydrofolate by dihydrofolate reductase during absorption. Methyltetrahydrofolate enters cells, where it is demethylated and converted back to folate polyglutamates. These are coenzymes in the synthesis of pyrimidines and purines and hence of DNA (see also Ch. 52)

FOLATE DEFICIENCY

The most obvious consequence of folate deficiency is a macrocytic anaemia with the presence of megaloblasts in the marrow, a feature it shares with vitamin B_{12} deficiency. Folate deficiency can arise for a number of reasons (Box 47.3). Unlike iron, folate cannot be recycled from old red cells that are removed from the circulation.

THERAPEUTIC USE OF FOLIC ACID

Folate deficiency almost always responds to oral folic acid supplements. Folic acid is a poor substrate for dihydrofolate reductase, and is largely absorbed unchanged and then converted to tetrahydrofolic acid in the plasma and liver. Most causes of folate deficiency are self-limiting, and folic acid treatment is usually given for 4 months to correct the anaemia and replace folate stores.

Folic acid is given prophylactically in pregnancy. It is given in higher doses if there is a history of neural tube defect in a previous pregnancy, when it may protect against recurrence. Folic acid is also given prophylactically to premature infants, during renal dialysis, and in chronic haemolytic anaemia.

Box 47.3 Causes of folate deficiency

- Poor diet: folate stores are adequate for a few weeks only. Lack of folate is uncommon in Western diets, but may be more common in the diet of elderly people or in alcoholism.
- Increased requirements: e.g. pregnancy, malignancies, haemolytic anaemias, exfoliative dermatitis.
- Malabsorption: e.g. coeliac disease, tropical sprue.
- Drugs that interfere with folate metabolism: anticonvulsants (especially phenytoin, Ch. 23), methotrexate (Ch. 52), pyrimethamine (Ch. 51).

Treatment of deficiencies in both vitamin B_{12} and folate using only folic acid may correct the anaemia, but neurological damage can be precipitated (see below). Therefore, vitamin B_{12} deficiency must be excluded before folic acid is used, or both vitamin B_{12} and folic acid should be administered if the extent of the deficiency is uncertain.

For folate deficiency produced by drugs that inhibit the enzyme dihydrofolate reductase (e.g. methotrexate; Ch. 52 and Fig. 51.4), it is necessary to 'bypass' this enzyme blockade by giving the synthetic tetrahydrofolic acid, folinic acid (5-formyl tetrahydrofolic acid). This is the basis of 'folinic acid rescue' discussed in Chapter 52. Folinic acid is formulated as a salt and given orally as calcium folinate, disodium folinate or calcium levofolinate.

VITAMIN B_{12}

Vitamin B_{12} has many roles in the body, including DNA synthesis. The term vitamin B_{12} refers to a group of cobalt-containing compounds, also known as cobalamins. Bacteria are the only organisms that can synthesise cobalamins de novo. Humans obtain vitamin B_{12} from meat (particularly liver), from animal products (milk, cheese, eggs, etc.) or from vegetables contaminated by bacteria. Absorption is by an unusual mechanism: dietary vitamin B_{12} binds in the stomach to a glycoprotein called intrinsic factor that is produced by gastric parietal cells. This complex is absorbed principally from the terminal ileum after binding to receptors on the luminal membranes of ileal cells.

Most vitamin B_{12} in plasma is bound to a glycoprotein, transcobalamin I, from which it is rapidly taken up by the tissues, especially the liver, which stores about 50% of the body content of vitamin B_{12}. A second protein, transcobalamin II, is mainly responsible for rapid transport to tissues, and for enhancing vitamin B_{12} uptake by the bone marrow via specific receptors. Vitamin B_{12} is essential as a coenzyme in nucleic acid synthesis, and in other metabolic pathways in conjunction with folate. Effects of vitamin B_{12} include isomerisation of methylmalonyl coenzyme A to succinyl coenzyme A, isomerisation of α-leucine to β-leucine, and methylation of homocysteine to methionine (a reaction that results in demethylation of methyltetrahydrofolate).

VITAMIN B_{12} DEFICIENCY

Impairment of vitamin B_{12}-dependent reactions affects DNA synthesis. The major organs affected by vitamin B_{12} deficiency are those with a rapid cell turnover, particularly the bone marrow and the gastrointestinal tract.

Vitamin B_{12} deficiency presents with a macrocytic anaemia and a megaloblastic bone marrow. The tongue becomes smooth, and changes to the lining of the small bowel can lead to malabsorption. Damage to the posterior and lateral neuronal tracts in the spinal cord can also occur, leading to a condition known as subacute combined degeneration of the cord. The biochemical basis for the neurological damage is poorly understood: it may not be fully reversible after correction of vitamin B_{12} deficiency.

Causes of vitamin B_{12} deficiency include:

- diet: strict vegetarians (vegans) only
- intestinal malabsorption due to damage to the terminal ileum – for example, Crohn's disease, lymphoma

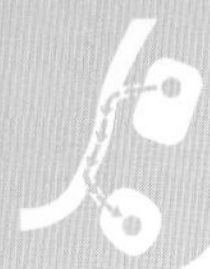

- deficiency of intrinsic factor: pernicious anaemia (destruction of gastric parietal cells with achlorhydria and failure of intrinsic factor production), total and subtotal gastrectomy.

THERAPEUTIC USE OF VITAMIN B_{12}

Most people with vitamin B_{12} deficiency have problems absorbing it from the gut, and treatment is usually by intramuscular injection of vitamin B_{12} in aqueous solution. Hydroxocobalamin is the form of vitamin B_{12} used for treating anaemia, and has completely replaced cyanocobalamin, because it is more highly bound to transcobalamins and less is excreted in the urine. Following initial injections on alternate days for 2 weeks to replenish stores, maintenance injections every 3 months for life are adequate. In the rare dietary causes of vitamin B_{12} deficiency, oral cyanocobalamin supplements can be given, but otherwise oral treatment is never indicated.

ERYTHROPOIETIN

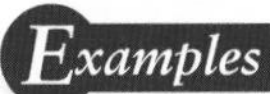

Examples

darbepoetin, epoetin

Erythropoietin is a glycosylated protein hormone, produced mainly by the kidney. It regulates red cell production by stimulating differentiation and proliferation of erythroid progenitor cells by reducing the levels of cell cycle inhibitors and increasing transcription of cyclins. Deficiency of erythropoietin in end-stage renal disease contributes to the anaemia that characterises this disorder. Interestingly, the hormone has also been found to have a protective effect on ischaemic neurons in the brain. Human erythropoietin has been synthesised using recombinant DNA technology (epoetin): it is produced in two forms, alfa and beta, which have identical clinical effects. Erythropoietin is also available as a hyperglycosylated derivative, darbepoetin alfa, which has a longer half-life.

Pharmacokinetics

Epoetin can be given intravenously or, more conveniently, subcutaneously, when a 25–50% lower dose can be used. The red cell response is more rapid after intravenous use, but ultimately greater after subcutaneous injection. Epoetin has a half-life of about 4–6 h, and is normally given two or three times a week. Darbepoetin has a long half-life of 20 h and is given once a week. Adequate iron stores are essential, since erythropoiesis demands large amounts of iron, and iron supplements may improve the response. The route of elimination is uncertain, but may be largely by receptor-mediated uptake in the bone marrow and subsequent intracellular degradation.

Unwanted effects

- Influenza-like symptoms early in treatment
- Hypertension, which is dose-dependent and can be severe, leading to encephalopathy with seizures
- Thrombosis of arteriovenous shunts
- Pure red cell aplasia (not affecting white cells or platelets) occurs rarely during subcutaneous administration in renal failure; this is usually associated with formation of antibodies to epoetin, and treatment must be discontinued if this occurs.

THERAPEUTIC USES OF EPOETIN

- Anaemia of end-stage renal disease. Other causes of anaemia should be excluded, and iron supplements, often given intravenously, may be needed to maximise the response. Anaemia can be corrected in more than 90% of those treated, and treatment improves quality of life. Epoetin also modulates lipid metabolism, creating a less atherogenic plasma lipid profile, which may reduce the high cardiovascular mortality in renal failure. However, recent evidence suggests that cardiovascular mortality and morbidity may be increased if the haemoglobin concentration is raised above 120 g L^{-1}.
- To increase red cell production prior to surgery. Autologous blood transfusion is becoming more popular to reduce the use of banked blood. Epoetin given twice weekly for 3 weeks before surgery can increase the number of units of blood that can be obtained.
- Anaemia associated with human immunodeficiency virus (HIV) infection or acquired immunodeficiency syndrome (AIDS).
- Anaemia associated with cytotoxic chemotherapy of non-myeloid malignant disease (Ch. 52).
- Epoetin is sometimes abused by athletes to increase haematocrit and improve performance. This abuse is associated with an increased risk of arterial and venous thromboses.

DRUG TREATMENT IN OTHER ANAEMIAS

Certain other anaemias require specific drug therapy.

Aplastic anaemia

Failure of haematopoietic stem cell production has many causes, including certain drugs (Box 47.4). Drugs do not have a major role in treatment. The anabolic steroid oxymetholone (Ch. 46; available in the UK only on a named-patient basis) is sometimes used, but its effectiveness is unpredictable. Antilymphocyte globulin is helpful in some acquired aplastic anaemias, and is sometimes used in combination with ciclosporin (Ch. 38).

Sideroblastic anaemia

This can also be caused by drugs (Box 47.5). It is characterised by accumulation of iron in the mitochondria of erythroblasts, which lie in a ring around the nucleus. Staining for iron reveals the characteristic ring sideroblasts. Pyridoxine supplements can increase the haemoglobin concentration in idiopathic acquired and hereditary forms of the disorder. They can also be useful for reversible sideroblastic anaemia associated with pregnancy, haemolysis, alcohol dependence or during treatment with the antituberculous drug isoniazid (Ch. 51).

Box 47.4 Causes of aplastic anaemia

Drugs:
- cytotoxic agents
- chloramphenicol
- sulphonamides
- NSAIDs
- gold salts
- carbimazole
- phenytoin
- carbamazepine
- phenothiazines
- chlorpropamide

Radiation
Infections, e.g. hepatitis, Epstein–Barr virus
Inherited, e.g. Fanconi anaemia
Malignant, e.g. myelodysplastic syndrome

Box 47.5 More common causes of sideroblastic anaemia

Congenital
Acquired
Myelodysplastic syndrome
Drugs and toxins:
- isoniazid
- chloramphenicol
- alcoholism
- lead poisoning

Autoimmune haemolytic anaemia

This can respond to immunosuppression with corticosteroids (Ch. 44).

β-Thalassaemia major

This is a genetic disorder of haemoglobin synthesis with a hyperplastic bone marrow and refractory anaemia. Blood transfusions or excessive iron supplements lead to iron overload, with damage to the liver, heart and pancreas. Iron overload can be prevented with infusions of desferrioxamine (Ch. 53) together with vitamin C, which enhances iron excretion. An oral iron chelator, deferiprone, is used when desferrioxamine is poorly tolerated or contraindicated, but it can cause neutropenia.

Sickle cell anaemia

This inherited disorder occurs when more than 80% of the haemoglobin is HbS; fetal haemoglobin (HbF) forms the remainder. Hydroxycarbamide (see Ch. 52) reduces the frequency and severity of sickle cell crises. It raises the HbF concentration and also reduces the number of young red cells, which are those most likely to adhere to endothelium and occlude blood vessels.

DRUGS AS A CAUSE OF ANAEMIA

- Iron deficiency: especially drugs causing bleeding from the upper gut, e.g. non-steroidal anti-inflammatory drugs (NSAIDs).
- Aplastic anaemia: see Box 47.4.
- Sideroblastic anaemia: see Box 47.5.
- Haemolysis in glucose-6-phosphate dehydrogenase (G6PD) deficiency: see Box 47.6. G6PD is involved in generating reduced glutathione, which protects red cells against oxidative stresses. Oxidant drugs produce haemolysis in deficient individuals, who are usually male (Ch. 53).

Box 47.6 Drugs causing haemolysis in glucose-6-phosphate dehydrogenase deficiency

Antimalarials
Primaquine
Pamaquine
Analgesics
Aspirin (high dose)
Others
Sulphonamides
Nalidixic acid
Dapsone

Box 47.7 Causes of neutropenia

Inherited
Congenital agranulocytosis
Cyclical neutropenia

Acquired
Viral infection, e.g. hepatitis, influenza, rubella, infectious mononucleosis
Bacterial infection
Radiotherapy
Drugs, especially cytotoxic drugs, carbimazole
Autoimmune
Hypersplenism
Marrow infiltration

NEUTROPENIA

Leucocytes are part of the first line of defence against pathogens. They include phagocytic cells (neutrophils, monocytes and eosinophils) and non-phagocytic cells (lymphocytes and basophils). In addition to their role in acute inflammation, all these cells participate in regulation of cellular and humoral immunity through the production of cytokines (Ch. 38). A reduction in the number of circulating neutrophils (neutropenia) in particular increases the risk of serious infection. There are several causes of neutropenia (Box 47.7). Neutropenia does not give rise to symptoms, but predisposes to infection, especially if the neutrophil count falls below $0.5 \times 10^9\ L^{-1}$.

DRUGS FOR NEUTROPENIA

Granulocyte colony-stimulating factors

Granulocyte colony-stimulating factors are produced by many cells, such as endothelial cells, monocytes and

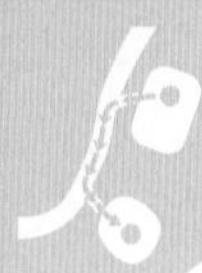

fibroblasts, and stimulate the maturation of pluripotent stem cells in the bone marrow. Granulocyte colony-stimulating factor (G-CSF) has now been produced by recombinant DNA technology. Therapeutic agents include:

- filgrastim (recombinant human G-CSF)
- lenograstim (glycosylated recombinant human G-CSF)
- pegfilgrastim (polyethylene glycol-conjugated [pegylated] filgrastim).

G-CSF is glycosylated in its natural state, but this does not seem to be a prerequisite for effectiveness. A transient fall in circulating neutrophils occurs within minutes of the injection, followed a few hours later by a substantial rise.

Pharmacokinetics

Granulocyte colony-stimulating factors are given by prolonged intravenous infusion or subcutaneous injection. After chemotherapy, daily injections are given until there is an adequate neutrophil response. Pegfilgrastim has a longer duration of action than filgrastim, and is only given once after chemotherapy. Filgrastim and lenograstim are eliminated both by the kidney and by neutrophil uptake. Pegfilgrastim is not eliminated by the kidney, and has a prolonged effect in neutropenia, since few neutrophils are available to contribute to its elimination.

Unwanted effects

- Musculoskeletal or bone pain
- Headache
- Fever
- Fatigue
- Anorexia, nausea, vomiting, diarrhoea
- Myeloproliferative disorders with long-term treatment
- Osteoporosis with long-term treatment.

THERAPEUTIC USE OF COLONY-STIMULATING FACTORS

The use of these drugs remains controversial in many indications.

Congenital neutropenia

Survival is prolonged by reduction of life-threatening infection, but 10% of subjects develop acute myeloid leukaemia as a result of treatment.

Chemotherapy-induced neutropenia

The duration of neutropenia may be reduced, with a limitation of associated sepsis. However, with many chemotherapy regimens there is no evidence that long-term survival is improved by G-CSF, and with some regimens the risk of acute myeloid leukaemia may be increased. G-CSF treatment is therefore reserved for those regimens that have greater than 20% historical risk of febrile neutropenia. It is also used when chemotherapy has previously been associated with a febrile neutropenic episode and the drug dosage cannot be reduced for subsequent courses.

Mobilisation of progenitor cells into peripheral blood for harvesting prior to bone marrow transplantation

The white blood cell count rises 7–12 days after treatment and is accompanied by an increase in haematopoietic stem cells, which are collected via a cell separation machine.

FURTHER READING

Cappellini MD, Fiorelli G (2008) Glucose-6-phosphate dehydrogenase deficiency. *N Engl J Med* 371, 64–74

Crawford J, Dale DC, Lyman GH (2004) Chemotherapy-induced neutropenia: risks, consequences and new directions for its management. *Cancer* 100, 228–237

Frewin R, Henson A, Provan D (1997) Iron deficiency anaemia. *BMJ* 314, 360–363

Henry DH, Bowers P, Romano MT et al (2004) Epoetin alpha. Clinical evolution of a pleiotropic cytokine. *Arch Intern Med* 164, 262–276

Hoffbrand V, Provan D (1997) Macrocytic anaemias. *BMJ* 314, 430–433

Hubell K, Engert A (2003) Clinical applications of granulocyte colony-stimulating factor: an update and summary. *Ann Haematol* 82, 207–213

Kaushansky K (2006) Lineage-specific hematopoietic growth factors. *N Engl J Med* 354, 2034–2046

Lyman GH, Shayne M (2007) Granulocyte colony-stimulating factors: finding the right indication. *Curr Opin Oncol* 19, 299–307

Macdougall IC, Eckardt K-U (2006) Novel strategies for stimulating erythropoiesis and potential new treatments for anaemia. *Lancet* 368, 947–953

Ng T, Marx G, Littlewood T et al (2003) Recombinant erythropoietin in clinical practice. *Postgrad Med J* 79, 367–376

Provan D, Weatherall D (2000) Red cells II: acquired anaemias and polycythaemias. *Lancet* 355, 1260–1268

Weatherall D, Provan D (2000) Red cells I: inherited anaemias. *Lancet* 355, 1169–1175

Weiss MJ (2003) New insights into erythropoietin and epoetin alpha: mechanisms of action, target tissues, and clinical applications. *Oncologist* 8(suppl 3), 18–29

SELF-ASSESSMENT

In questions 1–4, the first statement, in italics, is true. Are the accompanying statements also true?

1. *Pernicious anaemia is caused by reduced vitamin B_{12} absorption due to autoimmunity that inhibits intrinsic factor release from parietal cells.*
   a. Vitamin B_{12} is absorbed from the stomach.
   b. In vitamin B_{12} deficiency, treatment is required for life.
   c. The blood film in pernicious anaemia shows macrocytosis.
2. *The most common causes of megaloblastic anaemias are vitamin B_{12} or folate deficiency.*
   a. Both vitamin B_{12} and folate are essential for DNA synthesis.
   b. Folic acid cannot be given orally.

3. *Erythropoietin is a product of the kidney that stimulates progenitor cells to generate erythrocytes.* Chronic renal failure can result in a deficiency in erythropoietin.
4. *Colony-stimulating factors (CSFs) are formed from many cells and control the formation and survival of neutrophils, monocytes and eosinophils.* CSFs reduce the release of progenitor cells of neutrophils from bone marrow into the circulation.
5. Concerning the properties of erythropoietin, choose the one **correct** answer from the following.
   A. Erythropoietin is synthesised mainly by the adrenal glands.
   B. Erythropoietin can correct anaemia in end-stage renal disease.
   C. Erythropoietin is an effective sole treatment of anaemia even if iron levels are low.
   D. Erythropoietin can reduce athletic performance in long-distance runners.
   E. Erythropoietin can be given orally.
6. Concerning the usage and properties of folic acid and its metabolites, choose the one **incorrect** answer from the following.
   A. Tetrahydrofolate is a product of folic acid metabolism involved in the synthesis of the bases in DNA.
   B. Administration of folate to correct folate deficiencies requires months of treatment.
   C. Folate is absorbed in the stomach.
   D. Tetrahydrofolic acid is given rather than folic acid to correct the folate deficiency caused by methotrexate.
   E. Deficiency in vitamin B_{12} and folic acid both cause macrocytic megaloblastic anaemia.
7. Case history questions

A 40-year-old woman complained to her GP of fatigue and heavy menstrual periods lasting 7 days and occurring every 28 days. Her GP noted that she was pallid; her haemoglobin level was 67 g L^{-1} and mean cell volume (MCV) was 61 fl (normal 76–96). Other blood measurements of platelets and white cell counts were unremarkable.

   a. How would you interpret these data and what were the possible reasons?
   b. What biochemical tests could have helped the diagnosis?

The tests confirmed iron-deficiency anaemia.

   c. What pharmaceutical preparation should have been given?

Several iron formulations were tried, as the woman felt unwell taking ferrous sulphate.

   d. What unwanted effects might she have experienced?
   e. Where was the iron absorbed?
   f. In what dietary form would iron have been optimally absorbed?

After 2 months of oral iron therapy, the haemoglobin value was 80 g L^{-1}.

   g. Was this a sufficient response?

The woman was intolerant of oral iron.

   h. What could have been the reasons for the poor response?
   i. What alternative treatment could have been administered?

With the new treatment regimen her haemoglobin rose to 115 g L^{-1} over 2–3 weeks.

ANSWERS

1. a. **False**. Vitamin B_{12} is absorbed with the aid of intrinsic factor in the distal ileum.
   b. **True**. It is given by intramuscular injection every 2–3 months for life.
   c. **True**. Macrocytes (large red cells) are seen.
2. a. **True**. Folate is necessary for purine and pyrimidine synthesis, and vitamin B_{12} is also necessary for the formation of a cofactor in the synthesis of purines and pyrimidines.
   b. **False**. Folic acid is given daily orally for up to 4 months to replenish stores.
3. **True**. The main cause of erythropoietin deficiency is renal failure.
4. **False**. CSFs are used to enhance blood cell development, for example where damage to cell-producing systems has occurred due to cytotoxic drugs.
5. Answer **B**.
   A. Incorrect. The kidneys are the main producers of erythropoietin.
   B. Correct. Anaemia associated with renal disease is commonly treated with erythropoietin.
   C. Incorrect. Adequate iron stores are necessary for erythropoietin to be successful.
   D. Incorrect. Erythropoietin is sometimes abused by athletes to increase their red cell count and enhance performance.
   E. Incorrect. It is inactive orally and must be given by intravenous or subcutaneous routes.
6. Answer **C**.
   A. Correct. Tetrahydrofolate is utilised in the synthesis of the purine and pyrimidine bases in DNA.
   B. Correct. Treatment is required for 4 months to correct deficiencies and replenish stores.
   C. Incorrect. Folate is absorbed in the proximal jejunum, and absorption is deficient in coeliac disease.
   D. Correct. Methotrexate inhibits dihydrofolate reductase which converts dihydrofolate to tetrahydrofolate. Giving folinic acid (synthetic tetrahydrofolate) bypasses this block (see Ch. 52).
   E. Correct.
7. Case history answers
   a. The haemoglobin was low; it was less than 115 g L^{-1} and in a woman this indicates anaemia. The MCV was low at 61 fl. The common cause for low MCV is iron-deficiency anaemia. Iron-deficiency anaemia is common in menstruating women. The other common cause is gastrointestinal bleeding, including haemorrhoids.

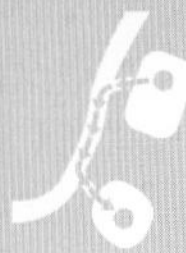

b. Serum ferritin should be low and iron-binding capacity elevated.
c. Oral ferrous salts (e.g. ferrous sulphate, the form most easily absorbed).
d. Gastrointestinal distension and loose bowel movements are common.
e. From the duodenum and upper jejunum.
f. It is optimally absorbed as haem.
g. No. The rise in haemoglobin should be about 10 g L^{-1} each week.
h. Lack of adherence; continued bleeding, malabsorption.
i. Slow intravenous injection or infusion of iron sucrose or iron dextran.

Drugs used to treat anaemias and neutropenia

Drug	Half-life (h) and kinetics	Comments
Drugs used in iron-deficiency anaemia		
Iron		
Oral formulations		
Ferrous sulphate Ferrous fumarate Ferrous gluconate Polysaccharide–iron complex Sodium feredetate	–	Often given as co-formulations with folic acid; extent of absorption depends on form, the presence of food, and iron status; water-soluble forms are the sulphate and gluconate, whereas the fumarate is only sparingly soluble
Parenteral formulations		
Iron dextran	– Extensive uptake by macrophage-rich spleen with effective release for erythrocyte formation	A complex of ferric hydroxide with dextran containing 5% iron; given by slow i.v. injection or infusion
Iron sucrose	– Extensive uptake by macrophage-rich spleen with effective release for erythrocyte formation	A complex of ferric hydroxide with sucrose containing 2% iron; given by slow i.v. injection or infusion
Drugs used in megaloblastic anaemias		
Hydroxocobalamin has completely replaced cyanocobalamin as the drug of choice		
Cyanocobalamin	6 days [B + R + M] Dose-dependent absorption and elimination; free cyanocobalamin is eliminated by glomerular filtration (and, like creatinine, can be used to determine GFR); the excretion increases with dose, from 5% after 25 mg to 85% after 1000 mg; metabolism gives cobalamin; incorporated into vitamin B_{12} which is eliminated in bile	Given orally or by intramuscular injection
Folic acid	Dose-dependent [R] About 70–80% absorption; low doses are retained in cells and higher doses are eliminated in urine; folic acid per se does not occur naturally in food	Has few indications for long-term therapy, since folate deficiency responds to a short course of treatment; usually given with hydroxocobalamin; given orally
Hydroxocobalamin	2–6 [R + M] Elimination by glomerular filtration, with 25% excreted at 500 mg and 29% at 1000 mg; excretion is complete by 24 h after dosage	Given by intramuscular injection
Drugs used in hypoplastic, haemolytic and renal anaemias		
Darbepoetin alfa	20 [M + R] Eliminated largely by undefined metabolism; half-life is longer after s.c. dosage (30–90 h)	Recombinant form of renal erythropoietin that is used for anaemia associated with chronic renal disease and anaemia in adults receiving chemotherapy for non-myeloid malignancies; a hyperglycosylated derivative of epoetin with a longer half-life; given by i.v. or s.c. injection

Drugs used to treat anaemias and neutropenia

Drug	Half-life (h) and kinetics	Comments
Epoetin alfa and beta	4–6 [M] Probably catabolised by target cells after internalisation	Used for anaemia associated with chronic renal disease, to increase autologous blood in normal subjects and for anaemia in adults receiving chemotherapy for malignancies; given by s.c. or i.v. injection
Oxymetholone	8–9 [M] Metabolised in the liver; metabolites excreted in urine	Used for 3–6 months for treatment of aplastic anaemia (see Ch. 47); given orally
Treatment of iron overload		
Deferasirox	8–16 [M] Metabolised by conjugation with glucuronic acid; conjugate excreted in bile	Used for iron overload in thalassaemia major, for people requiring frequent blood transfusions and for those intolerant to desferrioxamine; given orally
Deferiprone	1.5 [R + M] Eliminated by renal excretion plus some conjugation with glucuronic acid	Used for iron overload in thalassaemia major and for people intolerant to desferrioxamine; given orally
Desferrioxamine mesilate (deferoxamine mesilate)	6 [M + R] Eliminated unchanged in urine (15–65%) and by metabolism to inactive products	Chelating agent used for iron overload in thalassaemia major (or aluminium overload in people undergoing dialysis), and for haemochromatosis in people in whom repeated venesection is contraindicated; given by s.c. infusion
Drugs used in neutropenia		
All drugs are recombinant colony-stimulating factors which have to be given parenterally; all drugs are for specialist use only		
Filgrastim	3.5 [M+ neutrophil uptake] Pathways of metabolism have not been defined; metabolites eliminated by the kidneys (90% in animal studies)	Unglycosylated rhG-CSF; used for reduction in the duration of neutropenia, for example following cytotoxic chemotherapy of malignancy, and for severe congenital neutropenia; given by s.c. injection or by s.c. or i.v. infusion
Lenograstim	2.5–3.5 (s.c.); 1 (i.v.) [M+ neutrophil uptake] Pathways of metabolism have not been defined	Glycosylated rhG-CSF; used for reduction in the duration of neutropenia, for example following cytotoxic chemotherapy of malignancy; given by s.c. injection or i.v. infusion
Pegfilgrastim	15–80 [slow by neutrophil uptake] Clearance by neutrophil uptake depends on both the dose and the neutrophil count	Polyethylene glycol-conjugated (pegylated) derivative of filgrastim; used for reduction in the duration of neutropenia, for example following cytotoxic chemotherapy of malignancy; given by s.c. injection

[B], biliary excretion; [M], metabolism; [R], renal excretion; GFR, glomerular filtration rate; i.v., intravenous; rhG-CSF, recombinant human granulocyte colony-stimulating factor; s.c., subcutaneous.

48 Lipid disorders

LIPIDS AND LIPOPROTEINS

Lipid and lipoprotein metabolism is complex and the following account is a very brief summary, sufficient to establish the mechanism of action of drugs used to correct lipid abnormalities.

CHOLESTEROL AND TRIGLYCERIDES

Cholesterol is a vital structural component of cell membranes and a precursor of many steroids, including bile salts and steroid hormones. Cholesterol is a sterol, and about 20–25% of daily intake is synthesised in the liver; the rest is produced in other tissues or ingested in the diet. Its synthesis in the liver involves several enzymes, but the rate-limiting step is catalysed by HMG-CoA (β-hydroxy-β-methylglutaryl-coenzyme A) reductase. Intracellular cholesterol causes negative feedback on HMG-CoA reductase to reduce further hepatic cholesterol synthesis. Cholesterol leaves hepatocytes either by transport into the circulation (see below) or by secretion into the bile after incorporation into bile salt micelles (Figs 48.1 and 48.2). Virtually all of the cholesterol secreted in bile is reabsorbed and taken up by the liver, which also retains about 50% of cholesterol that is not incorporated into bile salts.

Triglycerides (fatty acids esterified with glycerol) are the major dietary fat, and can also be synthesised from intermediary metabolites formed in the liver from excess carbohydrate in the diet. Triglycerides are stored in adipose tissue, from which they can be mobilised as non-esterified free fatty acids to act as an energy substrate during periods of fasting.

THE BASIS OF LIPOPROTEIN METABOLISM

Lipids (triglycerides and esters of cholesterol) have low water solubility and therefore circulate in plasma encased in a coat of apolipoproteins, creating lipoproteins, thereby making them water soluble and therefore transportable. The lipoproteins can be differentiated according to the triglyceride/cholesterol ratio they carry, their apolipoprotein constituent and their density (Table 48.1). They are usually classified according to the density of the particles into very-low-density (VLDL), low-density (LDL), intermediate-density (IDL) and high-density (HDL) lipoproteins. There are specific receptors for processing different apolipoproteins and these will determine where and how that specific fraction of circulating cholesterol and triglyceride will be handled (Table 48.1). In healthy individuals, about 70% of plasma cholesterol is carried by LDL and 20% by HDL. The ratio of cholesterol to triglyceride carried is greatest in the highest density lipoprotein fraction. The least-dense and largest-diameter particles, known as chylomicrons, are exclusively concerned with the transport of dietary lipid from the intestine to the liver. Their low density and large size reflect their high content of triglycerides (Table 48.1), and they are almost completely removed from blood after a 12-h fast. VLDL carries about 60% of plasma triglyceride in the fasting state.

Processing of lipids absorbed from the gut (see Fig. 48.1)

Cholesterol and free fatty acids are solubilised by bile acids in the gut lumen to facilitate absorption into enterocytes. Soluble cholesterol is transported into the enterocyte from the intestinal lumen by a transmembrane protein that is inhibited by ezetimibe (see below). Cholesterol is incorporated into large lipoprotein particles called Chylomicrons in the enterocytes (see Table 48.1). Chylomicrons pass into the lymphatic system and then into the circulation. Hydrolysis of triglycerides in the chylomicrons is carried out by a lipoprotein lipase (LPL, attached to endothelium of capillaries perfusing muscle and adipose tissue) and requires the chylomicron-associated apolipoprotein C (the subtype C-II) as a cofactor (Table 48.1). Free fatty acids are released by hydrolysis from chylomicrons and also from VLDL (synthesised by the liver, see below), and can then be utilised by muscle and liver as an energy source or stored as triglycerides in adipose tissue. After removal of triglycerides from the chylomicrons, the remaining surface lipoprotein and lipid fractions leave the particles to enter the HDL pool as 'nascent HDL' (Fig. 48.1). The chylomicron remnants are taken into hepatocytes by specific chylomicron remnant (apo E) receptors.

Plasma transport and liver processing of lipids

Cholesterol is transported to tissues in chylomicrons, VLDL and LDL; it is transported from tissues to the liver by HDL. High levels of LDL are associated with atheromatous disease.

Liver cholesterol (as esters) and triglycerides in the liver that are surplus to synthetic and oxidative requirements are

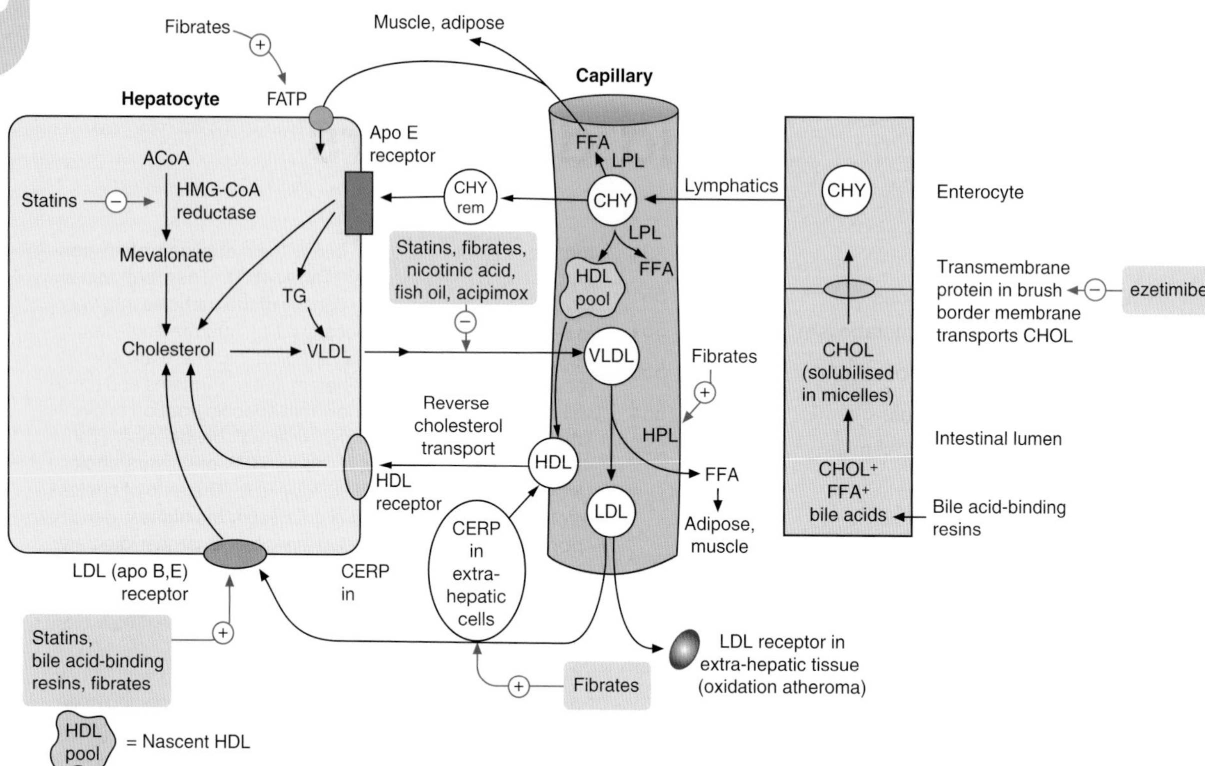

Fig. 48.1 **Some steps in lipoprotein formation and metabolism.** Apo, apolipoprotein; CERP, cholesterol efflux regulatory protein; CHOL, cholesterol; CHY, chylomicron; CHY rem, chylomicron remnant; FATP, fatty acid transport protein; FFA, free fatty acid; HPL, hepatic lipoprotein lipase; LDL, low-density lipoprotein; LPL, lipoprotein lipase; TG, triglycerides; VLDL, very-low-density lipoprotein; +, increases activity; –, decreases activity. The HDL pool is also referred to as nascent HDL and is an important source of mature HDL. It is derived from the chylomicrons following the action of LPL. Drugs used, their targets and their indirect effects are shown in red arrows. ACoA, acetyl coenzyme A. HmGCoA, β-hydroxyl-β-methylglutaryl-coenzyme.

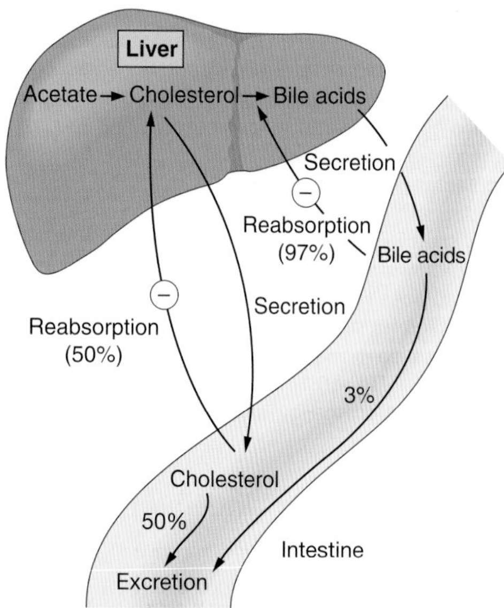

Fig. 48.2 **Enterohepatic cycling of cholesterol and bile acids.** They are secreted into the duodenum via the bile duct and are then returned to the liver by the portal circulation. ⊖, indicates negative feedback effect. Percentages are in relation to the amount excreted in bile.

released into the circulation complexed to VLDL. Peripheral LPL acts on VLDL to release free fatty acids, leaving IDL (not shown in Fig. 48.1); triglycerides in IDL are also hydrolysed by hepatic lipase to release free fatty acids, which generates LDL. LDL contains a higher concentration of cholesterol and a lower concentration of triglyceride compared with VLDL (Table 48.1). LDL is removed from the circulation by uptake into liver cells (75%) and peripheral tissues (25%). Some 70% of this uptake is by specific receptors for the apoproteins type B and E (Fig. 48.1), while the rest is by non-receptor-mediated pathways. The circulating levels of LDL rise if there is either excess production of LDL or deficient LDL receptor numbers. When plasma LDL rises, non-receptor-mediated uptake of cholesterol in peripheral tissues such as arterial walls will increase. Within arterial walls, oxidation of LDL cholesterol leads to formation of lipid-rich deposits in arterial walls and atheromatous plaques (see below).

HDL carries cholesterol mobilised from peripheral tissues, and transports it to the liver (reverse cholesterol transport). The efflux of cholesterol from peripheral cells is facilitated by cholesterol efflux regulatory protein (CERP). This cholesterol is bound to nascent HDL, and then the

Table 48.1 Apolipoprotein and lipid composition of some lipoproteins and their sources

Lipoprotein	Major associated apolipoproteins[a]	Cholesterol (%)	Triglycerides (%)	Source
Chylomicrons	Apo A/Apo B/Apo B_{48}/Apo C/Apo E	3	90	Intestine
VLDL	Apo C/Apo B_{100}/Apo E	20	50	Liver
LDL	Apo B_{100}	50	7	VLDL
HDL	Apo A	40	6	Chylomicrons, VLDL, liver, intestine

[a]The associated apolipoproteins supply essential structural integrity without which the lipoprotein cannot be synthesised or secreted. Individual apolipoproteins also have roles in controlling enzymes involved in lipoprotein metabolism and as receptor ligands. For example, Apo B_{100} and Apo E are the binding ligands for LDL and the chylomicron remnants, respectively (Fig. 48.1).
HDL, high-density lipoproteins; LDL, low-density lipoproteins; VLDL, very-low-density lipoproteins.

Table 48.2 The Fredrickson classification of dyslipidaemias

Type	Triglyceride	Total cholesterol	LDL cholesterol	Raised lipoprotein	Atheroma risk
I	+++	+	N	Chylomicrons	N
IIa	N	++	++	LDL	+++
IIb	++	++	++	LDL/VLDL	+++
III	++	+	N	VLDL and chylomicron remnants	++
IV	++	N/+	N	VLDL	++
V	+++	+	N	VLDL/chylomicrons	N

N = normal; + = slightly raised; ++ = moderately raised; +++ = extremely raised.

cholesterol is esterified by the circulating enzyme lecithin-cholesterol acyltransferase (LCAT) to create mature HDL. HDL is believed to protect against atheroma by this reverse cholesterol transport from peripheral tissues to the liver. The enzyme cholesterol ester transfer protein (CETP) can transfer cholesterol from HDL to VLDL in exchange for triglycerides. The extent of this exchange depends on the concentration of circulating triglycerides.

HYPERCHOLESTEROLAEMIA AND ATHEROMA

Abnormalities of plasma lipoprotein metabolism produce excessive concentrations of circulating cholesterol and/or triglyceride. Their clinical importance lies in their relationship to the production of atheroma (mainly raised LDL cholesterol with a contribution from triglycerides) and pancreatitis (triglycerides >12 mmol L^{-1}). Atheroma is focal thickening of the intima of arteries, produced by a combination of cells, elements of connective tissue, lipids and debris.

Excess LDL accumulates in the arterial wall, where its cholesterol undergoes oxidation to produce a cytotoxic and chemotactic lipid that can activate the endothelium. Activated endothelium (a state which is also initiated by other atherogenic factors such as smoking, diabetes or hypertension) expresses adhesion molecules that attract platelets, monocytes and some T-lymphocytes. These cells migrate into the sub-endothelial space, where the monocytes differentiate into macrophages under the influence of endothelial cytokines. The macrophages take up oxidised LDL cholesterol, which accumulates as droplets in the cytosol, creating lipid-rich foam cells. Foam cells initiate fatty streaks that are the precursor of atheroma. T-cells in the developing atheromatous lesion recognise lipid antigens, and release various cytokines that attract further inflammatory cells and initiate a T-helper cell type 1 inflammatory response (Ch. 38). These processes also result in formation of a cap of smooth muscle cells and collagen-rich matrix over the lesion. The extent of the inflammatory response determines whether the cap becomes fibrous and stable, or is destabilised by infiltration of inflammatory cells that make it prone to rupture or surface erosion. Plaque destabilisation underlies the development of acute coronary syndromes and many cases of ischaemic stroke (see Chs 5 and 9)

Atherogenic patterns of lipoproteins can result from the following.

- dietary factors.
- primary (inherited) disorders of enzymes or receptors involved in lipid metabolism. Most inherited hyperlipidaemias are polygenic, but an important inherited defect is familial hypercholesterolaemia, a single recessive gene disorder that affects 1 in 500 of the population, who have reduced synthesis of LDL receptors.
- secondary lipid disorders, when hyperlipidaemia results from diseases that affect lipid metabolism, for example liver disease, nephrotic syndrome, hypothyroidism.

A classification for the various phenotypic patterns of primary hyperlipidaemia adopted by the World Health Organisation is shown in Table 48.2.

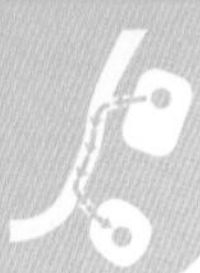

DRUGS FOR HYPERLIPIDAEMIAS

HMG-CoA reductase inhibitors ('statins')

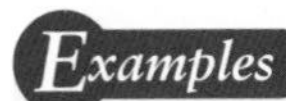

atorvastatin, pravastatin, rosuvastatin, simvastatin

Mechanism of action and effects

HMG-CoA reductase inhibitors competitively inhibit the enzyme that catalyses the rate-limiting step in the synthesis of cholesterol by the liver (Fig. 48.1). The fall in hepatic cholesterol levels produces a compensatory upregulation in the number of LDL receptors on hepatocytes, with increased clearance of circulating LDL cholesterol. The reduction of LDL cholesterol depends on the specific drug and the dose, and ranges from 25% to 50%. Statins also reduce the hepatic production of VLDL, and therefore reduce circulating triglycerides, although the mechanism of this effect is unclear. A modest increase in HDL cholesterol is often seen. Statins also have several other actions, which may be distinct from their ability to reduce plasma lipids (Box 48.1). There is increasing evidence that some of these may contribute significantly to the beneficial actions of statins.

Pharmacokinetics

The statins are well absorbed from the gut. Simvastatin is a prodrug (Ch. 2) which is activated in first-pass metabolism in the liver by cytochrome P450 (CYP3A4). Further metabolism inactivates the drug and only 5% of the active compound reaches the circulation. Atorvastatin undergoes first-pass metabolism, in part to active derivatives, and has a very long half-life. Pravastatin is a hydrophilic drug that is eliminated mainly by the kidneys; its half-life is 1–2 h. Rosuvastatin has a low oral bioavailability and is eliminated mainly in the bile, with a half-life of 20 h.

Unwanted effects

- Gastrointestinal upset, including nausea, vomiting, abdominal pain, flatulence and diarrhoea.
- Central nervous system effects, such as dizziness, blurred vision, headache.
- Transient disturbance of liver function tests, and, rarely, hepatitis.
- Myalgia or myositis, and, occasionally, rhabdomyolysis. The mechanism is uncertain but may involve reduced activation of muscle regulatory proteins that depend on the production of intermediates in the cholesterol synthetic pathway. There is an increased risk when a statin is used in combination with a fibrate, nicotinic acid or ciclosporin (Ch. 38).

Box 48.1 Non-lipid effects of statins

Not all statins share the same non-lipid-lowering effects

- Restored function to vascular endothelium that has been functionally damaged by hypercholesterolaemia. It is not known whether this is a direct effect or a consequence of reduction in plasma LDL cholesterol
- Stabilisation of atherosclerotic plaques by altered smooth muscle proliferation and migration
- Changes in haemostasis: decreased plasma fibrinogen and enhanced fibrinolysis
- Reduction of inflammatory cell infiltration into atherosclerotic plaques. Reduced inflammation is reflected in a reduction in plasma high-sensitivity C-reactive protein

Specific cholesterol absorption inhibitors

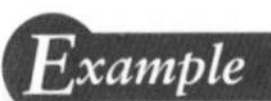

ezetimibe

Mechanism of action

Ezetimibe acts at the brush border of the small intestinal mucosa to specifically inhibit cholesterol absorption by about 50%. It has no effect on the absorption of triglycerides, bile acids or fat-soluble vitamins. Given alone, ezetimibe reduces plasma total cholesterol by about 15% and LDL cholesterol by about 20%. When taken with a low dose of statin, the combination is as effective as three doublings of the statin dose.

Pharmacokinetics

Ezetimibe is rapidly but incompletely absorbed from the gut, and metabolised in the gut wall and the liver. It undergoes enterohepatic circulation, which gives it a long half-life (about 22 h). About 80% is excreted in the faeces.

Unwanted effects

- Diarrhoea, abdominal pain
- Headache
- Angioedema.

Bile acid-binding (anion-exchange) resins

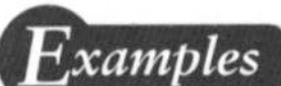

colesevelam, colestipol, colestyramine

Mechanism of action

Bile acid-binding resins are insoluble, non-absorbable polymers that bind bile salts in the gut and prevent enterohepatic circulation of bile acids. The taste and texture limit acceptability; consequently, they are no longer widely used. Bile acids are synthesised from cholesterol in the liver, and are secreted into the duodenum to aid absorption of dietary fat. They are then reabsorbed in the terminal ileum and returned to the liver in the portal circulation (Fig. 48.2).

When reabsorption of bile acids is impaired by binding to the resin, there is a compensatory increase in bile acid synthesis from cholesterol in the liver. This reduces intrahepatic cholesterol, and there is compensatory upregulation of hepatic LDL receptors in order to replenish liver cholesterol. LDL cholesterol is cleared more rapidly from plasma, with a fall in circulating levels of 15–20%. Stimulation of VLDL synthesis produces a small rise in plasma triglycerides. There is a small rise in HDL cholesterol, but the mechanism is unclear.

Unwanted effects

- Unpalatability. Sachets containing several grams of powder have to be taken, usually mixed with food.
- Constipation, or, occasionally, diarrhoea.
- Interference with the absorption of certain acidic drugs, for example digoxin (Ch. 7), warfarin (Ch. 11) and thyroxine (Ch. 41). These drugs should be given at least 1 h before or 4 h after taking a resin.

Fibrates

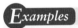

bezafibrate, fenofibrate, gemfibrozil

Mechanism of action

The main effect of these drugs is to activate a gene transcription factor known as peroxisome proliferator-activated receptor alpha (PPAR-α), which encodes for proteins that control lipoprotein metabolism. The mechanism of PPAR-mediated drug action is described in more detail in Chapter 40 (under thiazolidinediones). PPAR-α is expressed in several tissues, including the liver, heart and kidney. There are several consequences of PPAR-α activation:

- increased free fatty acid uptake by the liver due to induction of the fatty acid transport protein in the cell membrane. In the liver, conversion to acyl-coenzyme A derivatives is enhanced as a result of increased acyl-CoA synthetase activity. The esterified fatty acids are less available for hepatic triglyceride synthesis.
- increased mitochondrial free fatty acid uptake in the heart and skeletal muscle, with enhanced oxidation.
- increased lipoprotein lipase activity, which enhances the clearance of triglycerides from lipoproteins in the plasma (Fig. 48.1).
- increased plasma HDL because of enhanced apolipoprotein A-I and A-II production in the liver.

Pharmacokinetics

Fibrates are well absorbed from the gut and highly protein bound in the plasma. Fenofibrate is an ester prodrug that undergoes complete first-pass metabolism to the active form. Excretion is primarily by the kidney, although some metabolism occurs in the liver. The half-lives of bezafibrate and gemfibrozil are short (about 5 h), whereas other fibrates have long half-lives (20–30 h).

Unwanted effects

- Gastrointestinal upset
- Rash or pruritus
- Dizziness, headache
- Increased lithogenicity of bile theoretically increases the risk of gallstones, but this has not been a problem with the clinical uses of these drugs
- Myalgia and myositis are uncommon, unless there is impaired renal function or the fibrate is used in combination with a statin (especially gemfibrozil with simvastatin)
- Drug interactions include inhibition of the effect of warfarin (Ch. 11).

Nicotinic acid and derivatives

nicotinic acid (niacin), acipimox

Mechanism of action

Nicotinic acid is a B vitamin which has effects on lipids at pharmacological doses. It acts on adipocytes via an inhibitory G-protein-coupled membrane receptor, and reduces intracellular cAMP generation. This inhibits hormone-sensitive lipase and reduces lipolysis and, therefore, free fatty acid mobilisation. The decreased availability of free fatty acids to the liver reduces hepatic triglyceride synthesis and VLDL secretion. Nicotinic acid reduces circulating triglycerides by up to 35% and LDL cholesterol modestly by up to 15%. HDL cholesterol is increased by up to 25%, as a result of reduced hepatic uptake of the HDL molecule. A decrease in the activity of hepatic lipase also shifts the distribution of HDL subfractions, with a predominant elevation of HDL_2, which has greater protective effect than HDL_3.

Pharmacokinetics

Nicotinic acid is well absorbed from the gut. Hepatic metabolism occurs via two pathways. Oxidation is a high-affinity, low-capacity pathway that generates metabolites which are thought to be responsible for the hepatotoxicity that can occur with high doses of nicotinic acid. The other pathway is a low-affinity, high-capacity conjugation pathway. Large doses of nicotinic acid are excreted unchanged in the urine. Nicotinic acid has a very short half-life (<1 h).

Acipimox is a synthetic derivative of nicotinic acid that is longer-acting but less effective for lowering LDL cholesterol.

Unwanted effects

Nicotinic acid is often poorly tolerated, but unwanted effects can be reduced by gradual dosage increases. A modified-release formulation that minimises the risk of flushing, and acipimox, are better tolerated.

- Cutaneous vasodilation is particularly troublesome and causes flushing and itching. The action of nicotinic acid on specific G-protein-coupled receptors in the skin increases the production of prostaglandins (PGs) D_2 and E_2 which cause the flushing. The flushing can be reduced

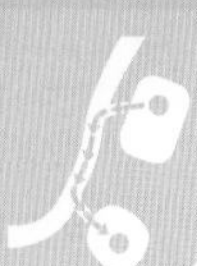

by taking a small dose of aspirin 30 min before nicotinic acid, taking the drug with food, or by using a modified-release formulation. A compound preparation of nicotinic acid with the PGD_2 receptor type 1 inhibitor laropiprant is now available with the prospect of further improving tolerability.

- Gastrointestinal upset and peptic ulceration.
- Headache, dizziness.
- Glucose intolerance with high doses of nicotinic acid (not with acipimox).
- Exacerbation of gout.
- Hepatotoxicity, which is less common with a modified-release formulation of niacin.

Omega-3 fatty acids

Omega-3 fatty acids are long-chain polyunsaturated acids such as alpha-linolenic acid, which is found in plants, and eicosapentaenoic acid (EPA) and docosahexaenoic acid (DHA), which are found in high quantities in oily fish such as mackerel and sardines. They have several potential cardioprotective effects.

- because they are poor substrates for the enzymes that synthesise triglycerides, they lead to the production of triglyceride-poor LDL and reduce triglycerides in plasma, although total cholesterol is increased. They also increase conversion of VLDL to LDL, and increase circulating HDL cholesterol.
- reduction of plasma fibrinogen, decreasing thrombogenesis.
- they substitute for arachidonic acid in platelet phospholipids, which results in the increased production of a prostanoid called thromboxane A_3 in platelets. This has a lower ability to induce platelet aggregation compared with the more usually formed prostanoid thromboxane A_2 (Ch. 11).
- retardation of growth of atherosclerotic plaques by reduced expression of endothelial adhesion molecules and an anti-inflammatory action.
- promotion of nitric oxide-mediated vasodilation.
- membrane stabilisation in heart muscle, with reduced susceptibility to ventricular arrhythmias and sudden cardiac death.

Unwanted effects

- Gastrointestinal upset with nausea, belching, diarrhoea or constipation at the higher intakes necessary to be effective
- Prolonged bleeding time.

MANAGEMENT OF HYPERLIPIDAEMIAS

Cardiovascular disease is the major risk associated with raised plasma LDL cholesterol. The relationship with raised LDL cholesterol is strongest for coronary atherosclerosis and peripheral vascular atherosclerosis, and to a lesser extent for cerebrovascular disease and atherothrombotic stroke. HDL cholesterol is protective against atherosclerosis and a low HDL cholesterol (<1.0 mmol L^{-1}) is associated with the highest risk of disease. The ratio of total cholesterol to HDL cholesterol provides a much more sensitive indicator of the relative risk of cardiovascular disease than does total cholesterol alone.

While a high total cholesterol : HDL cholesterol ratio predicts the relative risk of cardiovascular disease, the absolute risk (i.e. the overall number of individuals in the population under study who will develop disease in a particular time period) will be determined by the coexistence of other risk factors (see below).

Raised plasma triglycerides are an independent predictor of the risk of atherosclerosis, but less so than raised plasma cholesterol. Nevertheless, when raised triglycerides coexist with an atherogenic cholesterol profile, the overall risk is enhanced. A markedly raised plasma triglyceride concentration (>12 mmol L^{-1}) confers an increased risk of acute pancreatitis. Isolated hypertriglyceridaemia should be treated intensively for this reason alone.

Secondary cause of hyperlipidaemia, such as diabetes, hypothyroidism and nephrotic syndrome, should be excluded or treated before embarking on other aspects of management.

Primary prevention of cardiovascular disease

Atherothrombotic disease has a multifactorial aetiology, and any strategy for primary prevention must consider all relevant treatable factors. Drug treatment of hyperlipidaemia with drugs for primary prevention should only be considered if there is a sufficiently high absolute risk of disease, and should not be based on the cholesterol level alone. Important factors to consider in risk management include the following.

- smoking: smoking doubles the risk of coronary artery disease. Stopping smoking reduces the risk to that of a non-smoker in 3–5 years (see Ch. 5).
- physical activity: a physically active lifestyle reduces the risk of myocardial infarction by up to 50%, compared with a sedentary lifestyle.
- maintaining ideal body weight: Obesity (see Ch. 37) increases the risk of myocardial infarction by up to 50%.
- mild-to-moderate alcohol consumption: a modest alcohol intake (see Ch. 54) can reduce the risk of myocardial infarction by about one-third. A high alcohol intake increases blood pressure, and thus increases cardiovascular risk.
- hypertension (see Ch. 6): although treating hypertension is more effective for the prevention of stroke, it also reduces the risk of myocardial infarction, especially in older people.
- control of diabetes: there is conflicting evidence about whether close control of plasma glucose reduces vascular events. However, since the risk of ischaemic heart disease in diabetes is at least twice that of people without diabetes, intensive management of coexistent risk factors in diabetics should be undertaken.

- low-dose aspirin: this is less effective for primary prevention than for secondary prevention (Ch. 11) but is useful in selected high-risk individuals, especially those with hypertension or diabetes.
- cholesterol: this is a powerful predictor of future cardiovascular disease, especially in young people. The greatest risk is present when there is familial hypercholesterolaemia (FH), a dominantly inherited genetic defect that predisposes to premature coronary heart disease even in the absence of other risk factors. Heterozygous FH is associated with reduced LDL receptors on liver cells, and the total serum cholesterol is usually greater than 7.5 mmol L^{-1} in adult life. Lipid-lowering therapy in FH, usually with a statin, should normally begin in late teens in males and early twenties in females (because of the later onset of disease).

  For other forms of hypercholesterolaemia, the risk of cardiovascular disease should first be estimated using risk tables that assess the contribution of the cholesterol profile, systolic blood pressure, smoking, and preferably the presence of left ventricular hypertrophy on the electrocardiogram. The question exercising the minds of health economists is not whether treatment is effective, but when it becomes cost-effective. As part of a multiple risk factor intervention strategy, drug therapy has a role for those at higher absolute risk, usually because several other risk factors coexist or there is a history of premature coronary artery disease in a first-degree relative. In the UK, lipid-lowering drugs are recommended if the predicted 10-year coronary heart disease risk is greater than 15% (equivalent to a cardiovascular disease risk that includes stroke of 20%). Once treatment is started, the target should be greater than 50% reduction in LDL cholesterol for primary prevention, to minimise risk.

  The ability of cholesterol-lowering drugs (and particularly statins) to prevent ischaemic heart disease has been demonstrated in many trials. Reducing plasma total cholesterol by 25–30% (with a reduction in LDL cholesterol of 30–35%) with a statin reduces the subsequent risk of myocardial infarction or vascular death by about 30%.
- diet: dietary management should also be advised for all people with hypercholesterolaemia, with a reduction in saturated fat intake (which decreases hepatic LDL receptors) and an increase in monounsaturated fats (which decreases LDL cholesterol). Eating a diet containing fresh fruit and vegetables reduces oxidation of LDL cholesterol and therefore makes it less atherogenic.

Secondary prevention of cardiovascular disease

Once cardiovascular disease is clinically apparent, the subsequent risk of death from vascular events is high. Recent myocardial infarction or an episode of unstable angina confers the highest risk. People with clinical evidence of vascular disease are at much greater absolute risk of a further event than are those without clinical coronary artery disease but who have similar, or even higher, plasma cholesterol concentrations. At slightly lower absolute risk are those with stable angina pectoris, peripheral vascular disease or ischaemic stroke. Reduction of even 'normal' plasma cholesterol concentrations (as low as 4.0 mmol L^{-1}) in people with vascular disease reduces the subsequent risk of both fatal and non-fatal cardiovascular events.

Current evidence supports the use of statins as first-line therapy; trials with fibrates have shown less marked benefit unless the major lipid abnormality is low HDL cholesterol (see also Ch. 5). The target cholesterol concentration is total cholesterol <4.0 mmol L^{-1} (LDL cholesterol <2 mmol L^{-1}). When this is not achieved with a statin alone, then combinations of drugs, such as a statin with ezetimibe or a fibrate, may be used. There is also evidence that the use of omega-3 fatty acids after myocardial infarction has a cardioprotective effect, which may not entirely relate to their effects on plasma lipids.

Lowering plasma cholesterol for secondary prevention of coronary artery disease should be only one aspect of a comprehensive strategy for improving prognosis. This is discussed more fully in Chapter 5.

Mechanisms of prevention of coronary events by lipid-lowering drugs

There is a close relationship between the degree of LDL cholesterol reduction and the reduced risk of coronary events. Overall, there is a 2–3% reduction in risk for every 1% reduction in plasma total cholesterol concentration. Reducing plasma cholesterol probably stabilises existing atheromatous plaques by preventing lipid accumulation in their core and therefore reduces the risk of plaque rupture. Statins prevent the growth of existing coronary artery plaques and reduce the formation of new plaques; high doses may even produce regression of existing plaque. There is also evidence that an anti-inflammatory effect of statins may be important, measured by a reduction in plasma high-sensitivity C-reactive protein. Other actions of statins, such as reduction in thrombogenicity of blood and inhibition of smooth muscle proliferation in atheromatous plaques, may also contribute to the clinical benefit, but their roles remains speculative.

There is some uncertainty whether lipid-lowering drugs other than statins have the same protective effects. However, it is widely accepted that the evidence indicates that lowering LDL cholesterol alone, however it is achieved, should provide some protection against atheroma.

Management of hypertriglyceridaemia

When triglycerides are markedly raised, control of diabetes, weight loss and reduction of alcohol intake should be considered when appropriate. When drug therapy is necessary, modest hypertriglyceridaemia in association with hypercholesterolaemia will usually respond to a statin. Extremely high plasma triglyceride concentrations usually respond well to a fibrate or to nicotinic acid. Combination therapy with a statin and a fibrate may be necessary in some high-risk individuals, to achieve an acceptable lipid profile.

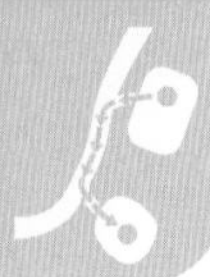

FURTHER READING

Afilalo J, Majdan AA, Eisenberg MJ (2007) Intensive statin therapy in acute coronary syndromes and stable coronary heart disease: a comparative meta-analysis of randomised controlled trials. *Heart* 93, 914–921

Almuti K, Rimawi R, Spevack D et al (2006) Effects of statins beyond lipid lowering: potential for clinical benefits. *Int J Cardiol* 109, 7–15

Armitage J (2007) Safety of statins in clinical practice. *Lancet* 370, 1781–1790

Baber U, Toto RD, de Lemos J (2007) Statins and cardiovascular risk reduction in patients with chronic kidney disease and end-stage renal failure. *Am Heart J* 153, 471–477

Cholesterol Treatment Trialists' Collaborators (2005) Efficacy and safety of cholesterol-lowering treatment: prospective meta-analysis of data from 90 056 participants in 14 randomised trials of statins. *Lancet* 366, 1267–1278

Cholesterol Treatment Trialists' Collaborators (2008) Efficacy of cholesterol-lowering therapy in 18 686 people with diabetes in 14 randomised trials of statins: a meta-analysis. *Lancet* 371, 117–125

Durrington P (2003) Dyslipidaemia. *Lancet* 362, 717–731

Gami AS, Montori VM, Erwin PJ et al (2003) Systematic review of lipid lowering for primary prevention of coronary heart disease in diabetes. *BMJ* 326, 528–529

Hachem SB, Mooradian AD (2006) Familial dyslipidaemias. An overview of genetics, pathophysiology and management. *Drugs* 66, 1949–1969

Harper CR, Jacobson TA (2001) The fats of life. The role of omega-3 fatty acids in the prevention of coronary heart disease. *Arch Intern Med* 161, 2185–2192

Lee C-H, Olson P, Evans RM (2003) Minireview: lipid metabolism, metabolic diseases, and peroxisome proliferator-activated receptors. *Endocrinology* 144, 2201–2207

McKenney J (2004) New perspectives on the use of niacin in the treatment of lipid disorders. *Arch Intern Med* 164, 697–705

Mudaliar S, Henry RR (2002) PPAR agonists in health and disease: a pathophysiological and clinical overview. *Curr Opin Endocrinol Diabetes* 9, 285–302

Nicholls SJ, Tuczu EM, Sipahi I et al (2007) Statins, high-density lipoprotein cholesterol, and regression of coronary atherosclerosis. *JAMA* 297, 499–508

Nissen SE, Tuzcu EM, Schoenhagen P et al (2005) Statin therapy, LDL cholesterol, C-reactive protein, and coronary artery disease. *N Engl J Med* 352, 29–38

Rallidis LS, Lekakis, J, Kremastinos DT (2007) Current questions regarding the use of statins in patients with coronary heart disease. *Int J Cardiol* 122, 188–194

Rizos ED, Mikhailidis DP (2002) Are high-density lipoprotein and triglyceride levels important in secondary prevention: impressions from the BIP and VA-HIT trials. *Int J Cardiol* 82, 199–207

Rosenson RS (2004) Current overview of statin-induced myopathy. *Am J Med* 116, 408–416

Schillinger M, Exner M, Mlekusch W et al (2004) Statin therapy improves cardiovascular outcome of patients with peripheral vascular disease. *Eur Heart J* 25, 742–748

Thompson PD, Clarkson P, Karas RH (2003) Statin-associated myopathy. *JAMA* 289, 1681–1690

Walsh JME, Pignone M (2004) Drug treatment of hyperlipidaemia in women. *JAMA* 291, 2243–2253

SELF-ASSESSMENT

In questions 1 and 2, the first statement, in italics, is true. Are the accompanying statements also true?

1. *Different drug classes available for treating hyperlipidaemia act at differing steps in the lipoprotein metabolic pathway.*
   a. In individuals with high HDL cholesterol, the risk of coronary disease will be lowered if the HDL cholesterol levels are reduced.
   b. An important contributor to the development of hypercholesterolaemia is a genetic defect.
   c. Anion-exchange resins act by enhancing the absorption of bile acids from the gut.
2. *Statins reduce cholesterol levels by inhibiting the rate-limiting enzymatic step (HMG-CoA reductase) in its synthesis.*
   a. Decreased hepatic cholesterol synthesis results in increased numbers of HDL receptors.
   b. Simvastatin lowers serum LDL cholesterol by 5%.
   c. Co-administration of bile acid-binding resins and statins has no greater effect than giving each drug separately.
3. Which one of the following statements concerning the physiological and pharmacological control of plasma lipids is **true**?
   A. In a lipoprotein, the outer coat is phospholipid in structure.
   B. VLDL has a greater percentage of cholesterol than does HDL.
   C. Lowering of plasma cholesterol by statins is not related to the dose of statin administered.
   D. Raising plasma cholesterol has a positive effect on liver cholesterol synthesis.
   E. Fibrates decrease the uptake of LDL cholesterol from the plasma.
4. Which one of the following statements concerning statins is **false?**
   A. Simvastatin is a prodrug that is activated by the liver.
   B. Statins can cause muscle pain.
   C. Statins reduce atherosclerotic plaques formation.
   D. Statins reduce cholesterol significantly within 3 days.
   E. Statins inhibit the activity of liver HMG-CoA reductase.
5. Which one of the following statements concerning hyperlipidaemias is **true?**
   A. If a person is at risk of coronary heart disease, total cholesterol levels should be reduced to 6 mmol L^{-1}.
   B. An increased intake of saturated fat is recommended in hypercholesterolaemia.
   C. Fish oils increase platelet aggregation.
   D. Increased intake of vegetables is recommended in hyperlipidaemias.
   E. Dietary modification of cholesterol intake can reduce plasma cholesterol by 50%.

6. Case history questions

A 58-year-old man recovered from an anterior myocardial infarction. His fasting plasma cholesterol was 7.8 mmol L^{-1}. You want to reduce his risk of a further myocardial infarction by lowering his cholesterol.

a. What advice should be offered?
b. What drug should be recommended and why?
c. What reduction in plasma cholesterol should be expected, and when should a response be expected?
d. How do statins work?
e. What target total cholesterol should be aimed for?
f. What unwanted effects should be looked out for?
g. If the target cholesterol was not attained with your chosen drug, what would be recommended and what is the rationale for this recommendation?

ANSWERS

1. a. **False**. The relationship is between high LDL cholesterol and coronary risk of atherosclerosis. High LDL cholesterol is associated with lipid peroxidation, take-up into macrophages and formation of fatty streaks.
   b. **True**. One in 500 of the population has a single recessive gene disorder causing reduced synthesis of LDL receptors.
   c. **False**. The resins sequester bile acids that contain cholesterol. The reduction in bile salts decreases absorption of ingested cholesterol and also increases bile acid–cholesterol synthesis in liver, leading to further reduction in cholesterol.
2. a. **False**. Reducing cholesterol synthesis results in increased LDL receptors in the liver and hence increased LDL clearance from plasma.
   b. **False**. Serum LDL cholesterol falls by 20–35%.
   c. **False**. The two classes of drugs act by different mechanisms. The combination of two drugs can be used where the response to the statins is inadequate.
3. Answer **A**.
   A. True. The outer coat is phospholipid; cholesterol and triglycerides together with the phospholipid and apolipoprotein constituents comprise a structure to carry the water-insoluble lipids in plasma.
   B. False. VLDL carries 20% cholesterol, whereas HDL has 40%.
   C. False. Statins reduce cholesterol dose-dependently.
   D. False. Cholesterol has a negative feedback effect on cholesterol synthesis.
   E. False. Fibrates act to enhance liver uptake of LDL.
4. Answer **D** is false. The explanations are given in the text.
5. Answer **D** is true. The explanations are given in the text.
6. Case history answers
   a. General advice would include avoidance of smoking, and have a low-fat diet and take exercise. Determine if there are problems with obesity, diabetes or hypertension.
   b. A statin would be recommended as first-choice drug in preventing cardiovascular events in people at increased risk. This man is at increased risk. Statins are of proven benefit using data from many outcome studies; they are also well tolerated (see f). Consider the use of aspirin where appropriate.
   c. The reduction would depend upon dosage of statins, but a reduction in the region of 25% should be aimed for. This could take more than a month to achieve.
   d. Statins inhibit HMG-CoA reductase and increase LDL receptors (Fig. 48.1).
   e. The target total cholesterol recommended is less than 4 mmol L^{-1} and an LDL cholesterol concentration of less than 2 mmol L^{-1}.
   f. Gastrointestinal upsets. Use of statins is not recommended in people with liver disease or in pregnancy. Liver function tests need to be performed.
   g. In addition to the statins, use fibrates, ezetimibe or anion-exchange resins. Because the sites of action are different to those of the statins, an additive effect should be expected: fibrates decrease VLDL production, increase hepatic LDL uptake and stimulate lipoprotein lipase; ezetimibe is a specific cholesterol absorption inhibitor; anion-exchange resins sequester bile salts in the intestine and reduce cholesterol uptake and increase the conversion of cholesterol to bile acids.

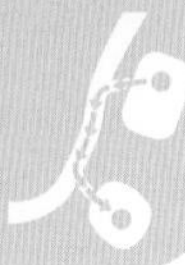

Drugs used to treat hyperlipidaemias (all drugs given orally unless otherwise stated)

Drug	Half-life (h) and kinetics	Comments
HMG-CoA reductase inhibitors		
Atorvastatin	32–36 [M] Bioavailability is 14% (as drug) and 30% (as HMG-CoA reductase inhibition) because the first-pass metabolites are active; bioavailability is lower if taken with food or in the evening; oxidised by CYP3A4 to metabolites that are responsible for much of the activity	Used for primary hypercholesterolaemia, heterozygous familial hypercholesterolaemia, or mixed hyperlipidaemia in individuals who have not responded to dietary measures
Fluvastatin	1 [M] Bioavailability is 30%; extensive hepatic uptake and oxidation; metabolites are conjugated and excreted in bile; parent drug is the active form	Used as an adjunct to diet in primary hypercholesterolaemia and mixed hyperlipidaemias in those who have not responded to dietary measures, and for prophylaxis of coronary atherosclerosis
Pravastatin	1–2 [R + M] Low oral bioavailability (17%), which is decreased by food and is due to poor absorption plus first-pass metabolism; eliminated by renal tubular secretion plus oxidative metabolism; parent drug is the active form	Used as an adjunct to diet in primary hypercholesterolaemia in those who have not responded to dietary measures, and for prophylaxis of coronary atherosclerosis
Rosuvastatin	20 [B + R] Bioavailability is 20% and nearly all activity is due to the parent compound; limited metabolism by CYP2C isoenzymes and little potential for drug interactions; about two-thirds of absorbed dose is eliminated in bile and the rest in faeces	Used in primary hypercholesterolaemia, mixed dyslipidaemia and homozygous familial hypercholesterolaemia in those who have not responded to diet or alternative treatments
Simvastatin	2 (activity) [M] Oral bioavailability as the acid is low (about 5%); a lactone prodrug which is metabolised by hepatic CYP3A4 to the active ring-opened acid analogue	Used as an adjunct to diet in primary hypercholesterolaemia and mixed hyperlipidaemias in those who have not responded to dietary measures, and for prophylaxis of coronary atherosclerosis
Drugs binding bile acids or inhibiting cholesterol absorption		
Colesevelam	Not relevant Not absorbed	A lipid-lowering polymer used for primary hypercholesterolaemia as an adjunct to dietary measures, given alone or with a statin. Improves glycaemic control in type 2 diabetes in adults
Colestipol	Not relevant Not absorbed	Anion-exchange resin that binds bile acids; used for hyperlipidaemias in people not responding to diet and other measures
Colestyramine	Not relevant Not absorbed	Anion-exchange resin that binds bile acids; used for hyperlipidaemias in individuals not responding to diet and other measures, for primary prevention in men aged 35–59 with primary hypercholesterolaemia not responding to other measures, and to treat pruritus associated with biliary obstruction
Ezetimibe	22 [M] Bioavailability has not been defined; metabolised to a glucuronide conjugate, which undergoes biliary excretion and hydrolysis in the lower bowel, thereby delivering drug to the site of cholesterol reabsorption (Fig. 48.2)	Inhibits intestinal absorption of cholesterol; used as an adjunct to dietary measures and a statin in primary and homozygous familial hypercholesterolaemia
Fibrates		
Used for hyperlipidaemias types IIa, IIb, III, IV and V in people who have not responded adequately to diet; most fibrates are carboxylic acid derivatives that are eliminated unchanged and as acyl glucuronides formed largely in the kidneys		
Bezafibrate	1–5 [R + M] Complete oral bioavailability; eliminated equally by renal excretion (unchanged) and by metabolism (conjugation and oxidation)	

Drugs used to treat hyperlipidaemias (all drugs given orally unless otherwise stated)

Drug	Half-life (h) and kinetics	Comments
Ciprofibrate	27–28 [M] Complete oral bioavailability; eliminated by glucuronidation; very low clearance (about 40 mL h^{-1}) causes long half-life	Not used in type V hyperlipidaemia
Fenofibrate	20–27 (FA) [M] Good oral bioavailability (60–90%) as FA (negligible ester absorbed intact); FA is eliminated mainly as the acyl glucuronide	Ester prodrug of fenofibric acid (FA)
Gemfibrozil	1–2 [R + M] Complete oral bioavailability; about one-half of the dose is excreted unchanged, with the remainder as hydroxylated metabolites and their conjugates	
Nicotinic acid and derivatives		
Acipimox	1–2 [R] Complete oral bioavailability; it is a polar pyridine-N-oxide derivative which has a low volume of distribution; undergoes limited reduction to the pyridine analogue (<5%) and is eliminated mostly by renal excretion	Used for hyperlipidaemia types IIa, IIb and IV in people who have not responded adequately to diet
Nicotinic acid (niacin)	0.3–0.8 [M + R] Rapidly and completely absorbed; at therapeutic doses, about one-third is excreted unchanged and the remainder is oxidised or conjugated with glycine	Used to reduce both cholesterol and triglycerides, but limited by vasodilation and hepatic effects
Other treatments		
Ispaghula	Not relevant	Soluble fibre which probably acts by reducing the reabsorption of bile acids in the bowel; acts as a bulk laxative (see Ch. 35)
Omega-3 acid ethyl esters	Not relevant	Used as an adjunct for treating hypertriglyceridaemias in those at a special risk of ischaemic heart disease
Omega-3 marine triglycerides	Not relevant	Used as an adjunct for treating hypertriglyceridaemias, but can aggravate hypercholesterolaemia

[B], biliary excretion; [M], metabolism; [R], renal excretion.

10

The skin and eyes

49 Skin disorders

TOPICAL APPLICATIONS

Topical preparations for the treatment of skin disorders usually have two components: a base and the active ingredient, such as a corticosteroid or an antifungal agent. Four types of base are used:

- ointments, which are greases such as white or yellow soft paraffin
- pastes, which are suspensions of powder in an ointment and will stay where they are put on the skin; their main use is to apply noxious chemicals that should be confined to one area of the skin
- creams, which are emulsions of water with a grease; they are less greasy than ointments, are absorbed more quickly into the skin, and are often used as a vehicle for active ingredients
- lotions, which are any kind of liquid; they are used on wet surfaces and hairy areas and their main advantage is that they do not make a mess.

The choice between an ointment and a cream depends on individual preference, unless the skin is very dry, when an ointment is better.

ATOPIC AND CONTACT DERMATITIS

Dermatitis describes eczematous inflammation with significant underlying genetic influences, which is triggered by external factors.

Atopic dermatitis (eczema)

This is associated with asthma and hayfever in about 30% of cases, and has a familial tendency. The pathogenesis is determined by a combination of genetic, environmental, pharmacological and immunological factors. There are two forms of atopic dermatitis: the extrinsic type (40% of cases) is associated with IgE-mediated sensitisation, while the intrinsic type is not. Many people with atopic dermatitis have an eosinophilia in the peripheral blood, with a raised plasma IgE concentration. Circulating mononuclear cells have a reduced ability to produce interferon gamma, which normally inhibits both IgE production and T-helper type 2 (Th2) lymphocyte proliferation. The function of T-regulator cells is also abnormal. Keratinocytes produce cytokines that stimulate eosinophil activation and adhesion to vascular walls.

As a result of the changes in the immune regulation, Th2-cells proliferate. Dominance of either a Th1 or Th2 response is partially programmed in early life, with exposure to microbial antigens promoting the normal Th1 dominance. Th1-cell responses, which are induced by infections, antagonise the development of Th2-cells, and therefore it is possible that the increasing use of antibacterial drugs in childhood may partially explain the rise in atopic dermatitis (Chs 38 and 39).

Affected skin is red, scaly and extremely dry, often affecting the flexures. The dryness is a consequence of the inflammation, but the permeability barrier function of the skin is also impaired, resulting in increased transepidermal water loss. There may be vesicles and weeping with crusting over the skin surface. Scratching produces excoriation and thickening of the skin. The affected skin is infiltrated with activated T-cells, with selective recruitment of Th2-cells, and eosinophils. Increased skin carriage of *Staphylococcus aureus* on the affected skin may also maintain skin inflammation by activating T-cells and macrophages.

Contact dermatitis

Two main types are recognised.

- due to an external agent inducing direct irritation.
- resulting from immunological sensitisation involving a delayed hypersensitivity response (Ch. 39). Once the skin has been sensitised, the potential for further reaction persists indefinitely. Sensitisation can arise in response to topical application of drugs.

Other types of dermatitis

These include nummular (discoid) eczema, photosensitive dermatitis and seborrhoeic dermatitis.

Treatment of atopic dermatitis

- emollients (substances that soften the skin) are helpful as hydrophobic agents that seal the surface of the skin and reduce water loss. Paraffin derivatives are most effective but are greasy and not well accepted by most people. Alternatives, such as aqueous creams, are more cosmetically acceptable.

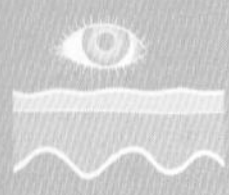

- avoidance of irritants, such as soaps, detergents, alcohols and astringents. Wet dressings may help to prevent skin fissuring and reduce scratching.
- identification of allergens by patch tests and their subsequent elimination.
- topical corticosteroid ointment (Ch. 44) is effective, but a low-potency corticosteroid should be chosen if there is continuous use, in order to minimise unwanted effects. The anti-inflammatory effect of these drugs makes them the mainstay of treatment, but tachyphylaxis (diminished effectiveness with prolonged use) limits their long-term value. Tachyphylaxis may be delayed by twice-weekly application of a more potent corticosteroid.
- topical calcineurin inhibitors, such as tacrolimus (Ch. 38), reduce activation of many of the inflammatory cells involved in the pathogenesis of the dermatitic lesions, including T-cells, dendritic cells, mast cells and keratinocytes. Local burning is the major unwanted effect, and skin malignancy has been reported. Tacrolimus is more effective than a potent corticosteroid for moderate to severe eczema.
- sedative antihistamines (Ch. 39) at night assist sleep, although they have little effect on itching. A topical formulation of the tricyclic antidepressant doxepin (see Ch. 22) is available to treat itch. It is uncertain whether its antihistamine activity is the major mode of action.
- immunosuppressant therapy with azathioprine, ciclosporin or mycophenolate mofetil (Ch. 38) can be tried for treatment-resistant dermatitis. Apart from unwanted effects, the main problem is rapid relapse when treatment is stopped.
- phototherapy with natural sunlight is helpful, but sweating can increase pruritus. Narrow-band ultraviolet B (UVB) is a useful alternative.
- tar bandages on the limbs are messy, but have anti-inflammatory and anti-pruritic effects.
- systemic antimicrobials are given for secondary infection. Anti-staphylococcal agents are often helpful if the skin lesions are poorly controlled.

Treatment of contact dermatitis

- Provision of a barrier to an irritant, for example wearing gloves, or removing an allergen may be sufficient.
- Dilute topical corticosteroid ointment (Ch. 44).
- Potassium permanganate soaks can help to dry up exudative lesions.

PSORIASIS

Psoriatic skin lesions are produced by a very rapid proliferation of epidermal cells. Cell turnover time is decreased from about 28 days to 3–4 days, which prevents adequate maturation. Instead of producing a normal keratinous surface layer, the skin thickens, forming a silvery scale with dilated upper dermal blood vessels. Psoriatic plaques (psoriasis vulgaris, accounting for 90% of cases) usually affect the elbows, knees, lower back, buttocks, scalp and nails. Various subtypes of the condition present with different clinical manifestations. An inflammatory arthritis occurs in up to 25% of people with psoriasis (see Ch. 30).

Inflammatory cells such as T-lymphocytes infiltrate into the dermis and then the epidermis. There is a genetic component to psoriasis, which interacts with unknown environmental factors to produce the immune reaction in the dermis. Antigen-presenting cells in the dermis mature after contact with the antigen, migrate to regional lymph nodes and activate T-cells. T-cells then proliferate and enter the circulation and extravasate into the skin at sites of inflammation, assisted by local chemokine production. In the dermis, interaction with the initiating antigen results in Th1 responses, with secretion of cytokines such as interferon gamma, IL-12 and IL-23 and tumour necrosis factor alpha (TNFα). The cytokines stimulate cell proliferation and impair maturation of keratinocytes, and produce vascular changes in the skin.

There are several treatments for the skin lesions, both topical and systemic, but none produce long-term remission. Increasingly, combinations of treatments have been found to be more effective than one agent alone. Psoriasis can be provoked or exacerbated by several drugs, including lithium, chloroquine, hydroxychloroquine, β-adrenoceptor antagonists, non-steroidal anti-inflammatory drugs and angiotensin-converting enzyme inhibitors.

Topical therapy

Emollients (see atopic dermatitis above)

These reduce scaling and itching and may be sufficient in mild psoriasis. They can also be used with a keratolytic.

Keratolytics

Keratolytics such as salicylic acid break down keratin and soften skin, which improves penetration of other treatments. Salicylic acid ointment is most frequently used.

Vitamin D analogues (e.g. calcipotriol, calcitriol)

Vitamin D regulates epidermal proliferation and differentiation. It also has immunosuppressant properties. Vitamin D analogues are clean and simple to apply and are particularly useful for chronic plaque psoriasis, although complete clearing of the plaques is unusual. Ointment has a greater emollient effect than has cream, but is messy to apply. Calcipotriol should not usually be used for the face, where it often causes irritation; calcitriol may be better tolerated on this site, although it is less effective elsewhere. Excessive use of vitamin D analogues can lead to hypercalcaemia, but this is not a problem at recommended dosages. The ease of use of these compounds makes them a popular choice if a keratolytic is insufficient.

Topical retinoids (e.g. tazarotene)

Retinoids are discussed more fully under systemic treatments. Tazarotene gel can be applied to plaque psoriasis and has minimal systemic absorption. Unlike other retinoids, tazarotene is selective for retinoic acid receptor (RAR) proteins, with no affinity for retinoid X receptors (RXR) (see below). This may reduce unwanted effects, which are mainly local irritation of healthy skin with pruritus. Tazarotene should be avoided for 1 month before conception, because of potential teratogenic effects.

Dithranol

This anthraquinone decreases cell division and is effective for healing psoriatic plaques. In hospital it is applied in a stiff paste to the plaque so that the dithranol does not burn normal skin, and left in contact with the plaque for 24 h. At home, dithranol is used as a cream that is applied to the plaque for 30 min and then washed off. The oxidation products of dithranol stain the skin brown, leaving discoloration of healed areas for a few days. They also stain bedding and clothes a mauve colour that will not wash out. Since dithranol irritates normal skin, it should not be used in flexures.

Coal tar preparations

Crude coal tar is a mixture of a large number of hydrocarbons that have a cytostatic action. It enhances the healing effect of UVB radiation on psoriatic lesions. The main disadvantage is messiness, and its efficacy when used alone is modest. More refined tar preparations have greater acceptability, but are even less effective.

Phototherapy

Ultraviolet light produces improvement by inhibiting DNA synthesis and depleting intra-epidermal T-cells. It should not be used on individuals with very fair skin who burn in the sun. Broad-band UVB ('sunburn' wavelength 270–350 nm) has largely been replaced by the more effective narrow-band UVB (311–313 nm). Long-wavelength UVA (320–400 nm) requires more specialised equipment and prior administration of an oral psoralen as a photosensitising drug (a process called photochemotherapy or PUVA). Psoralen probably locates between pyrimidine base pairs in the DNA helix and inhibits cell replication. PUVA is usually reserved for severe, resistant psoriasis and it is more effective than treatment with UVB. Psoralen can produce nausea and headache acutely. The long-term risks of PUVA include accelerated skin ageing and an increased incidence of skin cancer, and systemic treatments are increasingly preferred.

Topical corticosteroid preparations

These should be used sparingly on limited areas, since unwanted effects can be troublesome (Ch. 44). Withdrawal of a high-potency corticosteroid can produce a rebound exacerbation and even generalised pustular psoriasis.

Systemic treatments

Apart from emollients and corticosteroids, which are most useful for chronic plaque psoriasis, topical treatments should be avoided in more inflammatory forms of the condition because they can cause troublesome skin irritation. Systemic treatment is reserved for the most severe forms of disease.

Methotrexate (Chs 38 and 52)

This is a very effective treatment at low dosages for resistant and widespread disease. Its main actions are cytostatic and immunosuppressant. Oral or intramuscular dosing is commonly used once a week. Bone marrow depression and hepatotoxicity with liver fibrosis are the main complications; blood counts and serum procollagen III to identify liver toxicity must be checked every 3 months.

Retinoids

This term covers vitamin A (retinol) and therapeutically useful synthetic vitamin A derivatives, such as acitretin, the active metabolite of etretinate (which is no longer used). Given orally, they are anti-inflammatory and cytostatic. Vitamin A, and its metabolites all-*trans*-retinoic acid and 9-*cis*-retinoic acid, are involved in epithelial cell growth and differentiation. Retinoids enter cells by endocytosis and interact with two forms of retinoic acid nuclear receptor, RARs and RXRs, which are related to steroid/thyroid hormone receptors (Ch. 1). The retinoid–receptor complex initiates gene transcription and may affect cell growth and differentiation by modulation of growth factors and their receptors. Response of psoriatic lesions is delayed by up to 2 months. Elimination of retinoids is by hepatic metabolism, and the half-life of acitretin is about 2 days. Unwanted effects are almost universal and include dry lips and nasal mucosa, dryness of the skin with localised peeling over the digits, and transient thinning of hair. These effects are dose-dependent and reversible. Longer-term problems include ossification of ligaments, increased plasma triglycerides and, to a lesser extent, increased plasma cholesterol. There is a high risk of teratogenesis, and women must use adequate contraception during treatment and stop treatment for 2 years before conception.

Ciclosporin or tacrolimus (Ch. 38)

These immunosuppressants are effective in psoriasis at lower doses than those required for prevention of allograft rejection. However, remissions induced by these drugs are usually short-lived.

Biologic agents

Etanercept, infliximab and adalimumab (Chs 30 and 34) are intravenous therapies that block TNFα and are highly effective in treatment-resistant psoriasis. They inhibit the production of chemokines and endothelial adhesion molecules that attract activated lymphocytes into the skin. Infliximab produces a more rapid response than etanercept. Efalizumab is an inhibitor of T-cell activation that impairs adhesion of T-cells to endothelial cells and prevents them from entering the skin. It occasionally causes 'flu-like symptoms' and may precipitate an initial inflammatory flare of the psoriasis. Ustekinumab, an inhibitor of interleukins (IL)-12 and IL-23 has been shown to be effective for plaque psoriasis. IL-12 and IL-23 are products of dendritic cells and macrophages which activate T-cells involved in the inflammatory response in psoriasis.

Fumaric acid esters

This is an oral treatment for severe psoriasis that probably works by promoting a Th2-cell response in place of the Th1-dominant response found in psoriasis. This results from inhibition of nuclear factor kappa B (NF-κB) with enhanced T-cell apoptosis. Fumaric acid is poorly absorbed from the gut, and is therefore given as an ester. This is rapidly hydrolysed by esterases to monomethylfumarate, the active compound, and further metabolised in cells to water and carbon dioxide in the citrate cycle. Monomethylfumarate has a very long half-life of about 36 h. Unwanted effects include gastrointestinal upset in more than two-thirds of people, and flushing in one-third.

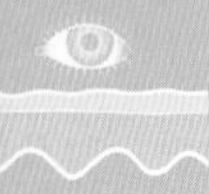

ACNE

Acne most commonly arises in adolescence and often regresses in the late teens or early twenties. Acne affects areas of skin with large numbers of sebaceous glands: the face, back and chest. There is increased production of sebum, which distends the pilosebaceous duct, producing a small closed papule (comedo) called a whitehead. Hyperkeratosis at the mouth of the hair follicle blocks the duct. If the duct then opens, compacted follicular cells at the tip give comedones the appearance of a blackhead. A resident anaerobic bacterium, *Propionibacterium acnes*, degrades triglycerides in sebum to free fatty acids and glycerol. It also produces chemotactic factors and inflammatory mediators. These, and the irritant free fatty acids, produce inflamed lesions of pustules, nodules, or multilocular cysts if the lesions coalesce. The inflammatory lesions can scar, leaving permanent disfigurement.

There is a genetic background to acne, which determines the rate of sebum production, particularly in response to androgens. Androgens, which are produced at puberty, induce hypertrophy of sebaceous glands, and the excess secretion rate in predisposed individuals triggers the acne. Acne can also be produced by systemic corticosteroids and anabolic steroids (Ch. 46). In women, it can be a manifestation of polycystic ovary syndrome (Ch. 43).

Treatment of acne

There are several effective treatments for acne. The choice will depend on the nature of the lesions and their severity. Topical treatments do not influence the rate of production of sebum.

Topical treatments

- *Benzoyl peroxide* has antibacterial activity against *P. acnes* and a keratolytic action, both of which reduce the numbers of comedones. It produces scaling and skin irritation, which may limit its use to short treatment periods.
- *Topical antibacterials*, for example clindamycin and erythromycin (Ch. 51), are less effective than oral antibacterials but have fewer unwanted effects. Their efficacy is similar to that of benzoyl peroxide, with less skin irritation. Combination therapy with benzoyl peroxide reduces the problem of bacterial resistance. Topical antibacterials are used for mild to moderate acne, and are particularly useful in pregnant women since there is no systemic absorption.
- *Isotretinoin* (13-*cis*-retinoic acid) is a vitamin A derivative that has a keratolytic action which unblocks the pilosebaceous follicles and allows flow of sebum to extrude the plug. The mechanism of action is similar to that of acitretin (see under psoriasis). It also reduces sebum production by up to 90% by decreasing sebocyte proliferation (this action is probably independent of effects on nuclear retinoid receptors). Topically, isotretinoin produces erythema and scaling, which can be minimised by starting with a low concentration. Adapalene is an extensively modified retinoid that has a faster onset of action and produces less skin irritation.
- *Azelaic acid* is an aliphatic dicarboxylic acid that has an antibacterial action against propionibacteria and is effective against bacteria that have become resistant to erythromycin and tetracycline. It also inhibits the division of keratinocytes, which may reduce follicular plugging and prevent the development of comedones. It is applied topically. The most frequent unwanted effects are local burning, scaling or itching, although hypopigmentation can also be a problem. Azelaic acid is most effective for mild to moderate non-inflammatory comedonal acne, especially of the face.
- *Nicotinamide* gel has equivalent efficacy to topical antibacterials. It has an anti-inflammatory action by inhibiting production of lipids in sebaceous secretions (Ch. 48). Unwanted effects include dryness, pruritus and burning of the skin.

Systemic treatments

- Oral antibacterials that are active against *P. acnes* are used for inflammatory acne (papules/pustules). Penetration into sebaceous follicles is poor, but they produce some improvement after 2–3 months, requiring 4–6 months of treatment for maximal benefit. Treatment should be given for extended periods, since relapse is common if it is stopped. Among the more useful antibacterial agents are tetracyclines, for example oxytetracycline and doxycycline. Alternatives include ciprofloxacin and cotrimoxazole (Ch. 51). Resistance to erythromycin makes it a less suitable choice than in the past.
- The anti-androgen cyproterone acetate (Ch. 46) is useful in women with moderate or severe acne and is usually given in combination with ethinylestradiol (Ch. 45). The combination reduces sebum flow by 40%. Alternatively, oestrogen can be given with a non-androgenic progestogen such as norgestimate or desogestrel. Improvement can take 2–4 months.
- Isotretinoin is used orally in severe acne and gives an almost 100% probability of complete remission. High doses can produce prolonged remission. Unwanted effects include dry lips, nose and eyes, increased plasma triglycerides, and, less commonly, myalgia. Teratogenesis is a major problem, and, although the half-life of the metabolites is less than 2 days, conception should be avoided during and for one menstrual cycle after stopping treatment.

Choice of treatment for acne

Initially, management of non-inflammatory comedones is by topical treatment such as azelaic acid or retinoids. For early inflammatory lesions, a topical antibacterial or benzoyl peroxide can be considered, alone or in combination. More severe inflammatory acne usually requires topical or systemic antibacterials with topical retinoid. Systemic treatment with isotretinoin is used for severe unresponsive acne. Oestrogen and anti-androgen therapy are alternatives for women, and oral contraceptives can be of benefit. Overall, the most common reason for treatment failure is probably non-adherence to the recommended regimen.

WOUND HEALING

Becaplermin

Mechanism of action and use

Becaplermin is a human recombinant platelet-derived growth factor (PDGF). Endogenous PDGF is synthesised by megakaryocytes, macrophages, fibroblasts, smooth muscle cells and endothelial cells. Platelets release PDGF after tissue injury. PDGF contributes to tissue healing by encouraging cell chemotaxis and activation of inflammatory cells, and by increasing extracellular matrix deposition, cell mitogenesis and cell protein synthesis. This enhances granulation tissue in wounds. Becaplermin can be used to enhance healing of chronic neuropathic diabetic foot ulcers.

Pharmacokinetics

Becaplermin is applied topically as a gel. There is negligible systemic absorption.

Unwanted effects

A local erythematous rash can occur. Concern over the possibility of local carcinogenesis appears unfounded.

FURTHER READING

Bieber T (2008) Atopic dermatitis. *N Engl J Med* 358, 1483–1494

Brown S, Reynolds NJ (2006) Atopic and non-atopic eczema. *BMJ* 332, 584–588

Haider A, Shaw JC (2004) Treatment of acne vulgaris. *JAMA* 292, 726–735

Menter A, Griffiths CEM (2007) Psoriasis 2. Current and future management of psoriasis. *Lancet* 370, 272–284

Naldi L, Rebora A (2009) Seborrheic dermatitis. *N Engl J Med* 360, 387–396

Purdy S, de Berker D (2006) Acne. *BMJ* 333, 949–953

Reynolds NJ, Al-Daraji WI (2002) Calcineurin inhibitors and sirolimus: mechanisms of action and application in dermatology. *Clin Exp Dermatol* 27, 555–561

Schön MP, Boehncke WH (2005) Psoriasis. *N Engl J Med* 352, 1899–1912

Smith CH, Barker JNWN (2006) Psoriasis and its management. *BMJ* 333, 380–384

Wasserbauer N, Ballow M (2009) Atopic dermatitis. *Am J Med* 122, 121–125

Williams HC (2005) Atopic dermatitis. *N Engl J Med* 352, 2314–2324

SELF-ASSESSMENT

In questions 1–3, the first statements, in italics, are true. Are the accompanying statements also true?

1. *Atopic dermatitis is the most common form of dermatitis and is an inflammatory condition with a familial tendency. It involves acute and chronic inflammation.*
   a. Topical corticosteroids should not be used in atopic dermatitis.
   b. Antihistamines given orally can reduce itching in atopic dermatitis.
2. *Dominance of Th1-type lymphocytes is important in psoriasis.*
   a. Immunosuppressant drugs are contraindicated in severe resistant psoriasis.
   b. Retinoids reduce cell growth and differentiation.
3. *Severe inflammatory acne should be treated with topical or systemic antibacterials and a topical retinoid.*
   a. Suitable topical antibacterials for inflammatory acne are erythromycin and clindamycin.
   b. Antibacterial resistance in *Propionibacterium acnes* is rare.
4. You have discussed with 50-year-old Mr PP the treatment options for his widespread psoriasis. He was also taking medication for high blood pressure. Choose the one **correct** option from the following.
   A. Mr PP thought that the atenolol he was taking as part of the regimen to lower his blood pressure did not affect his psoriasis.
   B. Mr PP would not go on holiday to Spain because he had heard that sunshine would make his psoriasis worse.
   C. Mr PP was pleased that he had been prescribed methotrexate; it helped his condition and he had read that it had few unwanted effects.
   D. Topical application of the vitamin D analogue calcipotriol applied topically would help improve his condition.
   E. Using a TNFα antibody would be of little benefit in psoriasis resistant to other treatments.
5. Case history questions

A 7-year-old girl with a history of asthma developed a red, scaly and dry rash in her knee and elbow flexures and on her arms and cheeks. The rash was extremely itchy and she was scratching the affected areas, causing excoriation and weeping. Her mother had had atopic dermatitis when she was young.

   a. What was the possible diagnosis?
   b. What treatments should be tried initially?
   c. What other factors should have been considered in the treatment of this young girl?

ANSWERS

1. a. **False**. Topical corticosteroids (e.g. hydrocortisone cream) are the mainstay of treatment of atopic dermatitis, used for up to 4 weeks.
   b. **True**. One of the sedative antihistamines (e.g. promethazine) may be of value, although direct effect on itching may be limited. Other topical antihistamines and topical doxepin (an antidepressant) are also available.

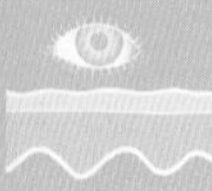

2. a. **False**. In severe psoriasis, ciclosporin or methotrexate can be used.
   b. **True**. Oral retinoids such as vitamin A and derivatives reduce cell growth and can be used in psoriasis, but they can be teratogenic. Oral and topical retinoids are also useful in acne.
3. a. **True**.
   b. **False**. Resistance is increasing. There is cross-resistance between erythromycin and clindamycin, and, when possible, drugs with an antibacterial action such as benzoyl peroxide or azelaic acid should be used.
4. Answer **D**.
   A. Incorrect. β-Adrenoceptor antagonists can exacerbate psoriasis.
   B. Incorrect. Regular short daily exposure doses of sunlight may benefit psoriasis. It increases production of vitamin D in the skin and ultraviolet rays fight psoriasis by slowing down the rapid proliferation of the skin cells. Sunburn should be avoided. Ultraviolet exposure is a treatment for psoriasis.
   C. Incorrect. Methotrexate can produce bone marrow depression and hepatoxicity and regular monitoring is required.
   D. Correct. Calcipotriol has several beneficial actions, including inhibition of T-cell proliferation and the release of inflammatory cytokines.
   E. Incorrect. Etanercept and infliximab have been shown to be of benefit in treatment of resistant psoriasis.
5. Case history answers
   a. Atopic dermatitis is possible because of the appearance of the rash and the child's atopy and the previous history of her mother.
   b. The following are the initial management approaches:
      - good skin hygiene with regular bathing but avoidance of soaps
      - emollients in bath water and topically applied to moisturise the skin and reduce water loss
      - short courses of topically applied hydrocortisone as the mainstay of treatment
      - if necessary, topically applied antihistamine or oral sedative antihistamine if the itch is severe, although there is not a consensus that antihistamines are beneficial; topical doxepin may also help reduce itch.
   c. Assessment of contributory factors such as food allergies and other allergens, psychological factors, and removal of irritants and allergens. Severe acute exacerbations may require rigorous topical measures and antibacterial treatment.

Drugs used in the treatment of skin disorders

Drug[a]	**Half-life (h)**[b] **and kinetics**	**Comments**
Corticosteroids		
Given topically for inflammatory skin conditions		
Alclometasone dipropionate	– [M] About 3% of the applied dose is absorbed across the skin over a period of 8 h; fate of absorbed compound has not been defined	Synthetic corticosteroid
Betamethasone esters	– [M] Poor absorption; little is absorbed from the forearm but higher absorption occurs from the forehead, scrotum, eyelids and from inflamed skin; hydration of the skin increases drug uptake and absorption	Use is restricted to severe conditions, such as eczemas unresponsive to less potent drugs
Clobetasol propionate	– [M] Very poor absorption (see betamethasone esters)	Use is restricted to short-term treatment of severe resistant conditions, such as eczemas unresponsive to less potent drugs; suppression of adrenocortical function is possible in people with psoriasis
Clobetasone butyrate	– [M] Poorly absorbed (see betamethasone esters)	Used for eczemas and dermatitis of all types
Diflucortolone valerate	– [M] Transdermal absorption is probably similar to betamethasone esters	Use is restricted to severe conditions, such as eczemas unresponsive to less potent drugs, and for psoriasis; few data available; only weak adrenocortical effects compared with clobetasol propionate
Fludroxycortide	– [M] The route of elimination is predicted as no data are available	No published data have been identified
Fluocinolone acetonide	– [M] Poorly absorbed (see betamethasone esters); eliminated by hepatic metabolism	

Drugs used in the treatment of skin disorders

Drug[a]	Half-life (h)[b] and kinetics	Comments
Fluocinonide	– [M] Poorly absorbed (see betamethasone esters); the route of elimination is predicted as no data are available	Use is restricted to severe conditions, such as eczemas unresponsive to less potent drugs, and for psoriasis
Fluocortolone	1.5 [M] Few data available after topical dosing	Use is restricted to severe conditions, such as eczemas unresponsive to less potent drugs, and for psoriasis
Fluprednidene acetate	? [?] No human kinetic data identified	
Fluticasone propionate	2–5 [M] Poorly absorbed transdermally (see betamethasone esters); half-life is following inhalation exposure	Use is restricted to severe conditions, such as eczemas unresponsive to less potent drugs, and for psoriasis
Hydrocortisone	1.5 [M] Poorly absorbed transdermally (see betamethasone esters); probably undergoes metabolism within the skin; see Ch. 44	
Hydrocortisone butyrate	1.5 [M] Poorly absorbed transdermally (see betamethasone esters); the ester group is completely hydrolysed during transdermal absorption; half-life is for hydrocortisone	Use of the butyrate ester is restricted to severe conditions, such as eczemas unresponsive to less potent drugs
Mometasone furoate	5 [M] Very poor absorption (see betamethasone esters); extensively metabolised, with metabolites eliminated in urine and bile	Use is restricted to severe conditions, such as eczemas unresponsive to less potent drugs, and for psoriasis
Triamcinolone acetonide	2–5 [M] Poorly absorbed from the skin (see betamethasone esters); rapidly eliminated from the blood by oxidation and then conjugation	Use is restricted to severe conditions, such as eczemas unresponsive to less potent drugs, and for psoriasis
Drugs for eczema and/or seborrhoeic dermatitis		
(Topical corticosteroids may also be given)		
Ichthammol	–	A sulphonated shale oil that is used as an ointment or cream
Pimecrolimus	30–40 (oral) [M] Very limited absorption across the skin and no skin-mediated metabolism; absorbed drug is metabolised by CYP3A	Calcineurin inhibitor; used for mild to moderate atopic eczema
Tacrolimus	9 (oral) [M] Limited absorption across the skin; see Ch. 38	Calcineurin inhibitor; used topically for moderate to severe atopic eczema unresponsive to other treatment
Drugs for psoriasis		
Acitretin	50 [M] Long half-life owing to low hepatic extraction and metabolism	Retinoid used for severe extensive and resistant psoriasis; teratogenic risk; given orally
Calcipotriol (calcipotriene)	– [M] About 5% absorbed after topical application; few data available (very short plasma half-life in animal studies)	Vitamin D analogue used for plaque psoriasis; given topically
Calcitriol	3–6 [M] Metabolised by hydroxylation and conjugation	Vitamin D analogue used for mild to moderate plaque psoriasis; given topically; see Ch. 42
Ciclosporin	27 [M] Oral bioavailability is about 30%; oxidised by intestinal and hepatic CYP3A4; see also Ch. 38	Used for short-term treatment of severe atopic dermatitis and severe psoriasis; given orally

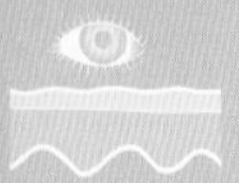

Drugs used in the treatment of skin disorders

Drug[a]	**Half-life (h)**[b] **and kinetics**	**Comments**
Coal tar	– [M] High transdermal absorption; coal tar contains polycyclic aromatic hydrocarbons which are oxidised (and activated) by CYP1A2	Also used occasionally for chronic atopic eczema; applied topically
Dithranol (anthralin)	– [M] Poorly absorbed across the skin; metabolised within the skin	Used for subacute and chronic psoriasis; given topically
Efalizumab	– [M] 50% bioavailability after subcutaneous injection; few kinetic data available	Used for moderate to severe chronic plaque psoriasis; given by subcutaneous injection
Methotrexate	8–10 [M] Good oral absorption (20–95%); metabolised by the formation of polyglutamates (which are active and retained intracellularly) and by oxidation	Folate antagonist used in the treatment of severe uncontrolled psoriasis, rheumatoid arthritis (see Ch. 30) and malignant disease (see Ch. 52); given orally or by intravenous or intramuscular injection
Salicylic acid	– See Ch. 29	Used with coal tar and dithranol preparations as a keratolytic in scaly psoriasis; applied as a paste containing zinc oxide
Tacalcitol	– [M] Negligible absorption after topical dosage	Vitamin D_3 analogue (1,24-dihydroxyvitamin D_3) used for plaque psoriasis; applied as an ointment
Tazarotene	18 (TA) [M] Poorly absorbed across the skin; hydrolysed in skin to tazarotenic acid (TA), which is further metabolised; TA is responsible for binding to retinoid receptors	Retinoid used for mild to moderate plaque psoriasis; given topically
Ustekinumab	15–32 days. Metabolism unknown.	Antibody directed at IL-12, IL-23; used for moderate to severe psoriasis resistant to other therapy; unwanted effects include arthralgia, cough, headache, respiratory tract infection; given by subcutaneous injection
Drugs for acne and rosacea		
In addition to the topical preparations given below, antibiotics such as clindamycin, doxycycline, erythromycin, minocycline, oxytetracycline, tetracycline and trimethoprim may be given in the treatment of acne		
Adapalene	– [B] Very low topical absorption; eliminated in bile; very few data available	Retinoid-like drug; binds to nuclear but not cytosolic retinoid receptors; given topically
Azelaic acid	0.75 [R] Low absorption (about 4%); eliminated unchanged in the urine (plus some limited β-oxidation); as for most topical drugs, absorption rate-limited kinetics result in a half-life after topical dosage (2 h) that is considerably longer than the elimination half-life	Antimicrobial and anticomedonal actions; given topically
Benzoyl peroxide	– [M] About 5% of the benzoic acid is absorbed	Powerful oxidising agent that is reduced to benzoic acid; given topically
Co-cyprindiol	NA	A mixture of cyproterone acetate and ethinylestradiol used for the treatment of severe acne unresponsive to antibiotics and for hirsutism in women at low risk of thromboembolism (which is increased by this treatment)
Isotretinoin	10–20 [M] Metabolised by oxidation and formation of an acyl glucuronide; isomerises to all-*trans*-retinoic acid	Retinoid (13-*cis*-retinoic acid); given topically and may be given orally but known to be a human teratogen largely due to its conversion to all-*trans*-retinoic acid
Tretinoin	1–2 [M] Metabolised by oxidation and formation of an acyl glucuronide; systemic half-life is derived from studies following its formation from vitamin A	Retinoid (all-*trans*-retinoic acid); given topically

Drugs used in the treatment of skin disorders

Drug[a]	Half-life (h)[b] and kinetics	Comments
Drugs used to assist wound healing		
Becaplermin	Not absorbed	Recombinant human platelet-derived growth factor; enhances formation of granulation tissue; applied topically
Preparations for warts and calluses		
Preparations not suitable for application to face or anogenital areas		
All compounds are used topically to produce localised tissue destruction		
Formaldehyde	–	Used for warts, particularly plantar warts
Glutaraldehyde	–	Used for warts, particularly plantar warts
Salicylic acid	–	Used for plantar and mosaic warts, corns, verrucas and calluses
Silver nitrate	–	Used for warts, verrucas, umbilical granulomas and over-granulation tissue
Preparations suitable for application to anogenital areas		
All compounds are used topically for soft non-keratinised external warts; risk of severe systemic toxicity		
Imiquimod	2 (subcutaneous) [?] Minimal percutaneous absorption; half-life is about 20–30 h after dermal application, indicating retention within the skin	Left on treated area for a maximum of 8–10 h; also used for superficial basal cell carcinoma
Podophyllum	–	Left on treated area for a maximum of 6 h

[a]The majority of treatments are given topically and show very slow and limited absorption.
[b]The systemic half-lives (when given) are not an indication of duration of action of topical formulations.
[B], biliary excretion; [M], metabolism; [R], renal excretion; NA, not applicable, as the 'drug' is a combination preparation.

50 The eye

Vision depends upon the eye converting light falling on the retina into an electrical signal to be carried to the brain through the optic nerve. The eye must focus objects sharply on the retina, a process called accommodation. To adjust the innate focus to achieve this, the ciliary muscle alters the shape of the lens, allowing the eye to accommodate to objects at different distances. The iris determines the size of the pupil and the amount of light entering the eye. The autonomic nervous system innervates the ciliary muscles and the iris.

Accommodation

The ciliary muscle is a circular (constrictor) smooth muscle that is attached to the lens by suspensory ligaments. The ciliary muscle only has a parasympathetic nerve supply (mediated by acetylcholine acting through muscarinic receptors; Ch. 4) and contracts in response to parasympathetic stimulation. As a result, tension on the suspensory ligaments is reduced and the capsule of the lens is relaxed. The lens then becomes shorter and fatter and accommodates for near objects. In the absence of parasympathetic stimulation, the ciliary muscle is relaxed and tension on the suspensory ligaments increases. This pulls on the capsule, which flattens the lens and adjusts visual acuity for distant vision. Drugs that are agonists at muscarinic receptors fix the lens for near objects, blurring far vision. Drugs that block muscarinic receptors fix the lens for far objects, with blurring of near vision, a state known as cycloplegia (Fig. 50.1).

Pupil size

This is determined by the relative tone in the two smooth muscle layers of the iris. The circular (constrictor) muscle is the more powerful and receives parasympathetic nervous innervation, mediated by acetylcholine, which acts on muscarinic receptors. The radial (dilator) muscle is sympathetically innervated, and its effects are mediated by noradrenaline, acting on α_1-adrenoceptors. Constriction of the pupil is known as miosis and can occur in response to drugs that stimulate muscarinic receptors and constrict the circular muscle of the iris; dilation is called mydriasis and can occur in response to drugs that block muscarinic receptors in the circular muscle or that stimulate α_1-adrenoceptors in the radial muscle of the iris. The light reflex is the primary determinant of pupil size. Pupillary constriction also accompanies accommodation for near vision, a response mediated by the parasympathetic nervous system. Dilation of the pupil is caused by shortening of the radial muscle, which also has the effect of moving the iris towards the cornea and narrowing the anterior angle between the iris and the cornea. This can reduce aqueous humour outflow through the canal of Schlemm.

Drainage of aqueous humour

The space between the cornea, at the front of the eye (Fig. 50.1), and the iris is the anterior chamber and is filled with a clear liquid known as aqueous humour. Contraction of the ciliary muscle aids drainage of aqueous humour through the trabecular meshwork into the episcleral veins. Pressure in the eye is maintained by a balance between the production of aqueous humour and its drainage. The intraocular pressure rises if drainage of the aqueous humour is impaired. High intraocular pressure is one of the factors that can damage retinal ganglion cells, leading to progressive loss of vision in the disease known as glaucoma. If the anterior chamber of the eye is abnormally shallow, this results in a narrow anterior angle (Fig. 50.1), and dilation of the pupil may narrow the angle to an extent where it impedes drainage of aqueous humour through the trabecular meshwork. This can result in an acute rise in pressure (acute angle-closure glaucoma) (Fig. 50.1). Conversely, constriction of the circular muscle of the iris makes the pupil smaller and moves the iris away from the trabecular meshwork to the canal of Schlemm, widening the anterior angle and facilitating drainage.

TOPICAL APPLICATION OF DRUGS TO THE EYE

Drugs applied in solution to the anterior surface of the eye can penetrate to the anterior chamber and the ciliary muscle, principally via the cornea. The high water content of the cornea makes lipid solubility less important for adequate penetration of a drug than is the case for transdermal drug delivery, but formulation of the carrier is important to avoid irritation of the conjunctiva. There is little diffusion to the more posterior structures of the eye.

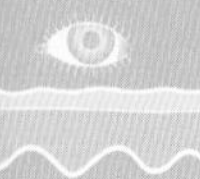

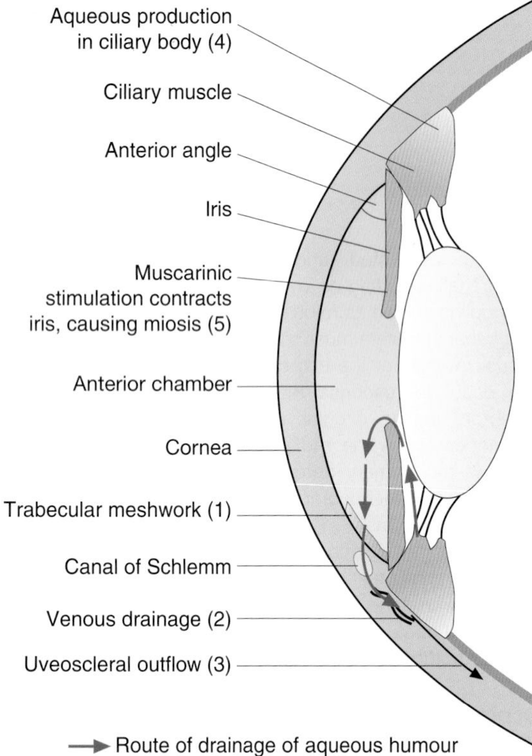

Fig. 50.1 **The route of drainage of aqueous humour from the eye, and the sites and mechanisms of action of drugs used in the treatment of glaucoma.** The mechanisms by which several drugs benefit glaucoma are still uncertain but are thought to include the following:

- In angle-closure glaucoma, muscarinic agonists, e.g. pilocarpine, constrict iris circular constrictor pupillae (5), widening the anterior angle and facilitating aqueous humour drainage (1,2).
- Carbonic anhydrase inhibitors, e.g. acetazolamide, decrease aqueous humour production (4).
- Beta-adrenoceptor antagonists, e.g. timolol, reduce aqueous humour production (4) and increase outflow (1).
- Selective α_2-adrenoceptor agonist, e.g. apraclonidine, brimonidine, decrease aqueous humour production (4).
- Prostaglandin analogues selective for stimulation of the prostaglandin $F_{2\alpha}$ (FP) receptor, e.g. latanoprost, enhance aqueous humour outflow (1,2,3) and may improve ocular blood flow.

Systemic absorption of drug following topical application to the surface of the eye can occur either via conjunctival vessels or from the nasal mucosa after drainage of excess drug via the tear ducts. Topical administration of drugs to the eye may therefore produce systemic effects. Drainage can be reduced by shutting the eyes for at least 1 min after putting the drops in and by compressing the nasolacrimal duct at the medial corner of the eye with a finger. Both eye-drops and ointments are usually administered into the pocket that can be formed by gently pulling the lower eyelid downwards (the lower fornix).

Microbial contamination is a potential problem once eye preparations have been opened. Multiple-application containers have preservative added to reduce the risk, but it is not advisable to use any eye preparation more than a month after it has been opened.

GLAUCOMA

Glaucoma is a group of disorders characterised by loss of retinal ganglion cells. In some cases, the intraocular pressure is raised, and ischaemia of the optic nerve head may be the cause. In many cases, however, the pressure in the anterior chamber of the eye is normal and a genetic susceptibility to ganglion cell apoptosis is responsible. Progressive visual defects occur, initially as scotomas (blind spots) in the peripheral visual field. These scotomas enlarge, resulting in tunnel vision and finally total blindness. Glaucoma is the second most common cause of blindness in the UK.

Aqueous humour is constantly secreted by the ciliary body. Most aqueous humour flows through the pupil to the anterior chamber, and leaves the eye via the trabecular meshwork that drains to the episcleral veins through the canal of Schlemm (Fig. 50.1). Some drains through the sclera (uveoscleral outflow). Production of aqueous humour is influenced by innervation from the autonomic nervous system. Alpha$_2$-adrenoceptor stimulation of the ciliary body reduces the production of aqueous humour, while β_1-adrenoceptor stimulation increases its production. Outflow of aqueous humour is also influenced by innervation from the autonomic nervous system, and by prostaglandins. **Open-angle glaucoma** is caused by obstruction in the trabecular meshwork. **Angle-closure glaucoma** is less common, usually acute in onset, and results from the iris blocking the drainage angle and preventing drainage through the trabecular meshwork. This usually arises when there is a shallow anterior chamber, such as occurs in long-sighted individuals. There is a greater prevalence of angle-closure glaucoma in Asians and Inuit compared with Caucasians. Chronic angle-closure glaucoma is rare.

DRUGS FOR GLAUCOMA

Beta-adrenoceptor antagonists

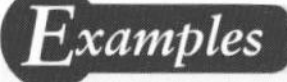

betaxolol, timolol

Beta-adrenoceptor antagonists reduce the formation of aqueous humour. They have no effect on accommodation or pupil size. Systemic absorption can produce the typical unwanted effects associated with these compounds, particularly bronchospasm, bradycardia and worsening of uncontrolled heart failure (Ch. 5). The contraindications for topical use in the eye are the same as those for oral use. Timolol is a non-selective β-adrenoceptor antagonist, while betaxolol is 'cardioselective'; they have similar efficacy in the eye.

Sympathomimetics

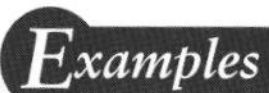

brimonidine, dipivefrine

Dipivefrine is converted to adrenaline (epinephrine) in the eye, and has greater penetration through the cornea than has adrenaline (epinephrine). It is mydriatic (dilates the pupil) by stimulating α_1-adrenoceptors in the radial muscle of the iris, and should not be used in angle-closure glaucoma. It improves drainage through the trabecular meshwork and decreases aqueous humour production by α_2-adrenoceptor stimulation. Dipivefrine should be used with care in people with hypertension and heart disease, because of the potential to cause systemic vasoconstriction.

Brimonidine is a selective α_2-adrenoceptor agonist that decreases ciliary body aqueous humour production and is not mydriatic.

Carbonic anhydrase inhibitors

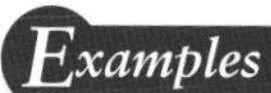

acetazolamide, brinzolamide, dorzolamide

The mechanism of action of the carbonic anhydrase inhibitors is discussed in Chapter 14. Carbonic anhydrase in the eye plays a key role in controlling aqueous humour production. It is responsible for secreting about 70% of the Na^+ that enters the anterior chamber, which is followed by water to maintain isotonicity. Therefore, inhibition of the enzyme reduces aqueous humour production.

Acetazolamide is taken orally. Dorzolamide and brinzolamide are topical preparations for the eye, with fewer systemic unwanted effects; their duration of action in the eye is 6–12 h, but they have extremely long plasma half-lives (≥2 weeks) due to retention within erythrocytes.

Prostaglandin analogues

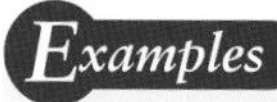

latanoprost, travoprost

These drugs are analogues of prostaglandin $F_{2\alpha}$. Their precise mechanism of benefit in glaucoma remains uncertain; however, they increase uveoscleral outflow of aqueous humour. This may result in part from an increase in extracellular matrix metalloproteinases in ciliary smooth muscle cells, and from remodelling of the uveal meshwork. The prostaglandin analogues also increase blood flow to the optic nerve, and this may contribute to neuroprotection in the retina. The reduction in intraocular pressure is greater than that achieved by β-adrenoceptor antagonists. The major disadvantage of prostaglandin analogues is an increase in brown pigmentation of the iris and growth of eyelashes. A rare complication in people who have no lens in the eye (aphakia) is the development of cystoid macular oedema, which responds to treatment with non-steroidal anti-inflammatory drugs. The prostaglandin analogues have a long duration of action of 1–2 days that is not a reflection of their half-lives.

Miotic drugs (muscarinic agonists)

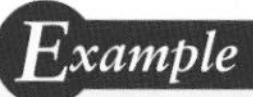

pilocarpine

Pilocarpine (see also Ch. 4) is usually given for angle-closure glaucoma to contract the circular sphincter muscle of the iris to produce miosis and open up the drainage channels in the anterior chamber of the eye. The miotic effect lasts for about 4 h, and more prolonged miosis can be achieved by the use of a gel delivery system. Ciliary muscle spasm is an undesirable consequence and produces blurred vision and an ache over the eye (especially in younger people). Pilocarpine can be used together with other drugs in simple open-angle glaucoma.

TREATMENT OF GLAUCOMA

In open-angle glaucoma, reducing intraocular pressure can slow the rate of disease progression sufficiently to prevent significant visual impairment. A target pressure reduction of at least 30% below the presenting pressure is usually set.

In primary open-angle glaucoma, a topical β-adrenoceptor antagonist or a prostaglandin analogue is the treatment of choice, because of their relative lack of ocular unwanted effects, providing there are no contraindications. If either treatment alone is insufficient, then a combination can give an additive effect. If these agents cannot be used, then the choice of a second-line drug lies between pilocarpine, a topical carbonic anhydrase inhibitor or an α_2-adrenoceptor stimulant. Surgery may also be considered at this point. Laser burns applied to the trabecular meshwork can produce a temporary increase in aqueous humour outflow, but drug treatment may still be required. Drainage surgery is the alternative and can often bring about long-term pressure control. Several potentially neuroprotective drugs are under investigation to retard neuronal degeneration in the retina.

Angle-closure glaucoma is treated by laser peripheral iridotomy or surgical peripheral iridectomy to provide a channel for aqueous humour to flow through the iris. If drug therapy is required after surgery, then topical treatment with a prostaglandin analogue or a β-adrenoceptor antagonist can be used.

MYDRIATIC AND CYCLOPLEGIC DRUGS

Antimuscarinics

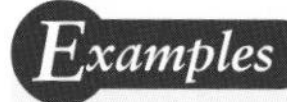

atropine, cyclopentolate, homatropine, tropicamide

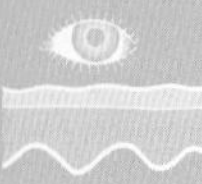

Antimuscarinic drugs (see also Ch. 4) are both mydriatic (dilating the pupil) and cycloplegic (paralysing the ciliary muscle). Tropicamide is weak and short-acting (about 3 h), which makes it useful for dilating the pupil for fundal examination. Cyclopentolate and homatropine both last for up to 24 h and are more powerful; the former has a more rapid onset of action. Atropine is long-acting, the effect persisting for up to 7 days. The longer-acting compounds are used to prevent adhesions (posterior synechiae) in anterior uveitis (often in combination with phenylephrine). Dark irises are more resistant to pupillary dilation with these drugs, as the pigments adsorb the applied drug.

The degree of cycloplegia will depend on the dose of drug; small doses produce pupil dilation with insufficient diffusion to reach the ciliary muscle and have much affect on accommodation. The law does not specifically prohibit driving after pupil dilation, but many people find that their vision is impaired for several hours. Care must be taken when using these drugs in individuals predisposed to acute angle-closure glaucoma. Local irritation in the eye is the most common unwanted effect, but systemic effects occasionally occur in children or the elderly (see Ch. 4).

Sympathomimetics

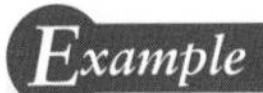

phenylephrine

Phenylephrine is a relatively selective α_1-adrenoceptor agonist that stimulates the radial muscle of the iris and produces mydriasis. It does not affect the ciliary muscle, and therefore does not affect accommodation. It is a vasoconstrictor, and can decrease vascular congestion of the conjunctiva and eyelid oedema in allergic conjunctivitis. In this role, it is often combined with an antihistamine in over-the-counter preparations. Local irritation is the most common unwanted effect, although systemic vasoconstriction with hypertension or coronary artery spasm can occur occasionally. It is often given together with muscarinic receptor blocking drugs to produce pupil dilation for procedures such as cataract operations.

OTHER TOPICAL APPLICATIONS FOR THE EYE

Several other drugs are used topically in the eye.

Antibacterial agents (Ch. 51)

These are given for local infections such as blepharitis, conjunctivitis or trachoma (caused by chlamydial infection). Aqueous solutions are rapidly diluted or flushed away by lacrimation and should initially be used every 1–2 h; ointments are often given for longer action, for example at night. Examples of broad-spectrum agents are gentamicin, chloramphenicol, ciprofloxacin, fusidic acid, neomycin and chlortetracycline (the last for trachoma).

Antiviral agents (Ch. 51)

These are mainly used for herpes simplex infection, which causes dendritic corneal ulcers. Aciclovir is most frequently used.

Corticosteroids

Local inflammatory conditions of the anterior part of the eye, such as uveitis and scleritis, are treated with corticosteroids, for example dexamethasone or prednisolone (Ch. 44). Care must be taken to exclude a viral dendritic ulcer and glaucoma before using them, since these conditions can be exacerbated by corticosteroids. Prolonged use of corticosteroids can lead to thinning of the sclera or cornea, or formation of a ‘steroid cataract’.

Antiallergic agents

Topical antihistamines such as antazoline (usually given in combination with the sympathomimetic xylometazoline) or levocabastine (Ch. 39) can be given for allergic conjunctivitis. Topical sodium cromoglicate or nedocromil (Ch. 12) are generally less effective than antihistamines.

Local anaesthetics

Oxybuprocaine or lidocaine eye-drops provide surface anaesthesia (Ch. 18) for tonometry (measurements of pressure in the anterior chamber). For minor surgical procedures, such as removal of cataracts, tetracaine gives more profound anaesthesia and may be combined with injection of a small amount of lidocaine into the anterior chamber.

Non-steroidal anti-inflammatory drugs

Diclofenac, flurbiprofen and ketorolac (Ch. 29) can be applied topically for pain following surgery or laser treatment in the eye.

Artificial tears

Hypromellose (hydroxypropyl-methylcellulose) is most commonly used to treat dry eyes, such as occurs in Sjögren’s syndrome. It may need to be reapplied every hour. The surface mucin in the eye is often abnormal when there is tear deficiency, and the mucolytic agent acetylcysteine is often added to hypromellose. Carbomers, synthetic high-molecular-weight polymers of acrylic acid, cling better to the surface of the eye than hypromellose and need less frequent application.

AGE-RELATED MACULAR DEGENERATION (ARMD)

Age-related macular degeneration is the main cause of irreversible visual loss in the Western world. Damage to the macula, the central part of the retina, leads to partial or complete loss of central vision. There are two clinical types:

- dry (non-exudative) form that involves hypertrophic changes in the retinal pigment epithelium under the macula, with formation of yellow deposits called drusen
- wet (exudative) form with development of new blood vessels (choroidal neovascularisation) under the macula, with leakage of blood and fluid.

Non-exudative maculopathy is common (85–90% of all macular pathology) and is associated with minor visual disturbance. By contrast, exudative ARMD produces severe visual loss in 70% of eyes within 2 years. The non-exudative form of ARMD can progress to the exudative form.

TREATMENT OF ARMD

Treatment is only available for exudative ARMD. Options include:

- High-dose antioxidants.
- Laser photocoagulation of neovascular tissue.
- Photodynamic therapy using the photosensitising agent verteporfin. Verteporfin is infused intravenously and activated in the eye by non-thermal red light, producing cytotoxic derivatives.
- Intravitreal injection of a vascular growth factor inhibitor such as the monoclonal antibodies bevacizumab or ranibizumab, or the pegylated oligonucleotide pegaptanib. These agents inhibit vascular endothelial growth factor (VEGF), a protein that induces angiogenesis and increases vascular permeability.

Treatment of exudative ARMD slows the loss of visual acuity in 20–30% of eyes compared to no treatment.

FURTHER READING

Bielory L (2002) Ocular allergy guidelines. *Drugs* 62, 1611–1634

Coleman AL (1999) Glaucoma. *Lancet* 354, 1803–1810

Ghate D, Edelhauser HF (2008) Barriers to glaucoma drug delivery. *J Glaucoma* 17, 147–156

Hylton C, Robin AL (2003) Update on prostaglandin analogs. *Curr Opin Ophthalmol* 14, 65–69

Ishida N, Odani-Kawabata N, Shimazaki A et al (2006) Prostanoids in the therapy of glaucoma. *Cardiovasc Drug Rev* 24, 1–10

Jager RD, Mieler WF, Miller JW (2008) Age-related macular degeneration. *N Engl J Med* 358, 2606–2617

Saw S-M, Gazzard G, Friedman DS (2003) Interventions for angle-closure glaucoma. An evidence-based update. *Ophthalmology* 110, 1869–1879

Singh A (2005) Medical therapy of glaucoma. *Ophthalmol Clin North Am* 18, 397–408

Takeda AL, Colquitt J, Clegg AJ et al (2007) Pegaptanib and ranibizumab for neovascular age-related macular degeneration: a systematic review. *Br J Ophthalmol* 91, 1177–1182

SELF-ASSESSMENT

In questions 1 and 2, the first statement, in italics, is true. Are the accompanying statements also true?

1. *The production of aqueous humour is not altered in glaucoma but drainage is reduced.*
   a. Dipivefrine is the drug of choice in patients with angle-closure glaucoma.
   b. Stimulation of α_2-adrenoceptors in the ciliary body reduces aqueous humour production.
   c. Tropicamide should be avoided in people with glaucoma.
2. *Accommodation of the lens is controlled by the parasympathetic autonomic nervous supply to the ciliary muscle.*
   a. Cocaine is a local anaesthetic that does not alter pupil size when administered topically.
   b. Cyclopentolate is a longer-acting mydriatic drug than tropicamide.
   c. Pilocarpine causes accommodation for near vision.
3. Extended-matching questions
   Which is an appropriate drug A–H in response to the statements 3.1–3.5? Each option may be used more than once or not at all.
   A. Cocaine
   B. Pilocarpine
   C. Dipivefrine
   D. Phenylephrine
   E. Tetracaine
   F. Tropicamide
   G. Timolol
   H. Atropine
   3.1. An antagonist of receptors in the ciliary body that will reduce aqueous production in glaucoma and has no effect on pupil size.
   3.2. An agonist of receptors in the ciliary body that will reduce aqueous production in glaucoma and affects pupil size.
   3.3. A drug that will dilate the pupil without affecting accommodation or aqueous humour production.
   3.4. A relatively short-acting drug that will dilate the pupil and is weakly cycloplegic.
   3.5. A long-acting drug that can be used to prevent adhesions (posterior synechiae) in anterior uveitis and is strongly cycloplegic.
4. Case history questions

During a routine eye examination, the optician noted a chronically raised intraocular pressure in a 56-year-old woman. Further tests revealed she had open-angle (simple) glaucoma.

   a. What is the most common cause of open-angle glaucoma?
   b. What drugs could have been used for this condition?
   c. What precautions should have been taken when using these drugs?

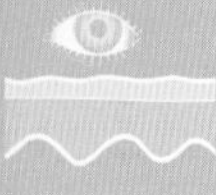

ANSWERS

1. a. **False**. Dipivefrine is used in open-angle not angle-closure glaucoma. It is converted to adrenaline (epinephrine) in the eye and can cause mydriasis, which serves to narrow even further the angle between the iris and the cornea.
   b. **True**.
   c. **True**. Tropicamide blocks the muscarinic receptors in the circular muscle of the iris, causing mydriasis, which narrows the anterior angle and may reduce aqueous draining in angle-closure glaucoma.
2. a. **False**. Cocaine causes mydriasis as well as having a local anaesthetic effect. It prevents the reuptake of released noradrenaline, which contracts the radial muscle, narrowing the drainage angle.
   b. **True**. Cyclopentolate acts for 12–24 h, whereas tropicamide has a duration of action of about 3 h.
   c. **True**. Pilocarpine is a muscarinic receptor stimulant; it contracts the ciliary muscle, causing the lens to shorten and bulge and accommodate for near vision.
3. Extended-matching answers
   3.1. Answer **G**. A β-adrenoceptor antagonist such as timolol reduces aqueous production but does not affect the pupil size, which is controlled by muscarinic and α_1-adrenergic receptors on the circular and radial muscles, respectively, of the iris.
   3.2. Answer **C**. Dipivefrine is converted to adrenaline which decreases aqueous humour by an α_2-adrenoceptor action and dilates the pupil by an α_1-adrenoceptor stimulation of the radial muscle of the iris.
   3.3. Answer **D** and **A**. Phenylephrine will dilate the pupil (α_1-adrenoceptor stimulation of the iris) but not the ciliary muscle (muscarinic receptors). Cocaine will also dilate the pupil by preventing reuptake of released noradrenaline.
   3.4. Answer **F**. Tropicamide is a relatively short-acting muscarinic antagonist with only a relatively weak blocking action on muscarinic receptors on the ciliary muscle. Atropine is very long-acting.
   3.5. Answer **H**. Atropine is a long-acting mydriatic that can be used to prevent adhesions but has a marked effect to block accommodation for near vision (cycloplegia).
4. Case history answers
   a. Reduced drainage of aqueous humour through the trabecular meshwork into the canal of Schlemm and the episcleral veins.
   b. Beta-adrenoceptor antagonists or prostaglandin analogues are the drugs of first choice. Alpha$_2$-adrenoceptor stimulants, inhibitors of carbonic anhydrase, or muscarinic agonists could also be used.
   c. Beta-adrenoceptor antagonists: avoid if asthma, bradycardia, heart block, heart failure. Prostaglandin analogues: avoid in pregnancy and asthma. Alpha$_2$-adrenoceptor stimulants: avoid if severe cardiovascular disease. Carbonic anhydrase inhibitors: can cause hypokalaemia and electrolyte imbalance; they should be avoided in pregnancy. Muscarinic agonists: avoid if conjunctival or corneal damage, cardiac disease, asthma.

Drugs used in the eye

Drug[a]	Half-life (h)[b] and kinetics	Comments
Treatment of infections		
Antibacterials		
See Ch. 51– systemic treatment may be necessary in some cases		
Chloramphenicol	5 (2–12) [M] Eliminated mainly by glucuronidation	Broad spectrum; used for a wide range of infections; drug of choice for superficial eye infections
Ciprofloxacin	3–4 [R + M] Eliminated by glomerular filtration, renal tubular secretion plus metabolism (15%)	Broad spectrum; used for a wide range of infections, including *Pseudomonas aeruginosa*; used for corneal ulcers
Fusidic acid	9 [M] Metabolised in liver and metabolites excreted in bile	Used for staphylococcal infections
Gentamicin	1–4 [R] Eliminated by glomerular filtration	Broad spectrum; used for a wide range of infections, including *Pseudomonas aeruginosa*
Levofloxacin	6–8 [R + M] Almost 90% is excreted unchanged in urine by glomerular filtration and renal tubular secretion	Active against Gram-positive and especially Gram-negative organisms
Neomycin	2 [R] Eliminated by glomerular filtration	Broad spectrum; used for a wide range of infections

Drugs used in the eye

Drug[a]	Half-life (h)[b] and kinetics	Comments
Ofloxacin	6–7 [R + M] Eliminated by kidneys plus limited metabolism (<5%)	Broad spectrum; used for a wide range of infections, including *Pseudomonas aeruginosa*
Polymyxin B	4–6 [R] Elimination is prolonged in subjects with renal impairment	Used for Gram-negative organisms
Propamidine isetionate	? [?] No relevant kinetic data available	Principal use is for treatment of the rare but devastating condition *Acanthamoeba* keratitis
Antivirals		
Aciclovir	3 [R + M] Eliminated largely by renal tubular secretion + filtration; only about 10% is metabolised to inactive excretory products	Used for local treatment of herpes simplex infections; see Ch. 51
Ganciclovir	4 [R] Eliminated largely by glomerular filtration	Used as slow-release implants inserted surgically for sight-threatening CMV retinitis; see Ch. 51
Treatment of inflammation		
Corticosteroids		
The drugs shown below are used locally for short-term treatment of inflammation (oral corticosteroids are given for treating anterior segment inflammation – see. Ch. 44)		
Betamethasone	35–55 [M] Phosphate ester hydrolysed to betamethasone, which is inactivated by metabolism	
Dexamethasone	2–4 [M] Metabolised in the liver by CYP3A4-mediated oxidation to the 6-hydroxy compound	
Fluorometholone	? [M] Metabolism probably occurs locally in the eye; systemic disposition has not been defined	Only used topically
Hydrocortisone acetate	1–2 [M] Metabolised by oxidation to cortisone and reduction to dihydro- and tetrahydrocortisol	
Prednisolone	2–4 [M] Extensively metabolised, but all pathways have not been defined	
Rimexolone	1–2 [M + B] The elimination half-life has been estimated by the fact that steady-state levels are achieved after 5–7 h; few other data available	Only used topically
Other anti-inflammatory preparations		
Many are histamine H_1 receptor antagonists – see also Ch. 39		
Antazoline	? [?] Metabolised by in vitro liver preparations; no relevant kinetic data are available	Used for allergic conjunctivitis; histamine H_1 receptor antagonist
Azelastine	17 [M] Metabolised by hepatic P450 to active desmethyl metabolite	Used for allergic conjunctivitis; histamine H_1 receptor antagonist
Emedastine	3–4 [M] Eliminated in urine largely as oxidised metabolites plus about 5% as the unchanged drug	Used for seasonal allergic conjunctivitis; histamine H_1 receptor antagonist
Epinastine	12 [R + M] About 50% is eliminated unchanged in urine and 30% in faeces; only limited (10%) metabolism	Used for seasonal allergic conjunctivitis; histamine H_1 receptor antagonist

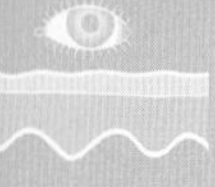

Drugs used in the eye

Drug[a]	Half-life (h)[b] and kinetics	Comments
Ketotifen	22 [M] Metabolised by formation of an N-glucuronide	Used for seasonal allergic conjunctivitis; antihistamine and mast cell stabiliser; rapid onset of action after application to the eye and negligible systemic exposure
Lodoxamide	8 [R] Eliminated largely in the urine as the parent drug; few data available	Used for allergic conjunctivitis; mast cell stabiliser
Nedocromil	2 [R] Highly polar compound showing slow absorption across membranes; once in the blood it is eliminated rapidly by renal excretion (a slower late phase with a half-life of 14 h has been reported but this is probably of little clinical relevance)	Used for allergic conjunctivitis; mast cell stabiliser
Olopatadine	3 [R + M] Detectable plasma levels after administration into the eye which persist for up to 2 weeks	Used for seasonal allergic conjunctivitis; antihistamine and mast cell stabiliser
Sodium cromoglicate	1–1.5 [R] Highly polar drug that shows limited absorption across cell membranes; absorbed drug is eliminated largely in the urine	Used for allergic conjunctivitis; mast cell stabiliser
Mydriatics and cycloplegics		
Atropine	2–5 [M + R] Probably well absorbed; undergoes limited hydrolysis, plus oxidation and conjugation; about 30% of the dose is excreted unchanged in the urine	Used for refraction procedures in children and for anterior uveitis; longer-acting antimuscarinic
Cyclopentolate	2 [?] Peak plasma concentrations occur about 30 min after giving eye-drops; method of elimination has not been described	Used for refraction procedures in children; longer-acting antimuscarinic
Homatropine	– Probably well absorbed; no relevant kinetic data are available	Used for treatment of anterior segment inflammation; antimuscarinic
Phenylephrine	2–3 [M + R] Eliminated in urine as glucuronic acid and sulphate conjugates and as parent compound (15–20% after intravenous dosage)	Sympathomimetic α_1-selective adrenoceptor agonist
Tropicamide	0.3 (or less) [?] Rapidly absorbed after ophthalmological dosage; peak plasma concentration occurs at 5 min, decreasing rapidly to undetectable levels by 2 h	Used to facilitate examination of the fundus; short-acting antimuscarinic
Local anaesthetics		
See Ch. 18		
Lidocaine	2 [M] Metabolised by dealkylation, catalysed by CYP3A4, followed by hydrolysis	
Oxybuprocaine (benoxinate)	– [M] Few kinetic data available; about 90% recovered in urine as parent drug and metabolites within 9 h (therefore half-life is 3 h or less)	Widely used
Proxymetacaine	– Few kinetic data available	Causes less initial stinging and is useful for children

Drugs used in the eye

Drug[a]	Half-life (h)[b] and kinetics	Comments
Tetracaine	Very short (?) [M] Any absorbed drug would be very rapidly hydrolysed by pseudocholinesterase (butyrylcholinesterase, plasma cholinesterase)	Widely used; produces more profound anaesthesia and is suitable for minor procedures
Treatment of glaucoma		
Beta-adrenoceptor antagonists		
Effective in chronic simple glaucoma		
Betaxolol	13–24 [M] Oxidised in liver, and metabolites eliminated in urine	Selective for β_1-adrenoceptors
Carteolol	3–7 [R + M] Mostly eliminated in urine unchanged; the main metabolite (8-hydroxycarteolol) is a more potent β-adrenoceptor antagonist	
Levobunolol	5–8 [M + R] Eliminated in urine as parent drug (about 15%), as a reduced metabolite and as conjugates of the parent drug and metabolite	
Metipranolol	5 [M] Various pathways of metabolism, including deacetylation, giving a highly active metabolite (which is responsible for in vivo activity on cardiac β-adrenoceptors); the role of local metabolism in relation to ocular effect is not known	
Timolol	2–5 [M + R] Eliminated by metabolism and renal excretion (20%)	Non-selective β-adrenoceptor antagonist
Miotics		
Carbachol	– No relevant kinetic data are available	Muscarinic agonist
Pilocarpine	1 [M] Few details available; oxidised to an acid analogue	Muscarinic agonist; ocular effects persist for 4–14 h
Sympathomimetics		
Apraclonidine	8 [M] Measurable systemic absorption	Used short term before or after surgery; agonist at α_2-adrenoceptors
Brimonidine	3 [M] Metabolised by human liver preparations to oxidised products; relative importance of metabolism and other routes of elimination have not been defined	Used alone or in combination with a β-adrenoceptor antagonist for ocular hypertension and alone for open-angle glaucoma if β-adrenoceptor antagonists are ineffective or inappropriate; agonist at α_2-adrenoceptors
Dipivefrine	? [M] The majority is converted to adrenaline (epinephrine); limited systemic absorption	A prodrug of adrenaline (epinephrine) that passes more rapidly through the cornea
Carbonic anhydrase inhibitors		
Acetazolamide	6–9 [R] Eliminated in urine without detectable metabolism	Used for open-angle, and secondary and preoperative angle-closure glaucoma; given orally or by intravenous injection as an adjunct to other treatments; not recommended for long-term use
Brinzolamide	11 days [R + M] Distributes into erythrocytes, where it has a very long half-life (111 days)	Used topically in combination with a β-adrenoceptor antagonist for ocular hypertension and open-angle glaucoma if β-adrenoceptor antagonists alone are ineffective, or alone if β-adrenoceptor antagonists are inappropriate

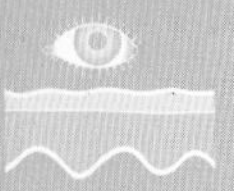

Drugs used in the eye

Drug[a]	Half-life (h)[b] and kinetics	Comments
Dorzolamide	Weeks [R + M] Blood concentrations are not detectable after ophthalmological use; an active de-ethylated metabolite has been reported; retained in red blood cells, which gives rise to an elimination half-life on cessation of the treatment of weeks	Used topically in combination with a β-adrenoceptor antagonist for ocular hypertension, and open-angle and pseudo-exfoliative glaucoma if β-adrenoceptor antagonists alone are ineffective, or alone if β-adrenoceptor antagonists are inappropriate
Prostaglandin analogues		
Used to reduce pressure in ocular hypertension and open-angle glaucoma		
Bimatoprost	45 min (intravenous) [M] Rapid absorption with peak blood levels within 10 min, which decrease rapidly over the next hour; metabolised by oxidation and conjugation	Used alone or as adjunctive therapy
Latanoprost	0.3 (acid) [M] The parent compound can be measured in the plasma during the first hour after ophthalmological administration; metabolised to an active acid metabolite, which has a half-life of 0.3 h	Analogue of $PGF_{2\alpha}$; the reduction of intraocular pressure occurs at about 8–12 h (systemic disposition gives no indication of therapeutic effect)
Travoprost	– [M] A prodrug that is hydrolysed by esterases in the eye to the active form, travoprost acid	A synthetic analogue of $PGF_{2\alpha}$

[a]Drugs are usually given topically to reduce unwanted systemic effects.
[b]The half-life data in this table refer to the systemic fate following absorption into the general circulation – the duration of action locally will depend on the rate of uptake by, and removal from, the eye.
[B], biliary excretion; [M], metabolism; [R], renal excretion.

11

Chemotherapy

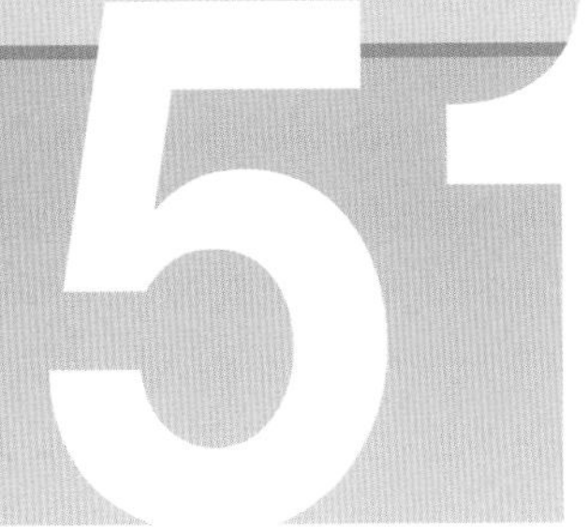

Chemotherapy of infections

Antimicrobial drugs are natural or synthetic chemical substances that suppress the growth of, or destroy, microorganisms, including bacteria, fungi and viruses. The term antibiotic is widely used, but strictly should be reserved for those antimicrobial drugs that are derived from microorganisms. The term antimicrobial or the more restrictive terms antibacterial, antifungal and antiviral are used in this book.

Effective antimicrobial drugs have certain key attributes. In order to avoid unwanted effects in humans, most are designed to have actions on processes that are unique to the target pathogen. They must also be able to penetrate human tissues to reach the site of infection. Many microorganisms can acquire resistance to various antimicrobial drugs and will then no longer be affected by the drug, and there is a continuing effort to discover and develop antimicrobial drugs that avoid or overcome the evolving mechanisms of resistance.

BACTERIAL INFECTIONS

CLASSIFICATION OF ANTIBACTERIAL DRUGS

Antibacterial drugs can be classified in several overlapping ways.

First, they can be **bacteriostatic** or **bactericidal**. This categorisation depends largely on the concentration of drug that can be achieved safely in plasma without causing significant toxicity in the person who takes the drug. Bacteriostatic antibacterials inhibit bacterial growth but do not destroy the bacteria at concentrations in plasma that are safe for humans; following inhibition of growth, the natural immune mechanisms of the body are used to eliminate the bacteria. Such drugs will be less effective in immunocompromised individuals or when the bacteria are dormant and not dividing. Bactericidal antibacterials kill bacteria at plasma concentrations that are safe for humans, but even then, immune mechanisms will play a role in the final elimination of the bacteria. Some bactericidal drugs are more effective when bacterial cells are actively dividing, and may therefore be less effective if taken together with a bacteriostatic drug. For antibacterials to be bactericidal they must be present at adequate concentration; too low a concentration may render them bacteriostatic.

Secondly, antibacterials can be grouped according to their **mechanisms of action** (Fig. 51.1):

- drugs can inhibit the synthesis of peptidoglycans of the cell wall of the bacterium, or activate enzymes that disrupt the cell wall (e.g. β-lactams).

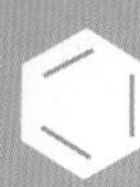

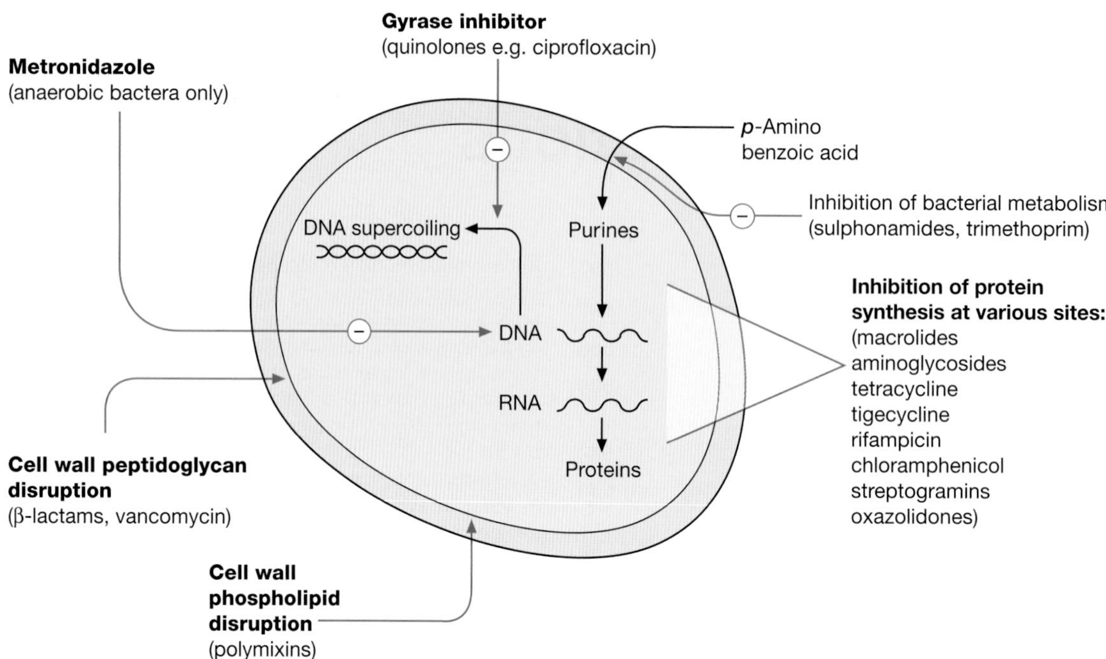

Fig. 51.1 **A simplified scheme of the sites of action of the main classes of antibacterial drugs.**

- drugs can act directly on the cell phospholipid membrane and affect its permeability, leading to leakage of intracellular contents (e.g. polymyxins).
- drugs can alter ribosomal function, producing a reversible inhibition of protein synthesis (e.g. aminoglycosides, macrolides). Such drugs can show a high degree of selectivity for bacteria because bacterial 70S ribosomes differ structurally from the 80S ribosomes in humans.
- drugs can block metabolic pathways that are essential for the life of the bacteria (e.g. trimethoprim).
- drugs can interfere with replication of DNA or RNA in the bacteria (e.g. quinolones).

Thirdly, antibacterials may be classified according to whether their **spectrum of activity** against bacteria is limited (narrow spectrum) or extensive (broad spectrum).

Finally, they can be classified by **chemical structure**.

In the following text, the antimicrobial drugs are grouped according to their mechanism of action and then by their chemical structure. However, cross-referencing to other methods of classification is necessary. The drug compendium is organised to accord with the *British National Formulary* (BNF).

ANTIMICROBIAL RESISTANCE

When an antibacterial is ineffective against a bacterium at doses that have historically been effective, the organism is said to be resistant to the antibacterial drug. Resistance to antibacterial drugs can be intrinsic to the bacterium (innate resistance) or can be acquired by modification of its genetic structure (acquired resistance).

Resistance is a major problem for infections with bacteria, and also for many protozoa (e.g. malaria) and viruses (e.g. HIV), but is less significant in fungal infections (unless the person is immunodeficient).

Antibacterial drug resistance

There are four general processes by which a bacterium can acquire resistance to antibacterial drugs (Fig. 51.2):

- modification of the bacterium such that it produces enzymes that inactivate the drug; examples are β-lactamase enzymes, which inactivate some penicillins, and acetylating enzymes, which can inactivate aminoglycosides
- modification of the bacterium so that penetration of the drug is reduced; an example is the absence of the membrane protein D2 porin in resistant *Pseudomonas aeruginosa*, which prevents penetration of the β-lactam antibacterial imipenem
- acquisition of efflux pumps that remove the antibacterial drug from the cell faster than it can enter; an example is quinolone efflux pumps in *Staphylococcus aureus*
- structural change in the target molecule for the antibacterial drug; examples are mutated penicillin-binding proteins in resistant enterococci that have a low affinity for binding of cephalosporins and mutant dihydrofolate reductase that is not inhibited by trimethoprim (see Fig. 51.4).

The major mechanisms by which bacteria acquire resistance to antibacterial drugs are spontaneous mutation, conjugation, transduction and transformation.

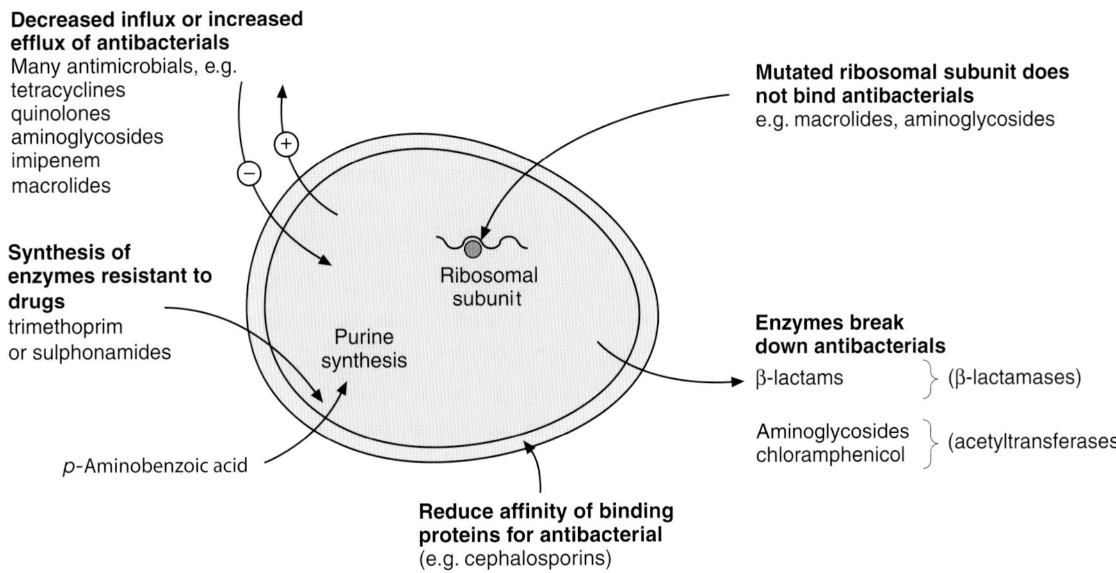

Fig. 51.2 **Mechanisms by which bacteria can resist antibacterial drugs.**

Spontaneous mutation

In this process, a single-step genetic mutation in a bacterial population leads to resistant organisms that selectively survive and grow while sensitive bacteria are killed by an antibacterial drug. This is termed *vertical evolution*.

The other mechanisms involve acquisition from other resistant organisms of genetic material that confers resistance. This is termed *horizontal evolution*. A transposon may facilitate transfer of sections of DNA from one organism to another.

Conjugation

Direct cell-to-cell contact is a way of exchanging genetic material that confers antibacterial resistance. It usually involves transfer of self-replicating circular fragments of DNA called plasmids, which can contain multiple resistance genes. Transfer occurs via a connecting structure called a pilus. The plasmid can remain outside the genome of the bacterium or can be incorporated into it, when it is more stable but less transmissible. Conjugation is by far the most important source of extrinsic DNA transfer between bacteria.

Transduction

Bacteria are susceptible to infection by viruses known as bacteriophages. During replication of the bacteriophages, the host cell's DNA (containing resistance genes) may be replicated along with viral DNA and taken into the virus. The phage carrying the resistance genes can then infect other bacterial cells and spread resistance. This is a rare method of acquired resistance.

Transformation

Uptake of DNA from dead bacteria by live bacteria can spread resistance genes.

ANTIBACTERIAL DRUGS

The antibacterial drugs in this section are grouped by their mechanism of action and then by their chemical structure.

DRUGS AFFECTING THE CELL WALL: β-LACTAM ANTIBACTERIALS

The drugs in this class each have a β-lactam ring; the intact nature of this ring structure is responsible for their activity (Fig. 51.3). The β-lactams include penicillins, cephalosporins and cephamycins, monobactams and carbapenems. Some are susceptible to attack by bacterial enzymes that split the β-lactam ring (β-lactamases, also known as penicillinases) but some are structurally modified to confer resistance to β-lactamase inactivation.

Penicillins

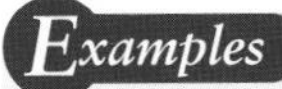

Penicillins: benzylpenicillin, phenoxymethylpenicillin
Aminopenicillins: amoxicillin, ampicillin, flucloxacillin
Ureidopenicillins: piperacillin
Amidinopenicillin: pivmecillinam
Carboxypenicillin: ticarcillin

Mechanism of action

The β-lactam antibacterials bind to penicillin-binding proteins and inhibit synthesis of the peptidoglycan layer of the cell wall which surrounds certain bacteria and is essential for their survival. Cross-linking in the cell wall utilises transpeptidases which are inhibited by β-lactam

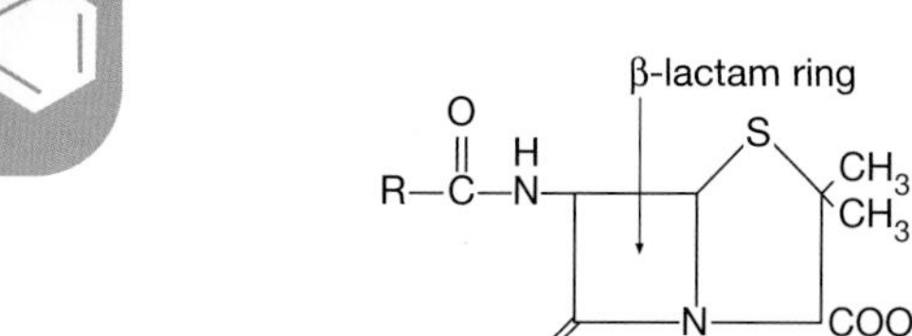

Fig. 51.3 **The structural backbone of β-lactam antibacterial drugs and the β-lactamase inhibitor clavulanic acid.**

antibacterials; the transpeptidases are amongst a number of penicillin-binding proteins in bacterial cells (see below). The antibacterial effect of β-lactam antibacterials is confined to dividing cells, which are unable to maintain their transmembrane osmotic gradient. This leads to cell swelling, which is followed by rupture and death of the bacterium.

Some bacterial cells also contain enzymes that, when activated, cause cell lysis. The β-lactam antibacterials bind to a variety of specific penicillin-binding proteins within bacteria, which reduces the natural inhibitors of lysis-inducing enzymes, thereby leading to lysis of the bacterial cell wall.

Penicillins consist of a thiazolidine ring connected to a β-lactam ring, to which is attached a side-chain (Fig. 51.3). The side-chain determines many of the antibacterial and pharmacological characteristics of particular penicillins.

Spectrum of activity

There is a range of penicillins that differ considerably in their spectra of activity (Table 51.1).

Benzylpenicillin (penicillin G) and phenoxymethyl penicillin (penicillin V) are active against many aerobic Gram-positive bacteria, a more limited range of Gram-negative bacteria, for example cocci (e.g. gonococci and meningococci), and many anaerobic micro-organisms. Gram-negative bacilli are not sensitive to benzylpenicillin. They are only effective against organisms that do not produce β-lactamases (see below).

The addition of an acyl side-chain to the β-lactam ring, to produce derivatives such as flucloxacillin, prevents access of β-lactamase to the β-lactam ring. However, flucloxacillin is generally less effective than benzylpenicillin against those bacteria that do not produce β-lactamase. Therefore, flucloxacillin is usually reserved for treating β-lactamase-producing staphylococci, which are particularly common in hospitals.

Ampicillin and amoxicillin are aminopenicillins that have an extended spectrum of activity to include many Gram-negative bacilli. However, they are less effective than benzylpenicillin against Gram-positive cocci. Both drugs are inactivated by β-lactamase.

Other extended-spectrum penicillins include ureidopenicillins (e.g. piperacillin), which are active against *Pseudomonas aeruginosa*, and amidinopenicillins (e.g. pivmecillinam), which are active mainly against Gram-negative bacteria. Carboxypenicillins (e.g. ticarcillin) are not widely used now, but have activity against *Pseudomonas* species, *Proteus* species and *Bacteroides fragilis*.

Clavulanic acid is a potent inhibitor of β-lactamase that is structurally related to the β-lactam antibiotics, although it has little intrinsic antibacterial activity (Fig. 51.3). When given in a combined formulation with penicillins that are destroyed by β-lactamase, such as amoxicillin (as co-amoxiclav) or ticarcillin (Table 51.1), it can be used to treat infections caused by some β-lactamase-producing organisms that would otherwise be resistant. Tazobactam has similar properties to clavulanic acid, and is used in combination with piperacillin.

Resistance

Resistance to penicillins is most often due to the production of β-lactamases which hydrolyse the β-lactam ring (Fig. 51.3). There are hundreds of β-lactamases, many of which are closely related to penicillin-binding proteins, but some are structurally different metalloenzymes. The β-lactamases produced by various organisms have widely differing spectra of activity. Some bacteria release extracellular β-lactamases, particularly *Staphylococcus aureus*. In Gram-negative bacteria, the β-lactamases are located between the inner and outer cell membranes in the periplasmic space. The genetic information for β-lactamase

Table 51.1 Examples of penicillins and their properties

	GRAM-POSITIVE STAINING			GRAM-NEGATIVE STAINING		
	Streptococci	***Staphylococcus aureus***		**Enterobacteriaceae (coliforms)**	***Pseudomonas aeruginosa***	***Bacteroides fragilis***
		β-Lactamase negative	***β-Lactamase positive***			
Benzylpenicillin/ phenoxymethylpenicillin	+	+	0	0	0	++
Broader spectrum						
Amoxicillin/ampicillin	+	+	0[a]	++	0	0
β-Lactamase resistant						
Flucloxacillin	+	+	+[b]	0	0	0
Antipseudomonal						
Ticarcillin	+	+	0[c]	+	+	+/0
Piperacillin	+	+	0[c]	+	+	+/0

[a]Can be used combined with a β-lactamase inhibitor, e.g. amoxicillin plus clavulanic acid (co-amoxiclav).
[b]Resistance is developing.
[c]Ticarcillin only available with clavulanic acid. Piperacillin is combined with the β-lactamase inhibitor tazobactam.
+, active; +/0, variable activity; 0, inactive or poor activity.

production is often encoded in a plasmid and this may be transferred to other bacteria by conjugation. By contrast, the broader-spectrum β-lactamases are often encoded by chromosomal genes.

An alternative type of penicillin resistance occurs in gonococci and in meticillin-resistant *Staphylococcus aureus* (MRSA), which develop mutated penicillin-binding proteins that do not bind β-lactam antibacterials. Meticillin has now been discontinued, but the name is still used.

Pharmacokinetics

Benzylpenicillin and phenoxymethylpenicillin

Only about one-third of an orally administered dose of benzylpenicillin is absorbed; the rest is destroyed by acid in the stomach. Benzylpenicillin is, therefore, restricted to intramuscular or intravenous administration. The phenoxymethyl derivative (penicillin V) is more stable in an acid environment and is better absorbed from the gut; it has a similar spectrum of activity as benzylpenicillin but is generally less active. Maximum concentrations of oral penicillins in blood occur rapidly after 30–60 min. Penicillins are widely distributed throughout the body, although transport across the meninges is poor unless they are acutely inflamed (e.g. in meningitis), when penetration by the antibacterial is improved. The half-lives of benzylpenicillin and phenoxymethylpenicillin, in common with most penicillins, are short (about 1 h) because they are very rapidly eliminated by the kidney, mainly by active tubular secretion at the proximal tubule. Effective plasma concentrations of penicillins are usually maintained by frequent dosing.

Flucloxacillin, amoxicillin and ampicillin

Flucloxacillin and amoxicillin are rapidly and almost completely absorbed from the gut, but ampicillin is incompletely absorbed. These drugs are eliminated by the kidney in a similar way to benzylpenicillin and have short half-lives (about 1 h). They can also be given intramuscularly or intravenously.

Other penicillins

The amidinopenicillin pivmecillinam is a prodrug for oral use which is hydrolysed to mecillinam. The carboxypenicillin ticarcillin is only available in combination with clavulanic acid for intravenous use. These drugs are renally excreted. The ureidopenicillin piperacillin is given intravenously in combination with the β-lactamase inhibitor tazobactam. Biliary excretion is responsible for the elimination of about a quarter of piperacillin, with the rest eliminated by the kidney.

Unwanted effects

Penicillins are normally well tolerated with a high therapeutic index.

- Nausea, vomiting.
- Hypersensitivity reactions in 1–10% of exposed individuals. Manifestations of allergy to penicillins include rashes, fever, vasculitis, serum sickness, exfoliative dermatitis, Stevens–Johnson syndrome and anaphylactic shock. Cross-allergy is widespread among various penicillins and to a lesser extent with cephalosporins. Penicillins and their breakdown products bind to proteins and act as haptens, stimulating the production of antibodies that mediate the allergic response (Chs 38 and 53).
- Aminopenicillins (e.g. amoxicillin) frequently produce a non-allergic maculopapular rash in people with glandular fever. This does not recur if another type of penicillin is given.
- Reversible neutropenia and eosinophilia can occur with prolonged high doses.

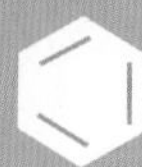

- Encephalopathy with excessively high cerebrospinal fluid (CSF) concentrations of penicillin. This occurs in severe renal failure, or after inadvertent intrathecal injection (which should never be given).
- Diarrhoea or *Clostridium difficile*-related colitis can occur as a result of disturbance of normal colonic flora, especially with broad-spectrum penicillins.
- Cholestatic jaundice can occur, especially with flucloxacillin or clavulanic acid.

Cephalosporins

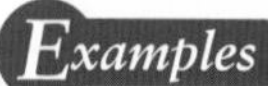

'First generation': cefadroxil, cefalexin
'Second generation': cefaclor, cefuroxime
'Third generation': cefotaxime, cefixime, ceftazidime, ceftriaxone

Mechanism of action

Cephalosporins, like penicillins, have a β-lactam ring, to which is fused a dihydrothiazine ring, which makes them more resistant to hydrolysis by β-lactamases (Fig. 51.3). They inhibit bacterial cell wall synthesis in a manner similar to that of the penicillins.

Spectrum of activity

Cephalosporins are often classified by 'generations'. The members within each generation share similar antibacterial activity. Succeeding generations tend to have increased activity against Gram-negative bacilli, usually at the expense of Gram-positive activity, and an increased ability to cross the blood–brain barrier (Table 51.2).

- First-generation oral cephalosporins (e.g. cefadroxil or cefalexin) have activity against staphylococci and most streptococci, but not enterococci.
- Second-generation oral cephalosporins (e.g. cefuroxime) have additional activity against some Gram-negative bacteria such as *Haemophilus influenzae* and *Neisseria gonorrhoeae*. They are able to penetrate the blood–brain barrier.
- Third-generation oral cephalosporins have improved β-lactamase stability and are able to penetrate the CSF in useful quantities. They also have greater Gram-negative activity than the other two generations. Cefixime adds *Proteus* and *Klebsiella* species to its spectrum, but it has no activity against staphylococci (Table 51.2). Ceftazidime has good activity against *Pseudomonas* species.

Resistance

The earlier generations are more sensitive to β-lactamase-mediated enzymatic hydrolysis of the β-lactam ring than are the later generations (Table 51.2). However, extended-spectrum β-lactamase (ESBL) can be acquired by *Escherichia coli* and confer resistance to third-generation cephalosporins.

Pharmacokinetics

First-generation oral cephalosporins are usually well absorbed from the gut. Several second- and third-generation drugs, for example cefuroxime and cefotaxime, are acid-labile and must be given by a parenteral route. Cefuroxime has also been formulated as a prodrug (cefuroxime axetil) for oral use, which has good absorption and is hydrolysed at first pass through the liver to cefuroxime. Most cephalosporins are primarily excreted by the kidney and have short half-lives (mostly less than 3 h). Cefixime is mainly eliminated by biliary excretion and has a half-life of 3–4 h, while ceftriaxone has a longer half-life (6–9 h), probably as a result of extensive plasma protein binding.

Unwanted effects

- Nausea, vomiting, abdominal discomfort.
- Headache.
- Skin rashes, including erythema multiforme and toxic epidermal necrolysis.
- Cephalosporins can produce hypersensitivity reactions similar to those observed with the penicillins. Less than 10% of people who are allergic to penicillins show cross-allergy to cephalosporins. A history of a serious reaction to penicillins precludes the administration of cephalosporins.
- Diarrhoea or *Clostridium difficile*-related colitis can be caused by disturbance of normal bowel flora. This is more common with oral cephalosporins.

Monobactams

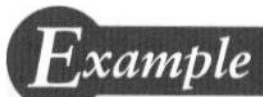

aztreonam

Aztreonam is a β-lactam antibacterial related to the penicillins but with a single ring structure ('monocyclic β-lactam') (Fig. 51.3). It has little cross-allergenicity with the penicillins and has been successfully given to people with proven penicillin allergy. Its spectrum of activity is limited to Gram-negative bacteria, including *Pseudomonas aeruginosa*, *Neisseria meningitidis*, *Neisseria gonorrhoeae* and *Haemophilus influenzae*, with no activity against Gram-positive bacteria or anaerobes. Aztreonam is given intramuscularly or intravenously and is usually β-lactamase-resistant. However, ESBL can be acquired by *Escherichia coli* and confer resistance to aztreonam. Aztreonam is excreted by the kidney and has a half-life of about 2 h. Unwanted effects are similar to those of other β-lactam antibacterials.

Carbapenems

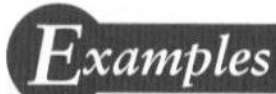

ertapenem, imipenem, meropenem

Imipenem is a β-lactam drug that has an extremely broad spectrum of bactericidal activity. It has potent activity against Gram-positive cocci, including some β-lactamase-producing pneumococci (Table 51.2), Gram-negative bacilli,

Table 51.2 Examples of β-lactams other than penicillins and their spectra of activity

	Staphylococcus aureus	***Haemophilus influenzae***	**Enterobacteriaceae (coliforms)**	***Pseudomonas aeruginosa***	***Bacteroides fragilis***	**Ability to cross blood–brain barrier**	**Resistance to β-lactamase**
Cephalosporins							
First generation							
Cefadroxil/ cefradine (oral)	+	0	+/0	0	0	+/0	+
Cefalexin (oral)	+	0	+/0	0	0	+/0	+
Second generation							
Cefuroxime axetil (oral)	+	+	+	0	+	+	+
Cefuroxime (parenteral)	+	+	+	0	+	+	+
Third generation							
Cefixime (oral)	0	+	+	0	0	+	+
Cefotaxime (parenteral)	+	+	+	0	+	+	+
Ceftazidime (parenteral)	0	0	+	+	0	+/0[a]	+
Monobactams (aztreonam)	0	+	0	+	+	+	+/0
Carbapenems (imipenem)	+	+	+	+	+	+	+

This table is only a general guide to individual drugs, and susceptibilities of organisms can vary widely.
Staphylococcus aureus is a Gram-positive staining organism. Other illustrative bacteria are Gram-negative staining.
[a]Some cephalosporins penetrate better into the CNS in the presence of inflamed meninges.
+, active; +/0, variable activity; 0, inactive or poor activity.

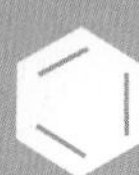

including *Pseudomonas aeruginosa*, *Neisseria suppurans* and *Bacteroides* species, and also many anaerobic bacteria. Imipenem can penetrate the blood–brain barrier and is resistant to β-lactamases. Narrow-spectrum resistance to imipenem in *Pseudomonas aeruginosa* occurs from a mutation that results in loss of a specific cell membrane uptake pathway. Imipenem is rapidly metabolised by dihydropeptidases in the kidney and so is given in combination with cilastatin, a compound that inhibits dihydropeptidase-induced hydrolysis. Meropenem is not inactivated by the renal enzyme and can be given alone. Both imipenem and meropenem are given intravenously; imipenem can also be given by deep intramuscular injection. Ertapenem has a broad spectrum of activity against Gram-positive and Gram-negative bacteria, but is inactive against *Pseudomonas* species. It is given intravenously.

These drugs are mainly excreted by the kidney and have short half-lives (1–5 h). Unwanted effects are similar to those of other β-lactam antibacterials, except for neurotoxicity with seizures, which is more common with imipenem than with other carbapenems.

OTHER DRUGS AFFECTING THE CELL WALL

Glycopeptides

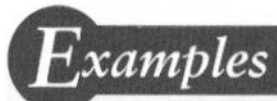

teicoplanin, vancomycin

Mechanism of action

Vancomycin and teicoplanin are high-molecular-weight glycopeptide compounds that act by inhibiting bacterial cell wall synthesis. They achieve this by inhibiting the linkages of peptidoglycan constituents (Fig. 51.1). Glycopeptides are bactericidal.

Spectrum of activity

Vancomycin and teicoplanin are active only against Gram-positive bacteria, particularly multi-resistant staphylococci. They do not penetrate the cell wall of Gram-negative bacteria. Both are usually reserved for treatment of serious staphylococcal infection or for bacterial endocarditis that is not responding to other treatments. Vancomycin given orally is also effective against *Clostridium difficile,* which colonises the colon when the normal gut flora is disturbed by antibacterial drugs causing diarrhoea and colitis. Metronidazole (see later) is preferred for this indication, but resistance to metronidazole is now relatively common.

Resistance

Acquired resistance to vancomycin can occur but is uncommon. Vancomycin-resistance in *Staphylococcus aureus* arises as a result of a multi-step genetic acquisition of a thickened peptidoglycan cell wall. This traps the drug and prevents it reaching its target on the cytoplasmic membrane. For other bacteria, plasmid-mediated resistance involves incorporation of D-lactate into the cell wall in place of D-alanine. This modification prevents binding of the glycopeptide.

Pharmacokinetics

Both vancomycin and teicoplanin are very poorly absorbed orally and are given by intravenous infusion for systemic infection. Teicoplanin can also be given by intramuscular injection. Oral vancomycin is only used for treating *Clostridium difficile*-related colitis. Both drugs are excreted by the kidney; vancomycin has a shorter half-life (5–11 h) than teicoplanin (32–176 h).

Unwanted effects

- Ototoxicity, often starting with tinnitus
- Nephrotoxicity, which may be enhanced if vancomycin or teicoplanin are used in combination with an aminoglycoside
- Thrombophlebitis at the site of infusion
- Rashes, including Stevens–Johnson syndrome and toxic epidermal necrolysis; rapid intravenous injection of vancomycin produces upper body flushing, the 'red man' syndrome
- Blood disorders, including neutropenia, thrombocytopenia
- Nausea.

Daptomycin

Mechanism of action

Daptomycin is a lipopeptide antibacterial with a unique mode of action. It binds to the cell wall of Gram-positive bacteria, and forms transmembrane channels that allow leakage of intracellular ions, destroying the membrane potential across the cell.

Spectrum of activity

Daptomycin does not penetrate the membrane of Gram-negative cells. Daptomycin is bactericidal against a similar spectrum of organisms as vancomycin, and is used to treat complicated skin and soft tissue infections.

Resistance

Resistance occurs when the bacterial membrane structure is changed to prevent binding of the drug.

Pharmacokinetics

Daptomycin is given intravenously, and eliminated unchanged by the kidneys. It has a half-life of about 8 h.

Unwanted effects

The most common unwanted effects are gastrointestinal upset and injection site reactions.

Polymyxins

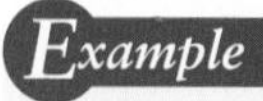

colistin (colistimethate sodium)

Mechanism of action

Polymyxins bind to bacterial membrane phospholipids and alter the permeability of the membrane to K^+ and Na^+. The cell's osmotic barrier is lost, and susceptible bacteria are killed by lysis (Fig. 51.1).

Spectrum of activity

Polymyxins have bactericidal action against Gram-negative bacteria, including *Pseudomonas* species, but are inactive against Gram-positive bacteria.

Resistance

Acquired resistance is rare.

Pharmacokinetics

Colistin is very poorly absorbed from the gut and is usually given by inhalation or topically to the skin. Penetration into joint spaces or CSF is poor. It is excreted unchanged by the kidney and has a half-life of 4–8 h. It is occasionally given by mouth for bowel sterilisation.

Unwanted effects

Substantial toxicity limits the use of polymyxins by systemic administration.

- Nephrotoxicity with dose-related reversible renal impairment.
- Neurotoxicity produces dizziness, circumoral and peripheral paraesthesiae, and confusion. Rarely, neuromuscular blockade can produce respiratory paralysis with apnoea.
- Bronchospasm or sore throat after inhalation.

DRUGS AFFECTING BACTERIAL DNA

Quinolones (fluoroquinolones)

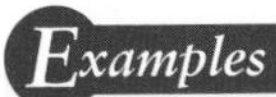

ciprofloxacin, moxifloxacin, norfloxacin

Mechanism of action

Quinolones inhibit replication of bacterial DNA. They block the activity of bacterial DNA gyrase and DNA topoisomerase, the enzymes that form DNA supercoils and are essential for DNA replication and repair (Fig. 51.1). The effect is bactericidal.

Spectrum of activity

Ciprofloxacin has a broad spectrum of activity and is active against many micro-organisms resistant to penicillins, cephalosporins and aminoglycosides. Its spectrum includes Gram-positive bacteria, but with only moderate activity against *Streptococcus pneumoniae* and *Enterococcus faecalis*. It is active against most Gram-negative bacteria, including *Haemophilus influenzae*, *Pseudomonas aeruginosa*, *Neisseria gonorrhoeae*, and *Enterobacter* and *Campylobacter* species. Its spectrum extends to chlamydia and some mycobacteria, but not anaerobes.

Moxifloxacin has a broad spectrum of activity against Gram-positive and Gram-negative bacteria, but is inactive against *Pseudomonas aeruginosa*. It has greater activity than ciprofloxacin against pneumococci. Norfloxacin is mainly useful for urinary tract pathogens.

Resistance

Resistance to quinolones is relatively uncommon but can be produced by a mutation that results in a DNA gyrase that is less susceptible to the drug's action, or by increased active drug efflux from the cell (Fig. 51.2).

Pharmacokinetics

Oral absorption of ciprofloxacin is variable but adequate. An intravenous formulation is available. Ciprofloxacin is widely distributed in body tissues and fluids, but CSF penetration is poor unless there is meningeal inflammation. The majority of the drug is eliminated unchanged by the kidney, partly by tubular secretion, but about 20% is excreted in the bile and a similar amount is metabolised in the liver. Ciprofloxacin has a short half-life (3–4 h). Moxifloxacin is well absorbed from the gut, is metabolised in the liver and partially excreted unchanged in the urine, and has a longer half-life of 12 h. Norfloxacin is moderately well absorbed from the gut, is eliminated by a combination of metabolism and renal excretion, and has a short half-life (3 h).

Unwanted effects

- Nausea, vomiting, abdominal pain, diarrhoea.
- Central nervous system (CNS) effects: dizziness, headache, tremor, seizures (especially in those with a prior history of epilepsy).
- Rashes.
- Pain and inflammation in tendons, occasionally with tendon rupture (especially in the elderly or with concomitant use of corticosteroids).
- Moxifloxacin prolongs the Q–T interval on the electrocardiogram (ECG) and predisposes to ventricular arrhythmias. The risk is greater if it is used in combination with other pro-arrhythmic drugs (Ch. 8).
- Drug interactions: inhibition of hepatic cytochrome P450 by ciprofloxacin and norfloxacin increases the plasma concentrations of theophylline (Ch. 12), warfarin (Ch. 11) and ciclosporin (Ch. 38), which can produce toxicity. The absorption of quinolones from the gut is decreased by oral iron salts.

Metronidazole and tinidazole

Mechanism of action

Metronidazole is bactericidal only after it has been degraded to an intermediate transient toxic metabolite, which inhibits bacterial DNA synthesis and breaks down existing DNA. Only some anaerobes and some protozoa contain the oxidoreductase enzyme that converts metronidazole to its antibacterial derivative. The intermediate metabolite is not produced in human cells, or in aerobic bacteria. Metronidazole is equally active against dividing and non-dividing cells.

Spectrum of activity

Metronidazole and tinidazole are mainly active against anaerobic bacteria and protozoa, including *Bacteroides*

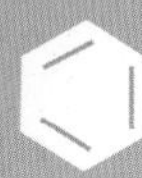

fragilis, *Clostridium* species, *Gardnerella vaginalis* and *Giardia lamblia*. Metronidazole is an important drug for treating *Clostridium difficile*-related colitis (pseudomembranous colitis) caused by broad-spectrum antimicrobial use. Metronidazole or tinidazole are important constituents of the triple or quadruple therapy utilised for the elimination of *Helicobacter pylori* (Ch. 33). They are also amoebicidal, with activity against *Entamoeba histolytica*.

Resistance

Acquired resistance is becoming more common. For example, in some countries, a significant percentage of strains of *Helicobacter pylori* are resistant to metronidazole, as are some strains of *Clostridium difficile*. Resistance can result from development of oxidoreductases that do not act on metronidazole, or from the induction of oxidative stress mechanisms that inhibit the action of the drug. Resistance to tinidazole is less common.

Pharmacokinetics

Metronidazole is well absorbed orally and can also be given intravenously, or by rectal suppositories. Rectal absorption is high, and this route is often preferable to intravenous administration if the drug cannot be taken by mouth. Metronidazole penetrates well into body fluids, including vaginal, pleural and cerebrospinal fluids, and can cross the placenta. Metronidazole and tinidazole are eliminated mainly by metabolism in the liver, and have half-lives of 6–9 h and 12–14 h, respectively.

Unwanted effects

- Nausea, vomiting, metallic taste
- Intolerance to alcohol can occur by a mechanism that is similar to the disulfiram reaction (Ch. 54)
- Rash.

Nitrofurantoin

Mechanism of action

Nitrofurantoin is activated by reduction via the flavoprotein nitrofurantoin reductase to unstable metabolites inside bacteria, which disrupt ribosomal RNA, DNA and other intracellular components. It is bactericidal, especially to bacteria present in acid urine.

Spectrum of activity

Nitrofurantoin is active against most Gram-positive cocci and *Escherichia coli*. *Pseudomonas* species are naturally resistant, as are many *Proteus* species. Its use is confined to infections of the lower urinary tract.

Resistance

Chromosomal resistance occurs by inhibition of nitrofurantoin reductase, but is not common.

Pharmacokinetics

Nitrofurantoin is well absorbed from the gut. The half-life in plasma is very short (<1 h) and therapeutic plasma concentrations are not achieved. It is excreted unchanged in the urine by both glomerular filtration and tubular secretion, but also undergoes some metabolic reduction. Urinary concentrations are high enough to treat lower urinary tract infections, but the low tissue concentrations are inadequate for the treatment of acute pyelonephritis.

Unwanted effects

- Gastrointestinal upset is common, including anorexia, nausea and vomiting
- Pulmonary toxicity with long-term use produces acute allergic pneumonitis or chronic interstitial fibrosis
- Peripheral neuropathy.

DRUGS AFFECTING BACTERIAL PROTEIN SYNTHESIS

Macrolides

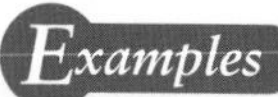

Examples

azithromycin, clarithromycin, erythromycin, telithromycin

Mechanism of action

Macrolides interfere with bacterial protein synthesis by binding reversibly to the 50S subunit of the bacterial ribosome. This causes dissociation of the peptidyl transfer RNA (tRNA) from its translocation site. The action is primarily bacteriostatic (Fig. 51.1).

Spectrum of activity

Erythromycin has a similar spectrum of activity to broad-spectrum penicillins, and is often used for treating individuals who are penicillin-allergic. It is effective against Gram-positive bacteria and gut anaerobes, but has poor activity against *Haemophilus influenzae*. It is also used for infections by *Legionella*, *Mycoplasma*, *Chlamydia*, *Mycobacterium* and *Campylobacter* species and for *Bordetella pertussis*. Although erythromycin is primarily bacteriostatic, it is bactericidal at high concentrations for some Gram-positive species, such as group A streptococci and pneumococci.

Azithromycin has less activity than erythromycin against Gram-positive bacteria, but enhanced activity against *Haemophilus influenzae*. Clarithromycin has slightly greater activity than erythromycin and is also used as part of the multidrug treatment of *Helicobacter pylori* (Ch. 33). Telithromycin is a ketolide derivative of erythromycin that is active against penicillin- and erythromycin-resistant *Streptococcus pneumoniae*.

Resistance

Bacteria become resistant to macrolides by activation of an efflux mechanism. To a lesser extent, there is also a gene mutation that encodes for a methyltransferase that modifies the target site on the ribosome.

Pharmacokinetics

Erythromycin is adequately absorbed from the gut. It is destroyed at acid pH and is therefore given as an enteric-coated tablet or as an ester prodrug (erythromycin ethyl succinate) which is acid-stable. Erythromycin can also be administered intravenously. Clarithromycin is acid-stable and well absorbed from the gut, but undergoes first-pass metabolism in the liver. Erythromycin and clarithromycin are metabolised in the liver and have short half-lives (1–3 h).

Azithromycin is poorly absorbed from the gut. It is widely distributed and released slowly from the tissues. Azithromycin is excreted unchanged in the bile and has a very long half-life of about 2 days. Telithromycin is well absorbed from the gut, is metabolised in the liver, partly by CYP3A4, and has a half-life of 10 h.

Unwanted effects

- Epigastric discomfort, nausea, vomiting and diarrhoea are common with the oral preparation of erythromycin. Azithromycin and clarithromycin are better tolerated.
- Rashes.
- Cholestatic jaundice with erythromycin, usually if treatment is continued for more than 2 weeks.
- Prolongation of the Q–T interval on the ECG, with a predisposition to ventricular arrhythmias (Ch. 8).
- Drug interactions: erythromycin and clarithromycin inhibit P450 drug-metabolising enzymes (CYP1A2, CYP3A4) and can elevate levels of drugs requiring these enzymes for metabolism (see Table 2.9). Examples include carbamazepine (Ch. 23) and ciclosporin (Ch. 38).

Aminoglycosides

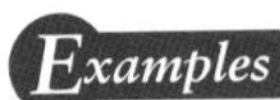

gentamicin, netilmicin, streptomycin, tobramycin

Mechanism of action

The aminoglycosides are similar in their properties, but there are some important differences that can be exploited in particular clinical circumstances, as illustrated below. Aminoglycosides inhibit protein synthesis in bacteria by binding irreversibly to the 30S ribosomal subunit (Fig. 51.1). This inhibits translation from messenger RNA (mRNA) to protein and also increases the frequency of misreading of the genetic code. Aminoglycosides are bactericidal.

Spectrum of activity

Aminoglycosides are active against many Gram-negative bacteria (including *Pseudomonas* species) and some Gram-positive bacteria. They are inactive against anaerobes, which are unable to take up the aminoglycosides. Aminoglycosides are particularly useful for serious Gram-negative infections, when they have a complementary and synergistic action with drugs that disrupt cell wall synthesis (e.g. penicillins). Gentamicin is the most widely used aminoglycoside. Streptomycin is rarely used, but is occasionally part of the drug regimen to treat *Mycobacterium tuberculosis* (see below).

Resistance

Resistance is increasingly a problem with the aminoglycosides and can occur by several mechanisms. It is transferred by plasmids and is principally caused by the production of enzymes that acetylate, phosphorylate or adenylyl aminoglycosides in the bacterial periplasmic space. Bacterial uptake of the modified drug is poor (Fig. 51.2). Resistance resulting from reduced penetration of the drug can be overcome by co-administration of antibacterials that disrupt cell wall synthesis, such as penicillins. Netilmicin is less susceptible to these enzymes, and is effective against many gentamicin-resistant bacteria. Changes in the ribosomal proteins in resistant bacteria can also reduce drug binding and antibacterial effectiveness, particularly for streptomycin.

Pharmacokinetics

Aminoglycosides are poorly absorbed from the gut, and, therefore, are given parenterally. They have short half-lives (1–4 h) and are rapidly excreted by the kidney. They do not cross the blood–brain barrier; however, they do cross the placenta. Blood concentrations should always be measured to guide dosing. Peak concentrations, measured 1 h after dosing, and trough concentrations immediately before the next dose are important, both to ensure bactericidal efficacy and to minimise the risk of toxic effects. Once-daily dosage regimens for aminoglycosides are increasingly used and are no more toxic than multiple daily dosages.

Tobramycin is also available as a preservative-free solution for administration by nebuliser for the management of people with bronchiectasis (including cystic fibrosis) whose respiratory tracts are colonised by *Pseudomonas aeruginosa*.

Unwanted effects

Most unwanted effects of aminoglycosides are dose-related and many are reversible; they are most closely related to high trough concentrations of the drug.

- Ototoxicity can lead to both vestibular and auditory dysfunction. Prolonged treatment or high plasma drug concentrations lead to accumulation of the aminoglycoside in the inner ear, resulting in disturbances of balance or deafness that are often irreversible. Mutations in the mitochondrial 12S ribosomal RNA gene predispose to ototoxicity. Netilmicin causes less ototoxicity than the other aminoglycosides.
- Renal damage occurs through retention of aminoglycosides in the proximal tubular cells of the kidney. It is usually reversible and is manifest initially by a defect in the concentrating ability of the kidney, with mild proteinuria followed by a reduction in the glomerular filtration rate.
- Acute neuromuscular blockade can occur, usually if the aminoglycoside is used with anaesthetic drugs (Ch. 17), and aminoglycosides can enhance the effects of other neuromuscular-blocking drugs (Ch. 27). This action is the result of inhibition of pre-junctional acetylcholine release, and also reduced postsynaptic sensitivity. It is reversed by intravenous Ca^{2+} salts.

Tetracyclines

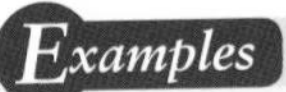

doxycycline, minocycline, oxytetracycline

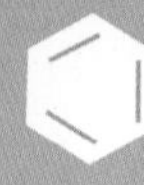

Mechanism of action

Tetracyclines enter bacteria mainly by an active uptake mechanism that is not found in human cells. They are bacteriostatic and inhibit bacterial protein synthesis by binding reversibly to the 30S subunit of ribosomes.

Spectrum of activity

Tetracyclines have a broad spectrum of activity against many Gram-positive and Gram-negative bacteria and in infections caused by rickettsiae, amoebae, *Chlamydia psittaci*, *Chlamydia trachomatis*, *Coxiella burnetii*, *Vibrio cholerae* and *Mycoplasma*, *Legionella* and *Brucella* species. They are useful in acne (Ch. 49). Minocycline is active against *Neisseria meningitidis*, unlike other tetracyclines.

Resistance

Resistance is carried by plasmids and is usually due to increased transport of the drug out from the bacterium (Fig. 51.2). An alternative mechanism is decreased binding of tetracyclines to bacterial ribosomes. Resistance to the tetracyclines develops slowly, but in the UK is now widespread among most Gram-positive and several Gram-negative bacteria. Micro-organisms that have developed resistance to one tetracycline frequently display resistance to the others.

Pharmacokinetics

Tetracyclines are incompletely absorbed from the gut, particularly if taken with food. Absorption of oxytetracycline is further impaired by milk, aluminium, calcium or magnesium salts (antacids; Ch. 33), iron and increased intestinal pH; tetracyclines bind to divalent and trivalent cations, forming inactive chelates (Ch. 56).

The tetracyclines diffuse reasonably well into sputum, urine, and peritoneal and pleural fluid, and cross the placenta. They have poor penetration into CSF. All of the tetracyclines have half-lives within the range 8–22 h. Tetracyclines are concentrated in the liver and some drug is excreted via the bile into the small intestine, from where it is partially reabsorbed. Drug concentrations in the bile may be three to five times higher than in the plasma.

Tetracyclines are mainly eliminated unchanged in the urine, with the exception of doxycycline, which is largely eliminated in the bile.

Unwanted effects

- Nausea, vomiting, epigastric discomfort and diarrhoea.
- In children, tetracyclines produce permanent yellow–brown discoloration of the growing teeth by chelating with Ca^{2+}, and can also cause dental hypoplasia. Tetracyclines should be avoided during the latter half of pregnancy and in children in the first 12 years of life.
- Anti-anabolic effects can occur in human cells from inhibition of protein synthesis (not seen with doxycycline or minocycline). If there is pre-existing impairment of renal function, this can lead to uraemia.
- Benign intracranial hypertension, with headache and visual disturbances.

Tigecycline

Mechanism of action

Tigecycline is a glycylcycline antibacterial that has structural similarities with the tetracyclines, and also binds to the 30S ribosomal subunit of bacteria.

Spectrum of activity

Tigecycline has a broad spectrum of activity against Gram-positive and Gram-negative bacteria, including some anaerobes. It is used for complicated skin and soft tissue infections, and complicated abdominal infections caused by resistant bacteria. Tigecycline is active against MRSA, vancomycin-resistant enterococci, *Proteus* species and *Pseudomonas aeruginosa*.

Resistance

Many strains of *Proteus* species and *Pseudomonas aeruginosa* are resistant, usually as a result of possessing a drug efflux pump.

Pharmacokinetics

Tigecycline is given intravenously and is mainly excreted unchanged, about two-thirds in bile and the remainder by the kidneys. It has a long half-life of about 27 h.

Unwanted effects

The most common unwanted effects are similar to those of tetracyclines.

Chloramphenicol

Mechanism of action

Chloramphenicol inhibits protein synthesis in bacteria by binding reversibly to the 50S subunit of bacterial ribosomes (Fig. 51.1). It inhibits peptide bond formation by impairing the translation of mRNA. The effect is mainly bacteriostatic, but can be bactericidal in some bacteria.

Spectrum of activity

Chloramphenicol is a broad-spectrum antibacterial, active against many Gram-positive cocci (both aerobic and anaerobic) and Gram-negative bacteria. The sensitivities of all these bacteria are variable, but it has a bactericidal effect on *Escherichia coli*, *Streptococcus pneumoniae*, *Haemophilus influenzae*, *Neisseria meningitidis*, *Bordetella pertussis*, *Vibrio cholerae*, and *Salmonella*, *Shigella* and *Bacteroides* species. It is bacteriostatic for some streptococci and staphylococci.

Because of its toxicity, chloramphenicol is reserved for life-threatening infections, particularly with *Haemophilus influenzae* or *Salmonella typhi*. It is used topically for conjunctivitis (Ch. 50).

Resistance

Resistance is caused by the production of a plasmid-mediated enzyme that inactivates the drug by acetylation. The enzyme is produced by many Gram-negative bacteria but can also be induced in Gram-positive bacteria. Resistant bacteria may also show reduced uptake of the drug.

Pharmacokinetics

Chloramphenicol is well absorbed orally, and can also be given intravenously. It is widely distributed into many tissues, including CSF and the biliary tree; it crosses the placenta and is present in breast milk. Chloramphenicol is almost completely metabolised by glucuronidation in the liver and has a half-life of about 5 h (2–12 h).

Unwanted effects

- The most important unwanted effect is bone marrow toxicity. Reversible anaemia, thrombocytopenia or neutropenia can occur, particularly in those receiving high or prolonged dosing. Aplastic anaemia is rare, but usually fatal.
- Peripheral neuritis, optic neuritis, headache.
- Rashes.
- Premature infants and babies of less than 2 weeks of age have immature glucuronyl transferase, and reduced renal drug elimination. Chloramphenicol can accumulate in neonates, causing the 'grey baby syndrome'. Initial symptoms include vomiting and cyanosis, followed by hypothermia, vasomotor collapse and an ashen grey discoloration of the skin. There is a high mortality.

Lincosamides

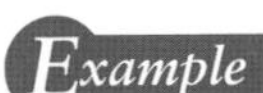

clindamycin

Mechanism of action

Clindamycin inhibits bacterial protein synthesis in a similar manner to the macrolide antibacterials.

Spectrum of activity

Clindamycin is used for staphylococcal bone infection such as osteomyelitis, and as prophylaxis for endocarditis in people who cannot take penicillins. It is also effective against Gram-positive cocci.

Resistance

Resistance develops by modification of the ribosomal binding site.

Pharmacokinetics

Clindamycin is well absorbed orally. It eliminated largely by metabolism in the liver and has a half-life of 2.5 h.

Unwanted effects

- Nausea, vomiting, abdominal discomfort, diarrhoea and, rarely, *clostridium difficile*-related colitis
- Rashes
- Jaundice and abnormal liver function tests
- Neutropenia, thrombocytopenia.

Fusidic acid

Mechanism of action

Fusidic acid is a steroid compound that inhibits bacterial protein synthesis. It forms a complex with the ribosome and inhibits translocation of peptidyl-tRNA.

Spectrum of activity

Fusidic acid is a narrow-spectrum antibacterial, mainly active against Gram-positive bacteria. It is most commonly used for treatment of penicillin-resistant *Staphylococcus aureus*, especially in the treatment of osteomyelitis. It is bactericidal.

Resistance

Resistance occurs usually by plasmid conjugation that alters the target binding site for the drug. Resistance develops rapidly when fusidic acid is used alone; consequently, it is usually given in combination with another drug.

Pharmacokinetics

Oral absorption is complete, but an intravenous formulation is available. Penetration into synovial fluid and soft tissues is good, and the drug concentrates in bone. Fusidic acid is extensively metabolised in the liver and has a half-life of 9 h.

Unwanted effects

- Thrombophlebitis with intravenous infusions
- Cholestatic jaundice
- Nausea, vomiting.

Streptogramins

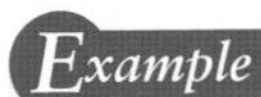

quinupristin with dalfopristin

Mechanism of action

Streptogramins are isolated from *Streptomyces pristinaespiralis*. Quinupristin and dalfopristin are synergistic streptogramins that are given in combination. They bind to the 50S subunit of the bacterial ribosome and inhibit the late phase of protein synthesis.

Spectrum of activity

The combination of quinupristin with dalfopristin acts synergistically and is effective against aerobic Gram-positive bacteria, including MRSA and vancomycin-resistant *Enterococcus faecium*, but not *Enterococcus faecalis*. It should be reserved for serious infections. There is little activity against Gram-negative bacteria.

Resistance

This occurs by modification of the ribosomal binding site.

Pharmacokinetics

The streptogramins are given intravenously; their metabolism is complex and several active metabolites are formed

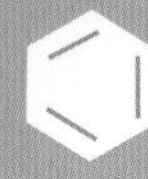

by cytochrome P450 enzymes. The main route of elimination is faecal. The half-lives of both quinupristin and dalfopristin are very short (0.5–1 h).

Unwanted effects

- Nausea, vomiting, diarrhoea
- Headache
- Arthralgia, myalgia
- Injection site reactions
- Hepatitis
- Prolongation of the Q–T interval on the ECG, with a risk of ventricular arrhythmias (Ch. 8).

Oxazolidinones

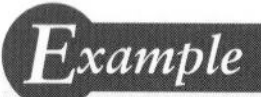

linezolid

Mechanism of action

The oxazolidinones are active against non-replicating bacteria. They have a unique mechanism of action, inhibiting protein synthesis through binding to the ribosomal 50S subunit and preventing initiation of tRNA transcription.

Spectrum of activity

Linezolid is active against a range of Gram-positive organisms, including MRSA and also vancomycin-resistant *Enterococcus faecium*.

Resistance

Resistance is due to mutation, leading to modification of the ribosomal target for the drug. This can develop with prolonged treatment, or with inadequate doses.

Pharmacokinetics

Linezolid is well absorbed orally. It is mainly metabolised in the liver, but one-third is excreted by the kidney. Linezolid has a half-life of 5 h.

Unwanted effects

- Headache
- Nausea, vomiting, taste disturbances, diarrhoea.

DRUGS AFFECTING BACTERIAL METABOLISM

Sulphonamides

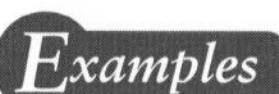

sulfadiazine, sulfamethoxazole

The global therapeutic importance of the sulphonamides has diminished because of the spread of resistance, and there are now only a few situations (nonetheless important) in which they are first-choice drugs. Sulfamethoxazole is only used in combination with trimethoprim, as co-trimoxazole (see below).

Mechanism of action

Folate is a nutrient that is essential for cell growth and is used to manufacture purines for incorporation into DNA. Unlike humans, bacteria cannot utilise pre-formed folate, and must synthesise it from *p*-aminobenzoic acid (PABA). Sulphonamides are structurally similar to PABA and inhibit the enzyme dihydropteroate synthetase in the synthetic pathway for folic acid (Fig. 51.4).

Spectrum of activity

Sulphonamides have a bacteriostatic action against a wide range of Gram-positive and Gram-negative bacteria and are also active against *Toxoplasma*, *Chlamydia* and *Nocardia* species. Because of the frequency of resistance with many of these micro-organisms, sulphonamides are given as sole therapy only for the treatment of nocardiosis or toxoplasmosis.

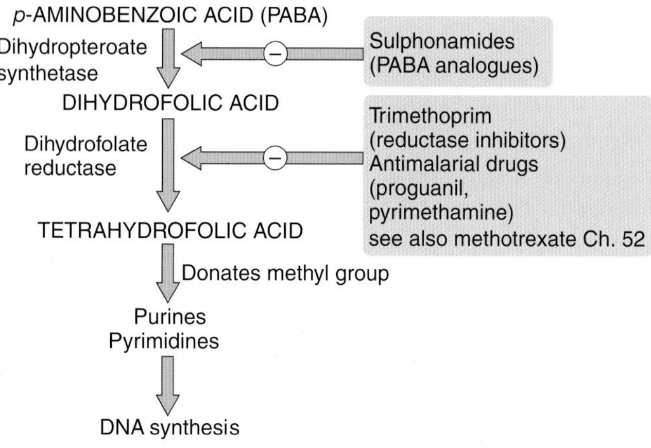

Fig. 51.4 **Mechanism of action of the sulphonamides, trimethoprim and antimalarial drugs in the folic acid pathway.**

Resistance

Resistance is common and occurs through the production of a mutated dihydropteroate synthetase that has reduced affinity for binding of sulphonamides (Figs 51.2 and 51.4). Resistance is transmitted among Gram-negative bacteria by plasmids. Resistance in *Staphylococcus aureus* occurs as a result of excessive synthesis of PABA. Some resistant bacteria have reduced uptake of sulphonamides.

Pharmacokinetics

Sulphonamides are well absorbed orally; a parenteral preparation of sulfadiazine is available. They are widely distributed in the body and cross the blood–brain barrier and placenta.

Sulphonamides are metabolised in the liver, initially by acetylation, which shows genetic polymorphism (Ch. 2). The acetylated product has no antibacterial action but retains toxic potential. Substantial amounts of parent drug and N-acetyl metabolite are excreted by the kidney. Most sulphonamides have half-lives of about 12 h.

Unwanted effects

- Nausea and vomiting
- Rashes, including toxic epidermal necrolysis and Stevens–Johnson syndrome
- Haemolysis in individuals with glucose-6-phosphate dehydrogenase deficiency (Chs 47 and 53)
- Neutropenia, thrombocytopenia
- Sulphonamides should not be used in the last trimester of pregnancy or in neonates, because the drug competes for bilirubin-binding sites on albumin; this can raise the concentration of unconjugated bilirubin and increases the risk of kernicterus.

Trimethoprim

Trimethoprim can be used alone, or less commonly combined with the sulphonamide sulfamethoxazole, as co-trimoxazole.

Mechanism of action

Trimethoprim inhibits dihydrofolate reductase, which converts dihydrofolate to tetrahydrofolate (Fig. 51.4). The bacterial enzyme is inhibited at much lower concentrations than its mammalian counterpart. The combination of trimethoprim with sulfamethoxazole (co-trimoxazole) acts synergistically to prevent folate synthesis by bacteria. However, resistance to the sulfamethoxazole component, and the incidence of unwanted effects, limit the value of this combination.

Spectrum of activity

Trimethoprim has broad-spectrum bacteriostatic activity against Gram-positive and Gram-negative bacteria. In many urinary and respiratory tract infections, trimethoprim alone gives results similar to the combination with sulfamethoxazole (co-trimoxazole). Co-trimoxazole is effective against the protozoan *Pneumocystis jirovecii*, which causes pneumonia in people with AIDS or other immunodeficiencies, and this is now its major indication (see below).

Resistance

Resistance to trimethoprim occurs in a variety of ways, including the production of mutated dihydrofolate reductases that are insensitive to trimethoprim.

Pharmacokinetics

Trimethoprim is well absorbed from the gut. Most is eliminated unchanged by the kidney and it has a half-life of 9–17 h. Both trimethoprim and co-trimoxazole are available for intravenous use.

Unwanted effects

- Nausea, vomiting and diarrhoea, which are usually mild
- Rashes
- Bone marrow depression
- Folate deficiency, leading to megaloblastic changes in the bone marrow, is rare, except in people with depleted folate stores.

DRUGS USED FOR TUBERCULOSIS

Tuberculosis is usually treated with a multidrug regimen because of the rapid development of resistance.

Rifamycins

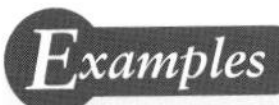

rifabutin, rifampicin

Mechanism of action and spectrum of activity

Rifamycins act by inhibition of DNA-dependent RNA polymerase and inhibit transcription in the bacterium. They have a bactericidal action. Rifampicin (rifampin) has a broad spectrum of activity and is used in the treatment of mycobacterial infections (*M. tuberculosis* and *M. leprae*), brucellosis, *Legionella* infections and serious staphylococcal infections. In the UK, it is considered an essential drug for treatment of tuberculosis. Rifabutin is also used for prophylaxis against *Mycobacterium avium complex* infection, most commonly occurring in people who are infected with HIV.

Resistance

Resistance develops rapidly, which limits the wider use of rifampicin as an antibacterial drug, other than for the treatment of tuberculosis. It is acquired by a one-step genetic mutation of the DNA-dependent RNA polymerase.

Pharmacokinetics

Oral absorption is good, and an intravenous formulation of rifampicin is also available. The bioavailability of rifabutin is low (20%) compared with rifampicin. Rifampicin and rifabutin are metabolised in the liver and have half-lives of 1–6 h and 35–40 h, respectively.

Unwanted effects

- Nausea and anorexia
- Pseudomembranous colitis with rifampicin

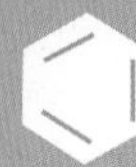

- Hepatotoxicity, usually only producing a transient rise in plasma transaminases; regular monitoring is recommended
- Orange coloration of tears, sweat, urine
- Various 'toxicity syndromes' occur, commonly with intermittent use, owing to sensitisation; they include renal failure, a shock-like syndrome and acute haemolytic anaemia
- Drug interactions: induction of drug-metabolising enzymes in the liver (Ch. 2) can reduce the levels of plasma oestrogen in those taking oral contraceptives (Ch. 45), and reduce plasma levels of phenytoin (Ch. 23), warfarin (Ch. 11) and sulphonylureas (Ch. 40).

Isoniazid

Mechanism of action

Isoniazid is an important and specific drug for the treatment of *Mycobacterium tuberculosis*. It is a prodrug that is activated by catalase–peroxidase activity within susceptible cells. Isoniazid acts on enzymes in the cell to inhibit the synthesis of long-chain mycolic acids, which are unique to the cell wall of mycobacteria. It is bactericidal against dividing organisms, but bacteriostatic on resting organisms. In the UK, it is considered an essential drug for treatment of tuberculosis along with rifampicin.

Resistance

Resistance may be due to mutations in enzymes responsible for the synthesis of mycolic acids, making them less susceptible to the drug. Resistance occurs rapidly through mutation if isoniazid is used alone. Resistance is currently uncommon in developed countries, but can be troublesome in developing countries.

Pharmacokinetics

Oral absorption is good but is reduced by food. Isoniazid is metabolised by acetylation in the liver, which is subject to genetic polymorphism (Ch. 2). Rapid acetylators show extensive first-pass metabolism, and blood isoniazid concentrations in slow acetylators are twice those in rapid acetylators. The half-life is 0.5–2 h in rapid acetylators and 2–6.5 h in slow acetylators.

Unwanted effects

- Nausea, vomiting, constipation.
- Peripheral neuropathy with high doses. This can be prevented by prophylactic use of oral pyridoxine supplements in people at high risk, for example those with diabetes, alcoholism, chronic renal failure, malnutrition, or HIV infection. Neuropathy is more common in slow acetylators.
- Hepatitis is rare, but regular monitoring with liver function tests is recommended.
- Systemic lupus erythematosus-like syndrome. Positive antinuclear antibodies are found in 20% of people during long-term treatment, but fewer develop symptoms.

Pyrazinamide

Mechanism of action

Pyrazinamide is a prodrug that acts through metabolites formed by the enzyme pyrazinamidase, which is found in *Mycobacterium tuberculosis*. The product pyrazinoic acid lowers intracellular pH, inactivates a vital enzyme in fatty acid synthesis and destroys the bacterium. It is bactericidal to semi-dormant cells.

Resistance

Resistance results from a point mutation in the gene which codes for pyrazinamidase. It develops rapidly if pyrazinamide is used as a sole treatment for tuberculosis.

Pharmacokinetics

Oral absorption is good and metabolism occurs in the liver. Pyrazinamide has a long half-life (10–24 h).

Unwanted effects

- Hepatotoxicity: a rise in plasma bilirubin usually requires cessation of treatment; regular monitoring is recommended
- Nausea and vomiting
- Arthralgia
- Sideroblastic anaemia.

Ethambutol

Mechanism of action

Ethambutol probably functions as an arabinose analogue, and inhibits arabinosyl transferase, resulting in impaired synthesis of the cell wall of mycobacteria. Ethambutol is primarily bacteriostatic. It is effective against *Mycobacterium tuberculosis* and several other mycobacteria, including *Mycobacterium avium* complex, which can cause lung infections.

Resistance

Resistance may be due to gene mutations that inhibit the binding of ethambutol to its target enzyme. It develops slowly, but is common during prolonged treatment of tuberculosis if ethambutol is used alone.

Pharmacokinetics

Oral absorption is good. It is mainly eliminated unchanged by the kidney. The half-life is long (10–15 h).

Unwanted effects

- Optic neuritis produces initial red/green colour blindness, then reduced visual acuity; it is dose-related but usually reversible
- Peripheral neuritis.

Other drugs used in the treatment of tuberculosis

Other drugs can be used as second-line treatments in multidrug-resistant tuberculosis. These include cycloserine, capreomycin, amikacin, ciprofloxacin, moxifloxacin, azithromycin, clarithromycin and *p*-aminosalicylic acid. Drugs used in countries other than the UK include thiacetazone, protionamide and streptomycin.

DRUGS USED FOR LEPROSY

The drugs recommended for treatment of leprosy, which is caused by *Mycobacterium leprae*, are rifampicin (see above), dapsone and clofazimine.

Dapsone

Mechanism of action and use

Dapsone is similar to the sulphonamides and acts by inhibition of folate synthesis. It is the most active drug against *Mycobacterium leprae*. Dapsone is also used to treat pneumocystis pneumonia and dermatitis herpetiformis.

Resistance

Resistance can develop as for sulphonamides (see above).

Pharmacokinetics

Dapsone is well absorbed from the gut. It is metabolised in the liver by oxidation and acetylation and undergoes enterohepatic cycling. It has a long half-life (27 h).

Unwanted effects

- Blood disorders: haemolysis and methaemoglobinaemia (Ch. 53), although these are rare at the doses used for treatment of leprosy
- Neuropathy
- Anorexia, nausea, vomiting
- Allergic dermatitis.

Clofazimine

Mechanism of action and use

Clofazimine is a dye that interferes with DNA and is used as a second-line drug in the event of dapsone intolerance in people with leprosy. It is given orally.

Pharmacokinetics

Clofazimine has a variable oral bioavailability and is eliminated slowly in the bile. It has a long half-life (10 days), and can accumulate in the body.

Unwanted effects

- Gastrointestinal upset
- Brownish-black discoloration of the skin
- Acne.

PRINCIPLES OF ANTIBACTERIAL THERAPY

The following guidelines outline the principles that should be considered in the choice of a safe and effective therapy.

'Blind' or empirical treatment

Most antibacterial therapy is started 'blind' without prior identification of the organism and its antibacterial drug sensitivities. Such treatment should be guided by the clinical diagnosis and knowledge of the most common pathogenic bacteria in the infection to be treated. Local information about patterns of antibacterial resistance should be considered.

Spectrum of antibacterial activity

A drug with a narrow spectrum of activity should be used in preference to a broad-spectrum drug whenever possible. The unnecessary use of broad-spectrum antibacterials encourages the development of resistant bacteria. This can present problems for the person treated, by the selection of resistant pathogens or colonisation by resistant bacteria from the environment. For the community, the selection of resistant pathogens can create problems by rendering standard antibacterial therapy less reliable. Broad-spectrum antibacterial cover is sometimes appropriate, for example in a seriously ill person when the infecting bacterium is unknown and a variety of bacteria could be causing the condition being treated.

Combination therapy

Treatment with more than one antibacterial drug should not be used routinely. It may, however, be valuable to provide broad-spectrum cover in serious illness when the organism is unknown, for example the combination of cefotaxime and metronidazole to cover aerobic and anaerobic organisms in suspected Gram-negative septicaemia. When resistance is likely to develop readily to the first-choice drug during prolonged treatment, the use of combination therapy can minimise that risk, for example in the treatment of infective endocarditis or tuberculosis.

Bactericidal versus bacteriostatic drugs

In some situations, bactericidal drugs are preferred to bacteriostatic drugs, for example for the treatment of infective endocarditis or when the person being treated is immunocompromised. In most other situations, the choice is not important.

Site of infection

This may determine the choice of drug; for example, some antibacterials only achieve low concentrations in the biliary tree, urine, bone or CSF.

Mode of administration

Oral therapy is usually preferred to parenteral treatment. Exceptions include the treatment of serious infections when reliable blood concentrations are essential, when the drug is only available in parenteral formulation, or when gastrointestinal absorption may be unreliable, for example after abdominal surgery.

Duration of therapy

This should be as short as is compatible with adequate treatment of the infection. The decision is often arbitrary,

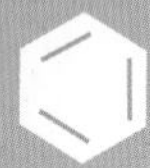

for example 7–10 days in many infections. Some infections can be effectively treated over much shorter periods; for example, courses of 1–3 days are usually adequate for uncomplicated lower urinary tract infections in women. There is evidence that the conventional longer courses of treatment for many other infections may be unnecessary. For a few infections, long periods of treatment may be essential to eliminate semi-dormant organisms or those in 'privileged sites' to which antibacterial drug penetration is poor. Examples include infective endocarditis, osteomyelitis and tuberculosis. Some antibacterials produce a 'post-antibiotic effect', in which there is delayed regrowth of surviving bacteria following exposure to the drug. This is marked with aminoglycosides such as gentamicin, but also occurs with other drugs, including β-lactam antibacterials.

Chemoprophylaxis

The use of chemoprophylaxis to prevent infection is important in many situations. Common examples include prevention of meningococcal meningitis in close contacts of an infected person, prevention of infective endocarditis in people with diseased or artificial heart valves undergoing surgery or dental treatment, and pre-operative prophylaxis before gut, biliary, thoracic or orthopaedic surgery.

TREATMENT OF SELECTED BACTERIAL INFECTIONS

This section is not intended to be comprehensive. It will outline the approach to antibacterial therapy in several common bacterial infections. The choice of antibacterial drug for these infections will depend on factors such as local patterns of bacterial resistance or the risk of *Clostridium difficile* infection, which make universal recommendations impossible.

Upper respiratory tract infections

Most upper respiratory tract infections are caused by viruses, producing symptoms of the common cold. Symptomatic treatment is all that should be offered, with an antihistamine (e.g. chlorphenamine; Ch. 39) or an antimuscarinic spray (e.g. ipratropium; Ch. 12) to reduce rhinorrhoea and sneezing. An α-adrenoceptor agonist given orally or nasally (e.g. xylometazoline) can reduce nasal congestion, but prolonged use can provoke a rebound effect (rhinitis medicamentosa) (Ch. 39). A non-steroidal anti-inflammatory drug (NSAID; Ch. 29) can be used to reduce associated headache and malaise. Antibacterial drugs are widely prescribed for upper respiratory tract symptoms but have no benefit.

Sinusitis and otitis media

Sinusitis and otitis media accompany catarrhal conditions in childhood and frequently follow an upper respiratory tract infection. Sinusitis produces headache, facial pain, fever and purulent rhinorrhoea. A nasal decongestant such as an α-adrenoceptor agonist can be helpful, in conjunction with an analgesic. An antibacterial is often not beneficial in acute sinusitis unless there is marked facial swelling and pain, or failure to resolve after 10–14 days. The most common infecting organisms are *Haemophilus influenzae* (which often produces β-lactamase), *Streptococcus pneumoniae* and *Moraxella catarrhalis*. Suitable antibacterial drugs include co-amoxiclav (amoxicillin plus clavulanic acid), cefuroxime axetil and erythromycin. Chronic sinusitis usually requires correction of an anatomical obstruction in the nose.

Otitis media is very common in childhood. When associated with an effusion in the middle ear, increased pressure causes pain and perforation of the eardrum. The organisms responsible are similar to those causing acute sinusitis. In more than 80% of affected children, the condition is self-limiting over 2–3 days without treatment. An antibacterial should be used for protracted episodes of otitis media. Surgery is occasionally necessary for recurrent infections.

Lower respiratory tract infections

Acute bronchitis

This is characterised by new-onset, often productive, cough without evidence of pneumonia. It is usually caused by a viral infection, and the cough often takes 2–4 weeks to resolve without treatment. Antibacterial treatment is inappropriate and does not alter the course of the illness. Even if there is underlying chronic obstructive airways disease, the evidence for benefit from antibacterial drugs is small, although they may slightly shorten the duration of symptoms. In such cases, *Streptococcus pneumoniae* (pneumococcus), *Haemophilus influenzae* or *Moraxella catarrhalis* are commonly found in the sputum, but are often isolated in remissions as well. If an antibacterial drug is used, then amoxicillin, co-amoxiclav, doxycycline or erythromycin will be effective against the most likely pathogens. Quinolones other than ciprofloxacin (which is poorly active against pneumococci) are an alternative.

Pneumonia

Primary community-acquired pneumonia is most commonly caused by *Streptococcus pneumoniae*, and less commonly by *Haemophilus influenzae* and staphylococci. 'Atypical' micro-organisms can also cause pneumonia, such as *Legionella* species, *Mycoplasma pneumoniae* or *Chlamydia pneumoniae*. Appropriate antibacterial treatment will be dictated by the most likely infecting agent.

Amoxicillin is the treatment of choice if pneumococcus is suspected. For people who are penicillin-allergic, erythromycin will cover most likely micro-organisms, including 'atypical' micro-organisms. Oral amoxicillin combined with erythromycin is often used for community-acquired pneumonia requiring admission of the person to hospital. Doxycycline is increasingly used as an alternative oral treatment because of a lower risk of *Clostridium difficile*-related colitis. Severe community-acquired pneumonia (defined by the CURB-65 score; Table 51.3) is often treated with intravenous therapy comprising a β-lactamase-resistant antibacterial, such as co-amoxiclav or cefuroxime, with intravenous clarithromycin. A quinolone with activity against pneumococci, such as moxifloxacin, would be an alternative choice. Adjunctive treatment of pneumonia may include supplemental oxygen via a facemask, pain relief for pleurisy, and ensuring adequate hydration.

Table 51.3 CURB-65 score: one point for each risk factor

■ Confusion (abbreviated mental test score ≤8/10 or new disorientation in place and time)
■ Serum urea >7 mmol L^{-1}
■ Respiratory rate ≥30 breaths min^{-1}
■ Systolic blood pressure <90 mmHg or diastolic blood pressure ≤60 mmHg
■ Age ≥65 years

Total score: 0–1, mortality 1.5%; 2, mortality 9.2%; ≥3, mortality 22%.

Secondary pneumonias occur in patients with other concurrent diseases, often during a stay in hospital (nosocomial or hospital-acquired pneumonia). A wide range of pathogens may be involved and parenteral drug treatment is usually necessary. A cephalosporin such as cefotaxime, an antipseudomonal penicillin (e.g. azlocillin) or ciprofloxacin is usually used. An aminoglycoside such as gentamicin is added for severe infection.

Chronic lung sepsis

This encompasses lung abscess, empyema and bronchiectasis. The pathogens in lung abscesses vary according to the immune status of the individual. Ideally, the antibacterial treatment should be directed by isolation and sensitivity testing of the bacteria. Empyema requires drainage, and then specific antibacterial therapy directed at the cultured pathogen. Bronchiectasis is most frequently associated with colonisation by *Haemophilus influenzae*, and less often *Pseudomonas* species or *Streptococcus pneumoniae*. A quinolone such as moxifloxacin or a macrolide such as azithromycin are reasonable empirical treatment choices. Increasing use is being made of inhaled nebulised antibacterial drugs, such as tobramycin, to treat frequent exacerbations. Adjunctive treatment with bronchodilators, mucolytics and physiotherapy may be useful (see also cystic fibrosis Ch. 13).

Urinary tract infections

Urinary tract infections are more common in women than men, because of their shorter urethra. Infections can occur in structurally normal urinary tracts or in association with a structural genitourinary abnormality that impairs drainage of urine or acts as a focus for infection, such as a stone in the urinary tract. An indwelling urinary catheter is often associated with bacterial colonisation of the urine that is almost impossible to eradicate.

The most frequent bacterial cause of urinary tract infection is *Escherichia coli*. Hospital-acquired infections are often caused by *Klebsiella*, *Enterobacter* and *Serratia* species or by *Pseudomonas aeruginosa*, because these organisms can be selected as resistant bacteria following antibacterial usage. *Proteus mirabilis* is often found if there are stones in the urinary tract. Less commonly, staphylococci, especially *Staphylococcus saprophyticus*, are responsible.

Uncomplicated urinary tract infection is confined to the bladder (cystitis) and can be treated by a short course (3 days) of an aminopenicillin such as amoxicillin or co-amoxiclav, the choice depending on local resistance patterns. Alternative drugs include a first-generation cephalosporin (e.g. cefalexin), trimethoprim and nitrofurantoin. A quinolone such as ciprofloxacin can be useful for *Pseudomonas aeruginosa* infections.

Complicated urinary tract infections also involve the kidney (pyelonephritis), or the prostate in males, and require longer courses of treatment. For pyelonephritis, initial intravenous therapy is usually started with broad-spectrum drugs such as aztreonam, ciprofloxacin or cefuroxime, sometimes with an initial dose of gentamicin; treatment is usually continued for 14 days. If there is associated prostatitis, oral treatment with trimethoprim or ciprofloxacin for at least 4 weeks is recommended.

If infection occurs with an indwelling urinary catheter, then treatment is only recommended if there are systemic symptoms of infection such as fever or rigors.

Long-term antibacterial prophylaxis against urinary tract infections may be necessary to prevent recurrent infection if there are underlying urinary tract abnormalities. Suitable drugs, usually given at low dosage, include trimethoprim, nitrofurantoin and cefalexin.

Gastrointestinal infection

In the UK, diarrhoea is usually caused by viruses and is self-limiting. However, gastroenteritis (a syndrome that includes nausea, vomiting, diarrhoea and abdominal discomfort) can result from ingestion of bacterial pathogens.

'Food poisoning' of bacterial origin can occur from ingestion of a pre-formed bacterial toxin (e.g. from *Clostridium botulinum* or *Staphylococcus aureus*), with onset of symptoms usually within hours, or it can be caused by ingested bacteria in the bowel (e.g. *Campylobacter* or *Salmonella* species). Severe bacterial infection of the large intestine can cause dysentery, an inflammatory disorder often associated with fever, abdominal pain, and blood and pus in the faeces.

The most common cause of bacterial diarrhoea (especially in children in developing countries) is *Escherichia coli*, which produces powerful enterotoxins. In other circumstances, *Salmonella* species, *Campylobacter* species, *Vibrio cholerae*, *Shigella* species or various other organisms are responsible.

If diarrhoea is severe, fluid replacement is often necessary. Antibacterial treatment is not usually recommended even if bacterial infection is suspected, unless there are systemic symptoms such as fever, rigors and hypotension. Ciprofloxacin and erythromycin are effective for *Campylobacter* enteritis. Salmonella infections and shigellosis can be treated with ciprofloxacin or trimethoprim, unless *Salmonella typhi* is suspected, when ciprofloxacin, cefotaxime or chloramphenicol is used.

Antibacterial drugs can cause diarrhoea due to alteration of bowel flora, which usually resolves rapidly when the drug is withdrawn. However, if it is complicated by colonisation with *Clostridium difficile*, then oral metronidazole or oral vancomycin will be necessary to eliminate the pathogen.

Biliary tract infection

Acute cholecystitis and cholangitis are often caused by *Escherichia coli* and most often occur if there is biliary

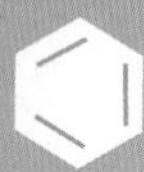

obstruction. Supportive treatment with fluid and electrolyte replacement is usually required. Antibacterial therapy with a cephalosporin or gentamicin is usually effective. Combination therapy with both drugs is recommended if the infection is severe; alternatively, a ureidopenicillin such as piperacillin can be given alone. Treatment is usually given for 7–10 days.

Osteomyelitis

Infection of bone produces necrotic tissue and generates an avascular privileged site for bacteria that antibacterial drugs penetrate to only a limited extent. Organisms involved include *Staphylococcus aureus*, which adheres readily to bone matrix, various streptococci, *Serratia* species, *Pseudomonas aeruginosa* and enteric Gram-negative rods.

Early antibacterial treatment is essential, with intravenous therapy for 6 weeks to achieve a cure. Surgical intervention may be necessary to remove necrotic tissue. The choice of drug depends on the suspected organisms. First-line treatment is often with clindamycin or flucloxacillin, combined with fusidic acid if a prosthesis is present or the infection is severe. If *Haemophilus influenzae* is identified, then amoxicillin or cefuroxime is usually used. Acute infections are treated for 4–6 weeks, but chronic infections for at least 12 weeks. If long-term therapy is necessary for chronic refractory osteomyelitis, then an oral quinolone such as ciprofloxacin can be substituted.

Septic arthritis

The standard treatment is with flucloxacillin together with fusidic acid or rifampicin. Clindamycin is used alone for individuals who are penicillin-allergic. Vancomycin is used for MRSA, combined with fusidic acid or rifampicin if a prosthesis is present or the infection is severe. Treatment should be continued for 6–12 weeks.

Cellulitis

This usually complicates a wound, ulcer or dermatosis. In most cases the infecting organism is *Staphylococcus aureus* or streptococci. Treatment is usually with β-lactam antibacterials, including one that is active against β-lactamase-producing *Staphylococcus aureus*. Benzylpenicillin (or phenoxymethylpenicillin for oral use) with flucloxacillin is normally used. Erythromycin is used alone for individuals who are penicillin-allergic.

Septicaemia

Septicaemia is a bacterial infection involving the bloodstream and can present with fever or, if more severe, can result in circulatory collapse from vasodilation, capillary leak and impaired myocardial contractility. Gram-positive organisms are a more frequent cause than Gram-negative organisms, with about 60% of infections arising from respiratory, intra-abdominal and urinary tract sources. Septicaemia is a medical emergency requiring intensive fluid replacement, plasma volume expansion and electrolyte correction. Noradrenaline (norepinephrine) or other vasopressors may be used to support the blood pressure (Ch. 4). There have been many advances in our understanding of the pathogenesis of sepsis and the associated immune activation, but little improvement in our ability to manage the complications of sepsis. The anti-inflammatory and anticoagulant drug recombinant activated protein C blocks the interaction between the coagulation system and the inflammatory cascade. However, it is unclear whether it produces any advantage even when there is severe sepsis and multi-organ compromise. Adrenal insufficiency is common in severe sepsis, and treatment with low-dose hydrocortisone may reduce the duration of shock.

If the source of the infection is not clinically apparent, then empirical antibacterial therapy is given to cover as wide a range of potential infecting organisms as possible. The prognosis is much worse if first-line drugs are ineffective. Suitable treatment would be with an aminoglycoside such as gentamicin combined with a broad-spectrum penicillin (e.g. amoxicillin) or a broad-spectrum cephalosporin (e.g. cefotaxime, or ceftazidime if pseudomonal infection is suspected). Alternatively, a carbapenem such as meropenem or imipenem (with cilastatin) can be used alone; metronidazole is added if anaerobic infection is suspected.

Immunocompromised and neutropenic individuals are at particularly high risk from septicaemia. A combination of gentamicin with a broad-spectrum penicillin or cephalosporin could be given in this situation. Other authorities recommend gentamicin combined with either piperacillin (plus tazobactam) or meropenem. Metronidazole is usually added if anaerobic infection is suspected; flucloxacillin or vancomycin is added if Gram-positive infection is suspected. Failure to respond to such triple therapy within 48 h may indicate a fungal infection, for which amphotericin can be added (see below).

Infective endocarditis

The majority of cases of infective endocarditis are caused by bacterial pathogens, most commonly oral streptococci, followed by enterococci, *Staphylococcus aureus* and coagulase-negative staphylococci. Endocarditis usually arises on the endothelial surface of a pre-existing heart defect (e.g. valvular heart defect, ventricular septal defect) or on a prosthetic heart valve. It arises when micro-organisms enter the bloodstream and become established on the endocardium, where they may adhere to pre-existing fibrin–platelet vegetations. Bacteria enter the blood during dental procedures, vigorous teeth cleaning or during some surgical procedures.

Untreated infection can destroy the infected heart valve and produce severe haemodynamic disturbance. Systemic complications can also arise from embolisation of vegetation from the valve, from bacteraemia, or through immune complexes that form in response to the infection.

When infection is suspected, treatment should be started and blood cultures taken. Prior to identification of the organism, treatment is usually started with intravenous benzylpenicillin combined with low-dose gentamicin. If the organism is sensitive to penicillin, then the benzylpenicillin is continued for 4 weeks and the gentamicin stopped after 2 weeks. Vancomycin is substituted for benzylpenicillin in

Table 51.4 Organisms causing bacterial meningitis

Age	Organism
<1 month	Group B streptococci
1 month to 4 years	*Haemophilus influenzae*
>4 years to young adult	*Neisseria meningitidis* (meningococcus)
Older adults	*Streptococcus pneumoniae* (pneumococcus)

people with penicillin allergy. Ceftriaxone is often used as single therapy if renal function is impaired. For staphylococcal endocarditis, flucloxacillin is given in combination with either gentamicin or fusidic acid; vancomycin is used alone for those who are allergic to penicillin.

Antibacterial prophylaxis is no longer recommended prior to procedures such as dental treatment, since there is no good evidence that it prevents endocarditis.

Meningitis

Bacterial meningitis is a medical emergency. The most likely organism depends on the age of the person (Table 51.4). Empirical selection of therapy is usually necessary, and treatment should be started at the first suspicion of bacterial meningitis. A single dose of benzylpenicillin can be given if the person is outside hospital, but cefotaxime is the preferred treatment in hospital. Chloramphenicol is an option for those who have an allergy to both penicillin and cephalosporins. Treatment is given for 5 days for meningococcus, and 10 days for *Haemophilus influenzae* or pneumococcus. Rifampicin is given for 2–4 days before hospital discharge if the meningitis was caused by meningococcus or *Haemophilus influenzae*. Close contacts of subjects with meningococcal or *Haemophilus influenzae* meningitis are usually given rifampicin as prophylaxis against infection.

Tuberculosis

Mycobacterium tuberculosis readily develops resistance to single-drug therapy. Three or four drugs are used for the first 2 months ('initial phase') to rapidly reduce the bacterial population prior to information on bacterial sensitivities becoming available, following which treatment is continued with two drugs for a further 4 months ('continuation phase') to achieve a cure. In some cases, more prolonged treatment may be necessary, especially for tuberculous meningitis or for resistant mycobacteria. A standard regimen in the UK includes rifampicin, isoniazid, ethambutol and pyrazinamide for 2 months (or until bacterial sensitivities are known) (*initial phase*), followed by rifampicin and isoniazid for a further 4 months. More prolonged treatment is sometimes necessary for cavitating lung disease or slow clearance of sputum cultures. Ethambutol is not used for treatment of young children because of difficulty in monitoring for eye toxicity.

Streptomycin is used in some countries in the initial phase of treatment. Thiacetazone is often used with isoniazid and initially streptomycin in countries that cannot afford rifampicin. Adherence to the treatment regimen can be a major problem in the treatment of tuberculosis, and combination tablets are often used to maximise this. In developed countries, directly observed treatment (DOT) has been instituted to improve adherence. This can result in major improvements in eradication rates.

Multidrug-resistant tuberculosis (resistance to at least rifampicin and isoniazid) is becoming more common, and new treatment strategies are needed to deal with emerging strains of *M. tuberculosis*. There are also increasing problems with the treatment of tuberculosis in people with HIV infection. This reflects the propensity for interactions among the antiretroviral drugs and antituberculous therapy, and overlapping unwanted effects.

FUNGAL INFECTIONS

Fungi usually infect skin or superficial mucous membranes, but can, more rarely, involve internal organs. Most fungal infections occur because of an underlying defect in host resistance. Fungi grow more readily in immunosuppressed individuals or following the suppression of normal flora with antibacterials. Good hygiene and the avoidance of sources of infection are important complementary approaches to the use of antifungal drugs.

Compared with antibacterial drugs, fewer drugs have been developed that have activity against fungi, and many of these are toxic to humans. A simplified outline of the ways in which antifungal drugs work is shown in Figure 51.5.

ANTIFUNGAL DRUGS

Polyenes

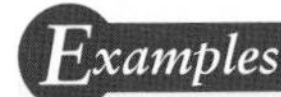

amphotericin, nystatin

Mechanism of action

Polyenes bind to ergosterol in the cell wall of fungi and form aqueous pores that promote leakage of intracellular ions and disruption of membrane active transport mechanisms. They can be fungistatic or fungicidal.

Spectrum of activity

Nystatin is particularly effective against infections with *Candida* species. Amphotericin is active against all common fungi that cause systemic infection (*Candida*, *Aspergillus*, *Mucor* and *Cryptococcus* species).

Resistance

Acquired resistance is rare but can occur in immunosuppressed people. Moulds and yeasts develop a mutation that permits synthesis of the cell membrane without using ergosterol.

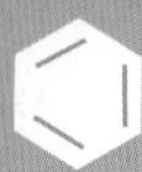

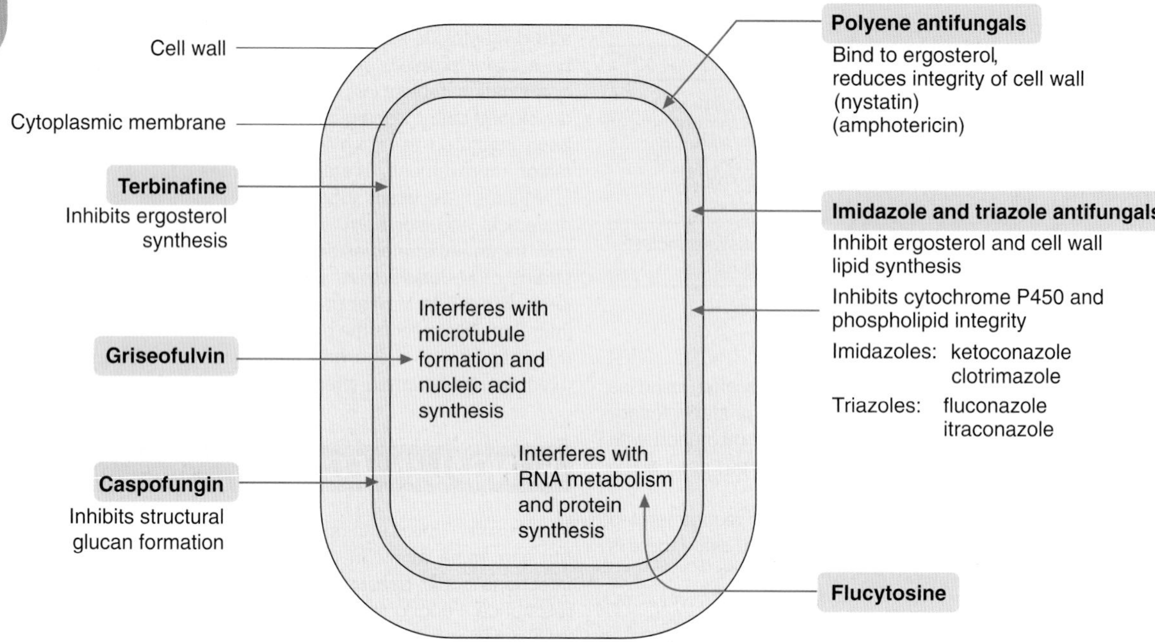

Fig. 51.5 **Sites at which antifungal drugs exert their actions on fungi.**

Pharmacokinetics

Nystatin is too toxic for systemic use and is not absorbed from the gastrointestinal tract. It is therefore used topically for *Candida albicans* infections, for example as cream for skin infection, as vaginal pessaries, or orally for buccal and bowel infections.

Amphotericin is poorly absorbed from the gut and is usually given intravenously for treatment of serious systemic fungal infections. An oral formulation is used for buccal and intestinal candidal infections. Amphotericin can also be given intrathecally for fungal meningitis. Amphotericin binds to steroid molecules in human tissue, and is released slowly and eliminated via the biliary tract and kidney. It has a very long half-life (about 2 days). Lipid delivery vehicles for amphotericin have been developed to reduce its nephrotoxicity. These formulations alter drug distribution and help to concentrate the drug at the site of infection. Formulations include liposomal spheres (in which the drug is dissolved in phospholipid membrane vesicles), lipid complexes (in which the lipid exists in ribbons interspersed with amphotericin), and a colloidal dispersion of lipid discs that incorporate the drug. The lipid component is probably cleared from the blood by mononuclear phagocytes.

Unwanted effects

Nystatin is virtually free of both toxic and allergic unwanted effects when used topically. Used orally for intestinal infection, it can cause gastrointestinal upset. Host toxicity with amphotericin is due to binding to cholesterol rather than ergosterol. Intravenous infusion of amphotericin is commonly associated with the following:

- Fever and rigors during the first week of therapy.
- Anorexia, nausea, vomiting, diarrhoea.
- Muscle and joint pain.
- Dose-related nephrotoxicity, which is the major limiting factor in treatment. It presents with reduced glomerular filtration rate and produces hypokalaemia and hypomagnesaemia through tubular leakage of K^+ and Mg^{2+}. Lipid formulations substantially reduce the risk of nephrotoxicity and are particularly useful to treat people with pre-existing renal impairment.

Imidazoles

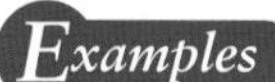

clotrimazole, ketoconazole, miconazole

Mechanism of action

The imidazoles alter the cell membrane fluidity of fungi by inhibiting lanosterol 14α-demethylase, which is a form of cytochrome P450 that participates in the conversion of lanosterol to ergosterol. This alters cell membrane synthesis, reduces the activity of membrane-associated enzymes, and increases cell wall permeability. Accumulation of ergosterol precursors in the cell causes growth arrest. Although the equivalent human enzyme is much less sensitive to the effects of the drug, inhibition of cytochrome P450 isoenzymes can occur in human tissues, especially with ketoconazole (Ch. 2).

Spectrum of activity

The imidazoles are active against a wide variety of filamentous fungi and yeasts, including *Candida* species. They are less active against *Candida krusei*. Clotrimazole is used for vaginal candidiasis and for dermatophyte infections (e.g. ringworm [tinea]; causative species vary geographically, but generally are *Trichophyton*, *Microsporon* or *Epidermophyton* species). Ketoconazole can be used for systemic mycoses, resistant mucocutaneous candidiasis, resistant vaginal candidiasis and resistant dermatophyte infections.

Resistance

The development of resistance is rare, except during long-term use in people with AIDS. The mechanism involves a point mutation in the target enzyme, or development of an active pump that removes drug from the cell, especially in *Candida* species.

Pharmacokinetics

Absorption of imidazoles from the gastrointestinal tract is poor, but oral ketoconazole achieves blood concentrations that are high enough to treat systemic infection. Clotrimazole is only used in topical formulations for superficial infections, for example skin and vagina. The imidazoles are metabolised in the liver. Ketoconazole has a half-life of about 6–10 h.

Unwanted effects

These are unusual with topical formulations, although oral miconazole can cause gastrointestinal upset. Oral ketoconazole can cause the following:

- Nausea, vomiting, abdominal pain
- Rash, urticaria, pruritus
- Hepatitis: asymptomatic elevation of liver enzymes is common; more severe hepatic reactions are unusual but can be fatal; liver function tests must be monitored during systemic use of ketoconazole
- High doses of ketoconazole suppress androgen production in males and can cause oligospermia or gynaecomastia
- Drug interactions: ketoconazole can inhibit metabolism of drugs that are eliminated by cytochrome P450 (see Table 2.9); examples of drugs affected include ciclosporin, tacrolimus (Ch. 38) and warfarin (Ch. 11).

Triazoles

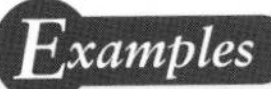

fluconazole, itraconazole, voriconazole

Mechanism of action and spectrum of activity

The triazoles have a similar mechanism of action and spectrum of activity to the imidazoles (see above). Fluconazole is used for candidiasis and for cryptococcal infection. Itraconazole is used for mucocutaneous candidiasis and for dermatophyte infections, such as pityriasis versicolor (caused by an organism known as *Malassezia furfur* or *Pityosporum orbiculare*) and tinea corporis or pedis (ringworms). Voriconazole is an 'extended-spectrum' triazole used for invasive aspergillosis, and serious infections caused by *Scedosporium* species, *Fusarium* species, or invasive fluconazole-resistant *Candida krusei* and *glabrata*.

Pharmacokinetics

Oral absorption is good. Intravenous (fluconazole, voriconazole) and topical (itraconazole) formulations are also available. The triazoles are metabolised in the liver and have long half-lives (6–30 h). Fluconazole penetrates well into cerebrospinal fluid, which is useful for treatment of fungal meningitis.

Unwanted effects

- Nausea, abdominal pain and diarrhoea.
- Headache, dizziness.
- Abnormalities of liver function and, occasionally, hepatitis or cholestasis. These are more common during prolonged treatment with itraconazole. Monitoring of liver function tests during systemic treatment is essential.
- Increased risk of heart failure with itraconazole. The mechanism of its negative inotropic effect is not known.
- Rashes, including Stevens–Johnson syndrome.

Terbinafine

Mechanism of action and use

Terbinafine is an allylamine that inhibits squalene epoxidase, an enzyme that converts squalene to ergosterol in the cell wall. It impairs cell wall synthesis, and the intracellular accumulation of squalene is probably cytotoxic (Fig. 51.5). It is used topically for treatment of dermatophyte infections of the nails, and systemically for ringworm infections.

Resistance

Resistance is rare, but similar to that for imidazole antifungals.

Pharmacokinetics

Terbinafine penetrates well into the stratum corneum and hair follicles after topical use. After oral administration, it is metabolised in the liver and has a long half-life (about 15 h).

Unwanted effects

These are unlikely with topical use of the drug. Unwanted effects include:

- Nausea, taste disturbance, abdominal discomfort and diarrhoea
- Headache
- Rashes, which are occasionally severe.

Echinocandins

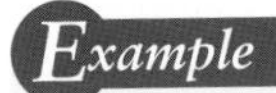

caspofungin

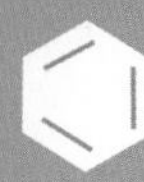

Mechanism of action

Caspofungin inhibits fungal cell wall synthesis, targeting the glucans that are found in fungal but not human cell walls (Fig. 51.5). It inhibits the enzyme 1,3-β-glucan synthase, and prevents production of the main structural polymer in the fungal cell wall. Caspofungin is used to treat invasive aspergillosis as a second-line drug, and invasive candidiasis.

Resistance

This is uncommon at present, but can occur from a point gene mutation coding for a structural change in the enzyme, which no longer binds the drug.

Pharmacokinetics

Caspofungin is only given by intravenous infusion. It is metabolised in the liver and has a very long half-life (40–50 h).

Unwanted effects

- Nausea, vomiting, abdominal pain, diarrhoea
- Dyspnoea
- Flushing, fever
- Headache
- Rashes
- Hypokalaemia, hypomagnesaemia.

Flucytosine

Mechanism of action and use

Flucytosine is converted to 5-fluorouracil (5-FU) selectively in fungal cells by the enzyme cytosine deaminase. This acts as an antimetabolite that competes with uracil for incorporation into fungal RNA. 5-FU is metabolised to compounds that inhibit enzymes involved in DNA synthesis (Fig. 51.5).

Flucytosine is only active against yeasts such as *Candida*, *Aspergillus* and *Cryptococcus* species. It is used for systemic infections.

Resistance

Resistance occurs readily and arises through a mutation that produces a deficiency of the enzyme which metabolises flucytosine or through excessive synthesis of uracil, which competes with the antimetabolite. For this reason, flucytosine is only used in combination with amphotericin or fluconazole.

Pharmacokinetics

Flucytosine is only available for intravenous use. It is mainly eliminated unchanged in the urine and has a short half-life (3 h).

Unwanted effects

- Nausea, abdominal pain, diarrhoea
- Rashes.

Griseofulvin

Mechanism of action and use

Griseofulvin inhibits dermatophyte mitosis by impairing the polymerisation of microtubule protein (Fig. 51.5). It is active against dermatophytes such as *Microsporum*, *Epidermophyton* and *Trichophyton* species.

Resistance

Resistance has not been shown.

Pharmacokinetics

Griseofulvin shows variable absorption from the gut. It is selectively concentrated in skin and nail beds; only low concentrations are found in plasma. Elimination is by metabolism in the liver and the half-life is long (10–21 h).

Unwanted effects

- Nausea, vomiting, diarrhoea
- Headache.

TREATMENT OF SPECIFIC FUNGAL INFECTIONS

Aspergillus

Aspergillus species can cause an invasive fungal infection that most commonly affects the lung. However, in immunocompromised individuals, it can invade more widely and infect the heart, brain, sinuses and skin. The treatment of choice is voriconazole, which is more effective and less toxic than amphotericin. If this fails, then itraconazole can be used. Caspofungin is reserved for infections that have failed to respond to standard treatments, or for those people who cannot tolerate the other drugs.

Candida

Amphotericin or nystatin is often used for oral candidiasis. If there is oropharyngeal disease that is refractory to topical treatment, then an absorbed drug such as fluconazole or itraconazole is used. Vulvovaginal infection is treated with cream and pessaries, and imidazole drugs, such as clotrimazole, are usually the first choice. Nystatin is an alternative for vulvovaginal candidiasis, but stains clothing yellow. For recurrent vulvovaginal infections, oral fluconazole or itraconazole should be taken once a week for 6 months. Superficial candidal infections of the skin are treated topically with cream, usually containing an imidazole. Terbinafine or nystatin can also be used topically.

Invasive candidiasis mainly occurs as a hospital-acquired infection, particularly in people who have had abdominal surgery, parenteral nutrition, antibacterial drugs or central vascular lines. *Candida albicans* is still the single most common organism, but *C. krusei*, *C. glabrata* and *C. parapsilosis* are increasingly common. Amphotericin is the treatment of choice, sometimes combined with fluconazole. Caspofungin is an alternative.

Cryptococcus

Infection with *Cryptococcus* species usually occurs in people who are immunocompromised. It can cause life-threatening meningitis, and is treated with intravenous amphotericin with flucytosine. Fluconazole is an alternative, and can be given orally for prophylaxis against relapse.

Skin and nail infections

Topical therapy is usually suitable for infections with most dermatophytes. Fungal infection of the scalp (tinea capitis), body (tinea corporis), groin (tinea cruris), hand (tinea manuum), foot (tinea pedis) or nail (tinea unguium) will respond to most azoles. Griseofulvin is usually reserved for treatment of scalp infections. Nail infection usually requires systemic treatment, with terbinafine or itraconazole.

Pityriasis versicolor can be treated topically or orally with itraconazole, or with oral fluconazole.

Prophylaxis in immunocompromised individuals

Individuals who are immunocompromised are at greater risk of fungal infection. Prophylaxis is often given with oral fluconazole, since this has better oral absorption than most azoles, and is less toxic than ketoconazole.

VIRAL INFECTIONS

Viruses are small infective particles consisting of either DNA or RNA, inside a protein coating (capsule), which in some viruses may be further surrounded by a lipoprotein coating. The proteins can have antigenic properties. Viruses lack any inherent metabolic machinery and must use the host cells' metabolic processes to attach to and enter host cells and to replicate. Viruses access host cells after binding to recognition sites that are endogenous receptors for normal cellular constituents, for example adrenoceptors, cytokine receptors, glycoproteins, etc (Fig. 51.6). Drugs that interfere with host cell membrane cytokine receptors, such as CCR5, and surface glycoproteins will inhibit viral entry and interrupt the virus replication.

The host will normally eliminate the virus by killing the infected cell. Cytotoxic T-lymphocytes recognise the viral surface proteins that are expressed by infected cells. The host can also produce antibodies that bind to and inactivate virus particles extracellularly. Vaccination is designed to generate this response.

Since viruses share many of the host's metabolic processes, this makes it difficult to damage the virus without damaging the host. Importantly, antiviral drugs are only effective while the virus is replicating, so the earlier they are given in the course of the infection the more likely they are to work. An outline of the replication of RNA and DNA viruses is shown in Figures 51.6 and 51.7. Since the replicative mechanisms involved may be distinctive to one type of virus, some antiviral drugs are specific for a particular class of virus.

New antiviral drugs are being introduced into clinical practice at an increasing rate. Drugs are available to treat

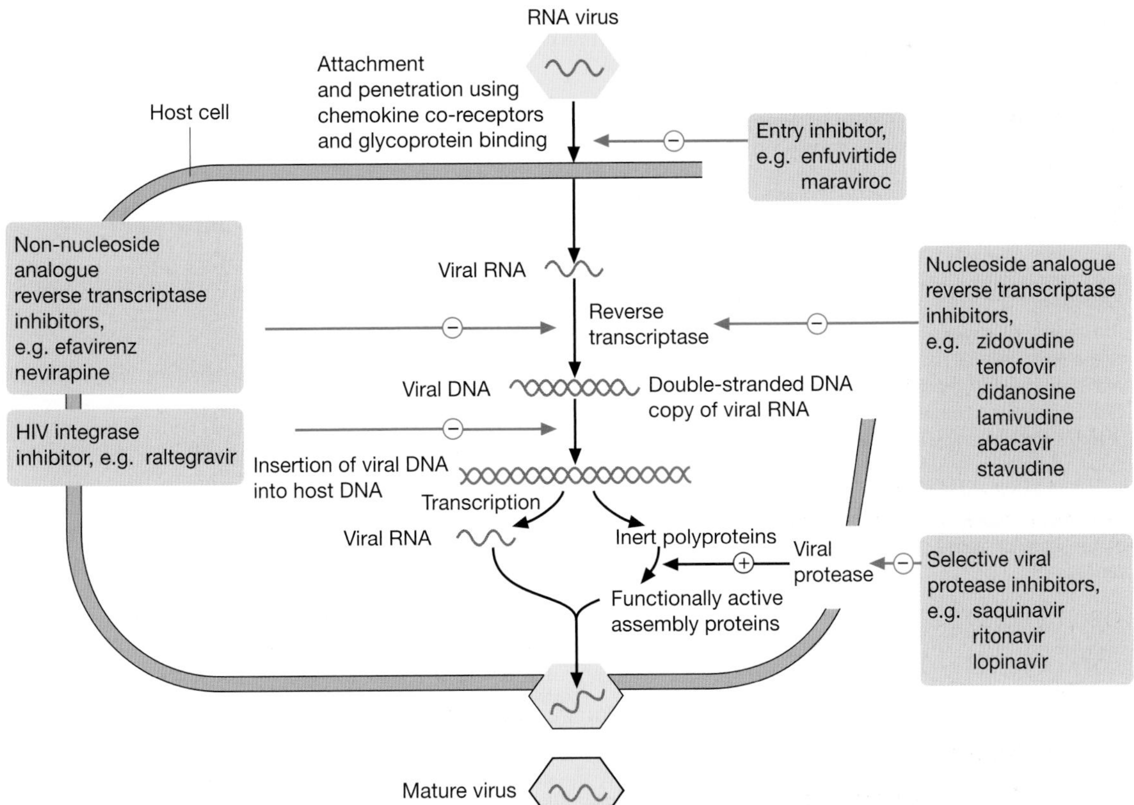

Fig. 51.6 **Principles of RNA virus replication and sites of action of antiviral drugs.** For details, see text.

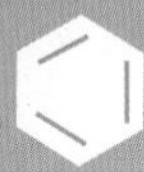

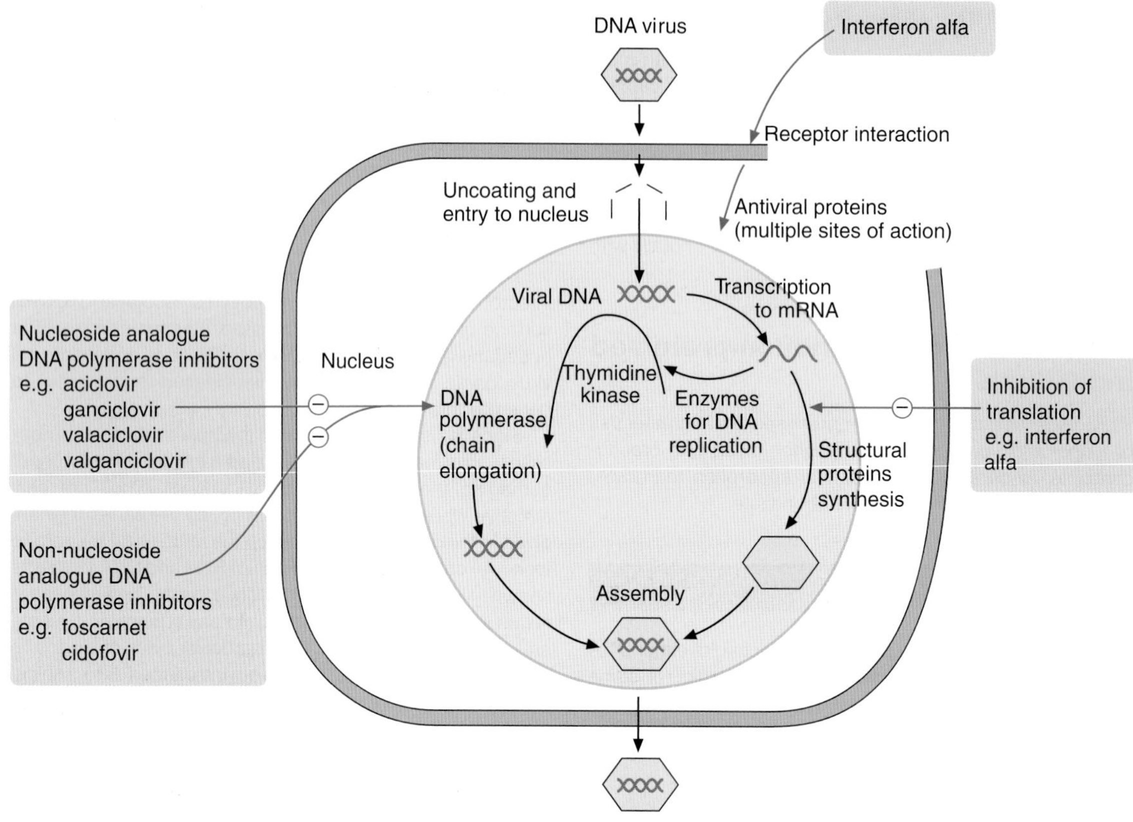

Fig. 51.7 **Principles of DNA virus replication and sites of actions of antiviral drugs.** For details, see text.

infection by RNA viruses (e.g. HIV, hepatitis C and influenza viruses) and DNA viruses (e.g. herpes viruses, cytomegalovirus [CMV] and hepatitis B virus). Drugs work by disturbing various steps in the replicative pathways of the virus. Because of the development of resistance and the variability in viral sensitivity to drugs, it is sometimes necessary to use concurrently drugs targeting different points in the virus replication.

Resistance to antiviral drugs occurs readily. This relates to the high rate of natural occurrence of mutations in the viral genome and production of quasi-species of the virus. Viral polymerases have a high inherent error rate (especially RNA viruses) and viruses tolerate a large number of nucleoside mutations without losing their infectivity. Normally, the large variety of viral quasi-species will be dominated by the variant most selected for survival, and, therefore, use of an antiviral drug will select for growth of resistant variants.

ANTIVIRAL DRUGS

HIV REVERSE TRANSCRIPTASE INHIBITORS

The reverse transcriptase inhibitors are active against the RNA virus human immunodeficiency virus (HIV). They prevent viral RNA being transcribed as viral DNA in the host cell (Fig. 51.6).

Nucleoside analogue HIV reverse transcriptase inhibitors

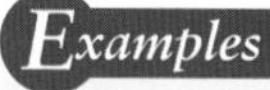

abacavir, emtricitabine, lamivudine, tenofovir, zidovudine

Mechanism of action

These drugs inhibit RNA virus replication by reversible inhibition of the viral enzyme HIV reverse transcriptase, which generates viral DNA for insertion into the host DNA sequence. The HIV reverse transcriptase inhibitor drugs (Fig. 51.6) are activated by phosphorylation inside the virus to the 5′-triphosphate form. The inhibition is achieved by competitive binding of the activated drug to the enzyme–template–primer complex in place of the natural 5′-deoxynucleoside triphosphates, thus terminating further DNA chain elongation.

The nucleoside reverse transcriptase inhibitors are analogues of precursors of the natural purines and pyrimidines involved in DNA transcription initiated by the virus. Zidovudine is an analogue of thymidine, one of the constituents of the base pairs in DNA (Fig. 51.6). Emtricitabine and lamivudine are analogues of cytidine, abacavir an analogue of deoxyguanosine, and tenofovir an analogue of adenosine.

Resistance

Resistant quasi-species emerge rapidly, within weeks or months, through mutation of the drug-binding site on the transcriptase enzyme, which results in an increase in the affinity for the natural substrate compared with the drug. Because of the rapid development of resistance, multiple drug therapy is used for treatment of HIV infection.

Pharmacokinetics

These drugs are almost completely absorbed from the gut. Elimination of abacavir, didanosine and zidovudine is mainly by hepatic metabolism and the half-lives are short (1–2 h). Emtricitabine, lamivudine, stavudine and tenofovir (the metabolite of tenofovir disoproxil) are mainly eliminated unchanged by the kidney, with half-lives in the range 1–17 h.

Unwanted effects

These are often so severe that they lead to withdrawal of therapy. They are probably related to inhibition of host mitochondrial enzymes, with impaired generation of intracellular adenosine triphosphate (ATP).

- Neutropenia and anaemia are the most frequent unwanted effects (usually occurring in individuals with advanced AIDS)
- Nausea, vomiting, diarrhoea, abdominal pain
- Headache, insomnia
- Myalgia or myositis, especially with high doses
- Severe potentially life-threatening hepatomegaly with steatosis and lactic acidosis
- Pancreatitis
- Lipodystrophy syndrome with fat redistribution (loss of subcutaneous fat, buffalo hump, breast enlargement), insulin resistance and dyslipidaemia; this may be due to inhibition of regulatory proteins in adipocytes.

Non-nucleoside reverse transcriptase inhibitors

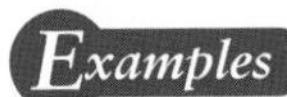

efavirenz, nevirapine

Mechanism of action and resistance

These drugs inhibit HIV reverse transcriptase by binding remotely from the active site to produce a conformational change in the enzyme that prevents substrate binding. They have greater antiviral activity than nucleoside analogue inhibitors, and are better tolerated. Resistance still emerges rapidly by single point gene mutations, unless they are used in combination with at least two other antiretroviral drugs.

Pharmacokinetics

Oral absorption of nevirapine is very good, while that of efavirenz is variable and incomplete. They are metabolised by hepatic CYP3A4, and also induce the enzyme. They have very long half-lives of about 2 days.

Unwanted effects

- Rash (severe in 10%), especially with nevirapine
- Nausea, vomiting, abdominal pain, diarrhoea
- Headache, drowsiness, fatigue
- Hepatotoxicity with nevirapine, which can cause potentially fatal fulminant hepatitis
- Drug interactions with drugs that are metabolised by hepatic cytochrome P450.

HIV PROTEASE INHIBITORS

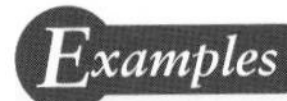

atazanavir, lopinavir, ritonavir

Mechanism of action

In HIV infection, there are some steps in viral replication that differ from the processes in host cells. RNA is translated into inert polyproteins rather than the functional proteins that are the products of host cells. Proteases that are found only in viruses cleave the polyproteins to the functionally active proteins required by the viruses for their continued existence (Fig. 51.6). Protease enzyme inhibitors are specific for the enzymes found in HIV. They block the infectivity of the virus but do not affect virus activity in host cells that are already infected.

Resistance

Resistance occurs by mutation in the amino acid sequence of the HIV protein that forms the target for the enzyme. Multiple mutations are required for high-level resistance, but over one-third of the amino acid residues in HIV protein can be changed without altering viral function. High plasma drug concentrations delay the onset of resistance, as does the combination of a protease inhibitor with two reverse transcriptase inhibitors. Sequential use of more than one protease inhibitor encourages high-level resistance.

Pharmacokinetics

Oral absorption differs between drugs (see compendium at the end of the chapter). They are all metabolised by CYP3A4 in the liver and have half-lives in the range 2–10 h. They are inhibitors of human CYP3A4 (see below).

Unwanted effects

- Nausea, vomiting, abdominal pain, diarrhoea.
- Lipodystrophy syndrome (see nucleoside analogue reverse transcriptase inhibitors).
- Hepatic dysfunction.
- Pancreatitis.
- Circumoral and peripheral paraesthesiae with ritonavir.
- Drug interactions (Ch. 56): inhibition of the P450 enzyme CYP3A4 (Table 2.9) can enhance the unwanted effects of protease inhibitors; the concurrent use of inducers of CYP3A4 can lower plasma concentrations of the protease inhibitor and encourage viral resistance. Inhibition

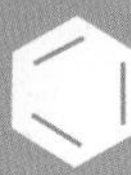

of the enzyme CYP3A4 by a low dose of ritonavir can increase the clinical effect of other protease inhibitors (boosted protease inhibition), a useful action that allows less frequent dosing with the other drug. Ritonavir also inhibits the metabolism of drugs such as warfarin (Ch. 11) and carbamazepine (Ch. 23). The use of protease inhibitors with simvastatin (Ch. 48) should be avoided because of an increased risk of myopathy.

HIV BINDING–FUSION–ENTRY INHIBITORS

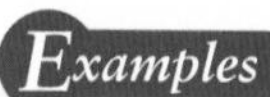

enfuvirtide

Mechanism of action

In order to enter a host cell, HIV fuses with the host cell membrane. This fusion is facilitated by a conformational change in a glycoprotein in the viral cell membrane. Enfuvirtide is a 36-amino-acid peptidomimetic that binds to the glycoprotein and prevents the conformational change. Enfuvirtide is used when there is resistance or intolerance to other antiretroviral drugs.

Resistance

This occurs by gene mutation that modifies the glycoprotein target.

Pharmacokinetics

Enfuvirtide is given by subcutaneous injection. It is expected to undergo catabolism to its constituent amino acids, but the metabolic fate has not been elucidated. The half-life is 4 h.

Unwanted effects

- Injection site reactions
- Pancreatitis, gastro-oesophageal reflux disease, anorexia
- Peripheral neuropathy, tremor, anxiety, nightmares.

CCR5 CO-RECEPTOR ANTAGONISTS

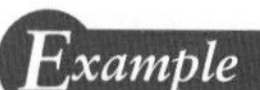

maraviroc

Mechanism of action

CCR5 (chemokine (C-C motif) receptor 5) is a receptor for several chemokines, including RANTES, MIP-1α and MIP-1β. It is expressed on many cells, including T-cells, macrophages, dendritic cells and microglia. CCR5 acts as a viral co-receptor that facilitates entry of the virus into the cell. Other chemokine receptors such as CCR4 or both CCR4 and CCR5 are also used by some HIV viruses to access cells. HIV viruses which use CCR5 are predominant early in the infection, but some viruses use CCR4 or both receptors for entry. Maraviroc selectively binds to CCR5 and prevents interaction with CCR5-tropic strains of HIV, inhibiting their entry into the cell. It has no effect on viruses that use CCR4 or are dual-tropic (use both CCR4 and CCR5). Maraviroc is used in combination with other antiretroviral drugs for individuals who have already received antiretroviral treatment.

Pharmacokinetics

Maraviroc is only partially absorbed from the gut. It is metabolised in the liver and has a long half-life of 14–18 h.

Unwanted effects

- Gastrointestinal disturbances
- Cough
- Dizziness, paraesthesiae, sleep disturbances, headache, muscle spasm.

HIV INTEGRASE INHIBITORS

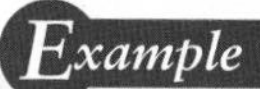

raltegravir

Mechanism of action

Once inside a host cell, HIV integrates its DNA into the host genome. This requires the action of a specific viral integrase. Raltegravir inhibits the integrase and prevents DNA strand transfer from the viral genome. Raltegravir is used when there is resistance to other antiretroviral drugs.

Resistance

This occurs when there is amino acid substitution in the integrase enzyme.

Pharmacokinetics

Raltegravir is well absorbed from the gut, and is excreted in the bile after glucuronide conjugation and unchanged in the urine. It has a half-life of 9 h.

Unwanted effects

- Nausea, diarrhoea
- Headache
- Fever.

VIRAL DNA POLYMERASE INHIBITORS

Nucleoside analogue DNA polymerase inhibitors

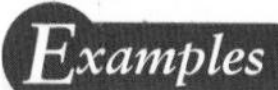

aciclovir, ganciclovir, valaciclovir, valganciclovir

Mechanism of action

Aciclovir and the other drugs in this class are guanosine analogues that inhibit the synthesis of viral DNA (Fig. 51.7). They all require phosphorylation by viral enzymes that are not present in uninfected host cells, before they can exert their antiviral activity. This dependency on viral enzymes prevents cytotoxic effects in human tissue. The phosphorylating enzymes, however, are not present in all DNA viruses.

Aciclovir is activated by conversion to a monophosphate by phosphorylation of the drug using viral thymidine kinase. The monophosphate is then converted to a triphosphate derivative by other intracellular enzymes. The triphosphate derivatives are potent inhibitors of viral DNA polymerase. This terminates viral DNA synthesis and thus inhibits viral replication (Fig. 51.7).

Ganciclovir also suppresses viral DNA replication by inhibiting viral DNA polymerase but does not act as a DNA chain terminator.

Spectrum of activity

Aciclovir is most active against herpes viruses (both simplex and zoster). It is only active against CMV at high doses. Ganciclovir has much greater activity than aciclovir against CMV, possibly because it is a better substrate for the CMV protein kinase, which activates it by phosphorylation.

Resistance

Viral mutants are selected that are unable to phosphorylate the drugs. Thymidine kinase-deficient mutants of herpes virus usually develop in immunocompromised individuals, for example those with AIDS or after bone marrow transplantation, when resistance rates average 5–10% of treated individuals.

Pharmacokinetics

Aciclovir can be given orally, intravenously, or topically to the skin or eye. Absorption from the gut is poor. The drug is widely distributed, but concentrations in the cerebrospinal fluid are low compared with those in plasma. Most is eliminated by the kidney, and the half-life is 3 h. Valaciclovir is an ester of aciclovir with higher oral bioavailability. Ganciclovir is given intravenously for acute infections since it is poorly absorbed from the gut; it penetrates into the CSF moderately well. It is eliminated by the kidney and has a half-life of 4 h. Valganciclovir is an oral prodrug of ganciclovir with better absorption. Famciclovir undergoes essentially complete first-pass metabolism to the active form, penciclovir, which has a half-life of 2 h.

Unwanted effects

Most unwanted effects occur with intravenous use, and are much more frequent with ganciclovir than with aciclovir.

- Severe local phlebitis at an infusion site.
- Nausea, vomiting, abdominal pain, diarrhoea.
- Rashes.
- Encephalopathy.
- Nephrotoxicity is caused by crystallisation of the drug in the kidney. It can be limited by a high fluid intake.
- Bone marrow suppression is the most frequent serious unwanted effect with ganciclovir, with neutropenia occurring in up to 40% of people, and thrombocytopenia less frequently. The neutropenia can be prevented by the use of granulocyte colony-stimulating factor (Ch. 47).
- Azoospermia with ganciclovir.

Non-nucleoside analogue DNA polymerase inhibitors

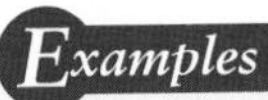

cidofovir, foscarnet sodium

Mechanism of action

Foscarnet is an inorganic pyrophosphate compound that binds to the pyrophosphate-binding sites of viral DNA polymerase, preventing DNA chain elongation. Affinity for the viral DNA polymerase is a hundred times greater than for the host cell DNA polymerase. Cidofovir is similar in structure to aciclovir but contains a phosphate moiety. Its action is similar to that of foscarnet. Foscarnet and cidofovir do not rely on intracellular activation for their antiviral activities (Fig. 51.7). These drugs are reversible inhibitors of CMV and herpes simplex replication.

Pharmacokinetics

Because both foscarnet and cidofovir are highly polar molecules, they are only given intravenously. Foscarnet and cidofovir are eliminated by the kidney and have half-lives of about 5 h and 3 h, respectively. Cidofovir is given with probenecid (Ch. 2) (and adequate hydration), which inhibits renal tubular secretion of cidofovir and minimises its nephrotoxicity.

Unwanted effects

- Nausea, vomiting
- Neutropenia
- Headache, tremor, dizziness, mood disturbances with foscarnet
- Both drugs are highly nephrotoxic, causing a rise in plasma creatinine; good hydration reduces kidney damage
- Iritis or uveitis with cidofovir.

DRUGS FOR TREATING VIRAL HEPATITIS

Ribavirin, adefovir and lamivudine are used in the treatment of infections with hepatitis B and C viruses and respiratory syncytial virus (RSV). They are discussed in Chapter 36.

DRUGS FOR TREATING INFLUENZA VIRUS

M2 ion channel inhibitors

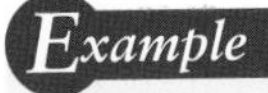

amantadine

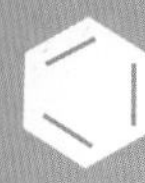

Amantadine is active against influenza A only, and inhibits the transmembrane M2 ion channel that permits H^+ entry into the viral cell. This is required for uncoating of the virus once it has penetrated the host cell, so viral replication is inhibited. Amantadine is discussed in Chapter 24.

Neuraminidase inhibitors

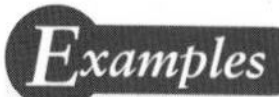

oseltamivir, zanamivir

Mechanism of action

Influenza viruses carry two surface glycoproteins, a haemagglutinin and a neuraminidase. The haemagglutinin mediates entry of the virus into the host cell. Neuraminidase cleaves cellular-receptor sialic acid residues to which newly formed viruses are attached as they bud from the infected cell. The released virions can then infect new cells. Neuraminidase inhibitors inhibit the neuraminidases of both influenza A and B, and are effective against isolates resistant to amantadine.

Pharmacokinetics

Zanamivir is administered by inhalation, when systemic absorption is low. Only 2% of the inhaled drug is absorbed, and then excreted unchanged. Oseltamivir is a more lipophilic molecule that is taken orally, and is converted by hepatic esterases to the active oseltamivir carboxylate, which is excreted by the kidneys and has a half-life of 6–10 h.

Unwanted effects

- Gastrointestinal disturbance with oseltamivir
- Headache, fatigue, insomnia, dizziness with oseltamivir
- Bronchospasm with zanamivir.

IMMUNOMODULATORS

Interferon alfa

Interferon alfa is most often used in the treatment of hepatitis B infection, and is discussed in Chapter 36. Clinical uses of interferon alfa include the treatment of:

- chronic hepatitis B infection
- condylomata acuminata
- AIDS-related Kaposi's sarcoma
- hairy cell leukaemia
- recurrent or metastatic renal cell carcinoma (Ch. 52).

Palivizumab

Mechanism of action and use

Palivizumab is a humanised monoclonal antibody with human and murine antibody sequences; it is produced by recombinant DNA technology. It has potent neutralising and fusion-inhibiting activity against respiratory syncytial virus (RSV). It reduces the ability of RSV to replicate and infect cells by binding to an antigenic site on the surface of RSV. RSV is a common cause of mild respiratory illness in infants but can produce more severe illness in premature infants or those with congenital heart disease or bronchopulmonary dysplasia. Palivizumab can be given to at-risk children under the age of 2 years prior to commencement of the RSV season (October to April in the Northern Hemisphere) and monthly thereafter.

Pharmacokinetics

Palivizumab is given intramuscularly into the anterolateral aspect of the thigh. The routes of elimination are unknown; it has a long half-life of about 20 days.

Unwanted effects

- Fever
- Injection site reactions.

TREATMENT OF SPECIFIC VIRAL INFECTIONS

HIV infection

There are several principles of antiviral therapy for HIV (retroviral) infection which are now widely adopted. The most frequently used treatment regimens include a protease inhibitor (e.g. atazanavir or lopinavir) or a non-nucleoside reverse transcriptase inhibitor (e.g. efavirenz or nevirapine) combined with two nucleoside analogue reverse transcriptase inhibitors (e.g. tenofovir with emtricitabine, abacavir with lamivudine, or zidovudine with lamivudine). A low dose of ritonavir is often added to this regimen to prolong the action of the other drugs and simplify the dosing regimen. Such combinations are referred to as highly active antiretroviral therapy (HAART). HAART involves complex regimens that require adherence by the individual and careful assessment of the progress of viral suppression. Key principles include the following:

- Combination drug treatment should be started before substantial immunodeficiency is present. The goal is to suppress the virus before resistant mutants emerge or irreversible immune damage occurs. The optimal time to start treatment is not known, but should definitely be started when the CD4+ T-lymphocyte count falls to less than $200 \times 10^6 L^{-1}$. If this does not occur, then treatment is given when symptoms arise as a result of HIV infection.
- When resistance occurs, modification in drug therapy should involve the addition or change of at least two drugs. Resistance of the HIV virus persists indefinitely. However, if toxicity limits the tolerability of one drug, a single substitution of a similar drug is a reasonable option.
- Optimal treatment should reduce the viral load to below detectable limits, and achieve a rise in CD4+ lymphocyte count. This may take 6 months of adequate therapy to achieve.
- Failure to achieve full suppression of viral load should prompt a change in therapy if adherence is believed to be good. Poor adherence with therapy is likely to encourage the development of drug resistance (see

above) and thus treatment failure. Drug therapy is ideally guided by patterns of resistance in the virus.
- The optimal duration of treatment is unclear, but withdrawal even when the CD4+ T-cell count rises is probably associated with less favourable long-term outcomes.

New drug classes are under investigation for HIV infection, and some are available on expanded-access pre-licensing programmes. These include etravirine, a second-generation non-nucleoside reverse transcriptase inhibitor.

Prophylaxis after accidental exposure to the virus is now recommended. The regimen depends on the level of risk: two drugs are often used for moderate risk exposures, or three drugs if the risk is high.

Varicella–zoster virus infections

Varicella–zoster virus (VZV) is a herpes virus responsible for both chickenpox and shingles (zoster). Shingles arises from reactivation of the virus, which lies dormant in a dorsal root ganglion after the primary chickenpox infection. Chickenpox is rarely treated with antiviral therapy, although the use of oral aciclovir reduces lesion formation and results in quicker healing.

Zoster is most commonly found in the elderly and in immunosuppressed people. The rash is often preceded by pain for 1–4 days. Oral antiviral drug therapy reduces pain and accelerates healing, but must be given while the virus is still replicating. Oral aciclovir or valaciclovir are often used and are particularly indicated for those over 50 years (who are at greater risk of complications), for ophthalmic infections, or in immunosuppressed people. Treatment should be started within 72 h of the onset of the rash. Complications occur in 15–20% of people with zoster and include meningoencephalitis, motor nerve paralysis, ocular complications and postherpetic neuralgia. The use of aciclovir has little effect on the risk of developing postherpetic neuralgia but does reduce the risk of motor nerve damage. Corticosteroids such as prednisolone as an adjunctive treatment to antiviral therapy reduce pain and produce more rapid healing of lesions, but do not prevent the development of neuralgia. Analgesics are often required in the early phases of zoster, and postherpetic neuralgia may require specific therapy (Ch. 19).

Herpes simplex virus infections

Herpes simplex virus exists in two forms: type 1 produces either oral or genital ulceration, and type 2 produces genital ulceration. Oral herpes infection will respond to early topical application of aciclovir. Primary genital herpes produces multiple painful lesions and responds to oral aciclovir or valaciclovir given for 7–10 days. Recurrent lesions occur from reactivation of latent virus in the dorsal root ganglia, producing symptoms that are usually less severe than with primary episodes. After initial therapy with aciclovir or valaciclovir for up to 3 days, continuous suppressive therapy can be given to prevent further relapses.

Cytomegalovirus infection

CMV infection is common and usually produces mild symptoms. However, it can be devastating in immunosuppressed individuals. Troublesome complications in this group include retinitis (which can threaten sight), gastrointestinal manifestations (including oesophagitis, gastritis, cholecystitis or colitis), pneumonia and CNS involvement.

Intravenous ganciclovir is the treatment of choice for severe manifestations of CMV infection. Foscarnet can be used as an alternative to ganciclovir, or cidofovir if both are contraindicated. For CMV retinitis, oral valganciclovir is used both for treatment and to prevent relapse. Oral valganciclovir or valaciclovir may be of particular value for the prevention of CMV infection, especially in renal transplant recipients and bone marrow transplant recipients, in whom CMV pneumonia is a major potential complication. Combined therapy with ganciclovir and CMV immunoglobulin may be more effective than ganciclovir alone for treatment of pneumonia in this situation.

Influenza

The use of a neuraminidase inhibitor, such as zanamivir or oseltamivir, reduces the duration of uncomplicated influenza by about 1 day. Treatment must be started within 48 h of the onset of an influenza-like illness. People who are at greater risk of complications of influenza include those with chronic respiratory disease, significant cardiovascular disease, chronic renal disease, diabetes mellitus or who are immunocompromised. However there is little evidence on the ability of these drugs to prevent the complications of influenza. Neuraminidase inhibitors are also effective for the prevention of influenza during an epidemic, reducing the likelihood of developing the illness by 70–90%. They should be considered for high-risk individuals who have not been vaccinated and who can be treated within 48 h of contact with someone who has an influenza-like illness. Such prophylaxis is not a substitute for an effective vaccination campaign.

PROTOZOAL INFECTIONS

MALARIA

Four species of the protozoan *Plasmodium* produce malaria in humans: *P. vivax*, *P. ovale*, *P. malariae* and *P. falciparum*. Sporozoites are formed by repeated division of oocysts in the body of the infected female *Anopheles* mosquito (the vector) and are transferred in the mosquito's saliva into host blood during a subsequent blood meal. The parasite is sequestered in the liver and divides to form tissue schizonts (Fig. 51.8). When the pre-erythrocytic (liver) sexual cycle is complete, the liver cells rupture and 20 000–40 000 merozoites escape into the blood and invade erythrocytes. They then undergo the erythrocytic cycle, multiplying asexually in the erythrocytes. Infected red cells then rupture and release merozoites to invade other red cells. Merozoites in the plasma at this stage are termed gametocytes. A mosquito biting an infected individual ingests gametocytes, which then go through a development cycle in the mosquito to form sporozoites.

At the pre-erythrocytic stage in the liver, some schizonts from *P. vivax* and *P. ovale* remain in the liver, rather than

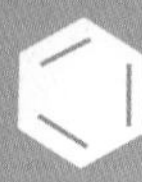

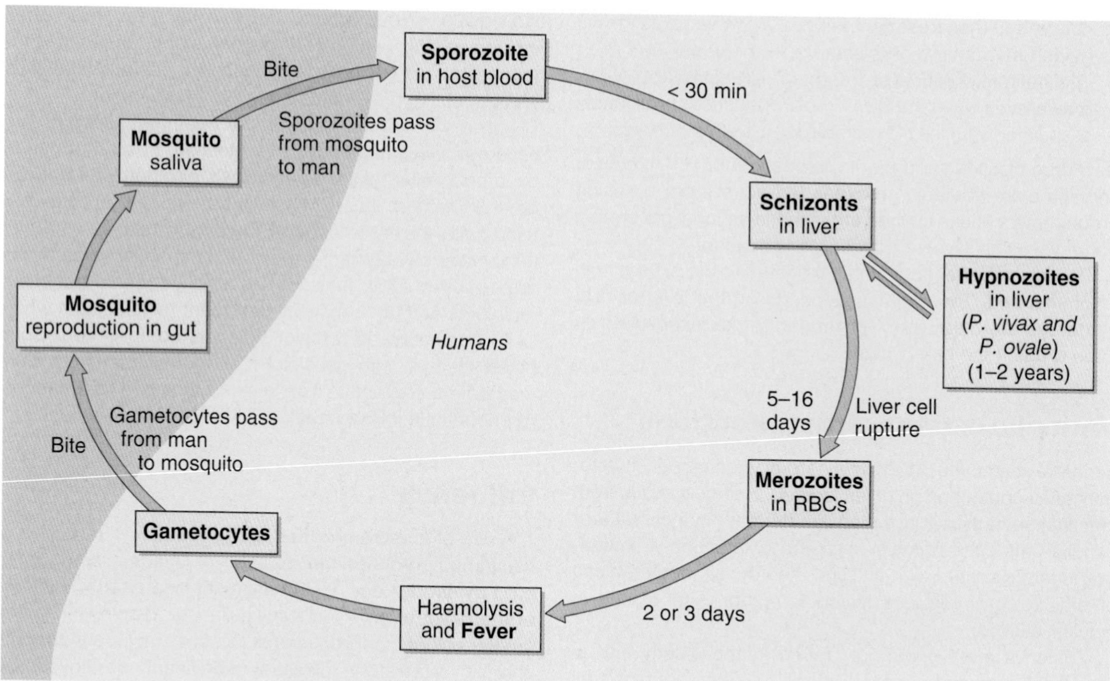

Fig. 51.8 **Life-cycle of the malarial parasite.**

being released as merozoites, remain in the liver, forming hypnozoites. These form a reservoir of parasites that are difficult to eradicate and can emerge to give relapses months or years after the initial infection. Release of merozoites in humans every 2–3 days causes repeated bouts of tertian or quartan fever. The duration of the infection varies with the parasite. Because *P. vivax* and *P. ovale* continue to multiply in the liver as hypnozoites, drugs that treat only the erythrocytic phase will not produce a radical cure (elimination of all parasites), and relapsing infection can occur.

P. falciparum and *P. malariae* multiply only in erythrocytes, but disease can recrudesce if parasites are not completely eliminated from the blood.

Clinical symptoms include chills as merozoites enter blood from ruptured erythrocytes. Nausea, vomiting and headache are common. A fever follows, and the attack concludes with sweating. *P. falciparum* produces the most severe symptoms because it causes agglutination of red cells, which produces capillary thrombosis, especially in the brain, leading to cerebral malaria.

ANTIMALARIAL DRUGS

Chloroquine

Mechanism of action

Erythrocytes infected by malaria parasites concentrate chloroquine more than 100-fold, since it binds to a breakdown product of haemoglobin induced by the parasite, and interferes with the haem degradative pathway.

- Chloroquine is digested by the erythrocyte-resident parasite, and this raises lysosomal pH, which reduces the ability of the parasite to digest haemoglobin and thereby inhibits its growth.
- Chloroquine interacts with ferriprotoporphyrin IX, which is formed during digestion of haemoglobin, an action that prevents further degradation of haemoglobin by the parasite.

Chloroquine (and its close relative hydroxychloroquine) also possesses slow-onset anti-inflammatory activity, which is useful in the treatment of rheumatoid arthritis (Ch. 30).

Pharmacokinetics

Chloroquine is a 4-aminoquinoline that is completely absorbed from the gut, or it can be given intravenously. It has a very high volume of distribution because of selective concentration in melanin-containing tissues, for example the retina of the eye, and in the liver, spleen and kidney. Approximately half is converted in the liver to active metabolites; the rest is excreted unchanged by the kidney. The half-life is very long during chronic dosing; an initial half-life of up to 6 days is followed by a second slow phase of tissue elimination with a half-life of greater than 1 month.

Unwanted effects

- Nausea, vomiting, diarrhoea and abdominal pain, which may be caused by anticholinesterase activity (Chs 27 and 28).
- Cardiovascular depression after intravenous use, with hypotension and heart block; these are quinidine-like effects (Ch. 8).

- Seizures.
- Retinopathy with cumulative doses, producing retinal pigmentation and visual field defects. Visual function should be monitored.
- Rashes and pruritus, hair loss and skin depigmentation.

Mefloquine

Mechanism of action

Mefloquine has a similar mode of action to that of chloroquine.

Pharmacokinetics

Mefloquine is an amino alcohol that is well absorbed from the gut and has a high affinity for lung, liver and lymphoid tissue. Extensive metabolism occurs in the liver, but the elimination half-life is extremely long (2–4 weeks).

Unwanted effects

- CNS effects: dizziness, vertigo, headache, sleep disorders. Less commonly, severe psychiatric disturbance can occur, and mefloquine should not be given to people with a previous history of psychiatric disorder.
- Gastrointestinal effects occur that are similar to those seen with chloroquine.
- Myalgia, arthralgia.
- Chest pain, tachycardia, hypotension.

Primaquine

Mechanism of action

Unlike structurally related drugs, primaquine only affects the exoerythrocytic parasite. It enters the parasite in the liver and may inhibit mitochondrial respiration. It is used after treatment with chloroquine, to eradicate *P. vivax* or *P. ovale* from the liver.

Pharmacokinetics

Primaquine is an 8-aminoquinolone that is completely absorbed from the gut and rapidly metabolised in the liver, producing active compounds. The half-life is 4–10 h.

Unwanted effects

- Intravascular haemolysis in people with glucose-6-phosphate dehydrogenase (G6PD) deficiency (Ch. 47). G6PD activity in erythrocytes produces NADPH, which keeps glutathione in the reduced state, thereby maintaining cell wall integrity and preventing haemolysis (see Ch. 53). G6PD activity should be checked before initiating treatment.
- Gastrointestinal effects are similar to those seen with chloroquine.

Quinine

Mechanism of action

Quinine is similar to chloroquine in its action.

Pharmacokinetics

Quinine is well absorbed from the gut but can also be given by intravenous infusion. Metabolism in the liver is extensive and the half-life is about 6 h in healthy people, becoming much longer in severe malaria.

Unwanted effects

- 'Cinchonism': tinnitus, headache, nausea, flushing, visual disturbances with vertigo, and, if severe, hearing loss
- Stimulation of insulin secretion, producing hypoglycaemia
- Quinidine-like effects on the heart (Ch. 8), with bradycardias, heart block or ventricular tachycardia; this occurs most often with intravenous loading doses.

Pyrimethamine

Mechanism of action

Selective inhibition of dihydrofolate reductase in the parasite reduces folic acid synthesis (Fig. 51.4). Pyrimethamine should only be given in combination with the sulphonamide sulfadoxine.

Pharmacokinetics

Pyrimethamine is well absorbed from the gut and undergoes extensive hepatic metabolism. The half-life is very long, approximately 2–6 days.

Unwanted effects

Pyrimethamine is usually well tolerated; occasional effects are:

- Photosensitive rashes
- Insomnia
- Megaloblastic anaemia due to inhibition of human folate metabolism (with high doses).

Proguanil

Mechanism of action

Proguanil inhibits plasmodial dihydrofolate reductase (Fig. 51.4), mainly through its active metabolite, cycloguanil, which inhibits folate production in both pre-erythrocytic and erythrocytic parasites. It is usually used for malaria prophylaxis in combination with chloroquine. It can also be used in the prophylaxis and treatment of *P. falciparum* in combination with atovaquone.

Pharmacokinetics

Absorption of proguanil from the gut is good, and extensive metabolism occurs in the liver to cycloguanil, a potent active derivative. The half-life of proguanil is long (12–24 h); the plasma profile of cycloguanil reflects its slow formation from proguanil, despite it having a short half-life (2 h) (see Ch. 2).

Unwanted effects

- Mouth ulcers
- Epigastric discomfort, diarrhoea.

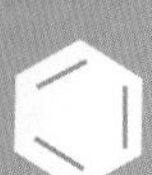

Artemether with lumefantrine

Mechanism of action

Artemether is a herb extract that is activated by complexing with iron in the haem ingested by the parasite. The resulting compound produces reactive oxygen species that disrupt Ca^{2+} transporter function in malarial trophozoites. It is used with lumefantrine, an amino alcohol (see mefloquine above) which reduces resistance.

Pharmacokinetics

Artemether is well absorbed from the gut and rapidly hydrolysed to an active metabolite that has a short half-life of 2–3 h.

Unwanted effects

- Abdominal pain, nausea, anorexia, diarrhoea
- Headache, dizziness, sleep disturbance, fatigue.

TREATMENT OF MALARIA

Chemotherapy of malaria falls into three categories:

- rapid-acting blood schizonticides (to kill schizonts in acute malaria): chloroquine, quinine, mefloquine
- slow-acting blood schizonticides (to prevent blood infections): pyrimethamine, proguanil
- tissue schizonticides (to eliminate liver parasites): primaquine.

The recommended drug to use within each category depends on the type of parasite and the pattern of resistance where the infection was acquired. If the infecting organism is unknown, it is assumed to be *P. falciparum*, which carries the greatest risk. The latest drug recommendations should be obtained from tropical disease advisory centres.

Examples are given for current recommended treatments for acute attacks of high- and low-risk malaria.

For *P. falciparum*, chloroquine and mefloquine resistance is common. Oral quinine (or intravenous quinine for serious infections) for 5–7 days is followed by pyrimethamine with sulfadoxine for 7 days or by doxycycline or clindamycin (see Antibacterials above) if the plasmodia are resistant to sulfadoxine. Alternatively, proguanil with atovaquone (see below) or artemether with lumefantrine (see compendium) are used for 3 days.

For benign malaria, chloroquine is taken for 3 days. For *P. vivax* and *P. ovale*, primaquine is then taken for 14 days to destroy hepatic parasites.

PROPHYLAXIS AGAINST MALARIA

The recommendations for prophylaxis depend on patterns of resistance in the area to be visited. Chloroquine or proguanil is often recommended for areas where resistance is low. For many areas, a combination of both drugs is desirable. Mefloquine, doxycycline, or proguanil with atovaquone are recommended in some areas where there is a high risk of chloroquine-resistant malaria. Prophylaxis must also take into account the unwanted effects of the drugs and other factors such as pregnancy and renal or hepatic impairment. Prophylaxis must be started 1 week before travel (3 weeks for mefloquine) and continued for 1 month after leaving a malarious area (7 days for proguanil with atovaquone), to protect against infection acquired immediately prior to departure.

OTHER PROTOZOAL INFECTIONS

Details of the natural history of other protozoal infections are not given in this book. Important drugs available in the UK for these conditions are discussed below. An outline of therapeutic uses is given in Table 51.5.

Atovaquone

Indications

Atovaquone is used as a second-line drug for treatment of *Pneumocystis jirovecii* infections and for treating *Toxoplasma gondii* infection. It is also active against *Plasmodium* species, *Entamoeba histolytica* and *Trichomonas vaginalis*.

Table 51.5 Selected protozoan infections and antiprotozoal drugs

Protozoa	Disease	Drug examples
Plasmodium	Malaria	Chloroquine, mefloquine, primaquine, quinine, proguanil, pyrimethamine, atovaquone
Entamoeba histolytica	Amoebic dysentery	Metronidazole, tinidazole, diloxanide
Trichomonas vaginalis	Vaginitis	Metronidazole, tinidazole
Giardia lamblia	Gastrointestinal dysfunction	Metronidazole, tinidazole, mepacrine
Leishmania	Cutaneous or visceral (kala-azar) leishmaniasis	Stibogluconate, pentamidine
Trypanosoma	Trypanosomiasis, Chagas' disease, sleeping sickness	Suramin*, nifurtimax*, benznidazole*, eflornithine, pentamidine, melarsoprol*
Toxoplasma gondii	Encephalomyelitis, toxoplasmosis	Pyrimethamine plus sulfadiazine, trimetrexate
Pneumocystis jirovecii	Pneumocystis pneumonia	Co-trimoxazole, pentamidine, atovaquone, trimetrexate

*not available or used in the UK for protozal infection.

Mechanism of action

Atovaquone interferes with DNA synthesis by inhibiting pyrimidine synthesis. It is selective for protozoa that cannot utilise pre-formed pyrimidines. It affects mitochondrial electron transport and ATP synthesis.

Pharmacokinetics

Oral absorption of atovaquone is poor but is improved with food, and most of the dose is eliminated in the faeces. The absorbed fraction is excreted in the urine and bile, which results in enterohepatic cycling, giving it a very long half-life of about 3 days.

Unwanted effects

- Diarrhoea, nausea, vomiting
- Rash
- Headache, insomnia
- Neutropenia.

Pentamidine

Indications

Pentamidine is used in pneumocystis pneumonia, leishmaniasis and trypanosomiasis.

Mechanism of action and use

Pentamidine undergoes active uptake into the cell, where it probably inhibits DNA synthesis and ribosomal synthesis of protein and phospholipid. It is cytotoxic to *Pneumocystis jirovecii* in the non-replicating state. Because of its toxicity, pentamidine is usually reserved for people who are intolerant of co-trimoxazole, which is the drug of first choice for pneumocystis pneumonia.

Pharmacokinetics

Pentamidine is given intravenously or inhaled as an aerosol for pneumocystis pneumonia. It can be given by deep intramuscular injection for leishmaniasis or trypanosomiasis. Inhalation is particularly useful for pneumocystis pneumonia (which affects immunocompromised people, especially those with AIDS), since lung concentrations are low after intravenous administration. Pentamidine is metabolised in the liver and has a very long half-life (13 days).

Unwanted effects

- Inhaled pentamidine produces bronchial irritation with cough and bronchospasm.
- Intravenous pentamidine is nephrotoxic, and can produce irreversible hypoglycaemia and life-threatening arrhythmias such as ventricular tachycardia.

Sodium stibogluconate

Indications

Sodium stibogluconate is used to treat visceral leishmaniasis.

Mechanism of action

Sodium stibogluconate is an organic pentavalent antimony derivative that may act by binding to thiol groups in the parasite and inhibiting the formation of high-energy phosphates.

Pharmacokinetics

Sodium stibogluconate must be given parenterally, either by intramuscular injection or slow intravenous infusion. It has a half-life of 6 h and is eliminated by the kidney.

Unwanted effects

- Anorexia, nausea, vomiting
- Headache
- Lethargy
- Myalgia
- Cough and substernal pain during intravenous infusion.

Diloxanide furoate

Indications

Diloxanide is used to treat chronic amoebiasis in asymptomatic individuals who are excreting cysts of *Entamoeba histolytica* in the stool. Acute infection is treated with metronidazole or tinidazole (Table 51.5).

Mechanism of action

The mechanism of action is unknown.

Pharmacokinetics

It is given orally and hydrolysed in the gut to diloxanide and furoic acid; 90% of the diloxanide is then absorbed and rapidly conjugated in the liver. There is little information about its fate in the body. The unabsorbed fraction of diloxanide may contribute to the drug's effectiveness in amoebic dysentery.

Unwanted effects

- Flatulence, anorexia, nausea and diarrhoea
- Urticaria, pruritus.

HELMINTHIC INFECTIONS

Details of the natural history of helminth infections are not given here, but an outline of the more commonly encountered conditions is given in Table 51.6. Drugs specifically for helminth infections are discussed below.

ANTIHELMINTHIC DRUGS

Ivermectin

Indications

Ivermectin is used to treat filariasis (especially onchocerciasis), hookworm and *Strongyloides stercoralis* infection. Treatment with a single dose reduces microfilarial levels for several months, and it can be repeated every 6–12 months if necessary. In the UK, it is an unlicensed drug, available on a 'named-patient' basis only. It is the drug of choice for onchocerciasis.

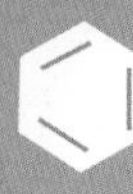

Table 51.6 Helminth infections

Helminth	Common name	Drug examples
Enterobius vermicularis	Threadworm	Mebendazole, piperazine
Ascaris lumbricoides	Roundworm	Mebendazole, piperazine, levamisole
Toxocara canis	Dog roundworm	Tiabendazole, diethylcarbamazine
Taenia species	Tapeworm	Niclosamide, praziquantel
Ancylostoma species, *Necator* species	Hookworm	Mebendazole, ivermectin, albendazole
Microfilariae (e.g. *Loa loa, Wuchereria bancrofti, Brugia malayi*)		Diethylcarbamazine, ivermectin
Strongyloides stercoralis		Tiabendazole, albendazole, ivermectin
Echinococcus granulosa	Hydatid disease	Albendazole

Mechanism of action

Ivermectin is a macrocyclic lactone. It produces an influx of Cl^- via an action on glutamate-gated membrane ion channels, generating hyperpolarisation of the filariae and muscle paralysis.

Pharmacokinetics

Ivermectin is well absorbed from the gut and is excreted mainly in the faeces. It undergoes some hepatic metabolism and has a long half-life (12 h).

Unwanted effects

- Itching
- Rash.

Diethylcarbamazine

Indications

Diethylcarbamazine is used to treat filariasis.

Mechanism of action

The mechanism of action of diethylcarbamazine is not well understood. It may inhibit arachidonic acid metabolism in the filariae. It also triggers exposure of antigens on the surface coat, leading to antibody-mediated phagocytosis. Diethylcarbamazine is not marketed in the UK but is a first-line drug for filariae. Treatment is usually required for 2–3 weeks to eliminate the microfilariae.

Pharmacokinetics

Oral absorption is good, and approximately half the drug is metabolised in the liver; the rest is excreted unchanged by the kidney. The half-life is not well established.

Unwanted effects

Most problems are caused by release of antigens from dying filariae. The onset is about 2 h after dosing and is almost diagnostic of the disease. The reaction is occasionally severe and life-threatening. The reaction includes:

- Fever
- Headache
- Nausea
- Muscle and joint pains
- Itching
- Postural hypotension.

Benzimidazoles

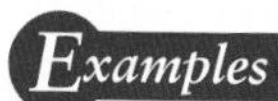

albendazole, mebendazole, tiabendazole

Indications

Tiabendazole: *Strongyloides stercoralis*, hookworm (cutaneous larva migrans). Tiabendazole is available in the UK on a 'named-patient' basis.
Mebendazole: threadworm, roundworm, hookworm.
Albendazole: hydatid cysts, *Strongyloides stercoralis*.

Mechanism of action

The benzimidazoles bind to tubulin, preventing its polymerisation into the cytoskeletal microtubules. The effect is selective for parasitic tubulin and the drugs are active against the adults, larvae and eggs.

Pharmacokinetics

Oral absorption of tiabendazole is almost complete; metabolism in the liver is extensive and the half-life is very short (about 1 h). The oral absorption of mebendazole and albendazole are very poor; the little drug that is absorbed is metabolised in the liver, and they have half-lives of 3–9 h and 8–12 h, respectively. These drugs act principally from within the gut.

Unwanted effects

- Gastrointestinal effects are common with tiabendazole and include anorexia, nausea, vomiting and diarrhoea; they are less severe with the other drugs.
- Dizziness and drowsiness can occur with tiabendazole.

Piperazine

Indications

Piperazine is given orally to treat threadworm and roundworm infections.

Mechanism of action

Piperazine competitively inhibits the effect of acetylcholine on the smooth muscle of the worm, producing a reversible flaccid paralysis.

Pharmacokinetics

Absorption of piperazine is rapid from the gut; up to 30% of the dose is eliminated unchanged in urine but little is known about the fate of the remainder.

Unwanted effects

Gastrointestinal upset can occur.

Niclosamide

Indications

Niclosamide is given orally to treat tapeworm infection. Niclosamide is available in the UK on a 'named-patient' basis.

Mechanism of action

Niclosamide inhibits generation of ATP by preventing phosphorylation of adenosine diphosphate (ADP) in mitochondria. It is ineffective against larval worms. Purgatives are usually given after niclosamide to remove viable ova from the gut.

Pharmacokinetics

Some oral absorption (up to 20%) occurs, with subsequent liver metabolism. The half-life is not known.

Unwanted effects

- Gastrointestinal upset, nausea, abdominal pain
- Lightheadedness
- Pruritus.

Praziquantel

Indications

Praziquantel is given orally to treat tapeworm infection and schistosomiasis. Praziquantel is unlicensed in the UK and is available only on a 'named-patient' basis.

Mechanism of action

It is not well understood how praziquantel acts; it is known to increase the permeability of the cell membrane of sensitive helminths to Ca^{2+}, causing muscular contraction and paralysis. It may also reduce cellular transport of adenosine, which cannot be synthesised by the parasites.

Pharmacokinetics

Praziquantel is well absorbed from the gut and penetrates well into most tissues; it is extensively metabolised by the liver and has a plasma half-life of 2 h.

Unwanted effects

- Dizziness, headache, lassitude
- Gastrointestinal upset.

FURTHER READING

Antibacterial drugs

Bartlet JG (2002) Antibiotic-associated diarrhoea. *N Engl J Med* 346, 334–339

Blumberg HM, Leonard MK Jr, Jasmer RM (2005) Update on the treatment of tuberculosis and latent tuberculosis infection. *JAMA* 293, 2776–2784

Calhoun JH, Manring MM (2005) Adult osteomyelitis. *Infect Dis Clin North Am* 19, 765–786

Durrington HJ, Summers C (2008) Recent changes in the management of community acquired pneumonia. *BMJ* 336, 1429–1433

Fihn SD (2003) Acute uncomplicated urinary tract infection in women. *N Engl J Med* 349, 259–266

Fitch MT, Abrahamian FM, Moran GJ et al (2008) Emergency department management of meningitis and encephalitis. *Infect Dis Clin North Am* 22, 33–52

Garcia D, Torre I (2003) Advances in the management of septic arthritis. *Rheum Clin North Am* 29, 61–75

Grant A, Gothard P, Thwaites G (2008) Managing drug resistant tuberculosis. *BMJ* 337, 564–569

Gruchella RS, Pirmohamed M (2006) Antibiotic allergy. *N Engl J Med* 354, 601–609

Hirschmann JV (2002) Antibiotics for common respiratory tract infections in adults. *Arch Intern Med* 162, 256–264

Hoare Z, Shen Lim W (2006) Pneumonia: update on diagnosis and management. *BMJ* 332, 1077–1079

Jacoby GA, Munoz-Price LS (2005) The new β-lactamases. *N Engl J Med* 352, 380–391

Li JZ, Winston LG, Moore DH et al (2007) Efficacy of short-course antibiotic regimens for community-acquired pneumonia: a meta-analysis. *Am J Med* 120, 783–790

Lode HM (2007) Managing community-acquired pneumonia: a European perspective. *Respir Med* 101, 1864–1873

Maartens G, Wilkinson RJ (2007) Tuberculosis. *Lancet* 370, 2030–2043

Mackenzie I, Lever A (2007) Management of sepsis. *BMJ* 335, 929–932

Mansharamani NG, Koziel H (2003) Chronic lung sepsis: lung abscess, bronchiectasis and empyema. *Curr Opin Pulm Med* 9, 181–185

Moreillon P, Que Y-A (2004) Infective endocarditis. *Lancet* 363, 139–149

Niederman MS (2007) Recent advances in community-acquired pneumonia: inpatient and outpatient. *Chest* 131, 1205–1215

Picazo JJ (2004) Management of the febrile neutropenic patient: a consensus conference. *Clin Infect Dis* 15(suppl 1), S1–S6

Rovers MM, Schilder AGM, Zielhuis GA et al (2004) Otitis media. *Lancet* 363, 465–473

Swartz MN (2004) Cellulitis. *N Engl J Med* 350, 904–912

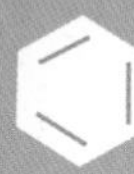

ten Hacken NHT, Wijkstra PJ, Kerstjens HAM (2007) Treatment of bronchiectasis in adults. *BMJ* 335, 1089–1093

Tenover FC (2006) Mechanisms of antimicrobial resistance in bacteria. *Am J Med* 119(suppl 1), S3–S10

Turnidge J (2001) Responsible prescribing for upper respiratory tract infections. *Drugs* 61, 2065–2077

Westphal J-F, Brogard J-M (1999) Biliary tract infections. *Drugs* 57, 81–91

Antifungal drugs

Balkis MM, Leidich SD, Mukherjee PK et al (2002) Mechanisms of fungal resistance. *Drugs* 62, 1025–1040

Hart R, Bell-Syer SE, Crawford F et al (1999) Systematic review of topical treatments for fungal infections of the skin and nails of the feet. *BMJ* 319, 79–82

Kontoyiannis DP, Lewis RE (2002) Antifungal drug resistance of pathogenic fungi. *Lancet* 359, 1135–1144

Leather HL, Wingard JR (2002) Prophylaxis, empirical therapy, or pre-emptive therapy of fungal infections in immunocompromised patients; which is better for whom? *Curr Opin Infect Dis* 15, 369–375

Patterson TF (2005) Advances and challenges in management of invasive mycoses. *Lancet* 366, 1013–1025

Rubin EA, Somani J (2004) New options for the treatment of invasive fungal infections. *Semin Oncol* 31(suppl 2), 91–98

Sobel JD (2003) Management of patients with recurrent vulvovaginal candidiasis. *Drugs* 63, 1059–1066

Antiviral drugs

Clavel F, Hance AJ (2004) HIV drug resistance. *N Engl J Med* 350, 1023–1035

Deeks SG (2006) Antiretroviral treatment of HIV infected adults. *BMJ* 332, 1489–1493

Deeks SG, Phillips AN (2009) HIV infection, antiretroviral treatment, ageing and non-AIDS related mortality. *BMJ* 338, 288–292

Esté JA, Telenti A (2007) HIV entry inhibitors. *Lancet* 370, 81–88

Glezen WP (2008) Prevention and treatment of seasonal influenza. *N Engl J Med* 359, 2579–2585

Gupta R, Warren T, Wald A (2007) Genital herpes. *Lancet* 370, 2127–2137

Moscana A (2005) Neuraminidase inhibitors for influenza. *N Engl J Med* 353, 1363–1373

Simon V, Ho DD, Karim QA (2006) HIV/AIDS epidemiology, pathogenesis, prevention and treatment. *Lancet* 368, 489–504

Wareham DW, Breuer J (2007) Herpes zoster. *BMJ* 334, 1211–1215

Antiparasitic drugs

Freedman DO (2008) Malaria prevention in short-term travellers. *N Engl J Med* 359, 603–612

Antiprotozoal drugs

Kremsner PG, Krishna S (2004) Antimalarial combinations. *Lancet* 364, 285–294

Montoya JG, Liessenfeld O (2004) Toxoplasmosis. *Lancet* 363, 1965–1977

Stanley SL Jr (2003) Amoebiasis. *Lancet* 361, 1025–1034

Whitty CJM, Lalloo D, Ustianowski A (2006) Malaria: an update on treatment of adults in non-endemic countries. *BMJ* 333, 241–245

Antihelminthic drugs

de Silva N, Guyatt H, Bundy D (1997) Antihelminthics. *Drugs* 53, 769–788

SELF-ASSESSMENT

In questions 1–7, the first statements, in italics, are true. Are the accompanying statements also true?

1. *Resistance to an antibacterial can be generated in bacteria by:*
   - *a decrease in the uptake or increase in the efflux of the drug*
   - *an increased production of enzymes that metabolise the drug*
   - *replacement of enzymes that are essential for microbial survival by mutated enzymes that have a similar function to the non-mutated enzymes but are not inhibited by drug*
   - *development of mutated ribosomal subunits that do not bind antibacterials.*

   a. Benzylpenicillin has a short half-life as it is rapidly excreted by the kidneys.
   b. Broad-spectrum penicillins do not disturb normal colonic flora.
   c. The antipseudomonal penicillin ticarcillin is resistant to β-lactamase.
   d. Penicillins are bactericidal by binding to bacterial ribosomal-binding sites.
2. *Cephalosporins are traditionally grouped into generations and show a range of activities against Gram-positive and Gram-negative bacteria, variable resistance to β-lactamase and variable ability to penetrate the CNS.*
   a. Cefotaxime is a third-generation cephalosporin. It crosses the blood–brain barrier and is not broken down by β-lactamases.
   b. Individuals who are allergic to penicillins cannot be given cephalosporins.
3. *Imipenem is a broad-spectrum drug that is effective against many Gram-positive and Gram-negative bacteria and is resistant to some β-lactamases.*
   a. Imipenem is rapidly metabolised.
   b. Imipenem shows only bacteriostatic activity.
4. *The quinolone ciprofloxacin is active against many Gram-negative and Gram-positive bacteria but has weak activity against streptococci and staphylococci. It has a relatively low incidence of unwanted effects.*
   a. Ciprofloxacin can be used for *Pseudomonas aeruginosa* infections in people with cystic fibrosis.
   b. Ciprofloxacin can safely be given together with theophylline in people with asthma.
5. *Macrolide antibiotics (e.g. erythromycin, clarithromycin) can be used as part of the regimen to eliminate Helicobacter pylori and Legionella infection.*
   a. Erythromycin commonly causes gastrointestinal disturbances.
   b. Gentamicin has a low incidence of unwanted effects.
   c. Gentamicin is not active when given orally.

6. *Metronidazole can be used as part of the regimen for eradicating Helicobacter pylori and for treatment of Clostridium difficile-related colitis resulting from overgrowths with Clostridium difficile.*
   a. Antibacterials do not reduce the development of serious illness for the majority of people with sore throat.
   b. Tetracyclines should be avoided during pregnancy and in young children.
   c. Vancomycin is active against β-lactamase-producing Gram-positive bacteria.
7. *Because of problems with resistance, Mycobacterium tuberculosis is always treated with at least two drugs with different antimicrobial mechanisms.*
   a. Rifampicin is an important drug for the treatment of tuberculosis and also severe Legionnaire's disease and leprosy.
   b. Isoniazid is active against a wide range of bacteria.
   c. Co-trimoxazole is the drug of choice for hospital-acquired acute urinary tract infection.
   d. Trimethoprim administration can result in folate deficiency.
8. Regarding HIV, choose the one **correct** statement from the following options:
   A. Binding of the virus to the chemokine receptor CCR5 in the host cell membrane inhibits attachment and entry of the virus.
   B. Low doses of the protease inhibitor ritonavir reduce the activity of other protease inhibitors.
   C. Once resistance of HIV has developed, it persists indefinitely.
   D. The nucleoside analogue zidovudine acts in HIV by preventing viral entry to the host cells.
   E. The non-nucleoside reverse transcriptase inhibitors treat HIV by preventing insertion of the viral DNA into the host genome.
9. Regarding the treatment of malaria, choose the one **incorrect** statement from the following options:
   A. Primaquine is used to treat the reservoir of parasites in the liver in *Plasmodium falciparum* infections.
   B. Chloroquine concentrates in erythrocytes and prevents the erythrocytic stage of malarial parasite reproduction.
   C. In many areas, prophylaxis against malaria requires administration of two drugs.
   D. Primaquine can induce haemolysis in people with glucose-6-phosphate dehydrogenase deficiency.
   E. Proguanil acts to inhibit malarial parasite folate production.
10. Case history 1 questions

> Mr JW, age 40 years, living at home was previously healthy, but saw his GP in August, 5 days after returning from a conference abroad, where he had stayed in a large hotel and indulged his passion for frequent whirlpool baths. He had characteristic symptoms of pneumonia, including pleuritic chest pain and sudden development of fever and cough, producing yellow sputum. He was disorientated. Physical examinations and chest radiograph supported the diagnosis.

   a. Before the results of the microbiological test were available, what treatment would you have commenced and what route of administration would you have used?
   b. How do the drugs that you are proposing to give work?
11. Case history 2 questions

> Mr RH, age 80 years, had influenza and was admitted to hospital when he developed symptoms similar to Mr JW (see above) and became seriously ill. A chest radiograph showed multiple abscesses.

   a. What treatment would you have commenced before microbiological results were available?
   b. What antibacterial could be used if the organism was not treatable by β-lactamase-resistant penicillins?
12. Case history 3 questions

> A 31-year-old man suffering from AIDs was admitted with shortness of breath, cough and generalised chest discomfort. Chest radiograph revealed diffuse bilateral opacities and a blood gas analysis demonstrated an arterial partial oxygen pressure (PaO_2) of 8.0 kPa (normal range 11.0–14.0). Sputum culture was uninformative. A bronchoalveolar lavage was performed and transbronchial biopsies taken.

   a. What was the likely clinical diagnosis?
   b. What microscopic investigation could have been useful and what might it have shown?
   c. How could this man have been managed and what factors needed to be considered?
   d. What drug treatment unrelated to the infection could have further exposed him to the increased risk of opportunistic infection.
   e. What prophylactic treatment could be commenced?
13. Case history 4 questions

> Twenty-four hours after attending a convention, a 36-year-old man became ill with a temperature, abdominal pain, vomiting and diarrhoea. Faeces were collected and inoculated onto culture plates with several different types of culture medium. Pale-coloured colonies that were non-lactose fermenting were identified.

   a. What organisms might have been causing this infection?
   b. *Salmonella enteritidis* phage type 4 was eventually identified. How should this man be managed?
   c. What food was most likely to have caused this infection?

ANSWERS

1. a. **True**. Benzylpenicillin is actively secreted into the proximal tubule by the organic acid transporter (Ch 2). This can be inhibited by probenecid or by other drugs that use the same secretory mechanism, such as aspirin.

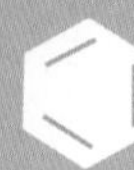

b. **False**. Broad-spectrum penicillins in particular can alter the balance of gut flora, potentially allowing overgrowth of pathogenic bacteria such as *Clostridium difficile*.
c. **False**. Ticarcillin is broken down by β-lactamase.
d. **False**. Penicillins are bactericidal and bind to penicillin-binding proteins and disrupt cell membrane peptidoglycans.

2. a. **True**. Cefotaxime is a third-generation cephalosporin antibacterial that penetrates the CNS and is resistant to β-lactamases.
b. **False**. But cephalosporins should be given carefully. Between 8% and 16% of patients who are allergic to penicillins will exhibit allergy to cephalosporins.

3. a. **True**. Imipenem is rapidly metabolised by dihydropeptidases in the kidney and is always given in combination with cilastatin, which inhibits the metabolising enzyme; in this combination it is rapidly eliminated in the urine.
b. **False**. Like all β-lactam antibacterials given in correct doses, imipenem is bactericidal.

4. a. **True**. The quinolones have good activity against *Pseudomonas* species.
b. **False**. Ciprofloxacin inhibits the hepatic metabolism of theophylline and can increase its toxicity.

5. a. **True**. Erythromycin often causes nausea and diarrhoea. Azithromycin is better tolerated.
b. **False**. Gentamicin is nephrotoxic and ototoxic, and its plasma levels should be monitored.
c. **True**. Gentamicin is poorly absorbed from the gastrointestinal tract and is given parenterally.

6. a. **True**. Most sore throats are caused by viruses; those with bacterial causes usually resolve without antibacterials. The selection of increasingly resistant organisms relates to unnecessary use of antibiotics.
b. **True**. Tetracyclines can chelate with Ca^{2+} and form permanent yellow–brown deposits on developing teeth.
c. **True**. It is reserved for MRSA and metronidazole-resistant *Clostridium difficile*, which causes colitis.

7. a. **True**. Rifampicin is a broad-spectrum antibiotic and can be utilised in some serious diseases caused by Gram-negative bacteria such as legionella and mycobacteria and also for MRSA. Resistance develops rapidly to rifampicin when given alone.
b. **False**. Isoniazid has a highly selective action to inhibit the production of mycolic acids, which are unique to the cell wall of *Mycobacterium* species.
c. **False**. There is a high degree of resistance to co-trimoxazole in the bacteria causing hospital urinary tract infections.
d. **True**. Trimethoprim inhibits the conversion of folate to products used in the construction of DNA. Deficiency can result in megaloblastic anaemia and this can be prevented by giving additional folinic acid.

8. Answer **C**.
A. Incorrect. The virus binds to a number of natural molecules including CCR5 receptors as well as other natural receptors and glycoproteins to facilitate entry.
B. Incorrect. Ritonavir inhibits CYP3A4 enzymes and is used to enhance the activity of other protease inhibitors.
C. Correct. Resistance persists indefinitely and drug treatment should be modified.
D. Incorrect. Zidovudine is an RNA reverse transcriptase inhibitor and prevents the formation of viral DNA from viral RNA.
E. Incorrect (see D).

9. Answer **A**.
A. Incorrect. Only infections by *P. vivax* and *P. ovale* result in schizonts that remain in the liver as hypnozoites and require primaquine for their eradication.
B. Correct. Chloroquine concentrates 100-fold in red cells and interferes with the ability of the parasite to digest haemoglobin.
C. Correct. Resistance is a problem in many areas where prophylaxis with chloroquine plus proguanil or atovaquone plus one of either mefloquine, doxycycline or proguanil is recommended.
D. Correct. Toxic metabolites of primaquine can induce haemolysis in people with G6PD deficiency.
E. Correct (see Fig 51.4).

10. Case history 1 answers
a. The most common cause of community-acquired infection is *Streptococcus pneumoniae*, but other 'atypical' organisms could be involved. In JW, who was previously well, a recent stay in a hotel abroad might indicate the involvement of *Legionella*, which multiplies in warm water, for example in the tanks of air-conditioning systems. (The incubation time is 5–10 days.) Co-amoxiclav (amoxicillin + clavulanic acid) plus erythromycin or another macrolide should be given orally before the diagnosis is confirmed. If his condition is severe, rifampicin should also be given. The treatment should be reviewed immediately the microbiology sensitivities are known.
b. Amoxicillin is bactericidal and acts by interfering with bacterial cell wall peptidoglycan synthesis. It also allows greater activity of enzymes that lyse bacterial cells. Clavulanic acid inhibits β-lactamase, thus extending the spectrum of activity of amoxicillin. Erythromycin inhibits bacterial protein synthesis by acting on the bacterial ribosome. Rifampicin, perhaps better known for its role in treating tuberculosis, inhibits DNA-dependent RNA polymerase in many Gram-positive and Gram-negative bacteria.

11. Case history 2 answers
a. *Staphylococcus aureus* is a likely cause of acute pneumonia following an attack of influenza. Although the treatment must be guided by the sensitivity tests, most *S. aureus* strains are sensitive to flucloxacillin and this is the most appropriate antibiotic to start with. In the circumstances, it may be combined with fusidic acid or gentamicin. *S. aureus* commonly produces abscesses in the lungs. Pulmonary infection with *S. aureus* may also occur in people with cystic fibrosis. A Gram stain of the sputum would demonstrate Gram-positive cocci in clusters – typical of staphylococci. The production of coagulase and DNAse would identify the organism as *S. aureus*. Many different species of coagulase-negative staphylococci exist and are found as part of the normal skin flora. The coagulase-negative staphylococci are typical causes of prosthetic valve endocarditis, joint prostheses and

infected venous catheters. Of concern is the large number of antibacterial-resistant staphylococci (MRSA), which pose a threat to people who are frail or immunocompromised.

b. A range of other second-choice antibacterials effective against β-lactamase-producing *S. aureus* might be useful. For example, fusidic acid, gentamicin, a cephalosporin, a quinolone or erythromycin may be effective. There are increasing concerns about MRSA. Vancomycin, a bactericidal glycopeptide that inhibits cell wall synthesis, is effective against some MRSA. A new group of drugs, the streptogramins, have recently become available, and quinupristin with dalfopristin is effective against MRSA.

12. Case history 3 answers
   a. Clinically, the man is likely to have *Pneumocystis jirovecii* pneumonia (PCP), which is the predominant respiratory illness in people with AIDS. This organism, which is a protozoan, is believed to be acquired at a young age and reactivates with waning immunity. The organism is endemic in the community and multiplies within the lungs and causes symptoms. There is often a seasonal prevalence of PCP. Symptoms can be scant, and, if present, consist of breathlessness and cough. Induced sputum or bronchoalveolar lavage specimens should be sent to laboratory for detection of PCP and routine culture.
   b. PCP can be detected in sputum or lavage by staining with methenamine silver stain for typical casts. It can also be detected by use of the polymerase chain reaction, and on lung biopsy.
   c. The treatment of choice is high-dose co-trimoxazole. Many people with AIDS have hypersensitivity reactions to sulphonamides and are on multiple drug combinations. Alternative treatments for PCP are aerosolised or parenteral pentamidine, dapsone and trimethoprim, primaquine, etc.
   d. Long-term treatment with corticosteroids or other immunosuppressants.
   e. After an attack of PCP, a prophylactic regimen should be taken, for example nebulised pentamidine or oral trimethoprim 3 days per week.
13. Case history 4 answers
   a. *Salmonella*, *Shigella*, *Proteus* and *Pseudomonas* species are non-lactose fermenting and produce pale-coloured colonies on this medium. All were contenders. *Salmonella enteritidis* phage type 4 was eventually identified.
   b. Antibacterials have no role to play in the management of the majority of cases of salmonella gastroenteritis. Exceptions are if the gastroenteritis occurs in an individual who is immunocompromised or if there is evidence of systemic invasion. Ciprofloxacin would be the antibiotic of choice; it can be given orally and is cheaper than intravenous preparations. Dehydration and electrolyte imbalance should be corrected by fluid replacement. Control of the diarrhoea by antidiarrhoeal drugs is contraindicated because of the risk of inducing paralytic ileus and causing septicaemia.
   c. Food poisoning, as this case would seem to be from the history, is a notifiable condition and should be reported to the consultant in Communicable Disease Control. Because the man has attended a convention, it is possible that this is part of an outbreak and all persons attending the convention should be contacted to find out if they have been symptomatic and to collect faecal specimens for culture. Specimens of food, if still available, should also be collected for culture.

Drugs used for infections

Drug	Half-life (h) and kinetics	Comments
Antibacterial drugs		
Penicillins		
Amoxicillin	1 [R + M] Good oral bioavailability (90%) not influenced by food; rapid renal excretion	Used for urinary tract infections, otitis media, sinusitis, bronchitis, uncomplicated community-acquired pneumonia, *Haemophilus influenzae* infections, invasive salmonellosis and listerial meningitis; broad-spectrum penicillin; given orally, by intramuscular injection, or by intravenous injection or infusion
Ampicillin	1–2 [R + M] Low oral bioavailability which is reduced if taken with food; eliminated largely by renal clearance	See amoxicillin for uses; broad-spectrum penicillin; given orally, by intramuscular injection, or by intravenous injection or infusion
Benzylpenicillin (penicillin G)	0.5–1 [R + M] Unreliable oral absorption owing to hydrolysis by gastric acid; rapidly eliminated by renal excretion	Used for throat infection, otitis media, streptococcal endocarditis, meningococcal disease, pneumonia and anthrax; given by intramuscular injection, slow intravenous injection or infusion; depot formulation (procaine benzylpenicillin) is available as intramuscular injection

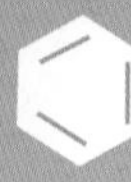

Drugs used for infections

Drug	Half-life (h) and kinetics	Comments
Flucloxacillin (floxacillin)	0.8–1.2 [R + M] High oral bioavailability (80%); absorption delayed by food; cleared largely by the kidneys	Used for infections caused by β-lactamase-resistant staphylococci; given orally, by intramuscular injection, or by intravenous injection or infusion
Phenoxymethyl penicillin (penicillin V)	0.5 [R + M] Rapidly but incompletely (60%) absorbed from the gut; eliminated equally by renal excretion unchanged and as the penicilloic acid metabolite	Used for tonsillitis, otitis media, erysipelas, rheumatic fever and pneumococcal infection prophylaxis; given orally
Piperacillin	0.7–1.3 [R + B] Poorly absorbed from the gut, therefore not given orally; not metabolised	Antipseudomonal used for infections of lower respiratory tract, urinary tract, abdomen and skin; given by intramuscular injection, or by intravenous injection (over 3–5 min) or infusion
Pivmecillinam	– [M] Rapidly and extensively hydrolysed prodrug for mecillinam; mecillinam has a half-life of 1–2 h	Antipseudomonal and active against many Gram-negative bacteria; used for urinary tract infections; given orally
Temocillin	5 [R] Eliminated largely unchanged in urine	Used for infections caused by Gram-negative bacteria; given by intramuscular or intravenous injection or by intravenous infusion
Ticarcillin	1 [R] Excreted mostly in the urine unchanged	Antipseudomonal active also against *Proteus* species; given by intravenous infusion in combination with clavulanic acid
Cephalosporins and other β-lactams		
Aztreonam	1.7 [R] Not given orally because of very poor absorption (<1%); rapidly eliminated by renal clearance without metabolism	Active only against Gram-negative bacteria and used for infections by *Pseudomonas aeruginosa*, *Haemophilus influenzae* and *Neisseria meningitides*; given by deep intramuscular injection, or by intravenous injection (over 3–5 min) or infusion
Cefaclor	0.5–1 [R + M] Rapidly and extensively absorbed; eliminated largely by the kidneys plus limited metabolism (15%)	Used for sensitive Gram-negative or Gram-positive infections of urinary tract (unresponsive to other drugs), respiratory tract and soft tissues, and for otitis media and sinusitis; given orally
Cefadroxil	1–2 [R] Rapidly and completely absorbed (not affected by food); eliminated unchanged (>90%)	For uses, see under cefaclor; given orally
Cefalexin	1 [R] Rapidly and completely absorbed; eliminated unchanged	For uses, see under cefaclor; given orally
Cefixime	2.5–3.8 [R + B] Absorbed slowly and incompletely (50%); excreted more slowly than other cephalosporins (not eliminated by renal tubular secretion)	For uses, see under cefaclor (but acute infections only), also used for gonorrhoea; given orally
Cefotaxime	0.9–1.3 [R + M] Renal excretion (with some tubular secretion) is major route of elimination but metabolism accounts for 20% of dose	For uses, see under cefaclor; also used for gonorrhoea, surgical prophylaxis, *Haemophilus epiglottitis* and meningitis; given by deep intramuscular injection, or by intravenous injection (over 3–5 min) or infusion
Cefpirome	1.4–2.3 [R] Eliminated by glomerular filtration with negligible secretion	For uses, see under cefaclor; given by intravenous injection or infusion
Cefpodoxime	1.9–3.2 [R] The proxetil derivative is a prodrug, which is absorbed rapidly and quantitatively hydrolysed to cefpodoxime; only about 50% of the dose is absorbed and the fraction absorbed is increased by low gastric pH; cefpodoxime is eliminated by glomerular filtration and secretion	Used for upper and lower respiratory tract infections, skin and soft tissue infections, uncomplicated urinary tract infections and uncomplicated gonorrhoea; given orally as the proxetil derivative

Drugs used for infections

Drug	Half-life (h) and kinetics	Comments
Cefradine	1.3 [R] Completely absorbed but rate affected by food; eliminated unchanged in urine	For uses, see under cefaclor; also used for surgical prophylaxis; given orally, by deep intramuscular injection, or by intravenous injection (over 3–5 min) or infusion
Ceftazidime	1.8–2.2 [R] Eliminated unchanged by glomerular filtration	For uses, see under cefaclor; also used for surgical prophylaxis; given by deep intramuscular injection, or by intravenous injection (over 3–5 min) or infusion
Ceftriaxone	6–9 [R + B] Eliminated unchanged; long half-life is probably a result of extensive plasma protein binding (95%)	For uses, see under cefaclor; also used for surgical prophylaxis and prophylaxis of meningococcal meningitis; given by deep intramuscular injection, or by intravenous injection (over 3–5 min) or infusion
Cefuroxime	1.2 [R] The axetil derivative is a prodrug, which is quantitatively hydrolysed to cefuroxime and absorbed better if taken after food; cefuroxime is eliminated equally by renal filtration and secretion	For uses, see under cefaclor; also used for surgical prophylaxis; given orally (as cefuroxime axetil), by deep intramuscular injection, or by intravenous injection (over 3–5 min) or infusion; the oral formulation is the axetil derivative
Ertapenem	4.5 [R + M] Eliminated in urine as equal amounts of parent drug and an inactive metabolite	Broad-spectrum active against both Gram-negative and Gram-positive organisms; used for abdominal and acute gynaecological infections and for community-acquired pneumonia; given by intravenous infusion
Imipenem (with cilastatin)	1 [R + M] Eliminated unchanged in urine and also hydrolysed by a renal enzyme; always given with cilastatin, which inhibits the renal enzyme (although this does not have a major impact on half-life or clearance)	Active against aerobic and anaerobic Gram-negative and Gram-positive organisms; used for hospital-acquired septicaemia and for surgical prophylaxis; given by deep intramuscular injection or intravenous infusion
Meropenem	1 [R + M] Eliminated by kidneys (80%) and hepatic metabolism (20%)	Used for aerobic and anaerobic Gram-negative and Gram-positive infections; given by intravenous injection (over 5 min) or intravenous infusion
β-Lactamase inhibitors		
Given with some β-lactam antibacterial agents that are susceptible to hydrolysis		
Clavulanic acid	1 [M + R] Undergoes extensive metabolism (pathways are not known) and glomerular filtration	Given orally, or by slow intravenous injection or infusion in combination with amoxicillin, or intravenously with ticarcillin
Tazobactam	0.7–1.5 [R + M] Eliminated via renal tubular secretion and filtration; the one identified metabolite is inactive	Given by slow intravenous injection or infusion in combination with piperacillin
Quinolones		
Ciprofloxacin	3–4 [R + B + M] Good bioavailability (50–80%); eliminated by glomerular filtration, renal tubular secretion, plus biliary excretion and metabolism (15%); the relatively long half-life results from a high apparent volume of distribution (3 L kg^{-1}), not low clearance	Active against Gram-positive and especially Gram-negative organisms, including *Salmonella*, *Shigella*, *Campylobacter*, *Neisseria* and *Pseudomonas* species, and used for infections of respiratory tract (but not pneumococcal pneumonia), of the urinary and gastrointestinal tracts, chronic prostatitis and gonorrhoea and septicaemia; given orally or by intravenous infusion
Levofloxacin	6–8 [R + M] Complete bioavailability (unaffected by food); eliminated largely unchanged by the kidneys	Similar activity to ciprofloxacin, but more active against pneumococci; used for bronchitis, community-acquired pneumonia, and infections of urinary tract, skin and soft tissues; given orally or as an intravenous infusion
Moxifloxacin	12 [M + R] High bioavailability (90%); metabolised by conjugation with glucuronic acid and sulphate	Similar activity to ciprofloxacin but more active against pneumococci and not active against *Pseudomonas aeruginosa* or MRSA; used for bronchitis, community-acquired pneumonia, and sinusitis; given orally
Nalidixic acid	1.5 [M] Essentially complete bioavailability; eliminated by hepatic metabolism (oxidation + conjugation)	Used in uncomplicated urinary tract infections; given orally

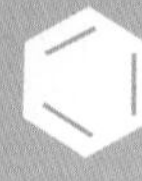

Drugs used for infections

Drug	Half-life (h) and kinetics	Comments
Norfloxacin	3 [R + M] Bioavailability has not been defined, but absorption is reduced by 30% if taken with food; eliminated by kidneys (filtration + secretion) plus metabolism (about 10%)	Used in uncomplicated urinary tract infections; given orally
Ofloxacin	6–7 [R + M] Rapid and complete oral absorption; eliminated by kidneys plus limited metabolism (<5%)	Used for infections of the urinary tract and lower respiratory tract, and for gonorrhoea, and non-gonococcal urethritis and cervicitis; given orally or as intravenous infusion
Macrolides		
Azithromycin	40–60 [B] Bioavailability is 37% (owing to poor absorption) and is reduced by food; eliminated largely by biliary excretion of the parent drug (mol. wt. 785 Da); does not affect P450 isoenzymes	Used for respiratory tract infections, otitis media, skin and soft tissue infections, uncomplicated chlamydial infections, non-gonococcal urethritis, and moderate typhoid due to multiple antibacterial-resistant organisms; given orally
Clarithromycin	3 [M + R] Bioavailability is 55% (owing to first-pass metabolism); eliminated by metabolism and renal excretion; half-life increased to 9 h at high doses; inhibits CYP3A4	Used for respiratory tract infections, otitis media, mild to moderate skin and soft tissue infections, and for *Helicobacter pylori* eradication; given orally or by intravenous infusion
Erythromycin	1–1.5 [M + R + B] Oral formulations are as ester prodrugs that are rapidly hydrolysed; erythromycin is eliminated largely by CYP3A4 in the liver (plus gut wall after oral dosage?); inhibits CYP3A4	Spectrum is similar to penicillins and used for people hypersensitive to these drugs; used for campylobacter enteritis, pneumonia, Legionnaires' disease, syphilis, non-gonococcal urethritis, chronic prostatitis, diphtheria and whooping cough prophylaxis, and for acne vulgaris and rosacea; given orally or by intravenous infusion
Spiramycin	6–8 [B + R] Total clearance is about 6 times renal clearance; pathways have not been defined but high concentrations are found in bile	Used on a 'named-patient' basis for toxoplasmosis
Telithromycin	10 [M + R + B] Good bioavailability (60%); metabolised by CYP3A4 and other enzymes	Used for community-acquired pneumonia, bronchitis, sinusitis, β-haemolytic streptococcal pharyngitis, or tonsillitis when β-lactams are inappropriate; given orally
Aminoglycosides		
All are bactericidal and active against Gram-negative and Gram-positive organisms; gentamicin is the aminoglycoside of choice in the UK and is used for serious infections		
Amikacin	2 [R] Eliminated by glomerular filtration	Used for serious Gram-negative infections resistant to gentamicin; given by intramuscular injection, slow intravenous injection, or intravenous infusion
Gentamicin	1–4 [R] Eliminated by glomerular filtration	Used for septicaemia and neonatal sepsis, CNS infections (including meningitis), biliary tract infections, acute pyelonephritis and prostatitis, endocarditis, pneumonia in hospital, and as an adjunct in listerial meningitis; given by intramuscular injection, slow intravenous injection, intravenous infusion or by intrathecal injection
Neomycin	2 [R] Very poor absorption (<5%); eliminated by glomerular filtration	Too toxic for parenteral use and restricted to skin infections and for bowel sterilisation before surgery; given orally
Netilmicin	2.5 [R] Eliminated by glomerular filtration	Used for serious Gram-negative infections resistant to gentamicin; given by intramuscular injection, slow intravenous injection, or intravenous infusion
Tobramycin	2–3 [R] Eliminated by glomerular filtration	For uses, see under gentamicin; given by intramuscular injection, slow intravenous injection, or intravenous infusion

Drugs used for infections

Drug	Half-life (h) and kinetics	Comments
Tetracyclines		
Broad-spectrum antibacterial but with increasing resistance; remain drugs of choice for infections caused by *Chlamydia*, *Rickettsia* or *Brucella* species, and for Lyme disease; all are given orally; no parenteral formulations are available		
Demeclocycline	10–15 [R + B] Oral bioavailability is 66% (owing to poor absorption); equal amounts excreted unchanged in urine and bile	Main uses are given above
Doxycycline	18–22 [B + R] High oral bioavailability (>90%); eliminated in bile (20–40%) and urine (20–26%)	Main uses are given above; also used for chronic prostatitis, sinusitis, syphilis, pelvic inflammatory disease, anthrax, malaria, rosacea and acne vulgaris; also used with quinine in the treatment of malaria (see below)
Lymecycline	8–10 [M] Degraded in gastrointestinal tract into tetracycline, lysine and formaldehyde	Main uses are given above
Minocycline	12–16 [B + R + M] Oral bioavailability is >90%; bile is major route of elimination; only 30% has been recovered in excreta (possibly chemical decomposition in vivo rather than metabolism?)	Main uses are given above; also used for meningococcal carrier state and acne vulgaris
Oxytetracycline	9 [R + B] Variable absorption (up to 60%); renal excretion is major route of elimination	Main uses are given above; also used for acne vulgaris and rosacea
Tetracycline	9 [B + R + M] Irregular and incomplete absorption; eliminated in bile and urine, with some metabolism	Main uses are given above; also used for acne vulgaris and rosacea
Tigecycline	27 [B + R] Eliminated unchanged in bile and urine, with only limited metabolism by conjugation	Structurally related to tetracyclines, with similar unwanted effects; used for complicated intra-abdominal, skin or soft tissue infections; given by intravenous infusion
Sulphonamides		
Their importance has decreased due to increasing resistance and the availability of better alternatives		
Sulfadiazine	7–12 [M + R] Completely absorbed from the gut, but first-pass metabolism reduces the bioavailability to 60–90%; metabolised by acetylation, and parent drug and acetyl metabolite are eliminated by kidney	Used for prevention of rheumatic fever recurrence; given orally or by intravenous infusion (silver sulfadiazine cream is available for topical use)
Sulfamethoxazole	9 (6–20) [M + R] Rapidly absorbed; eliminated mainly by acetylation and some glucuronidation	Used only in combination with trimethoprim (see below) and restricted to *Pneumocystis jirovecii* (where it is the drug of choice), toxoplasmosis, nocardiasis and for acute exacerbations of infections shown to be susceptible; given orally or by intravenous infusion
Trimethoprim	9–17 [R + M] Essentially complete absorption and bioavailability; eliminated largely by the kidneys (filtration + secretion) with some oxidative metabolism (20%)	Used with sulfamethoxazole (see above) and alone for urinary tract infections and bronchitis (when it is given orally)
Other antibacterial drugs		
Chloramphenicol	5 (2–12) [M] High oral bioavailability (80–90%); eliminated mainly by glucuronidation	Potent but toxic broad-spectrum compound with use limited to life-threatening infections, especially *Haemophilus influenzae* and typhoid fever; given orally or by intravenous injection or infusion
Clindamycin	2.5 [M + R] Rapidly and extensively absorbed after oral dosage; mostly eliminated by hepatic metabolism, with two of the metabolites being active; elimination in saliva may give a bitter taste	Use limited to staphylococcal bone and joint infections and for peritonitis, because of serious toxicity; given orally, by deep intramuscular injection or by intravenous infusion

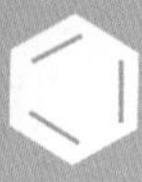

Drugs used for infections

Drug	Half-life (h) and kinetics	Comments
Colistin (colistimethate sodium)	4–8 [R] Not absorbed orally; eliminated by renal excretion	Used for infections by Gram-negative organisms, including *Pseudomonas aeruginosa*; given orally (for bowel sterilisation only), by intravenous injection or infusion, or by inhalation (nebuliser)
Daptomycin	8–9 [R] Mostly excreted unchanged in urine	Used for complicated skin and soft tissue infections by Gram-positive bacteria; given by intravenous infusion
Fusidic acid (sodium fusidate)	9 [M] Essentially completely bioavailable after oral dosage; metabolised in liver and metabolites excreted in bile	Narrow spectrum with use restricted to penicillin-resistant staphylococcal infections; given orally or by intravenous infusion
Linezolid	5 [M + R] Eliminated by oxidative metabolism (not P450) to inactive carboxylic acid metabolites; about 30% is excreted unchanged in urine	Used for pneumonia and complicated skin and soft tissue infections caused by Gram-positive organisms; given orally or by intravenous infusion
Methenamine	4 [M] Broken down in acid stomach contents, so given as enteric-coated formulation; gives rise to urinary excretion of formaldehyde	Used for prophylaxis and long-term treatment of lower urinary tract infections; given orally for urinary tract infections
Metronidazole	6–9 [M + R] Complete oral bioavailability; metabolites are eliminated slowly, primarily in the urine	Active against anaerobic bacteria and used for surgical and gynaecological sepsis, antibiotic-associated colitis and eradication of *Helicobacter pylori*; given orally, rectally or by intravenous infusion
Nitrofurantoin	0.3–1 [R + M] Complete oral bioavailability; over 40% is excreted rapidly unchanged by filtration and renal tubular secretion; about 20% metabolised by nitroreduction	Used for urinary tract infections, when it is given orally
Quinupristin plus dalfopristin	0.5–1.0 [M] Both drugs are rapidly cleared from the blood and converted into active metabolites which are eliminated in the bile	Used for serious Gram-positive infections where no alternative antibiotic is suitable; given by intravenous infusion; treatment reserved for MRSA or patients who cannot be treated with other regimens
Teicoplanin	32–176 [R] Slowly eliminated in urine without metabolism; slower elimination than vancomycin because its higher lipid solubility gives a higher volume of distribution, and because renal excretion is limited by extensive reabsorption and high plasma protein binding (90%)	Used for Gram-positive infections, including endocarditis, peritonitis and for prophylaxis in orthopaedic surgery; given by intramuscular injection, intravenous injection or infusion
Tinidazole	12–14 [M + R] Complete oral bioavailability; about 25% excreted unchanged and the remainder metabolised and eliminated via urine and bile	Uses and actions similar to metronidazole; given orally
Vancomycin	5–11 [R] Negligible absorption from the gut; eliminated by glomerular filtration	Used for prophylaxis and treatment of endocarditis and other serious infections of Gram-positive cocci and for *clostridium difficile*-related colitis; given orally (for colitis) or by intravenous infusion
Antituberculous drugs		
Capreomycin	? [R + ?] About 50% is eliminated by renal excretion; old drug with few data available	Used in combination with other drugs when resistance to first-line drugs occurs; given by deep intramuscular injection
Cycloserine	4–30 [R + M] High oral bioavailability (>90%); 60–70% excreted in urine and the remainder is metabolised	Used in combination with other drugs when resistance to first-line drugs occurs; given orally
Ethambutol	10–15 [R + M] Good oral bioavailability (80%); cleared by glomerular filtration + renal tubular secretion, plus <10% metabolism	First-line drug (initial phase only) which is included in treatment regimen if resistance to isoniazid is suspected; given orally

Drugs used for infections

Drug	Half-life (h) and kinetics	Comments
Isoniazid	0.5–2 RA, 2–6.5 SA [M] High oral bioavailability; eliminated largely by acetylation, with slow acetylators (SA) having higher blood concentrations than rapid acetylators (RA); other minor metabolites may be linked to hepatotoxicity	First-line drug; given orally or by intramuscular or intravenous injection
Pyrazinamide	10–24 [M + R] High oral bioavailability; metabolised in liver to the active compound pyrazinoic acid, which is eliminated in urine	First-line drug (initial phase only) which is particularly useful in tuberculous meningitis; given orally
Rifabutin	35–40 [M + R] Bioavailability is 20%, decreasing to 12% (owing to autoinduction); eliminated largely by CYP3A, which it induces during chronic treatment; only about 5% is excreted unchanged	New drug that is an analogue of, and an alternative to, rifampicin (see below); given orally
Rifampicin (rifampin)	1–6 [M + R + B] High oral bioavailability (percentage not defined); eliminated by a number of routes; potent inducer of CYP3A4	Key component of any regimen (also used for brucellosis, Legionnaires' disease and serious staphylococcal infections); given orally or by intravenous infusion
Streptomycin	2–3 [R] Eliminated by kidney (50–60%) but the fate of the remainder not known (metabolites?)	Use is mainly restricted to resistant organisms (also used as an adjunct in the treatment of brucellosis); given by deep intramuscular injection because of poor and highly variable oral bioavailability
Drugs used in leprosy		
Clofazimine	10 days [B] Bioavailability is variable (20–85%), dependent on formulation and food (which enhances absorption); slowly eliminated unchanged in bile; urinary excretion is negligible (but enough to make urine red)	Given orally
Dapsone	27 [M + R] Bioavailability is >90%; undergoes polymorphic acetylation and N-glucuronidation (a rare reaction); metabolites undergo enterohepatic circulation; about 10% eliminated in urine unchanged	Given orally
Rifampicin	–	See above
Antifungal agents		
Amorolfine	? [?] Limited transdermal absorption (<10% across 100 cm^2); very slow elimination may be because of a build-up of drug in the skin	Used for fungal infections of skin and nails; applied as a cream or nail lacquer
Amphotericin	24–48 [R] Negligible oral absorption; slow renal excretion; the half-life given is following a single dose; the elimination half-life after chronic administration is up to 2 weeks, probably reflecting detectable plasma concentrations due to drug released from the tissues	Active against most fungi and yeasts; given orally (for intestinal candidiasis) or by intravenous infusion for systemic infections
Caspofungin	40–50 [M] Metabolised by hydrolysis and N-acetylation in the liver; metabolites are eliminated in bile	Used for invasive aspergillosis unresponsive to amphotericin or itraconazole and for invasive candidiasis; given by intravenous infusion
Clotrimazole	– [M] Negligible absorption across the skin; 5–10% is absorbed after vaginal use and fungicidal concentrations are maintained locally for up to 3 days	Used for fungal skin infections and vaginal candidiasis; applied as a cream, powder or spray

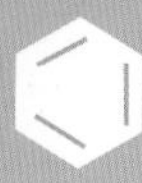

Drugs used for infections

Drug	Half-life (h) and kinetics	Comments
Econazole	– [M] Negligible absorption across the skin; data on absorption after vaginal use are not available (see clotrimazole)	Used for fungal skin infections and vaginal candidiasis; applied as a cream
Fluconazole	30 [R + M] High oral bioavailability (90%); renal excretion accounts for 80% of clearance, with oxidation and conjugation a further 11%; weak inhibitor of CYP3A4	Used for local and systemic fungal infections; good penetration of blood–brain barrier makes it useful for fungal meningitis; given orally or by intravenous infusion
Flucytosine	3 [R] Eliminated by glomerular filtration; about 1% is deaminated to 5-fluorouracil (which may explain the bone marrow toxicity)	Used for systemic fungal and yeast infections, used in combination with amphotericin or fluconazole; given by intravenous infusion
Griseofulvin	10–21 [M] Variable absorption, which is increased by ingestion with fatty foods (bioavailability not defined); eliminated by glucuronidation	Used for widespread or intractable dermatophyte infections of the skin, scalp and nails where topical treatment has been ineffective; given orally
Itraconazole	20 [M] Oral bioavailability is 55%; eliminated by hepatic metabolism followed by biliary excretion; metabolised by and is a competitive inhibitor of CYP3A4	Used for numerous local and systemic fungal infections; given orally
Ketoconazole	6–10 [M + B] Incomplete bioavailability owing to first-pass metabolism (absolute bioavailability has not been reported); metabolised by CYP3A4 and inhibits CYP3A4 metabolism of other drugs	Used for systemic mycoses and for a range of serious and resistant infections; given orally or topically
Miconazole	24 [M] Poorly absorbed from the gut; data indicate that up to 50% is absorbed from the gut but blood levels are too low to give a therapeutic effect	Used for oral and intestinal infections; given orally
Nystatin	– Not absorbed from the gastrointestinal tract or from intact skin	Principally used for *Candida albicans* infections of skin and mucous membranes; given orally or topically (for vaginal and skin infections)
Posaconazole	35 [R + M + B] Absorption is slow and incomplete but increased three-to-fourfold if taken with a meal; eliminated mostly in faeces, probably due to biliary excretion and poor absorption; limited glucuronidation and some renal excretion	Used in patients unresponsive to amphotericin or other suitable treatments; given orally
Sulconazole	– [R] Limited absorption across the skin (5–15%); absorbed drug is eliminated in the urine; half-life will be limited by the absorption rate	Used for fungal skin infections; applied as a cream
Terbinafine	11–17 [M] Good oral bioavailability (80%); numerous pathways of metabolism; does not inhibit P450 isoenzymes	Drug of choice for fungal nail infections (also used for ringworm infections); given orally or topically
Tioconazole	– Negligible systemic absorption after topical treatment	Used for fungal nail infections; applied as a solution
Voriconazole	6 [M] High oral bioavailability (96%); metabolised mainly by the polymorphic enzyme CYP2C19; poor metabolisers have fourfold higher blood levels	Used for invasive aspergillosis and other serious infections; given orally or by intravenous infusion

Drugs used for infections

Drug	**Half-life (h) and kinetics**	**Comments**
Antiviral agents		
Reverse transcriptase inhibitors		
Each drug is used for the treatment of HIV infection in combination with other antiretroviral drugs (any other indications are given under the individual drug)		
Abacavir	1.5 [M] Good oral bioavailability (80%); metabolised by alcohol dehydrogenase and glucuronidation; does not inhibit P450 isoenzymes	Given orally
Didanosine	0.6–1.4 [R + M] Absorption is approximately 20–40% but affected by gastric acidity and food; about one-half of the absorbed fraction is excreted unchanged in the urine and the remainder metabolised (pathways not known)	Given orally
Efavirenz	40–70 [M] Variable and incomplete absorption; metabolised by CYP3A4 and CYP2B6, which it induces, so that the half-life is slightly shorter after regular dosage	Non-nucleoside drug; given orally
Emtricitabine	10 [R + M] Rapidly and essentially completely absorbed; forms an intracellular triphosphate which has a half-life of about 40 h; eliminated largely by renal secretion and by S-oxidation and conjugation with glucuronic acid	Given orally
Lamivudine	5–7 [R + M] Rapid and nearly complete absorption as parent drug (90%); eliminated largely in the urine unchanged; the intracellular half-life of the active triphosphate metabolite (11–16 h) is longer than that of the parent drug in the plasma	Also used for chronic hepatitis B with evidence of viral replication; given orally
Nevirapine	45 [M] High bioavailability (90%); eliminated by hepatic metabolism via CYP3A4; half-life is reduced to 25–30 h after chronic treatment, owing to induction of its own metabolism	Non-nucleoside drug; used in advanced disease in combination with at least two other drugs; given orally
Stavudine	1–1.6 [R + M] High oral bioavailability (>80%); approximately equal amounts eliminated unchanged and by metabolism through normal pathways of pyrimidine biochemistry	Given orally
Tenofovir disoproxil	17 [R] Rapidly converted to tenofovir in the gut, giving a bioavailability of 25%; forms active intracellular diphosphate metabolite; eliminated by glomerular filtration and renal tubular secretion	Given orally
Zidovudine	1 [R + M] Oral bioavailability is about 65% owing to first-pass metabolism; most of the dose is metabolised by glucuronidation, with limited excretion unchanged (about 20%); intracellular phosphorylation may be saturable, which may explain the apparent non-linear dose–response relationship	Also used for prevention of maternal–fetal HIV transmission; given orally or by intravenous infusion
Protease inhibitors		
Each drug is used for the treatment of HIV infection in combination with other antiretroviral drugs (any other indications are given under the individual drug); all are given by oral route only		

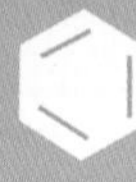

Drugs used for infections

Drug	Half-life (h) and kinetics	Comments
Amprenavir	7–10 [M] Rapidly absorbed; metabolised by CYP3A4 to numerous metabolites that are eliminated in bile	Used in individuals treated previously with other antiretroviral drugs
Atazanavir	7 [M] Oral bioavailability is 70%; eliminated by hepatic CYP3A4-mediated metabolism	Used in individuals treated previously with other antiretroviral drugs
Fosamprenavir	7–10 (amprenavir) [M] Rapidly and completely hydrolysed to amprenavir in gut mucosa	A phosphate ester prodrug for amprenavir
Indinavir	2 [M] Oral bioavailability is only 18–20% owing to metabolism by CYP3A4 in gut wall and liver, and by efflux from enterocytes back into the gut lumen by the P-glycoprotein transporter (saturation of which results in increased absorption at high doses); eliminated solely by CYP3A4 metabolism; metabolites eliminated via the faeces	Used in combination with nucleoside reverse transcriptase inhibitors
Lopinavir (with ritonavir)	5–6 [M] The extent of absorption is increased markedly by a high-fat meal; metabolised by CYP3A4 to numerous metabolites that are eliminated in bile	
Nelfinavir	3.5–5 [M + B] Oral bioavailability in humans is not known; metabolised in liver by CYP3A4, with a major metabolite as active as the parent drug; metabolites plus parent drug (about 20%) are eliminated via the faeces	
Ritonavir	3–5 [M] Oral bioavailability in humans is not known, but is very high (>70%) in test animals; metabolised by CYP3A4 and is an inhibitor of the enzyme (more potent than other protease inhibitors); one of the metabolites is as active as the parent drug; metabolites eliminated in the faeces	Used for progressive and advanced HIV infection in combination with nucleoside reverse transcriptase inhibitors, and low doses are used to increase the effect of some protease inhibitors
Saquinavir	5–7 [M] Oral bioavailability is low and variable (1–30%) (see indinavir for reasons) and is considerably influenced by food; metabolised by CYP3A4, and metabolites are eliminated in the faeces (different papers have reported average half-lives of between 1 and 7 h after oral dosage, and 10–15 h after intravenous dosage, which suggests this inconsistency is an artefact of analytical sensitivity)	
Tipranavir	6 [M] The extent of absorption is increased markedly by a meal; metabolised by CYP3A4	Used for HIV infection resistant to other protease inhibitors and in those treated previously with other antiretroviral drugs
Viral DNA polymerase inhibitors		
Aciclovir	3 [R + M] Slowly and poorly absorbed from the gut (bioavailability is 10–20%); eliminated largely by renal tubular secretion + filtration; only about 10% is metabolised to inactive excretory products	Used for herpes simplex and varicella-zoster infections; given orally, topically or by intravenous infusion
Cidofovir	3 [R] Undergoes further intracellular phosphorylation to mono-, di- and triphosphates, which have longer half-lives; eliminated by renal tubular secretion + filtration	Used for CMV in people with AIDS; phosphorylated analogue of aciclovir; given by intravenous infusion

Drugs used for infections

Drug	Half-life (h) and kinetics	Comments
Famciclovir (prodrug for penciclovir)	2 (penciclovir) [M] Inactive prodrug for penciclovir; negligible oral absorption intact, but extensive conversion to penciclovir (77%); penciclovir is eliminated largely by renal excretion; triphosphate formed intracellularly has a longer half-life	Used for treatment of herpes zoster, acute genital herpes simplex and suppression of recurrent genital herpes infections; given orally
Foscarnet	3–7 [R] Eliminated by glomerular filtration and renal tubular secretion + filtration	Used for CMV retinitis in people with AIDS and for mucocutaneous herpes simplex infections unresponsive to aciclovir in immunocompromised people; highly polar compound; given by intravenous infusion
Ganciclovir	4 [R] Eliminated largely by glomerular filtration	Used for life-threatening or sight-threatening CMV infections in immunocompromised people only; given by intravenous infusion
Valaciclovir	3 (aciclovir) [M] Rapidly and well absorbed (bioavailability 55%); rapidly and extensively metabolised to aciclovir; aciclovir is eliminated by the kidneys	Uses similar to aciclovir; given orally
Valganciclovir	4 (as ganciclovir) [M] Nearly completely converted to ganciclovir by intestinal and hepatic esterases, giving a 'bioavailability' as ganciclovir of 60% (compared with 3–7% when the parent drug itself is given)	Used for CMV retinitis in people with AIDS and for prevention of CMV infection following transplantation from an infected donor; L-valyl ester prodrug of ganciclovir; given orally
Other antivirals		
Adefovir dipivoxil	8 (adefovir) [M] After oral dosage, diester prodrug extensively converted to adefovir, which is eliminated by filtration plus active renal tubular secretion	Used for chronic hepatitis B infection with either compensated liver disease and evidence of viral replication or decompensated liver disease; given orally
Amantadine	10–15 [R] Slowly but completely absorbed from the gut; eliminated by active renal tubular secretion plus filtration	Used for herpes zoster and influenza A; given orally
Enfuvirtide	4 [M] A peptide that probably undergoes hepatic hydrolysis	Used for the treatment of HIV infection in combination with other antiretroviral drugs for resistant infection or in people intolerant to other drugs; given by subcutaneous injection
Idoxuridine	? Few data available	Used for topical infections with herpes simplex and herpes zoster, but is of little value; given as a 5% solution; the phosphorylated metabolite of idoxuridine is incorporated into viral DNA and impairs transcription; it is now little used; for use on the skin, penetration is enhanced by dissolving it in dimethyl sulfoxide (DMSO); not recommended for children under 12 years of age
Inosine pranobex	? Very few data available; complex that probably decomposes to *p*-acetamidobenzoic acid, N,N-dimethylamino-2-propanol and inosine	Used for mucocutaneous herpes simplex, genital warts and subacute sclerosing panencephalitis; given orally
Maraviroc	14–18 [M] Partially absorbed from the gut; metabolised in the liver	Used for the treatment of HIV infection in combination with other antiretroviral drugs for resistant infection; given orally
Oseltamivir	1–3 [M] Undergoes almost complete first-pass metabolism to the carboxylic acid analogue (the active form), which has a longer half-life (6–10 h) and is excreted by the kidneys	Used to treat influenza in at-risk people if started within 48 h of onset of symptoms; given orally

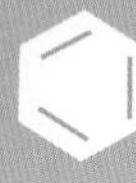

Drugs used for infections

Drug	Half-life (h) and kinetics	Comments
Palivizumab	20 days [?] Very few published kinetic data available; probably eliminated by peptide hydrolysis	Used for prevention of serious lower respiratory tract infection by RSV in neonates and children under 2 years; humanised monoclonal antibody; given by intramuscular injection
Raltegravir	9 [M + R] Good oral absorption; eliminated by conjugation and excretion unchanged in urine	Used for the treatment of HIV infection when there is resistance to other antiretroviral drugs; given orally
Ribavirin (tribavirin)	7–21 days [M + R] Oral bioavailability is 50%; metabolised by hydrolysis of ribosyl group from triazole moiety, which is then excreted in urine; very slowly cleared from erythrocytes and tissue compartments (shorter half-lives are reported after single doses)	Used for severe RSV bronchiolitis in infants and children, and with interferon alfa or peginterferon alfa for chronic hepatitis C infection; given orally or by inhalation
Zanamivir	2–5 [R] Very low oral absorption (1–5%), therefore not given by this route; eliminated in urine	Used to treat influenza in at-risk subjects if started within 48 h of onset of symptoms; given by inhalation for influenza
Antiprotozoal drugs		
Antimalarials		
Artemether with lumefantrine	2–3 [M] Rapidly absorbed and hydrolysed to an active metabolite	Used for the treatment of acute uncomplicated falciparum malaria; given orally
Atovaquone	3 days [R] Poor and variable absorption influenced by food; most eliminated unabsorbed in faeces	Given orally with proguanil for the treatment of acute uncomplicated falciparum malaria and for prophylaxis of falciparum malaria; also used for mild to moderate pneumocystis pneumonia
Chloroquine	30–60 days [R + M] Complete oral bioavailability; limited metabolism (about 20%) but metabolite retains activity; mostly eliminated by filtration in the kidney; the very long half-life results from the very high volume of distribution (200 L kg^{-1}) and low renal clearance	Used for chemoprophylaxis and treatment of malaria and also used for rheumatoid arthritis and lupus erythematosus; given orally or by intravenous infusion
Mefloquine	15–33 days [M + R] Good bioavailability (80%); metabolised by hydrolysis, and metabolites eliminated in urine and bile; renal clearance accounts for about 10% of total	Used for chemoprophylaxis and treatment of uncomplicated falciparum and chloroquine-resistant vivax malaria; given orally
Primaquine	4–10 [M] Rapidly absorbed, with almost complete bioavailability; metabolised to carboxyprimaquine, which retains antimalarial activity and is implicated in haemolysis	Used as an adjunct for eradication of the liver stages of vivax and ovale malaria; given orally
Proguanil (prodrug for cycloguanil)	12–24 [M] High oral bioavailability; it is a prodrug for cycloguanil (which accounts for 19% of an oral dose), which has a short half-life (2 h), so plasma concentrations of the active metabolite are usually less than those of the parent drug	Used for chemoprophylaxis of malaria; given orally (alone or with atovaquone)
Pyrimethamine	2–6 days [M] Well absorbed (human bioavailability is not known); numerous metabolites eliminated mainly in the faeces	Used for malaria but only in combination with sulfadoxine; given orally
Quinine	6–47 [M] High oral bioavailability (80–90%); eliminated largely by metabolism by CYP3A4; also binds to and inhibits CYP2D6; may also be metabolised by CYP1A2, because smoking (which does not induce CYP3A4) increases its clearance	Used for treatment but not chemoprophylaxis of falciparum malaria, or when the infection is either mixed or not known; also used in combination with doxycycline (see above); given orally or by intravenous infusion

Drugs used for infections

Drug	Half-life (h) and kinetics	Comments
Sulfadoxine	10 days [M] Metabolised by acetylation	Used for malaria but only in combination with pyrimethamine (see above); given orally
Other antiprotozoals		
Diloxanide furoate	? [M] Completely hydrolysed in the gut lumen and mucosa to diloxanide, which is incompletely absorbed; absorbed diloxanide is conjugated with glucuronic acid; few kinetic data available	Used for amoebiasis and is drug of choice for asymptomatic *Entamoeba histolytica* infections; given orally
Mepacrine	? Few published data available; very slowly eliminated by metabolism	Used for giardiasis and discoid lupus erythematosus; given orally
Metronidazole	6–9 [M + R] Complete oral bioavailability; metabolites are eliminated slowly in urine	Used for intestinal and extra-intestinal amoebiasis and for urogenital trichomoniasis and giardiasis; also has antibacterial actions (see above); given orally
Pentamidine	13 days [M + R] Metabolised by oxidation, and conjugation with sulphate and glucuronic acid	Used for pneumocystis pneumonia, leishmaniasis and trypanosomiasis; given by inhalation (nebuliser), by deep intramuscular injection or by intravenous infusion
Stibogluconate	6 (as pentavalent antimony) [R] Pentavalent antimony is eliminated in urine; very slow minor late elimination phase reported (half-life of 76 h) but chemical form of pentavalent antimony not defined	Used for leishmaniasis; pentavalent antimony compound; given by intramuscular injection or slow intravenous infusion (over at least 5 min)
Tinidazole	12–14 [M + R] Complete oral bioavailability; about 25% excreted unchanged and the remainder metabolised and eliminated via urine and bile	Uses are similar to those of metronidazole; also has antibacterial actions (see above); given orally
Antihelminthic drugs		
Albendazole	8–12 [M] Low oral bioavailability (parent drug not usually detectable); metabolised by S-oxidation; the parent compound and sulphoxide (SO) are active, while the sulphone (SO_2) is inactive	Used on a 'named-patient' basis either alone or as an adjunct to surgery for echinococcal infections and for cutaneous hookworm larval infections; given orally
Diethylcarbamazine	? [M + R] Good oral absorption; eliminated by hepatic metabolism and renal excretion	First line drug for use against filariae (not approved) in UK; given orally
Ivermectin	12 [M] Well absorbed but bioavailability has not been defined; eliminated as metabolites in faeces	Used on a 'named-patient' basis as the drug of choice for onchocerciasis; also used for cutaneous hookworm larval infections and for chronic *Strongyloides* infections; given orally
Levamisole	4–6 [M] Bioavailability 60–70%; oxidised in liver and conjugated with glucuronic acid	Used on a named-patient basis as the drug of choice for *Ascaris lumbricoides* infection; given orally
Mebendazole	3–9 [M] Low bioavailability (20% for solutions, 2% for tablets); metabolites excreted in urine	Used for threadworm, roundworm, whipworm and hookworm infections; given orally
Niclosamide	? [M] Some oral absorption (up to 20%) occurs, with subsequent liver metabolism; few kinetic data available	Used on a 'named-patient' basis for tapeworm infections; given orally; not used in the USA
Piperazine	? [R] Few data available; about 5–30% of an oral dose is excreted in urine unchanged within 24 h	Used for threadworm and roundworm infections; given orally

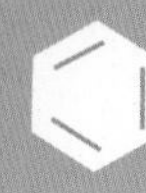

Drugs used for infections

Drug	Half-life (h) and kinetics	Comments
Praziquantel	2 [M] Probably extensive first-pass metabolism; rapidly metabolised and excreted	Used on a 'named-patient' basis for tapeworm infections and bilharziasis; given orally
Tiabendazole	1.2 [M] Rapidly and extensively absorbed; metabolised by oxidation and conjugation	Used on a 'named-patient' basis as the drug of choice for *Strongyloides* infection and used for cutaneous hookworm larval infections; given orally

[B], biliary excretion; [M], metabolism; [R], renal excretion; CMV, cytomegalovirus; MRSA, meticillin-resistant *Staphylococcus aureus*; RSV, respiratory syncytial virus.

52 Chemotherapy of malignancy

Approximately 20–25% of people in the Western world die from cancer. Surgery and radiotherapy are valuable for treating localised cancers but are less effective in prolonging life once the tumour has spread to produce metastases. The introduction of cytotoxic chemotherapy to kill rapidly proliferating neoplastic cells has had a major impact on the treatment of malignant disease, especially diffuse tumours. The successful treatment of cancer frequently involves a multidisciplinary approach, which also includes necessary psychological and social support.

A wide range of different chemicals to treat cancer, with a variety of mechanisms and sites of action within the cell, has been introduced into clinical practice since the 1970s. Although the drugs may differ in their specific cellular targets, they nearly all rely on the rapid rate of growth and division of cancer cells to provide a degree of selectivity between normal and malignant tissue. Recent developments in molecular biology are resulting in the discovery of new potential targets for drug action, and a resurgence of cytotoxic drug development. The ability of molecular biological approaches to define the mechanisms of cell–cell communication, apoptosis, angiogenesis, etc., will undoubtedly prove a major stimulus for the production of new drugs with greater selectivity for cancer cells. There are a number of in vivo animal tests for detecting antineoplastic activity, but these frequently overpredict the likely effectiveness of a compound in clinical use, because the animal tumours used as models have a much higher growth fraction (see below). A placebo-controlled clinical trial (Ch. 3) of a new antineoplastic drug given as sole treatment is now unethical if an effective drug is already available. Therefore, the efficacy of any new drug usually has to be assessed by its addition to the best available current therapy. A successful new drug would have to show a clinically significant benefit above that of current treatment. As a result, many recent advances in cancer chemotherapy have arisen from the more effective use of existing drugs, by optimising drug combinations and regimens, and by minimising toxicity, rather than the introduction of novel compounds.

Cytotoxic drugs share a number of generic properties and characteristics, both beneficial and adverse, which will be discussed first. The major classes of drug will then be discussed, with information on mechanisms of action and general toxic effects.

MOLECULAR ORIGINS OF CANCER

Most cancers probably arise from a combination of genetic mutations in a cell, with sequential gene defects resulting in progressive changes in the cell through initial metaplastic and dysplastic phases, and then to invasive and ultimately metastatic cancer. Normal cells are regulated by numerous external factors that control cell growth and death. These include growth factors, cytokines and hormones that activate or suppress the genes controlling cell division. Cancers develop as a result of abnormalities in the control of cell function.

Exposure to environmental factors such as viruses and chemicals, and to inherited mutations can change gene expression and cell cycle control by altering the following:

- **Activation of proto-oncogenes to oncogenes:** proto-oncogenes are normal gene sequences that control cell proliferation and differentiation. They are capable of being activated to oncogenes, the expression of which leads to tumour development. Oncogene activation occurs as a result of chromosomal rearrangement, gene mutations or gene amplification. Products of oncogene activation include transcription factors, chromatin remodellers, growth factors, altered growth factor receptors, intracellular signal transducers and apoptosis regulators. Gene mutations that activate oncogenes lead

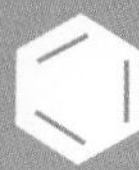

to the excessive production of proteins that inhibit cell death, and that allow cell growth in the absence of stimulation by an external regulator.

- **Suppression or deletion of tumour suppressor genes** or changes in microRNA genes (genes that encode RNA which regulates gene expression): as a result, there is unregulated cell proliferation, and also a delay in programmed cell death (apoptosis).

Growth factors secreted by cancer cells promote angiogenesis and increase blood supply to the tumour. Other secreted factors can impede the host's immune response to the cancer cells. Genetic changes in cancer cells can give rise to metabolic changes or transporters such as P-glycoprotein that confer resistance to chemotherapy.

ANTINEOPLASTIC DRUGS

MECHANISMS OF ACTION

The majority of antineoplastic drugs act on the process of DNA synthesis within the cancer cell, as summarised in Figure 52.1; selectivity of these drugs for cancer cells compared with normal tissues is determined by the rate of DNA synthesis and cell division. Resting cells in the G_0 phase (Fig. 52.2) are resistant to many antineoplastic drugs. *Cell cycle-specific antineoplastic drugs*, such as the antimetabolites (Fig. 52.2), work effectively only when the cells are in the appropriate phase of the cell cycle at the time of treatment. *Non-cell cycle-specific antineoplastic drugs*, such as the alkylating drugs, nitrosoureas and cisplatin, have a 'hit and run' action on the DNA, and it is not critical

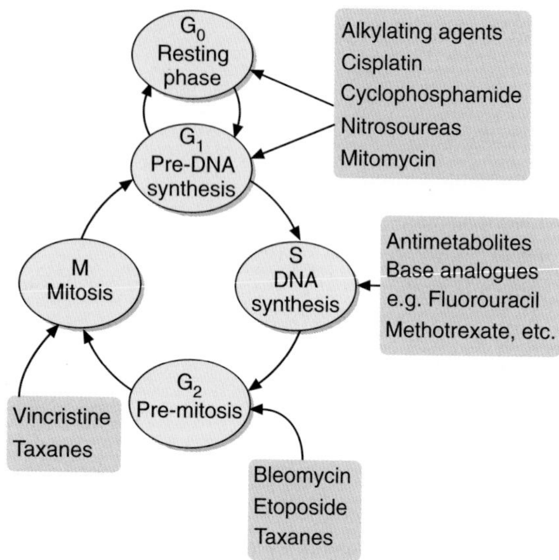

Fig. 52.2 **Sites of action for the main groups of cell cycle-specific anticancer drugs.**

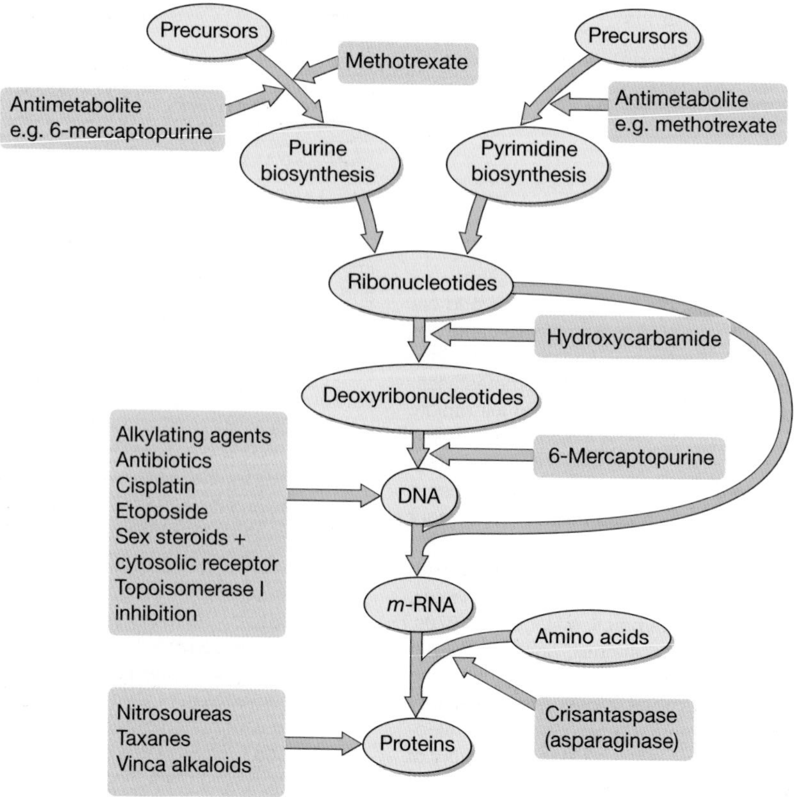

Fig. 52.1 **Sites of action for the main groups of anticancer drugs.**

when the cell is exposed, because the drug effect becomes apparent later when the cells attempt to divide.

The sensitivity of a cancer to treatment depends on its growth fraction – that is, the fraction of cells undergoing mitosis at any time. For example, in Burkitt's lymphoma, almost 100% of neoplastic cells are undergoing division, and it is very sensitive to chemotherapy, showing a dramatic response to a single dose of cyclophosphamide. In contrast, the growth fraction in a carcinoma of the colon represents less than 5% of cells, resulting in its relative resistance to chemotherapy. However, metastases from colonic carcinoma deposited in the liver and elsewhere initially have a high growth fraction and are sensitive to anticancer drugs.

Using in vitro cancer cell lines, it has been shown that:

- antineoplastic drugs produce a proportional cell kill; in other words, a proportion, such as 95% of the cells present, may be eliminated during a single course of treatment; consequently, multiple treatments may be necessary to eradicate the cancer, with each treatment producing an exponential decrease in the number of residual viable cancer cells
- essentially complete eradication of tumour cells is necessary to prevent regrowth
- efficacy of chemotherapy is increased if treatment with cell cycle-specific drugs is timed to coincide with the appropriate phase of cell division within the cell population.

In vivo, the immune system probably contributes to the final removal of residual malignant cells; however, most antineoplastic drugs compromise immunoresponsiveness, which will reduce this removal process. The periodicity of doses is probably less critical in vivo because cancer cell cycles are not synchronised within the target cell population between treatments; in practice, dose intervals are often established to allow recovery from toxic effects of the treatment. Therefore, while these concepts apply to in vivo cancer treatment, risk–benefit considerations may change with successive treatments and preclude complete eradication of the tumour.

RESISTANCE

Resistance to chemotherapeutic drugs may develop in a number of ways (further explanations are given later in the text under the individual drugs):

- Reduced drug uptake into cancer cells, e.g. methotrexate enters cells by the high-affinity transport system (the reduced folate carrier) for tetrahydrofolic acid, and downregulation of the transporter limits the uptake of methotrexate and confers resistance to the drug.
- Use of alternative metabolic pathways and salvage mechanisms to circumvent a blocked biochemical process; such mechanisms are usually drug-specific, e.g. induction of asparagine synthesis in cells exposed to crisantaspase (asparaginase).
- Alteration of intracellular drug targets, e.g. production of topoisomerase II with reduced sensitivity to the inhibitory effects of anthracyclines.
- Increased inactivation of the compound within the cancer cell, e.g. high intracellular levels of glutathione S-transferase inactivate cisplatin and alkylating drugs.
- Reduced activation of prodrugs, e.g. low intracellular levels of deoxycytidine kinase reduces activation of cytarabine (cytosine arabinoside); reduced activity of thiopurine S-methyltransferase impairs activation of mercaptopurine and tioguanine.
- Increased removal of the drug from the cancer cell. This involves the possibility of increased transcription of the gene for proteins which act as carriers for the elimination from the cell of complex foreign chemicals (see Fig 2.1), including a number of cytotoxic compounds. There are several such proteins (see Table 2.1), including P-glycoprotein and the multidrug resistance-related proteins (MRPs). The increased production of the carrier confers multidrug resistance to a number of structurally unrelated natural compounds, or their derivatives, including vinca alkaloids, etoposide, taxanes, anthracyclines, dactinomycin (actinomycin D), mitomycin C and mitoxantrone. The carrier can be inhibited by calcium channel blockers, such as nifedipine or verapamil, by ciclosporin, or by tamoxifen. These drugs may be added to cytotoxic drug regimens to prevent resistance.

UNWANTED EFFECTS

Cytotoxic antineoplastic drugs are among the most toxic compounds given to humans. Many have a therapeutic index (see Ch. 53) of approximately 1 – that is, the therapeutic dose is approximately the same as the toxic dose. Because drug action is usually greater in tissues with a high growth fraction, it is not surprising that a number of normal non-malignant tissues are also affected. In addition to effects that occur in all rapidly dividing tissues, many chemotherapeutic drugs also have specific toxic effects on other tissues. Dosage regimens are usually designed so that normal tissues, especially bone marrow and gut, can recover between doses (Fig. 52.3).

Gastrointestinal tract

Mucosal cells have a rapid turnover. Toxicity can produce anorexia, mucosal ulceration or diarrhoea. Nausea and vomiting are common, especially with alkylating drugs and cisplatin, and this may limit an individual's ability to tolerate an optimal dosage regimen.

Bone marrow

Myelosuppression is a serious consequence of treatment and can lead to severe leucopenia, thrombocytopenia and sometimes anaemia. These haematological consequences may limit the drug dosage that the person is able to tolerate. There is a high risk of both infection and haemorrhage following cytotoxic chemotherapy (see the drug compendium at the end of this chapter).

Hair follicle cells

Partial or complete alopecia may occur, but this is usually temporary.

Reproductive organs

Both sexes are affected and sterility can result, particularly after therapy with cyclophosphamide or cytarabine; women

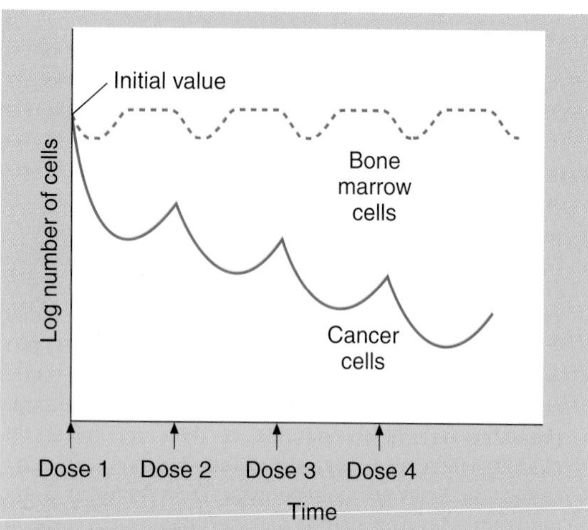

Fig. 52.3 **Hypothetical dosing schedule to allow recovery of normal tissues.** The malignant cells show a greater proportional kill because a greater fraction is in division at any time. Theoretically, the response of the malignant cells to dose 2 would be greater than for dose 1 if cell cycles became synchronised and dose 2 was given during the correct phase of the growth cycle. A typical dose interval would be 3–4 weeks. A minimum of 10^9 tumour cells are usually present when tumours are first detectable.

frequently have dysmenorrhoea or amenorrhoea. Because of the mechanisms of action of cytotoxic drugs, most would be expected to exhibit teratogenic activity. Pregnant women should not be exposed to cytotoxic drugs for treatment or as members of the healthcare team. Drugs that mimic or affect the activity of sex hormones are frequently used for the treatment of breast or prostate cancer, and these inevitably produce adverse effects on sexual function.

Growing tissues in children

Of particular concern in children is the possibility that intensive cytotoxic chemotherapy can impair growth. Children treated with cytotoxic drugs for malignancy also have an increased risk of the subsequent development of a second malignancy (about 10%), which is often leukaemia.

DRUG COMBINATIONS

It is common practice to treat many cancers with a combination of different antineoplastic drugs simultaneously, and there are numerous permutations used clinically. Combinations of drugs are investigated using in vitro and in vivo experiments before they are subjected to clinical evaluation. The most successful combinations are those that show synergism in their actions on cancer cells, rather than a simple additive interaction, while showing no interaction or simple additivity in relation to systemic toxicity. Criteria for selecting ideal combinations are:

- each drug should be an active antineoplastic drug in its own right; a second drug would not be given simply to increase the formation of an active metabolite of the first, although sometimes drugs are given to reduce the development of toxicity or resistance
- each drug should have a different mechanism of action and target site within the cancer cell; this will increase efficacy while reducing the likelihood of resistance
- each drug should have a different site for any organ-specific toxicity (some common toxicity is almost inevitable because nearly all drugs affect tissues with a high growth fraction).

SPECIFIC ANTINEOPLASTIC DRUGS

The drug compendium at the end of this chapter gives the uses of individual drugs and notes any unusual or limiting toxicity.

DRUGS AFFECTING NUCLEIC ACID FUNCTION

Alkylating drugs

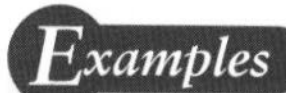

busulfan, chlorambucil, cyclophosphamide, melphalan

Mechanism of action

The nitrogen mustards were developed from the sulphur mustard gases used in the trenches in World War I. These chemical warfare gases caused bone marrow suppression in addition to the respiratory toxicity for which they were developed. Replacement of the divalent sulphur atom by trivalent nitrogen allowed the introduction of a complex side-chain, which resulted in a range of more stable non-volatile drugs that could be given therapeutically under controlled conditions. Alkylating drugs contain side-chains (for example $-CH_2CH_2Cl$) which undergo a metabolic activation step that involves loss of part of the molecule (for example the Cl is lost from $-CH_2CH_2Cl$) and yields a highly reactive product which binds to DNA or proteins. Many alkylating drugs are bifunctional (i.e. have two reactive groups).

The reactive alkylating group(s) in the molecule may be:

- nitrogen mustard $N-CH_2CH_2Cl$ (Cl is the leaving group), e.g. carmustine (BCNU), chlorambucil, chlormethine, cyclophosphamide, estramustine, ifosfamide, lomustine (CCNU), melphalan
- sulphonate ester $-CH_2OSO_2CH_3$ (SO_2CH_3 is the leaving group), e.g. busulfan, treosulfan
- nitrosourea –NNO, e.g. carmustine, lomustine
- cyclic nitrogen derivative (a three-membered ring with CH_2, CH_2 and N as the three components), e.g. thiotepa (which has three of these rings attached to a central P-S group).

The mechanism of action is by covalent binding to DNA (nitrogen mustards, sulphonate esters and cyclic nitrogen compounds), which prevents DNA and RNA synthesis, or by covalent binding to proteins (nitrosoureas), which blocks DNA repair processes.

When alkylating drugs bind to DNA, such as to N-7 of guanine, the alkylated guanine may either be repaired, in which case the cell survives, or it may interfere with DNA replication by:

- being misread
- undergoing further metabolism via ring opening
- cross-linking to another guanine via the remaining reactive group (this applies to bifunctional drugs).

Because of the covalent nature of the product, these effects are not cell cycle-specific (Fig. 52.2). Alkylating drugs have numerous clinical uses in cancer chemotherapy.

Pharmacokinetics

The pharmacokinetic characteristics of the alkylating drugs depend on the nature of the reactive group(s) and the third non-reactive substituent on the N-atom. A major advance in the use of nitrogen mustards was achieved with the introduction of cyclophosphamide, which is a chemically stable, solid chemical that can be given orally. It is a prodrug that undergoes metabolic activation to produce two toxic metabolites: acrolein (CH_2–CHCHO) and phosphoramide mustard, which contains the N–$(CH_2CH_2Cl)_2$ group. Ifosfamide undergoes similar metabolism to cyclophosphamide, and toxic metabolites of both cyclophosphamide and ifosfamide are excreted in the urine. Melphalan and chlorambucil, which have an aromatic substituent, undergo rapid metabolism. Most of the drugs have half-lives of less than 6 h, but the duration of action on DNA is very long.

Unwanted effects

- Alkylating drugs are highly cytotoxic and cause bone marrow suppression and neutropenia. Amifostine is a compound used to reduce the severity of cyclophosphamide- (and cisplatin-) induced neutropenia in advanced ovarian cancer (see cisplatin below). It is a prodrug that is metabolised in neutrophils by alkaline phosphatase to a free thiol metabolite that binds to the reactive metabolites of the cytotoxic drugs.
- Fertility is reduced through impaired gametogenesis.
- A particular problem with the long-term use of alkylating drugs, especially if combined with radiotherapy, is the development of acute myeloid leukaemia.
- Busulfan, carmustine and treosulfan can cause pulmonary fibrosis.
- Busulfan and treosulfan commonly cause skin pigmentation.
- Cyclophosphamide and ifosfamide cause bladder toxicity with haemorrhagic cystitis; this is due to acrolein and can be prevented by prior treatment with mesna (mercaptoethane sulphonic acid; Ch. 53), which provides free thiol groups in the urinary bladder. Bladder cancer may develop years after cyclophosphamide therapy.

Cytotoxic antibiotics

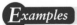

bleomycin, dactinomycin, doxorubicin, epirubicin, mitomycin, mitoxantrone

Mechanisms of action

The cytotoxic antibiotics represent a diverse range of chemical structures.

- The 'rubicin' drugs are all quinone-containing four-ringed structures (planar anthraquinones) that contain an amino sugar group (anthracyclines).
- Mitoxantrone has a three-ringed planar quinone structure with amino-containing side-chains (anthracycline derivative), and mitomycin is a non-planar tricyclic quinone.
- Bleomycin and dactinomycin are complex peptide or glycopeptide derivatives.

Although these antibacterials affect normal nucleic acid function, and also have other mechanisms of action.

- Intercalation. This is shown particularly by the rubicins, with the planar ring system intercalating between DNA bases, and the amino sugar part binding to the deoxyribose phosphate groups. Intercalation blocks reading of the DNA template and also stimulates topoisomerase II-dependent DNA double-strand breaks.
- Free radical attack. The metabolism of the drugs gives rise to superoxide and hydroxyl radicals and hydrogen peroxide, which cause DNA damage and cytotoxicity.
- Membrane effects. Interference with membrane function can occur either directly or via oxidative damage.

In general, the mechanisms of action are not cell cycle-specific, although some members of the class are reported to show greatest activity at certain phases of the cycle, for example S phase (doxorubicin, mitoxantrone), G_1 and early S phase (mitomycin), and G_2 phase and mitosis (bleomycin).

Pharmacokinetics

The cytotoxic antibiotics are poorly absorbed from the gut and are given intravenously. They are eliminated by metabolism, and some have very long half-lives (mostly 12 h or longer – see the drug compendium at the end of this chapter).

Unwanted effects

Many of these drugs have radiomimetic properties. They should not be used at the same time as radiotherapy, since toxicity can be greatly increased.

- General cytotoxicity
- Doxorubicin, epirubicin and mitoxantrone produce dose-related irreversible myocardial damage leading to cardiomyopathy, through free radical release and oxidative stress; liposomal formulations of doxorubicin may reduce the cardiac toxicity, as may infusion of the iron chelator antidote, dexrazoxane (see the drug compendium at the end of this chapter)
- Painful skin eruptions with liposomal doxorubicin
- Bleomycin often causes skin pigmentation
- Bleomycin and mitomycin produce dose-related pulmonary fibrosis
- Tissue extravasation during infusion of anthracyclines produces severe necrosis, which can be minimised by subsequent intravenous infusion of dexrazoxane.

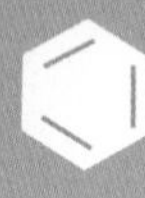

ANTIMETABOLITES

Folic acid antagonists

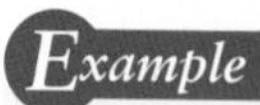

methotrexate

Mechanism of action and uses

An astute clinical observation, that the administration of folic acid to children with leukaemia exacerbated their condition, led to the development of a folate antagonist, methotrexate. This represented an important landmark in cancer chemotherapy.

Folic acid in its reduced form (tetrahydrofolic acid; THF) is an important biochemical intermediate. It is essential for synthetic reactions that involve the addition of a single carbon atom during a biochemical reaction, such as the introduction of the methyl group into thymidylate and the synthesis of the purine ring system. During such reactions, THF is oxidised to dihydrofolic acid (DHF), which has to be reduced by dihydrofolate reductase back to THF before it can accept a further 1-carbon group, and be reused.

Methotrexate has a very high affinity for, and inhibits the active site of, mammalian dihydrofolate reductase. This blocks purine and thymidylate synthesis and inhibits the synthesis of DNA, RNA and protein. Methotrexate blocks dihydrofolate reductase and the 1-carbon cycle. It may show selectivity for cancer cells because these rely more on de novo synthesis of purines and pyrimidines, whereas normal tissues use salvage pathways (that reutilise preformed purines and pyrimidines) to a greater extent. Methotrexate is specific for S phase and slows G_1 to S phase.

Methotrexate is given for acute lymphoblastic leukaemia, non-Hodgkin's lymphomas and various other malignancies. It is also used in non-malignant conditions such as inflammatory joint diseases and psoriasis (Chs 30 and 49).

Pharmacokinetics

Methotrexate is well absorbed from the gut but can also be given intravenously or intrathecally. It is eliminated by renal excretion, but a small amount may be retained for longer periods both strongly bound to the dihydrofolate reductase and intracellularly as polyglutamate conjugates.

Unwanted effects

- Toxicity to normal rapidly dividing tissues (especially the bone marrow)
- Hepatotoxicity can follow chronic therapy (as in psoriasis).

Toxicity is increased in the presence of reduced renal excretion, and methotrexate should be avoided if there is significant renal impairment. Folinic acid (leucovorin) is frequently administered shortly after high-dose methotrexate, to reduce mucositis and myelosuppression. Non-steroidal anti-inflammatory drugs such as aspirin can reduce the renal excretion of methotrexate and increase its toxicity.

Base analogue antimetabolites

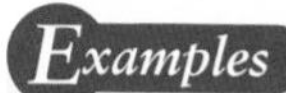

capecitabine, cladribine, clofarabine, cytarabine, fludarabine, fluorouracil, gemcitabine, mercaptopurine, raltitrexed, tegafur, tioguanine (6-thioguanine)

Mechanism of action

A number of useful chemotherapeutic drugs have been produced by simple modifications to the structures of normal purine and pyrimidine bases (Fig. 52.4). These act in a number of ways to interfere with DNA synthesis (Table 52.1).

Pharmacokinetics

Base analogues tend to be absorbed and metabolised by the pathways involved with the corresponding normal (unmodified) base. Oral absorption is often erratic, and

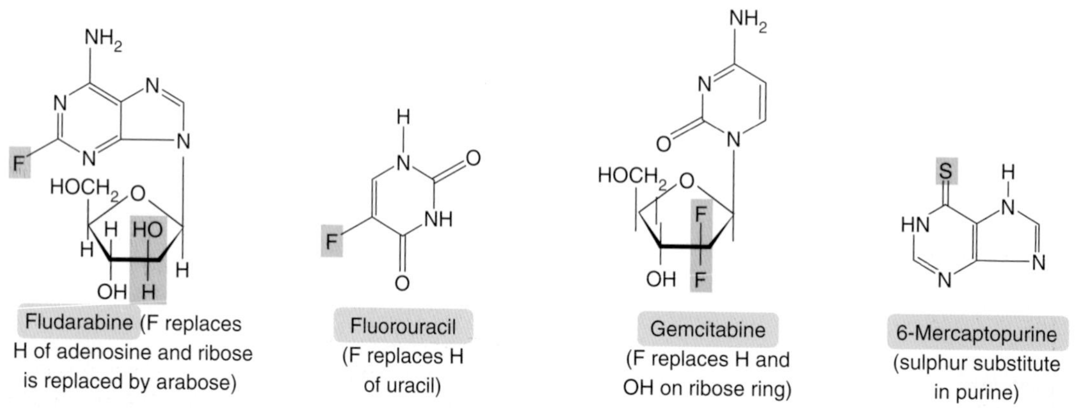

Fludarabine (F replaces H of adenosine and ribose is replaced by arabose)

Fluorouracil (F replaces H of uracil)

Gemcitabine (F replaces H and OH on ribose ring)

6-Mercaptopurine (sulphur substitute in purine)

Fig. 52.4 The structure of some antimetabolites, illustrating their similarity to normal bases and nucleotides (structural changes are highlighted).

Table 52.1 Mechanisms of action of base analogues

Analogue	Metabolism	Action	Cell cycle effect
Cladribine	Phosphorylated intracellularly by deoxycytidine kinase	The main action is by incorporation of the triphosphate into DNA and blocking DNA polymerase and DNA ligase	Not specific
Clofarabine	Phosphorylated intracellularly by deoxycytidine kinase	Inhibits DNA synthesis by inhibition of ribonucleotide reductase, and by terminating DNA chain elongation	Not specific
Cytarabine	Phosphorylated intracellularly by deoxycytidine kinase	The main action is by incorporation of the triphosphate into DNA and blocking DNA polymerase and DNA ligase	Specific: mostly active in S phase
Fludarabine	Phosphorylated intracellularly by deoxycytidine kinase	The main action is by incorporation of the triphosphate into DNA and blocking DNA polymerase and DNA ligase	Specific: mostly active in S phase
Fluorouracil	Phosphorylated intracellularly to fluorouridine monophosphate (FUMP) and the deoxy analogue (FdUMP)	FdUMP inhibits thymidylate synthase, is converted to the triphosphate and is incorporated into DNA FUMP is converted to the triphosphate and is incorporated into RNA	Some selectivity for G_2 and S phases
Gemcitabine	Converted to a triphosphate	Triphosphate is incorporated into DNA and blocks elongation and promotes apoptosis	Specific for S phase
6-Mercaptopurine	Phosphorylated to mono- and triphosphate	Monophosphate inhibits de novo purine synthesis Triphosphates are incorporated into DNA and/or RNA, giving cytotoxicity	Specific for S phase
Tegafur	Metabolised to fluorouracil (5FU)	See fluorouracil	
Tioguanine	Converted to intracellular nucleotides	Main action arises from incorporation of triphosphates into DNA and RNA The nucleotides cause 'pseudo' feedback inhibition of the synthesis of other purines and inhibit purine nucleotide interconversions	Active in G_1 and S phases

most are given intravenously. The urine is a minor route of elimination (up to 1% of the parent drug) and most half-lives are in the range 1–8 h. Tegafur is a prodrug of 5-fluorouracil, and is given in combination with uracil, which inhibits the breakdown of 5-fluorouracil.

Unwanted effects

- Typical cytotoxic effects are common; myelosuppression, in particular, can be severe and prolonged after cladribine, cytarabine, fludarabine and tioguanine
- Drug interaction: allopurinol (Ch. 31) interferes with the metabolism of 6-mercaptopurine, and the dose should be reduced if these drugs are used concurrently.

ANTIMITOTICS

Vinca alkaloids and etoposide

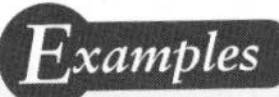

etoposide, vinblastine, vincristine, vindesine, vinorelbine

Mechanism of action and uses

The vinca alkaloids are complex natural chemicals isolated from the periwinkle plant (*Vinca rosea*). Etoposide is a synthetic derivative of a compound that is extracted from the mandrake root (*Podophyllum peltatum*) and is sometimes called a 'podophyllotoxin'.

Vinca alkaloids bind to tubulin and cause depolymerisation of microtubules, thus producing metaphase arrest. They are therefore cycle-specific. The vinca alkaloids are used for various lymphomas and for acute leukaemia. They are also effective in some solid tumours.

Etoposide is active during the G_2 phase and binds to the complex of DNA and topoisomerase II (an enzyme involved in the uncoiling and coiling of DNA during repair). The etoposide-bound complex prevents DNA replication and causes strand breaks.

Pharmacokinetics

The absorption of oral doses of vinca alkaloids is unpredictable and they are usually given intravenously. Etoposide can be given orally. Elimination is largely by metabolism, with little renal excretion. They have long half-lives.

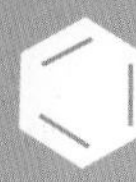

Unwanted effects

The spectrum of unwanted effects differs between different drugs, despite their close structural similarities.

- General cytotoxicity. Myelosuppression is dose-limiting for vinblastine, vindesine and vinorelbine, but unusual with vincristine.
- Neurotoxicity is dose-limiting with vincristine. It causes peripheral paraesthesiae, loss of tendon reflexes, abdominal pain and constipation; motor weakness occasionally accompanies the sensory neuropathy.
- Severe tissue damage if the drugs extravasate from the infusion site.

Taxanes

docetaxel, paclitaxel

Mechanism of action and uses

The clinically used drugs are produced from taxane, which is a diterpenoid extracted from the bark of the Pacific yew tree (*Taxus brevifolia*).

Taxanes promote the assembly of microtubules and inhibit their depolymerisation, leading to the formation of stable and non-functional microtubular bundles in the cell. They bind to a different site to that used by vinca alkaloids. Microtubules are essential for numerous cellular functions, including maintenance of cell shape, motility, transport between organelles and cell division.

The cell is inhibited during the G_2 and M phases of the cell cycle. Taxanes are also radiosensitisers, since cells in the G_2 and M phases are more sensitive to radiation. The drugs are used for ovarian and breast cancer.

Pharmacokinetics

These drugs are given intravenously because of poor oral absorption. They are extensively metabolised in the liver and have half-lives of 10–20 h.

Unwanted effects

- General cytotoxicity.
- Severe hypersensitivity reactions can occur, with hypotension, angioedema and bronchospasm. Routine premedication with histamine (H_1 and H_2) receptor antagonists (Chs 33 and 39) combined with a corticosteroid (Ch. 44) is recommended.
- Neutropenia is dose-limiting.
- Arthralgia/myalgia syndrome.
- Paclitaxel causes peripheral sensory neuropathy, with motor neuropathy at high dosages.
- Docetaxel causes persistent leg oedema due to fluid retention.

PLATINUM COMPOUNDS

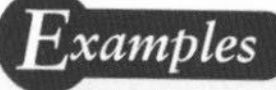

carboplatin, cisplatin, oxaliplatin

Mechanism of action and uses

The platinum drugs enter cells and generate a reactive complex that cross-links between guanine units in DNA. The result is similar to that of alkylating drugs that break the DNA chain. Cisplatin and carboplatin are particularly useful for ovarian and testicular tumours. Oxaliplatin is used for advanced colorectal cancer.

Pharmacokinetics

These drugs are poorly absorbed from the gut and are given by intravenous infusion. They are mainly excreted by the kidney as platinum compounds. Cisplatin and oxaliplatin have long half-lives (20–60 h), largely owing to extensive protein binding.

Unwanted effects

- Severe nausea and vomiting
- Nephrotoxicity with irreversible renal impairment; hydration is important to minimise the risk
- Hypomagnesaemia
- Ototoxicity with hearing loss and tinnitus
- Peripheral neuropathy (especially with oxaliplatin)
- Myelosuppression (more marked for carboplatin).

Most effects are more marked for cisplatin than for carboplatin. Amifostine (see unwanted effects of alkylating agents) is used to reduce the severity of cisplatin-induced neutropenia in advanced ovarian cancer. It also reduces the nephrotoxicity of cisplatin.

TOPOISOMERASE I INHIBITORS

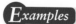

irinotecan, topotecan

Mechanism of action and uses

These are semi-synthetic derivatives of a cytotoxic alkaloid isolated from the Chinese tree *Camptotheca acuminata*.

The drugs inhibit topoisomerase I, which is important in DNA transcription and translation. The enzyme relieves the torsional strain in DNA by producing single-strand breaks that, under normal cell conditions, are then religated. The drugs bind to the DNA–topoisomerase I complex and prevent religation. Although this binding is readily reversible, the consequences are irreversible, because cell death occurs when a double-strand break is produced at the DNA replication fork during S phase. Inhibition of DNA repair increases the sensitivity of the cell to ionising radiation. Topoisomerase I inhibitors are given as second-line treatments for metastatic colorectal or ovarian cancer.

Pharmacokinetics

They are large complex molecules that are given by intravenous infusion and are eliminated mainly by hepatic metabolism.

Unwanted effects

- General cytotoxicity, with dose-limiting myelosuppression
- Diarrhoea; cholinergic stimulation produces early diarrhoea, but other toxicity can result in delayed onset.

DRUGS AFFECTING TYROSINE KINASE FUNCTION

These can be subdivided into monoclonal antibodies that act at the cell surface receptor and small organic molecules acting intracellularly on the tyrosine kinase enzyme.

Tyrosine kinase receptor inhibitors

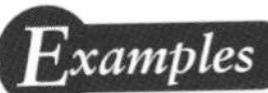

bevacizumab, cetuximab, trastuzumab

Mechanism of action and uses

The products of activated oncogenes include various cell surface receptors, including vascular endothelial growth factor receptor (VEGFR – of which there are three types) and human Epidermal Growth Factor Receptors: HER1 (often called EGFR) and HER2, HER3 and HER4. These are transmembrane receptors that activate a variety of intracellular tyrosine kinases which autophosphorylate the receptor (see Ch. 1). Autophosphorylation triggers a series of intracellular pathways that stimulate cancer cell proliferation and block apoptosis.

VEGFR activity affects the microenvironment of the tumour by angiogenesis; bevacizumab is a monoclonal antibody that inhibits VEGFR. Bevacizumab is given by intravenous infusion as part of the first-line treatment of metastatic colorectal cancer Unwanted effects include mucocutaneous bleeding, gastrointestinal perforation and impaired wound healing.

The EGFR (HER1) responds to stimulation by EGF, amphiregulin, epiregulin, transforming growth factor alpha (TGFα) and other ligands. Cetuximab is a monoclonal antibody that binds to the extracellular domain of the EGFR and blocks ligand-induced activation of tyrosine kinase. It is given by intravenous infusion in cases of colorectal tumour expressing EGFR and in combination with radiotherapy for locally advanced squamous cell cancer of the head and neck. Unwanted effects may occur with the infusion, including chills, fever and hypersensitivity reactions.

Trastuzumab is a monoclonal antibody used for metastatic breast cancer when the tumour overexpresses human epidermal growth factor receptor 2 (HER2). It binds to HER2 and prevents activation of tyrosine kinase. Unwanted effects may occur with the infusion, including chills, fever and hypersensitivity reactions. Cardiotoxicity occurs if trastuzumab is used with anthracyclines, leading to heart failure.

Tyrosine kinase inhibitors

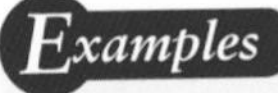

dasatinib, erlotinib, imatinib, sorafenib, sunitinib

These drugs block tyrosine kinase enzyme activity intracellularly, preventing transduction of signals from a variety of tyrosine kinase-linked cell surface receptors, and inhibiting cell growth and enhancing apoptosis. The drugs compete with ATP for binding to the enzyme and inhibit autophosphorylation of the receptor (see Ch. 1).

- Dasatinib inhibits multiple tyrosine kinases, including those associated VEGFR, platelet-derived growth factor receptor (PDGFR), stem cell factor receptors (KITs) and BCR-ABL kinase (BCR-ABL is a fusion protein that has serine/threonine kinase activity and is encoded by *BCR* and *ABL* genes; it is often found in those with chronic myeloid leukaemia). Dasatinib is used for chronic myeloid leukaemia and acute lymphoblastic leukaemia.
- Erlotinib inhibits signals from the EGFR (HER1). It is used for small-cell cancer of the lung.
- Imatinib inhibits signals from the PDGFR, KITs and BCR-ABL kinase. It is used for chronic myeloid leukaemia, acute lymphoblastic leukaemia and a variety of rare tumours.
- Sunitinib and sorafenib inhibit signals from several receptors, including VEGFR (types 2 and 3), PDGFR and KITs. They are used for renal cell carcinoma; sunitinib is also used for gastrointestinal stromal tumours and sorafenib also for hepatocellular cancer.

Pharmacokinetics

These drugs are well absorbed from the gut. They are metabolised in the liver, sometimes to active metabolites. The half-lives are about 1–2 days (except for dasatinib, which is 3–5 h). For more details, see the drug compendium at the end of this chapter.

Unwanted effects

Apart from characteristic cytotoxic effects, unwanted effects include:

- Gastrointestinal upset
- Dizziness, headache, insomnia
- Oedema with dasatinib and imatinib.

PROTEASOME INHIBITORS

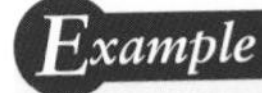

bortezomib

Mechanism of action

Proteasomes are large protein complexes that degrade ubiquinated proteins. They are involved in regulating the intracellular content of specific proteins and maintaining cell homeostasis. Inhibition of the 26S proteasome by bortezomib interferes with several signalling processes in the cell and can lead to cell death.

Pharmacokinetics

Bortezomib is given intravenously. It is metabolised in the liver and has a long half-life of 9–15 h.

Unwanted effects

Apart from characteristic cytotoxic effects, unwanted effects include:

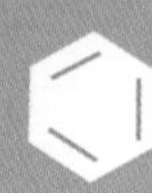

- peripheral neuropathy, fatigue
- gastrointestinal disturbances
- pyrexia
- postural hypotension.

DRUGS ACTING ON STEROID RECEPTORS AND STEROID METABOLISM

Some drugs used in cancer therapy act to suppress cell division by actions at intracellular steroid receptors or by influencing the metabolism of steroidal hormones; examples include corticosteroids or drugs that control the division of cells sensitive to sex hormones. Cancers that arise from cell lines possessing steroid receptors that promote their growth and cell division are frequently susceptible to inhibitory steroids.

Glucocorticoids

Glucocorticoids (Ch. 44) suppress lymphocyte mitosis and are used in leukaemia and lymphoma; they are also helpful in reducing oedema around a tumour.

Oestrogens

Oestrogens (Ch. 45) suppress prostate cancer cells, both locally and in metastases, and provide symptomatic improvement; gynaecomastia is a common unwanted effect.

Progestogens

Progestogens (Ch. 45) suppress endometrial cancer cells and kidney cancer metastases.

Oestrogen receptor antagonists

Breast cancer can be suppressed by oestrogen antagonists (e.g. tamoxifen). Tamoxifen is active orally and binds competitively to oestrogen receptors. It shows both oestrogenic effects (on bone) and anti-oestrogenic effects (on breast tissue). Tamoxifen inhibits oestrogen-regulated genes and reduces the secretion of growth factors by tumour cells. Tumour cells are affected mainly in the G_2 phase of the cell cycle. Tamoxifen is extensively metabolised in the liver and has active metabolites with long half-lives; therefore, several weeks of treatment are necessary to achieve steady-state concentrations. Unwanted effects include hot flushes and amenorrhoea in premenopausal women and vaginal bleeding in postmenopausal women. Tamoxifen inhibits CYP3A4 and, therefore, reduces the metabolism of other substrates, such as warfarin.

Androgen receptor antagonists

These drugs (e.g. flutamide; Ch. 46) suppress prostate cancer cells.

Gonadorelin analogues

These drugs (e.g. buserelin; Ch. 43) suppress prostate cancer cells.

Aromatase inhibitors

Aromatase is the enzyme that converts androgens to oestrogens. Inhibitors of aromatase (e.g. anastrazole and letrozole, which are non-steroidal, or exemestane, which is a steroid) reduce oestrogen production in postmenopausal women, who produce oestrogen mainly from androstenedione and testosterone in many tissues such as adipose tissue, skin, muscle and liver. Aromatase is also present in the cells of two-thirds of breast carcinomas, and many breast cancers are oestrogen-dependent.

MISCELLANEOUS ANTICANCER DRUGS

These drugs represent a mixture of compounds with a variety of mechanisms of action. Further details (including therapeutic uses and adverse effects) are given in the drug compendium at the end of this chapter.

Mechanisms of action and uses

Most potential biochemical sites within cells have been investigated as targets for anticancer drugs. Actions of different drugs include the following:

- removal of asparagine required for protein synthesis (crisantaspase)
- inhibition of incorporation of thymidine and adenine into DNA (procarbazine)
- inhibition of adenosine deaminase, which causes a build-up of deoxyadenosine triphosphate (dATP), which inhibits the formation of other deoxyribonucleotide triphosphates (pentostatin)
- inhibition of reduction of ribonucleotides to deoxyribonucleotides (hydroxycarbamide)
- intercalation between DNA base pairs (amsacrine)
- alkylating action, especially on thiol groups, to inhibit DNA repair (dacarbazine and temozolomide)
- superoxide production causing DNA backbone cleavage and cell apoptosis (trabectedin)
- increased cell differentiation and inhibition of proliferation by action on retinoid receptors (RAR and RXR) (bexarotene, tretinoin) (Ch. 49)
- photodynamic activation in superficial tumours by laser light to produce cytotoxic oxygen free radicals (porfimer sodium, temoporfin)
- immunomodulation (by inhibition of TNFα and several other pro-inflammatory chemokines) and inhibition of angiogenesis (lenalidomide and thalidomide – neither of which are currently licensed for this use in the UK); interferon alfa (see Ch. 36) has proved to be a disappointing drug for cancer treatment; it is not the 'natural, side-effect-free' drug that was hoped for when it was first isolated
- activation of cytotoxic killer cells (Ch. 38); interleukin-2 (aldesleukin) is a lymphokine produced by T-lymphocytes that is made by recombinant DNA technology
- antibody activity: several monoclonal antibodies have been developed that have highly specific effects on lymphocytes, e.g. alemtuzumab (which produces lysis of B-lymphocytes in treatment-resistant or rapidly relapsing chronic lymphocytic leukaemia) and rituximab (which produces lysis of B-lymphocytes in chemotherapy-resistant advanced follicular lymphoma) (see also Ch. 49).

Pharmacokinetics

The drugs show a diverse array of pharmacokinetic characteristics (see the drug compendium at the end of this chapter).

Unwanted effects

See the drug compendium at the end of this chapter.

CLINICAL USES OF ANTINEOPLASTIC DRUGS

Different forms of cancer vary in their sensitivity to chemotherapy. The most responsive include lymphomas, leukaemias, choriocarcinoma and testicular carcinoma, while solid tumours such as colorectal, adrenocortical and squamous cell bronchial carcinomas generally show a poor response. An intermediate response is shown by other cancers, for example those of the bladder, head and neck, oat cell bronchogenic tumours and sex-related cancers (breast, ovary, endometrium and prostate). In addition, the sensitivity of an individual tumour can change during treatment with antineoplastic drugs, because of the development of resistance.

Chemotherapy can be used alone to treat cancer, or in combination with surgery or with radiation (chemoradiation). Chemotherapy may be given as a curative or a palliative treatment, or to reduce the risk of relapse after tumour removal. Adjuvant chemotherapy refers specifically to treatment following a surgical procedure that appears to have removed all the tumour, with the intention of preventing relapse from occult disease.

Neoadjuvant chemotherapy is given before surgery to reduce tumour size.

ANTICANCER DRUG THERAPY FOR SPECIFIC MALIGNANCIES

The following discussion selects certain important cancers and outlines the role of chemotherapeutic drugs in their management. The choice of specific regimens is a complex process involving an assessment of prognosis, frailty, toxicity and the wishes of the individual. Clinical trials are producing a continuing flow of improved therapeutic options, and this is a field of medicine that changes rapidly.

Oesophageal cancer

Oesophageal cancer usually presents with advanced disease, with 50% being unresectable or having radiological metastases at presentation. If the disease is localised, then surgical resection is the treatment of choice. Therapy with cisplatin and fluorouracil before surgery improves short-term survival. Chemotherapy alone after surgery has no benefit, but chemotherapy with cisplatin and fluorouracil given concurrently with radiotherapy may improve long-term survival.

Gastric cancer

Surgery can be curative for early disease, but about 90% of people present with advanced disease. For these individuals, neoadjuvant chemotherapy in order to reduce tumour bulk before surgical resection is undergoing trials; an example of the drugs chosen is a combination of epirubicin, cisplatin and intravenous infusion of fluorouracil. Adjuvant chemotherapy after surgery has not yet been shown to improve survival; however, fluorouracil combined with cisplatin or methotrexate and doxorubicin can be palliative in advanced disease (response rate of 65%). Radiotherapy is used for palliation of bone metastases.

Pancreatic cancer

Most pancreatic cancers present late and 5-year survival is rare because of liver metastases. Surgical resection is the treatment of choice. Chemotherapy with fluorouracil plus radiotherapy may shrink larger tumours and make subsequent surgery possible. Adjuvant chemotherapy combined with radiotherapy after resection in cases where the resection margins are free of tumour only produces a marginal improvement in survival. In cases with liver metastases, chemotherapy with gemcitabine may offer greater palliation than with fluorouracil. Several trials of more intensive adjuvant chemotherapy are underway.

Colorectal cancer

Surgery is the treatment of choice for people with colorectal cancer without metastatic disease, and palliative surgery is often used, even if spread has occurred. About 50% of colorectal tumours are cured by surgery; the recurrence rate of rectal tumour is higher than that of colonic tumour. For colon cancer, adjuvant postoperative chemotherapy is often given, with fluorouracil modulated by the use of folinic acid, and perhaps oxaliplatin. This regimen has improved survival by 10–15% for locally invasive tumours. Pre-operative chemotherapy with fluorouracil plus radiotherapy is preferred for rectal cancer. The major benefit of these adjuvant treatments is reduction of metastatic spread rather than of local recurrence. In rectal cancer, chemotherapy can be combined with radiotherapy. Once an individual has survived for 5 years, life expectancy is similar to that in the general population.

In advanced and metastatic colorectal cancer, bevacizumab with fluorouracil, with or without irinotecan, is the preferred regimen and more than doubles survival and improves quality of life. Oxaliplatin with fluorouracil has also been used. Cetuximab is available for use with irinotecan for tumours that express EGFR (HER1).

Lung cancer

There are four principal types of lung cancer. Non-small-cell cancers (adenocarcinoma, squamous cell cancer and large-cell cancer) account for about three-quarters of cases, with small-cell cancer responsible for the remainder.

For non-small-cell lung cancer, superficial lesions are amenable to several treatments, including photodynamic therapy with porfimer sodium. Surgical resection can be curative in the early stages. Radiotherapy is used after surgery when the tumour is not fully resectable, or for palliation of metastases. Neoadjuvant therapy is under investigation. Chemotherapy has a limited place for advanced or recurrent disease and is mainly palliative; regimens including drugs such as cisplatin, doxorubicin and cyclophosphamide produce only a small survival advantage. Current interest is focusing on chemoradiotherapy, which is a combination of cyclical multidrug chemotherapy followed by radiotherapy. In these studies, cisplatin is often combined with one or more additional drugs.

Small-cell lung cancer is more sensitive to chemotherapy, and has an initial response rate of 60–70%, with complete remission in 20–30% of cases. Cisplatin combined

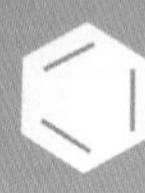

with etoposide is often used, and various other combinations are being studied. The use of pemetrexed, although licensed for this situation, is not widely endorsed. Radiotherapy is also given for limited-stage disease.

Melanoma

Survival in melanoma is related to tumour thickness, with 5-year survival falling from >95% with superficial tumours to <50% survival if the depth is greater than 4 mm. Wide surgical excision is the treatment of choice. Postsurgical adjuvant chemotherapy does not improve survival or disease-free outcome. Immunotherapy with Bacillus Calmette-Guérin (BCG) may produce a benefit if there is a negative tuberculin skin test before therapy. The use of granulocyte–macrophage colony-stimulating factor (GM-CSF) has shown promising preliminary results. Currently, interferon alfa is the only drug shown to increase disease-free survival. For metastatic disease, current therapy rests mainly on single-drug chemotherapy with dacarbazine or the vinca alkaloids (vincristine or vinblastine), which produces responses in 10–20% of patients. Combination chemotherapy increases toxicity with no improvement in response. Immunotherapy with interferon alfa has produced similar response rates to chemotherapy, and a combination of interferon alfa and dacarbazine may have additive or synergistic effects.

Renal cancer

Nephrectomy is the treatment of choice for early-stage renal cancer, but up to one-third of people have metastases at the time of diagnosis. The response to medical treatment in advanced disease is poor. Options for chemotherapy include the following.

- chemotherapy with a combination of the antimetabolites fluorouracil and gemcitabine; the response is generally low, with fewer than 15% partial or complete responses.
- progestogens produce a response in about 10% of those treated.
- immunotherapy with interferon alfa produces a response rate of about 10%; aldesleukin (interleukin-2) has a slightly higher success rate of about 15%. Combination therapy with low doses of both drugs is used for disseminated disease.
- renal cancer is very vascular. Protein kinase inhibitors of EGFR (HER1) function, such as sorafenib and sunitinib, are used for advanced disease.

Bladder cancer

Superficial bladder tumours are removed surgically, but recurrence rates are high. Intravesical immunotherapy with BCG vaccine is used to limit recurrence in superficial disease. For more advanced disease, neoadjuvant chemotherapy with gemcitabine and cisplatin improves survival. Several other regimens have been used or are under investigation. A bladder-sparing approach, using transurethral resection followed by concurrent chemotherapy (cisplatin, methotrexate and vinblastine) and irradiation, has given promising results for those who do not want cystectomy.

Prostate cancer

Treatment is largely determined by the extent of spread of the cancer. There are several options.

- 'watchful waiting' for localised disease confined to the prostate. This is usually used for individuals with a life expectancy under 10 years, since many tumours do not progress in this time.
- radical prostatectomy for localised disease, usually in men under 70 years, in whom the risk of subsequent metastases is reduced from 25% to 15%. Impotence is a common sequel, occurring in 35–60% of cases.
- radiotherapy for localised disease or locally advanced disease in older men. Impotence follows therapy in 40–60% of cases.
- interstitial implantation of radioactive pellets for localised disease or locally advanced disease (brachytherapy).
- hormonal therapy for lymph node involvement or distant metastases. Prostate cancer is hormone-dependent for growth. Testosterone reduction can be achieved by bilateral orchidectomy or the use of gonadotrophin-releasing hormone (GnRH) analogues such as leuprolide or goserelin (Ch. 43). Tumour flare reactions are prevented by the use of anti-androgen therapy (e.g. with flutamide or cyproterone acetate; Ch. 46) for the first few weeks to block adrenal androgen activity.
- hormone-refractory disease can be treated by combination chemotherapy with drugs such as estramustine with vinblastine, etoposide, docetaxel or paclitaxel. Response rates of about 50% can be achieved. Painful metastatic deposits can be treated with radiotherapy or with strontium-89, which is taken up by sclerotic metastases.

Testicular cancer

Testicular tumours are either seminomas or non-seminomatous germ cell tumours, depending on the tissue of origin. Cure rates are now greater than 95%.

For *seminomas*, treatment choice includes:

- orchidectomy then follow-up for recurrence or chemotherapy with carboplatin if the recurrence risk is high
- for locally advanced disease, surgery is followed by radiotherapy, perhaps combined with carboplatin
- for metastatic disease, chemotherapy with bleomycin, etoposide and cisplatin (BEP) is used.

For *non-seminomatous germ cell tumours*, treatment choice includes:

- orchidectomy for early disease, which may be followed by chemotherapy with a regimen containing cisplatin
- for more advanced or recurrent disease, combination chemotherapy with bleomycin, etoposide and cisplatin (BEP), which produces an 85% complete remission rate when combined with surgery.

Ovarian cancer

Initial surgery for ovarian cancer is followed by chemotherapy for all disease that is not localised to the ovary (which occurs in 80% of cases). About 70% of these women respond to chemotherapy, with complete remission in 10–20%. Options include:

- carboplatin or cisplatin alone: this is the most widely used first-line treatment
- for tumours that are refractory to standard chemotherapy, the addition of paclitaxel achieves palliation in 25–35% of cases.

The role of intraperitoneal drug delivery and more intensive combination chemotherapy is the subject of several current studies.

Cervical cancer

Surgery is the mainstay for local disease, but chemoradiation is used if there are poor prognostic predictors or advanced disease. Cisplatin is most frequently used, and improves survival by 30%. For recurrent disease, the combination of cisplatin and paclitaxel has a small advantage over cisplatin alone.

Endometrial cancer

Surgery is the usual initial treatment for endometrial cancer. Adjuvant radiotherapy is given to the pelvis, and radiotherapy is also used for extrauterine metastases. Disseminated disease can be treated by hormone therapy with progestogens, but responses are low (less than one-third of those treated) and depend on the presence of progesterone receptors on the tumour cells. Adjuvant chemotherapy with drugs such as carboplatin plus paclitaxel has a palliative role in advanced disease.

Breast cancer

Breast-conserving surgery is the treatment of choice for very early disease and for oestrogen receptor-positive tumours; it is usually followed by local radiotherapy. The risk of invasive recurrence is low; if this occurs, it is treated by mastectomy followed by chemotherapy. Chemotherapy or hormonal therapy is used for larger locally invasive tumours or distant spread, or as neoadjuvant treatment for recurrence.

Determination of the hormone receptor status of the tumour is an important guide to the most appropriate hormonal therapy or chemotherapy.

Oestrogen receptor-positive tumours

Options for adjuvant hormonal therapy for *postmenopausal* women with oestrogen receptor-positive tumours include the following:

- Non-steroidal aromatase inhibitors such as anastrazole or letrozole or the steroidal aromatase inhibitor exemestane are more effective than tamoxifen, which was long considered the treatment of choice. They can also be used as neoadjuvant therapy to reduce the extent of surgical resection.
- Anti-oestrogen therapy, e.g. with tamoxifen, is often considered second-line treatment for hormone-responsive cancer. If tamoxifen is used, then switching to an aromatase inhibitor after 2–3 years further improves disease-free survival.
- The selective oestrogen receptor downregulator (SERD) fulvestrant is an alternative second-line treatment for locally advanced or metastatic disease.
- Progestogens such as megestrol acetate are used as a third-line treatment.
- GnRH analogues such as goserelin (Ch. 43) are a fourth-line treatment.

For *premenopausal* women with oestrogen receptor-positive tumours:

- Tamoxifen remains the cornerstone of treatment, with or without chemotherapy. Aromatase inhibitors are ineffective before the menopause
- Tamoxifen can be combined with ovarian ablation using a GnRH analogue such as goserelin.

Hormonal treatment is usually given for 5 years and reduces mortality by 30%, with continuing benefit after stopping treatment for 15 years. The benefit of extending treatment beyond 5 years is unproven. The 10–20% of women who become unresponsive to one hormonal treatment may still respond to the use of an alternative class of drug.

Oestrogen receptor-negative tumours

Chemotherapy (treatment which does not involve hormonal manipulation) is used for oestrogen receptor-negative tumours, HER2-positive tumours, and younger women (especially under 35 years but up to 70 years of age) or for hormonally unresponsive disease, An example of a current regimen is doxorubicin or epirubicin with cyclophosphamide, combined with docetaxel for node-positive disease, which produces response rates of up to 40%. Trastuzumab can be added to chemotherapy for cancers that express HER2; it reduces early recurrence by 50% and improves survival by 25%. Trastuzumab can also be used as first-line therapy without cytotoxic drugs.

Acute myeloid leukaemias

The acute myeloid leukaemias are a heterogeneous group of disorders (Box 52.1) that are differentiated on morphological grounds. Acute myeloid leukaemia is responsible for up to 15% of childhood leukaemias and is the commonest leukaemia of adult life. Complications usually result from bone marrow failure, and management of serious infection or bleeding are important issues in supportive care. The risk of infection is amplified by chemotherapy. The initial aim of chemotherapy is to reduce 'blast' cells in the marrow to below 5% of the total cell population (remission) with induction therapy and then to eradicate the leukaemic cells with consolidation therapy.

Box 52.1 Simplified classification of acute myeloid leukaemias

Acute myeloid leukaemia
Acute myeloblastic leukaemia
Acute promyelocytic leukaemia
Acute myelomonocytic leukaemia
Acute monocytic/monoblastic leukaemia
Acute erythroleukaemia
Acute megakaryoblastic leukaemia

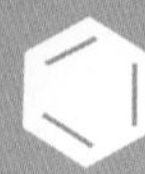

Intravenous chemotherapy with two or more drugs is used in the induction phase, to reduce the development of resistance. A typical regimen consists of daunorubicin with cytarabine, which produces remission in 65–70% of individuals under 60 years old; older people have a less favourable response. Consolidation is achieved with further courses of similar therapy for 3–4 cycles. Haematopoietic stem cell transplantation may be considered after remission is achieved. In children, treatment for the central nervous system is also given with intrathecal methotrexate. Salvage treatment is used for failure to enter remission or for relapse, with high-dose cytarabine alone or combined with fludarabine.

For acute promyelocytic leukaemia, the best initial response is obtained with tretinoin, a vitamin A derivative (see Ch. 49), and consolidation achieved by the addition of daunorubicin.

Acute lymphoblastic leukaemia

Acute lymphoblastic leukaemia is most common in children under 10 years of age, with a few cases occurring after age 40 years. Supportive therapy is similar to that for acute myeloid leukaemia.

Remission induction (eradication of 99% of leukaemic cell burden) is achieved with combinations of three or more drugs. In children, vincristine and prednisolone or dexamethasone with crisantaspase, doxorubicin or daunorubicin is often used. Four or more drugs are used for children with high-risk disease and most adults. Cyclophosphamide is often used for T-cell leukaemias, and imatinib if the cells are Philadelphia chromosome-positive. Consolidation therapy is initially with at least two multidrug intensification modules, using various combinations of corticosteroid with vincristine, crisantaspase, methotrexate and mercaptopurine. Continuation therapy is used after the first 5 months with mercaptopurine and methotrexate for at least 2 years. Eradication of cranial disease is important, using intrathecal methotrexate, cytarabine and hydrocortisone; cranial irradiation is less commonly used. Selective use of haematopoietic stem cell transplantation can further improve outcome.

The results of treatment in childhood are excellent, with about 80% 5-year survival; 5-year survival is 40% if the disease occurs in adult life.

Chronic myeloid leukaemia

Chronic myeloid leukaemia occurs in all age groups but is rare in children. Most disease follows an initial chronic course, lasting 3–4 years, with subsequent transformation to an accelerated phase, when survival is just 3–6 months. Imatinib is standard treatment for the chronic phase, and achieves cytogenetic remission in up to 87% of people. Interferon alfa, usually given with cytarabine or hydroxycarbamide, is an alternative for those who do not tolerate imatinib. In younger people, allogeneic stem cell transplantation is the treatment of choice after failed chemotherapy.

For advanced disease with blast crisis, combination chemotherapy can be considered, such as the regimen used for acute myeloid leukaemia.

Chronic lymphocytic leukaemia

Chronic lymphocytic leukaemia is predominantly a disease of the elderly. Cure is unusual and median survival is 5–8 years. Treatment may not be necessary if the disease is causing few problems, but oral chlorambucil, often combined with prednisolone, can be given for up to 6 months to regress the disease. Transformation of the disease to a more aggressive form can occur after several years, with increasing disease bulk, lymphoma-related symptoms or bone marrow failure. Standard therapy in these situations is either oral or intravenous fludarabine or oral chlorambucil, with the goal of reducing leukaemic cells in the marrow to below 30%. The monoclonal antibody rituximab and cyclophosphamide both enhance the efficacy of fludarabine. Optimal drug combinations are still under investigation.

Malignant lymphomas

The malignant lymphomas are a diverse group of disorders comprising Hodgkin's disease and a variety of non-Hodgkin's lymphomas, which are classified by histopathological and cytochemical techniques. Low-grade non-Hodgkin's lymphomas are managed in a similar way to chronic lymphocytic leukaemia and have a similar prognosis. Non-Hodgkin's lymphomas of intermediate grade are curable in about 40% of cases, using courses of combination chemotherapy with cyclophosphamide, doxorubicin, vincristine and prednisolone ('CHOP' therapy, named after a combination of the initials of the generic and proprietary names of the drugs). Rituximab may improve survival when added to standard chemotherapy, and radiotherapy is sometimes used as adjunctive treatment, or for relapsed disease. More frequent, intensive therapy is required for high-grade, aggressive non-Hodgkin's lymphomas.

For Hodgkin's disease, radiotherapy is curative if the tumour is localised; combination chemotherapy is the usual approach for more extensive disease. The most frequently used regimen is doxorubicin, bleomycin, vinblastine and dacarbazine (ABVD).

Multiple myeloma

Multiple myeloma is mainly a disorder of the elderly. Treatment is aimed at suppression of the monoclonal protein in the blood. Supportive therapy is often required to treat hypercalcaemia, renal impairment and infection. Rehydration and analgesia for bone pain are often required.

Chemotherapy is usually with oral melphalan and prednisolone in pulses for 4–6 weeks. This reduces the myeloma protein in blood by more than 50% in half of those treated. Median survival with this treatment is 3 years.

High doses of intravenous melphalan or combination therapy with vincristine, doxorubicin and dexamethasone, or cyclophosphamide, vincristine, doxorubicin and methylprednisolone, produce a response rate of up to 70% and may be justifiable in younger people who tolerate the associated toxicity better. Bortezomib, lenalidomide or thalidomide may be used for the treatment of relapsed disease.

Autologous stem cell transplantation is increasingly used as salvage therapy after intensive chemotherapy and can produce 30–50% complete remission.

FURTHER READING

Drugs and drug action

Ambudkar SV, Dey S, Hrycyna CA, Ramachandra M, Pastan I, Gottesman MM (1999) Biochemical, cellular, and pharmacological aspects of the multidrug transporter. *Annu Rev Pharmacol Toxicol* 39, 361–398

Ciardiello F, Tortora G (2008) EGFR antagonists in cancer treatment. *N Engl J Med* 358, 1160–1174

Croce CM (2008) Oncogenes and cancer. *N Engl J Med* 358, 502–511

Dubowchik GM, Walker MA (1999) Receptor-mediated and enzyme-dependent targeting of cytotoxic anticancer drugs. *Pharmacol Ther* 83, 67–123

Eccles SA, Welch DR (2007) Metastasis: recent discoveries and novel treatment strategies. *Lancet* 369, 1742–1757

Efferth T, Volm M (2005) Pharmacogenetics for individualized cancer chemotherapy. *Pharmacol Ther* 107, 155–176

Gottesman MM (2002) Mechanisms of cancer drug resistance. *Annu Rev Med* 53, 615–627

Griffioen AW, Molema G (2000) Angiogenesis: potentials for pharmacologic intervention in the treatment of cancer, cardiovascular diseases, and chronic inflammation. *Pharmacol Rev* 52, 237–268

Hofseth LJ, Hussain SP, Harris CC (2004) p53: 25 years after its discovery. *Trends Pharmacol Sci* 25, 177–181

Links M, Lewis C (1999) Chemoprotectants: a review of their clinical pharmacology and therapeutic efficacy. *Drugs* 57, 293–308

Marsh S, McLeod HL (2004) Cancer pharmacogenetics. *Br J Cancer* 90, 8–11

Bowel cancer

Allum WH, Griffin SM, Watson A et al (2002) Guidelines for the management of oesophageal and gastric cancer. *Gut* 50(suppl V), v1–v23

Ballinger AB, Anggiansah C (2007) Colorectal cancer. *BMJ* 335, 715–718

Enzinger PC, Mayer RJ (2003) Esophageal cancer. *N Engl J Med* 349, 2241–2252

Hartgrink HH, Jansen EPM, van Grieken NCT et al (2009) Gastric cancer. *Lancet* 374, 477–490

Hohenberger P, Gretschel S (2003) Gastric cancer. *Lancet* 362, 305–315

Meyerhardt JA, Mayer RJ (2005) Systemic therapy for colorectal cancer. *N Engl J Med* 352, 476–487

Roch Lima CMS, Centeno B (2002) Update on pancreatic cancer. *Curr Opin Oncol* 14, 424–430

Lung cancer

Booton R, Jones M, Thatcher N (2003) Lung cancer 7: management of lung cancer in elderly patients. *Thorax* 58, 711–720

Cullen M (2003) Lung cancer 4: chemotherapy for non-small cell lung cancer: the end of the beginning. *Thorax* 58, 352–356

Jackman DM, Johnson BE (2005) Small-cell lung cancer. *Lancet* 366, 1385–1396

Price A (2003) Lung cancer 5: state of the art radiotherapy for lung cancer. *Thorax* 58, 447–452

Spira A, Ettinger DS (2004) Multidisciplinary management of lung cancer. *N Engl J Med* 350, 379–392

Urogenital cancer

Amant F, Moerman P, Neven P et al (2005) Endometrial cancer. *Lancet* 366, 491–505

Borden LS, Clark PE, Hall MC (2003) Bladder cancer. *Curr Opin Oncol* 15, 227–233

Bott SR, Birtle AJ, Taylor CJ et al (2003) Prostate cancer management: 2. An update on locally advanced and metastatic disease. *Postgrad Med J* 79, 643–645

Cohen HT, McGovern FJ (2005) Renal cell carcinoma. *N Engl J Med* 353, 2477–2490

Dahut N, Gulley JL, Dahut WL (2005) Androgen deprivation therapy for prostate cancer. *JAMA* 294, 238–244

Feldman DR, Bosl GJ, Sheinfeld J et al (2008) Medical treatment of advanced testicular cancer. *JAMA* 299, 672–684

Harris KA, Reese DM (2001) Treatment options in hormone-refractory prostate cancer. *Drugs* 61, 2177–2192

Hellerstedt BA, Pienta KJ (2002) Testicular cancer. *Curr Opin Oncol* 14, 260–264

Hernandez J, Thompson IM (2004) Diagnosis and treatment of prostate cancer. *Med Clin North Am* 88, 267–279

Horwich A, Shipley J, Huddart R (2006) Testicular germ-cell cancer. *Lancet* 367, 754–765

Kaufman DS, Shipley WU, Feldman AS (2009) Bladder cancer. *Lancet* 374, 239–249

Petignat P, Roy M (2007) Diagnosis and management of cervical cancer. *BMJ* 335, 765–768

Waggoner SE (2003) Cervical cancer. *Lancet* 361, 2217–2225

Walsh PC, DeWeese TL, Eisenberger MA (2007) Localized prostate cancer. *N Engl J Med* 357, 2696–2705

Wilt TJ, Thompson IM (2006) Clinically localized prostate cancer. *BMJ* 333, 1102–1106

Breast cancer

Smith IE, Dowsett M (2003) Aromatase inhibitors in breast cancer. *N Engl J Med* 348, 2431–2442

Turner NC, Jones AL (2008) Management of breast cancer – Part 1. *BMJ* 337, 107–110

Turner NC, Jones AL (2008) Management of breast cancer – Part 2. *BMJ* 337, 164–169

Melanoma

Eggermont AMM (2002) European approach to the treatment of malignant melanoma. *Curr Opin Oncol* 14, 205–211

Acute leukaemias

Estey E, Döhner H (2006) Acute myeloid leukaemia. *Lancet* 368, 1894–1907

Pui C-H, Robinson LL, Look AT (2008) Acute lymphoblastic leukaemia. *Lancet* 371, 1030–1043

Ravandi F, Kantarajian H, Giles F et al (2004) New drugs in acute leukemia and other myeloid disorders. *Cancer* 100, 441–454

Chronic leukaemias

Dighiero G, Hamblin TJ (2008) Chronic lymphocytic leukaemia. *Lancet* 371, 1017–1029

Goldman JM, Melo JV (2003) Chronic myeloid leukemia – advances in biology and new approaches to treatment. *N Engl J Med* 349, 1451–1464

Hehlmann R, Hochhaus A, Baccarani M et al (2007) Chronic myeloid leukaemia. *Lancet* 370, 342–350

Shanafelt TD, Byrd JC, Call TG et al (2006) Narrative review: initial management of newly diagnosed, early-stage chronic lymphocytic leukaemia. *Ann Intern Med* 145, 435–447

Lymphomas

Evans LS, Hancock BW (2003) Non-Hodgkin lymphoma. *Lancet* 362, 139–146

Yung L, Linch D (2002) Hodgkin's lymphoma. *Lancet* 361, 943–951

Multiple myeloma

Sirohi B, Powles R (2004) Multiple myeloma. *Lancet* 363, 875–887

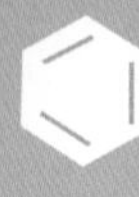

SELF-ASSESSMENT

1. What are the criteria for combination chemotherapy of cancer? How well do the following treatment regimens meet the criteria?
   a. Acute lymphoblastic leukaemia (ALL; initial phase for induction of remission): intravenous vincristine, subcutaneous crisantaspase (asparaginase) and oral prednisolone.
   b. Non-Hodgkin's lymphoma: cyclophosphamide, doxorubicin, vincristine and prednisolone (CHOP regimen).
   c. Testicular teratoma (in an adult): intravenous etoposide, intravenous bleomycin and intravenous cisplatin.
2. a. Why are the doses of anticancer drugs corrected to surface area rather than simply body weight (e.g. mg kg^{-1} body weight)?

Table 52.2 Examples of surface area calculation

Age (years)	Body weight (kg)	Height (cm)	Body surface area (m^2)
0.5	7.4	65.8	0.350
1.0	9.9	74.7	0.434
3	14.5	96.0	0.613
6	21.5	116.8	0.835
Adult			
Male	72.1	175.3	1.874
Female	60.3	167.6	1.681

   b. Does the use of surface area correction result in higher or lower doses for children compared with simple body weight correction (Table 52.2)?

   Surface area can be calculated using a nomogram or by the equation:

$$A = 71.84\, W^{0.425} H^{0.725}$$

   where A is surface area (in cm^2), W is weight (in kg) and H is height (in cm).

ANSWERS

1. The criteria for combination therapy in cancer treatment are:
   - each drug should be active as a single agent (ethics of clinical trials means that new drugs are not usually tested for this criterion in clinical studies)
   - each drug should have a different target within the cell (increases cell kill and decreases drug resistance)
   - each drug should show different unwanted effects (ideally this will give additivity for effect [previous criteria] but not of toxicity, and hence an increase in therapeutic index)

   For each of the three drug regimens, the first criterion can be assumed to be met because all the agents are well-used drugs. Table 52.3 summarises the sites of action and side-effects of the drugs in each regimen. As can be seen, all three use drugs that have different actions, although regimen (c) is targeted only at DNA function. Regimen (b) contains three drugs that have bone marrow toxicity. This will need careful monitoring during therapy.

Table 52.3 Effects of three treatment regimens

	Site of action	Principal toxicity
(a) Acute lymphoblastic leukaemia		
Vincristine	Binds to tubulin/metaphase arrest	BMS + peripheral neuropathy
Crisantaspase	Depletes asparagine in blood	↓ Clotting factors/insulin/albumin
Prednisolone	DNA transcription of cytokines (etc.)	Glucocorticoid actions
(b) Non-Hodgkin's lymphoma (CHOP regimen)		
Cyclophosphamide	Alkylates DNA	BMS + nausea/vomiting
Doxorubicin	Intercalation into DNA + oxygen radicals	BMS + cardiotoxicity
Vincristine	Binds to tubulin/metaphase arrest	BMS + peripheral neuropathy
Prednisolone	DNA transcription of cytokines (etc.)	Glucocorticoid actions
(c) Testicular teratoma		
Etoposide	↑ DNA cleavage by topoisomerase II	BMS, nausea, alopecia
Bleomycin	Oxidative damage to DNA	Pulmonary fibrosis 'allergy'
Cisplatin	Cross-links DNA	Nausea, BMS, nephrotoxicity, ototoxicity

BMS, bone marrow suppression.

2. a. Because many of the drugs used in cancer therapy have a therapeutic index of 1 (i.e. toxic dose is the therapeutic dose), it is important to tailor the dosage to the individual patient. Children have a higher cardiac output and greater hepatic and renal blood flows than adults on a body weight basis. (Such parameters are related to body weight (BWt) to the power 0.65–0.75 [i.e. $BWt^{0.7}$].) Therefore, the clearance of drugs tends to be faster in children than in adults and a proportional higher dose is necessary to give the same blood levels. Surface area also correlates to $BWt^{0.7}$; therefore, it is usual to correct the doses to surface area (calculated by the formula given or by nomogram).

   b. For example, if an adult male (BWt = 72.1 kg) is given 100 mg of a drug, how much would you give a 1-year-old child (BWt = 9.9 kg)? Simple correction for BWt would suggest 13.7 mg (100 ± 9.9/72.1), but correction using $BWt^{0.7}$ gives a calculated dose of $100 \times 9.9^{0.7}/72.1^{0.7} = 100 \times 4.98/19.98 = 24.9$ mg. Interestingly, this goes against what you may have assumed, i.e. that children would be 'more sensitive' and would have to be given lower doses. The main organs of elimination, the liver and kidneys, are essentially mature by about 6–9 months of age.

Drugs used in the treatment of cancer

Drug	Half-life (h) and kinetics	Comments	Unusual or limiting toxicity[a]
Anticancer drugs			
Alkylating agents			
Widely used drugs; act by damaging DNA and thereby interfering with cell division; chlormethine (mustine) was one of the earliest examples and has been replaced by less toxic drugs			
Busulfan	2–3 [M] Metabolism is largely by interaction with thiol groups, such as cysteine, the products of which are further metabolised and eliminated	Mainly used for effects on the bone marrow (e.g. chronic myeloid leukaemia); given orally or by intravenous infusion	Myelosuppression and irreversible bone marrow aplasia; rare pulmonary fibrosis
Carmustine (BCNU)	0.4–0.5 [M] Crosses blood–brain barrier; metabolites eliminated in urine	Used for myeloma, lymphoma and brain tumours; unstable reactive molecule that cross-links DNA and the nitroso function inactivates DNA repair; given intravenously	Renal damage; delayed pulmonary fibrosis
Chlorambucil	1–2 [M] Metabolised at alkylating groups owing to reactivity and in the liver by β-oxidation of the carboxylic acid side-chain	Used mainly in lymphocytic leukaemia, non-Hodgkin's lymphoma and Hodgkin's disease; given orally, usually after fasting	Vomiting
Cyclophosphamide	4–10 [M] Good penetration of blood–brain barrier; metabolic oxidation by CYP2B1 and CYP3A4 leads to bioactivation; wide inter-subject variability	Widely used for leukaemias, lymphomas and solid tumours; given orally or by intravenous injection	Haemorrhagic cystitis (see mesna antidote)
Estramustine	20–24 [M] The phosphate ester, which is given orally, is dephosphorylated to the active drug, which is oxidised in the steroid ring	Used for prostate cancer; (an oestrogen molecule linked to a nitrogen mustard group); acts as an alkylating agent, especially on microtubule proteins, and increases circulating oestrogen levels; given orally	–
Ifosfamide	4–15 [M] Metabolic fate is similar to cyclophosphamide	Uses similar to cyclophosphamide; given by intravenous injection	Cystitis (see mesna antidote)

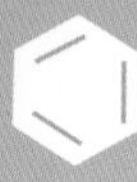

Drugs used in the treatment of cancer

Drug	Half-life (h) and kinetics	Comments	Unusual or limiting toxicity[a]
Lomustine (CCNU)	1–5 (4-OH) [M] Oxidised to 4-hydroxy compound (4-OH) completely in the gut wall and liver during first-pass metabolism	Mainly used for Hodgkin's disease and some solid tumours; bifunctional drug similar to carmustine; given orally	Permanent bone marrow damage
Melphalan	1.5 [M] Oral absorption is incomplete and variable; does not cross blood–brain barrier in useful amounts; pathways of metabolism are not well defined	Used mainly for multiple myeloma, ovarian adenocarcinoma, advanced breast cancer and neuroblastoma; given orally or by intravenous injection	–
Thiotepa	1–3 thiotepa, 10–21 TEPA [M] Extensively absorbed from bladder lumen; bioactivated by CYP2B and CYP2C to TEPA (the active form), in which sulphur is replaced by oxygen	Used for bladder cancer; given by intravesicular injection	–
Treosulfan	1–2 [Non-enzymatic] High oral bioavailability; 'metabolised' by loss of reactive groups through non-enzymatic reactions; leaving groups are eliminated as methylsulphonic acid	Used mainly for ovarian cancer; given orally or by intravenous injection	Allergic alveolitis; pulmonary fibrosis
Cytotoxic antibiotics			
Widely used drugs; many act as radiomimetics and should be avoided if overall treatment includes simultaneous radiotherapy			
Bleomycin	2–4 [M + R] Slow uptake by tissues; hydrolysed by enzyme 'bleomycin hydrolase', which largely inactivates the drug; low levels of the hydrolase correlate with cytotoxicity	Used for testicular cancer, lymphomas and squamous cell carcinoma; given intravenously or intramuscularly	Dermatological effects; progressive pulmonary fibrosis
Dactinomycin (actinomycin D)	36 [R + B] Negligible metabolism; eliminated in urine and bile	Mainly used for paediatric solid tumours; given intravenously	Bone marrow toxicity; gastrointestinal toxicity
Daunorubicin	24–48 [M + B] Undergoes metabolic reduction and redox cycling, giving toxic superoxide radicals and H_2O_2; long half-life owing to slow release from tissues; metabolite retains activity	Used for acute leukaemias and AIDS-related Kaposi's sarcoma (as a liposome preparation which has a half-life of 5 h); given intravenously	Bone marrow toxicity
Doxorubicin	2–10 [M] Reduced in liver to doxorubicinol, which is further metabolised and excreted, largely in the bile; does not cross blood–brain barrier	Widely used for leukaemias, lymphomas and a variety of solid tumours; given intravenously	Myelosuppression; cardiotoxicity
Epirubicin	11–69 [M + R] Reduced to epirubicinol and also conjugated in amino sugar ring; very wide inter-subject variability in kinetics; does not cross blood–brain barrier	Uses are similar to doxorubicin; given intravenously	Myelosuppression; cardiotoxicity (less than with doxorubicin)
Idarubicin	12–35 [M] Oral bioavailability is low and variable (4–50%); metabolised by reduction to idarubicinol (which has a longer half-life of 50–70 h and retains activity) and by hydrolysis of the amino sugar moiety	Used mainly for acute leukaemias and advanced breast cancer (non-responsive to first-line treatments); given orally or intravenously	Myelosuppression

Drugs used in the treatment of cancer

Drug	Half-life (h) and kinetics	Comments	Unusual or limiting toxicity[a]
Mitomycin	0.5–1.5 [M] Reduced to a hydroquinone, which gives rise to a highly unstable alkylating species that cross-links DNA; metabolism gives toxic superoxide and hydroxyl radicals	Mainly used for upper gastrointestinal and breast cancers and by bladder instillation for superficial bladder tumours; given intravenously	Myelosuppression; nephrotoxicity; lung fibrosis
Mitoxantrone	4–220 [R + M] Metabolised in the liver by side-chain oxidation to inactive metabolites; extremely wide inter-individual variability in half-life; long half-life may result from high tissue uptake and affinity	Used to treat metastatic breast cancer and non-Hodgkin's lymphoma and non-lymphocytic leukaemia; given by intravenous infusion	Myelosuppression; cardiotoxicity
Antimetabolites			
Incorporated into nucleic acids or combine irreversibly with cellular enzymes essential for normal cell division			
Capecitabine	0.5–1 [M] Hydrolysed to fluorouracil	Used as monotherapy for metastatic colorectal cancer; a prodrug of fluorouracil; given orally	–
Cladribine	7 [M] Undergoes intracellular phosphorylation to the active triphosphate form	Used for hairy cell leukaemia; chlorine-substituted purine; given by intravenous infusion	Myelosuppression; neurotoxicity
Clofarabine	5 [R] Eliminated unchanged in urine	Used for acute lymphoblastic leukaemia in refractory or relapsed patients aged 1–21 years old; a chlorine- and fluorine-substituted purine analogue; given by intravenous infusion	
Cytarabine (cytosine arabinoside)	1–3 [M] Undergoes intracellular phosphorylation to the active triphosphate form; metabolism to uracil arabinoside gives inactivation	Main use is for induction of remission in acute myeloblastic leukaemia; given intravenously, subcutaneously or intrathecally	Myelosuppression
Fludarabine phosphate	7–20 [R + M] Phosphate is rapidly hydrolysed to give fludarabine, which enters the cell and is phosphorylated to a triphosphate	Used for B-cell chronic lymphocytic leukaemia; fluorine-substituted purine riboside; given orally or by intravenous injection or infusion	Myelosuppression
Fluorouracil	0.25 [M] Converted to fluorouracil monophosphate intracellularly and then to di- and triphosphates; catabolised in the liver by dihydropyrimidine dehydrogenase	Used for cancers of the gastrointestinal tract and malignant and pre-malignant skin lesions; fluorine-substituted uracil; given topically or by intravenous injection or infusion or intra-arterial infusion	Relatively low toxicity (not usually the limiting drug given in a combination)
Gemcitabine	0.2–0.5 [M] Bioactivated by intracellular conversion to the active triphosphate; inactivated by deamination to difluorodeoxyuridine	Used for palliative treatment of non-small-cell lung and pancreatic cancer; deoxycytidine analogue with two fluorine atoms in the deoxyribose moiety; given intravenously	Limited toxicity
Mercaptopurine	1–1.5 [M] Poor oral bioavailability owing to first-pass metabolism (about 20%); bioactivated by intracellular phosphorylation; inactivated by xanthine oxidase (interaction with allopurinol)	Used almost exclusively for maintenance therapy for acute leukaemias (also used in inflammatory bowel disease); sulphur-substituted purine; given orally	Limited toxicity

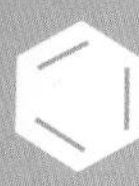

Drugs used in the treatment of cancer

Drug	Half-life (h) and kinetics	Comments	Unusual or limiting toxicity[a]
Methotrexate	8–10 [R + M] Taken up into cells by the reduced folate carrier and undergoes polyglutamate formation (like folate); the polyglutamates are retained for months (the half-life refers to the non-glutamate form); eliminated mainly by the kidneys with some as a hydroxy metabolite; contraindicated in renal impairment	Used for maintenance therapy for childhood acute lymphoblastic leukaemia, choriocarcinoma, non-Hodgkin's lymphoma and some solid tumours (also used for rheumatoid arthritis and psoriasis); folate analogue; given orally, intravenously, intramuscularly or intrathecally	Myelosuppression (folinic acid is an 'antidote'– see below)
Pemetrexed	3.5 [R] Eliminated unchanged by glomerular filtration and tubular secretion; a minor pathway of metabolism is to polyglutamates that retain activity	Used with cisplatin for malignant pleural mesothelioma; inhibits folate-dependent enzymes; substituted purine compound; given by intravenous infusion	
Raltitrexed	10–12 days [R + M] Prolonged retention within cells gives prolonged inhibition of thymidylate synthase and 3-weekly dosage intervals; forms polyglutamates intracellularly	Used for palliation of metastatic colon cancer when fluorouracil cannot be used; chemically related to folic acid; given intravenously	Myelosuppression
Tegafur with uracil	8 [M] A racemate that is metabolised to fluorouracil; the R-isomer is more rapidly metabolised and determines the formation rate-limited half-life of fluorouracil; the half-life of the parent compound is determined by the S-isomer	Used with folinate for management of metastatic colorectal cancer; given orally	–
Tioguanine	3–6 [M + R] Bioavailability is 25–50%; rapidly taken up by cells; converted to corresponding nucleotide intracellularly, which is retained within cells; methylation of the 6-thio group is the major route of metabolism	Used for acute leukaemia and chronic myeloid leukemia; thio-substituted guanine; given orally	Myelosuppression
Vinca alkaloids and etoposide			
Used for a variety of cancers			
Etoposide	4–8 [M] Oral absorption is 25–75%; eliminated in urine and bile mainly as metabolites	Used for small-cell carcinoma of the bronchus, lymphomas and testicular cancer; given orally or by slow intravenous infusion	Myelosuppression; alopecia
Vinblastine	20–80 [M] Metabolised by hepatic CYP3A4, and metabolites are eliminated in bile and urine	Used for acute leukaemias, lymphomas and non-solid tumours (e.g. breast and lung); given by intravenous injection	Myelosuppression
Vincristine	85 [M] Metabolised in liver; metabolites eliminated mainly in the bile	Used for acute leukaemias, lymphomas and non-solid tumours (e.g. breast and lung); given by intravenous injection	Neurotoxicity – peripheral and autonomic neuropathy (recovery is slow but complete)
Vindesine	25 [M + R] Metabolised by CYP3A4, and metabolites are eliminated in bile and urine; up to 10% excreted unchanged in urine	Used for acute leukaemias, lymphomas and non-solid tumours (e.g. breast and lung); given by intravenous injection	Myelosuppression

Drugs used in the treatment of cancer

Drug	Half-life (h) and kinetics	Comments	Unusual or limiting toxicity[a]
Vinorelbine	28–44 [M] Metabolised by CYP3A4, and metabolites are eliminated in bile and urine	Used for advanced breast and non-small-cell lung cancer; semi-synthetic vinca alkaloid made from vinblastine; given intravenously	Myelosuppression
Taxanes			
Docetaxel	11 [M + R] Metabolised by CYP3A4-mediated oxidation; metabolites eliminated in the bile; a small amount (<10%) excreted unchanged in urine	Used for advanced or metastatic anthracycline-resistant breast cancer; given by intravenous infusion	Hypersensitivity reactions; myelosuppression; peripheral neuropathy; fluid retention
Paclitaxel	19 [M] Metabolised by CYP2C8 and CYP3A4 to different metabolites, which are eliminated in bile	Used for advanced ovarian cancer and as secondary treatment for breast and non-small-cell lung cancer; given by intravenous infusion	Hypersensitivity reactions; myelosuppression; peripheral neuropathy
Platinum compounds			
Carboplatin	1.5 [R] Eliminated by glomerular filtration; good correlation between AUC in blood (see Ch. 2), creatinine clearance and myelosuppression; the excretion of total platinum (Pt) (equivalent to 'metabolites') is much slower than that of the parent compound	Used for ovarian cancer and some other solid tumours; active form produced by interaction with water; given by intravenous injection	Myelosuppression (plus some nausea and vomiting – less than with cisplatin)
Cisplatin	24–60 [R] Eliminated by kidney; some sources give the half-life as up to 60 h, and these values relate to total Pt not cisplatin per se	Used for solid tumours such as ovarian cancer and metastatic seminoma and testicular teratoma; active form produced by interaction with water; given by intravenous injection	Nausea and vomiting; nephrotoxicity; myelosuppression; ototoxicity
Oxaliplatin	27 [R] Half-life relates to free Pt because the parent drug undergoes rapid hydration and ligand-exchange reactions	Used for metastatic colorectal cancer; has a 1,2-diamino-cyclohexane ligand (which increases the formation of DNA adducts) and an oxalate ligand on the Pt atom; given intravenously	Neurotoxicity
Topoisomerase I inhibitors			
Topoisomerase I is involved in maintaining the topographic structure of DNA during translation, transcription and mitosis			
Irinotecan	6 [M + R] Metabolised by esterase to a highly active metabolite and by CYP3A4 to largely inactive metabolites; activity resides in parent drug and esterase product; some renal excretion (10–20%)	Used for metastatic colorectal cancer; given by intravenous infusion	Myelosuppression; gastrointestinal effects
Topotecan	2–3 [R + M] Undergoes pH-dependent hydrolysis of the lactone ring, which results in inactivation; enzymatic metabolism is only a minor route of elimination	Used for metastatic ovarian cancer when first-line treatment has failed; given by intravenous infusion	Myelosuppression; gastrointestinal effects

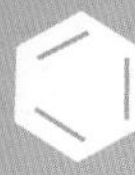

Drugs used in the treatment of cancer

Drug	Half-life (h) and kinetics	Comments	Unusual or limiting toxicity[a]
Porfimer sodium and temoporfin			
Used in photodynamic treatment of various tumours. Drugs accumulate in tumour tissue and are activated by laser light			
Porfimer sodium	40–50 [B] Breakdown products eliminated in bile; the photosensitising product has a very long half-life (250 h)	Used in photodynamic treatment of small-cell lung cancer and for oesophageal cancer; given by intravenous injection	Photosensitivity
Temoporfin	Days? [?] Few data available; animal studies indicate kinetics may be similar to porfimer	Used in photodynamic treatment of advanced refractory head and neck squamous cell carcinoma; given by intravenous injection	Photosensitivity
Tyrosine kinase receptor inhibitors			
Bevacizumab	≈20 days [M] Peptide drug, the clearance of which is higher in men than in women and is proportional to the tumour burden of the individual	Used as part of first-line treatment of metastatic colorectal cancer; inhibitor of vascular endothelial growth factor; given by intravenous infusion	Mucocutaneous bleeding and arterial thromboembolism
Cetuximab	≈100 [M] Peptide drug that is largely restricted to the vascular space	Used for metastatic colorectal cancer where tumour expresses epidermal growth factor receptor; monoclonal antibody that binds to and blocks epidermal growth factor receptors on the surface of normal and tumour cells; given by intravenous infusion	Hypersensitivity reactions such as rash and airways obstruction; skin reactions
Trastuzumab	25 days [M?] Few details available but probably cleared by the reticuloendothelial system	Used for metastatic breast cancer; recombinant DNA-derived humanised monoclonal antibody against the HER2 protein that acts on tumor cells that overexpress HER2; binds to the HER2 receptor on the surface of tumour cells, which causes accumulation of the cyclin-dependent kinase inhibitor p27 and cell cycle arrest; given by intravenous infusion	Cardiotoxicity, especially if used with anthracyclines (cytotoxic antibiotics – see above)
Tyrosine kinase enzyme inhibitors			
Inhibit tyrosine kinases (except sorafenib, which inhibits multiple kinases)			
Dasatinib	3–5 [M] Rapidly absorbed; metabolised by hepatic CYP3A4 to various metabolites that are eliminated in faeces	Used for chronic myeloid leukaemia in those resistant to or intolerant of imatinib; given orally	Numerous, including gastrointestinal effects
Erlotinib	36 [M] Slowly absorbed with a bioavailability of 60%, which increases to almost 100% if given with food; metabolised by hepatic CYP3A4 to various metabolites that are eliminated in faeces	Used for advanced or malignant small-cell lung cancer after failure of previous therapy; selective inhibitor of epidermal growth factor receptor-tyrosine kinase; given orally	Numerous, including gastrointestinal effects
Imatinib	18 [M] Rapidly and completely absorbed; metabolised by CYP3A4 to an active metabolite which has a longer half-life (40 h) and contributes to in vivo activity	Used for newly diagnosed chronic myeloid leukaemia (under special circumstances); a protein-tyrosine kinase inhibitor; given orally	Numerous, including gastrointestinal effects

Drugs used in the treatment of cancer

Drug	Half-life (h) and kinetics	Comments	Unusual or limiting toxicity[a]
Sorafenib	25–48 [M] Slowly absorbed with a bioavailability of 40%; metabolised by hepatic CYP3A4 to numerous metabolites that are eliminated in urine and faeces	Used for advanced renal cell carcinoma; given orally	Numerous, including gastrointestinal effects
Sunitinib	40–60 [M] Slowly absorbed; metabolised by hepatic CYP3A4 to an active metabolite that has a half-life of 80–110 h and accounts for about 30% of the plasma AUC; the metabolites are eliminated in faeces	Used for malignant gastrointestinal stromal tumours; given orally	Numerous, including gastrointestinal effects
Proteasome inhibitors			
Bortezomib	9–15 [M] Undergoes removal of boron and subsequent hydroxylation by hepatic CYP3A4, CYP2C19 and CYP1A2	Used for progressive multiple myeloma; a boron-containing proteasome inhibitor (a proteasome is a large multiprotein particle present in the cytosol and cell nucleus which is critical for activation or suppression of cellular functions); given by intravenous injection	Nausea, vomiting and diarrhoea
Drugs for breast cancer			
See also 'Miscellaneous anticancer drugs' listed below			
Anastrozole	40–50 [M + R] Metabolised by oxidation and formation of an N-glucuronide (rare reaction); a small amount is excreted unchanged	Used as adjunct for oestrogen receptor-positive early breast cancer, and for advanced metastatic breast cancer in postmenopausal women; selective aromatase inhibitor; given orally	Hot flushes; vaginal dryness and bleeding; gastrointestinal effects
Exemestane	24 [M] Bioavailability is about 40% and increased markedly by a fatty meal; metabolised by CYP3A4-mediated oxidation and by reduction to essentially inactive metabolites	Used for advanced breast cancer in postmenopausal women in whom anti-oestrogen therapy has failed; irreversible aromatase inhibitor; given orally	Nausea and gastrointestinal effects; hot flushes
Fulvestrant	40 days [M] Eliminated by oxidation and conjugation with glucuronic acid or phosphate on the steroid nucleus, and by oxidation of the sulphoxide side-chain; half-life is probably dependent on the rate of uptake from injection site	Used for receptor-positive breast tumours; oestrogen receptor antagonist that causes receptor downregulation; given by deep intramuscular depot injection	Hot flushes; nausea; gastrointestinal effects
Letrozole	2 days [M] High oral bioavailability; oxidised in the liver by CYP3A4 to an inactive metabolite	Used for advanced metastatic breast cancer in postmenopausal women that is not responsive to other anti-oestrogens; selective non-steroidal aromatase inhibitor; given orally	Hot flushes; nausea; gastrointestinal effects

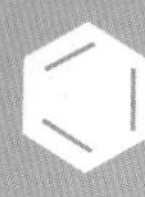

Drugs used in the treatment of cancer

Drug	Half-life (h) and kinetics	Comments	Unusual or limiting toxicity[a]
Tamoxifen	7 days [M] High bioavailability; oxidised by hepatic CYP3A and CYP2C9 isoenzymes; the N-desmethyl metabolite (which has similar activity to the parent compound) has a half-life of 14 days; metabolites are excreted in faeces	Used for oestrogen receptor-positive breast cancer; non-steroidal anti-oestrogen; given orally	Exacerbation of pain from bone metastases
Toremifene	5 days [M] Well absorbed; metabolised by CYP3A4-mediated demethylation; metabolite retains weak activity; undergoes enterohepatic circulation	Used for hormone-dependent metastatic breast cancer in postmenopausal women; non-steroidal oestrogen receptor antagonist; given orally	Hot flushes; vaginal bleeding and discharge plus numerous other effects
Trastuzumab	25 days [M?] See above	Used for metastatic breast cancer; see above	See above
Drugs for prostate cancer			
See also 'Miscellaneous anticancer drugs' listed below			
Bicalutamide	7–10 days [M] Well absorbed; the active R-isomer undergoes oxidation and conjugation; the inactive S-isomer is cleared more rapidly so that steady-state blood levels reflect the active form; metabolites are excreted in urine and bile	Used for advanced prostate cancer to cover the 'flare' associated with administration of gonadorelin analogues; anti-androgen; given orally	Hot flushes; pruritus; gynaecomastia plus rare serious hepatic and cardiovascular effects
Buserelin	1–1.5 [M + R] Metabolism plus some excreted in urine	Used for advanced prostate cancer; peptide hormone; gonadorelin analogue; given by subcutaneous injection for 7 days and then nasally	May cause tumour 'flare' leading to spinal cord compression; ureteric obstruction and bone pain
Cyproterone acetate	2 days [M] Hydrolysed and conjugated with glucuronic acid and sulphate; metabolites eliminated in urine and bile	Used for prostate cancer and to cover 'flare' of gonadorelin analogues; anti-androgen; given orally	See bicalutamide
Degarelix	23–61 days [M] Peptide hydrolysis	A gonadotrophin-releasing hormone inhibitor used to treat advanced hormone dependent prostate cancer. Given by subcutaneous injection	Unlike gonaderelin analogues (see Ch. 43), does not induce a testosterone surge or tumour flare. Susceptibility to QT-interval prolongation
Flutamide	8 [M] Complete bioavailability; rapid oxidation in the liver to an active hydroxy metabolite	Used for advanced prostate cancer and to cover the 'flare' of gonadorelin analogues; anti-androgen; given orally	See bicalutamide
Goserelin	4 [M + R] Metabolised by hepatic hydrolysis; about 20% excreted unchanged in urine	Used for prostate cancer and advanced breast cancer; gonadorelin analogue; potent LHRH agonist; given by subcutaneous implant into the anterior abdominal wall	See buserelin
Leuprorelin acetate (leuprolide)	3–4 [M] Metabolised by proteases	Used for advanced prostate cancer; gonadorelin analogue; given by subcutaneous or intramuscular injection	See buserelin; plus muscle weakness, hypertension, palpitations

Drugs used in the treatment of cancer

Drug	Half-life (h) and kinetics	Comments	Unusual or limiting toxicity[a]
Triptorelin	3 [M] Metabolised but routes have not been defined	Used for advanced prostate cancer (and endometriosis); gonadorelin analogue; given by intramuscular injection	See buserelin
Miscellaneous anticancer drugs			
The drugs given below are those that affect the cancer per se; other drugs used in the management of people with cancer (e.g. antiemetics) are described in the appropriate chapters			
Aldesleukin (interleukin-2)	0.5–6 [M] Taken up and degraded by the kidneys; the half-life is that seen after intravenous dosage; subcutaneous dosage gives prolonged low plasma levels with a half-life of 3–12 h	Use is restricted to metastatic renal cell carcinoma; recombinant interleukin-2; given by subcutaneous injection	Severe toxicity; pulmonary oedema; hypotension; bone marrow, hepatic, renal, thyroid and CNS toxicity
Alemtuzumab	12 days [?] Few data available; probably eliminated by metabolism, possibly by the reticuloendothelial system	Unconjugated, humanised monoclonal antibody against antigen CD52; causes lysis of B-lymphocytes; used for chronic lymphocytic leukaemia unresponsive to an alkylating agent; given by intravenous infusion	Cytokine release syndrome (characterised by severe dyspnoea)
Amsacrine	4–7 [M] Metabolites formed in the liver and eliminated in bile	Used for acute myeloid leukaemia; action and toxicity similar to doxorubicin; planar fused ring system that intercalates into DNA; given as intravenous infusion	Myelosuppression (fatal arrhythmias when there is hypokalaemia)
Arsenic trioxide	? [M] Kinetics have not been defined; metabolised by reduction and methylation	Used for acute promyelocytic leukaemia in patients who have relapsed or failed with other treatment; mechanism of action is not defined; given by intravenous infusion	Leucocyte activation syndrome (requires immediate treatment)
Bacillus Calmette-Guérin (BCG)	? [?] No kinetic data available	Used for primary or recurrent bladder carcinoma; immunostimulant that produces a non-specific, localised immune reaction with histocyte and leucocyte infiltration; given by bladder instillation	
Bexarotene	7 [M] Oxidised in the liver by CYP3A4, and products conjugated and excreted	Used for skin manifestations of cutaneous T-cell lymphoma; an agonist at retinoid X receptors; given orally	Leucopenia
Crisantaspase (asparaginase)	7–13 [M] Taken up by reticuloendothelial system and degraded	Used for acute lymphoblastic leukaemia; enzyme isolated from *Erwinia chrysanthemi* that hydrolyses circulating L-asparagine to aspartic acid and ammonia, causing depletion of L-asparagine; given by intramuscular or subcutaneous injection	Anaphylaxis; CNS depression; nausea; hyperglycaemia
Dacarbazine	5 [R + M] Activated by P450-mediated metabolism to a cytotoxic and alkylating metabolite; about 50% is excreted in the urine unchanged	Used for metastatic melanoma and soft tissue sarcomas; alkylating agent that interacts primarily with -SH groups and inhibits cellular functions; given intravenously	Myelosuppression; intense nausea and vomiting

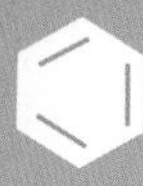

Drugs used in the treatment of cancer

Drug	Half-life (h) and kinetics	Comments	Unusual or limiting toxicity[a]
Diethylstilbestrol	2–3 days [M] Eliminated by conjugation with glucuronic acid; undergoes enterohepatic cycling	Used (but very rarely) for prostate cancer, and occasionally for breast cancer; oestrogen that acts by inhibition of the hypothalamic–pituitary axis through negative feedback; given orally	Nausea; fluid retention; thrombosis; impotence and gynaecomastia in men; hypercalcaemia and bone pain in women
Ethinylestradiol	8–24 [M] See contraceptive hormones (Ch. 45)	May be used for breast cancer (unlicensed indication in the UK); given orally	See contraceptive hormones (Ch. 45)
Hydroxycarbamide (hydroxyurea)	2–6 [R] Eliminated unchanged by glomerular filtration	Used for chronic myeloid leukaemia; blocks ribonucleotide reductase (the rate-limiting enzyme of DNA synthesis); given orally	Myelosuppression
Interferon alfa	3–4 [M] Catabolised by kidney; slow absorption from subcutaneous dosage with peak concentrations at 4–8 h	Used for certain lymphomas and solid tumours; given by subcutaneous or intravenous injection	Nausea; lethargy; ocular effects; depression; myelosuppression; cerebrovascular, liver and kidney problems
Medroxyprogesterone acetate	30 days [M] Complete oral bioavailability; eliminated as conjugated metabolites; half-life is longer after intramuscular injection (50 days)	Used for endometrial and breast cancer, and rarely for prostate and renal cancer; progestogen; given orally or by deep intramuscular injection	Glucocorticoid effects at high doses
Megestrol acetate	15–20 [M] Complete oral bioavailability; metabolised largely by oxidation followed by conjugation	Used for endometrial and breast cancer; progestogen; given orally	
Mitotane	0.5–6 months [B + M] 30–40% is absorbed; highly lipid-soluble compound that is related chemically to DDT; most is eliminated unchanged in bile	Used for advanced or inoperable adrenocortical carcinoma; selectively toxic to the adrenal cortex (mechanism is unknown); given orally	Gastrointestinal effects; CNS disturbances
Norethisterone (norethindrone)	5–12 [M] Complete oral bioavailability; metabolised by reduction of the ketone group to an alcohol, which is conjugated	Used for endometrial cancer and to a limited extent for renal and breast cancer; progestogen; given orally	–
Pentostatin	3–15 [R] Eliminated by kidneys with negligible metabolism; clearance correlates with creatinine clearance	Used for hairy cell leukaemia; inhibitor of adenosine deaminase which regulates intracellular adenosine levels; given intravenously	Myelosuppression; immunosuppression
Prednisolone	2–4 [M] High oral bioavailability (70–80%); extensively metabolised but all pathways have not been defined	Used for its marked antitumour effect in acute lymphoblastic leukaemia, Hodgkin's disease and non-Hodgkin's lymphoma (also used in palliative care); given orally, topically and by intramuscular injection; injectable form is the acetate ester as an aqueous suspension	See corticosteroids (Ch. 44)
Procarbazine	0.1 [M + R] Very rapidly eliminated by hepatic metabolism via CYP1A2, which gives rise to reactive methyl radicals; limited renal excretion (5% of dose); crosses blood–brain barrier	Used in Hodgkin's disease; exact mechanism is unclear, but probably related to the cytotoxicity of its metabolites and chemical decomposition products; given orally	Nausea; myelosuppression; rash; ingestion with alcohol may give a disulfiram-like effect

Drugs used in the treatment of cancer

Drug	Half-life (h) and kinetics	Comments	Unusual or limiting toxicity[a]
Rituximab	60 [M] The elimination of the peptide has a shorter half-life for the first infusion compared with subsequent dosage	Used for chemotherapy-resistant advanced follicular lymphoma; monoclonal chimeric mouse/ human antibody that causes lysis of B-lymphocytes; given by intravenous infusion	Fever; chills; nausea; allergic reactions; cytokine release syndrome (characterised by severe dyspnoea)
Temozolomide	2 [M] Converted to the same active compound as dacarbazine but non-enzymatically; eliminated as metabolites	Used as a second-line treatment for malignant glioma; structural analogue of dacarbazine (see above); given orally	Myelosuppression
Tretinoin (all-*trans*-retinoic acid)	1–2 [M] Eliminated by oxidation, conjugation with glucuronic acid, and isomerisation to the less active *cis*-isomer	Used for remission of acute promyelocytic leukaemia; agonist at both RAR and RXR receptors; given orally	Numerous symptoms (highly teratogenic)
Antidotes			
Chemoprotectants – each agent is used reduce the toxicity of a specific anticancer drug or of a group of related anticancer drugs			
Amifostine	<0.2 [M] Rapid uptake by normal tissues, where it is dephosphorylated to the active thiol form	Used prior to cytotoxic treatment to reduce the risk of neutropenia-related infection in people treated with cisplatin or cyclophosphamide, and to reduce cisplatin nephrotoxicity; given by intravenous infusion	Hypotension
Dexrazoxane	2–4 [M] Metabolised in the liver by hydrolysis to EDTA-like compounds	Used for anthracycline-induced extravasation; acts as a chelating agent that protects against anthracycline-induced free radical damage; given by intravenous infusion	–
Folinate (leucovorin) and levofolinate	0.75 [M] Formyl group is used for thymidate synthesis and folate enters body pool	Given 24 h after methotrexate to speed recovery from myelosuppression; given orally or by intramuscular or intravenous injection	–
Mesna (mercaptoethane sulphonic acid)	1 [R + M] Eliminated in the urine; some dimerisation of SH group to a disulphide, which is eliminated in the urine and reduced back to mesna	Given either before (oral) or with (intravenous) cyclophosphamide or ifosfamide treatment, to prevent urothelial toxicity; highly polar molecule that contains a sulfhydryl (SH) group; given orally or by intravenous injection	–
Palifermin	3–5 [?] Peptide, therefore probably eliminated by peptidase activity or reticuloendothelial system	Used for oral mucositis in treated patients with haematological malignancies; human keratinocyte growth factor; acts on epithelial cells to aid cellular defences; given by intravenous injection	–

[a]The toxicity that is typical for a class of drug is described in the general text for the class; toxicity given in this table represents 'non-class' effects and/ or severe dose-limiting toxicity.

[M], metabolism; [R], renal excretion; AUC, area under the curve for plasma concentration versus time; CNS, central nervous system; LHRH, luteinising hormone releasing hormone.

12

General features: toxicity and prescribing

53 Drug toxicity and overdose

Most therapeutic drugs alter human homeostatic mechanisms in order to produce a beneficial response; only antimicrobial agents and parasiticides have the theoretical possibility of a therapeutic response without some direct action on human metabolic or physiological processes. Several therapeutic agents, for example atropine (belladonna), tubocurarine (curare), ergot alkaloids (causing St. Anthony's fire), digoxin (digitalis) and dicoumarol (causing haemorrhagic disease in cattle), have pharmacological properties that were first recognised as a result of either accidental or intentional poisonings. It is hardly surprising that all drugs are capable of producing adverse effects if the dosage is high enough. The relationship between a potentially beneficial drug and a poison was recognised five centuries ago when Paracelsus stated: '*All things are toxic and it is only the dose which makes something a poison.*'

Many of the medicines prescribed today were first used as relatively crude plant extracts, for example digitalis glycosides and opium extracts. It was the identification and isolation of the active chemical entities in plant extracts that allowed the dose and purity of the active ingredient to be controlled sufficiently to optimise the ratio between benefit and risk. In this respect, the current vogue for 'natural, herbal remedies' should be considered to represent a backward step in relation to controlling the safety and efficacy of drugs.

Drug toxicity can develop at normal therapeutic doses of a drug or as a result of an acute overdose. In some cases, toxicity occurs in the majority of treated individuals because of the nature of the drug, for example cytotoxic agents used for cancer chemotherapy, but significant toxicity is rare with the majority of commonly prescribed drugs when used at recommended dosages. There is considerable inter-individual variability in the development of adverse reactions, and toxicity may be reduced by taking into account factors that are known to increase susceptibility, such as age, concurrent disease or body weight, when selecting both the drug and the dosage. Usually, a reduction in dosage or a change of drug during chronic treatment will reduce the severity of adverse effects (but see immunological mechanisms discussed below).

Toxicity following an acute overdose usually produces predictable adverse reactions, which may be life-threatening and/or prejudice long-term health. Rapid treatment is then required and this may be aimed at preventing further drug absorption, increasing drug elimination/inactivation and managing the adverse effects produced.

This chapter is, therefore, divided into two main sections:

- *drug toxicity*, which discusses mechanisms for adverse effects produced both during normal drug therapy and after an overdose
- *self-poisoning and drug overdose*, which is concerned with the management of drug overdose.

DRUG TOXICITY

This section provides a framework for classifying adverse effects, rather than an exhaustive catalogue of drugs and their toxicities. The adverse effects caused by different drugs are listed in the *British National Formulary* (BNF), and it is apparent that for most drugs, potential toxic effects are more numerous than beneficial properties. Prescribers should be alert to both predicted and unexpected reactions to medicines, and should consider the risk–benefit ratio for each individual and the suitability of alternative drugs and/or treatments. People who are prescribed drugs should also be informed of the risk–benefit balance inherent in their treatment. The patient information leaflet (PIL) included with the dispensed medicine represents a useful way of providing such advice.

It should be appreciated that all drugs are associated with some risk of toxicity, although both the severity and incidence differ widely between drugs. In general, the acceptability of a risk of toxicity is inversely related to the severity of the disease being treated; for example, serious idiosyncratic reactions with incidences of 1 in 10 000 have led to the withdrawal of some non-steroidal anti-inflammatory drugs (NSAIDs), whereas some cancer chemotherapeutic agents can cause significant toxicity in nearly all individuals. In addition, '*one man's cure is another man's poison*', because the beneficial effects of a drug in one situation (e.g. the antidiarrhoeal effect of opioids) may be an adverse effect in other circumstances (e.g. constipation, when an opioid is used for pain relief). Therefore, even classification of the nature of effect into beneficial or adverse may depend on the condition being treated.

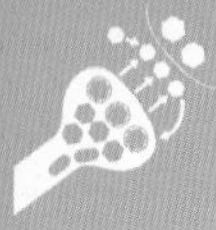

A useful indication of the safety margin available for a drug is given by the therapeutic index (TI):

$$\text{Therapeutic index} = \frac{\text{Dose resulting in toxicity}}{\text{Dose giving therapeutic response}}$$

Drugs such as diazepam have a TI of about 50 and it is difficult for even the most inept doctor to cause serious adverse effects with diazepam. In contrast, digoxin has a TI of only about 2, and for such drugs, toxicity may be precipitated by relatively small changes in dosage regimen, the bioavailability of the formulation (a problem in the past that led to the introduction of bioavailability testing requirements) or the clearance of the drug from the body. The TI relates to serious adverse effects and does not indicate the potential for minor unwanted effects, which may inconvenience the person enough for him or her to stop treatment but are not considered to represent drug toxicity.

For many effects, the response increases with increase in dose, with low sub-therapeutic doses giving an inadequate response, therapeutic doses giving the desired response, but very high doses giving an excessive response that can be regarded as a form of toxicity (response 1 in Fig. 53.1). A good example is warfarin (Ch. 11), where inadequate doses are associated with a lack of effect and a risk of thrombosis remains, whereas at excessive doses there is a risk of haemorrhage. The increase in response with increase in dose has given rise to the concept of a 'therapeutic window', which is a range of doses or blood/plasma concentrations within which most individuals should show a beneficial response with minimal risk of adverse effects (response 1 in Fig. 53.1). This concept is particularly valuable in the interpretation of measurements of drug

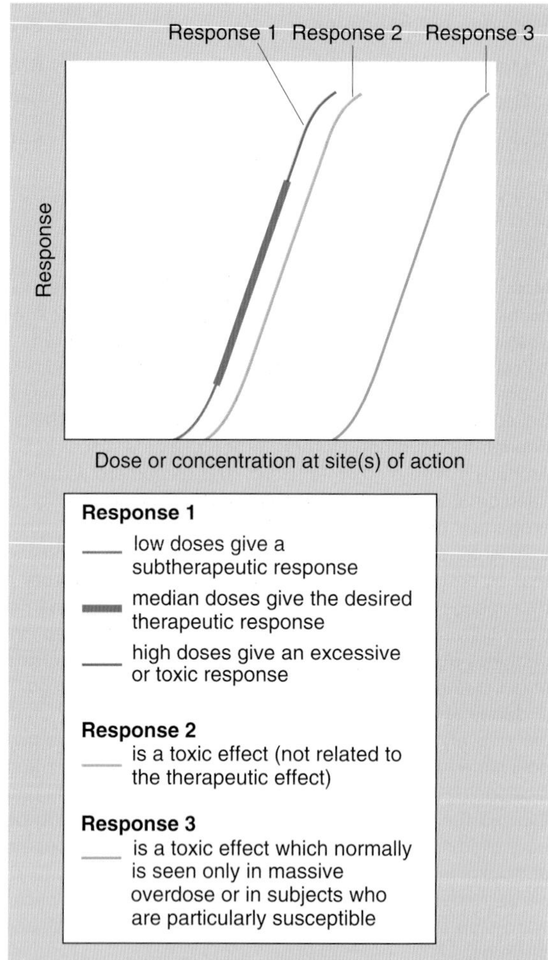

Fig. 53.1 **Dose–response relationships in relation to toxicity.** Response 1 is the primary therapeutic effect, which shows an increase in the magnitude of response with increase in dose from sub-therapeutic, through therapeutic, to potentially toxic. Response 2 is an undesired effect seen at a dose only slightly greater than those producing the therapeutic effect. Response 3 is an adverse effect normally seen only in overdose.

TYPES OF DRUG TOXICITY

Toxicity is usually divided into two main types:

Type A: these effects are dose-related and largely predictable.

Type B: these effects are not dose-related and are idiosyncratic and unpredictable.

Our understanding of the mechanisms involved in drug toxicity has increased greatly in recent years, and this provides a useful framework for students to integrate future knowledge:

- pharmacological: type A
- biochemical: type A and some type B
- immunological: type B
- unknown: mostly type B?

PHARMACOLOGICAL TOXICITY

In 'pharmacological toxicity', the toxic reaction is a predictable extension of the known pharmacology of the drug at its site(s) of action (Table 53.1), and should be recognised readily when monitoring the individual's response to treatment. There are numerous examples in this book where the adverse effect is really an excessive therapeutic action.

Table 53.1 Drugs with adverse effects that are related to their primary therapeutic properties

Drug	Adverse effect
Warfarin	Haemorrhage
Insulin	Hypoglycaemia
β-Adrenoceptor antagonists	Heart block when used as an antiarrhythmic
Loop diuretics	Hypokalaemia
General anaesthetics	Medullary depression
Acetylcholinesterase inhibitors	Muscle weakness

Table 53.2 Therapeutic windows based on plasma concentrations

Drug	Therapeutic concentration range[a]		Toxic response
	Minimum	*Maximum*[b]	
Aspirin (analgesia) (μg mL^{-1})	20	300	Tinnitus, metabolic acidosis
Carbamazepine (μg mL^{-1})	4	10	Drowsiness, visual disturbances
Digitoxin (ng mL^{-1})	15	30	Bradycardia, nausea
Digoxin (ng mL^{-1})	0.8	3	Bradycardia, nausea
Gentamicin (μg mL^{-1})	2	12	Ototoxicity, renal toxicity
Kanamycin (μg mL^{-1})	10	40	Ototoxicity, renal toxicity
Phenytoin (μg mL^{-1})	10	20	Nystagmus, lethargy
Theophylline (μg mL^{-1})	10	20	Tremor, nervousness

[a]The values given represent average values only; individuals will vary in their inherent sensitivity and response to particular concentrations. The concept of a therapeutic window also applies to situations where the response can be measured directly (e.g. blood clotting control with warfarin and hypoglycaemia with oral hypoglycaemics).
[b]The maximum concentration may be based on toxicity related to the primary therapeutic response (e.g. carbamazepine) or an unrelated effect (e.g. gentamicin).

Table 53.3 Examples of drugs with adverse effects unrelated to their primary therapeutic use

Drug	Adverse effects
β-Adrenoceptor agonists	Increase in heart rate when used in asthma
β-Adrenoceptor antagonists	Reduction in heart rate when used for hypertension
Anticancer drugs	Myelosuppression
Anticonvulsants	Sedation when used for epilepsy
Antipsychotics	Dystonias or parkinsonism
Drugs for Parkinson's disease	Hallucinations and confusion
Opioid analgesics	Respiratory depression when used for analgesia
Thiazides	Glucose intolerance

concentrations in plasma, which can be used to monitor compliance and to assess likely response (Table 53.2).

In many other cases, the toxic reaction may be unrelated to the primary therapeutic effect (examples are given in Table 53.3), and may be caused by a secondary effect that is not the primary aim of the treatment given (response 2 in Fig. 53.1). This toxicity will often be present to a limited extent at appropriate therapeutic doses.

The separation of therapeutic and toxic dose–response curves is a measure of the TI. If these are very close (e.g. response 2 in Fig. 53.1), then there is a low safety margin and most individuals will exhibit some degree of toxicity, for example myelosuppression with cytotoxic anticancer drugs.

For drugs with widely separated dose–response curves for the therapeutic benefit (response 1 in Fig. 53.1) and for toxicity (response 3 in Fig. 53.1), i.e. those with high TIs, toxicity would not be seen at normal therapeutic doses, for example heart failure caused by myocardial depression in those with normal left ventricular function taking β-adrenoceptor antagonists. However, the toxic effect may occur in individuals who are uniquely sensitive because of their genetics or their physical condition, for example β-adrenoceptor antagonists may precipitate heart failure in people with pre-existing impaired left ventricular function.

Pharmacological toxicity is the most common cause of adverse effects. Such toxicity can be minimised by an assessment of the risk–benefit balance for the individual to be treated. This should take into account factors that may influence both pharmacokinetics and target-organ sensitivity, including age, physiological status (e.g. renal function), concurrent medication, disease processes, environmental aspects (e.g. smoking), etc.

Because of the predictable nature of pharmacological toxicity, for some treatments it is usual to co-prescribe drugs that will reduce the possibility of toxic effects; examples include antiemetics given with cancer chemotherapy, vitamin B_6 given with isoniazid, and leucovorin (folinic acid) given after methotrexate.

BIOCHEMICAL TOXICITY

In 'biochemical toxicity', the toxicity or tissue damage is caused by an interaction of the drug, or an active metabolite, with cell components, especially macromolecules such as structural proteins and enzymes. A generalised scheme is given in Figure 53.2. For most approved drugs, this form of toxicity is identified and characterised during preclinical studies in animals and monitored in clinical trials (Ch. 3), for example by measuring changes in serum enzyme levels.

In some situations, an understanding of the mechanism of toxicity has allowed the development of appropriate treatments or antidotes. An example is the key observation that the thiol (-SH) group of the tripeptide glutathione provides a cytoprotective mechanism for preventing cell

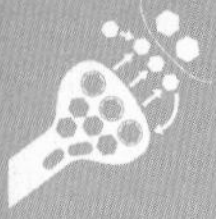

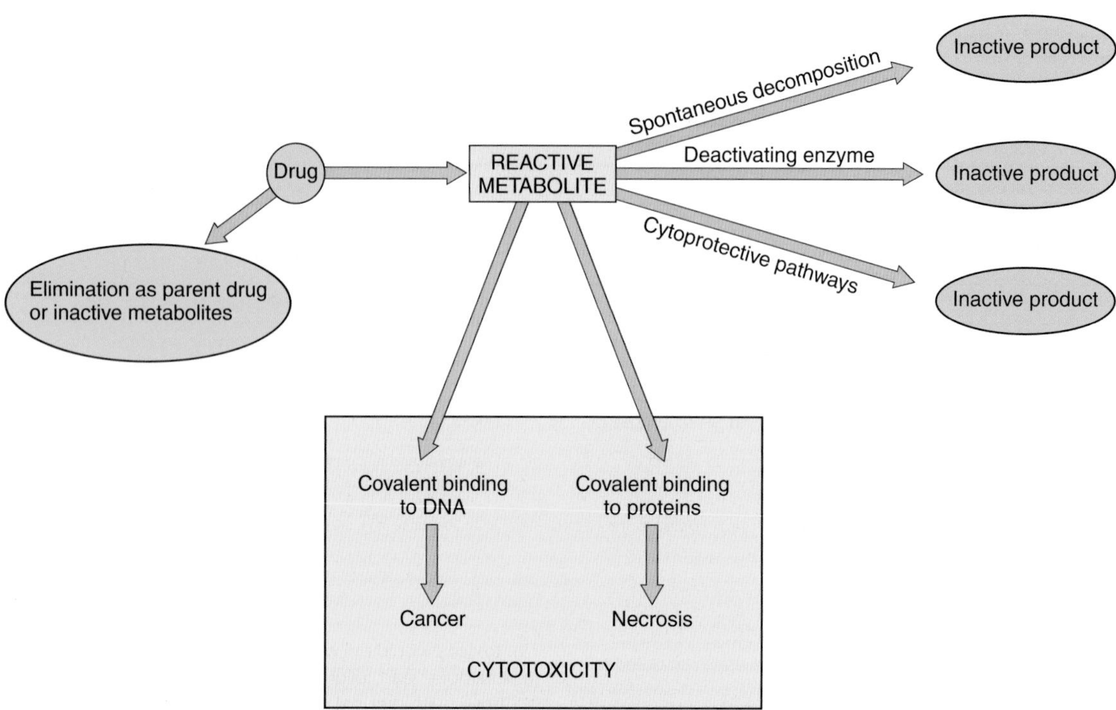

Fig. 53.2 **Metabolism and cytotoxicity.** The extent of cytotoxicity depends on (i) the balance between the activation process and alternative pathways of elimination of the parent drug to produce an inactive product, and (ii) the balance between inactivation of the reactive metabolite and the production of biochemically adverse effects. Therapeutic interventions are aimed at either increasing elimination of the parent drug or enhancing cytoprotective pathways to protect against the effects of cytotoxic products.

damage caused by highly reactive chemical species, such as the toxic metabolite of paracetamol (see below and Fig. 53.3). The nature of the cell damage is related to the stability of the toxic reactive chemical (metabolite); extremely unstable metabolites may bind covalently to and inactivate the enzyme that forms them, whereas more stable species may be able to diffuse to a distant site, for example DNA, and initiate changes, such as cancer. Examples of biochemical toxicity are given below.

Paracetamol

Paracetamol-induced hepatotoxicity represents the results of an imbalance between metabolic detoxication of paracetamol, via conjugation with glucuronic acid and sulphate, and metabolic activation to an unstable toxic metabolite, via oxidation by cytochrome P450. This metabolite binds covalently to proteins and causes cell necrosis. Low doses of paracetamol are safe because they are eliminated by conjugation with little oxidation; however, in overdose, the sulphate conjugation reaction is saturated and there is increased cytochrome P450-mediated oxidation to the toxic unstable quinone-imine metabolite (Fig. 53.3). Early after an overdose, much of the toxic metabolite is inactivated by a cytoprotective pathway involving glutathione, but there is increased covalent binding, oxidative stress and cell death once the available intracellular glutathione has been depleted. This biochemical mechanism explains:

- the site of toxicity (centrilobular necrosis in the liver because of the large amounts of cytochrome P450 present)
- the increased toxicity seen in individuals treated with inducers of cytochrome P450 (especially alcohol-related induction of CYP2E1)
- the increased toxicity seen in individuals with low hepatic stores of glutathione due to poor nutrition
- the development of treatment of paracetamol overdose with acetylcysteine, which enhances cytoprotective processes by providing an additional source of thiol groups for conjugation of the active metabolite and for the protection of thiol groups in proteins (see treatment of drug overdose, below).

The sulphur-containing amino acid methionine can also prevent paracetamol-induced hepatotoxicity, and a combination of paracetamol plus methionine (co-methiamol) is available. Such a formulation may prove to be of particular value to high-risk groups such as children (because of the greater risk of accidental overdose) and alcoholics (because of their induced levels of CYP2E1 and depressed hepatic glutathione stores).

Cyclophosphamide

Cyclophosphamide is an oxazaphosphorine anticancer drug that is converted to highly toxic metabolites which

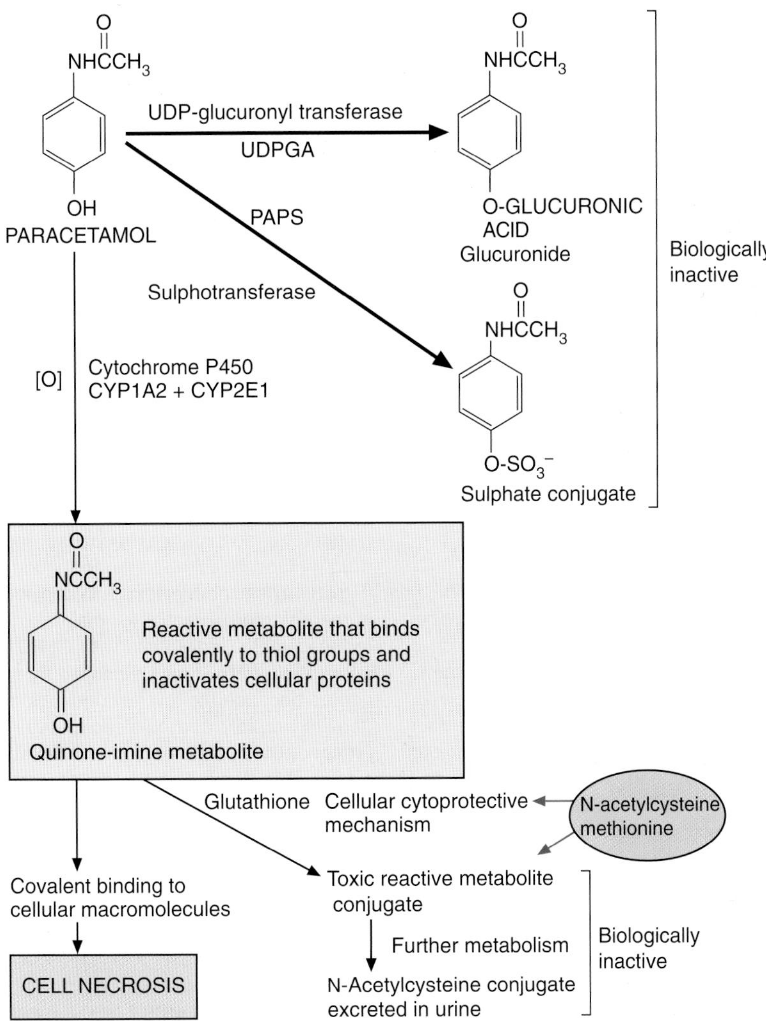

Fig. 53.3 **Pathways of paracetamol metabolism.** In overdose, the concentrations of 3′-phosphoadenosine 5′-phosphosulphate (PAPS) (for sulphation) and glutathione (for cytoprotection) are depleted, and extensive macromolecular binding leads to hepatocellular necrosis. UDPGA, uridine diphosphate glucuronic acid. N-acetylcysteine and methionine replenish glutathione in order to conjugate the toxic metabolite.

bind to DNA as part of their mechanism of action and which are also eliminated in the urine and cause haemorrhagic cystitis (Ch. 52). This adverse effect can be prevented by prior treatment with mesna (mercaptoethane sulphonic acid), which possesses both a thiol group for cytoprotection and a highly polar sulphonic acid group. This combination of functional groups results in high renal excretion and delivery of this cytoprotective molecule to the bladder epithelium. Because of its polarity, mesna is absorbed only slowly and incompletely from the gut, but is eliminated rapidly; therefore it is usually given either orally 2 h before the oxazaphosphorine anticancer drug or intravenously at the same time in order to cover the period of maximum urinary excretion of toxic metabolites. It is not yet known if mesna will also protect against bladder cancer, which can arise about 10–20 years after initial treatment with cyclophosphamide.

Isoniazid

Isoniazid, which is used for the treatment of tuberculosis (Ch. 51), causes hepatitis in about 0.5% of treated individuals. This is believed to result from the formation of a reactive metabolite, N-acetylhydrazine, which is produced by acetylation followed by oxidative metabolism. The biochemical basis for the susceptibility of some individuals to the hepatotoxic metabolite is not known. Fast acetylators (see Ch. 2) form more N-acetylhydrazine than do slow acetylators, but, unexpectedly, they are not more sensitive to isoniazid toxicity. Susceptibility may be related to the balance between further activation of N-acetylhydrazine (by cytochrome P450-mediated oxidation) and detoxification of N-acetylhydrazine (by further acetylation); if this is so, then fast acetylators may produce more active metabolite and also inactivate it more rapidly.

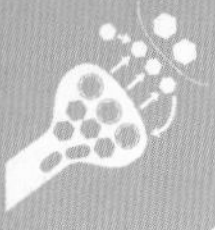

Spironolactone

Spironolactone (Ch. 14) is oxidised by cytochrome P450. The metabolite formed in the testes binds to and destroys testicular cytochrome P450 and this causes a decrease in the metabolism of progesterone to testosterone (which is also catalysed by a cytochrome P450). This effect, combined with an anti-androgenic action at receptor sites (pharmacological toxicity), results in gynaecomastia and decreased libido.

Aromatic amines and nitrites

Aromatic amines, such as the anti-leprosy drug dapsone and some antimalarials, are oxidised in the liver to active metabolites, which are released into the circulation, where they can affect erythrocytes, causing methaemoglobinaemia and/or haemolysis.

Methaemoglobinaemia

In the erythrocyte, the active metabolite interacts with molecular oxygen (O_2), which then oxidises haemoglobin (Fe^{2+}) to methaemoglobin (Fe^{3+}) and also oxidises the active metabolite itself (Fig. 53.4a). Because of the large amounts of haemoglobin compared with the amount of drug given, this would be inconsequential, were it not for the fact that the oxidised active metabolite can be recycled back to the active metabolite by reduction with NADPH (reduced nicotinamide adenine dinucleotide phosphate) in the erythrocyte. Consequently, each molecule of the metabolite undergoes repeated redox cycling and is able to oxidise many molecules of haemoglobin. The redox cycling depends on the presence of NADPH, which is formed during the metabolism of glucose-6-phosphate via the enzyme glucose-6-phosphate dehydrogenase (G6PD) (Fig. 53.4a). The activity of G6PD, and hence the amounts of NADPH, are determined genetically; the incidence of G6PD deficiency is high in black races and very high in Mediterranean races, such as the Kurds. Such subjects have limited NADPH reserves and, therefore, have a low ability to reduce the oxidised active drug metabolite (Fig. 53.4a) back to the active metabolite. In consequence, there is limited redox cycling of the active drug metabolite and such individuals are less susceptible to drug-induced methaemoglobinaemia.

Haemolysis

This arises from an increase in erythrocyte membrane permeability associated with accumulation of oxidised glutathione (GS–SG in Fig. 53.4b) in the erythrocyte. Oxidised glutathione accumulates because redox cycling of the drug metabolite linked to the formation of methaemoglobin (Fig 53.4a) (see above) results in depletion of NADPH, which is the cofactor essential for maintaining glutathione in the reduced state. Individuals with G6PD deficiency are very susceptible to haemolysis caused by aromatic amines and nitrites because the low endogenous levels of NADPH are depleted rapidly and oxidised glutathione cannot then be reduced. Given the geographical distribution of G6PD deficiency, it is ironic that the amino groups associated with this form of toxicity are often present in drugs used to treat tropical infections (primaquine for the treatment of malaria; see Ch. 51 and Box 47.6).

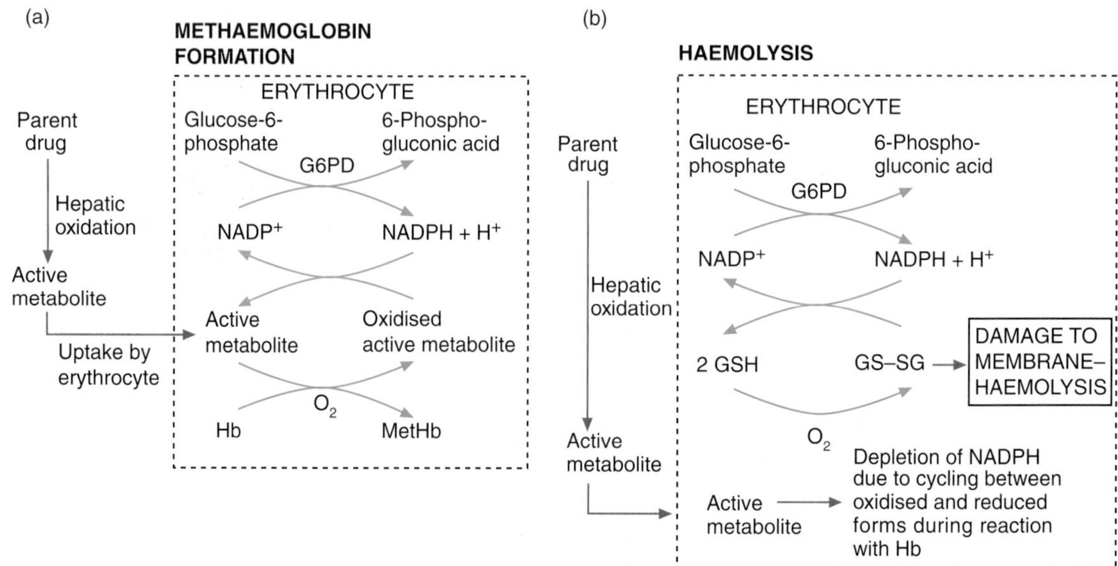

Fig. 53.4 **Mechanisms of methaemoglobinaemia (a) and haemolysis (b).** Hb, haemoglobin; G6PD, glucose-6-phosphate dehydrogenase; GS–SG, glutathione dimer (oxidised form); GSH, glutathione (reduced form); NADP, nicotinamide adenine dinucleotide phosphate. High concentrations of reduced glutathione are necessary for maintaining the erythrocyte cell membrane integrity; a build-up of oxidised glutathione is associated with haemolysis. The active metabolite may also react with glutathione directly to lower GSH concentrations.

IMMUNOLOGICAL TOXICITY

Immunological toxicity is frequently referred to as 'drug allergy' and is the form of toxicity with which people may be most familiar, for example penicillin allergy. Immunological mechanisms are implicated in a number of common adverse effects, such as rashes and fever, but may also be involved in organ-directed toxicity. Although the term 'allergy' may not be strictly correct for all forms of immunologically-mediated toxicity, it is probably better than 'hypersensitivity', which has also been used to describe an elevated sensitivity to any mechanism or effect.

Low-molecular-weight compounds (<1100 Da) are not able to elicit an allergic response as such, but can do so after the compound, or a metabolite, has formed a stable or covalent bond with a macromolecule. Covalent binding to a normal protein produces a 'novel protein' that is recognised as foreign by the immune system and can act as an antigen. This process has been recognised for many years and is summarised in Figure 53.5.

Immunologically mediated toxicity can show a wide range of characteristics.

- The effects are unrelated to pharmacological toxicity, but have been implicated in some forms of biochemical toxicity because immunological toxicity may arise if a reactive metabolite is formed which binds covalently to cellular proteins.
- Toxicity is unrelated to dose: once the antibody has been produced, even very small amounts of antigen can trigger a reaction.

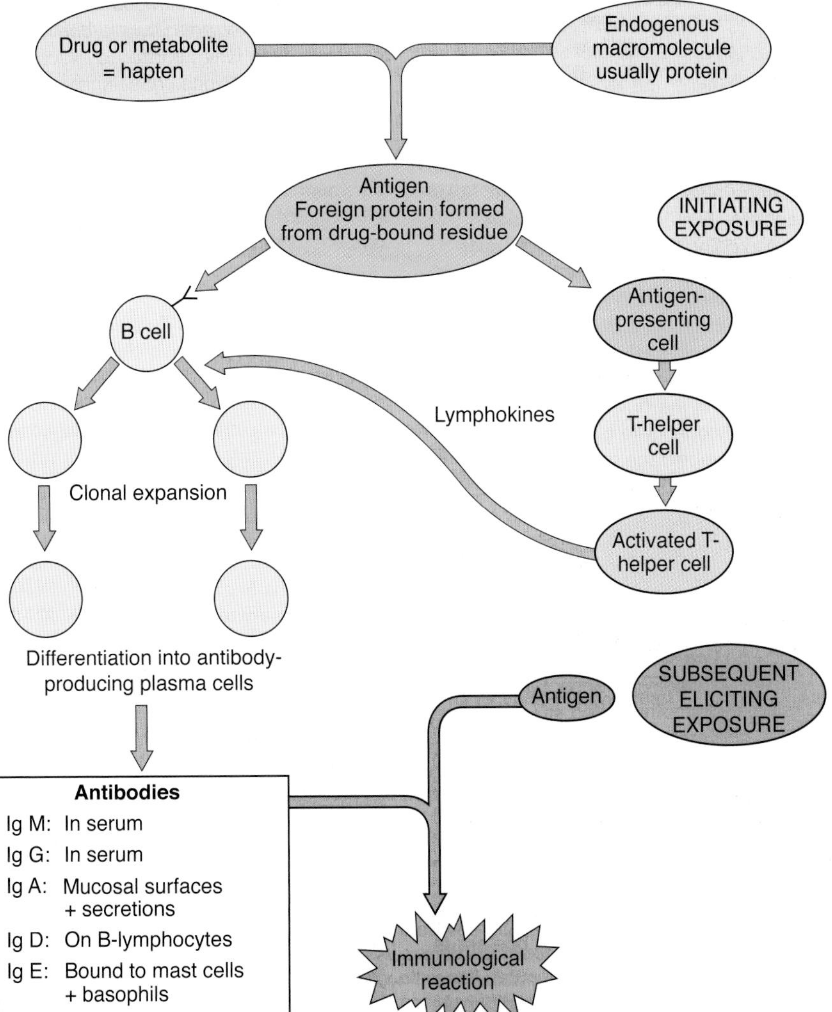

Fig. 53.5 **Mechanisms of drug allergy.** The initial exposure produces an antigen, which results in the production of antibodies via B-cell clonal expansion and differentiations; this is stimulated by cytokines from activated T-helper cells. The eliciting exposure occurs later (usually at least 3 days later, during which time therapy may or may not be continuing); antigen–antibody interaction then exposes a complement-binding site, which triggers the reaction. The nature of the immunological reaction depends on the nature of the antibody and/or localisation of the antigen. Treatment is with immunosuppressant drugs (Ch. 38).

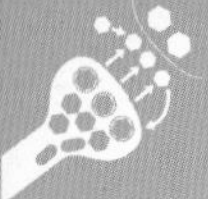

- There is normally a lag of at least 3 days between initial exposure and the development of symptoms; however, the first dose of a subsequent treatment may give an immediate reaction.
- Cross-reactivity is possible among different compounds that share the same antigenic determinant or structural component that is involved in antibody recognition, such as the penicilloyl group of the penicillin family.
- The incidence varies widely between different drugs – for example, from about 1 in 10 000 people for phenylbutazone-induced agranulocytosis to 1 in 20 for ampicillin-related skin rashes.
- The response is idiosyncratic but genetically controlled; individual responsiveness cannot be predicted, but individuals who have a history of atopic disease are more likely to develop a 'drug allergy'.

The effects produced may be subdivided into the classic four types of allergic reaction (see also Ch. 38).

- *Type 1: immediate or anaphylactic reactions*. These are mediated via IgE antibodies attached to the surface of basophils and mast cells; the release of numerous mediators, for example histamine, serotonin (5-HT) and leukotrienes, produces effects that include urticaria, bronchial constriction, hypotension, oedema and shock. A skin-prick challenge test usually produces an acute inflammatory response. Examples of drugs having this type of effect are penicillins and peptide drugs, such as crisantaspase (asparaginase).
- *Type 2: cytotoxic reactions*. The antigen is formed by the drug binding to a cell membrane; subsequent interaction of this antigen with circulating IgG, IgM or IgA antibodies activates complement and initiates cell lysis. Depending on the carrier cell to which the drug is bound, cell lysis can result in thrombocytopenia (e.g. digitoxin, cephalosporins, quinine), neutropenia (e.g. metronidazole) or haemolytic anaemia (e.g. penicillins, rifampicin [rifampin] and possibly methyldopa).
- *Type 3: immune-complex reactions*. The antigen–antibody interaction occurs in serum and the complex formed is deposited on endothelial cells, basement membranes, etc., to initiate a more localised inflammatory reaction, such as arteritis or nephritis. Examples include serum sickness (urticaria, angioedema, fever) with penicillins, lupus erythematosus-like syndrome with hydralazine and procainamide (especially in slow acetylators) and possibly NSAID-related nephropathy.
- *Type 4: cell-mediated delayed-type reactions*. Reaction to the eliciting exposure is delayed. The reactions occur mostly in skin through the formation of an antigen between the drug (hapten) and skin proteins. This is followed by an infiltration of sensitised T-lymphocytes, which recognise the antigen and release lymphokines to produce local inflammation, oedema and irritation, for example contact dermatitis.

In addition to true immunologically mediated toxicity, as described above, there are examples of so-called 'allergic' reactions, such as aspirin hypersensitivity, which show many of the characteristics given above (e.g. rashes, induction of asthma in susceptible individuals, cross-reactivity with other aromatic acids such as benzoates), but for which a true immunological basis has not been demonstrated.

It has been estimated that 'drug allergy' accounts for about 10% of adverse drug reactions but that severe reactions are rare. For example, only about 5 individuals in 10 000 develop an anaphylactic reaction to penicillins, but about one-half of these are sufficiently serious to warrant hospital treatment, which is aimed at reversing the effects on the airways and heart and preventing further mediator release (see Ch. 39). However, given the large numbers of subjects receiving drugs such as penicillins, 'drug allergy' is an important source of iatrogenic morbidity.

SELF-POISONING AND DRUG OVERDOSE

Self-poisoning can be either accidental or deliberate. Approximately a quarter of a million episodes are believed to occur each year in England and Wales, although less than 40% of these reach hospital. Deaths from self-poisoning still average about 2000 each year in England and Wales. Accidental poisoning is common in children under 5 years of age, when it often involves household products as well as medicines. A second peak of self-poisoning occurs in the teens and early twenties, when it is more frequent in girls. The incidence then progressively falls with increasing age. Most deliberate self-poisoning represents 'parasuicide' or attention-seeking behaviour. True suicide attempts comprise a minority of events, occurring most frequently in those over 45 years. About 30% of the deaths from deliberate overdose are in those over 65 years of age: self-poisoning at this age occurs most often in response to depression or specific life events such as bereavement. It is important to recognise that at any age the severity of poisoning bears little relationship to suicidal intent.

The drugs most frequently used for self-poisoning are benzodiazepines, analgesics and antidepressants. Alcohol is often taken together with these drugs. It is important to attempt to identify the cause of the poisoning because it may determine the most suitable treatment. However, it should be remembered that information from the person about which drug was taken, how much, and the time of overdosing, is frequently unreliable. TICTAC is a computerised database which aids the identification of tablets and capsules: **http://www.tictac.org.uk/Introduction/**

MANAGEMENT PRINCIPLES

The emergency treatment of poisoning is described in the introduction to the BNF. Additional sources of information include the UK National Poisons Information Service, and its computer database TOXBASE (which has information on household products and industrial and agricultural chemicals as well as drugs) which is available to registered users: *http://www.toxbase.co.uk*

The management of drug overdose, which is outlined below, has a number of principal aims (Fig. 53.6).

MANAGING ADVERSE EFFECTS

Immediate measures

There are certain immediate measures required when someone presents with a possible drug overdose or poisoning:

- remove the person from contact with the poison if appropriate, for example gases, corrosives
- assess vital signs, i.e. pulse, respiration and pupil size; inspect the person for injury
- ensure a clear airway; if breathing but unconscious, place in the coma position
- obtain a clear history if possible
- preserve any evidence, for example bottles, written notes, etc.

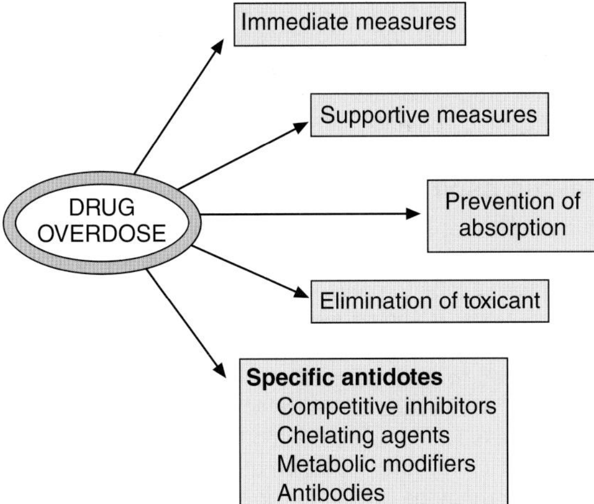

Fig. 53.6 **Principles underlying the management of drug overdose.**

Supportive measures

Examples of unwanted effects seen in drug overdose are shown in Table 53.4. A number of the effects will require supportive measures (Fig. 53.7).

Cardiac or respiratory arrest

This may result from a toxic effect of the drug on the heart, from depression of the respiratory centre or from metabolic disturbance. Assisted ventilation, ranging from mouth-to-mouth, or Ambu-bag inflation, to the use of a ventilator, may be required. In some circumstances, recovery is possible even after prolonged resuscitation.

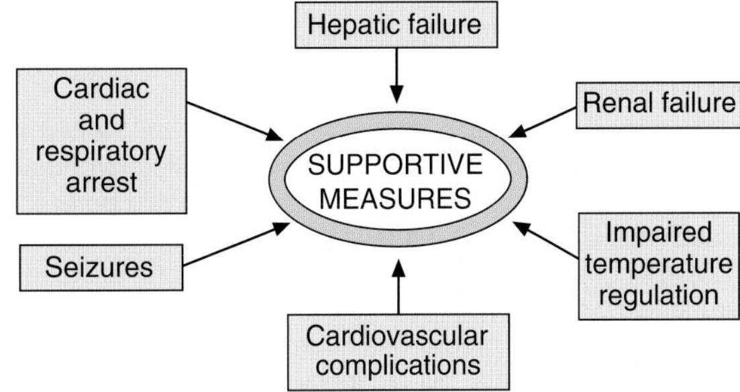

Fig. 53.7 **Main effects of overdose requiring supportive measures.**

Table 53.4 Complications of acute poisonings

Complication	Cause	Examples of poisons
Cardiac arrest	Direct cardiotoxicity	Many
	Hypoxia	Many
	Electrolyte/metabolic disturbance	Many
Central nervous system depression		Many
Seizures	Direct neurotoxicity	Tricyclic antidepressants, theophylline
	Hypoxia	Many
Hypotension	Myocardial depression	β-Adrenoceptor antagonists, tricyclic antidepressants (dextropropoxyphene[a])
	Peripheral vasodilation	Many
Arrhythmia	Direct cardiotoxicity	β-Adrenoceptor antagonists, tricyclic antidepressants, verapamil, digoxin
	Hypoxia	Many
	Electrolyte/metabolic disturbance	Many
Renal failure	Hypotension	Many
	Rhabdomyolysis	Opioids, hypnotics, ethanol, carbon monoxide
	Direct nephrotoxicity	Paracetamol, heavy metals
Hepatic failure	Direct hepatotoxicity	Paracetamol, carbon tetrachloride
Respiratory depression	Direct neurotoxicity	Sedatives, hypnotics, opioids

[a]Dextropropoxyphene has been withdrawn in the UK.

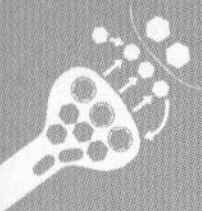

Hypotension

A low blood pressure is common in severe poisoning with central nervous system (CNS) depressants. A blood pressure below 70 mmHg systolic can cause irreversible brain damage, but any degree of low blood pressure should be treated if accompanied by poor tissue perfusion or low urine output. Depression of the vasomotor centre can cause arterial dilation and peripheral venous pooling, producing a low central venous pressure. This should be raised to 10–15 cmH_2O (measured from the midaxillary line) by intravenous infusion of a colloid solution, such as dextran polymers. A vasoconstrictor such as noradrenaline (norepinephrine; Ch. 4) may occasionally be required. If hypotension occurs with a normal or raised central venous pressure, this suggests myocardial depression. Positive inotropic drugs such as the β_1-adrenoceptor agonist dobutamine (Ch. 7) should then be used.

Arrhythmias

Disturbances of cardiac rhythm should only be treated if they are severe. Ventricular arrhythmias causing hypotension often require intervention, but caution should be exercised if there is a long Q–T interval on the electrocardiogram (ECG), since the tachycardia often fails to respond to standard antiarrhythmic drugs. It is essential to correct metabolic derangements that predispose to arrhythmias, for example hypothermia, hypoxia, hypercapnia, hypokalaemia, hyperkalaemia and acidosis.

Seizures

These may be caused by a treatable underlying change such as hypoxia, hypoglycaemia or hypocalcaemia, or they may be a direct toxic effect of the drug on neuronal function. The treatment of choice is lorazepam or diazepam intravenously, or rectal diazepam if the intravenous route is unavailable (Ch. 20). Artificial ventilation with neuromuscular blockade (Ch. 27) is used if the seizures cannot be controlled.

Renal failure

Kidney damage is usually a consequence of prolonged hypotension. Other causes include a direct nephrotoxic effect of the drug and renal damage produced by the products of toxic muscle necrosis (rhabdomyolysis).

Hepatic failure

This usually results from the direct toxic effects of specific agents, such as paracetamol.

Impaired temperature regulation

Hypothermia is common, and can be caused by depression of the metabolic rate with reduced heat production and by increased heat loss from cutaneous vasodilation. It is common with phenothiazines and barbiturates, but is seen with any prolonged coma. Rewarming, preferably by wrapping in a 'space blanket', reduces the risk of serious ventricular arrhythmias. By contrast, CNS stimulants such as ecstasy can produce hyperthermia, as can aspirin, which uncouples cellular oxidative phosphorylation.

REDUCING TOXICITY

The adverse effects can be reduced by:

- minimising further drug absorption
- maximising drug elimination
- negating effects with antidotes, etc.

Prevention of absorption of poisons

There are two principal methods of preventing further absorption of the drug: gastric aspiration and lavage, and activated charcoal. Inducing emesis with an irritant such as ipecacuanha is no longer recommended, since it has little effect on drug absorption and increases the risk of aspiration of gastric contents.

Gastric aspiration and lavage

This should not be considered in unconscious or drowsy persons without protection of the airways by a cuffed endotracheal tube to prevent aspiration of gastric contents into the lungs. It should never be used after ingestion of corrosives or petroleum products. A large-bore orogastric tube is used to aspirate gastric contents initially and then to lavage with doses of water at body temperature. Its effectiveness is unproven. Gastric lavage is normally used for up to 1 h only after ingestion of a significant amount of drug. There may be benefit for up to 4 h after aspirin and/or in unconscious persons, and for up to 4–6 h after a life-threatening overdose of tricyclic antidepressants, but activated charcoal is now preferred.

Activated charcoal

This formulation of charcoal has a large adsorbent area and is given as a suspension in water. Activated charcoal adsorbs or binds the drug and retains it in the gastrointestinal lumen. Not all drugs are adsorbed onto charcoal (see Table 53.5). About 10 g of charcoal is required for every 1 g of poison, which makes it impractical for poisons that are usually ingested in large quantities. For suitable drugs, an initial dose of 50 g of charcoal for adults can prevent absorption if given within 1 h of drug ingestion (later after poisoning with modified-release preparations, or drugs with antimuscarinic properties that delay gastric emptying).

Table 53.5 Drug adsorption onto activated charcoal

Drugs/compounds not adsorbed	Drugs/compounds adsorbed
Acids	Aspirin
Alkalis	Carbamazepine
Cyanide	Dapsone
DDT (insecticide)	Digoxin
Ethanol	Ecstasy
Ethylene glycol (antifreeze)	Paraquat (herbicide)
Ferrous salts	Phenobarbital
Lead	Quinine
Lithium	Sustained-release preparations
Mercury	Theophylline
Methanol	Tricyclic antidepressants
Organic solvents	

Charcoal should not be given to drowsy or comatose persons, because of the risk of aspiration into the lungs. Constipation is the major unwanted effect of charcoal; charcoal should not be given in the absence of bowel sounds, because of the risk of bowel obstruction.

Elimination of poisons

There are three principal methods of enhancing elimination of the drug: activated charcoal, renal elimination and haemodialysis/haemoperfusion.

Activated charcoal

Repeated administration of 50 g of activated charcoal every 4 h for up to 24–36 h achieves further retention of adsorbed drug in the small intestine. Drug is continuously being transferred in both directions across the gut wall, with the concentration gradient normally favouring net absorption, owing to the high concentration free in solution within the gut lumen. If drug in the bowel is bound onto the charcoal, this lowers the free concentration and can result in net transfer from the body into the gut and thereby enhance elimination of the compound. This is useful for overdose with barbiturates, carbamazepine, dapsone, quinine and theophylline.

Renal elimination

Forced diuresis with intravenous infusion of large quantities of fluid was advocated in the past for drugs or toxic metabolites that are mostly eliminated unchanged by the kidney. However, serious disturbances of fluid or electrolyte balance can occur, and therefore it is no longer recommended. Altering urine pH, while maintaining normal urine flow, can be effective in increasing the renal elimination of drugs that are weak electrolytes. Modification of urine pH to increase the extent of ionisation of the drug will reduce reabsorption from the renal tubule (Ch. 2). Only a modest increase in urinary flow rate is required. Weak acids, such as salicylates, are excreted more readily in alkaline urine (alkaline diuresis – achieved by giving sodium bicarbonate), while the converse is true for weak bases (acid diuresis – achieved by giving ammonium chloride).

Haemodialysis or haemoperfusion

These are reserved for the most severely poisoned individuals. The techniques are only successful if a large proportion of the body burden of the drug is retained in the plasma and available for removal (i.e. the drug has a low apparent volume of distribution; see Ch. 2). Haemodialysis relies on diffusion of the drug across a semi-permeable membrane from blood into the dialysis fluid; it is used for salicylates, phenobarbital, methanol, ethylene glycol and lithium. Haemoperfusion involves adsorption of drug from blood as it passes down a column containing activated charcoal or a resin; it is used for short- or medium-acting barbiturates, chloral hydrate, meprobamate and theophylline.

Specific antidotes

Antidotes are available only for a minority of the drugs that are commonly involved in poisoning cases. Some important examples are given below.

Competitive receptor antagonists

- Atropine acts at muscarinic receptors to block the parasympathetic effects of organophosphate insecticides. It is given by intravenous or intramuscular injection.
- Naloxone acts at opioid receptors to reverse the effects of opioid analgesics. Its short half-life, compared with those of most opioids, means that repeated injections or an infusion are usually needed.
- Flumazenil acts at benzodiazepine receptors. It is given intravenously, but is rarely needed for the treatment of intentional benzodiazepine overdose because fatalities are uncommon with this class of drug. Flumazenil can cause seizures in benzodiazepine-dependent subjects. It is used to reverse the effects of benzodiazepines when toxicity occurs in people with chronic liver disease.

Chelating agents

Chelating agents act by forming a complex with the drug or chemical, thereby reducing the free (active) drug concentration:

- desferrioxamine for iron salts; given by intravenous infusion
- dicobalt edetate for cyanide; given by intravenous injection
- dimercaprol for antimony, arsenic, bismuth, gold and mercury; it is used with sodium calcium edetate for lead; given by intramuscular injection
- sodium calcium edetate for lead; given by intravenous infusion
- sodium nitrite, together with sodium thiosulphate, for cyanide; both given by intravenous injection.

Compounds that affect drug metabolism

- Ethanol is used in the treatment of methanol poisoning, because it acts as a competitive substrate for alcohol dehydrogenase, preventing formation of the toxic metabolites formaldehyde and formic acid.
- Acetylcysteine provides a substrate for conjugation of the cytotoxic metabolite of paracetamol when the natural conjugating ligand, glutathione, is depleted (see below).

Antibodies

Digoxin can be neutralised in severe poisoning by specific antibody fragments. The antibodies are raised in sheep and cleaved to remove the antigenic crystalline (Fc) portion of the molecule while retaining the specific antigen-binding fragment (Fab).

SOME SPECIFIC COMMON POISONINGS

Paracetamol

Paracetamol overdose can be fatal, with about 200 deaths occurring each year in England and Wales. Metabolism of paracetamol takes place in the liver, mainly producing non-toxic conjugates (Fig. 53.3). A small amount is oxidised by the cytochrome P450 system to a reactive intermediate,

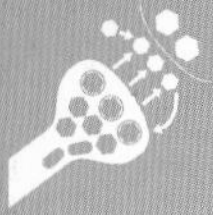

N-acetyl-*p*-benzoquinone imine (NAPBQI), which is inactivated by conjugation with the thiol group on glutathione. When hepatic glutathione is depleted, which occurs readily in overdose, oxidative stress coupled with NAPBQI-mediated denaturation of protein produces hepatic necrosis. Similar processes in the kidney can cause renal tubular necrosis.

In the first 24 h there are few symptoms apart from nausea, vomiting, abdominal pain and sweating, which usually resolve. Liver damage begins within 24 h after a large overdose, producing right upper quadrant pain and tenderness. Jaundice is apparent by 36–48 h and liver damage is maximal by 3–4 days. Severe liver failure, requiring transplantation for survival, can ensue. The most sensitive measures of liver damage are the prothrombin time, or the international normalised ratio (INR), and the plasma unconjugated bilirubin. Renal failure is seen in about a quarter of cases with severe liver damage.

Activated charcoal in large doses is recommended within 1 h of a potentially serious paracetamol overdose. Because antidotes are most effective when given early, blood should be analysed for paracetamol if there is any suspicion of poisoning. Blood should be taken at 4 h or more after the suspected overdose. Earlier sampling is not informative because a low plasma level at that time could reflect incomplete absorption of a large overdose, rather than ingestion of a small overdose. Antidotes used in paracetamol poisoning, such as acetylcysteine and methionine, are used to replace glutathione as a thiol donor in the liver; glutathione itself is not used, because it cannot enter liver cells from the blood.

Methionine can be given orally if acetylcysteine is not available, but not with or after activated charcoal, because methionine can compete with paracetamol for adsorption. Methionine should not be used if there is vomiting, or started more than 10–12 h after ingestion of paracetamol, since the efficacy of methionine in late poisoning is unknown. Intravenous acetylcysteine is the preferred treatment for potentially serious poisoning, and should be started prior to the analysis of a plasma paracetamol concentration. A graph is available (Fig. 53.8) to indicate the risk of liver damage for a given plasma paracetamol concentration related to the time after ingestion. Plasma concentrations after 15 h must be interpreted by extrapolation of the graph. Treatment is only necessary if potentially toxic paracetamol concentrations are detected. It is important to realise that toxicity can occur at much lower plasma paracetamol concentrations under certain circumstances:

- concurrent use of drugs such as alcohol or phenytoin that induce liver cytochrome P450 (Ch. 2) and hence increase the formation of the reactive metabolite
- pre-existing liver disease
- malnourished/anorexic persons
- infection with HIV.

All such individuals should be treated if plasma paracetamol concentrations are only one-half of those shown in Figure 53.8.

Treatment used to be confined to the first 15 h after overdose, but liver damage can be reduced even when the antidote is delayed for up to 20–30 h. It may be useful even later after ingestion to reduce the severity of established liver damage.

Salicylates

Although salicylate poisoning is becoming less common, there are still about 150 deaths each year in England and Wales. Aspirin is hydrolysed rapidly to salicylic acid after absorption, but further metabolism, by conjugation with glycine, is rate-limited. Symptoms of toxicity are nausea, vomiting, abdominal pain, tinnitus, deafness, hyperventilation and sweating. Agitation frequently occurs in adults, but children become comatose. The chain of metabolic events produced by aspirin is shown in Figure 53.9.

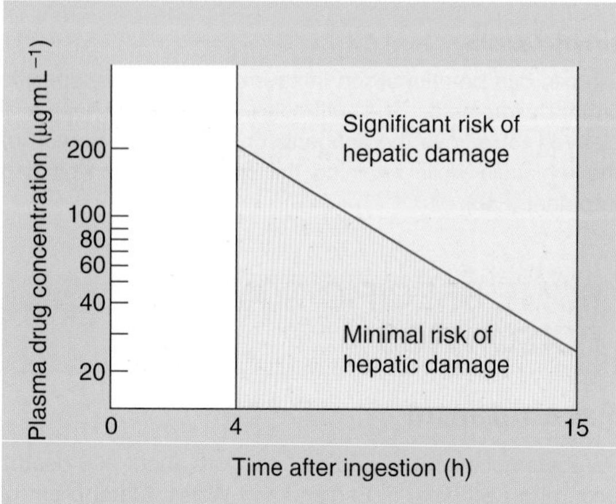

Fig. 53.8 **Relationship between plasma paracetamol concentration and the risk of liver damage.**

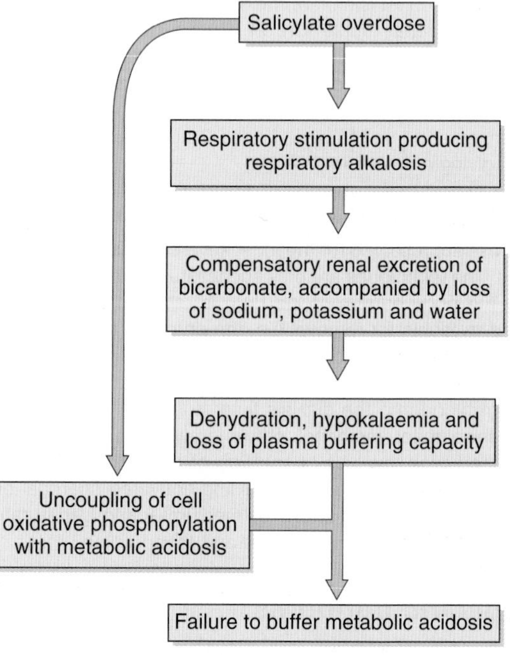

Fig. 53.9 **The metabolic consequences of salicylate overdose.**

Activated charcoal is recommended for reducing absorption if given early. Correction of fluid, electrolyte and acid–base balance is fundamental to successful management; a fluid deficit of 3–4 L is not unusual in severe poisoning. Forced alkaline diuresis is no longer advocated to enhance salicylate elimination (see above); simple alkalinisation of the urine with 1.26% sodium bicarbonate to raise the pH above 7.5 is effective and safer. Haemodialysis is the treatment of choice in severe poisoning, especially if there is severe metabolic acidosis.

Tricyclic antidepressants

Approximately 400 deaths per year occur in England and Wales from overdose with tricyclic antidepressants. Antimuscarinic effects delay gastric emptying and oral activated charcoal is used routinely for up to 4 h after the overdose. Drowsiness and confusion are followed by convulsions and coma in more severe poisoning. Cardiac depression can produce hypotension. Serious arrhythmias, such as ventricular tachycardia, can occur, and ECG monitoring is recommended for at least 24 h. Arrhythmias frequently respond to correction of acidosis or hypoxia; if this is not successful, phenytoin or direct current shock can be used. Antiarrhythmic drugs that depress cardiac contractility should be avoided.

Opioid analgesics

The triad of signs characteristic of opioid overdose are:

- respiratory depression
- pinpoint pupils
- impaired consciousness.

They can be reversed rapidly by administration of naloxone (Ch. 19), which is a competitive antagonist at opioid μ-receptors. After an initial intravenous bolus dose of naloxone, it is often necessary to give repeated boluses or a continuous infusion, because the half-life of naloxone is very short compared with those of most opioids. In poisoning with buprenorphine, the effect of naloxone is often incomplete, and assisted ventilation may also be needed. In poisoning with dextropropoxyphene, especially if taken with alcohol, acute cardiovascular collapse can occur within 30 min of ingestion. For this reason, dextropropoxyphene has been withdrawn from the market in the UK. Acute poisoning with organophosphorus insecticides can produce signs that are similar to those with opioids, but naloxone will have no effect.

Beta-adrenoceptor antagonists

Poisoning by β-adrenoceptor antagonists usually presents with bradycardia and hypotension. More severe effects, including coma and convulsions, can occur with some drugs in this class. Treatment of the bradycardia is with intravenous atropine, which may increase the blood pressure. Cardiogenic shock that does not respond to atropine should initially be treated with intravenous glucagon, which has a positive inotropic effect. A temporary cardiac pacemaker may be necessary.

Ecstasy

Ecstasy (3,4-methylenedioxymethamphetamine; MDMA) toxicity is characterised by tachycardia, hyperreflexia, hyperpyrexia, and initial hypertension followed by hypotension. In severe cases, delirium, seizures, coma and cardiac dysrhythmias may occur. MDMA is metabolised by CYP2D6 (Ch. 2), and genetic differences in this enzyme may result in wide inter-individual differences in susceptibility to the toxic effects of MDMA. Some subjects may present with hyponatraemia, possibly as a result of drinking excessive water as a precaution to prevent dehydration. Treatments include activated charcoal, but only for up to 2 h post ingestion, since MDMA is absorbed rapidly, and diazepam for agitation or seizures.

FURTHER READING

2003 Pharmaceutical drug overdose case reports. From the World Literature. *Toxicol Rev* 22, 191–197

Buckley NA, Dawson AH, Whyte IM, O'Connell DL (1995) Relative toxicity of benzodiazepines in overdose. *BMJ* 310, 219–221

Dargan PI, Jones AL (2003) Management of paracetamol poisoning. *Trends Pharmacol Sci* 24, 154–157

Dawson AH, Whyte IM (2001) Therapeutic drug monitoring in drug overdose. *Br J Clin Pharmacol* 52(suppl 1), 97S–102S

Edwards JG (1995) Suicide and antidepressants. Controversies on prevention, provocation, and self poisoning continue. *BMJ* 310, 205–206

Hawton K, Ware C, Mistry H et al (1995) Why patients choose paracetamol for self poisoning and their knowledge of its dangers. *BMJ* 310, 164

Heard KJ (2008) Acetylcysteine for acetominophen poisoning. *N Engl J Med* 359, 285–292

Henry JA, Alexander CA, Sener EK (1995) Relative mortality from overdose of antidepressants. *BMJ* 310, 221–224

Jick SS, Dean AD, Jick H (1995) Antidepressants and suicide. *BMJ* 310, 215–218

Lee WM (1995) Drug-induced hepatotoxicity. *N Engl J Med* 333, 1118–1127

Park BK, Kitteringham NR, Pirmohamed M, Tucker GT (1996) Relevance of induction of human drug-metabolising enzymes: pharmacological and toxicological implications. *Br J Clin Pharmacol* 41, 477–491

Park BK, Kitteringham NR, Powell H, Pirmohamed M (2000) Advances in molecular toxicology – towards understanding idiosyncratic drug toxicity. *Toxicology* 153, 39–60

Roujeau JC, Stern RS (1994) Severe adverse cutaneous reactions to drugs. *N Engl J Med* 331, 1272–1285

Sung J, Russell RI, Yeomans N et al (2000) Non-steroidal anti-inflammatory drug toxicity in the upper gastrointestinal tract. *J Gastroenterol Hepatol* 15(suppl), G58–G68

Vale JA, Proudfoot AT (1995) Paracetamol (acetaminophen) poisoning. *Lancet* 346, 547–552

Waring RH, Emery P (1995) The genetic origin of responses to drugs. *Br Med Bull* 51, 449–461

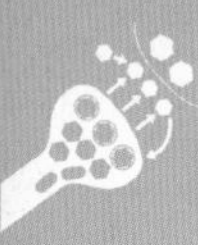

SELF-ASSESSMENT

1. Case history questions

A 70-year-old man with a history of depressive illness and alcohol abuse was prescribed a compound analgesic containing 500 mg paracetamol and 30 mg codeine phosphate (co-codamol 30/500) for back pain. Eight hours after collecting his prescription, he was seen as an emergency by his GP, who considered the man had taken an overdose and he was admitted to hospital.

a. What features might be seen soon after the overdosage and during the subsequent 24–48 h?
b. Outline what suitable pharmacological treatments should be undertaken.
c. Would co-dydramol have been a safer alternative to prescribe?

ANSWERS

1. Case history answers
   a. Initial features would be those of opioid overdosage caused by the codeine with possible symptoms of respiratory depression, pinpoint pupils, coma and cardiovascular collapse. Later-developing symptoms of nausea, abdominal pain and sweating, and, if untreated, jaundice, are those owing to liver damage caused by the toxic metabolite of paracetamol.
   b. The opioid antagonist naloxone is a rapid reversible antagonist of opioids at μ-, κ- and δ-receptors. It has a short half-life and may have to be given repeatedly. Acetylcysteine is given, which conjugates with the hepatotoxic metabolite of paracetamol, and is most effective when given early after an overdosage; the risk of liver damage is related to the time of ingestion before treatment and the plasma paracetamol concentrations. Chronic alcohol consumption would increase the toxic effects of codeine and paracetamol. It enhances the central depressant actions of the opioid. Alcohol also induces cytochrome P450 enzymes, increasing formation of the toxic metabolite of paracetamol and causing toxicity at lower levels of paracetamol ingestion. The toxicity of paracetamol would also be increased by intake of drugs such as carbamazepine or rifampicin, which would enhance P450 metabolising enzymes and increase formation of the toxic metabolite.
   c. Codydramol also contains the opioid dihydrocodeine together with paracetamol.

Drugs used to treat drug toxicity and drug overdose, and drugs used to treat toxicity due to environmental chemicals

Drug	Half-life (h) and kinetics	Comments
Drugs used to treat drug toxicity and drug overdose		
Acetylcysteine	5–6 [M] Deacetylated by the liver and incorporated as cysteine into cellular pools	Used for paracetamol overdose; given by intravenous infusion
Charcoal activated	Unabsorbed and passes down gastrointestinal tract	Taken orally for a range of drug overdoses (see Table 53.5); adsorbs drug and reduces absorption
Methionine	? [M] Metabolised by normal pathways of intermediary metabolism	Used for paracetamol overdose; given orally
Naloxone	1–1.5 [M] Half-life is shorter than that of morphine and repeated doses may be necessary; eliminated by conjugation with glucuronic acid	Opioid antagonist used to treat opioid overdose; administered by injection, giving a rapid onset of action (1–2 min)
Drugs used to treat toxicity due to environmental chemicals		
Iron poisoning/overload (see also Ch. 47)		
Desferrioxamine mesilate (deferoxamine mesilate)	6 [R + M] Slowly eliminated in urine and by metabolism and chelation	Given by continuous intravenous infusion
Cyanide poisoning		
Dicobalt edetate	? [?]	Given by intravenous injection
Sodium nitrite	? [R + ?] Fate is not well defined but includes oxidation to nitrate	Given by intravenous injection

Drugs used to treat drug toxicity and drug overdose, and drugs used to treat toxicity due to environmental chemicals

Drug	Half-life (h) and kinetics	Comments
Sodium thiosulphate	? [?] Thiosulphate acts as a sulphur donor for rhodanese-catalysed conversion of cyanide to thiocyanate which is excreted in urine	Given by intravenous injection
Heavy metals		
Dimercaprol	? [M] Excess that does not complex with heavy metals is rapidly inactivated by metabolism; drug–metal complexes are excreted in about 4 h	Used for various metals; given by intramuscular injection
Sodium calcium edetate	? [?]	Chelating agent; used for various metals, especially lead; given by intravenous infusion
Organophosphate pesticides		
Pralidoxime	1 [M + R] Undergoes both hepatic metabolism and renal excretion	Reactivates acetylcholine esterase (see Ch. 4); given by slow intravenous injection

[M], metabolism; [R], renal excretion.

54 Substance abuse and dependence

Substance abuse is characterised by compulsive drug-seeking and drug-taking behaviour addiction and an inability to control intake; there may also be symptoms of withdrawal when the drug becomes unavailable (dependence).

Dependence-inducing drugs are mind-modifying substances that are taken initially because of the pleasurable effect they produce, but also to avoid unpleasant withdrawal symptoms. Dependence produces different degrees of need for the drug, from mild desire to a craving.

THE BIOLOGICAL BASIS OF DEPENDENCE

The mechanisms of drug dependence are relatively poorly understood but involve complex dysfunctional adaptation of the neurocircuits in the brain that subserve physiological reward processes; the mesolimbic system is involved in motivation and reward processes, and, depending upon the particular stimulus and the functional status of the individual, its activation can result in a spectrum of response from slight mood elevation to intense pleasure or euphoria; stimulation can result from a plethora of factors that are very personal, for example food intake, sexual activity and the controlled and occasional use of lifestyle drugs such as alcohol and nicotine.

Acute activation of the mesolimbic dopamine reward pathways

The mesolimbic system is activated by impulses arising in the ventral tegmental area of the brain. These impulses are relayed through the medial forebrain bundle, via the nucleus accumbens, to the prefrontal cortex (Fig. 54.1). Stimulation of the reward pathways in the ventral tegmentum results in dopamine release in the nucleus accumbens and stimulation of postsynaptic D_2 receptors (acting via inhibitory G_i proteins to inhibit the generation of intracellular cyclic adenosine monophosphate [cAMP] – (see Ch. 1)). This is thought to be central to the processes of reward.

Occasional and limited administration of most drugs of potential abuse directly or indirectly releases dopamine in the nucleus accumbens (Fig. 54.1). For example, morphine enhances dopaminergic input to the nucleus accumbens by stimulating opioid receptors in the ventral tegmental area. This effect may eventually drive the processes resulting in drug dependence, because, with repeated drug taking, the drug becomes essential to maintain a 'normal' level of pleasure.

Chronic stimulation of the mesolimbic dopamine reward pathways

The complexities of the changes involved are daunting and only a limited description of these events is given here. Chronic exposure of the mesolimbic system to drugs such as opioids, alcohol and cocaine eventually leads to neuroadaptive changes and sensitisation of the mesolimbic system to further drug administration. *Upregulation of neuronal cAMP* results from chronic exposure to many drugs of abuse, with increased intraneuronal CREB (cAMP response element binding protein). Increased CREB in the nucleus accumbens is thought to be important for tolerance and dependence. CREB also activates dysphoria-inducing κ-opioid receptors that bind to the opioid peptide dynorphin (Ch. 19) on dopamine- and glutamate-releasing neurons in the prefrontal cortex. The long-term actions of dependence-inducing drugs also affect plasticity in the neural circuits of the reward pathway. Upregulation of transcription factors such as CREB and ΔFosB leads to long-term changes in the number of dendrites on various neurons in the pathway. Therefore, the changes in the reward and stress systems in the brain that arise with addiction may become 'imprinted' even if the causative drug is stopped for long periods. This would explain the vulnerability to relapse after detoxification. There are probably genetic influences on the neurochemical events involved in the reward pathways and stress systems that also increase susceptibility to addiction.

Drug craving is also influenced by neural inputs to the mesolimbic pathway from the amygdala, which are involved in emotion and conditioned responses. In particular, the amygdala is central to the reinforcing effects of drug binges and also the anxiety and negative effect involved in acute withdrawal. Conditioned responses provide powerful cues to drug-taking in specific social circumstances, and the conditioning is reinforced by aspects of the drug-taking process. Eventually, learning that a drug withdrawal can, for example, produce irritability that is relieved by the drug may lead to *any* source of stress or frustration becoming a cue for drug use. Dependence is associated with recruitment of stress systems in the brain, probably in an attempt to restore normal neuronal function. There is an elevation of corticotrophin-releasing factor and noradrenaline, with suppression of the anti-stress neuropeptide Y. These changes support the acute reinforcing effects of the dependence-inducing drug on CNS neurotransmitters.

Nicotine stimulates transiently then inhibits GABA release
Opioids and cannabis inhibit GABA release
Alcohol activates GABA receptors
GABA DYN inhibit ⊖
Ventral tegmentum
DA neuron
GABA DYN ⊖
DA
↓cAMP
↓CREB
Nucleus accumbens
Decreased cAMP and CREB results in pleasure and disposition to repeat reward behaviours. Chronic intake results in dysfunctional adaptation with upregulation of cAMP and CREB and DYN (a mechanism for dependence and tolerance)
⊕ GLU stimulates
Nicotine augments GLU release
Alcohol inhibits GLU release
Cocaine increases synaptic DA
Amfetamine enhances DA release

Fig. 54.1 **The role of dopamine/cAMP in reward pathways in the mesolimbic system and the possible relevance of these pathways to substance abuse.** This diagram illustrates only a small part of the complex and poorly understood molecular mechanisms involved in processes of reward and the ways that substances of abuse may influence these mechanisms. Many drugs of abuse alter gene transcription, which may contribute to their abuse potential and factors such as dependence and withdrawal. cAMP response element binding protein (CREB) is one such transcription factor and it is a major hypothesis that dopamine (DA) neurons in the ventral tegmentum release DA at the nucleus accumbens, which decreases cAMP and its effect on CREB; as shown, many substances of abuse **when administered acutely and in limited amounts** act in different ways to increase DA and consequently inhibit cAMP, providing the pleasurable and rewarding effects of the drug. However, **chronic persistent intake** of many drugs of abuse eventually seems to increase CREB and dynorphin, which will dampen reward mechanisms in the nucleus accumbens and provide a suggested mechanism for drug dependence and tolerance (see further explanations in the text). DYN, dynorphin; GABA, gamma-aminobutyric acid; GLU, glutamate.

In contrast, physical dependence on a drug is unrelated to activity in the mesolimbic system and arises from excessive noradrenergic output from the locus ceruleus, a structure in the base of the brain that is involved in arousal and vigilance.

This chapter covers drugs that are encountered in clinical practice primarily because of their abuse, such as ecstasy and cannabis, or because of their potential to cause dependence, such as nicotine and ethanol (Box 54.1).

Box 54.1 Drugs of abuse

- Psychomotor stimulants
  - Cocaine
  - Amfetamine and derivatives
  - Nicotine
- Psychotomimetic agents
  - Hallucinogens, e.g. LSD, mescaline, psilocybin
  - Cannabis
  - Dissociative anaesthetics, e.g. ketamine
- CNS depressants
  - Alcohol
  - Benzodiazepines
  - Gamma-hydroxybutyric acid (GHB)
  - Inhaled solvents

DRUGS OF ABUSE

PSYCHOMOTOR STIMULANTS

Several drugs that have central stimulant properties are abused and produce dependence. Those more commonly encountered are considered here.

Cocaine

Cocaine is usually taken as the hydrochloride salt. 'Crack' cocaine is the free-base form, named after the crackling sound produced when it is smoked.

Mechanism of action and effects

The psychomotor effects of cocaine are due to inhibition of the reuptake of catecholamines into presynaptic nerve terminals. This in turn may activate opioid systems in the brain, with upregulation of μ-receptors (Ch. 19). Cocaine binds strongly to the catecholamine reuptake transporters, particularly inhibiting dopamine, and to a lesser extent noradrenaline, reuptake. Reduced serotonin reuptake may contribute to wakefulness. Changes in various pituitary neuroendocrine functions occur with more prolonged use; in particular, the release of corticotrophin and luteinising hormone (LH) are enhanced. Tolerance to the psychomotor effects of cocaine is limited. One of the metabolites of cocaine, norcocaine, has direct vasoconstrictor activity.

Effects of cocaine include:

- intense euphoria
- alertness and wakefulness
- increased confidence and strength
- heightened sexual feelings
- indifference to concerns and cares
- severe psychological, but not physical, dependence, brought about by the reinforcing effect of the rapid onset and brief duration of action; this develops particularly rapidly with 'crack' cocaine
- despondency and despair rapidly follow withdrawal; after chronic use, withdrawal can produce a dysphoric mood with fatigue, vivid dreams, insomnia or excessive sleeping, increased appetite and either psychomotor retardation or agitation, irritability and aggressive and stereotyped behaviour
- toxic paranoid psychosis, with delusions of great stamina, occurs with chronic use
- in overdose, excessive catecholamine concentrations produce convulsions, hypertension, cardiac rhythm disturbances and hyperthermia (due to excessive muscle activity and reduced heat loss); if severe, death can occur from respiratory depression and circulatory collapse; the cardiovascular toxicity can be treated with combined α- and β-adrenoceptor blockade, and seizures by intravenous diazepam
- cocaine snuff produces necrosis of the nasal septum through its vasoconstrictor action
- exposure in utero leads to impaired brain development and other teratogenic effects.

Pharmacokinetics

Cocaine, as the hydrochloride salt, is used orally, intranasally (cocaine snuff) or by intravenous injection; the intravenous route gives an intense and rapid onset of effect. 'Crack' cocaine is prepared by mixing cocaine hydrochloride with sodium bicarbonate or ammonia and water, then heating to volatilise the free base; this method of use produces effects similar to intravenous use. Cocaine is metabolised by plasma esterases and its half-life is very short.

Management of cocaine dependence

There are no recognised drug treatments for cocaine dependence. Prolonged behavioural treatments remain the main approach. Tricyclic antidepressants (especially desipramine) are sometimes advocated for the severe depression that can occur on withdrawal.

Amfetamine and derivatives

Amfetamine, dexamfetamine, methamphetamine and 3,4-methylenedioxymethamphetamine (MDMA, 'ecstasy') are all drugs of abuse. Sustained-release dexamfetamine (Dexedrine®) has been used in Canada and the USA as a treatment for attention deficit hyperactivity disorder (ADHD).

Mechanism of action and effects

Amfetamine and related drugs have indirect sympathomimetic effects, releasing monoamines from central nervous system (CNS) neurons (Ch. 4). CNS stimulation by amfetamine is principally a consequence of dopamine and noradrenaline release and is most marked in the reticular formation although it also occurs in many other areas of the brain. The D-isomer (dexamfetamine) is twice as potent as the L-isomer of amfetamine in its central stimulant activity. Effects of amfetamine include:

- euphoria, similar to that experienced with cocaine; this is particularly intense after intravenous use
- reduced fatigue and increased alertness for repetitive tasks
- anorexia
- psychotic behaviour during repeated use over a few days or with acute intoxication, causing hallucinations, paranoia and aggressive behaviour and repetitive actions
- acute intoxication can cause hyperthermia, cerebral haemorrhage and the serotonin syndrome with panic, psychosis, convulsions and death
- peripheral sympathomimetic effects can lead to hypertension and cardiac arrhythmias
- tolerance develops rapidly to some of the central effects of amfetamine, such as anorexia, presumably through central monoamine depletion; tolerance to the euphoric effects and motor stimulation is slower
- withdrawal leads to prolonged sleep, followed by fatigue, depression, anxiety, craving, and increased appetite.

MDMA (ecstasy) is more selective than amfetamine for serotonin release, and produces euphoria similar to that of amfetamine but with less stimulant activity. Disturbance of thermoregulatory homeostasis occurs, leading to a syndrome resembling heat stroke with hyperthermia and dehydration, usually after exertion in hot environments. Stimulation of antidiuretic hormone release can cause thirst and water retention with subsequent water intoxication and hyponatraemia. The toxic effects of MDMA include cardiac arrhythmias, seizures, muscle damage and severe metabolic acidosis, which may be fatal. The long-term toxicity is unknown.

Pharmacokinetics

Although amfetamine is sometimes used intravenously or via nasal inhalation, absorption from the gut is rapid and complete. Amfetamine readily crosses the blood–brain barrier. About half is excreted unchanged in the urine, and the rest is metabolised in the liver. The half-life of amfetamine varies according to urine flow and pH; at low urine pH greater ionisation increases excretion to produce a shorter half-life, whereas at high urine pH the half-life is longer because of renal tubular reabsorption of the drug. Metabolites of amfetamine are believed to contribute to the psychotic effects seen with long-term use.

Ecstasy is usually taken orally. It undergoes hepatic metabolism via CYP2D6, and polymorphism of this enzyme may explain some of the serious intoxication that occurs with the drug, although the half-life does not differ much between poor and extensive metabolisers (about 5 h in both).

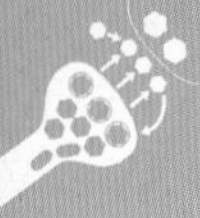

Nicotine and tobacco

Mechanism of action

Over 300 chemical compounds are present in tobacco smoke, but the actions of nicotine are central to the addictive pharmacological effects of smoking. Nicotine has dose-related peripheral actions. At low doses, stimulation of aortic and carotid chemoreceptors enhances sympathetic nervous system activity (Ch. 4). At higher doses, there is direct stimulation of the nicotinic N_1 receptors on autonomic ganglia (Ch. 4). At even higher doses, nicotine acts as a ganglion-blocking agent. Initial stimulation of autonomic nervous tissue is therefore followed by depression. Effects on the CNS are mediated by presynaptic nicotinic receptors structurally distinct from those in the periphery. Stimulation of CNS nicotinic receptors increases neuronal permeability to Na^+ and K^+, and inhibits the release of gamma-aminobutyric acid (GABA) and enhances the release of glutamate and dopamine. Nicotinic receptors are found in the mesocortical and mesolimbic dopaminergic systems, in projections from the ventral forebrain to the cortex that mediate arousal, and in hippocampal projections where stimulation enhances learning and short-term memory. Tolerance to the CNS effects of nicotine is rapid.

Effects of nicotine and tobacco

Tobacco components, including nicotine, have effects on a number of organ systems.

Respiratory effects

The lungs are the first area to be in contact with the chemical components of tobacco smoke and are also exposed to particles and gases. Tars and other irritants, rather than nicotine, are responsible for the chronic damage to the lungs.

- An increase in blood carboxyhaemoglobin concentration (from carbon monoxide in tobacco smoke) decreases oxygen-carrying capacity. This may be important in ischaemic heart disease, increasing the chance of provoking angina.
- Increased mucus secretion, with reduced activity of bronchial cilia and consequent decreased clearance of lung secretions, leads to chronic bronchitis.
- Progressive destruction of the supporting tissue in the bronchioles produces emphysema and chronic obstructive lung disease. Smoking is now the major cause of this condition.
- The risk of lung cancer is increased to about 20 times that of a non-smoker. Inhalation of tobacco smoke is a major contributory factor and explains the greater risk in cigarette smokers. Giving up smoking reduces the risk progressively over about 10 years of abstinence. The constituent of tobacco smoke responsible for altering DNA structure and initiating the cancer process remains controversial, but the relationship between smoking and lung cancer has been confirmed by numerous epidemiological studies. Compared with non-smokers, passive smokers also have a 20–25% increased risk of lung cancer.

Cardiovascular effects

- Stimulation of the autonomic nervous system and sensory receptors in the heart increases heart rate, blood pressure and cardiac output.
- The risk of cardiovascular disease is increased by smoking cigarettes, but not by pipe and cigar smoking, and it occurs at a younger age. The overall risk of death from coronary artery disease is doubled in smokers compared with non-smokers, and the magnitude of the effect is related to the numbers of cigarettes smoked. Peripheral vascular disease and stroke are also increased. Even passive smokers have an excess risk of vascular disease of 25%. The major reason for the excess of events is accelerated formation of atheromatous plaques, while contributory effects include increased plasma fatty acids and enhanced platelet aggregability. The risk of vascular disease falls over the first 3–5 years after stopping smoking to a level close to that of non-smokers.

Psychological effects

The psychological effects of smoking are substantial, as indicated by the difficulties experienced by those 'giving up' smoking.

- Decreased appetite, with weight gain on stopping smoking.
- Emotional dependence on nicotine and the physical act of smoking is powerful. Physical withdrawal is less marked than psychological withdrawal but includes restlessness, irritability, anxiety, depression, difficulty concentrating, sleep disturbance and increased appetite.

Other effects

Nicotine and smoking have a number of other effects.

- Peptic ulceration is twice as common in smokers.
- Smoking in pregnancy, especially during the second half, has several effects. The most important are an increased risk of a low-birthweight child, and increased perinatal mortality. The vasoconstrictor effects of nicotine are responsible. Physical and mental development is slowed in children born to mothers who smoked during pregnancy.
- Smoking induces several hepatic cytochrome P450 isoenzymes (Ch. 2), and increases the clearance of CYP1A2 substrates such as theophylline (Ch. 12) and imipramine (Ch. 22).

Pharmacokinetics of nicotine

Nicotine is absorbed from the mouth in its un-ionised form, which is found in the less acidic environment of cigar and pipe tobacco smoke. Cigarette smoke, which is acidic, ionises nicotine, which can then only be absorbed in significant amounts from the lungs. About 10% of the nicotine from a cigarette is absorbed, but at a faster rate than from cigars or a pipe owing to the larger surface area of the lungs, and results in a higher, but less prolonged, peak plasma concentration. Nicotine can also be absorbed transdermally. It is metabolised in the liver; the major metabolite, cotinine, has a much longer half-life (about

10–40 h) than nicotine (0.5–2 h) and its plasma concentration can be used as a monitor of smoking behaviour.

Dependence on and withdrawal from nicotine

Withdrawal is often difficult to achieve unless motivation is high. Patients should be supported by counselling about health benefits of quitting and advice on overcoming problems, such as weight gain. Behavioural therapy as an aid to quitting has a success rate of 20% at 1 year. Pharmacotherapy is often used to reduce the intensity of withdrawal symptoms.

Nicotine replacement therapy

Smokers usually adjust their smoking habit to maintain plasma nicotine concentrations just above a threshold that averts withdrawal symptoms. The plasma concentration falls rapidly within 1–2 h of the last cigarette, and rather more slowly after smoking a cigar or pipe. The resultant craving for nicotine can be reduced by nicotine replacement. This can be delivered via transdermal patches, sublingual tablets, chewing gum, an inhaler (with most absorption occurring in the mouth) or a nasal spray. The delivery method determines the rate at which plasma nicotine concentrations increase; this is most rapid after the nasal spray. The individual can choose the most appropriate vehicle for his or her needs and preferences. Established cardiovascular disease is a caution for, but not a contraindication to, nicotine replacement therapy. Behavioural therapy enhances the success rate achieved by nicotine replacement therapy. Use of nicotine replacement therapy doubles the chance of achieving abstinence.

Bupropion

This is an atypical antidepressant. Most antidepressants are ineffective for smoking cessation, but the use of bupropion gives smoking cessation rates equal to, or slightly greater than, nicotine replacement therapy. Treatment should be started 1–2 weeks before a 'quit date'. Used together with nicotine replacement therapy, bupropion produces a modest increase in the chance of stopping. An additional benefit is that smokers who use bupropion as an aid to quitting are less likely to gain weight. Bupropion is a weak inhibitor of neuronal reuptake of noradrenaline and dopamine, and probably works by enhancing mesolimbic dopaminergic activity. It is given as a modified-release formulation and has a long half-life (24 h). Elimination is by hepatic metabolism, which also generates active metabolites. Unwanted effects include anxiety, headache, insomnia and dry mouth. There is an increased risk of epileptic seizures, and bupropion should be avoided if there is a past history of seizures. Recent evidence indicates that, in contrast to other antidepressants that have been studied, nortriptyline is as effective as bupropion for smoking cessation.

Varenicline

This is a partial agonist at nicotine receptors, with high selectivity for the CNS receptor subtype involved in addiction. It produces about 30–45% of the response expected from nicotine, and blocks the effect of added nicotine. The modest release of dopamine reduces craving and nicotine withdrawal symptoms. Treatment should be started 1–2 weeks before a 'quit date', and combined with behavioural support. The oral bioavailability of varenicline has not been defined; it is excreted unchanged by the kidney and has a half-life of 24 h. Unwanted effects include gastrointestinal disturbances, dry mouth, headache, dizziness, drowsiness and sleep disturbance. Depression with suicidal thoughts has also been reported.

PSYCHOTOMIMETIC AGENTS

Hallucinogens

Lysergic acid diethylamide (LSD), psilocybin ('magic mushrooms'), mescaline (from peyote cactus) and the synthetic drug dimethyltryptamine (DMT) are adrenergic hallucinogens that have structural similarities to monoamine neurotransmitters. LSD is the most potent hallucinogen.

Mechanism of action and effects

The actions of hallucinogens on the brain are probably related to postsynaptic $5HT_2$ receptor stimulation in the cerebral cortex and locus ceruleus, a region of the midbrain that receives sensory signals. LSD also produces presynaptic $5HT_{1A}$ receptor blockade in the dorsal raphe neurons, inhibiting firing of neuronal projections to the forebrain. Tolerance to LSD occurs rapidly, and appears to be related to downregulation of these receptors. The actions of LSD, psilocybin and mescaline are similar, and they share several properties, including cross-tolerance.

- Visual hallucinations are frequent, especially with high doses, and auditory acuity is accentuated. There may be an overlap of sensory impressions such that music is 'seen' or colours 'heard', which can produce severe anxiety. Time appears to pass slowly. Emotions are altered, with either elation or depression, and rapid mood swings can occur. The overall experience can produce a 'good' or a 'bad' 'trip', and can vary in the same individual on different occasions.
- Serious psychotic reactions can occasionally occur, and long-term psychotic disorders can be precipitated. The other unpleasant persistent effect in some individuals is 'flashback', seeing bright flashes, or halos or trails attached to moving objects.
- Physical consequences of CNS stimulation include dizziness, weakness, drowsiness and paraesthesiae.
- Excessive sympathetic nervous system stimulation with large doses produces nausea, salivation, lacrimation, dizziness, mydriasis, tremor, hyperthermia, tachycardia and hypertension.
- Tolerance can occur within 5 days.
- Emotional dependence is frequent, but physical dependence is not seen.

Pharmacokinetics

Oral absorption of these drugs is good. Physical effects begin after about 20 min, but psychoactive effects are delayed for 2–4 h and then last up to 12 h. DMT has a rapid

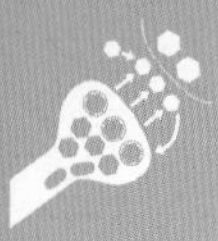

onset of hallucinogenic action, within 15–30 min, but the duration is only 1–2 h. Elimination is by hepatic metabolism and the half-lives are short.

Cannabis

Cannabis can be smoked as marijuana, which consists of dried leaves or flowers of the *Cannabis sativa* (hemp) plant, or as a resin extracted from the leaves of the plant and then dried, known as hashish. Solvent extraction of the resin produces cannabis oil, which can be added to tobacco. The hallucinogenic effects of cannabis are much less marked than those of the aminergic hallucinogens such as LSD.

Mechanism of action and effects

The constituent compounds (cannabinoids) interact with specific CB_1 receptors in the brain. These receptors are coupled to G_i proteins that reduce intracellular cAMP production, and inhibit cell membrane Ca^{2+} and K^+ channels. The natural ligands are the arachidonic acid derivatives anandamide, 2-arachidonylglycerol and noladin ether. CB_1 receptors are found in greatest density in areas of the brain involved in cognition and pain recognition (cerebral cortex), memory (hippocampus), reward (mesolimbic system) and motor coordination (substantia nigra and cerebellum).

- The psychomotor effects result largely from tetrahydrocannabinol (THC) and one of its metabolites, 11-hydroxy-THC, which produce euphoria, heightened intensity of sensations, and relaxation. Occasionally, panic reactions, hallucinations and depersonalisation can occur. Psychotic reactions are rare except in predisposed individuals, but recent evidence shows that the use of cannabis substantially increases the risk of developing schizophrenia. Recent memory is markedly impaired and complex mental tests are executed less well, although the user may perceive that their performance is enhanced. Motor incoordination may affect driving ability.
- Effects on the cardiovascular system include tachycardia and increased systolic blood pressure with a postural fall.
- The tars inhaled during chronic use predispose to heart disease, chronic bronchitis and lung cancer.
- THC has an antiemetic action (Ch. 32), which may be useful during cancer chemotherapy (Ch. 52).
- Cannabinoids have analgesic effects that are used by some people with multiple sclerosis to control neuropathic pain.
- Tolerance to the psychomotor effects of cannabis occurs with regular use, and there is recent evidence of dependence.

Pharmacokinetics

Metabolism of THC is extensive, with some active metabolites being produced. The high lipid solubility of THC means that absorption from the lung or gut is high, and it has a large apparent volume of distribution (Ch. 2); however, because of its very rapid metabolism, its half-life is only 1.5 h. The psychomotor effects last for 2–3 h after inhalation.

Dissociative anaesthetics

Phencyclidine (PCP) and ketamine differ from adrenergic hallucinogens in their mode of action. Both drugs were developed as anaesthetics, but PCP was withdrawn because of severe adverse effects (hallucinations, mania, delirium and disorientation).

Mechanism of action and effects

Both drugs block the excitatory effects of glutamate at NMDA (N-methyl-D-aspartate) receptors. These receptors are abundant in the cortex, basal ganglia and sensory pathways of the CNS. PCP also releases dopamine from nerve terminals in a manner similar to amfetamine. The term dissociative anaesthetic refers to the feelings of detachment (dissociation) from the environment and self that are produced by the drugs. These are not true hallucinations.

- Acute effects include euphoria, decreased inhibition, a feeling of immense power, analgesia, altered perception of time and space, and depersonalisation. Ketamine creates a ‘mellow, colourful wonderworld’.
- Catatonic rigidity can occur, followed by ataxia and slurring of speech.
- Adverse experiences include confusion, restlessness, disorientation and impaired judgement. Irritability, paranoia, depression and anxiety are also common. Psychotic reactions are precipitated in susceptible people.
- Ketamine can produce near-death experiences.
- Persistent abuse of PCP leads to memory loss, speech and thought difficulties, and depression that persist for months after the last use.
- Tolerance is unusual, but psychological dependence occurs.

Pharmacokinetics

PCP is rapidly absorbed from the gut, nose or lungs after smoking. Effects are seen within minutes of ingestion and usually last 4–6 h. It is a weak base that is excreted in the urine. It is also excreted into the stomach, and reabsorbed by the small intestine. The half-life is variable and can be up to 2 days. Ketamine is abused intravenously. It is metabolised in the liver and has a short half-life (see Ch. 17).

CNS DEPRESSANTS

Alcohol (ethyl alcohol, ethanol)

Mechanism of action and effects

Alcohol has multiple actions on the CNS. Non-specific actions such as increased fluidity of neuronal cell membranes (cf. general anaesthetics) may be important by reducing Ca^{2+} flux across the cell membrane, but several other actions have been described (Box 54.2). Overall, alcohol facilitates central inhibitory neurotransmission, particularly enhancing the effects of GABA, and therefore it is

Box 54.2 Possible mechanisms of action of alcohol

Inhibition of monoamine oxidase B in neurons
Inhibition of Na^+/K^+-ATPase in neuronal membranes
Increased neuronal adenylyl cyclase activity
Decreased intracellular phosphatidylinositol system activity, leading to reduced Ca^{2+} availability
Enhanced opioid δ-receptor activation

Table 54.1 The effects of alcohol at various plasma concentrations

Plasma concentration (mg 100 mL^{-1})	Effects
30	Mild euphoria owing to suppression of inhibitory pathways in the cortex; the individual is more talkative, emotionally labile with loss of self-control; the risk of accidental injury is increased
80	The legal limit for driving in the UK; the risk of serious injury in a road accident is more than doubled
100–200	Speech becomes slurred and motor coordination is impaired
>300	Often produces loss of consciousness
>400	Frequently fatal as a result of respiratory and vasomotor centre depression

Box 54.3 Alcoholic content of alcoholic drinks

1 unit of alcohol is about 10 g and is found in:

- ½ pint of normal-strength beer, lager, cider
- 1½ pints of low-alcohol beer, lager, cider
- ⅓ pint of strong beer, lager, cider
- ⅕ pint of extra-strong beer, lager, cider
- 1 glass of wine (8 units per 75 cl bottle)
- 1 small measure of sherry (13 units per bottle)
- 1 standard measure of spirits (30 units per bottle)
- ⅔ bottle of 'alcopop'

a general CNS depressant. With acute alcohol intake, there is an initial depression of inhibitory neurons, particularly in the mesolimbic system, which produces a sense of relaxation, but this is followed by progressive depression of all CNS functions. Mental processes that are modified by education, training and previous experience are affected first, while relatively 'mechanical' tasks are less impaired. Despite subjective impressions, there is no increase in mental or physical capabilities, unless anxiety has previously reduced performance. All effects are closely related to blood alcohol concentration (Table 54.1).

In people who regularly use large amounts of alcohol, tolerance is seen to many of its psychological effects. Alcohol increases dopamine release in the nucleus accumbens indirectly by activating GABA receptors or inhibiting NMDA receptors. Long-term use of alcohol produces long-lasting adaptive changes in the NMDA receptor that enhance their function. Opioid and serotonin receptor stimulation is also involved in the reinforcing effects of alcohol on the brain.

Alcohol intake is usually measured in units (Box 54.3).

Other effects of alcohol

Alcohol has a range of effects.

Cardiovascular effects

- A modest alcohol intake may have protective effects on the circulation, by inhibiting platelet aggregation and increasing high-density lipoprotein cholesterol. The form in which the alcohol is taken is probably not important. The extent of this beneficial effect is probably greatest at 1 unit per day and is lost when intake exceeds 3–4 units per day.
- Higher intake of alcohol has pressor effects that raise blood pressure, possibly through increased vascular sensitivity to catecholamines. This increases the risk of coronary artery disease and stroke.
- Cardiac arrhythmias can be provoked by high alcohol intake, particularly atrial fibrillation. This can occur after an alcoholic binge ('holiday heart' syndrome) or following more chronic abuse (Ch. 8).
- Alcoholic cardiomyopathy is a dilated cardiomyopathy that is only partially reversible with abstinence, and can lead to heart failure. An average intake of 10 units of alcohol daily for 8–10 years can produce this condition.

Liver

- Hypoglycaemia occurs as a consequence of the metabolism of alcohol in the liver. The metabolic process generates excess protons, which enhance the conversion of glucose, via pyruvate, to lactate and predisposes to lactic acidosis. Alcoholics often have a low-carbohydrate diet, which compounds the hypoglycaemia. Hypoglycaemia tends to occur several hours after heavy alcohol intake and can contribute to convulsions on alcohol withdrawal.
- The lactic acidosis created by alcohol metabolism in the liver impairs the renal excretion of uric acid, which predisposes to gout.
- Lactic acidosis also facilitates the synthesis of saturated fatty acids, which accumulate in the liver, leading to a fatty liver, possibly with altered liver function. Plasma triglycerides are also increased.
- Alcoholic hepatitis is usually a consequence of short-term heavy alcohol abuse. It can be fatal.
- Cirrhosis occurs with prolonged alcohol abuse, but individual susceptibility varies widely. On average, consumption of more than 8 units per day for at least 10 years is required for cirrhosis to occur in men. About two-thirds of this amount creates the same risk for women. Established cirrhosis reduces the first-pass metabolism and clearance of drugs eliminated by the liver (Ch. 56).
- Chronic intake of alcohol induces hepatic drug-metabolising enzymes, especially CYP2E1, which decreases the effectiveness of some therapeutic drugs, for example warfarin, phenytoin and carbamazepine.

Other gastrointestinal consequences

- Erosive gastritis can occur as a result of stimulation of gastric secretions.
- Pancreatitis is probably caused by raised triglycerides or by pancreatic duct obstruction by proteinaceous secretions induced by alcohol.

Sexual function

- Sexual desire is often increased by alcohol, but the ability to sustain penile erection is reduced, possibly because of the vasodilator actions of alcohol.
- Direct damage to the Leydig cells of the testis reduces the circulating testosterone, leading to reduced libido, infertility and a loss of the male distribution of body hair. Altered steroid metabolism in the liver leads to an increase in circulating oestrone in males, which causes gynaecomastia.

Neuropsychiatric effects

- A combination of alcohol toxicity with deficiencies of vitamin B_6 and thiamine in the diet of alcoholics predisposes to peripheral neuropathy and dementia. Specific mid-brain damage can result and produces the syndromes of Wernicke's encephalopathy and Korsakoff's psychosis.
- Alcohol has anticonvulsant properties and withdrawal predisposes to seizures, even in individuals without a history of epilepsy.
- Alcohol can disturb sleep patterns, with decreased rapid eye movement (REM) sleep and increased stage 4 sleep during intoxication. Withdrawal increases REM sleep, with associated nightmares (Ch. 20).
- Dose-related memory impairment can be caused by suppressed hippocampal function.
- Subdural haematoma is more common after head injury in heavy drinkers, perhaps as a consequence of cerebral atrophy.
- Depression or anxiety states are more common in heavy drinkers.

Carcinogenesis and teratogenesis

- Cancer of the mouth, oesophagus and liver are more common with heavy alcohol use. Colon and breast cancer may also be increased.
- The fetal alcohol syndrome is believed to be caused by the effects of alcohol on neuronal adhesion molecules that regulate neuronal migration. Heavy maternal drinking during pregnancy leads to impaired learning and memory in the child. Genetic factors may be involved in the susceptibility of the fetus to these problems.

Pharmacokinetics

Although ethanol is absorbed from the stomach, the majority is absorbed from the small intestine, due to its larger surface area. High concentrations of alcohol (above 20%) and large volumes inhibit gastric emptying and delay absorption, as do foods high in fat or carbohydrate. Peak blood alcohol concentrations, therefore, depend on the dose and strength of the alcohol and on whether or not it was taken with food. Following absorption, alcohol undergoes substantial first-pass metabolism in the liver. The extent of first-pass metabolism of alcohol is related to the speed of absorption; thus, with slower absorption, such as when alcohol is taken with food, less alcohol will reach the systemic circulation. Distribution of alcohol is fairly uniform and the ready passage across the blood–brain barrier and high cerebral blood flow ensure rapid access to the CNS. The effects on the brain are more marked when the concentration is rising, indicating a degree of acute tolerance.

Metabolism occurs mainly in the liver (Fig. 54.2), more than 90% being oxidised, mainly by alcohol dehydrogenase, while the rest is removed unchanged in expired air (in direct proportion to the blood concentration, which is the basis of the alcohol breath test) or in the urine. Alcohol metabolism shows saturation kinetics due to the limited supply of nicotine adenine nucleotide (NAD^+), which is the cofactor for the oxidative process. The maximum rate of alcohol metabolism averages 8 g h^{-1}. The initial metabolic reaction is mediated by alcohol dehydrogenase, producing acetaldehyde, which is subsequently metabolised by alde-

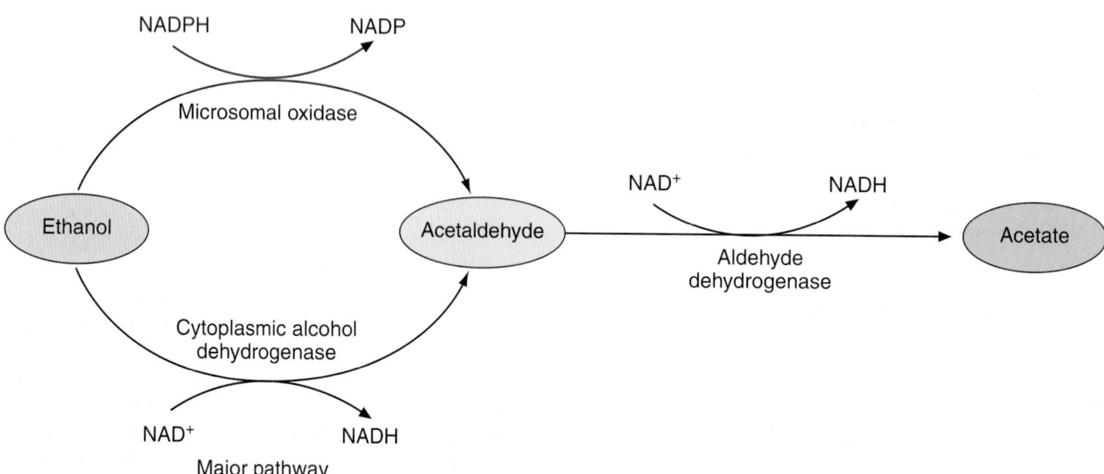

Fig. 54.2 **The metabolism of alcohol.** Alcohol dehydrogenase is responsible for 80–90% of the metabolism of ethanol.

hyde dehydrogenase to acetic acid (Fig. 54.2). Genetic variability in alcohol and aldehyde dehydrogenases occurs among ethnic groups, leading to different capacities for alcohol or aldehyde metabolism. Accumulation of acetaldehyde in the circulation is responsible for many of the unpleasant effects of a hangover. Small amounts of alcohol are metabolised via the microsomal ethanol oxidising system (CYP2E1), the activity of which is increased by enzyme inducers such as alcohol itself (which does not affect the activity of alcohol dehydrogenase) (Ch. 36).

Some drugs, such as metronidazole (Ch. 51) and chlorpropamide (Ch. 40), inhibit aldehyde dehydrogenase, leading to acetaldehyde accumulation if alcohol is taken with them. Typical 'hangover' effects of flushing, sweating, headache and nausea then occur after even small amounts of alcohol.

Alcohol abuse and dependence

There are no reliable estimates of the number of people in the UK with alcohol-related problems, although it has been suggested that 1–2% of the population are affected. The distribution curve for alcohol consumption is continuous but skewed at higher alcohol intakes. The risk of alcohol-related problems rises with the average alcohol intake. Up to 30% of hospital admissions are for alcohol-related problems, although the contribution of heavy drinking is often unrecognised. Screening for alcohol abuse can be carried out by obtaining a complete history of alcohol intake and, if necessary, using the CAGE questions (Box 54.4). Abnormal measurements of both the mean corpuscular volume (MCV) of red cells (which is raised with increasing alcohol intake because of an effect of alcohol on the cell membrane) and the liver enzyme γ-glutamyl transpeptidase (γGT) will identify about 75% of people with an alcohol problem.

Psychological dependence on alcohol is common, but physical dependence also occurs. Withdrawal symptoms occur 6–24 h after the last drink in dependent persons. If mild, these are related to autonomic hyperactivity and include anxiety, agitation, tremor, sweating, anorexia, nausea and retching. Convulsions can occur through neuronal excitation. Insomnia, tachycardia and hypertension are common with more severe withdrawal reactions. The most severe form of withdrawal is *delirium tremens*, with confusion, paranoia, and visual and tactile hallucinations. Delirium tremens can cause death from respiratory and cardiovascular collapse.

If an individual is drinking excessively, controlled drinking may be an option. However, if there is alcohol dependence or alcohol-related problems, then abstinence is usually preferable.

Controlled detoxification is usually undertaken with a sedative agent, such as a benzodiazepine (Ch. 20), to attenuate withdrawal symptoms. Chlordiazepoxide or diazepam is usually used, decreasing the dose over 7–10 days. Clonidine (a presynaptic α_2-adrenoceptor agonist at the vasomotor centre in the brain; Ch. 6) can be useful, by reducing the excessive sympathetic stimulation that accompanies withdrawal. Beta-adrenoceptor antagonists (Ch. 5) may be helpful for the same reason. Multivitamin preparations containing an adequate amount of thiamine should be given for 1 month to prevent Wernicke's encephalopathy. Relapse is common after withdrawal from alcohol.

Two drugs are licensed in the UK to assist in the management of chronic alcoholism. **Disulfiram**, an inhibitor of acetaldehyde dehydrogenase, causes unpleasant hangover symptoms after small amounts of alcohol. Given alone, or with psychosocial rehabilitation, it can help to maintain abstinence. **Acamprosate** inhibits the excitatory amino acid glutamate by antagonism at the NMDA receptor, although several other contributory effects have been suggested. It has few unwanted effects, is non-addictive and can be used to reduce the craving for alcohol. **Naltrexone**, a long-acting opioid receptor antagonist can reduce the craving associated with alcohol withdrawal. It is not licensed for this indication in the UK.

Box 54.4 The CAGE questionnaire for alcoholism

Have you ever felt you could Cut down on your drinking?
Have people Annoyed you by criticising your drinking?
Have you ever felt bad or Guilty about your drinking?
Have you ever had a drink first thing in the morning to steady your nerves or get rid of a hangover (Eye-opener)?

An answer of yes to one question or more should lead to further evaluation of the patient for alcoholism.

Gamma-hydroxybutyric acid (GHB)

Mechanism of action and effects

Gamma-hydroxybutyric acid was originally introduced as a general anaesthetic, but is now used illegally as an intoxicant, a 'date rape' drug, or by athletes to improve performance. GHB acts as an agonist at a specific inhibitory GHB receptor in the cortex and hippocampus of the brain, and also as an agonist at $GABA_B$ receptors, which mediate its sedative effects. GHB receptor activation stimulates dopamine release. GHB receptor stimulation also increases growth hormone release, which is the basis of its abuse by athletes and bodybuilders. In a similar manner to ethanol, GHB produces euphoria, increased libido and increased sociability. At high doses it produces nausea, dizziness, drowsiness, agitation, visual disturbances, amnesia and coma. Both psychological and physical dependence occur. Withdrawal can be treated with baclofen (Ch. 24).

Pharmacokinetics

GHB is usually taken orally, occasionally intravenously. It has low oral bioavailability, is metabolised in the liver, and has a short half-life of 30–60 min. The clinical effect lasts for 1.5–3 h, and longer if taken with alcohol.

Inhaled solvents

Various organic solvents are abused as recreational drugs. Examples include butane, toluene and diethyl ether. Inhalation via a plastic bag held over the mouth or from an open container produces rapid intoxication resembling that produced by alcohol. These compounds probably act in a similar way to volatile general anaesthetics (Ch. 17). Death can occur from asphyxiation during inhalation, while long-term use produces brain damage by increasing neuronal apoptosis.

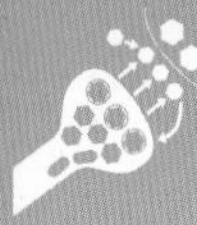

FURTHER READING

Anton RF (2008) Naltrexone for the management of alcohol dependence. *N Engl J Med* 359, 715–721

Aveyard P, West R (2007) Managing smoking cessation. *BMJ* 335, 37–41

Barlecchi CE, MacKenzie TD, Schrier RW (1994) The human cost of tobacco. *N Engl J Med* 330, 907–912, 975–980

Benowitz NL (2008) Neurobiology of nicotine addiction: implications for smoking cessation treatment. *Am J Med* 121(suppl 4A), S3–S10

Berke JD, Hyman SE (2000) Addiction, dopamine, and the molecular mechanisms of memory. *Neuron* 25, 515–532

Cami J, Farre M (2003) Drug addiction. *N Engl J Med* 349, 975–986

Gerdeman GL, Partridge JG, Lupica, CR et al (2003) It could be habit forming: drugs of abuse and striatal synaptic plasticity. *Trends Neurosci* 26, 184–192

Hall W, Solowij N (1998) Adverse effects of cannabis. *Lancet* 352, 1611–1616

Hatsukami DK, Stead LF, Gupta PC (2008) Tobacco addiction. *Lancet* 371, 2027–2038

Hays JT, Ebbert JO (2008) Varenicline for tobacco dependence. *N Engl J Med* 359, 2018–2024

Koob GF (2006) The neurobiology of addiction: a neuroadaptational view relevant for diagnosis. *Addiction* 101(suppl 1), 23–30

Kosten TR, O'Connor PG (2003) Management of drug and alcohol withdrawal. *N Engl J Med* 348, 1786–1795

Lancaster T, Hajek P, Stead LF et al (2006) Prevention of relapse after quitting smoking. *Arch Intern Med* 166, 828–835

Mendelson JH, Mello NK (1996) Management of cocaine abuse and dependence. *N Engl J Med* 334, 965–972

Moore THM, Zammit S, Lingford-Hughes A et al (2007) Cannabis use and risk of psychotic or affective mental health outcomes: a systematic review. *Lancet* 370, 319–328

Nides M (2008) Update on pharmacologic options for smoking cessation treatment. *Am J Med* 121(suppl 4A), S20–S31

Parker AJ, Marshall EJ, Ball DM (2008) Diagnosis and management of alcohol use disorder. *BMJ* 336, 496–501

Rigotti A (2002) Treatment of tobacco use and dependence. *N Engl J Med* 346, 506–512

Saitz R (2005) Unhealthy alcohol use. *N Engl J Med* 352, 596–607

Schippenberg TS, Zapata A, Chefer VI (2007) Dynorphin and the pathophysiology of drug addiction. *Pharmacol Ther* 116, 306–321

Schuckit MA (2009) Alcohol-use disorders. *Lancet* 373, 492–501

Snead OC, Gibson KM (2005) γ-Hydroxybutyric acid. *N Engl J Med* 352, 2721–2732

Sullivan LE, Fiellin DA (2008) Narrative review: Buprenorphine for opioid-dependent patients in office practice. *Ann Intern Med* 148, 662–670

SELF-ASSESSMENT

In the following questions, the first statement, in italics, is true. Are the following statements also true?

1. *Cocaine potently inhibits the uptake of noradrenaline into nerve terminals and this is the explanation for its mydriatic effect.*
   a. 'Crack' cocaine is the free-base form of cocaine.
   b. Cocaine can be given topically into the eye to test for Horner's syndrome.
   c. Prolonged cocaine use has little damaging effect on the cardiovascular system.
   d. Tolerance to the euphoric and anorexic effects of cocaine develops rapidly.
2. *MDMA (ecstasy) causes the release of serotonin from nerve endings while inhibiting serotonin uptake.*
   a. Adverse effects of taking ecstasy in some individuals are hyperthermia and dehydration.
   b. Ecstasy suppresses appetite.
   c. Amphetamines are used to treat ADHD.
3. *Cannabis may impair driving ability and the performance of complex mental tasks, and give rise to psychotic reactions in predisposed individuals.*
   a. The euphoria caused by cannabis lasts for 24 h.
   b. THC, the active ingredient of cannabis, causes nausea and vomiting.
   c. Cannabis acts on specific receptors in the brain.
4. *Nicotine induces very strong psychological and also a physical dependence.*
   a. Tolerance to the effects of nicotine develops very slowly.
   b. Nicotine causes tachycardia and reduced gut motility.
   c. Cotinine, a metabolite of nicotine, has a long half-life and can be measured in serum to determine smoking habits.
   d. Nicotine patches given alone are the optimum method for someone giving up smoking.
   e. A physical withdrawal symptom does not occur when giving up smoking.
5. *Ethanol is metabolised in the liver to a toxic substance, acetaldehyde, which is then further metabolised to acetic acid.*
   a. Chronic intake of alcohol induces hepatic drug-metabolising enzymes.
   b. A modest intake of alcohol increases the incidence of cardiovascular disease.
   c. Some individuals have a genetically determined low ability to metabolise ethanol.
6. *One approach to reduce alcohol intake is to inhibit acetaldehyde metabolism with disulfiram, which causes sickness, headache and hangover symptoms following a small amount of alcohol intake.*
   a. Acamprosate, which is used to encourage abstinence, acts to reduce alcohol metabolism in a similar way to disulfiram.
   b. The severity of symptoms of withdrawal from ethanol consumption (detoxification) cannot be controlled by pharmacological means.
7. *Up to one-third of hospital admissions are for alcohol-related problems.*
   a. Ethanol can cause a macrocytosis.
   b. Ethanol enhances antidiuretic hormone secretion.
   c. The plasma levels of the liver enzyme γ-glutamyl transpeptidase are depressed with heavy ethanol intake.

ANSWERS

1. a. **True**. Unlike the salt form of cocaine, the free base can be illicitly smoked.

b. **True**. In the absence of sympathetic supply to the iris in Horner's syndrome, cocaine will not cause mydriasis.
c. **False**. Acute actions are cardiac arrhythmias, and chronic use can lead to heart failure.
d. **True**. Tolerance develops to euphoria and appetite suppression in only a few days.

2. a. **True**. Malignant hyperthermia is observed in some individuals after ingesting ecstasy. This resembles heat stroke and dehydration.
b. **True**. Like other amphetamines, ecstasy has a short-term effect to suppress appetite.
c. **True**. Amphetamines can be used to treat ADHD (not an approved use in UK).

3. a. **False**. The euphoric effects last only 2–3 h.
b. **False**. The related cannabinoid, nabilone, is used to inhibit nausea and vomiting in patients taking cytotoxic drugs.
c. **True**. Cannabis acts on cannabinoid receptors in the brain and periphery. The natural ligands for these receptors include anandamide.

4. a. **False**. Tolerance develops rapidly.
b. **True**. These effects are caused by stimulation of autonomic ganglia.
c. **True**. Cotinine is stable and inactive, and can be measured.
d. **False**. Nicotine patches and counselling are required.
e. **False**. Irritability, sleep disturbances and reduced psychomotor test performance occur on giving up smoking.

5. a. **True**. The induction of CYP2E1 can decrease the effectiveness of some drugs such as warfarin and phenytoin.
b. **False**. Modest ethanol intake can increase high-density lipoprotein concentrations, which has cardiovascular protective effects. This is lost if consumption is greater than 3–4 units per day.
c. **True**. Some individuals have a genetically determined variant of alcohol dehydrogenase that has reduced ability to metabolise ethanol. This incidence is low in Caucasians but high in some Asian races.

6. a. **False**. Acamprosate acts to reduce craving for alcohol and not by affecting its metabolism.
b. **False**. Benzodiazepines or chlordiazepoxide can attenuate withdrawal symptoms but there is a risk of dependence to these agents.

7. a. **True**. Ethanol intake is a common cause of macrocytosis (increased red cell volume) in the absence of anaemia.
b. **False**. The diuresis resulting from ethanol intake is partly caused by inhibition of release of antidiuretic hormone.
c. **False**. Plasma γ-glutamyl transpeptidase is elevated.

Drugs of abuse and drugs used to treat drug dependence

Drug	Half-life (h) and kinetics	Comments
Drugs of abuse		
Alcohol (ethyl alcohol, ethanol)	Zero order [M + R] Oxidation by alcohol dehydrogenase is saturated at normal intakes	
Amfetamine	8–10 [R + M] Rapidly absorbed; half-life is dependent on the urine pH (basic drug)	The dextro-isomer (dexamfetamine) is the active form and is sometimes used for treatment of hyperactivity in children (especially in the USA)
Benzodiazepines	–	See Ch. 20
Cannabis (delta-9-tetrahydrocannabinol or THC)	1.5 [M] Oxidised in the liver to metabolites which have slightly longer half-lives and are eliminated in urine and faeces	Delta-9-tetrahydrocannabinol is the main active constituent
Cocaine	1–1.5 [M + R] Oral bioavailability is 30–40%; oxidised and hydrolysed in the liver; about 10% excreted unchanged in urine	Has very limited use as a non-injection local anaesthetic; abuse involves non-oral routes (mostly nasal or inhalation)
Ecstasy (3,4-methylenedioxy-methamphetamine; MDMA)	6 (*R*), 4 (*S*) [M + R] Peak plasma concentrations occur about 2 h after ingestion; half-lives differ slightly between the enantiomers; oxidised by CYP2D6 (polymorphism of which may explain in part the idiosyncratic cases of intoxication); saturation of metabolism may contribute to the risk of overdose	The amphetamine analogue (MDA) and ethylamphetamine analogue (MDE or 'Eve') show similar properties
Gamma-hydroxybutyric acid (GHB)	0.5–1 [M + R] Oral bioavailability is 25%; eliminated by hepatic oxidation with about 5% excreted unchanged	
Lysergic acid diethylamide (LSD)	3–5 [M + R] Eliminated by hepatic metabolism; 2-oxo-3-hydroxy-LSD is a major urinary metabolite; LSD is detectable in urine after oral dosage	

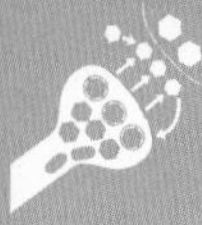

Drugs of abuse and drugs used to treat drug dependence

Drug	Half-life (h) and kinetics	Comments
Ketamine	2–4 [M]	See Ch. 17
Methamphetamine	10–12 [R + M] Rapidly absorbed after ingestion; about 40% excreted in urine unchanged; oxidised by CYP2D6; few data available; renal excretion is pH-dependent (methamphetamine is a metabolite of selegiline)	
Nicotine	0.5–2 [M + R] Very rapidly absorbed after inhalation; the main metabolite, cotinine, has a half-life of 10–40 h (and can be used to assess exposure)	
Opioids	–	See Ch. 19
Phencyclidine (PCP)	7–46 [M + R] Oral bioavailability is about 70%; oxidised in the liver to a number of metabolites; about 10% is excreted in urine unchanged	
Psilocybin	? (minutes) [M] Oxidised very rapidly by dephosphorylation to psilocin and also in the intestine to 4-hydroxyindole-3-acetic acid; few other data available	
Drugs used to treat drug dependence		
Cigarette smoking		
Bupropion	≈24 [M] Oral bioavailability is 5–20%; metabolised in the liver to the 3 major active metabolites; all active metabolites are present in higher concentrations in the plasma than is the parent compound	Used as an adjunct to smoking cessation; given orally
Nicotine	See above The kinetics are absorption rate-limited when given as a patch; peak nicotine plasma concentrations occur at 15–30 min with gum and 4–12 h after application of a patch compared with15 min after inhalation	Used as an adjunct to smoking cessation; given sublingually, as chewing gum, transdermally as a patch, or by inhaler or nasal spray
Varenicline	≈24 [R] Eliminated almost exclusively through glomerular filtration and active tubular secretion (by the transporter OCT2)	Used as an adjunct to smoking cessation; given orally
Alcohol dependence		
Acamprosate calcium	20–33 [R] Oral bioavailability is 11%; eliminated exclusively by renal excretion	Used for the maintenance of abstinence; given orally
Disulfiram	60–120 [M] About 20% excreted in faeces unchanged (due to incomplete absorption?); metabolised to diethylthiocarbamate and excreted slowly in expired air (as CS_2) and in urine	Used as an adjunct in the treatment of chronic alcohol dependence; given orally
Opioid dependence		
Opioid dependence is discussed in Ch. 19		
Buprenorphine	See Ch. 19	Used as an adjunct to treatment of dependence
Lofexidine	See Ch. 19	Used for management of symptoms of withdrawal
Methadone	See Ch. 19	Used as an adjunct to treatment of dependence
Naltrexone	See Ch. 19	Oral opioid receptor antagonist; longer duration of action than naloxone; used to prevent relapse in detoxified formerly opioid-dependent individuals

[M], metabolism; [R], renal excretion.

55 Prescribing, adherence and information about medicines

About 80% of medicines are prescribed in general practice (primary medical care). On average, men visit their general practitioners three to four times each year and women visit five times. A little over two-thirds of consultations end with the issuing of a prescription. Prescribing is particularly frequent for elderly people, who are likely to continue treatment for long periods of time. For these reasons, regular review of prescribed treatment should take place to determine whether it is still appropriate or necessary, and to ensure that important drug interactions and unwanted effects are not overlooked. Some drugs also require regular monitoring of efficacy (e.g. warfarin, antihypertensive treatment), blood concentrations (e.g. lithium) or for unwanted effects (e.g. amiodarone, thiazide diuretics).

DUTIES OF THE PRESCRIBER

There are certain legal requirements that must be met when a medicine is prescribed. The information to be recorded is:

- the name of the person for whom the drug is prescribed (surname and initial) and address; in the case of children up to 12 years, the person's age must be specified
- drug name (without abbreviation)
- dose
- route of administration (usually given on the manufacturer's product information rather than the prescription)
- frequency of administration (with minimum dose-interval for preparations to be taken 'as required')
- either the quantity to be supplied or the duration of therapy
- doctor's name, address and signature
- date.

Generic prescribing

In most situations, the generic name (the officially accepted chemical name) of the drug is preferred to the proprietary trade name (a 'brand' name approved for use by a specific pharmaceutical company). One advantage of the generic name is that it is likely to indicate the nature of the drug. For example, all β-adrenoceptor antagonist drugs (β-blockers) end with either -olol or –alol, such as atenolol, labetalol and metoprolol, but the trade names for these drugs, i.e. Tenormin®, Trandate® and Lopressor®, give little idea of the active ingredient. Another problem with trade names is that they rarely give any indication when there is more than one active ingredient; for example, Tenoret® contains both atenolol and chlortalidone. The generic names for many compound preparations have this indicated by the term 'co-'; for example, co-tenidone is the generic equivalent of Tenoret®. Because there are often different brand names for the same medicine, a person who is given a repeat prescription may become confused if prescribed their usual medicine under a different brand name.

Another advantage of generic prescribing is that pharmacists can dispense any product that meets the necessary specifications, rather than having to buy in a specific brand. This helps to simplify stock holding and avoids unnecessary delays when dispensing. However, different generic preparations of the same drug may differ in the tablet size, colour or scoring and therefore it is important to inform the person taking the drug if a different brand is dispensed.

Generic prescribing is sometimes cheaper than prescribing by trade name, although the difference depends on pack size and other commercial factors and is sometimes marginal. In recent years, there has been an increasing tendency for doctors to prescribe by generic name. It is likely that economic arguments have been the chief factor leading to this change.

Despite the advantages, generic prescribing can potentially create difficulties. For drugs with a narrow therapeutic index, such as anticonvulsants, oral anticoagulants and oral hypoglycaemic agents, drugs supplied from a different source could show differences in bioavailability of the active ingredient. Stringent controls have almost eliminated this problem, except for some modified-release formulations of drugs with a narrow therapeutic index, such as those for lithium or theophylline, for which different release characteristics can influence the plasma concentration profile of the drug. In these situations, prescribing by brand is recommended.

Dosage

The total exposure to a medicine during a course of treatment is related to the individual dose size, its frequency and the duration of therapy. The route of administration may also be important.

Dose

This is an essential item on all prescriptions and should be written in grams (g), milligrams (mg) or micrograms (which should not be abbreviated).

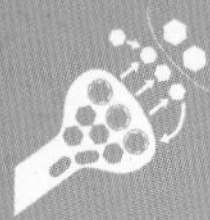

The route of administration

The route should be identified if there is any possibility of confusion. Confusion can arise with intravenous administration of drugs since there are numerous methods for delivery: drugs can be given by direct injection (either as a bolus or by slow injection) into a vein or can be infused, for example through the side-arm of a continuously running intravenous drip, via a motor-driven pump or added to the intravenous infusion fluid reservoir. It is particularly important when prescribing drugs for intravenous administration to make clear the precise intentions.

Frequency and times of administration

Sometimes, drugs are administered once only, while others must be given on a regular basis, in which case the frequency or times of administration should be specified, for example twice daily or at 12-h intervals.

The quantity to be supplied or the duration of therapy

Most general practice prescriptions specify the amount to be dispensed, for example the total number of tablets or capsules; the duration of therapy will then be determined by the amount dispensed and the frequency of dosage. Duration can be specified in a number of ways. When the medicine is to be dispensed by a health professional or by a carer in a sheltered environment, it can be specified on the prescription sheet. Alternatively, it can be written on the prescription to be dispensed by a pharmacist. Medicines are now dispensed in original packs with tablets individually packed by the pharmaceutical company. Specifying the duration of therapy is essential in the case of controlled drugs (preparations that are subject to the prescription requirements of the Misuse of Drugs Regulations 2001), such as opioids, for which there is a legal requirement that the total amount to be dispensed must be written in both figures and words.

Other items on a prescription

Other essential items on prescriptions include the doctor's signature and the address of his or her place of work. The latter is effectively waived for hospital prescriptions since it is assumed that the medical practitioner is based at the hospital in question. The prescription must be dated. Increasing use is now made of computer-issued prescriptions. The specific requirements for these are essentially similar to those outlined above. Computer-issued prescriptions avoid handwriting problems and assist in record keeping and in data accumulation and analysis.

Abbreviations

Directions for prescribing should preferably be in English (rather than Latin) without abbreviation. However, there are a number of abbreviations that are widely accepted. They include the following for route of administration: o or p.o., oral; i.v., intravenous; i.m., intramuscular; s.c., subcutaneous; and p.r., per rectum. Others, such as intrathecal, must not be abbreviated, because of the potential seriousness of inappropriate administration: inappropriate intrathecal administration of vincristine, for example, has caused the death of several people. Besides the abbreviations already listed for quantities, ml or mL is acceptable. Quantities of less than 1 g should be written in milligrams (e.g. 400 mg, rather than 0.4 g), whereas quantities of less than 1 mg should be written in micrograms (e.g. 500 micrograms [in full], rather than 0.5 mg; when handwritten, μg is easily mistaken for mg). Decimal points should be avoided wherever possible, but, if unavoidable, a zero should precede the decimal point when there is no figure (e.g. 0.5 mL, not .5 mL).

When indicating the timing of doses, od (omni die) is acceptable, but there is nothing wrong with saying once daily! The abbreviation om (omni mane) stands for in the morning and on (omni nocte) for at night; ac is short for ante cibum (before food) and pc for post cibum (after food). Twice daily can be abbreviated to bd (bis die), thrice daily to tds (ter die sumendus) and four times daily to qds (quater die sumendus).

ADHERENCE, CONCORDANCE AND COMPLIANCE

The term 'compliance' is used to describe the extent to which a person takes his or her medicine. However, other terms such as 'adherence' or 'concordance' are now preferred, because they emphasise the partnership between the person and health professions in the process of taking medicines, rather than simply following instructions. It is frequently assumed that once a prescription has been given, the recipient will automatically comply with the doctor's instructions. However, there is abundant evidence that this is often not the case. Indeed, many prescriptions are not even taken to the pharmacist for dispensing. Prescriptions are sometimes not presented to a pharmacist because of cost or because the doctor failed to discuss the 'hidden agenda' for which the presenting complaint was an excuse to see the doctor. In addition, a very substantial proportion of medicines collected are not taken in the manner intended.

The degree of adherence is affected by many factors, which include the duration of treatment. Less than 50% of people comply fully with long-term therapy, such as that for high blood pressure or psychotic illness. There is increasing evidence that adherence to prescribed therapy is associated with the outcome of treatment. For example, in treating hypertension, the control of blood pressure is substantially less good when adherence falls below 80% of prescribed doses.

The frequency of dosing has a major influence on adherence. Few people like taking their medicines with them to work. Therefore, adherence with twice-daily regimens tends to be much better than that for more frequent administration. There is a further improvement in the extent of adherence with once- rather than twice-daily dosing.

Unwanted effects can reduce the likelihood of a person complying with therapy, but at times this can be turned to an advantage. For example, giving the entire dose of a tricyclic antidepressant at night means that the sedation it produces can be used to aid sleep. Giving the person advanced warning of likely unwanted effects such as dry mouth with this compound may earn the person's trust and encourage him or her to continue therapy.

A proportion of non-adherence is caused by people forgetting whether or not they have taken their medicine on a particular day. The use of calendar packs or prepacked dispensing boxes can be helpful in this situation.

The individual's health beliefs are also particularly important. Adherence can be improved by involving the person in monitoring his or her disease and its control by therapy, for example home monitoring of blood pressure, blood sugar in diabetes mellitus, or peak flow measurements in people with asthma. Supplying accurate information about medicines can improve the level of satisfaction, and satisfied people are more likely to take their medicines.

INFORMING PEOPLE ABOUT THEIR MEDICINES

It is almost incredible to think that at one time doctors were reluctant to allow the name of a medicine to be shown on the container in which it was dispensed; however, paternalistic attitudes amongst the medical profession have been slow to disappear. Several surveys carried out in the early 1980s showed that most people felt that neither doctors nor pharmacists gave sufficient explanations about medicines. People are particularly keen to know:

- the name of the medicine
- the purposes of treatment
- when and how to take their medicine
- how long to take it for and what to do if a dose is missed
- unwanted effects and what to do about these
- any necessary precautions to take, such as possible effects on driving
- any problems with alcohol or with other drugs.

Manufacturers of pharmaceuticals now produce printed leaflets about medicines, which are included in original packs. However, leaflets are complementary to, and not a substitute for, discussion with the medical practitioner, pharmacist, practice nurse, etc. The Internet provides an increasingly rich source of information for people about their medicines and the variety of treatments available for their condition(s). However, advertising and the lack of peer-review of websites means that, in many cases, information the individual may have acquired before they first see their doctor may be incorrect and/or misunderstood.

RATIONAL PRESCRIBING

A definition of good prescribing has been proposed that encompasses four goals. These are to:

- maximise effectiveness
- minimise risks
- minimise costs
- respect the person's choice.

Irrational prescribing can take several forms, such as inappropriate polypharmacy (use of multiple drugs), the use of drugs that are not related to the diagnosis, the use of unnecessarily expensive drugs, the inappropriate use of antibiotics, or under-dosage with an appropriate drug.

The standards against which rational prescribing can be judged will depend on locally or nationally agreed treatment protocols or an agreed list of therapeutic alternatives. Ideally, prescribing should follow evidence-based guidelines, but it is often necessary to extrapolate these guidelines to situations not covered by the evidence. In the absence of evidence from clinical trials, it may be appropriate to use consensus guidelines produced by experts, and derived from a relevant evidence base.

There has been considerable debate about 'class effects' of drugs, and whether it is reasonable to extrapolate data from a clinical study with one drug to another in the same class. This is a complex area, and in part depends on the definition of a drug class (e.g. a group of drugs with similar chemical structure, a group of drugs with similar mechanisms of action, or a group of drugs with similar pharmacological effects). Class effect may be related to clinical outcome, effects on surrogate end-points, or unwanted effects. Many consensus guidelines assume that drug efficacy is related to a class effect when there is a large body of information about several drugs in a class that suggest similar outcomes.

The sequence of events leading to a rational prescription involves initially making a diagnosis and determining prognosis. This may not always be possible, and it may be necessary to substitute differential diagnoses and rank these in order of probability and/or importance to diagnose or exclude. The goal of treatment must then be determined. This may be curative, symptom-relief, prevention or, occasionally, an aid to the diagnostic process. The prescriber should then decide whether a treatment is necessary and select an appropriate first choice. The process is completed by monitoring the outcome, and reaching a decision to stop, to modify or to continue treatment.

Assuming that the choice of drug is appropriate for the condition that the prescriber believes he or she is treating, there will be several further considerations involved in individualising drug treatment.

- Is this drug licensed for use in this condition? If it is not, prescribing may still be appropriate but the prescriber should be familiar with the evidence to support its use.
- How does it compare with available alternatives in relation to published evidence, efficacy, safety, convenience and cost?
- Does the individual have any coexisting conditions that will compromise the efficacy of the drug?
- Are there co-morbidities that might benefit from the use of this or an alternative option?
- Are any other drugs being taken that might adversely interact with your choice?
- Are there any absolute contraindications to using the drug in this individual?
- Are there relative contraindications to use in this individual, including co-morbidities or common unwanted effects?
- Has the individual suffered previous adverse drug events that should make you cautious about using this particular drug?

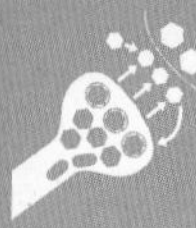

FURTHER READING

Burnier M (2006) Medication adherence and persistence as the cornerstone of effective antihypertensive therapy. *Am J Hypertens* 19, 1190–1196

Dans AL, Dans LF, Guyatt GH, Richardson S (1998) Users' guides to the medical literature: XIV. How to decide on the applicability of clinical trial results to your patient *JAMA* 279, 545–549

De Vries TPGM (1993) Presenting clinical pharmacology and therapeutics: a problem-based approach for choosing and prescribing drugs. *Br J Clin Pharmacol* 35, 581–586

Guyatt GH, Sinclair J, Cook DJ et al (1999) Users' guides to the medical literature: XVI. How to use a treatment recommendation. *JAMA* 281, 1836–1843

McAlister FA, Laupacis A, Wells GA et al (1999) Applying clinical trial results Part B. Guidelines for determining whether a drug is exerting (more than) a class effect. *JAMA* 282, 1371–1377

McAlister F, Strauss SE, Guyatt GH et al (2000) Users' guides to the medical literature: XX. Integrating research evidence with the care of the individual patient *JAMA* 283, 2829–2836

Osterberg L, Blaschke T (2005) Adherence to medication. *N Engl J Med* 353, 487–497

Santaguida PL, Helfand M, Raina P (2005) Challenges in systematic reviews that evaluate drug efficacy. *Ann Intern Med* 142, 1066–1072

Spinewine A, Schmader KE, Barber N et al (2007) Appropriate prescribing in elderly people: how well can it be measured and optimized? *Lancet* 370, 173–184

56 Drug therapy in special situations

PRESCRIBING IN PREGNANCY

Guidelines for prescribing during pregnancy are set out in the *British National Formulary* (BNF) and only general points are made below. Pregnancy can be associated with medical problems that require treatment (Ch. 45), but exposure of the fetus to any unnecessary drugs is undesirable, particularly in the first trimester, because of the risk of teratogenicity. The magnitude of the potential problem is illustrated by the fact that about 90% of women take medication during pregnancy, and an unrecorded number will take over-the-counter medication without guidance from a medical practitioner or a pharmacist.

Unequivocal teratogenic activity of drugs in humans is limited to a relatively small number of compounds, but the effects are irreversible and affect the whole life of the offspring. The potential catastrophic consequences of the administration of a teratogenic drug were highlighted by the thalidomide tragedy in the 1960s. Thalidomide was introduced as a sedative and hypnotic and was used for the treatment of pregnancy-associated morning sickness. Following its introduction there was a dramatic increase in the incidence of phocomelia (abnormal or absent development of limb buds). The drug was banned once the association had been recognised, and this resulted in the incidence of phocomelia decreasing to previous levels (Fig. 56.1). Thalidomide is not teratogenic in rodents but is in rabbits, although the doses necessary are about 100 times higher than those in humans or other primates; this observation resulted in the required use of rabbits in preclinical testing for teratogenicity. The recent use of thalidomide as an unlicensed treatment for leprosy raises the spectre of teratogenicity; the drug should never be given to women with childbearing potential.

The list of teratogenic drugs includes thalidomide, some anticonvulsants, some chemotherapeutic drugs (e.g. alkylating agents and antimetabolites), warfarin, androgens, danazol, diethylstilbestrol, lithium and retinoids (Table 56.1). Because of their long half-lives, some retinoids can result in teratogenesis even if the course of treatment in the mother is stopped before pregnancy occurs. Although teratogenesis is commonly thought of in terms of structural abnormalities or dysfunctional growth in utero, by definition it also refers to long-term functional defects. For example, maternal consumption of alcohol during pregnancy may cause behavioural and cognitive abnormalities in childhood, despite the birth of a seemingly unaffected infant. Some drugs may initially appear harmless yet exhibit a long latency period: diethylstilbestrol, which was given during pregnancy between the 1940s and early 1970s, resulted in abnormalities in the offspring when they reached adulthood.

Notwithstanding the limited list of drugs that are known to cause teratogenesis, there is a much larger number that should be avoided or used with caution in pregnancy because of their potential to produce pharmacological or biochemical dysfunction leading to detrimental effects in the fetus. Examples include warfarin-induced anticoagulation (Ch. 11), which may predispose to cerebral haemorrhage in the fetus during delivery; in contrast, heparin is an effective anticoagulant in the mother and does not cross the placenta. Non-steroidal anti-inflammatory drugs (NSAIDs; Ch. 29), can prevent closure of the ductus arteriosus after delivery. Adverse effects produced at therapeutic doses, such as tachycardia with tricyclic antidepressants and growth restriction with corticosteroids, may also affect the fetus or neonate.

Whenever a drug is given to a pregnant woman an assessment should be made, taking into account any risk to the fetus balanced against the benefit to the mother and any risk associated with not treating the mother. For example, treatment with anticonvulsants or antimalarials may be essential for the mother, despite the possible risk to the fetus/neonate. The risk to the fetus/neonate should be minimised whenever possible by selecting the drug with the least potential for teratogenicity. The BNF provides detailed information on potential adverse drug effects on the fetus and/or neonate.

Pharmacokinetics

The placenta provides a potential barrier to the transfer of drugs from the maternal circulation, but lipid-soluble drugs cross, particularly if they are of low molecular weight. Some metabolism of drugs can occur in the placenta, which may further restrict fetal exposure, although the placenta does not have a high drug-metabolising capacity. The fetal liver has only a modest ability to metabolise drugs. The fetus represents a slowly equilibrating maternal kinetic compartment, with transfer across the placenta being determined by the concentration gradient between fetal and maternal circulations.

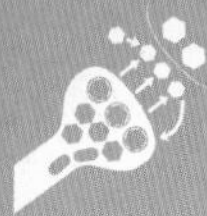

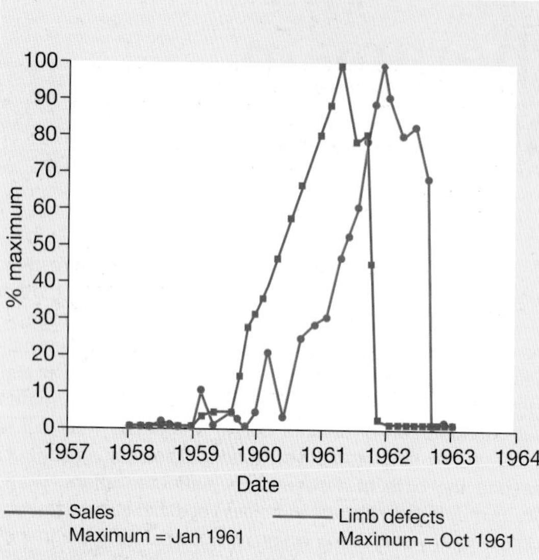

Fig. 56.1 **The relationship between the sales of thalidomide and the incidence of phocomelia (each is expressed as a percentage of the maximum reported).**

Maternal pharmacokinetics are affected by a number of physiological changes, especially in late pregnancy. These include:

- increased hepatic drug metabolism
- increased renal blood flow and glomerular filtration rate
- decreased plasma concentrations of albumin.

These changes mean that maternal drug concentrations are often lower than those in a non-pregnant woman given the same dose. Care needs to be taken in the interpretation of data from therapeutic drug monitoring using plasma samples, because the total concentration may be decreased, which could be interpreted as needing an increase in dosage, but if this is due to decreased binding to plasma proteins, then the free, and active, concentration may not have decreased.

DRUGS AND BREASTFEEDING

Almost any compound present in the maternal circulation will enter breast milk and be ingested by the suckling baby,

Table 56.1 Examples of drug-induced teratogenicity and fetal/neonatal toxicity (see current British National Formulary for detailed advice)

Therapeutic drug	Teratogenic and adverse effects in fetus and neonate
ACE inhibitors	Affect fetal and neonatal blood pressure control and renal function; oligohydramnios
Alcohol	Fetal alcohol syndrome; growth restriction (Ch. 54)
Aminoglycosides	Auditory or vestibular nerve damage
Amiodarone	Neonatal goitre
Androgens	Virilisation of female fetus
Anticancer drugs	Possibility of carcinogenic and teratogenic effects (avoid before and during pregnancy); this advice covers non-chemotherapeutic uses of drugs such as methotrexate; see BNF for individual agents
Barbiturates	Fetal abnormalities; withdrawal effects in neonates
Benzodiazepines	Withdrawal effects in neonates
Beta-adrenoceptor antagonists (β-blockers)	Intrauterine growth restriction, neonatal hypoglycaemia and bradycardia
Carbamazepine	Risk of neural tube defects
Carbimazole	Neonatal goitre
Corticosteroids	Intrauterine growth suppression if prolonged treatment is given
Dapsone	Neonatal haemolysis and methaemoglobinaemia
Diethylstilbestrol	High doses cause vaginal cancer in female offspring and risk of hypospadias in males
Fibrinolytics	Premature separation of placenta in first 18 weeks

Table 56.1 Examples of drug-induced teratogenicity and fetal/neonatal toxicity (see current British National Formulary for detailed advice) *(Continued)*

Therapeutic drug	Teratogenic and adverse effects in fetus and neonate
Lamotrigine	Teratogenicity
Leflunomide	Teratogenic in animals; effective contraception necessary for at least 2 years after end of treatment for women and 3 months for men
Lithium salts	Teratogenicity; cardiac abnormalities
NSAIDs	Premature closure of ductus arteriosus and possible pulmonary hypertension
Opioids	Neonatal respiratory depression and risk of withdrawal syndrome if the mother is habituated
Oral anticoagulants	Malformations and fetal or neonatal haemorrhage
Oxcarbazepine	Risk of neural tube defects
Phenytoin	Congenital malformations and risk of neonatal haemorrhage due to vitamin K deficiency
Primaquine	Neonatal haemolysis and methaemoglobinaemia
Retinoids and retinoid-like drugs (RAR and RXR agonists)	Teratogenic, craniofacial malformations; some have long half-lives and effective contraception is essential for prolonged periods after stopping treatment and before pregnancy, e.g. acitretin (2 years), bexarotene (1 month), isotretinoin (1 month) and tretinoin (1 month)
Ribavirin	Teratogenic in animals; effective contraception necessary for at least 6 months after treatment for both women and men
Statins	Decreased cholesterol synthesis affects fetal development
Sulphonamides	Neonatal haemolysis and methaemoglobinaemia
Sulphonylureas	Neonatal hypoglycaemia
Thiazide diuretics	Growth retardation; electrolyte disturbance
Valproate	Congenital malformations and developmental delay in offspring

Note – manufacturers of most drugs advise that they should be taken in pregnancy only if the potential benefit outweighs the possible risk; also, many recommend that prescribing to women of childbearing age should be carried out with pregnancy in mind and contraception should be adequate before, during and after cessation of treatment.
ACE, angiotensin-converting enzyme; NSAIDs, non-steroidal anti-inflammatory drugs; TCAs, tricyclic antidepressants.

and this concern has contributed to a decrease in the extent and/or duration of breastfeeding in Western societies (American Academy of Pediatrics, 2001). However, with a few exceptions there is little evidence that drug intake via breastfeeding is of concern because most drugs enter breast milk in quantities too small to affect the baby. Appendix 5 of the BNF states, '*The amount of drug transferred in breast milk is rarely sufficient to produce a discernible effect on the infant*.' In general, drugs licensed for use in children can be safely given to the nursing mother, whereas drugs known to have serious toxic effects in adults, or known to affect lactation, such as bromocriptine, should be avoided.

The American Academy of Pediatrics (2001) divides drugs into:

i. cytotoxic drugs that may interfere with cellular metabolism of the nursing infant (e.g. cyclophosphamide, ciclosporin, doxorubicin, methotrexate)
ii. drugs of abuse for which adverse effects on the infant during breastfeeding have been reported (e.g. amfetamine, cocaine, heroin, marijuana)
iii. radioactive compounds that require temporary cessation of breastfeeding (e.g. radio-iodine)
iv. drugs for which the effect on nursing infants is unknown but may be of concern (a list of about 40 miscellaneous drugs)
v. drugs that have been associated with significant effects on some nursing infants and should be given to nursing mothers with caution (e.g. acebutolol, atenolol, bromocriptine, aspirin, ergotamine, lithium, phenindione, phenobarbital/primidone)
vi. maternal medication usually compatible with breastfeeding (the vast majority of drugs).
vii. food and environmental agents.

The reader should refer to the up-to-date information in the BNF for detailed advice.

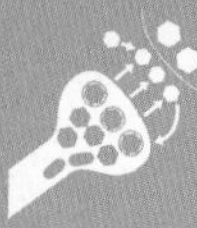

Pharmacokinetics

Several factors influence transfer from maternal circulation into breast milk, including the characteristics of the milk (which changes in the first few days of lactation), the physicochemical properties of the drug, and the amount of drug in the maternal circulation. The concentrations of drugs in breast milk are in equilibrium with those in the maternal circulation. At equilibrium, the free concentrations in milk and plasma will be the same, but the total concentrations will be influenced by the extent of protein binding and uptake into the lipid phase (see Fig. 2.3). Water-soluble drugs diffuse from plasma into milk, and the concentrations in breast milk are similar to the non-protein-bound fraction in the maternal plasma. Lipid-soluble compounds diffuse into breast milk and may concentrate because of the high fat content in milk. Highly lipid-soluble persistent organic pollutants (group vii of The American Academy of Pediatrics groupings – see above), such as dioxins, are present in maternal body fat, from where they are mobilised during lactation and transferred to the suckling infant. Despite this, the World Health Organisation (WHO) currently recommends that the benefits of breastfeeding while taking a drug are usually greater than any possible risk.

If drugs are given during breast feeding, compounds with short half-lives are preferred, because they are less likely to accumulate in neonates (who have lower drug clearance, see below). Neonatal exposure can be minimised if the feed is timed to coincide with the trough blood concentration in the mother, which is just before taking a dose.

PRESCRIBING FOR CHILDREN

Both the pharmacokinetics and responses to drugs may differ among neonates, infants and children compared with adults. There are considerable differences among neonates (<1 month), infants (1–12 months) and children, because many metabolic and physiological processes are immature at birth and develop rapidly in the first months of life. These differences may affect the absorption and distribution of drugs and the rate of elimination of the drug from the body, and also the sensitivity of tissues to the actions and/or adverse effects produced by the drug. Particular care is needed in prescribing drugs that may affect growing or maturing organ systems, such as the bones and teeth and the reproductive system. Box 56.1 shows some of the differences between the young and adults.

Although medicines should usually be used within the terms of the product licence (see Ch. 3), many of the drugs given to children have not undergone formal clinical evaluation in this age group, and are not specifically licensed for paediatric use. It is recognised that 'off-label' use (strictly speaking, an unlicensed use) may be necessary, and the Medicines Act (1968) does not prohibit such use. There is an increasing recognition of the need for formal clinical trials in the paediatric population, but such studies raise significant ethical issues. Further information on the regulation of medicines for children is available:

for the UK, at: *http://www.mhra.gov.uk/Howweregulate/Medicines/Medicinesforchildren/index.htm*
for the EU, at: *http://ec.europa.eu/enterprise/pharmaceuticals/paediatrics/medchild_en.htm*
for the USA, at: *http://www.fda.gov/oc/opt/default.htm*

The BNF for children (BNFC) give specific guidance for children.

Pharmacokinetics

In neonates, inefficient metabolism and renal clearance mean that lower doses of some drugs are needed after allowing for body weight, and doses need to be calculated with special care. In contrast, the processes of drug elimination are largely mature by a few weeks of age, after which drug clearance (adjusted to body weight) is similar to or higher than that in adults (see below). However, children may be more susceptible to effects on growing or maturing tissues and organs. Nevertheless, generalisations are difficult and each drug needs consideration in its own right.

Absorption

Slow rates of gastric emptying and intestinal transit may reduce the rate of drug absorption in neonates, but total absorption of poorly absorbed drugs may eventually be more complete because of longer contact with the intestinal mucosa. In the neonate, gastric pH is neutral and this can reduce the absorption of weak acids but increase the absorption of weak bases.

Distribution

Neonates and young children have a lower body fat content and higher total body water compared with adults; this influences the distribution of both lipid- and water-

Box 56.1 Developmental changes in the young compared with adults that have the potential to alter drug handling

- Gastric acid production is decreased during infancy
- Gastric emptying is erratic in the first year of life
- Smaller gut surface area/body mass ratio relative to adults but greater gut permeability to larger molecules than adults
- Relatively larger proportion of body fat and extracellular volume may alter the volumes of distribution of some drugs compared with adults
- Maturation of liver metabolising enzymes occurs in the first year and there are temporal differences in rates of maturation of different metabolic pathways
- Glomerular filtration rate and tubular functions including tubular transporting enzymes are relatively decreased in the first year of life
- Decreased maturation and function of some gut flora compared with adults

The maturation of these systems towards adult values occurs at different rates and final decisions on therapy require close monitoring of individual drugs in each child.

soluble drugs. Neonates have a lower plasma albumin concentration, which also has a lower affinity for drug binding. In addition, the higher plasma concentrations of free fatty acids and bilirubin compete with drugs for plasma protein binding sites and vice versa (Ch. 2). The overall effect is reduced plasma protein binding, which not only increases the apparent volume of distribution of the drug but also increases the proportion of drug able to cross the blood–brain barrier and also the amounts diffusing into the liver and therefore available for metabolism. Drugs that are strongly bound to albumin should not be used during neonatal jaundice because the drugs may displace bilirubin (which is mostly in the unconjugated form) from protein binding sites, and increase the risk of kernicterus.

Metabolism

The liver drug-metabolising enzyme systems are immature in the neonate, and first-pass metabolism and hepatic drug clearance are low, especially for substrates of CYP1A2, CYP3A4 and glucuronidation. The clearances for substrates for these enzymes are 2–6 times lower in neonates compared with adults. When the enzyme systems mature, drug metabolism processes become more extensive. Plasma drug clearance is often higher in young children than in adults, because of their higher relative liver mass and greater hepatic blood flow per kilogram body weight; hepatic blood flow is the rate-limiting step in the elimination of high-clearance drugs.

Renal elimination

Renal function in the neonate and infant is much less developed than in children or adults. The glomerular filtration rate in the newborn is about 40% of the adult level, and tubular secretory processes are poorly developed. Elimination of drugs such as digoxin, gentamicin and penicillin will therefore be slower until about 6–8 months of age.

In children, the larger volume of distribution and faster hepatic elimination mean that doses of metabolised drugs need to be higher than in adults after correcting for the difference in body weight. Prescribed doses are most accurately judged by considering both age and body surface area. In children, body surface area is a better guide to appropriate drug dosage than body weight (see Self-assessment section of Ch. 52). The dose for a child can be approximated as:

$$\frac{\text{Adult dose} \times \text{surface area of child (in m}^2\text{)}}{1.8}$$

where 1.8 is the average body surface area of a 70 kg adult.

PRESCRIBING FOR THE ELDERLY

The elderly (usually taken to mean those over 70 years old) comprise a heterogeneous group who show considerable variation in 'biological' age. Changes occur in both the pharmacodynamics and pharmacokinetics of drugs with increasing age.

The density or numbers of receptors may be reduced with age; for example, β-adrenoceptors are decreased in number, reducing the response to agonist drugs. The elderly are often more susceptible to sedatives and hypnotics, possibly because of changes in receptor numbers and/or changes in the efficiency of the blood–brain barrier.

Altered structure and function of target organs can also influence the effects of drugs. For example, baroreceptor function is impaired in the elderly and vasodilator drugs are more likely to provoke postural hypotension. The high peripheral resistance and less distensible arterial tree found with increasing age also respond less well to arterial vasodilators.

These changes reflect the ageing process itself; however, they are often complicated by the presence of chronic disease (frequently involving multiple pathological processes) and variation due to both genetic and environmental influences. The risks of unwanted effects are higher in the elderly as a consequence of these changes. Significant numbers of hospital admissions in the elderly are due to adverse drugs reactions, most of which are the more predictable type A effects (see Ch. 53). In addition, drug interactions are more common in the elderly because of the coexistence of different treatable conditions requiring the simultaneous use of several drugs. For all these reasons, it is usual to start drug treatment in the elderly with the smallest effective dose. Rational prescribing should also seek to minimise the numbers of drugs used.

Pharmacokinetics

Absorption

Drug absorption across the gut wall is not greatly affected by ageing, although bioavailability may be increased due to reduced first-pass metabolism.

Distribution

Older people have a lower lean body mass and a relative increase in body fat compared with young adults. The apparent volume of distribution of water-soluble drugs is therefore lower in the elderly and a smaller loading dose of a drug such as digoxin may be needed. Conversely, lipid-soluble drugs may be eliminated more slowly because of their increased volume of distribution due to the relative increase in body fat and because of reduced hepatic metabolism.

Metabolism

The size of the liver and its blood flow decrease with age. Although enzyme activity per hepatocyte probably shows little change, the overall capacity for drug metabolism, particularly phase 1 metabolic reactions (Ch. 2), is reduced. This is particularly important for lipid-soluble drugs, such as nifedipine or propranolol, which undergo extensive first-pass metabolism, because lower hepatic metabolism increases bioavailability and reduces systemic clearance.

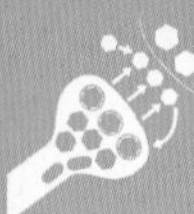

Renal elimination

Increasing age is also associated with a progressive reduction in glomerular filtration rate, so the elimination of polar drugs and metabolites is slower. This can produce toxicity when renally eliminated drugs with a low therapeutic index are prescribed in the elderly, for example lithium, digoxin or gentamicin. Creatinine clearance, which is an estimate of glomerular filtration rate, usually correlates well with the clearance of drugs that are eliminated in the urine unchanged (as the parent drug). Because the elderly have a lower muscle mass than younger people, the plasma creatinine concentration (which is dependent on lean body mass) is a poor guide to renal glomerular function. Plasma creatinine in the elderly frequently remains within the 'normal' laboratory reference range even when renal function is substantially reduced, because the reduced elimination is balanced by decreased production. The Cockcroft and Gault equation, which relates plasma creatinine to creatinine clearance, contains elements reflecting sex- and age-dependent differences in muscle mass.

Creatinine clearance (mL min^{-1}) for males equals:

$$\frac{1.23 \times (140 - \text{age in years}) \times \text{weight (in kg)}}{\text{plasma creatinine } (\mu\text{mol L}^{-1})}$$

and for females equals:

$$\frac{1.04 \times (140 - \text{age in years}) \times \text{weight (in kg)}}{\text{plasma creatinine } (\mu\text{mol L}^{-1})}$$

As an alternative, the eGFR (see below) is used to approximate GFR.

PRESCRIBING IN RENAL FAILURE

Individuals with renal failure show increased responses to many drugs, especially when the drug, or its active metabolite, is eliminated in the urine. The extent to which dose adjustment is necessary depends on the extent of renal impairment and also the proportion of total plasma clearance that is due to renal clearance. Increasingly, the estimated glomerular filtration rate (eGFR) is reported with laboratory estimations of serum creatinine. This is a useful guide to renal function, but does not consider weight as a variable that affects GFR. Nevertheless, for most drugs that are excreted by the kidney it is an adequate guide for dosage adjustment.

There are also pharmacodynamic changes; for example, there are altered responses to drugs in people with uraemia, and drugs acting on the central nervous system (CNS) in particular produce enhanced responses, possibly because of increased permeability of the blood–brain barrier.

The BNF gives advice on drug prescribing to those with renal impairment. Subjects with renal impairment may show an abnormal drug response due to one or more of the following factors:

- failure to excrete the drug or its metabolites may produce toxicity
- there may be increased sensitivity, even if elimination is unaltered
- many unwanted effects are poorly tolerated in such individuals
- some drugs cease to be effective in such individuals.

Pharmacokinetics

The kidneys provide the major route of elimination for water-soluble drugs and water-soluble metabolites (see Ch. 2). Renal elimination of drugs can be affected indirectly by abnormal renal perfusion, such as might occur in shock, or directly by changes in the kidney, for example renal tubular necrosis. Reduced renal function may increase the risk of toxicity from the parent drug and/or its metabolites due to their accumulation in the body, although in some cases sensitivity may be increased in renal failure in the absence of obviously impaired elimination of the drug per se. Impaired renal function does not affect the majority of drugs, because most drugs are eliminated by hepatic metabolism.

There are several other ways in which renal impairment may influence the handling of drugs:

- Metabolism in the liver can be altered in uraemic patients; although most oxidative metabolism is unchanged, other processes such as reduction, acetylation and ester hydrolysis are impaired.
- Metabolism in the kidney is important for the 1-α-hydroxylation of vitamin D and also for the degradation of insulin, both of which can be impaired in renal failure.
- The distribution of drugs can be affected by changes in fluid balances in renal failure, and more importantly by altered protein binding. Circulating concentrations of albumin are decreased in severe renal failure with proteinuria. In addition, retained endogenous metabolites, such as the tryptophan metabolite indican, may compete for drug-binding sites on plasma proteins. The increased concentrations of free drug can lead to an enhanced response.
- The greater concentration of free drug in the circulation can lead to increased elimination (by filtration and/or metabolism) so that the active unbound drug concentration may be unchanged (see 'Drug interactions', below).
- Tissue binding of digoxin is reduced in renal failure, so a lower loading dose should be given to compensate for the reduced volume of distribution.

The elimination of drugs by the kidney is significantly impaired only when the glomerular filtration rate is reduced below 50 mL min^{-1}. For some drugs, clinically important accumulation does not occur until much lower filtration rates. Changes in renal tubular secretion of drugs in renal disease are less well established.

A reduction in drug dosage in renal failure is usually necessary only if a high proportion of the drug is eliminated by the kidney and also the compound has a low therapeutic index. Maintenance dosage may be lowered by either reducing the dose or increasing the dose interval (see Ch. 2, Equation 2.24); loading doses do not usually require any modification. Large dose modifications are rarely needed for drugs that do not have dose-related unwanted effects. For the purposes of prescribing and dosage adjustment (Appendix 3 of the BNF), renal impairment can be divided into three grades:

1. mild – with a glomerular filtration rate of 60–89 mL min^{-1} 1.73 m^2
2. moderate – with a glomerular filtration rate of 30–59 mL min^{-1} 1.73 m^2
3. severe – with a glomerular filtration rate of 15–29 mL min^{-1} 1.73 m^2
4. established renal failure with a glomerular filtration rate of <15 mL min^{-1} 1.73 m^2.

For some drugs, only established renal failure needs to be considered (for example, a reduction in dosage is recommended for ampicillin), while for other drugs, even mild impairment may be important (for example, dosage reduction and haematological monitoring are recommended for carboplatin, whereas cisplatin should be avoided) (see the BNF for details).

A further important consideration is the avoidance of drugs that have toxic effects on the kidney. Use of these in renal impairment can sometimes produce an irreversible decline in renal function.

PRESCRIBING IN LIVER DISEASE

Changes in both drug responses and pharmacokinetics can occur in liver disease. The BNF lists six main potential problems in prescribing for individuals with liver disease:

- impaired drug metabolism
- hypoproteinaemia
- reduced clotting
- hepatic encephalopathy
- fluid overload
- hepatotoxic drugs.

The severity of the liver disease is important, as is whether the disease is decompensated and includes jaundice, hypoproteinaemia or encephalopathy. Many of the pharmacodynamic and pharmacokinetic changes in liver failure arise from decreased hepatic synthesis of proteins that perform essential functions within the hepatocyte, or which are released into the blood, such as albumin and clotting factors.

CNS depressant drugs, such as morphine and chlorpromazine, have an enhanced effect in people with liver failure. This is caused by increased sensitivity of neuronal tissue (although the mechanism is not known) and can provoke encephalopathy in susceptible patients. Decreased plasma protein binding may contribute to this greater sensitivity by increasing the percentage of free drug so that more drug crosses the blood–brain barrier. Benzodiazepines used during investigational procedures in individuals with liver failure can produce profound and long-lasting effects, which may require reversal by the administration of the benzodiazepine antagonist flumazenil.

Encephalopathy may be triggered by drugs that cause constipation (which increases the formation of potentially toxic metabolites, such as ammonia, by the intestinal bacteria). Diuretics that produce hypokalaemia can precipitate hepatic encephalopathy in chronic liver disease. Therefore, potassium-sparing diuretics such as spironolactone are usually used in preference to diuretics such as furosemide; an additional advantage of spironolactone is that it blocks the effects of circulating aldosterone, which is often increased in decompensated liver disease.

The reduced ability to synthesise vitamin K-dependent clotting factors makes people with chronic liver disease prone to clotting problems: they would be very sensitive to anticoagulant drugs, which are clearly contraindicated.

People with pre-existing liver disease are likely to be more susceptible to potentially hepatotoxic drugs. This raises a problem for pain relief, since paracetamol is hepatotoxic at high doses, whereas NSAIDs can increase the risk of gastrointestinal bleeding and cause fluid retention, and opioids can precipitate encephalopathy. In practice, lower doses of paracetamol are usually given, taking care that the amounts do not exceed the reduced threshold for hepatotoxicity shown by such individuals (see Ch. 53).

Pharmacokinetics

The rate of absorption of drugs from the gut lumen is not greatly affected, but other aspects of drug handling may be altered. Distribution may be affected if protein synthesis is reduced, because the plasma albumin concentrations are decreased, resulting in a higher percentage of free drug in plasma and a greater apparent volume of distribution. An elevated plasma bilirubin may displace some drugs from their plasma protein binding sites, and this would also increase the apparent volume of distribution; examples of drugs that can be affected are lidocaine and propranolol.

The liver has characteristics that facilitate the rapid and extensive uptake and metabolism of lipid-soluble drugs (Fig. 56.2). These include:

- fenestrations in the endothelium, allowing ready access to extracellular fluid
- rapid diffusion across the space of Disse (which is a matrix consisting primarily of type 4 collagen)
- a brush border on hepatocytes, allowing rapid uptake
- high intracellular enzyme activity for both phase 1 and phase 2 metabolism.

During chronic liver disease, a number of changes may occur that reduce the capacity of the liver to metabolise drugs (Fig. 56.3):

- fenestrations in the endothelium are lost
- diffusion across the space of Disse may be reduced in fibrosis/cirrhosis as type 4 collagen is replaced by type 1 and type 3 collagen (which can form dense fibrils)
- the brush border on hepatocytes is lost
- intracellular enzyme activity is reduced
- intrahepatic vascular shunts may reduce the perfusion of hepatocytes.

Reduced hepatic uptake and metabolism or decreased biliary excretion of drugs may result in a greater proportion of the drug and/or its metabolites being eliminated via other routes, such as the urine.

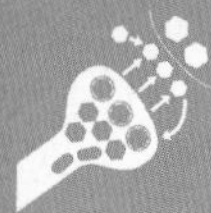

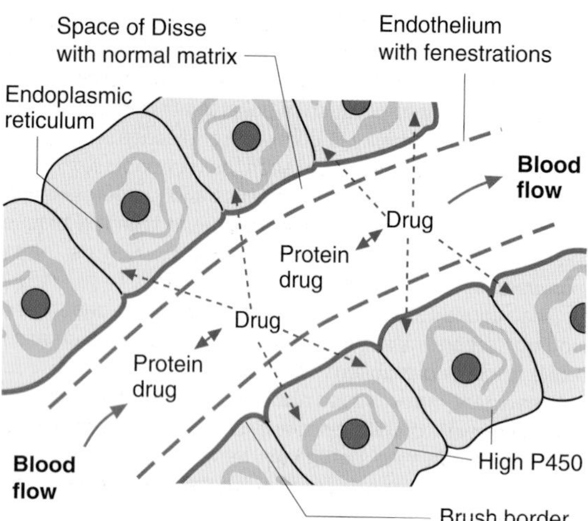

Fig. 56.2 **Schematic for the uptake of a drug from the sinusoid of a normal healthy liver.**

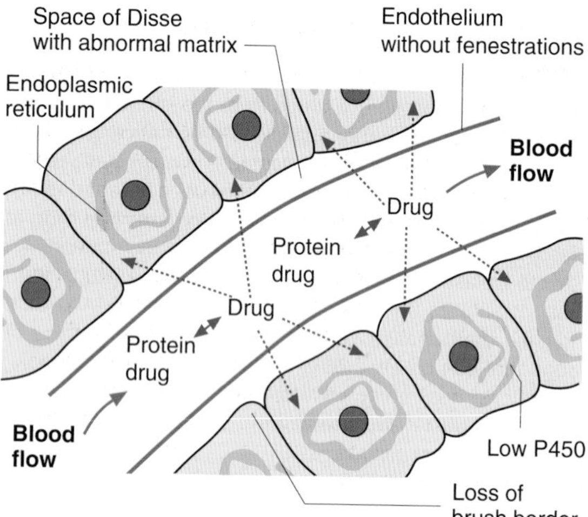

Fig. 56.3 **Schematic for the uptake of a drug from the sinusoid of a liver showing the features characteristic of cirrhosis.**

First-pass metabolism may be considerably reduced in conditions such as liver cirrhosis; the consequences are most apparent with drugs that undergo extensive hepatic first-pass metabolism in patients with normal liver function. In liver failure, bioavailability may increase considerably and approach 100%, such that the bioavailability could change fivefold or more (e.g. from <0.2 to 1.0).

Biliary excretion is impaired in conditions causing reduced formation of bile. A correlation between drug clearance and bilirubin would be expected for drugs eliminated unchanged in bile, such as rifampicin and fusidic acid. Reduced elimination of drug metabolites in bile could affect enterohepatic circulation (Ch. 2). Reduced bile production can affect the absorption of highly lipid-soluble molecules, such as the fat-soluble vitamins, that require micelle formation for effective absorption.

Systemic clearance may be reduced for drugs eliminated by hepatic metabolism. The changes that occur in liver disease affect both high-clearance drugs, where the elimination rate is dependent on effective liver blood flow, and low-clearance drugs, where it is dependent on hepatic extraction and enzyme activity.

Prescribing in liver disease should be undertaken with care, and drugs that are extensively metabolised by the liver should be given in smaller doses. The need for dose reduction arises primarily from an increase in bioavailability and a decrease in systemic clearance, both of which increase the average steady-state plasma concentration and the area under the plasma concentration–time curve for a single dose (Ch. 2). The BNF deals with liver disease, and there are numerous examples for which the advice is 'Reduce dose'.

DRUG INTERACTIONS

Many patients receive more than one drug during a course of treatment because:

- combination therapy is preferable or necessary for producing an adequate effect or response; important examples are the chemotherapy of malignant disease and the treatment of hypertension
- a single condition or pathology may give rise to a variety of symptoms that are controlled by different drugs
- the person may suffer from more than one condition or pathology requiring treatment with drugs that are unrelated pharmacologically.

The term 'interaction' implies that the response to the combination of drugs is different to that which could be predicted from a simple summation of the effects produced by each drug if given singly.

The consequences of treatment with a combination of drugs can be divided into four different types:

- **dose-addition** – where each drug produces the same response and the magnitude of response to a combination of both drugs is given by simple addition of the doses after allowing for any difference in potency (see below); this is the usual situation when more than one drug is used to treat a single condition, such as the control of hypertension
- **response-addition** – where each drug produces a different response and a combination of both drugs gives each response as if the other compound were not present; this is the usual situation when two drugs are used to treat two different conditions, e.g. one drug is to treat hypertension and the other is given for epilepsy, or a combination of antibacterials is used empirically to affect different types of organisms in an unspecified infection
- **synergism** – where each drug produces the same response and the magnitude of response to a combination of both drugs is greater than would be predicted by simple addition of the doses after allowing for any difference in potency (see below); synergism is often produced when each drug has a different mechanism or acts at a different step in the process leading to the overall response; synergism is the usual aim of using more than one drug in cancer chemotherapy
- **antagonism** – where each drug produces the same response and the magnitude of response to a combina-

tion of both drugs is lower than would be predicted by simple addition of the doses after allowing for any difference in potency (see below); this sort of interaction can occur if a partial agonist is given with a full agonist and reduces the overall activity.

Interactions may result in either a decrease in response (antagonism) or increase in response (synergism) compared with that predicted; this may be either beneficial, or potentially harmful because of a lack of clinical response or the risk of toxicity. Considerable research on drugs used in cancer chemotherapy (Ch. 52) is designed to identify synergistic interactions on cancer cells that give only dose-addition or response-addition at other sites. Simple summation of the responses to single doses does not define the nature of any interaction, and data on the shape of the dose–response relations for each drug alone and in combination are necessary to define whether synergism has occurred. For example, if 10 mg of drug A or 100 mg of drug B each gives a 25% response when given alone, it might be assumed that 10 mg of A + 100 mg of B would give a 50% response; BUT the response to the combination would depend on the shape and slope of the dose–response curve. The interpretation of drug combination data relies on comparisons of the doses of each compound alone and of different combinations *giving the same magnitude of response*. To extend the example above, the data for different mixtures of A and B can be analysed by the method of isoboles (Fig. 56.4) in which the doses giving the same magnitude of response are plotted. Thus, simple *dose-addition* would be shown if a 25% response is given by 10 mg of A, or 100 mg of B, or (5 mg of A + 50 mg of B). From the data plotted in Figure 56.4, *synergism* would be proven if a 25% response were produced by (5 mg of A + 12 mg of B) or (1.1 mg of A + 50 mg of B) – or any other combination that fitted the 'synergism' curve shown. The

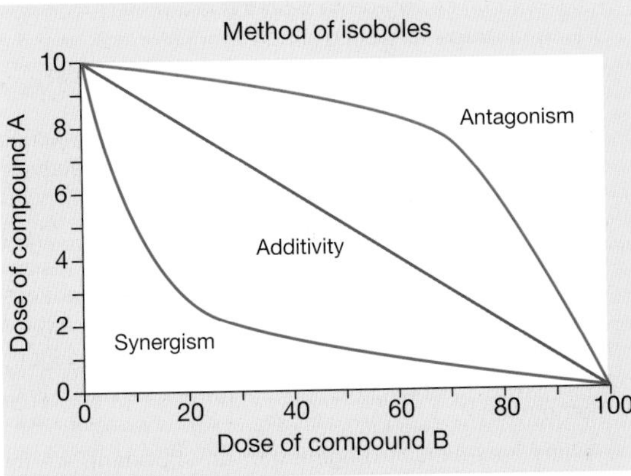

***Fig. 56.4* Analysis of drug interactions by the method of isoboles.** Dose–response data for each drug alone and for different combinations are plotted and analysed to define the doses giving the same magnitude of response. The doses of each drug (A and B above) alone and in different combinations *that give the same level of response* are plotted against each other.

extent of synergism is indicated by the magnitude to which the combination curve is displaced to the left or below the line of additivity. *Antagonism* is proven if the doses of A + B required to give a 25% response are above the line of additivity.

Beneficial interactions are usually well recognised – for example, combinations of different anticancer drugs, and levodopa plus carbidopa – and are part of prescribing recommendations. In consequence, the focus of this section, and of Appendix 1 of the BNF, is those interactions that may give rise to adverse effects, especially when the interaction would not be readily predicted based on a knowledge of the sites and mechanisms of action.

Interactions are of greatest importance for drugs that have a narrow therapeutic index and for groups at increased risk, such as the elderly (who are more likely to suffer multiple pathologies and may have decreased hepatic and renal function).

Drug interactions may arise at the site of the mechanism of action (pharmacodynamics) or from altered delivery of the drug to its site of action (pharmacokinetics).

Pharmacodynamic interactions

Pharmacodynamic interactions are usually predictable, based on the known mechanisms of action of the drugs. Interactions may relate to the principal site of action of the drug, or to secondary sites of action that are responsible for unwanted effects of the drug. In principle, drugs that are highly selective for a single site of action are less likely to produce pharmacodynamic interactions than are drugs that show low selectivity. An example of a serious adverse synergistic interaction is between an angiotensin-converting enzyme (ACE) inhibitor, such as enalapril (Ch. 6), and spironolactone (Ch. 14); the ACE inhibitor reduces the production of aldosterone, thereby reducing the excretion of K^+, an effect which is exaggerated by the action of spironolactone, and the combination can cause potentially life-threatening hyperkalaemia.

Pharmacokinetic interactions

Absorption

Co-administration of two drugs could give an interaction if one drug affected the rate or extent of absorption of the other drug. Changes in the rate of absorption, for example by increasing or decreasing gastric emptying or intestinal motility, will affect the peak concentration but not usually the extent of absorption. Interactions affecting the rate of absorption are less important than those that alter the extent of absorption. Examples of interactions affecting the extent of absorption include retention of the drug in the gut lumen (e.g. tetracycline antibiotics bind to divalent or trivalent metals, such as Ca^{2+} or Fe^{3+}, to form complexes that are not absorbed) and inhibition or induction of first-pass metabolism in the gut lumen, gut wall or liver.

Distribution

The main interactions affecting drug distribution arise from competition for the non-specific binding sites on plasma

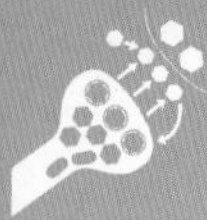

proteins, such as albumin (see Table 2.3). Interactions affecting plasma protein binding are of greatest importance when:

- the displaced drug is highly protein bound; for example, if competition for protein binding sites reduces binding from 98% to 96%, this will double the free drug concentration in plasma (from 2% to 4%); a 2% change in the binding of a drug which is 50% bound and 50% free would not be clinically or biologically significant
- the displaced drug has a narrow therapeutic index, so that a two- to three-fold change in free drug concentration gives an increase in drug activity
- the displaced drug has a low apparent volume of distribution, such that the plasma contains a significant proportion of the total body load; if the drug has a high apparent volume of distribution, the increase in free drug in the plasma volume (about 3 L) may be negligible after it has been distributed to (or 'diluted' in) a much higher apparent volume of distribution (for example 300 L)
- the displacing drug is of low potency, such that large doses (on a milligram basis) are given and protein binding sites become limiting.

In reality, such interactions are of limited clinical relevance even when the above criteria are fulfilled. For example, the potentially important interaction between warfarin and aspirin is due to their combined pharmacodynamic effects on haemostasis (Ch. 11), rather than the displacement of warfarin (which is 99% bound and has an apparent volume of distribution of 0.1 L kg^{-1}) from its protein binding sites. One reason for limited significance is that the additional free drug that has been displaced from protein binding sites may undergo rapid elimination by metabolism or glomerular filtration. When this occurs, a new 'steady state' will be established when the combination is given, with similar amounts of free (active) drug but reduced amounts of protein-bound (inactive) drug. Therefore, the total (free and bound) plasma concentration of the drug (which is measured in most drug assays) will be lower, and may misleadingly indicate an inappropriate increase in drug dose. Examples of drugs displaying this problem are theophylline and phenytoin.

Metabolism

At first sight it might be thought that an interaction would occur whenever drugs that share a common pathway of elimination are given simultaneously. However, the concentrations of drugs presented to metabolising enzymes, such as cytochrome P450, are usually far below the K_m values – in other words, there is a vast excess of enzyme over substrate and first-order kinetics (Ch. 2) apply. Therefore, the kinetic parameters, such as bioavailability and clearance, of one drug are not affected simply by the co-administration of a second drug that shares the same enzyme; the situation for the combination can be regarded as analogous to giving more of the first drug (see Ch. 2). Interactions arising from simple competition for the same enzyme would only be important if the combination resulted in saturation of the enzyme system. A clinically useful example is the administration of ethanol to prevent the metabolism of methanol (in overdose) to formate, in order to reduce the risk of blindness (Ch. 53).

Important interactions can occur when one drug in a combination induces or inhibits the enzymes involved in the metabolism of the other drug. This has been well recognised for drugs affecting the cytochrome P450 enzyme system, largely because of the importance of this enzyme system for the elimination of most drugs and the potential for inhibition or induction of different isoenzymes (Table 2.9). Enzyme inhibition occurs as soon as the drug concentration is sufficiently high, and inhibition can occur after a single dose (e.g. cimetidine). In contrast, enzyme induction requires the synthesis of additional enzyme and it takes a few days (or longer) before the elevated enzyme activity reaches a new equilibrium between synthesis and degradation. Induction or inhibition of hepatic enzymes can affect both systemic clearance and first-pass metabolism (bioavailability) after oral dosage.

Co-administration of two drugs, one of which is an enzyme inducer, will reduce the concentrations of the other drug. This may decrease the response to the second drug (if the parent compound is active), but could also increase the response to a prodrug, if the induced enzyme was responsible for this bioactivation. A problem can also arise when drug dosage has been optimised for the combination and treatment with the inducer is then stopped. Under such circumstances, the enzyme activity decreases (usually over a period of 2–3 weeks) and plasma levels of the still-prescribed drug will increase, possibly giving a risk of toxicity.

Excretion

Each of the three processes that are important in the renal elimination of drugs, i.e. glomerular filtration, pH-dependent reabsorption and renal tubular secretion (Ch. 2), could be a site for a drug interaction.

- Glomerular filtration depends on renal perfusion and removes free or non-protein-bound drug only. In consequence, drugs affecting renal perfusion or plasma protein binding (see above) could give rise to interactions.
- pH-dependent reabsorption could be altered by drugs that affect urine pH, either directly or via metabolic effects; the pH changes associated with aspirin overdose could affect the excretion of drugs taken concurrently.
- Renal tubular secretion can give rise to interactions when there is competition for the transporter. Aspirin can interfere with the transport of both endogenous compounds (e.g. uric acid) and drugs (e.g. methotrexate).

The biliary excretion of drugs is not an important site for drug interactions, but the enterohepatic cycling of drugs can be affected by the co-administration of poorly absorbed broad-spectrum antibacterials, which affect the hydrolysis of drug conjugates in the lower bowel (Fig. 2.13).

FURTHER READING

American Academy of Pediatrics (2001) Committee on Drugs. The transfer of drugs and other chemicals into human milk. *Pediatrics* 108, 776–789. Available online at: *http://aappolicy.aappublications.org/cgi/content/full/pediatrics;108/3/776*

Bressler R, Bahl JJ (2003) Principles of drug therapy for the elderly patient. *Mayo Clin Proc* 78, 1564–1577

Briggs GG, Freeman RK, Yaffe SJ (1998) Drugs in Pregnancy and Lactation. A Reference Guide to Fetal and Neonatal Risk, 5th edn. Baltimore: Williams and Wilkins

Cresswell KM, Fernando B, McKinstry B, Sheikh A (2007) Adverse drug events in the elderly. *Br Med Bull* 83, 259–274

Dickinson BD, Altman RD, Nielsen NH, Sterling ML; Council on Scientific Affairs, American Medical Association (2001) Drug interactions between oral contraceptives and antibiotics. *Obstet Gynecol* 98, 853–860

Dorne JLCM, Walton K, Renwick AG (2005) Human variability in xenobiotic metabolism and pathway-related uncertainty factors for chemical risk assessment: a review. *Food Chem Toxicol* 43, 203–216

Henderson L, Yue QY, Bergquist C, Gerden B, Arlett P (2002) St John's wort (*Hypericum perforatum*): drug interactions and clinical outcomes. *Br J Clin Pharmacol* 54, 349–356

Ito S (2000) Drug therapy for breast-feeding women. *N Engl J Med* 343, 118–126

Johnson TN (2003) The development of drug metabolising enzymes and their influence on the susceptibility to adverse drug reactions in children. *Toxicology* 192, 37–48

Koren G, Pastuszak A, Ito S (2000) Drugs in pregnancy. *N Engl J Med* 338, 1128–1137

Larimore WL, Petrie KA (2000) Drug use during pregnancy and lactation. *Primary Care* 27, 35–53

Mallet L, Spinewine A, Huang A (2007) Prescribing in elderly people 2. The challenge of managing drug interactions in elderly people. *Lancet* 370, 185–191

Nunn T, Williams J (2005) Formulation of medicines for children. *Br J Clin Pharmacol* 59, 674–676

O'Mahony D, Gallagher PF (2008) Inappropriate prescribing in the older population: need for new criteria. *Age Ageing* 37, 138–141

Patsalos PN, Froscher W, Pisani F, van Rijn CM (2002) The importance of drug interactions in epilepsy therapy. *Epilepsia* 43, 365–385

Patsalos PN, Perucca E (2003) Clinically important drug interactions in epilepsy: interactions between antiepileptic drugs and other drugs. *Lancet Neurol* 2, 473–481

Routledge PA, O'Mahony MS, Woodhouse KW (2004) Adverse drug reactions in elderly patients. *Br J Clin Pharmacol* 57, 121–126

Spina E, Scordo MG, D'Arrigo C (2003) Metabolic drug interactions with new psychotropic agents. *Fundam Clin Pharmacol* 17, 517–538

Spinewine A, Schmader KE, Barber N et al (2007) Prescribing in elderly people 1. Appropriate prescribing in elderly people: how well can it be measured and optimised? *Lancet* 370, 173–184

Stephenson T (2006) The medicines for children agenda in the UK. *Br J Clin Pharmacol* 61, 716–719

Strolin Benedetti M, Baltes EL (2003) Drug metabolism and disposition in children. *Fundam Clin Pharmacol* 17, 281–299

Thurmann PA, Steioff A (2001) Drug treatment in pregnancy. *Int J Clin Pharmacol Ther* 39, 185–191

Turnheim K (2003) When drug therapy gets old: pharmacokinetics and pharmacodynamics in the elderly. *Exp Gerontol* 38, 843–853

Index

Please note that page references relating to non-textual content such as Boxes, Figures or Tables are in *italic* print